Oral Pathology

Clinical-Pathologic Correlations

JOSEPH A. REGEZI, D.D.S., M.S.

Professor, Department of Oral Medicine/Pathology/Surgery
School of Dentistry and University Hospital
Associate Professor, Department of Pathology
School of Medicine
University of Michigan
Ann Arbor, Michigan

JAMES J. SCIUBBA, D.M.D., Ph.D.

Chairman, Department of Dentistry
Long Island Jewish Medical Center
New Hyde Park, New York
Professor, Department of Oral Biology and Pathology
School of Dental Medicine
State University of New York at Stony Brook
Stony Brook, New York

W. B. SAUNDERS COMPANY
Harcourt Brace Jovanovich, Inc.
Philadelphia London Toronto Montreal Sydney Tokyo

W. B. SAUNDERS COMPANY
Harcourt Brace Jovanovich, Inc.

The Curtis Center
Independence Square West
Philadelphia, PA 19106

Library of Congress Cataloging-in-Publication Data

Regezi, Joseph A.

Oral pathology: clinical-pathologic correlations /
Joseph A. Regezi, James J. Sciubba.

p.   cm.

Includes index.

1. Mouth—Diseases.   2. Teeth—Diseases.   I. Sciubba,
James J.   II. Title.   [DNLM: 1. Pathology, Oral.
WU 140 R333o]

RC815.R39   1989   617'.522—dc19
DNLM/DLC

ISBN 0–7216–2433–2   88-38204

Editor: John Dyson
Developmental Editor: Linda Mills
Designer: Nina McDaid Ikeda
Production Manager: Peter Faber
Manuscript Editor: Mimi McGinnis
Illustration Coordinator: Brett MacNaughton
Indexer: Diane Forti

Oral Pathology: Clinical-Pathologic Correlations   ISBN 0–7216–2433–2

© 1989 by W. B. Saunders Company. Copyright under the Uniform Copyright Convention. Simultaneously published in Canada. All rights reserved. This book is protected by copyright. No part of it may be reproduced, stored in a retrieval system, or transmitted in any form or by any means, electronic, mechanical, photocopying, recording, or otherwise, without written permission from the publisher. Made in the United States of America. Library of Congress catalog card number 88-38204.

Last digit is the print number: 9   8   7   6   5   4   3   2

Contributors

Frederick Burgett, D.D.S., M.S., M.S.
Professor of Dentistry in Periodontics, School of Dentistry, University of Michigan, Ann Arbor, Michigan
Periodontal Disease

Paul Crespi, D.D.S.
Professor of Pediatric Dentistry, State University of New York at Stony Brook, School of Dental Medicine, Stony Brook, New York; Chief of Pediatric Dentistry, Schneider Children's Hospital, Long Island Jewish Medical Center, New Hyde Park, New York
Metabolic and Genetic Jaw Diseases

Nathaniel Rowe, D.D.S., M.S.D.
Professor of Dentistry, School of Dentistry, Professor of Pathology, School of Medicine, University of Michigan, Ann Arbor, Michigan; University of Michigan Hospitals, Ann Arbor, Michigan
Dental Caries

Jeffery C. B. Stewart, D.D.S., M.S.
Lecturer in Oral Pathology, School of Dentistry, University of Michigan, Ann Arbor, Michigan; Attending Staff, Department of Hospital Dentistry, University of Michigan Hospitals, Ann Arbor, Michigan
Benign Non-odontogenic Tumors

Richard J. Zarbo, M.D., D.M.D.
Clinical Associate Professor of Pathology, Wayne State University School of Medicine, Detroit, Michigan; Senior Staff Pathologist, Section Chief, Immunohistochemistry Laboratory, Department of Pathology, Henry Ford Hospital, Detroit, Michigan
Malignant Non-odontogenic Neoplasms of the Jaws

Preface

The purpose of this book is to present to the reader a consistent and logical approach to the study of oral pathology. Its clinical orientation as evidenced by disease classifications, descriptions, and photographs should facilitate the identification and treatment of oral diseases. Microscopic correlations are also provided—an aspect that not only helps in the understanding of disease processes but also can provide an invaluable aid in clinical diagnosis and patient management. This text should help form a bridge between the didactic aspects of oral pathology and the practical clinical considerations.

This book is also designed to help enhance diagnostic skills through the use of differential diagnostic considerations. The development of a differential diagnosis is an effective academic teaching tool with considerable practical value in daily practice. An appreciation of the significance of all the possible diagnostic entities helps prevent needless delay or haste in treatment and helps eliminate the expense of unnecessary laboratory tests and consultations. Also, when a differential diagnosis is established, a more rational approach to biopsy and treatment can be followed.

Also presented in the text are current theories on etiology and pathogenesis, current therapeutic regimens, and a current bibliography. When pertinent to etiology or diagnosis, immunohistochemical, immunofluorescent, and ultrastructural materials have been included. An additional distinctive feature of this book is the clinical overview found at the beginning.

How to Use This Book

The narrative or latter part of this book provides the body of information that is oral pathology. It is the starting place for comprehensive study of oral pathology. The overview or front section is essentially a distillation of the clinical aspects found in the main text and is designed to be used as a quick chairside and laboratory reference or as a rapid review. The two sections are keyed together through the page numbers listed after the various diseases in the overview so that detailed information is readily available at the readers' fingertips.

JOSEPH A. REGEZI
JAMES J. SCIUBBA

Acknowledgments

Although this book is the product of the authors, it would not have come to fruition without the direct and indirect support of many others. First and foremost, appreciation must be expressed to Jane Folske for her highly competent efforts in manuscript typing. Her organizational skills and computer knowledge were also invaluable in this process. The photographic assistance provided by Kerry Campbell and the artwork done by Chris Jung were likewise important in the construction of this book.

Thank yous are due to our oral pathology colleagues, fellow faculty members, biopsy contributors, and referring clinicians, who provided patients, tissue, and photographs that were the foundation of the illustrative material in this book. Appreciation is also expressed for their ideas, opinions, and criticisms. A special thanks goes to friend and colleague Richard M. Courtney, who was particularly supportive and encouraging during the project. To John Dyson and his very capable staff at W. B. Saunders Publishing Company appreciation is also expressed for putting together all the skills and ingredients necessary to deliver the final product.

Our mentors Donald A. Kerr, John P. Waterhouse, and Leon Eisenbud must share some of the credit and responsibility for the commitment that the authors made in writing this book. As teachers and role models, they significantly contributed to the authors' professional and personal development. Other influential mentor/colleagues, John G. Batsakis and John T. Headington, deserve mention here also because of the sharing of their knowledge of pathology and of the example of their professional character.

Our families are especially deserving of recognition. It is, unfortunately, from them that much of the time necessary to write this text was stolen. For their support and understanding, we are grateful.

Finally, acknowledgment must be accorded to the many fine students and residents we have come to know and love over the many years of our careers. It is the curious and motivated student who provides the stimulus and challenge that makes teaching rewarding work. It is the energy, the questions, and the new ideas from the student that will maintain the vitality of the profession. We believe that all students young and old will find this text of value in their educational endeavors.

JOSEPH A. REGEZI
JAMES J. SCIUBBA

Contents

CLINICAL OVERVIEW

Vesiculo-Bullous Diseases (Chapter 1) O–2

Ulcerative Conditions (Chapter 2) O–8

White Lesions (Chapter 3) O–18

Red-Blue Lesions (Chapter 4) O–28

Pigmentations of Oral and Perioral Tissues (Chapter 5) O–36

Verrucal-Papillary Lesions (Chapter 6) O–42

Submucosal Swellings (By Region) (Chapters 7–9) O–48
    GINGIVAL SWELLINGS O–49
    FLOOR OF MOUTH SWELLINGS O–54
    LIP AND BUCCAL MUCOSA SWELLINGS O–56
    TONGUE SWELLINGS O–58
    PALATAL SWELLINGS O–60
    NECK SWELLINGS O–63

Jaw Lesions (Chapters 10–15) O–69

Cysts of the Oral Region (Chapter 10) O–71

Odontogenic Tumors (Chapter 11) O–79

Benign Non-odontogenic Tumors (Chapter 12) O–85

Inflammatory Jaw Lesions (Chapter 13) O–91

Malignant Non-odontogenic Neoplasms of the Jaws (Chapter 14) O–95

Metabolic and Genetic Jaw Diseases (Chapter 15) O–101

Chapter 1
Vesiculo-Bullous Diseases 1
   VIRAL DISEASES 1
   CONDITIONS ASSOCIATED WITH IMMUNOLOGIC
      DEFECTS 14
   HEREDITARY DISEASES 26

Chapter 2
Ulcerative Conditions 29
   REACTIVE LESIONS 29
   BACTERIAL CONDITIONS 34
   FUNGAL DISEASES 42
   CONDITIONS ASSOCIATED WITH IMMUNOLOGIC
      DYSFUNCTION 46
   NEOPLASMS 68

Chapter 3
White Lesions 84
   HEREDITARY CONDITIONS 84
   REACTIVE LESIONS 89
   OTHER WHITE LESIONS 94
   NON-EPITHELIAL WHITE-YELLOW LESIONS 110

Chapter 4
Red-Blue Lesions 125
   INTRAVASCULAR, FOCAL 125
   INTRAVASCULAR, DIFFUSE 141
   EXTRAVASCULAR—PETECHIAE AND ECCHYMOSES 146

Chapter 5
Pigmentations of Oral and Perioral Tissues 151
   BENIGN LESIONS OF MELANOCYTE ORIGIN 151
   NEOPLASMS 157
   PIGMENTATIONS CAUSED BY EXOGENOUS
      DEPOSITS 163

Chapter 6
Verrucal-Papillary Lesions 167
   REACTIVE LESIONS 167
   NEOPLASMS 175
   UNKNOWN ETIOLOGY 180

Chapter 7
Connective Tissue Lesions 184
    FIBROUS CONNECTIVE TISSUE LESIONS 184
    VASCULAR LESIONS 201
    NEURAL LESIONS 207
    LESIONS OF MUSCLE AND FAT 219

Chapter 8
Salivary Gland Diseases 225
    REACTIVE LESIONS (NON-INFECTIOUS) 226
    INFECTIOUS CONDITIONS 239
    METABOLIC CONDITIONS 243
    CONDITIONS ASSOCIATED WITH IMMUNE
        DEFECTS 243
    BENIGN NEOPLASMS 248
    MALIGNANT NEOPLASMS 263

Chapter 9
Lymphoid Lesions 284
    REACTIVE LESIONS 284
    DEVELOPMENTAL LESIONS 286
    NEOPLASMS 287

Chapter 10
Cysts of the Oral Region 301
    ODONTOGENIC CYSTS 301
    NON-ODONTOGENIC CYSTS 319
    PSEUDOCYSTS 323
    SOFT TISSUE CYSTS OF THE NECK 329

Chapter 11
Odontogenic Tumors 337
    EPITHELIAL TUMORS 337
    MESENCHYMAL TUMORS 353
    MIXED (EPITHELIAL AND MESENCHYMAL) TUMORS 363

Chapter 12
Benign Non-odontogenic Tumors 369
    Jeffery C. B. Stewart
    OSSIFYING FIBROMA 369
    FIBROUS DYSPLASIA 372
    OSTEOBLASTOMA 375
    OSTEOID OSTEOMA 377
    CHONDROMA 377
    OSTEOMA 378
    CENTRAL GIANT CELL GRANULOMA 379
    GIANT CELL TUMOR 381
    HEMANGIOMA OF BONE 382

IDIOPATHIC HISTIOCYTOSIS (LANGERHANS
   CELL DISEASE) 383
TORI AND EXOSTOSES 386
CORONOID HYPERPLASIA 387

Chapter 13
Inflammatory Jaw Lesions 390
   PULPITIS 390
   PERIAPICAL ABSCESS 393
   ACUTE OSTEOMYELITIS 394
   CHRONIC OSTEOMYELITIS 395

Chapter 14
Malignant Non-odontogenic Neoplasms of the Jaws 405
   Richard J. Zarbo
   OSTEOSARCOMA 405
   CHONDROSARCOMA 413
   EWING'S SARCOMA 417
   BURKITT'S LYMPHOMA 419
   PLASMA CELL NEOPLASMS 421
   METASTATIC CARCINOMA 424

Chapter 15
Metabolic and Genetic Jaw Diseases 427
   Paul Crespi
   METABOLIC CONDITIONS 427
   GENETIC ABNORMALITIES 437

Chapter 16
Abnormalities of Teeth 460
   ALTERATIONS IN SIZE 460
   ALTERATIONS IN SHAPE 461
   ALTERATIONS IN NUMBER 467
   DEFECTS OF ENAMEL 472
   DEFECTS OF DENTIN 477
   DEFECTS OF ENAMEL AND DENTIN 480
   ABNORMALITIES OF DENTAL PULP 480
   ALTERATIONS IN COLOR 484

Chapter 17
Dental Caries 488
   Nathaniel Rowe
   CLINICAL FEATURES 489
   MICROSCOPIC FEATURES 491
   CAUSATION 494

Chapter 18
Periodontal Disease 503
   Frederick Burgett
   ETIOLOGY AND PATHOGENESIS.. 504
   PERIODONTAL EXAMINATION 508
   GINGIVITIS.. 508
   PERIODONTITIS.. 512

Index 521

CLINICAL OVERVIEW*

CLINICAL CLASSIFICATION OF ORAL SOFT
    TISSUE DISEASES
Mucosal (Surface) Lesions
    Vesiculo-Bullous Diseases
    Ulcerative Conditions
    White Lesions
    Red-Blue Lesions
    Pigmentations of Oral and Perioral Tissues
    Verrucal-Papillary Lesions
Submucosal Swellings (by Region) (Chapters 7–9)
    Gingiva
    Floor of Mouth
    Lips and Buccal Mucosa
    Tongue
    Palate
    Neck
DIFFERENTIAL DIAGNOSIS APPROACH TO JAW
    LESIONS
Cysts of the Oral Region
Odontogenic Tumors
Benign Non-odontogenic Tumors
Inflammatory Jaw Lesions
Malignant Non-odontogenic Neoplasms of the Jaws
Metabolic and Genetic Jaw Diseases

*Photographs and text in Clinical Overview taken in modified form from Regezi J, Courtney R. *Clinical Oral Pathology*. University of Michigan, Ann Arbor, 1987. Reproduced by permission of the University of Michigan.

VESICULO-BULLOUS DISEASES

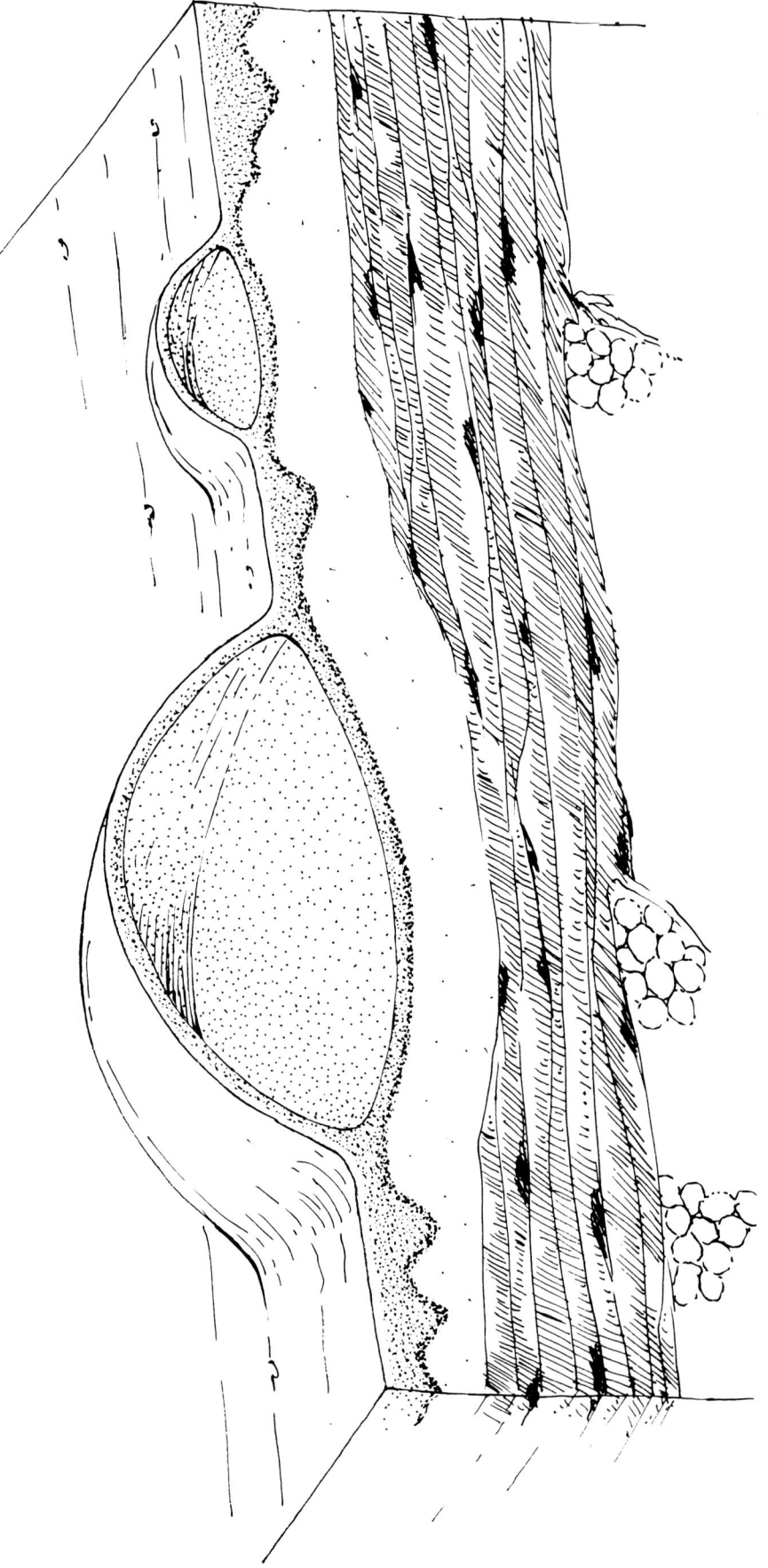

The presence of, or history of, vesicles or bullae places an oral disease into a distinct and limited group of lesions. These generally include viral diseases and oral manifestations of dermatologic diseases. It is uncommon clinically to see bullae or vesicles, since most become ulcers in a matter of hours. The important question to ask of patients with oral ulcers, therefore, is whether or not the lesions were preceded by blisters. In patients with a positive history, the presence of systemic signs and symptoms would favor a viral etiology.

Chapter 1

Vesiculo-Bullous Diseases

VIRAL DISEASES
Herpes Simplex Infections
Varicella-Zoster Infections
Hand, Foot, and Mouth Disease
Herpangina
Measles (Rubeola)
CONDITIONS ASSOCIATED WITH IMMUNOLOGIC
 DEFECTS
Pemphigus Vulgaris
Cicatricial Pemphigoid
Bullous Pemphigoid
Dermatitis Herpetiformis
HEREDITARY DISEASES
Epidermolysis Bullosa

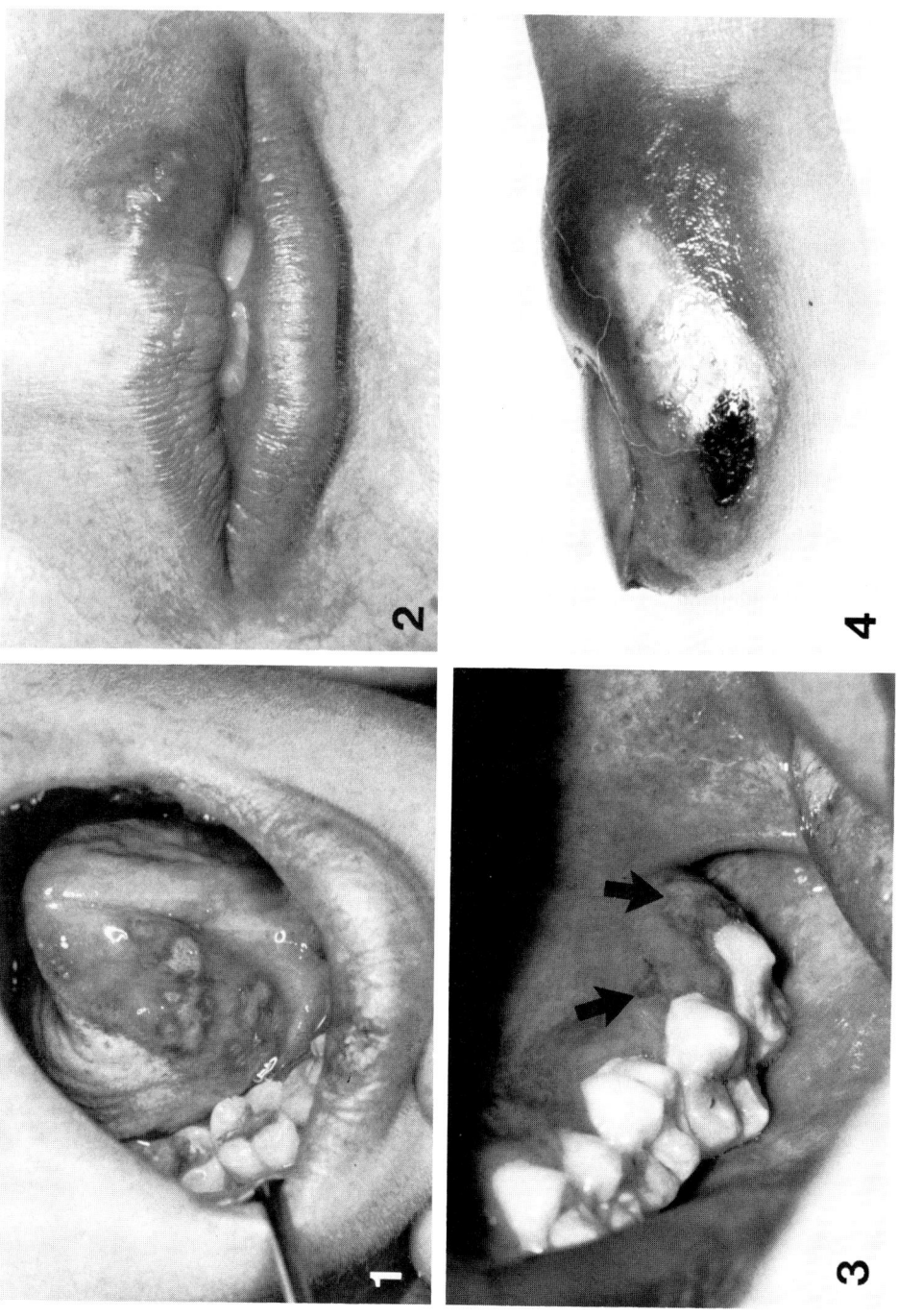

VESICULO-BULLOUS DISEASES

Disease	Clinical Features	Cause	Treatment	Significance
Herpes simplex infections Primary herpetic gingivostomatitis (Fig. 1) (p. 4)	Multiple painful oral ulcers preceded by vesicles; may have similar perioral and skin lesions; gingivitis usually present; usually affects children under 5 years; uncommon	Herpes simplex virus type I (rarely type II)	Supportive; acyclovir and other virus-specific drugs available for rare life-threatening infections	Self-limited, heals in about 2 weeks; reactivation of latent virus results in secondary infections; circulating antibodies provide only partial immunity
Secondary herpes simplex infection (Figs. 2–4) (p. 4–5)	Multiple small ulcers preceded by vesicles; prodromal symptoms of tingling, burning, or pain; most common on lip, intraorally on palate and attached gingiva; called herpetic whitlow when occurs around fingernail; adults and young adults usually affected; very common	Herpes simplex virus—represents reactivation of virus and not reinfection; commonly precipitated by stress, sunlight, cold temperature, low-resistance states	Symptomatic; the only virus-specific drug effective against oral herpes is acyclovir; topical or systemic	Self-limited; heals in 2 weeks without scar; occupational hazard; lesions infectious during vesicular stage; patient must be cautioned against autoinnoculation; herpes type I infections have not been convincingly linked to oral cancer
Varicella-zoster infections (p. 9)	Painful, pruritic vesicles and ulcers in all stages on trunk and face, few oral lesions; common childhood disease	Varicella-zoster virus	Supportive	Self-limited; recovery uneventful in several weeks
Herpes zoster (p. 9–11)	Unilateral multiple ulcers preceded by vesicles distributed along a sensory nerve course; very painful; usually on trunk, head, and neck, rare intraorally; adults	Reactivation of varicella-zoster virus	Supportive	Self-limited, but may have a prolonged painful course; sometimes seen with lymphomas
Hand, foot, and mouth disease (p. 11–13)	Painful ulcers preceded by vesicles on hands, feet, and oral mucosa; usually children; rare	Coxsackie virus	Supportive	Self-limited; recovery uneventful in about 2 weeks
Herpangina (p. 13)	Multiple painful ulcers in posterior oral cavity and pharynx; lesions preceded by vesicles; children most commonly affected; seasonal occurrence; rare	Coxsackie virus	Supportive	Self-limited; recovery uneventful in less than a week
Measles (Rubeola) (p. 13–14)	Oral Koplik's spots precede maculopapular skin rash; fever, malaise, plus other symptoms of systemic viral infection; children most commonly affected	Measles virus	Supportive	Self-limited; recovery uneventful in about 2 weeks

VESICULO-BULLOUS DISEASES

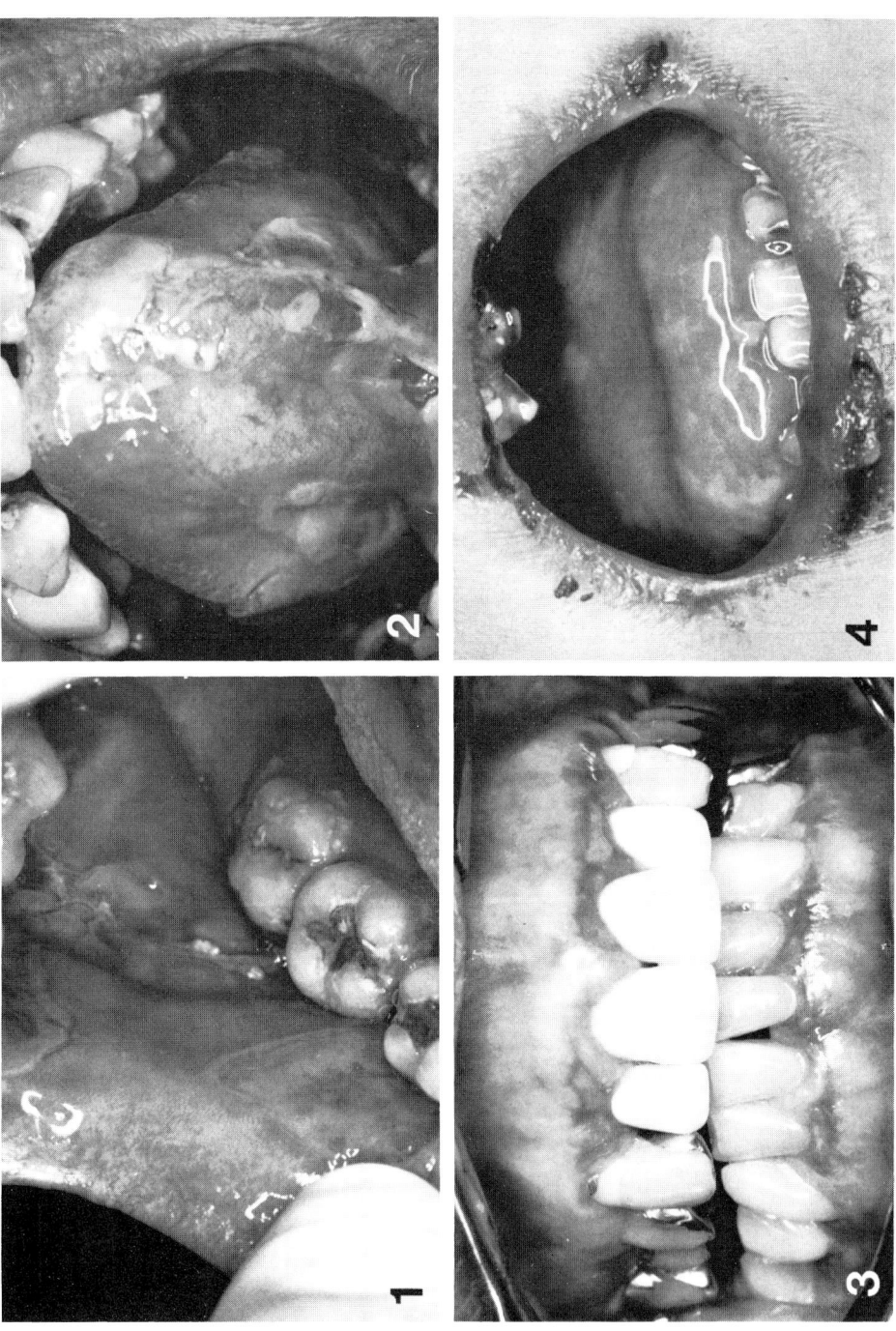

VESICULO-BULLOUS DISEASES (continued)

Disease	Clinical Features	Cause	Treatment	Significance
Pemphigus vulgaris (Figs. 1 and 2) (p. 14–19)	Multiple painful ulcers preceded by bullae; middle age; positive Nikolski's sign; progressive disease, remissions or control only with therapy; rare	Autoimmune; antibodies directed against desmosome-tonofilament complex	Systemic steroids; occasionally immunosuppressive drugs	May be fatal; significant morbidity from steroid therapy; oral lesions precede skin lesions in half the cases; prognosis improved if treated early
Cicatricial pemphigoid (Fig. 3) (p. 19–22)	Multiple painful ulcers preceded by bullae; lesion may heal with scar; positive Nikolski's sign; may affect mucous membranes of oral cavity, eyes, and genitals; when limited to attached gingiva only, may be called desquamative gingivitis or gingivosis; middle-aged or elderly females; uncommon; may be confused clinically with erosive lichen planus of gingiva	Autoimmune; antibodies directed against basement membrane area	Topical or systemic steroids	Protracted course; may cause significant debilitation if severe; death uncommon
Bullous pemphigoid (p. 22–24)	Skin disease (trunk and extremities) with infrequent oral lesions; ulcers preceded by bullae; no scarring; elderly people	Basement membrane autoantibodies are detected in tissue and serum	Systemic steroids/immunosuppressive drugs	Chronic course; remissions; uncommon
Dermatitis herpetiformis (p. 24–26)	Skin disease with rare oral involvement; vesicles and pustules; exacerbations and remissions are typical; young and middle-aged adults	Unknown; IgA deposits in site of lesions; may have an association with gluten sensitivity	Dapsone	Chronic course that may require diet restriction or drug therapy
Epidermolysis bullosa (Fig. 4) (p. 26–27)	Multiple ulcers preceded by bullae; positive Nikolski's sign; inheritance pattern determines age of onset during childhood and severity; may heal with scar; primarily a skin disease, but oral lesions often present; rare	Hereditary, autosomal dominant or recessive	Steroids, reduction of trauma, antibiotics	Severe debilitating disease that may be fatal in recessive form; simple operative procedures may elicit bullae

VESICULO-BULLOUS DISEASES

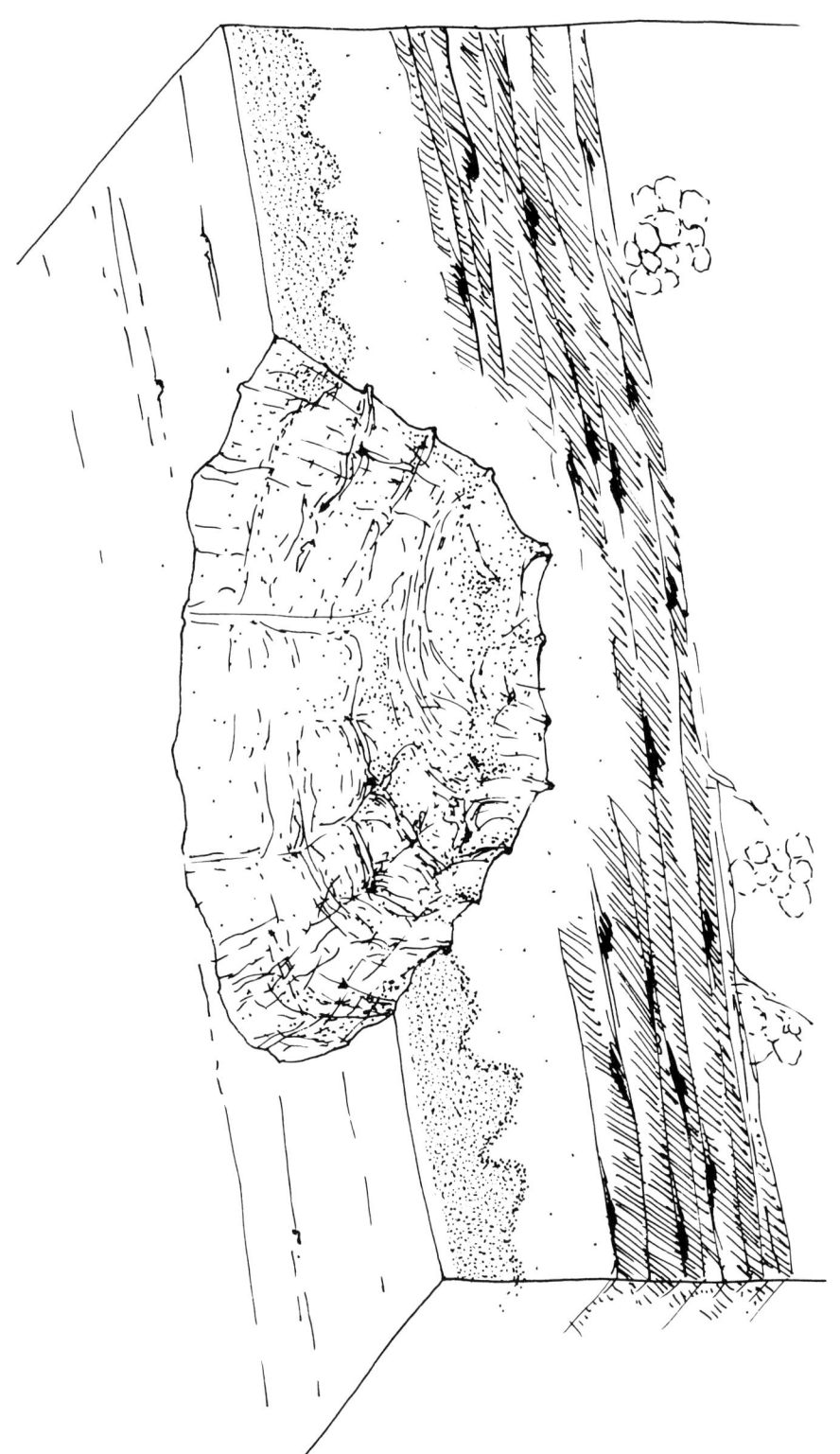

Ulcerative lesions are commonly encountered in dental patients. Lesions range from reactive to neoplastic to oral manifestations of dermatologic disease. Diagnosis is important not only for the patient but also for the clinician. Infectious ulcers are potentially contagious to dental personnel and should be approached with caution until definitive diagnosis is established.

Chapter 2

Ulcerative Conditions

REACTIVE LESIONS
BACTERIAL CONDITIONS
  Syphilis
  Gonorrhea
  Tuberculosis
  Leprosy
  Actinomycosis
  Noma
FUNGAL DISEASES
  Deep Fungal Diseases
  Subcutaneous Fungal Diseases—Sporotrichosis
  Opportunistic Fungal Infections—Phycomycosis
CONDITIONS ASSOCIATED WITH IMMUNOLOGIC
  DYSFUNCTION
  Aphthous Ulcers
  Behçet's Syndrome
  Reiter's Syndrome
  Erythema Multiforme
  Lupus Erythematosus
  Drug Reactions
  Contact Allergy
  Wegener's Granulomatosis
  Midline Granuloma
  Chronic Granulomatous Disease
NEOPLASMS
  Basal Cell Carcinoma
  Squamous Cell Carcinoma
  Carcinoma of the Maxillary Sinus

ULCERATIVE CONDITIONS

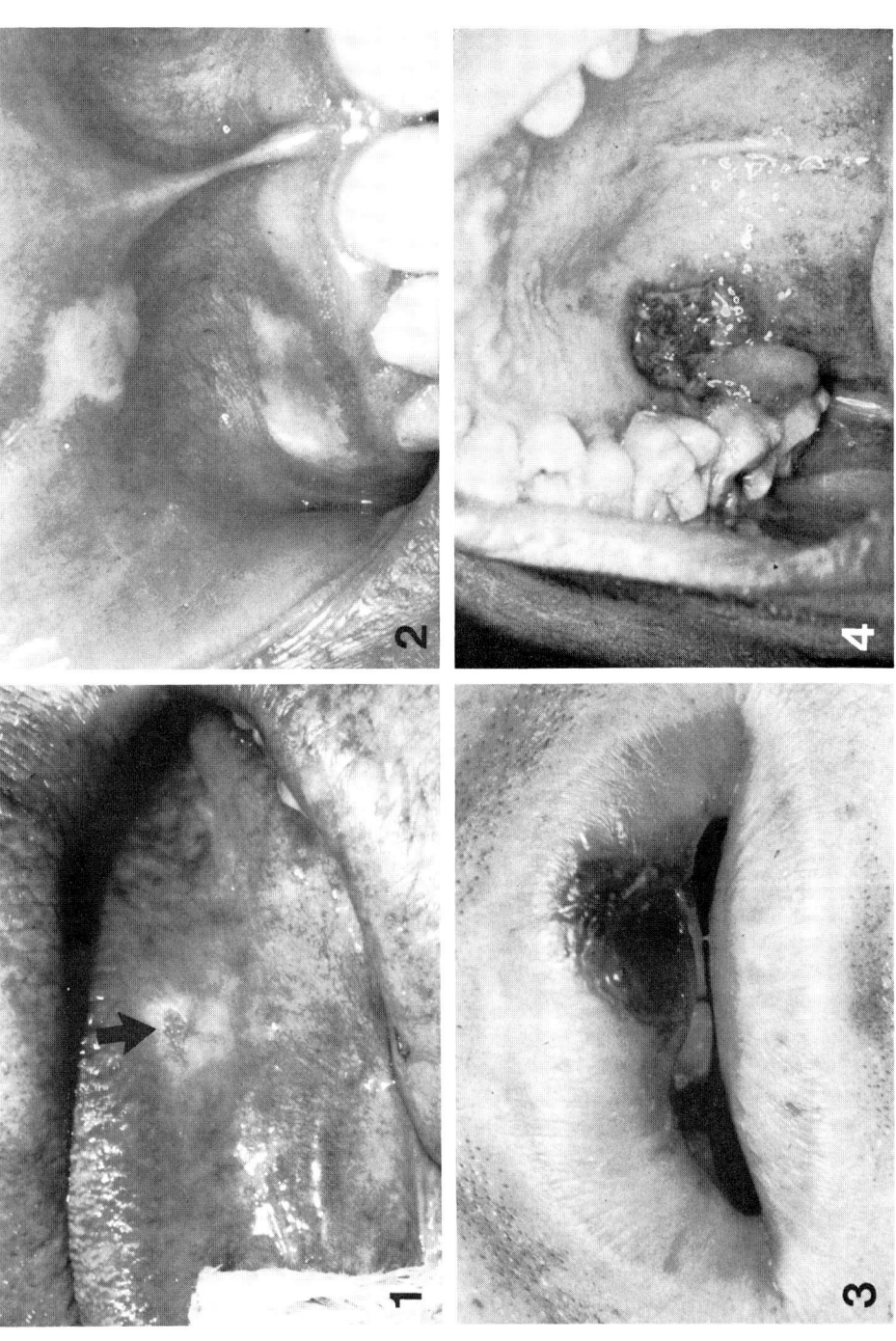

ULCERATIVE CONDITIONS

Disease	Clinical Features	Cause	Treatment	Significance
Reactive Lesions (Figs. 1 and 2) (p. 29–34)	Painful ulcer covered by yellow fibrin membrane; diagnosis usually evident from appearance, when combined with history; common; traumatic factitial injuries are diagnostic challenge	Trauma, chemicals, heat, radiation	Symptomatic; remove causative agent if still active	Self-limited; heals in days to weeks; factitial injuries follow unpredictable course
Syphilis (Fig. 3) (p. 34–37)	*Primary* (chancre)—single, indurated, non-painful ulcer at site of spirochete entry, spontaneously heals in 4 to 6 weeks; *secondary*—maculopapular rash on skin, multiple ulcers covered by membrane (mucous patches) orally; *tertiary*—glossitis, cardiovascular and central nervous system lesions; *congenital*—dental abnormalities (mulberry molars, notched incisors), deafness, interstitial keratitis (Hutchinson's triad)	Spirochete—*Treponema pallidum*	Penicillin	Occupational hazard; primary and secondary forms are highly infectious; mimics other diseases clinically; if untreated, secondary form develops in 2 to 10 weeks; a minority of patients develop tertiary lesions; latency periods, in which there is no clinically apparent disease, seen between primary and secondary, and secondary and tertiary stages
Gonorrhea (p. 37)	Typically genital lesions, with rare oral manifestations, painful erythema or ulcers, or both	*Neisseria gonorrhoeae*	Penicillin G, alternate antibiotics may be required because of penicillin resistance	May be confused with many oral ulcerative diseases
Tuberculosis (Fig. 4) (p. 38–39)	Indurated, chronic ulcer that may be painful	*Mycobacterium tuberculosis*	Isoniazid, ethambutol, streptomycin, others	Occupational hazard; lesions are infectious; oral lesions almost always secondary to lung lesions
Leprosy (p. 39–40)	Skin disease, with rare oral nodules/ulcers	*Mycobacterium leprae*	Dapsone, rifampin, clofazimine	Rare in the United States but relatively common in southeast Asia, India, South America
Actinomycosis (p. 40–41)	Typically seen in mandible, with draining skin sinus	*Actinomyces israelii*	Long-term, high-dose penicillin	Infection follows implantation resulting from a surgical procedure

ULCERATIVE CONDITIONS

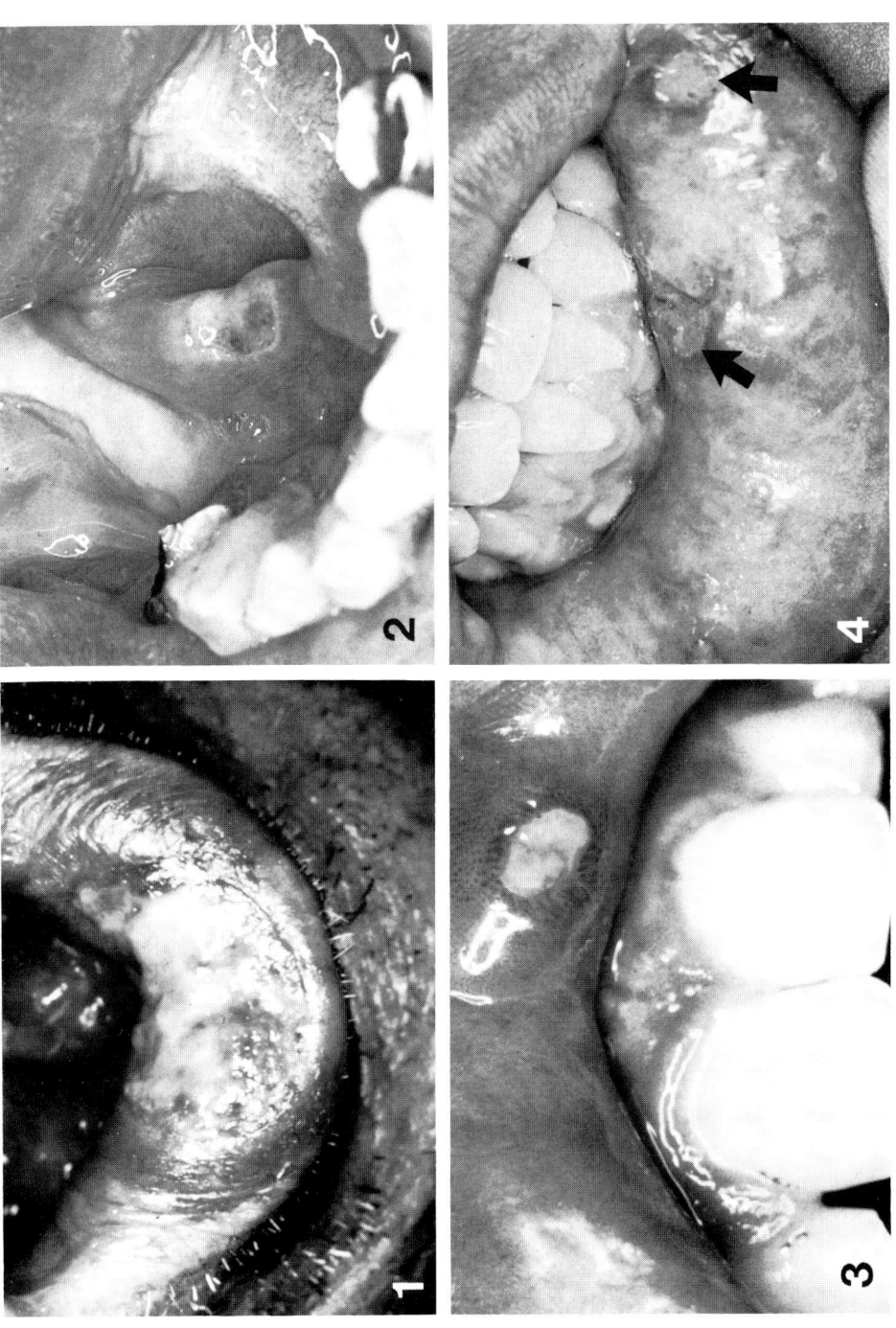

ULCERATIVE CONDITIONS (continued)

Disease	Clinical Features	Cause	Treatment	Significance
Noma (p. 41–42)	Necrotic, non-healing ulcer of gingiva or buccal mucosa; rare; affects children	Anaerobes in patient whose systemic health is compromised	Antibiotics and improve systemic health	Often associated with malnutrition; may result in severe tissue destruction
Deep fungal diseases (Fig. 1) (p. 42–45)	Indurated, non-healing, frequently painful, chronic ulcer, usually following implantation of organism from lung	*Histoplasma capsulatum, Coccidioides immitis*, others	Amphotericin B	Occupational hazard; oral lesions are secondary to systemic lesions
Subcutaneous fungal diseases (p. 45)	Non-specific ulcers of skin and, rarely, mucosa	Usually *Sporothrix schenckii*	Iodides or ketoconazole	Sporotrichosis usually follows inoculation via thorny plants
Opportunistic fungal infections (p. 45–46)	Occurs in compromised host; necrotic, non-healing ulcer(s)	*Mucor, Rhizopus*, others	Amphotericin B plus treat underlying disease	Known collectively as phycomycosis; may mimic syphilis, midline granuloma, others; frequently fatal
Aphthous ulcers (Figs. 2–4) (p. 46–53)	Recurrent, painful ulcers found on tongue, vestibular mucosa, floor of mouth, and faucial pillars; not found on skin, vermilion, attached gingiva, or hard palate; usually round or oval; ulcers not preceded by vesicles; *minor type*—usually solitary, less than 1 cm in diameter, common; *major type*—severe, heals in up to 6 weeks, with scar (Fig. 4); *herpetiform type*—multiple, recurrent crops of ulcers	Unknown; probably an immune defect mediated by T cells; not caused by virus; precipitated by stress, trauma, other factors	Symptomatic; most remedies contain either steroid or tetracycline	Painful nuisance disease; rarely debilitating, except in major type; recurrences are the rule and cures the exception
Behçet's syndrome (p. 53)	Minor aphthae; eye lesions (uveitis, conjunctivitis); genital lesions (ulcers); arthritis occasionally seen	Probably an immune defect	Steroids, immunosuppressives	Biopsy and laboratory studies give non-specific results; complications may be significant
Reiter's syndrome (p. 53–54)	Arthritis, urethritis, conjunctivitis or uveitis, oral ulcers; usually in white males in third decade	Unknown; ?immune response to bacterial antigen	Non-steroidal, anti-inflammatory drugs	Duration of weeks to month; may be recurrent

ULCERATIVE CONDITIONS

O-14

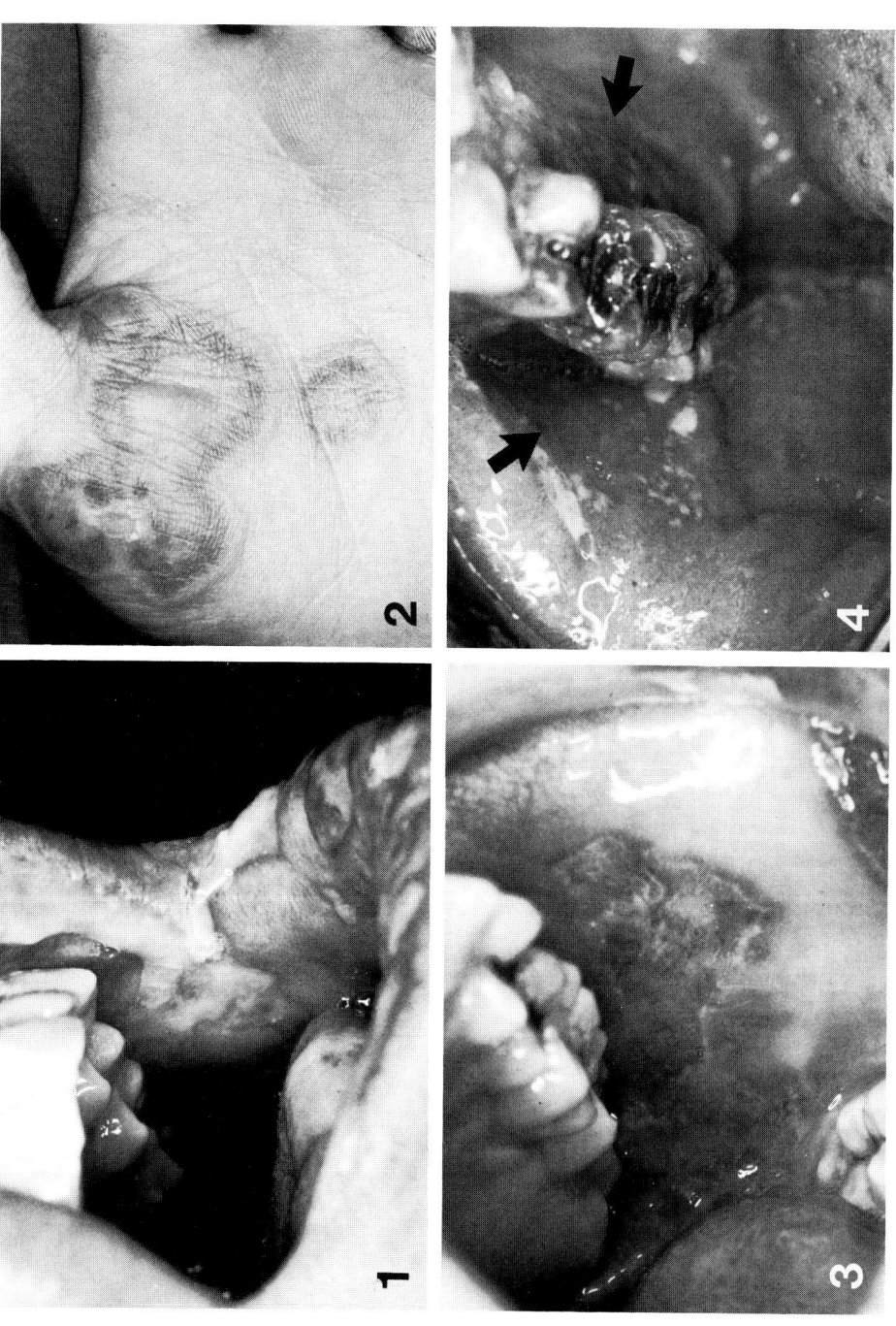

ULCERATIVE CONDITIONS (continued)

Disease	Clinical Features	Cause	Treatment	Significance
Erythema multiforme (Figs. 1 and 2) (p. 54–57)	Sudden onset; painful, widespread, superficial ulcers; usually self-limited; young adults; may also have target or iris lesions of skin; may be recurrent, especially in spring and fall; some cases become chronic; uncommon	Unknown; ?hypersensitivity; may follow drug ingestion or an infection such as herpes labialis	Symptomatic; systemic steroids in severe cases	Etiology should be investigated; can be debilitating, especially in severe forms (i.e., Stevens-Johnson syndrome)
Lupus erythematosus (Fig. 3) (p. 57–62)	Usually painful, erythematous and ulcerative lesions on buccal mucosa, gingiva, and vermilion; white, keratotic areas may surround lesions; *discoid type*—generally affects skin and mucous membrane only; *systemic type*—skin lesions may be erythematous with scale (classic sign is "butterfly" rash across bridge of nose); also may have joint, kidney, and heart lesions; middle-aged females, uncommon	Immune defect; patient develops autoantibodies, especially antinuclear antibodies	Steroids, immunosuppressive drugs, others	*Discoid type* may result in patient discomfort and cosmetic problems; *systemic type* has guarded prognosis
Drug reactions (p. 62–64)	May affect skin or mucosa; erythema, vesicles, ulcers may be seen; history of recent drug ingestion is important	Potentially any drug via stimulation of immune system or mast cells	Withdraw causative agent; antihistamines or corticosteroids	Reactions, such as anaphylaxis or angioedema, may require emergency care; highly variable clinical picture can make diagnosis difficult
Contact allergy (Fig. 4) (p. 64–66)	Lesion occurs directly under foreign antigen; erythema, vesicles, ulcers may be seen	Potentially any foreign antigen that contacts skin or mucosa	Eliminate offending material	Patch testing may be helpful for diagnosis; history is important
Wegener's granulomatosis (p. 66–67)	Inflammatory lesions (necrotizing vasculitis) of lung, kidney, and upper airway; may affect gingiva when intraoral; rare	Unknown; ?immune defect, ?infection	Cyclophosphamide	May become life threatening due to tissue destruction in any of the three involved sites

ULCERATIVE CONDITIONS

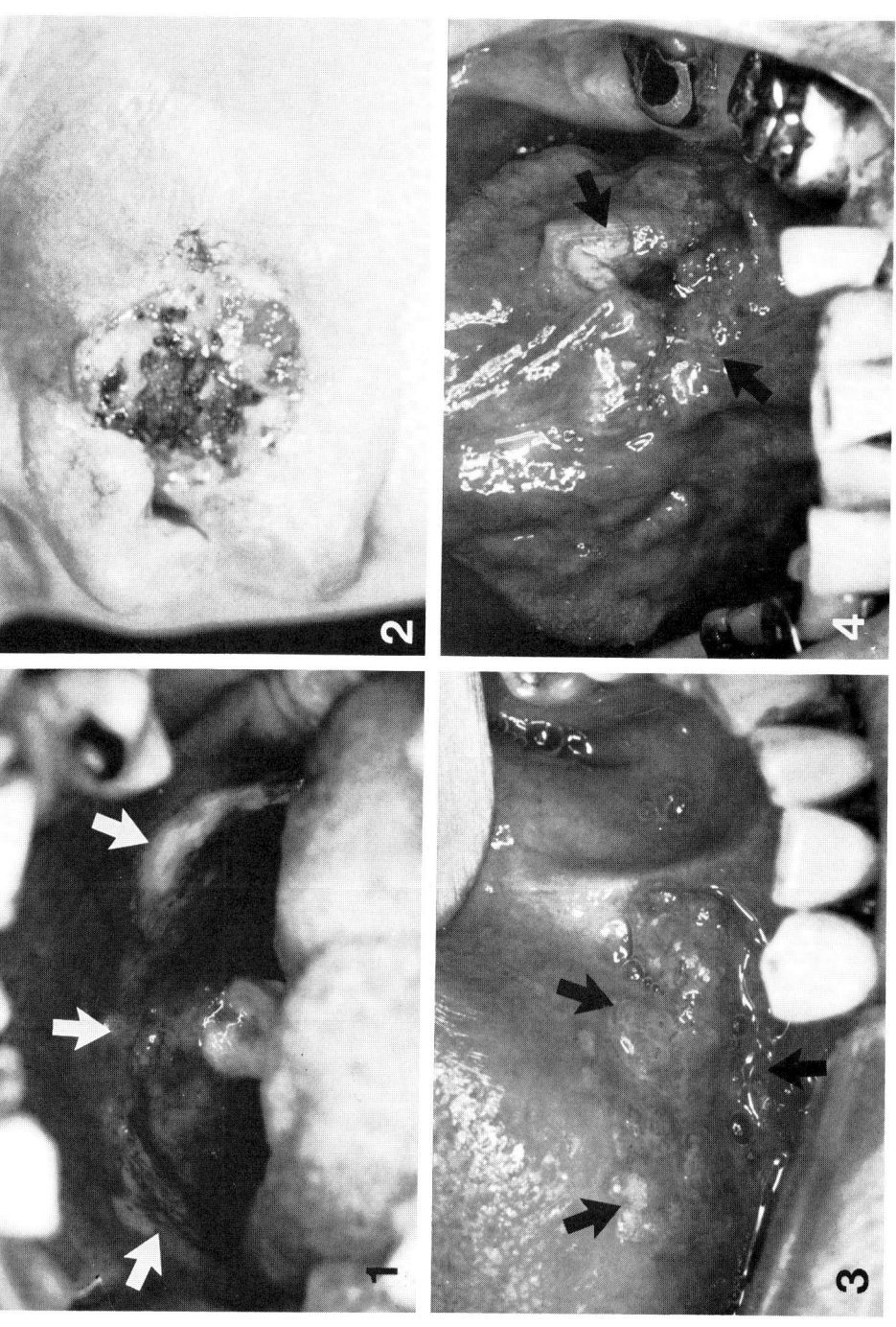

ULCERATIVE CONDITIONS (continued)

Disease	Clinical Features	Cause	Treatment	Significance
Midline granuloma (Fig. 1) (p. 67–68)	Destructive, necrotic, non-healing lesions of nose, palate, and sinuses; biopsy results in non-specific inflammation; distinct from Wegener's granulomatosis; rare	Unknown; ?immune defect	Steroids, radiation	Poor; death may follow erosion into major blood vessel
Chronic granulomatous disease (p. 68)	Recurrent infections in various organs; oral ulcers; males; rare	Genetic disease (X-linked)	Antimicrobials	Altered neutrophil and macrophage function results in inability to kill bacteria and fungi
Basal cell carcinoma (Fig. 2) (p. 68–70)	Non-healing ulcer with rolled margins; usually sun-exposed skin; does not occur orally or on vermilion	UV light, age	Surgery or radiation	Lesions are slow growing and rarely metastasize; excellent prognosis for lesions treated early
Squamous cell carcinoma (Figs. 3 and 4) (p. 70–81)	Indurated, non-painful ulcer with rolled margins; most commonly found on lateral tongue and floor of mouth; males affected twice as often as females; clinical appearance may also be as a white or red patch or mass	Mechanism unknown; tobacco, UV light; ?some microorganisms; alcohol and chronic irritation are co-carcinogens	Surgery or radiation	Overall 5-year survival rate is 45–50%; excellent prognosis if found in early stages, poor prognosis if metastasis to regional lymph nodes
Carcinoma of the maxillary sinus (p. 81–82)	Patient may have symptoms of sinusitis or referred pain to teeth; may cause malocclusion or mobile teeth; may appear as ulcerative mass in palate or alveolus	Unknown	Surgery or radiation	Prognosis only fair; metastases are not uncommon

WHITE LESIONS

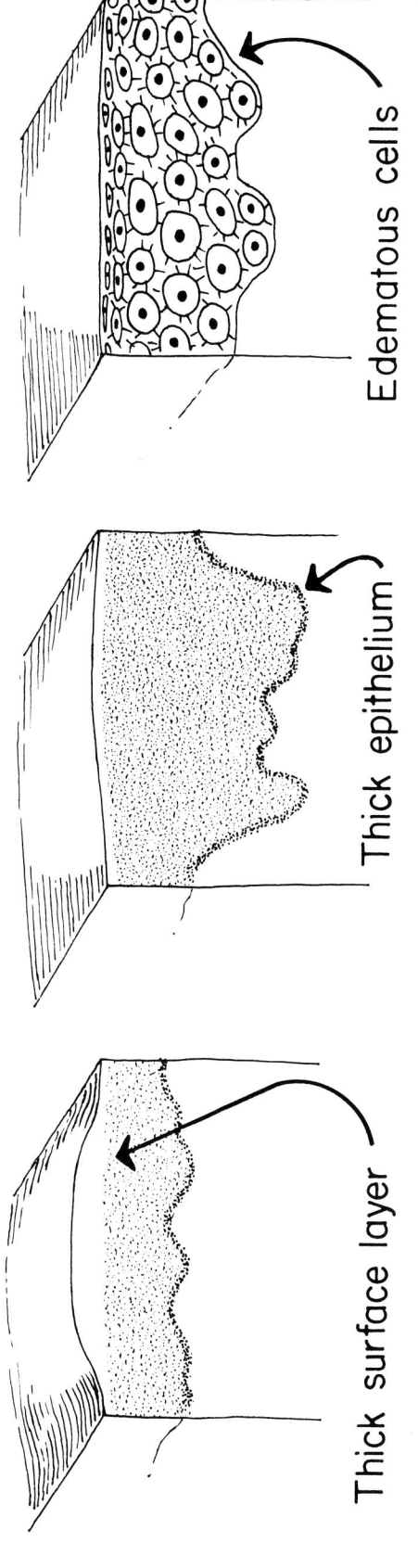

Lesions generally appear white intraorally for one of three reasons (assuming that the lesion cannot be rubbed off). A thickened surface layer of keratin, an acanthotic (increase in thickness of the prickle cell layer) epithelium, and edematous epithelial cells can all produce clinically white lesions. Exudates and adherent surface debris may also appear white. With experience, the reason for a lesion's white appearance can often be determined clinically, but final proof rests on microscopic examination. This becomes especially important for idiopathic leukoplakia, since some of these lesions represent squamous cell carcinomas.

The white lesions in the following list range from those that are genetically determined (genodermatoses) to those that are neoplastic. These lesions vary widely in their significance and treatment, making recognition an important clinical responsibility.

Chapter 3

White Lesions

HEREDITARY CONDITIONS
Leukoedema
White Sponge Nevus
Hereditary Benign Intraepithelial Dyskeratosis
Follicular Keratosis
REACTIVE LESIONS
Focal (Frictional) Hyperkeratosis
White Lesions Associated with Smokeless Tobacco
Nicotine Stomatitis
Solar Cheilitis
OTHER WHITE LESIONS
Idiopathic Leukoplakia
Hairy Leukoplakia
Hairy Tongue
Geographic Tongue
Lichen Planus
NON-EPITHELIAL WHITE-YELLOW LESIONS
Candidiasis
Mucosal Burns
Submucous Fibrosis
Fordyce's Granules
Ectopic Lymphoid Tissue
Gingival Cyst
Parulis
Lipoma

WHITE LESIONS

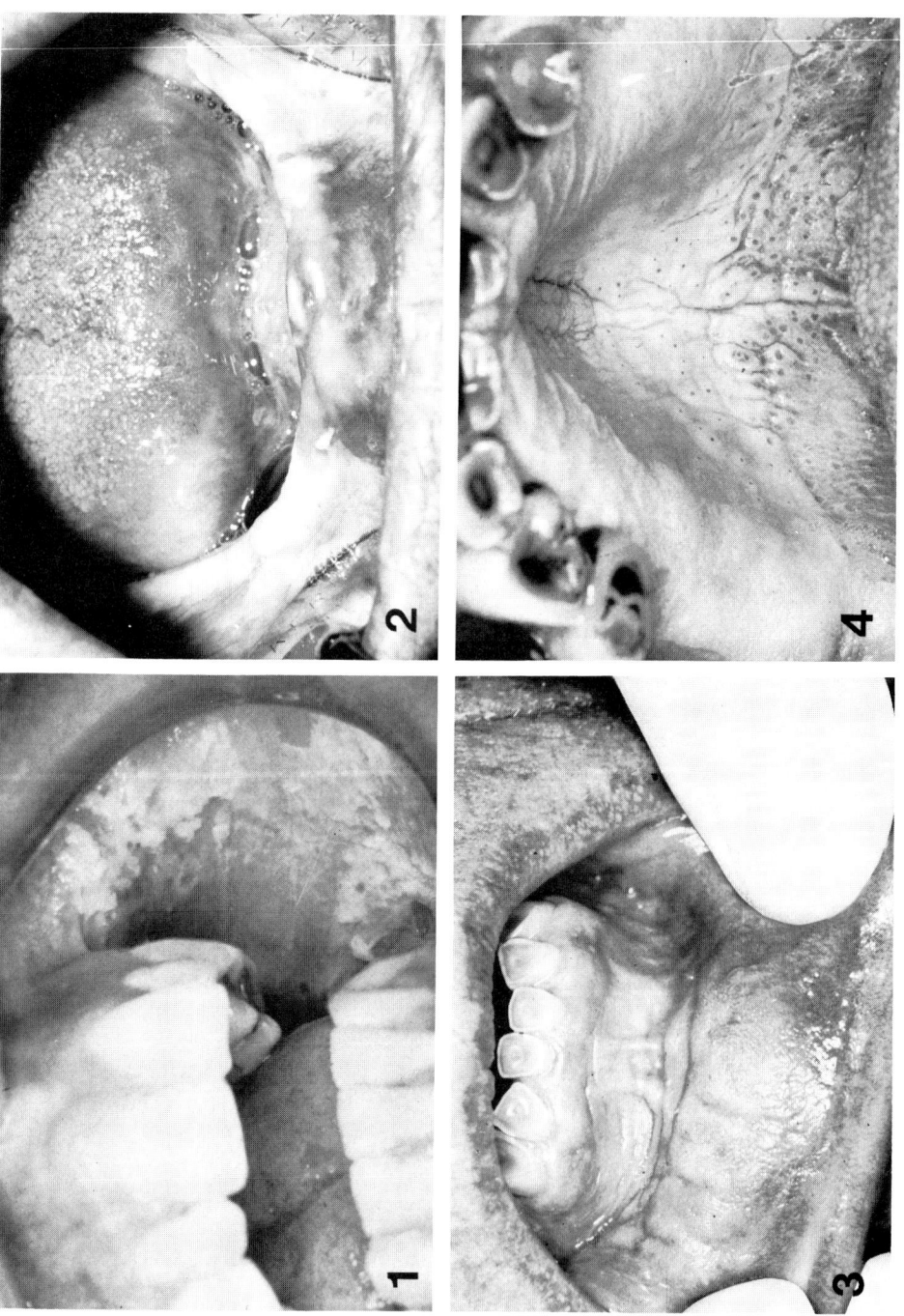

WHITE LESIONS

Disease	Clinical Features	Cause	Treatment	Significance
Leukoedema (p. 84–85)	50% of whites and 90% of blacks affected; uniform opacification of buccal mucosa bilaterally	Unknown	None	Remains indefinitely; no ill effects
White sponge nevus (Fig. 1) (p. 85–86)	Asymptomatic, bilateral, dense, shaggy, white or gray, generalized opacification; primarily buccal mucosa affected, but other membranes may be involved; rare	Hereditary, autosomal dominant	None	Remains indefinitely; no ill effects
Hereditary benign intraepithelial dyskeratosis (p. 86–87)	Asymptomatic, diffuse, shaggy, white lesions of buccal mucosa as well as other tissues; eye lesions—white plaques surrounded by inflamed conjunctiva; rare	Hereditary, autosomal dominant	None	Remains indefinitely
Follicular keratosis (p. 87–89)	Keratotic papular lesions of skin and, infrequently, mucosa; lesions are numerous and asymptomatic	Genetic, autosomal dominant	Retinoids	Chronic course with occasional remissions
Focal (frictional) hyperkeratosis (Fig. 2) (p. 89–90)	Asymptomatic, white patch, commonly on edentulous ridge, buccal mucosa, and tongue; does not rub off; common	Chronic irritation	Remove irritant	May regress if cause eliminated
White lesions associated with smokeless tobacco (Fig. 3) (p. 90–92)	Asymptomatic, white folds surrounding area where tobacco is held; usually found in labial and buccal vestibule; common	Chronic irritation from snuff or chewing tobacco	Discontinue habit; biopsy suspicious areas	May develop into verrucous carcinoma after many years
Nicotine stomatitis (Fig. 4) (p. 92–93)	Asymptomatic, generalized opacification of palate with red dots representing salivary gland orifices; common	Heat and smoke associated with combustion of tobacco	Discontinue smoking	Rarely develops into palatal cancer

WHITE LESIONS

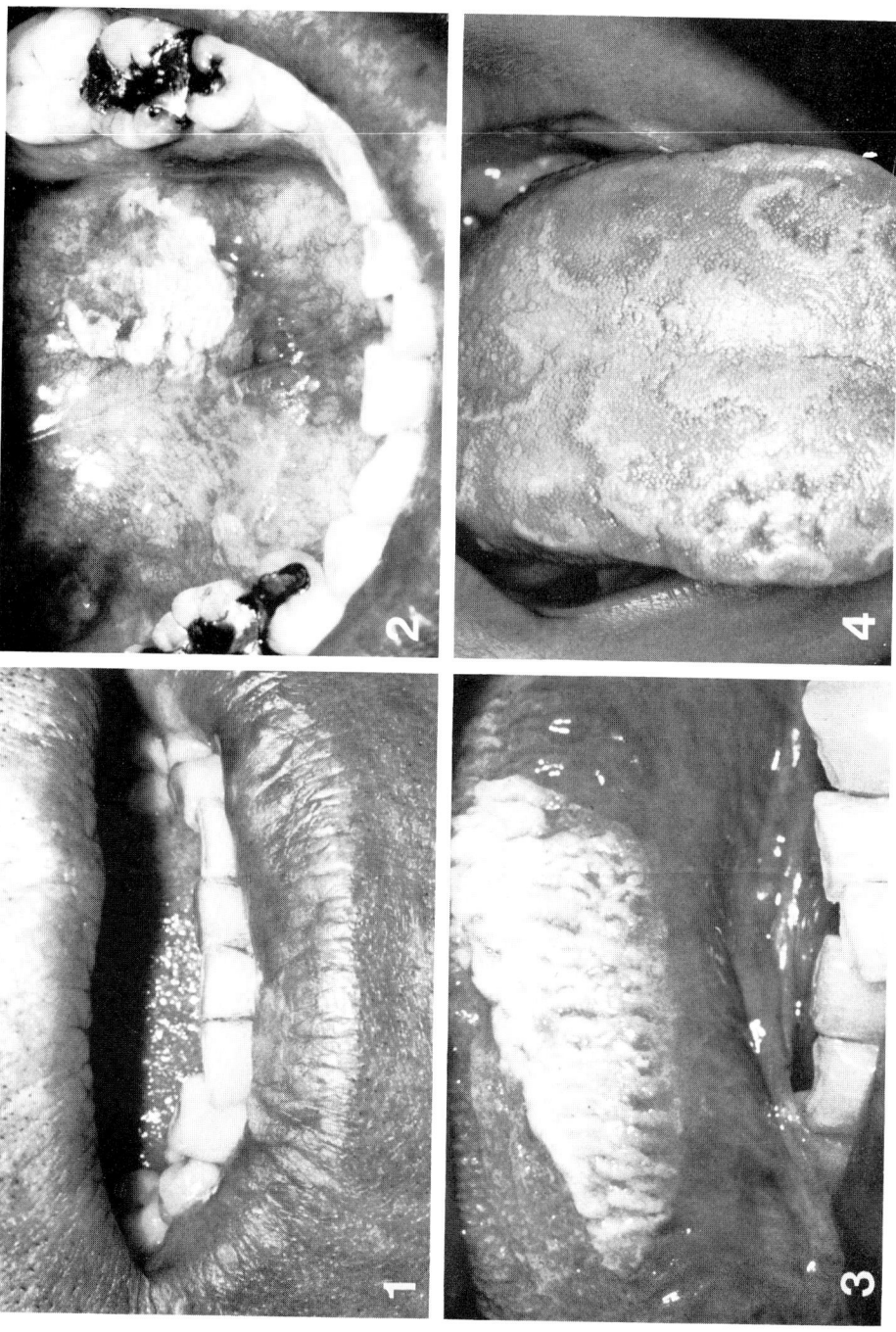

WHITE LESIONS (continued)

Disease	Clinical Features	Cause	Treatment	Significance
Solar cheilitis (Fig. 1) (p. 93–94)	Lower lip—atrophic epithelium, poor definition of vermilion-skin margin, focal zones of keratosis; common	UV light (especially UVB, 2900–3200 Å) and aging	Sun screens (PABA) and sun blockers (zinc oxide, titanium dioxide), surgery in severe cases	May result in chronic ulceration or squamous cell carcinoma
Idiopathic leukoplakia (Fig. 2) (p. 94–100)	Asymptomatic, white patch; cannot be wiped off; males affected more than females	Unknown; may be related to tobacco and alcohol use	Biopsy, excision	May recur after excision; 5% are malignant, 5% become malignant
Hairy leukoplakia (Fig. 3) (p. 100–102)	Filiform to flat patch on lateral tongue, often bilateral, occasionally on buccal mucosa; asymptomatic, found in *high-risk AIDS patients*	Unknown, probably Epstein-Barr virus	No specific treatment, evaluate for AIDS	Pre-AIDS sign in high-risk patients; many patients develops AIDS
Hairy tongue (p. 102–103)	Elongation of filiform papillae; asymptomatic	Unknown; may follow antibiotic or corticosteroid use	Improve oral hygiene; identify contributing factors	Benign process; may be cosmetically objectionable
Geographic tongue (Fig. 4) (p. 103–105)	White, annular lesions with atrophic red centers; pattern migrates over dorsum of tongue; varies in intensity and may spontaneously disappear; occasionally painful; common	Unknown	None, symptomatic treatment for painful lesions	Completely benign; spontaneous regression after months to years

WHITE LESIONS

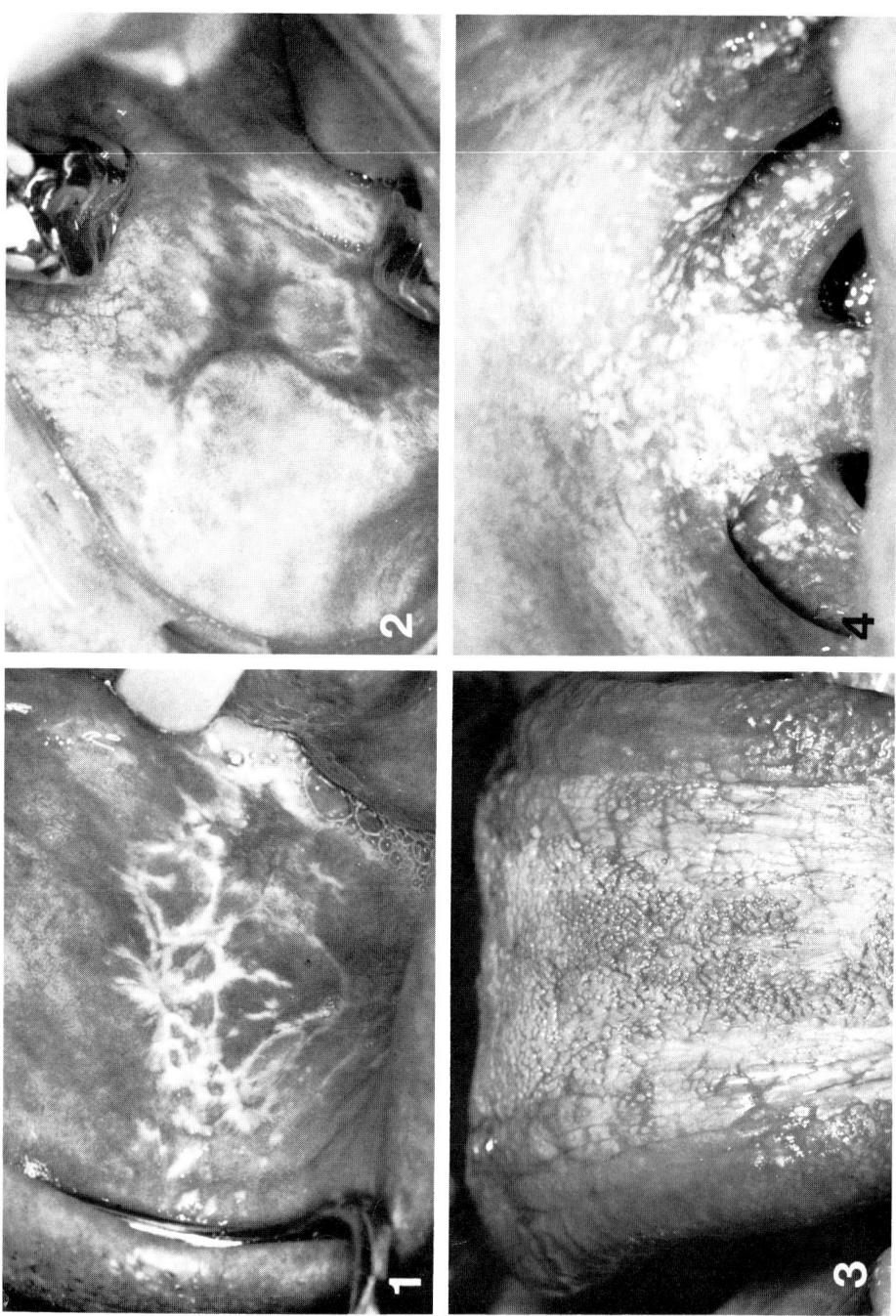

WHITE LESIONS (continued)

Disease	Clinical Features	Cause	Treatment	Significance
Lichen planus (Figs. 1–3) (p. 105–110)	Bilateral, white striae (Wickham's); asymptomatic except when erosions are present (Fig. 2); skin lesions occasionally present and are purple, pruritic papules; seen in middle age; buccal mucosa most commonly affected, with lesions occasionally on tongue, gingiva, and palate; forearm and lower leg most frequent skin areas; uncommon	Unknown; precipitated by stress; may be hyperimmune condition mediated by T cells	Topical or systemic steroids; retinoids may be helpful with or instead of steroids; follow-up examinations necessary	May regress after many years; treatment may only control disease; rare malignant transformation
Candidiasis (Fig. 4) (p. 110–116)	Painful, elevated plaques (fungus) can be wiped off, leaving eroded, bleeding surface; associated with poor hygiene, systemic antibiotics, systemic diseases, debilitation, reduced immune response; chronic infections may result in erythematous mucosa without obvious white colonies; common	Opportunistic fungus—*Candida albicans*	Clotrimazole troches or nystatin suspension and treatment of underlying disease if present	Usually disappears in 1 to 2 weeks after treatment; some chronic cases require long-term therapy

WHITE LESIONS

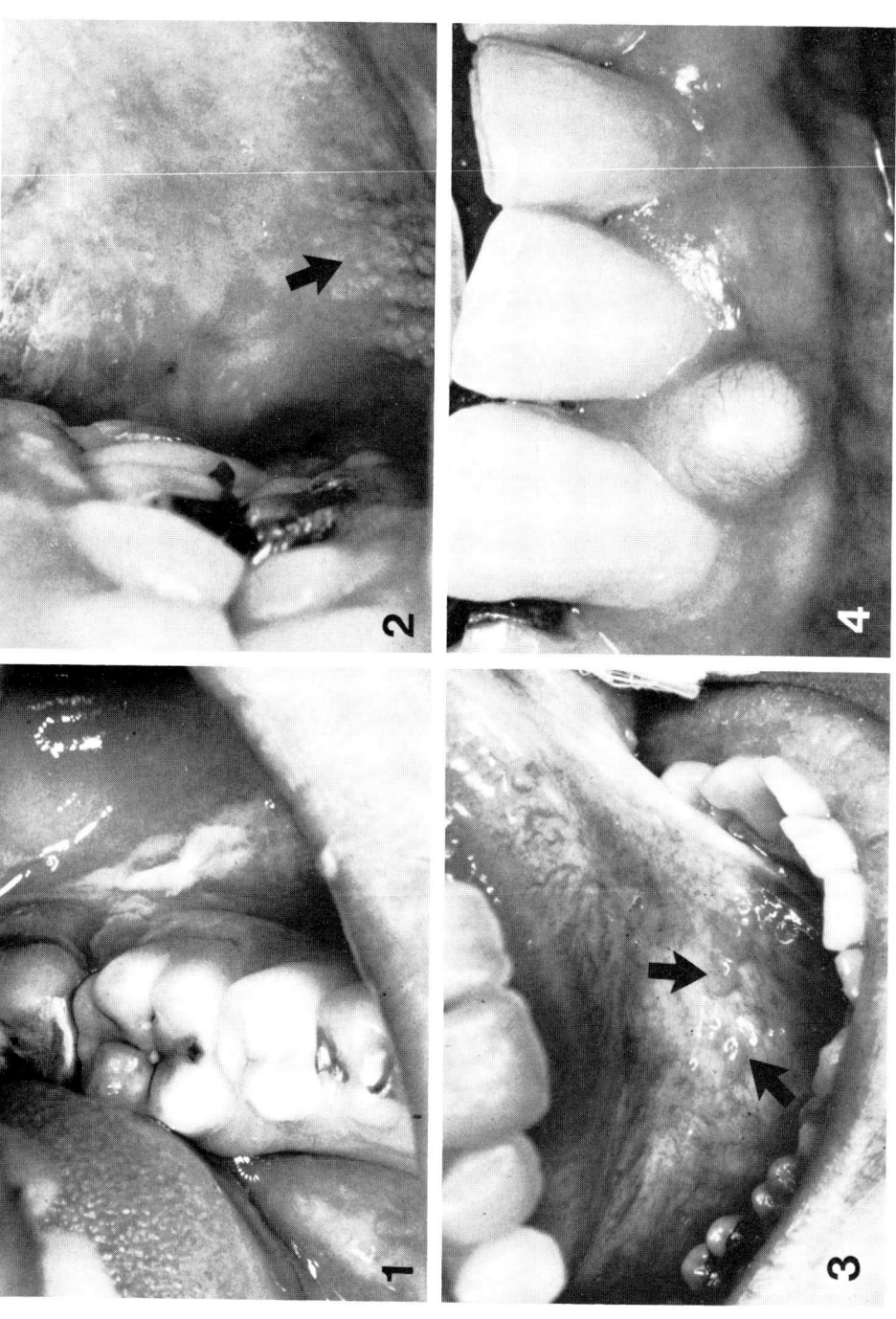

WHITE LESIONS (continued)

Disease	Clinical Features	Cause	Treatment	Significance
Mucosal burns (Fig. 1) (p. 116–117)	Painful, white fibrin exudate covering superficial ulcer with erythematous ring; common	Chemicals (aspirin, phenol), heat, electrical burns	Remove cause; symptomatic therapy	Heals in days to weeks
Submucous fibrosis (p. 117–118)	Areas of opacification with loss of elasticity; any oral region affected; rare	?Hypersensitivity to dietary constituents	None consistently effective	Irreversible; predisposes to oral cancer
Fordyce's granules (Fig. 2) (p. 118–119)	Multiple, asymptomatic, yellow, flat or elevated spots seen primarily in buccal mucosa and lips; seen in a majority of patients; many consider them to be a variation of normal	Developmental	None; lesions are diagnostic clinically and should not be biopsied	Ectopic sebaceous glands of no significance
Ectopic lymphoid tissue (Fig. 3) (p. 119–120)	Asymptomatic, elevated, yellow nodules less than 0.5 cm in diameter; usually found on tonsillar pillars, posterolateral tongue, and floor of mouth; covered by intact epithelium; common	Unknown	None	No significance; remain indefinitely and are usually diagnostic clinically
Gingival cyst (Fig. 4) (p. 120–122)	Small, usually white to yellow nodule; multiple in infants, solitary in adults; common in infants, rare in adults	Proliferation and cystification of dental lamina rests	None when in infants; excision when in adults	In infants, lesions spontaneously rupture or break when teeth erupt; recurrence not expected in adults
Parulis (p. 122–123)	Yellow-white gingival swelling due to submucosal pus	Periodontitis or tooth abscess	Treat periodontal pocket or non-vital tooth	Periodic drainage until primary cause is eliminated
Lipoma (p. 123)	Asymptomatic, slow-growing, well-circumscribed, yellow or yellow-white tumescence; rare, benign neoplasm of fat; occurs in any area	Unknown	Excision	Seems to have limited growth potential intraorally, recurrence not expected after removal

RED-BLUE LESIONS

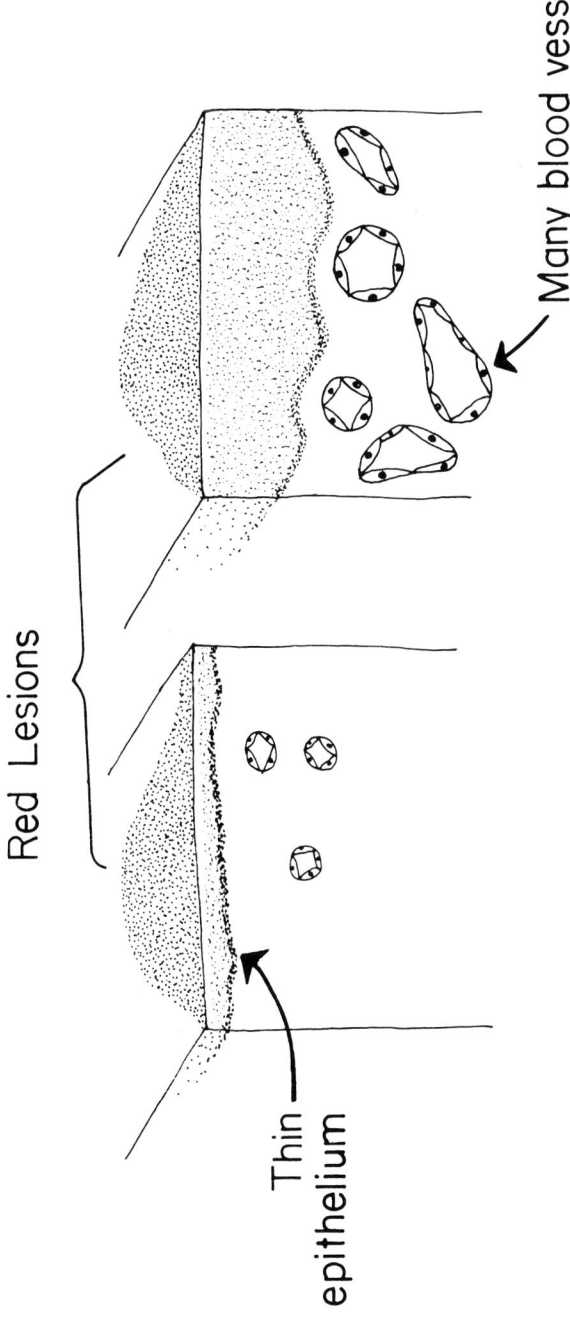

Red Lesions

Thin epithelium

Many blood vessels

Lesions may appear red either because of epithelial atrophy (allowing the submucosal vasculature to show, as in the tongue changes of pernicious anemia) or because of an actual increase in the number of submucosal blood vessels (hemangioma). They may also appear red because of extravasation of blood into soft tissues.

Chapter 4

Red-Blue Lesions

INTRAVASCULAR, FOCAL
Developmental Lesions
 Hemangioma
Reactive Lesions
 Pyogenic Granuloma
 Peripheral Giant Cell Granuloma
 Median Rhomboid Glossitis
Neoplasms
 Erythroplakia
 Kaposi's Sarcoma
Unknown Etiology
 Geographic Tongue
 Psoriasis
INTRAVASCULAR, DIFFUSE
Metabolic-Endocrine Conditions
 Vitamin B Deficiency
 Pernicious Anemia
 Iron Deficiency Anemia
 Burning Mouth Syndrome
Infectious Conditions
 Scarlet Fever
 Atrophic Candidiasis
Immunologic Abnormalities
 Plasma Cell Gingivitis
 Drug Reactions and Contact Allergies
EXTRAVASCULAR—PETECHIAE AND
 ECCHYMOSES

RED-BLUE LESIONS

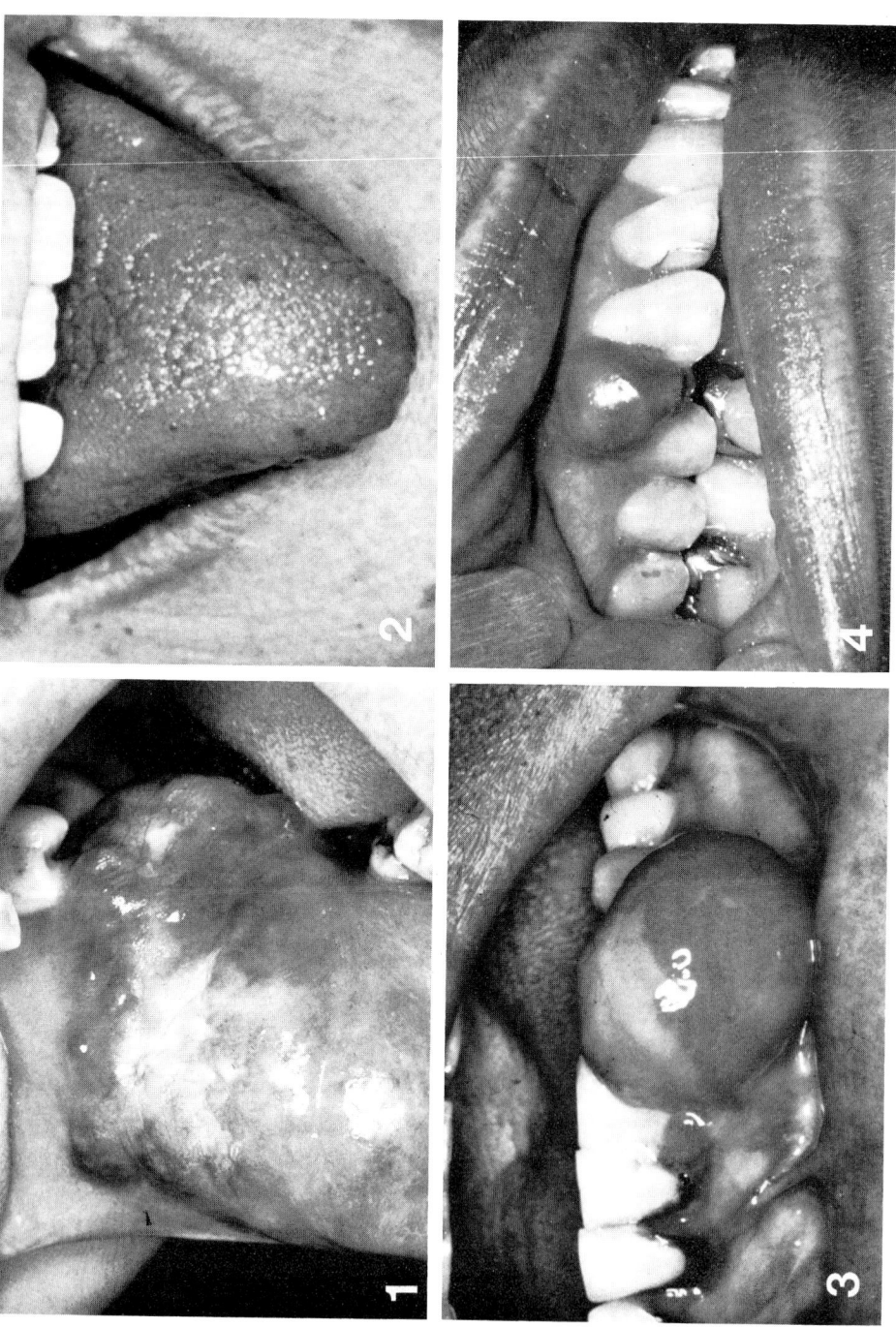

O-30

RED-BLUE LESIONS

Disease	Clinical Features	Cause	Treatment	Significance
Hemangioma (Figs. 1 and 2) (p. 125–130)	Red or blue lesion which blanches when compressed; extent of lesion usually difficult to determine; skin, lips, tongue, and buccal mucosa most commonly affected; common on skin, uncommon in mucous membrane, rare in bone; part of Sturge-Weber syndrome (intracranial calcifications, seizures, mental retardation); telangiectasias (small focal dilations of terminal blood vessels) blanch when compressed; commonly found in sun-damaged skin, and seen with Rendu-Osler-Weber syndrome or hereditary hemorrhagic telangiectasia (HHT) (Fig. 2); venous varix is a form of vascular malformation seen on lower lip and ventral tongue	Some are benign congenital neoplasms, others are due to abnormal vessel morphogenesis (vascular malformation); *HHT*—autosomal dominant; *venous varix*—congenital or induced by UV light	Most congenital lesions involute without treatment; vascular malformations require surgical removal; *HHT*—may be treated with surgery or cautery; *venous varix*—none	May remain quiescent or gradually enlarge; hemorrhage may be a significant complication; often a cosmetic problem; *HHT*—epistaxis may be a problem
Pyogenic granuloma (Fig. 3) (p. 131–132)	Asymptomatic, red tumescence composed of granulation tissue; most commonly seen in gingiva; periodontal ligament origin; may be secondarily ulcerated; common	Trauma or chronic irritation; size modified by hormonal changes	Excision	Remains indefinitely; recurrence if incompletely excised; reduction in size if cause removed or after pregnancy
Peripheral giant cell granuloma (Fig. 4) (p. 132–134)	Asymptomatic, red tumescence of gingiva composed of granulation tissue and multinucleated giant cells; found mostly in adults in the former area of deciduous teeth; produces cup-shaped lucency when found in edentulous areas; uncommon	Trauma or chronic irritation	Excision	Remains indefinitely if untreated, a reactive lesion

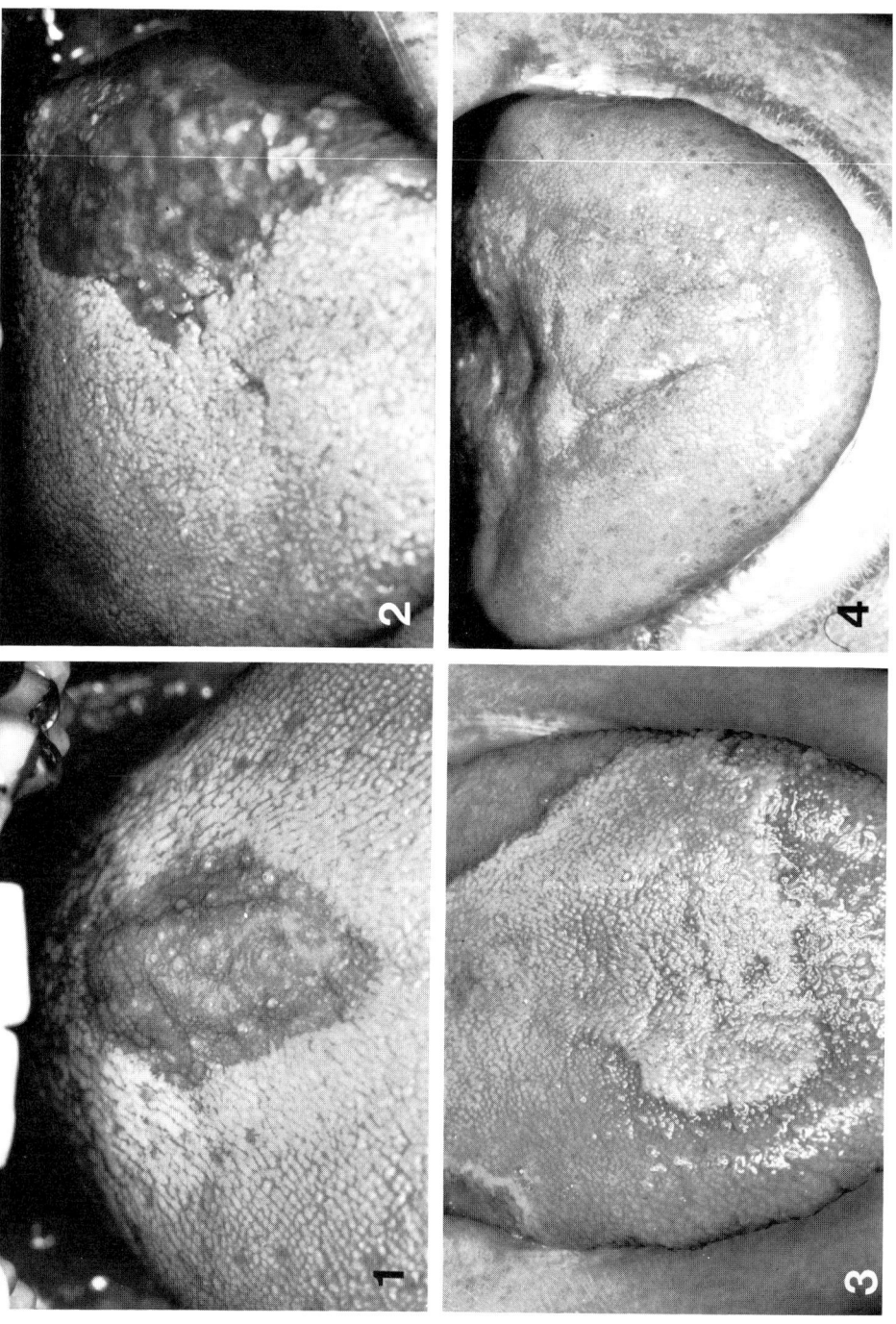

RED-BLUE LESIONS (continued)

Disease	Clinical Features	Cause	Treatment	Significance
Median rhomboid glossitis (Fig. 1) (p. 134–135)	Red, lobular elevation anterior to circumvallate papillae in midline	?Congenital versus acquired	None	May support growth of *Candida albicans*
Erythroplakia (Fig. 2) (p. 135–137)	Asymptomatic, red "velvety" patch found usually in floor of mouth or retromolar area in adults; seen in older adults; red lesions may have foci of white hyperkeratosis (speckled erythroplakia)	Unknown	Excision	Most (90%) are *in situ* or invasive squamous cell carcinoma
Kaposi's sarcoma (p. 137–139)	Malignant neoplasm of capillaries may be part of AIDS; usually on extremities but may be oral, especially in palate; reddish-brown or red to blue nodules; rare	Unknown	Surgery, radiation, chemotherapy	Good prognosis except when part of AIDS
Geographic tongue (Fig. 3) (p. 139)	White, annular lesions with atrophic, red centers; white (keratotic) areas may be poorly developed, leaving red patches on dorsum of tongue; occasionally painful; common	Unknown	None; symptomatic treatment	Little significance except when painful; not premalignant
Psoriasis (p. 139–141)	Chronic skin disease with rare oral lesions; red skin lesions covered with silvery scales; oral lesions red to white patches	Unknown	Topical or systemic drugs; photochemotherapy	Must have skin lesions to confirm oral disease; exacerbations and remissions are typical
Vitamin B deficiency (Fig. 4) (p. 141–142)	Generalized redness of tongue due to atrophy of papillae; may be painful; may have an associated angular cheilitis; rare in U.S.	B complex deficiency	Vitamin B supplements	Remains until therapeutic levels of vitamin B are administered
Anemia (pernicious and iron deficiency) (p. 142–143)	May result in generalized redness of tongue due to atrophy of papillae; may be painful; may have angular cheilitis; females more commonly affected than males; Plummer-Vinson syndrome—anemia (iron deficiency), mucosal atrophy, predisposition for oral cancer	Some forms acquired, some hereditary	Diagnosis and treatment of specific type of anemia	Some types may be life threatening; oral manifestations disappear with treatment; complication of oral cancer with Plummer-Vinson syndrome

RED-BLUE LESIONS

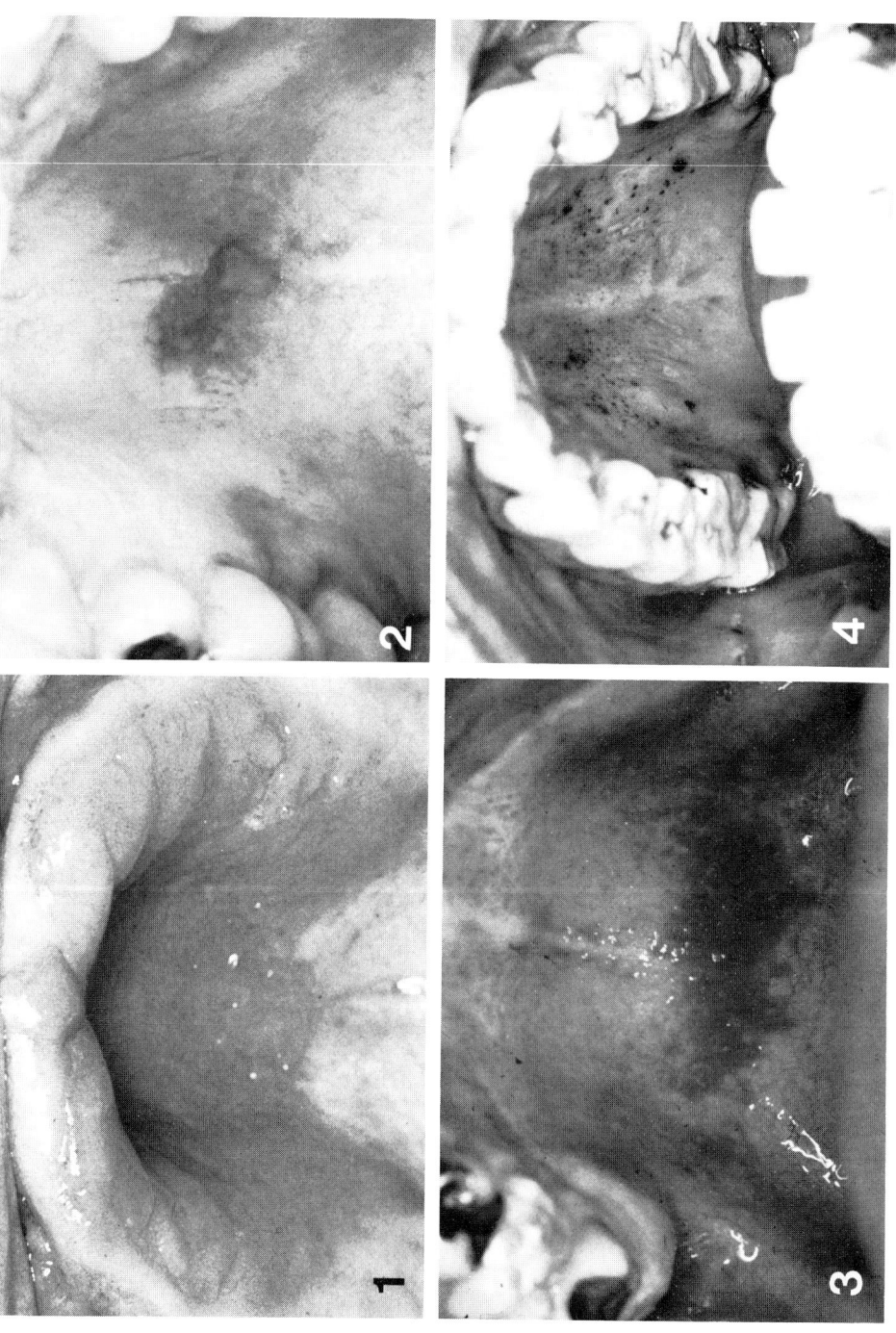

RED-BLUE LESIONS (continued)

Disease	Clinical Features	Cause	Treatment	Significance
Burning mouth syndrome (p. 143–145)	Wide range of oral complaints, usually without any visible tissue changes; especially middle-aged females; uncommon	Multifactorial—e.g., *Candida albicans*, vitamin B deficiency, anemias, xerostomia, idiopathic	Antifungal, steroid, vitamin B, iron; symptomatic; empathy and careful explanation required	May persist in spite of treatment
Scarlet fever (p. 145)	Pharyngitis, systemic symptoms, strawberry tongue	Group A streptococci	Penicillin	Complications of rheumatic fever and glomerulonephritis
Atrophic candidiasis (Fig. 1) (p. 145)	Painful, hyperemic palate under denture; angular cheilitis; red, painful mucosa	Chronic *Candida albicans* infection; poor oral hygiene, ill-fitting denture are frequent predisposing factors	Nystatin, instruction on good oral hygiene, new denture	Discomfort may prevent wearing of denture; not allergic or premalignant
Plasma cell gingivitis (p. 145–146)	Red, painful tongue; angular cheilitis; red gingiva	Allergic reaction to ?dietary antigen	Eliminate allergen	Gingival lesions similar to lupus, lichen planus, and pemphigoid lesions
Drug reactions and contact allergies (Fig. 2) (p. 146)	Red, vesicular, or ulcerative eruption	Immune reaction to allergen	Identify and remove cause	May simulate lesions of vitamin B deficiency and anemia
Petechiae and ecchymoses Traumatic lesions (Fig. 3) (p. 146–149)	Hemorrhagic spot (red, blue, purple, black) composed of extravasated blood in soft tissue; does not blanch with compression; may be seen anywhere in skin or mucous membranes after trauma; changes color as blood is degraded and resorbed	Follows traumatic insult such as tooth extraction, tooth bite, fellatio, chronic cough	Observe	Resolves in days to weeks; no sequelae
Blood dyscrasias (Fig. 4) (p. 149)	Hemorrhagic spots (small—petechiae, large—ecchymoses) on mucous membranes due to extravasated blood; may be spontaneous or follow minor trauma; spots do not blanch with compression; color varies with time; uncommon in general practice but dental personnel may be first to observe	Lack of clotting factor, reduced numbers of platelets for various reasons, or lack of vessel integrity	Treatment of underlying blood disease	May be life threatening; must be investigated, diagnosed, and treated

PIGMENTATIONS OF ORAL AND PERIORAL TISSUES

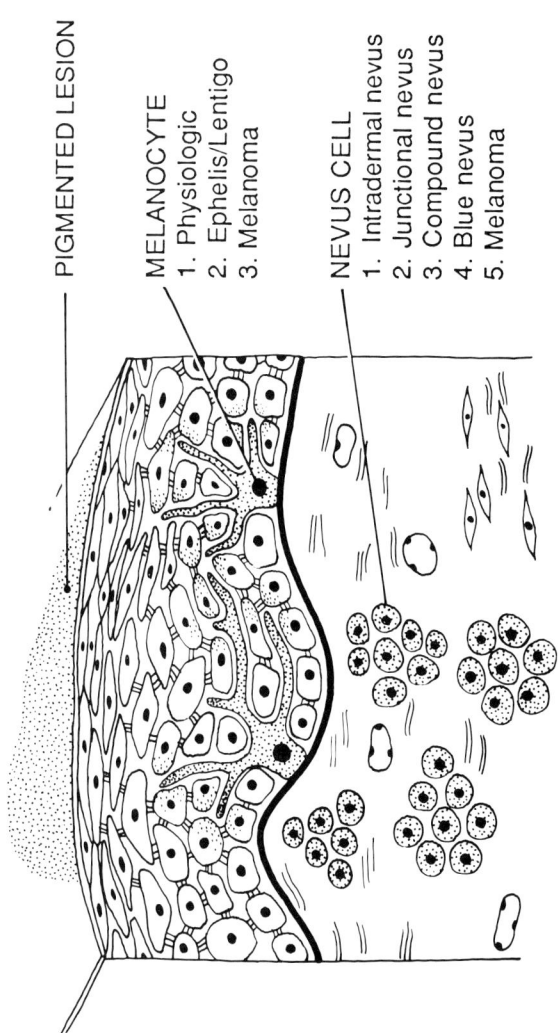

PIGMENTED LESION

MELANOCYTE
1. Physiologic
2. Ephelis/Lentigo
3. Melanoma

NEVUS CELL
1. Intradermal nevus
2. Junctional nevus
3. Compound nevus
4. Blue nevus
5. Melanoma

Oral lesions of abnormal color can generally be divided into two large groups, pigmented lesions and vascular lesions, with a third small group of yellow lesions.

Pigmented lesions appear dark because of melanin production by either the melanocyte or its close relative, the nevus cell. Physiologic pigmentation, ephelides, and lentigines are due to melanocyte stimulation; the various types of nevi are due to pigment production by nevus cells. Malignant melanoma may theoretically arise from either cell.

Chapter 5

Pigmentations of Oral and Perioral Tissues

BENIGN LESIONS OF MELANOCYTE ORIGIN
Physiologic Pigmentation
Smoking-Associated Melanosis
Ephelis
Lentigo
Café-au-lait Macule
Oral Melanotic Macule
Vitiligo
NEOPLASMS
Nevus
Melanoma
Neuroectodermal Tumor of Infancy
PIGMENTATIONS CAUSED BY EXOGENOUS DEPOSITS
Amalgam Tattoo
Heavy-Metal Pigmentation
Minocycline Pigmentation

PIGMENTATIONS OF ORAL AND PERIORAL TISSUES

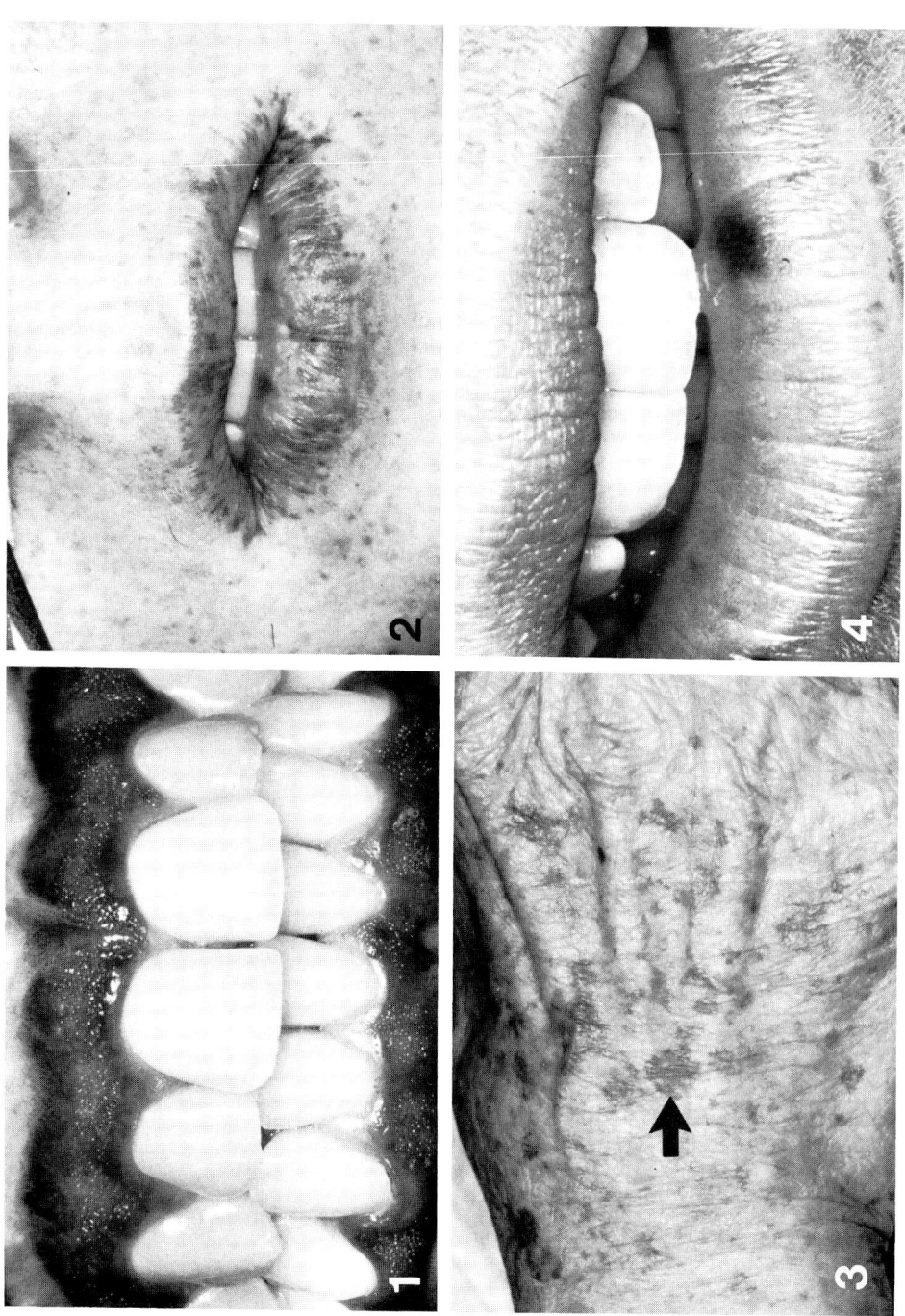

PIGMENTATIONS OF ORAL AND PERIORAL TISSUES

Disease	Clinical Features	Cause	Treatment	Significance
Physiologic pigmentation (Fig. 1) (p. 151–153)	Symmetric distribution; does not change in intensity; does not alter surface morphology	Normal melanocyte activity	None	None
Smoking-associated melanosis (p. 153)	Gingival pigmentation; especially females on birth control pills	Component in smoke stimulates melanocytes	Reversal after cessation of smoking	Cosmetic
Ephelis (Fig. 2) (p. 153–155)	Macule, asymptomatic, tan or brown; perioral ephelides associated with Peutz-Jeghers syndrome (intestinal polyposis) and Addison's disease (adrenal cortex insufficiency); common lesions of skin, rare intraorally	Melanocyte activity stimulated by UV light	None; if intraoral, excision may be indicated to rule out melanoma	Remain indefinitely; may darken if exposed to UV light
Lentigo (Fig. 3) (p. 155)	Brown macules on face or dorsa of hands (sun-exposed skin) of middle-aged or elderly; common skin lesion	Melanocyte activity	None	Remain indefinitely; cosmetic significance only
Café-au-lait macule (p. 156)	Large, brown skin macules; six or more may indicate neurofibromatosis (von Recklinghausen's disease of nerve); may be part of fibrous dysplasia (Albright's syndrome); uncommon	Melanocyte activity	None	Remain indefinitely
Oral melanotic macule (Fig. 4) (p. 156)	Flat, oral pigmentation less than 1 cm in diameter; lower lip, gingiva, buccal mucosa, palate usually affected; may represent oral ephelis	Unknown; post-inflammatory; trauma	Excision may be required to rule out melanoma	Remains indefinitely, not known to be premalignant
Vitiligo (p. 156–157)	Patches of depigmentation on skin or mucosa	Unknown; ?immunologic abnormality	Use of tanning or other creams	Cosmetically objectionable

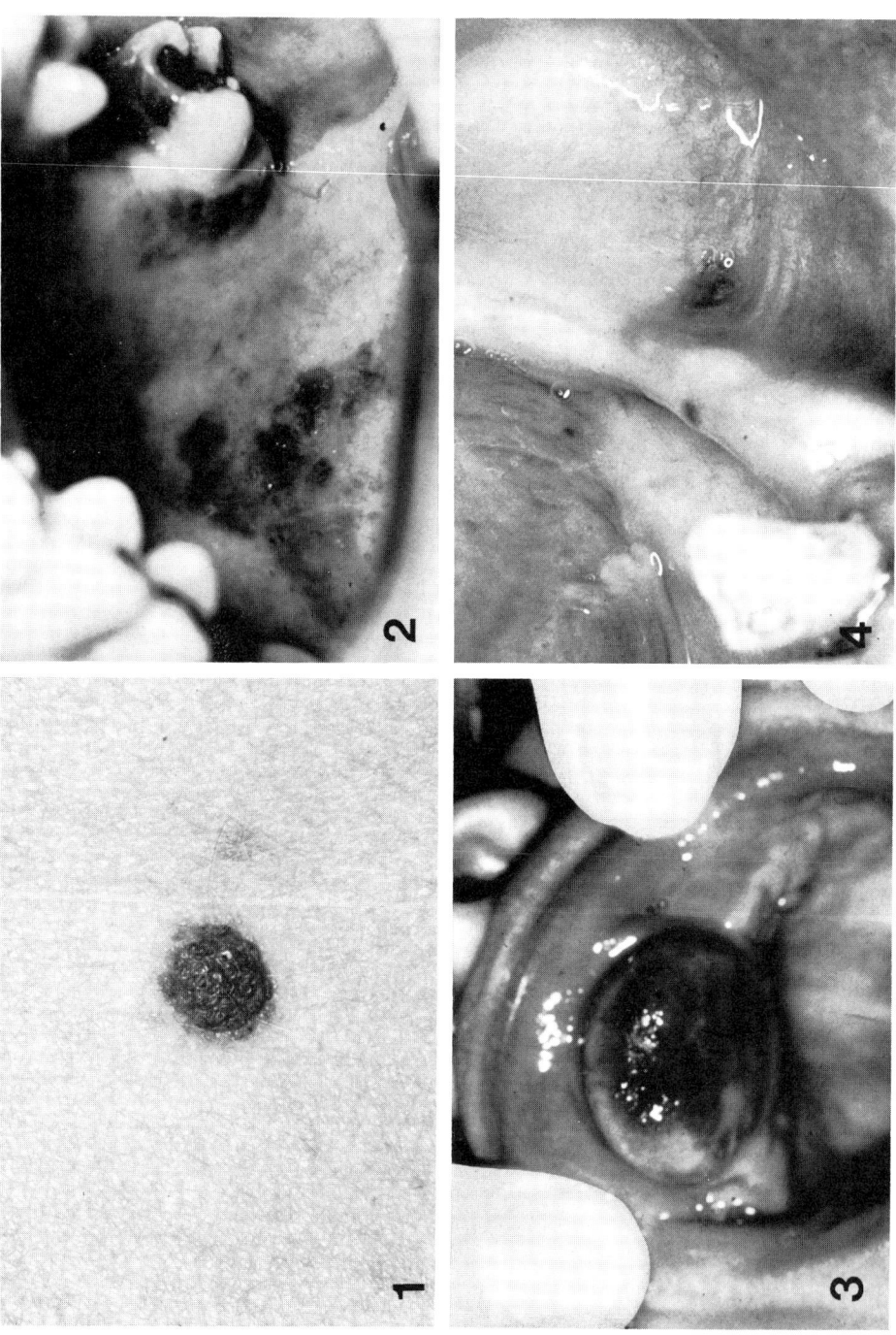

PIGMENTATIONS OF ORAL AND PERIORAL TISSUES (continued)

Disease	Clinical Features	Cause	Treatment	Significance
Nevus (Fig. 1) (p. 157–160)	Elevated pigmentations; often non-pigmented when intraoral; 15 per person on skin, uncommon orally; blue nevi seen in palate; cannot clinically separate various microscopic types	Unknown, due to nests of nevus cells	Skin—excision of irritated or suspicious lesions to rule out melanoma; oral—excise all nevi to rule out melanoma	Remains indefinitely
Melanoma (Fig. 2) (p. 160–163)	Malignancy of pigmentary system; many develop from pre-existing pigmented spot; some have a radial growth phase of years' duration (superficial type) before vertical growth phase, but nodular type has only vertical growth phase; oral melanomas may appear first as insignificant spot, especially on palate and maxillary ridge; adults affected	UV light may be carcinogenic; chronic irritation and trauma probably co-carcinogens	Wide surgical excision	Skin—65% five-year survival; oral—20% five-year survival; superficial melanomas have better prognosis than nodular melanomas; bad reputation because of unpredictable metastatic behavior
Neuroectodermal tumor of infancy (Fig. 3) (p. 163)	Pigmented, radiolucent, benign neoplasm in maxilla of newborns; pigment is melanin; rare	Unknown; tumor cells of neural crest origin	Excision	Recurrence unlikely
Amalgam tattoo (Fig. 4) (p. 163–164)	Asymptomatic, gray-pigmented macule found in gingiva, tongue, palate, or buccal mucosa adjacent to amalgam restoration; may be seen radiographically if particles are large; no associated inflammation; common	Traumatic implantation of amalgam	Observe or excise if melanoma cannot be ruled out on clinical basis	Remains indefinitely and changes little; no ill effects
Heavy-metal pigmentation (p. 165–166)	Dark line along marginal gingiva due to precipitation of metal; rare	Intoxication by metal vapors (lead, bismuth, arsenic, mercury) from occupational exposure	Treat systemic problem	Exposure may affect systemic health; gingiva pigmentation of cosmetic significance
Minocycline pigmentation (p. 166)	Gray pigmentation of palate, skin, scars, bone, and, rarely, of formed teeth	Ingestion of minocycline	None	Must differentiate from melanoma

VERRUCAL-PAPILLARY LESIONS

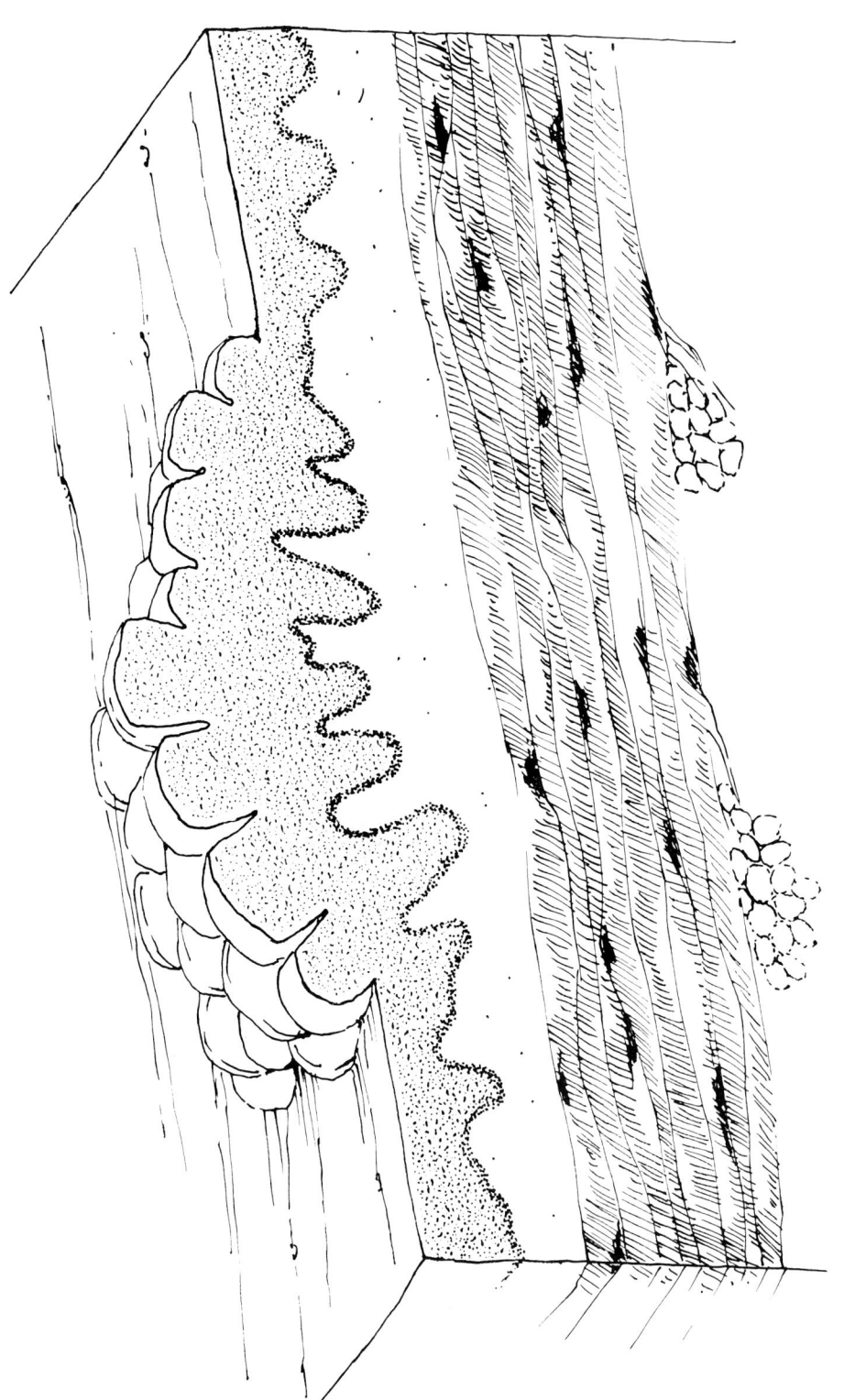

Lesions in this rather small group present as outgrowths from mucous membranes. They range from insignificant lesions of limited growth potential to verrucous carcinoma.

Chapter 6
Verrucal-Papillary Lesions

REACTIVE LESIONS
Papillary Hyperplasia
Condyloma Latum
Squamous Papilloma/Oral Verruca Vulgaris
Condyloma Acuminatum
Focal Epithelial Hyperplasia
NEOPLASMS
Keratoacanthoma
Verrucous Carcinoma
UNKNOWN ETIOLOGY
Pyostomatitis Vegetans
Verruciform Xanthoma

VERRUCAL-PAPILLARY LESIONS

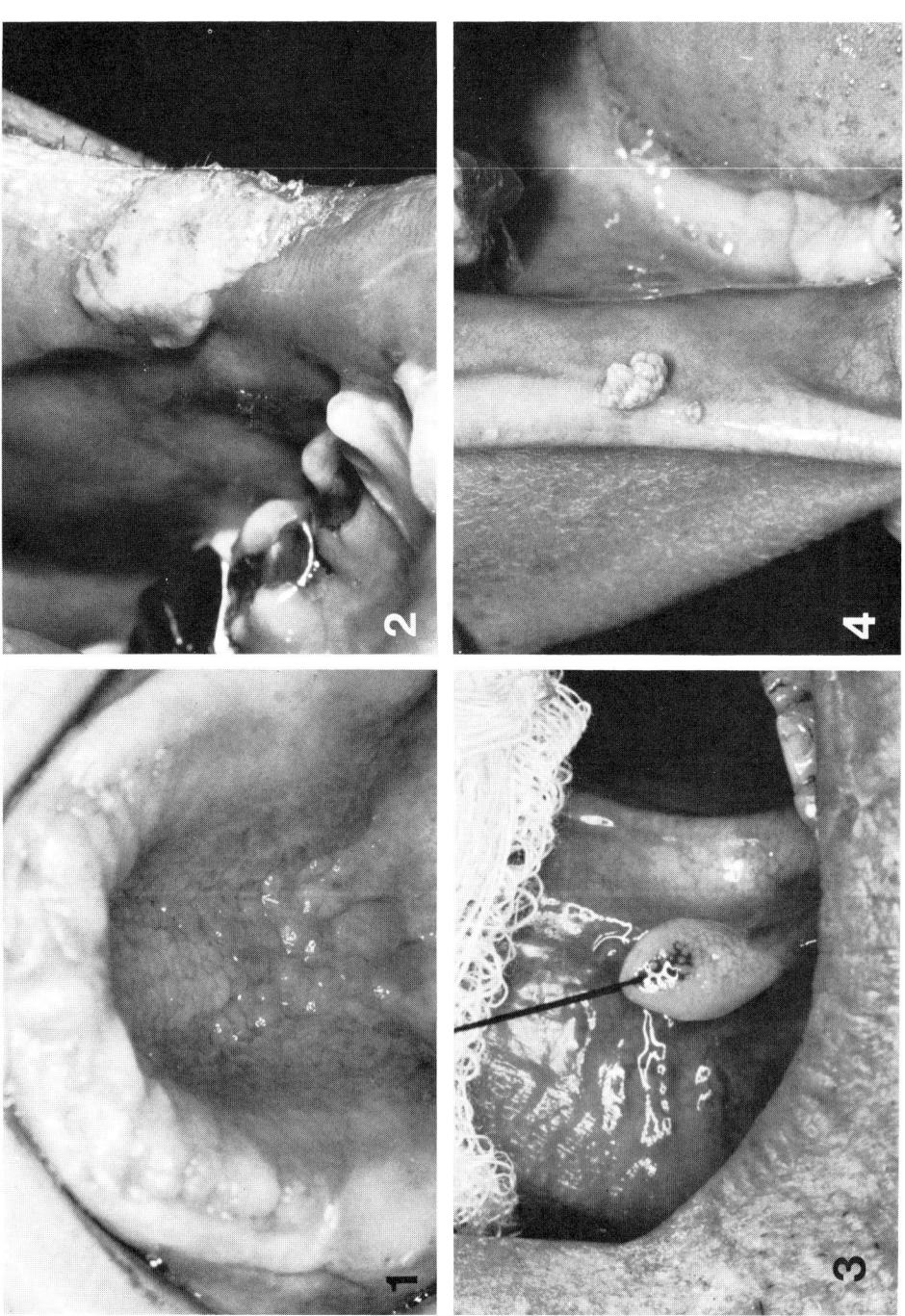

VERRUCAL-PAPILLARY LESIONS

Disease	Clinical Features	Cause	Treatment	Significance
Papillary hyperplasia (Fig. 1) (p. 167–168)	Painless, papillomatous, "cobblestone" lesion of hard palate in denture wearers; usually red due to inflammation; common	Soft tissue reaction to ill-fitting denture	Excision; construction of new denture	Lesion is not premalignant; may show significant regression if denture taken away from patient
Condyloma latum (Fig. 2) (p. 169)	Clinically similar to papillary hyperplasia; part of secondary syphilis	*Treponema pallidum*	Penicillin	Prognosis good with treatment
Squamous papilloma (Fig. 3) (p. 169–172)	Painless, exophytic granular to cauliflower-like lesions; predilection for tongue, floor of mouth, palate, uvula, lips, faucial pillars; generally solitary; soft texture; color is white or same as surrounding tissue; young adults and adults; common	Some due to papillomavirus, some unknown	Excision	Lesion has no known malignant potential; recurrences rare
Oral verruca vulgaris (Fig. 4) (p. 169–172)	Painless, papillary lesion usually with white surface projections because of keratin production; may be clinically indistinguishable from papilloma; children and young adults; common on skin, uncommon intraorally	Papillomavirus	Excision	Little significance; may be multiple and a cosmetic problem
Condyloma acuminatum (p. 172–174)	Painless, pedunculated to sessile, exophytic, papillomatous lesion; adults; same color as or lighter than surrounding tissue; patient or sexual partner will have similar lesions; rare in oral cavity	Papillomavirus	Excision	Oral lesions acquired through autoinoculation or sexual contact with infected partner; recurrences common

VERRUCAL-PAPILLARY LESIONS

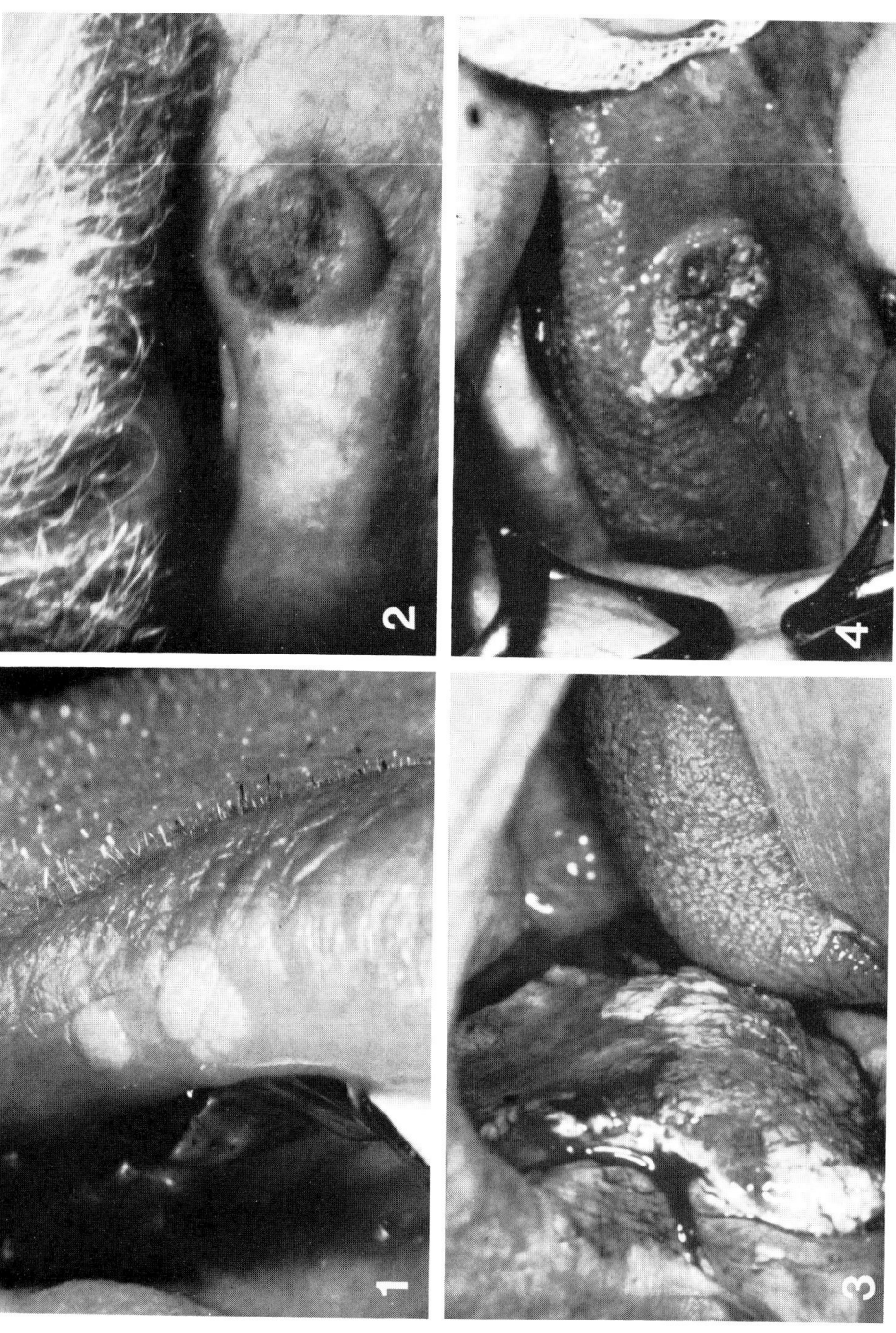

VERRUCAL-PAPILLARY LESIONS (continued)

Disease	Clinical Features	Cause	Treatment	Significance
Focal epithelial hyperplasia (Fig. 1) (p. 174–175)	Multiple soft nodules on lips, tongue, buccal mucosa; asymptomatic	Papillomavirus likely	Excision	Little significance, may be included in differential diagnosis of mucosal nodules
Keratoacanthoma (Fig. 2) (p. 175–177)	Well-circumscribed, firm, elevated lesion with central keratin plug; may cause pain; develops rapidly over 4 to 8 weeks and involutes in 6 to 8 weeks; found on sun-exposed skin and lips; rare intraorally; predilection for adult males	Unknown	Excision or observation	Difficult to differentiate clinically and microscopically from squamous cell carcinoma; may heal with scar
Verrucous carcinoma (Figs. 3 and 4) (p. 178–180)	Broad-based, exophytic, indurated lesion; usually found in buccal mucosa or vestibule; adult males most frequently affected; uncommon	Most are associated with use of tobacco, especially smokeless tobacco	Excision; radiation may be inappropriate	Slow-growing malignancy; well differentiated with better prognosis than usual squamous cell carcinoma; growth pattern is more expansile than invasive; metastasis uncommon
Pyostomatitis vegetans (p. 180)	Multiple, small pustules in oral mucosa; males more than females	Unknown	Topical preparations plus control of inflammatory bowel disease	May be associated with bowel disease such as ulcerative colitis or Crohn's disease
Verruciform xanthoma (p. 180–182)	Solitary, pebbly, elevated or depressed lesion occurring anywhere in oral mucous membrane; color ranges from white to red; rare	Unknown	Excision	Limited growth potential; does not recur

SUBMUCOSAL SWELLINGS (BY REGION)

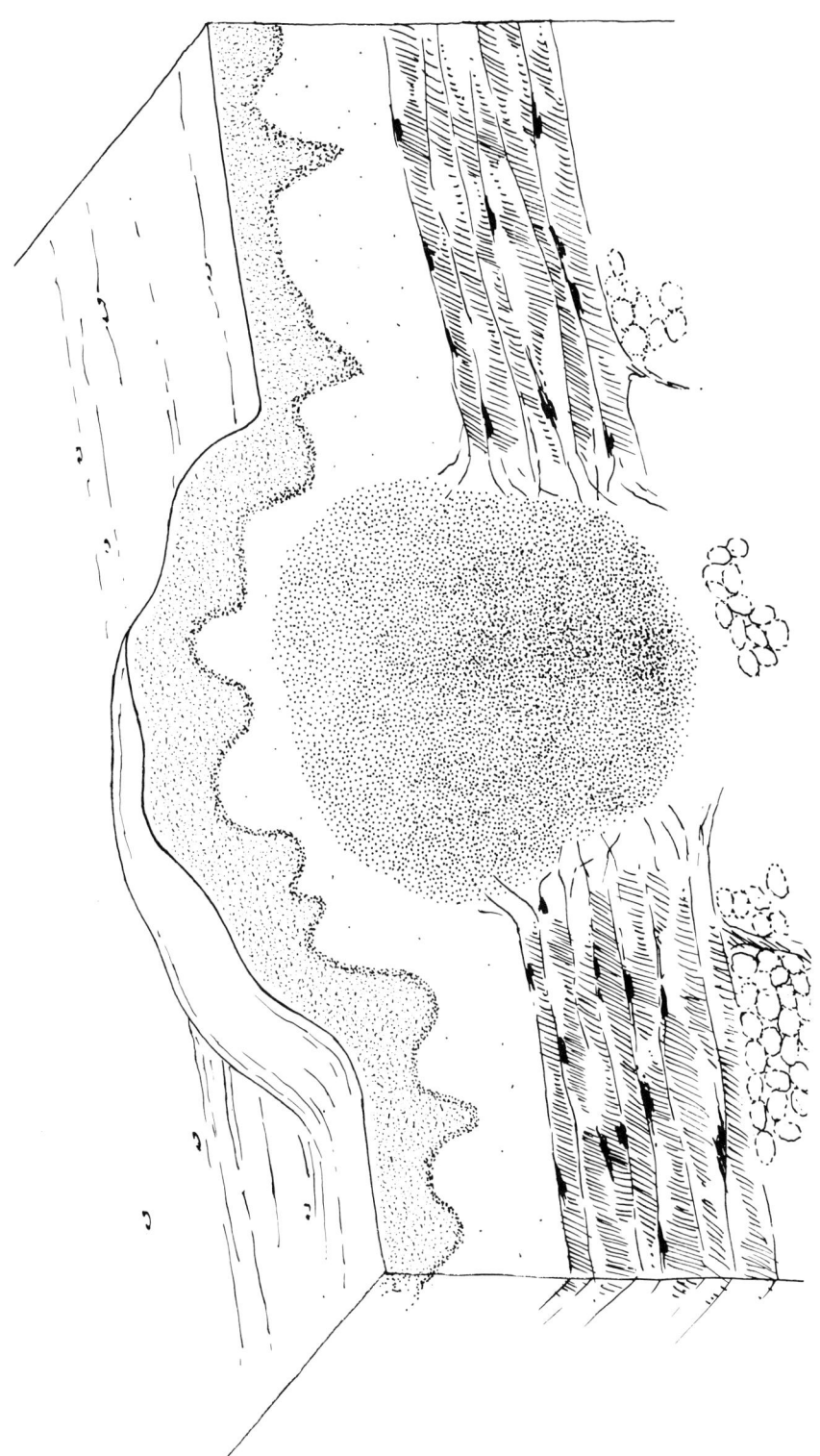

This group of lumps and bumps characteristically presents as asymptomatic swellings covered by normal, intact epithelium. A differential diagnosis is dependent upon the region in which they are found. Many entities and disease subtypes not listed in this section are described in detail in Chapters 7, 8, and 9, on connective tissue, salivary gland, and lymphoid lesions.

Chapters 7–9

Submucosal Swellings (By Region)

GINGIVAL SWELLINGS
Focal
*Pyogenic Granuloma
Peripheral Giant Cell Granuloma
Peripheral Fibroma
Parulis
Exostosis
Gingival Cyst
Eruption Cyst
Congenital Epulis of the Newborn*
Generalized Hyperplasia
*Non-specific Hyperplastic Gingivitis
Dilantin-Induced Hyperplasia
Hormone-Modified Hyperplasia
Leukemia-Induced Hyperplasia
Idiopathic (Genetically Influenced?) Fibrous Hyperplasia*

GINGIVAL SWELLINGS

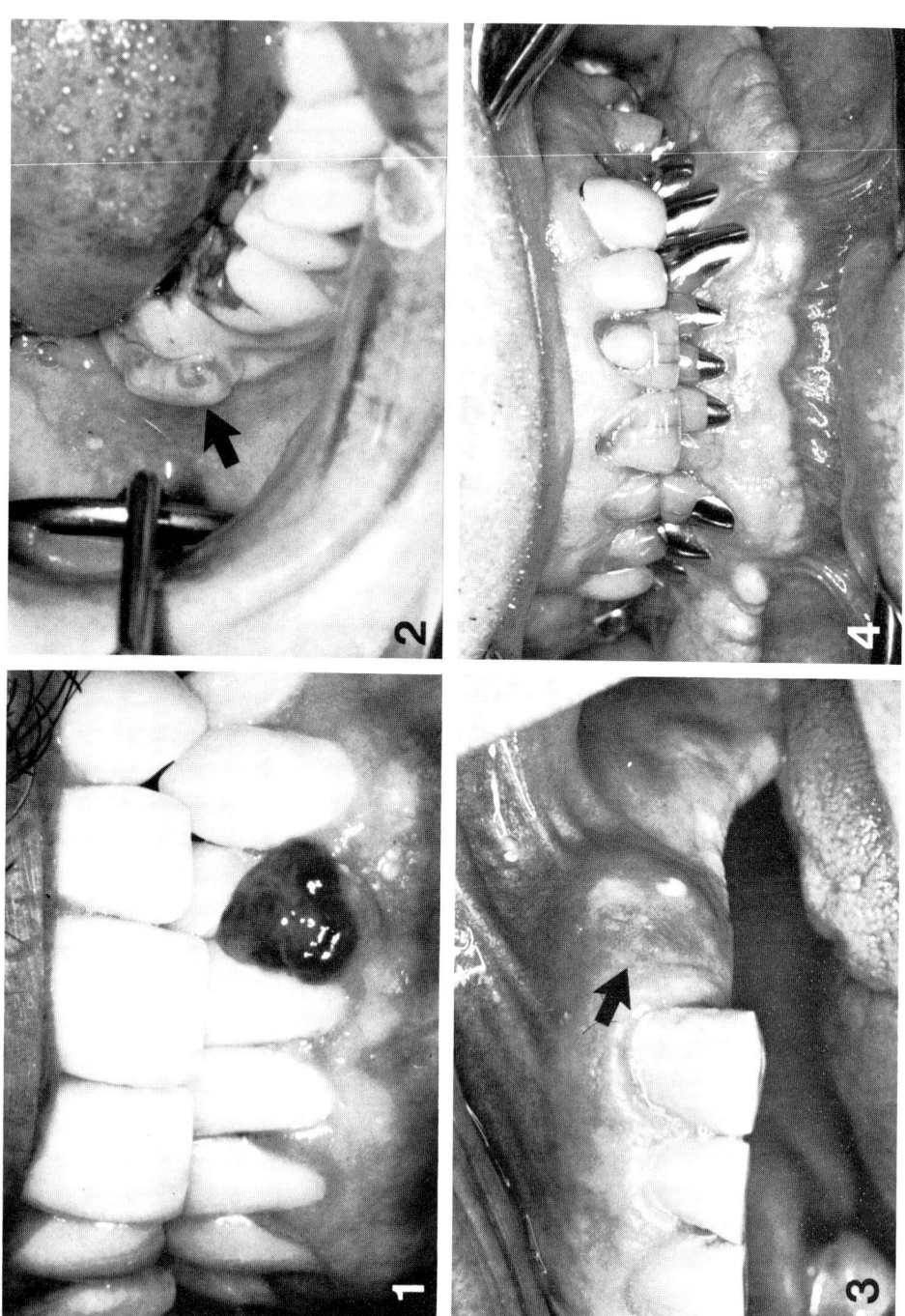

GINGIVAL SWELLINGS

Disease	Clinical Features	Cause	Treatment	Significance
Pyogenic granuloma (Fig. 1) (p. 131–132)	Asymptomatic, red tumescence found primarily on gingiva but may be found anywhere on skin or mucous membrane where trauma has occurred; common	Reaction to trauma or chronic irritation	Excision	May recur if incompletely excised; usually does not cause bone resorption
Peripheral giant cell granuloma (p. 132–134)	Asymptomatic, red tumescence of gingiva; cannot be clinically separated from pyogenic granuloma; uncommon	Reaction to trauma or chronic irritation	Excision	Completely benign behavior; unlike central counterpart; recurrence not anticipated
Peripheral fibroma (Fig. 2) (p. 185–186)	Firm tumescence; color same as surrounding tissue; no symptoms; common; may be pedunculated or sessile	Reaction to trauma or chronic irritation	Excision	Represents overexuberant repair process with proliferation of scar; recurrence not anticipated
Parulis (Fig. 3) (p. 122–123)	Red tumescence (or yellow if pus filled) occurring usually on buccal gingiva of children and young adults; usually without symptoms	Sinus tract from periodontal or periapical abscess	Treatment of periodontal or periapical condition	Cyclic drainage occurs until underlying problem is eliminated
Exostosis (Fig. 4) (p. 386–387)	Bony, hard nodule(s) covered by intact mucosa found attached to buccal aspect of alveolar bone; asymptomatic; common; usually appears in adulthood	Unknown	None; may require removal for denture construction	No significance except in denture construction

GINGIVAL SWELLINGS

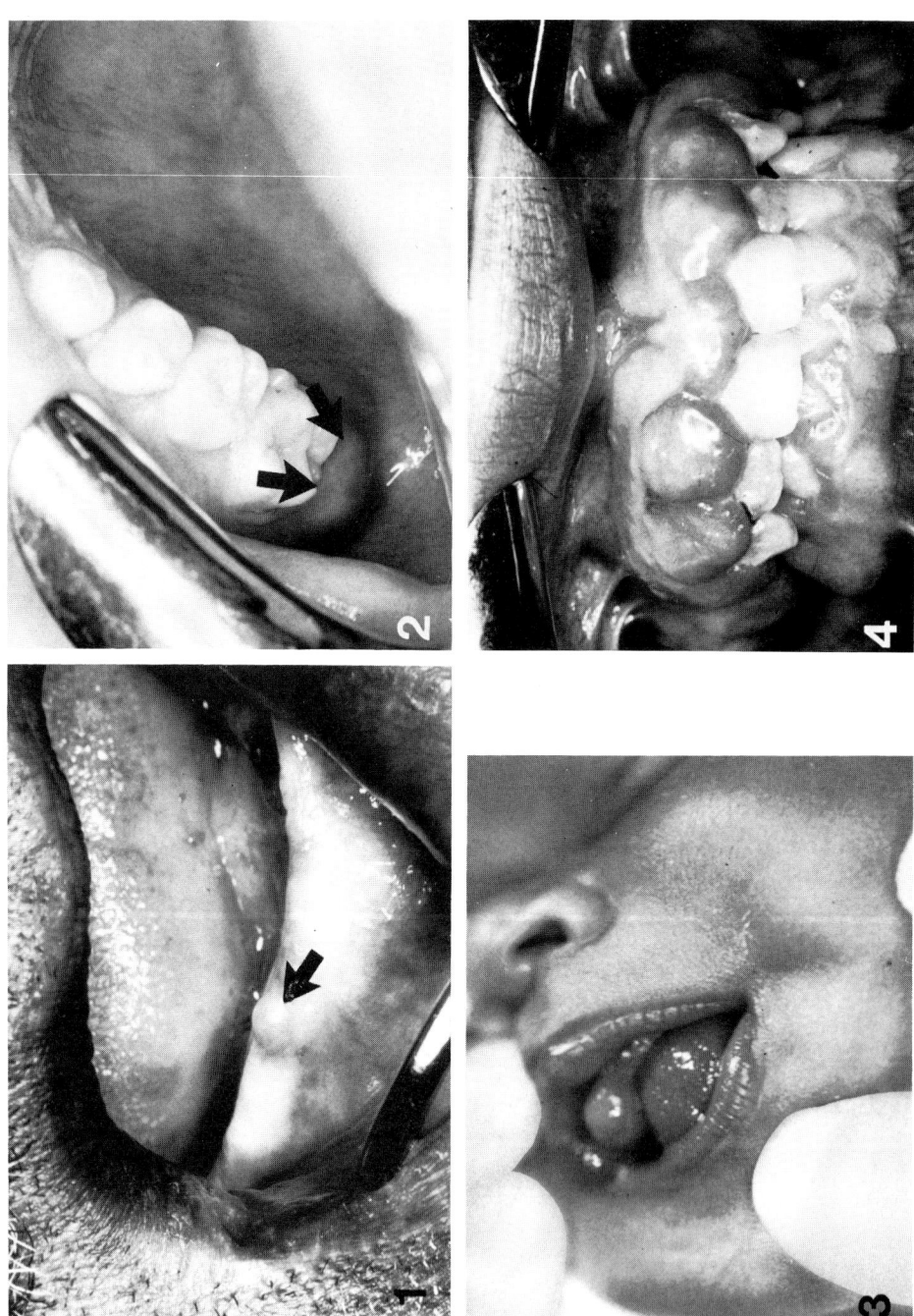

GINGIVAL SWELLINGS (continued)

Disease	Clinical Features	Cause	Treatment	Significance
Gingival cyst (Fig. 1) (p. 313)	Small, elevated, yellow to pink nodule(s); multiple in infants, solitary in adults; common in infants, rare in adults	Proliferation and cystification of dental lamina rests	None when in newborns; excision when in adults	Known as Bohn's nodules or Epstein's pearls in infants, lesions are unroofed during mastication; adult lesions do not recur
Eruption cyst (Fig. 2) (p. 310)	Bluish (fluid- or blood-filled) sac over the crown of an erupting tooth; uninflamed and asymptomatic; uncommon	Hemorrhage into follicular space between tooth crown and reduced enamel epithelium	None, tooth erupts through lesion	None, should not be confused with something else
Congenital epulis of the newborn (Fig. 3) (p. 207–208)	Firm, pedunculated or sessile mass attached to gingiva in infants; same color as or lighter than surrounding tissue; rare	Unknown	Unknown	A benign neoplasm of granular cells similar to the granular cell tumor of the adult; does not recur; may regress spontaneously
Generalized hyperplasia (Fig. 4) (p. 187–191)	Firm, increased bulk of free and attached gingiva; usually asymptomatic; pseudopockets; non-specific type common, others (Dilantin induced, hormone modified, leukemia induced, genetically influenced) uncommon to rare	Local gingival irritants, plus systemic Dilantin, hormone imbalance, leukemia, or hereditary factors	Improve oral hygiene, prophylaxis, gingivoplasty	Cosmetic as well as hygienic problem; causative factors should be eliminated if possible; improvement can be made by control of local factors

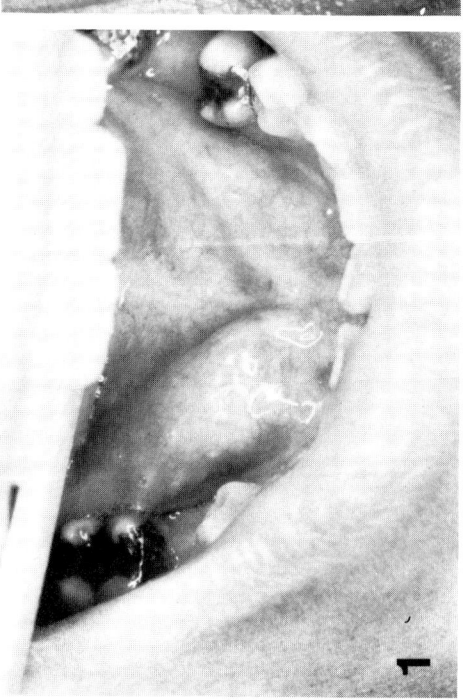

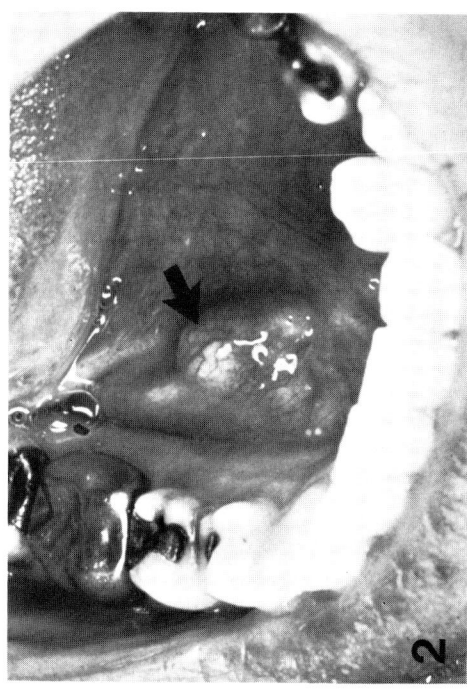

FLOOR OF MOUTH SWELLINGS
Mucus Retention Phenomenon (Ranula)
Dermoid Cyst
Lymphoepithelial Cyst
Salivary Gland Tumor
Mesenchymal Neoplasm

FLOOR OF MOUTH SWELLINGS

Disease	Clinical Features	Cause	Treatment	Significance
Mucus retention phenomenon (ranula) (Fig. 1) (p. 231–233)	Elevated, fluctuant, bluish-white mass in lateral floor of mouth; cyclic swelling often; usually painful; uncommon	Sialolith blockage of duct or traumatic severance of duct	Removal of stone or salivary gland extirpation	Most are due to sialoliths, some due to severance of duct with extravasation of mucin into soft tissues; recurrence not uncommon
Dermoid cyst (p. 330–331)	Asymptomatic mass in floor of mouth (usually midline) covered by intact epithelium of normal color; young adults; feels "doughy" on palpation; rare	Proliferation of multipotential cells; stimulus unknown	Excision	Recurrence not expected; called teratoma when tissues from all three germ layers are present, and dermoid when secondary skin structures are dominant
Lymphoepithelial cyst (Fig. 2) (p. 286–287)	Asymptomatic nodules covered by intact epithelium less than 1 cm in diameter; any age; characteristically found on faucial pillars, floor of mouth, ventral and posterolateral tongue; yellowish-pink in color; uncommon within oral cavity, common in major salivary glands	Developmental defect	Excision	Ectopic lymphoid tissue of no significance; recurrence not expected
Salivary gland tumor (p. 248–282)	Solitary, firm, asymptomatic mass usually covered by epithelium; malignant tumors may cause pain, paresthesia, or ulceration; young adults and adults; most frequent intraorally in palate, followed by tongue, upper lip, and buccal mucosa; uncommon	Unknown	Excision; may be extensive for some malignant tumors	Approximately half of minor salivary gland tumors are malignant (mucoepidermoid carcinoma and adenocystic carcinoma); malignancies metastasize more commonly to bones and lungs than to regional lymph nodes; pleomorphic adenoma is most common benign neoplasm
Mesenchymal neoplasm (p. 184–223)	Firm, asymptomatic tumescence covered by intact epithelium; may arise from any connective tissue cell	Unknown	Excision	Benign tumors not expected to recur; malignancies rare

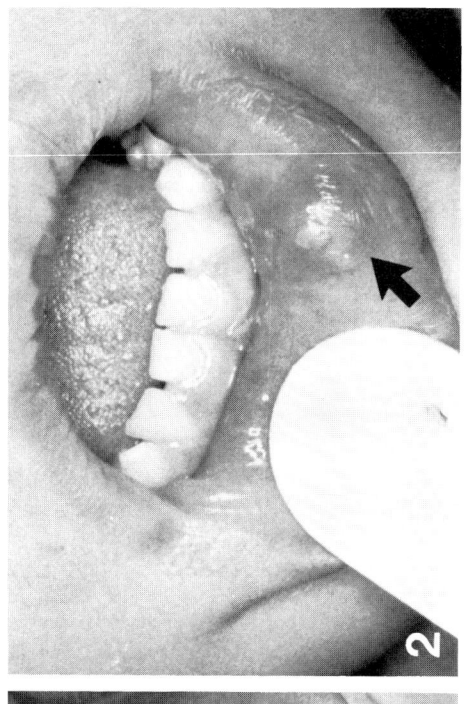
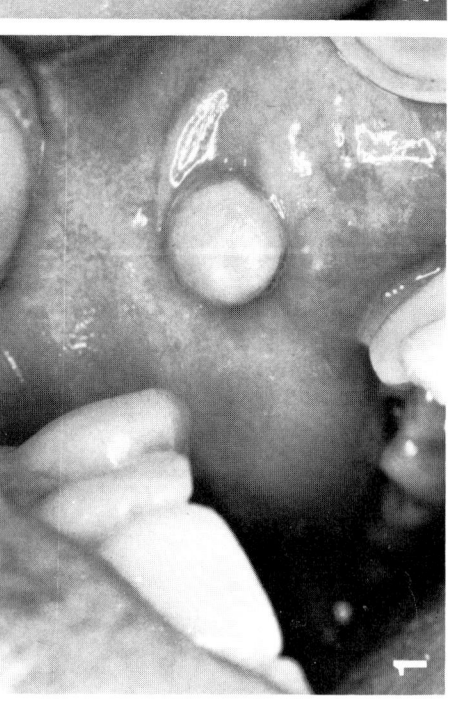

LIP AND BUCCAL MUCOSA SWELLINGS
Upper Lip
 Salivary Gland Tumor
 Mucus Retention Cyst
Lower Lip
 Traumatic Fibroma
 Mucus Extravasation Phenomenon (Mucocele)
Buccal Mucosa
 Traumatic Fibroma
 Mucus Extravasation Phenomenon
 Salivary Gland Tumor
 Mesenchymal Neoplasm

LIP AND BUCCAL MUCOSA SWELLINGS

Disease	Clinical Features	Cause	Treatment	Significance
Salivary gland tumor	See Floor of Mouth Swellings			
Mucus retention cyst (p. 229–230)	Solitary, usually asymptomatic, mobile, non-tender; covered by intact epithelium; color same as surrounding tissue; adults over 50 years of age; common in palate, cheek, floor of mouth, uncommon in upper lip, rare in lower lip	Blockage of salivary gland excretory duct by sialolith	Excision	Recurrence not anticipated if associated gland removed; clinically indistinguishable from more significant salivary gland neoplasms
Traumatic fibroma (Fig. 1) (p. 191–193)	Firm, asymptomatic nodule covered by epithelium unless secondarily traumatized; usually found along line of occlusion in buccal mucosa and lower lip; common	Reaction to trauma or chronic irritation	Excision	Represents hyperplastic scar; limited growth potential and no malignant transformation seen
Mucus extravasation phenomenon (Fig. 2) (p. 226–229)	Bluish nodule (normal color if deep) usually covered by epithelium; may be slightly painful and have associated acute inflammatory reaction; most frequently seen in lower lip and buccal mucosa, rare in upper lip; adolescents and children; common	Traumatic severance of salivary gland excretory duct	Excision	Recurrence expected if contributory salivary gland not removed or if adjacent ducts are cut
Mesenchymal neoplasm	See Floor of Mouth Swellings			

TONGUE SWELLINGS

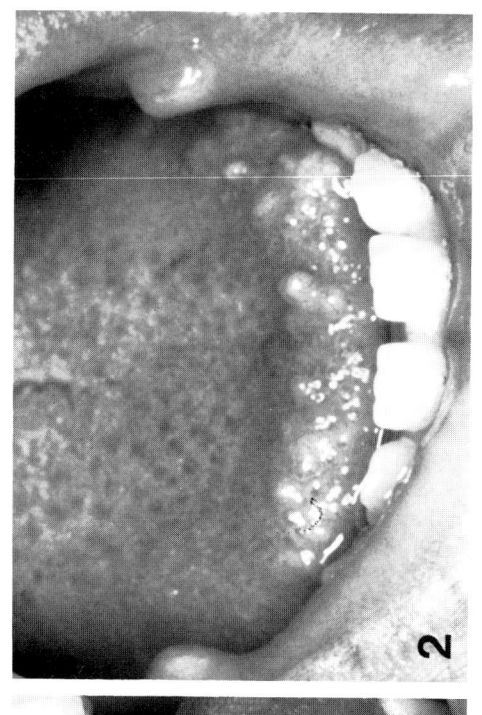

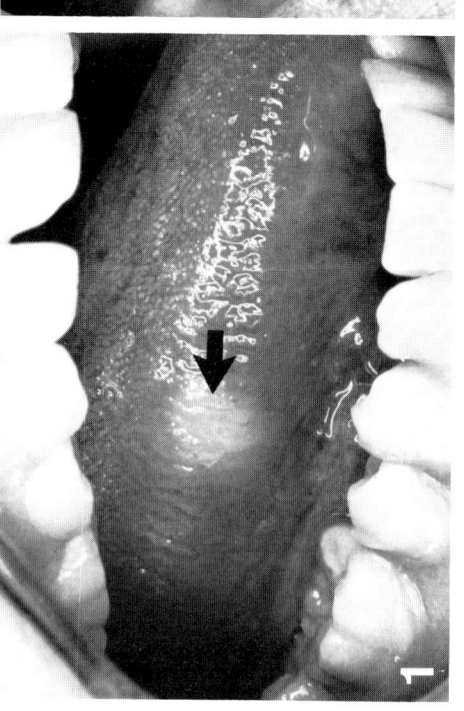

TONGUE SWELLINGS
Traumatic Fibroma
Pyogenic Granuloma
Granular Cell Tumor (Granular Cell Myoblastoma)
Neurofibroma
Salivary Gland Tumor
Lingual Thyroid

TONGUE SWELLINGS

Disease	Clinical Features	Cause	Treatment	Significance
Traumatic fibroma	See Lip and Buccal Mucosa Swellings			
Pyogenic granuloma	See Gingival Swellings			
Granular cell tumor (Fig. 1) (p. 207–210)	Painless, elevated tumescence covered by intact epithelium; color same as or lighter than surrounding tissue; strong predilection for dorsum of tongue but may be found anywhere; any age; uncommon	Unknown; cell of origin undetermined; Schwann cell; granularity due to cytoplasmic autophagosomes	Excision	Does not recur; of significance in that it must be differentiated from other lesions; no malignant potential
Neurofibroma (Fig. 2) (p. 214–215)	Soft, single or multiple, asymptomatic nodules covered by epithelium; same color as or lighter than surrounding mucosa; most frequently seen on tongue, buccal mucosa, and vestibule, but may be seen anywhere; any age; uncommon	Unknown; cell of origin is probably Schwann cell	Excision	Recurrence not expected; multiple lesions should suggest von Recklinghausen's disease of nerve (neurofibromas with malignant potential plus café-au-lait spots) or MEN III syndrome (pheochromocytoma, medullary carcinoma of the thyroid, and mucosal neuromas)
Salivary gland tumor	See Floor of Mouth Swellings			
Lingual thyroid (p. 331)	Nodular mass in base of tongue, may cause dysphagia; young adults; rare	Incomplete descent of thyroid anlage to neck	Excision only after demonstration of normal functioning thyroid tissue elsewhere	Lingual thyroid may be patient's only thyroid tissue

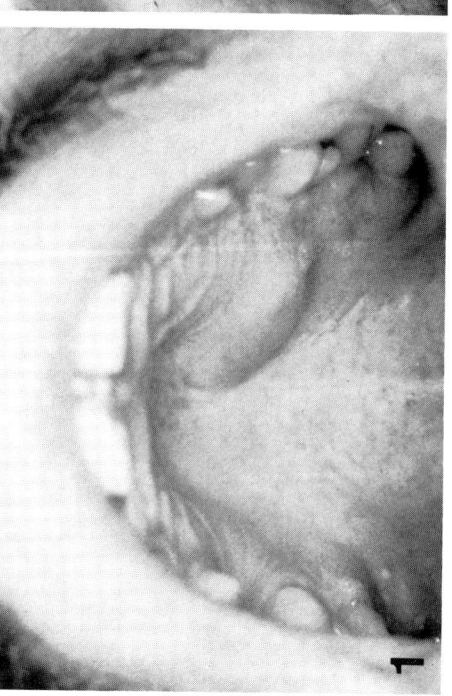

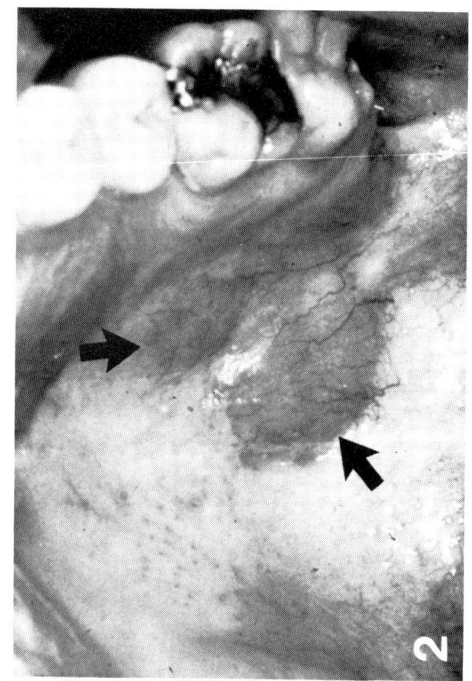

PALATAL SWELLINGS
Mucus Extravasation Phenomenon
Salivary Gland Tumor
Palatal Abscess from Periapical Lesion
Lymphoma
Torus
Neoplasm of Maxilla or Maxillary Sinus

PALATAL SWELLINGS

Disease	Clinical Features	Cause	Treatment	Significance
Mucus extravasation phenomenon	See Lip and Buccal Mucosa Swellings			
Salivary gland tumor (Fig. 1)	See Floor of Mouth Swellings			
Palatal abscess from periapical lesion	Painful, pus-filled, fluctuant tumescence of hard palate; color same as or redder than surrounding tissue; associated with non-vital tooth	Extension of periapical abscess through palatal bone	Incise and drain, treat non-vital tooth; antibiotics may be necessary	Pus may spread to other areas, seeking path of least resistance
Lymphoma (Fig. 2) (p. 287–297)	Asymptomatic, spongy to firm tumescence of hard palate; adults; rare	Unknown	Evaluation of other reticuloendothelial tissues for lymphoma; radiation; follow-up examinations	May represent primary lymphoma (non-Hodgkin's type); lymphoma work-up indicated
Torus (p. 386–387)	Asymptomatic, bony, hard swelling of hard palate (torus palatinus); bony, exophytic growths along lingual aspect of mandible (torus mandibularis); torpid growth; young adults and adults; affects up to 25% of population	Unknown	None; may be excised for prosthetic considerations	No significance; should not be confused with other palatal lesions
Neoplasm of maxilla or maxillary sinus	Palatal swelling with or without ulceration; pain or paresthesia; may cause loosening of teeth or malocclusion; denture may not fit; any age; rare	Unknown	Surgery or radiation	May represent benign or malignant jaw neoplasm or carcinoma of maxillary sinus; poor prognosis for malignant lesions

NECK SWELLINGS

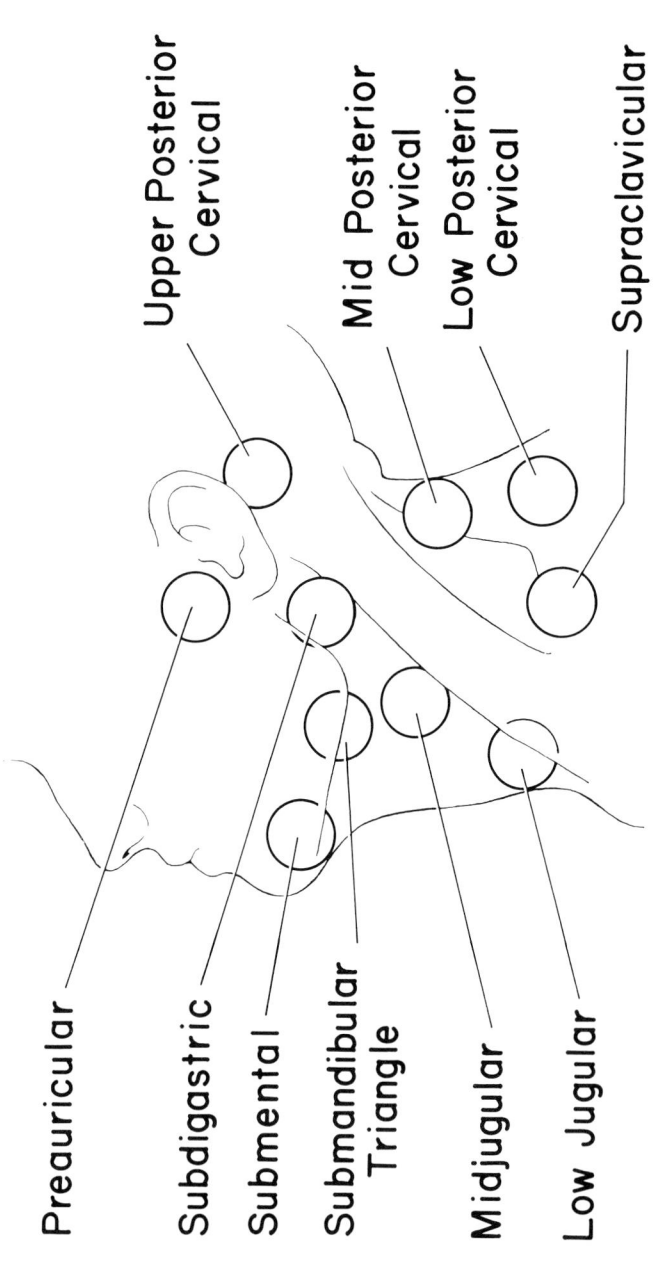

NECK SWELLINGS

Lateral Neck
  Branchial Cyst
  Lymphadenitis—Non-specific, Bacterial, Fungal
  Metastatic Carcinoma to Lymph Nodes
  Lymphoma
  Parotid Lesion—Neoplasm, Sjögren's Syndrome, Infection, Metabolic Disease
  Carotid Body Tumor (Paraganglioma, Chemodectoma)
  Epidermal Cyst
  Lymphangioma (Cystic Hygroma)
Midline
  Thyroglossal Tract Cyst
  Thyroid Gland Tumor
  Dermoid Cyst

NECK SWELLINGS

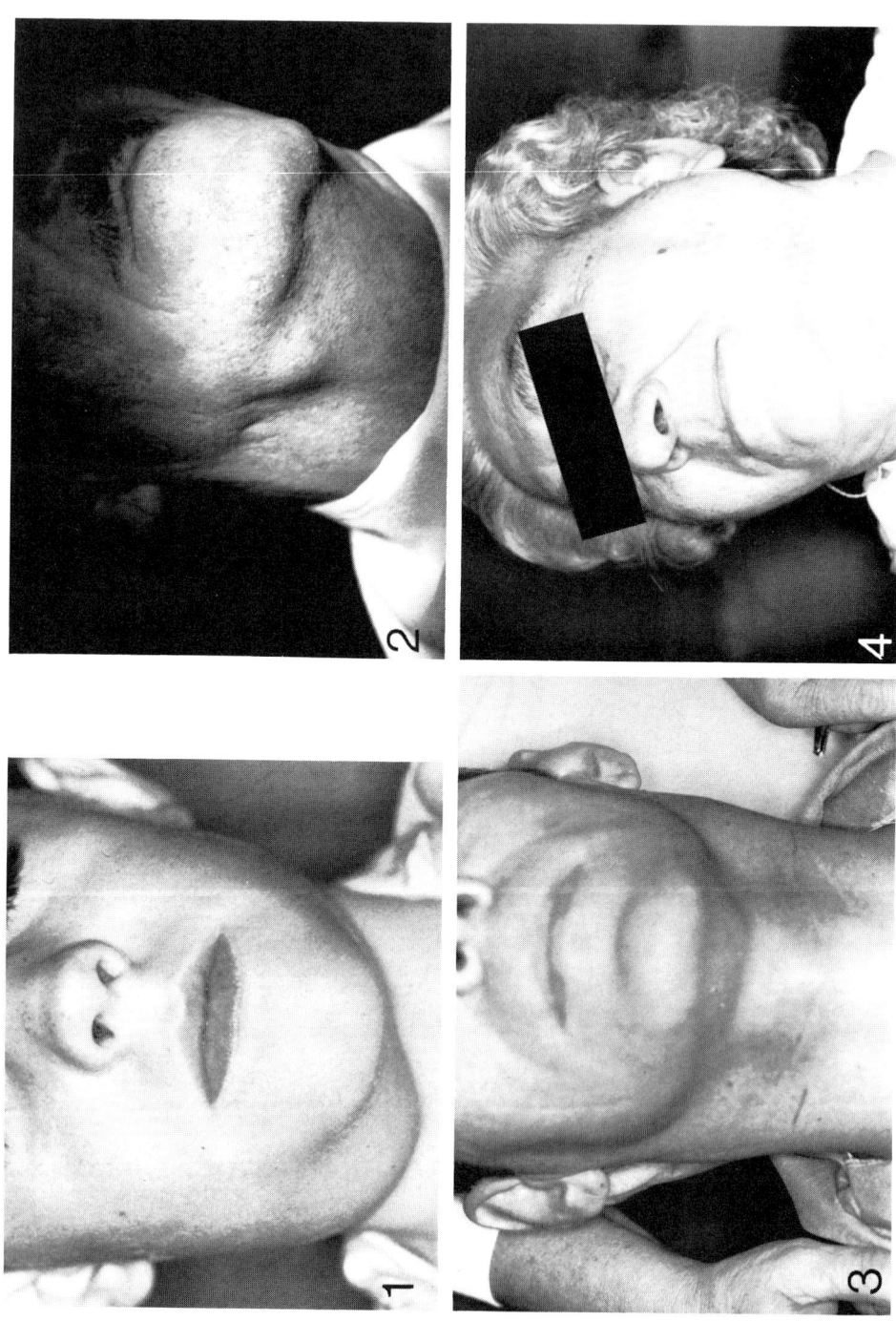

O-64

NECK SWELLINGS

Disease	Clinical Features	Cause	Treatment	Significance
Branchial cyst (Fig. 1) (p. 329–330)	Asymptomatic, non-inflamed swelling in lateral neck; soft or fluctuant; children and young adults; rare	Developmental, proliferation of epithelial remnants within lymph nodes	Excision	Clinical diagnostic problem
Lymphadenitis—non-specific, bacterial, fungal	Single or multiple, painful nodules (lymph nodes) in neck, especially submandibular and jugulodigastric areas; lesions are usually soft when acute and usually not fixed to surrounding tissue; non-specific type common	Any oral inflammatory condition, especially dental abscess; oral tuberculosis, syphilis, or deep fungus may affect neck nodes	Treat specific cause	Neck disease often reflects in oral cavity
Metastatic carcinoma to lymph nodes (Fig. 2)	Usually single but may be multiple (rarely bilateral), indurated masses; fixed and non-painful; most frequently affects submandibular and jugulodigastric nodes; adults; uncommon	Metastatic oral cancer; may occasionally come from nasopharynx lesion	Find primary lesion; surgery or radiation	Signifies advanced disease with poor prognosis
Lymphoma (Fig. 3) (p. 287–297)	Single or bilateral swellings in lateral neck; indurated, asymptomatic, and often fixed; may have weight loss, night sweats, and fever; young adults and adults; uncommon	Unknown	Radiation or chemotherapy	After diagnostic biopsy, staging procedures are done; prognosis fair to excellent depending on stage and classification
Parotid lesion (Fig. 4)	When tail of parotid affected, neck mass may occur; *neoplasm*—indurated, asymptomatic, single lump (Warthin's tumor—may be bilateral); *Sjögren's syndrome*—bilateral, diffuse, soft swelling plus sicca complex, affects primarily older women; *infection*—unilateral, diffuse, soft, painful mass	*Neoplasm*—unknown; *Sjögren's syndrome*—autoimmune; *infection*—viral, bacterial, or fungal; *metabolic disease*—diabetes, alcoholism	Treat cause	Requires diagnosis and treatment by experienced clinician
Carotid body tumor	Firm, movable mass in neck at carotid bifurcation; bruit and thrill may be apparent; adults; rare	Neoplastic transformation of carotid body (chemoreceptor) cells	Excision	Morbidity from surgery may be profound because of tumor attachment to carotid sheath

NECK SWELLINGS

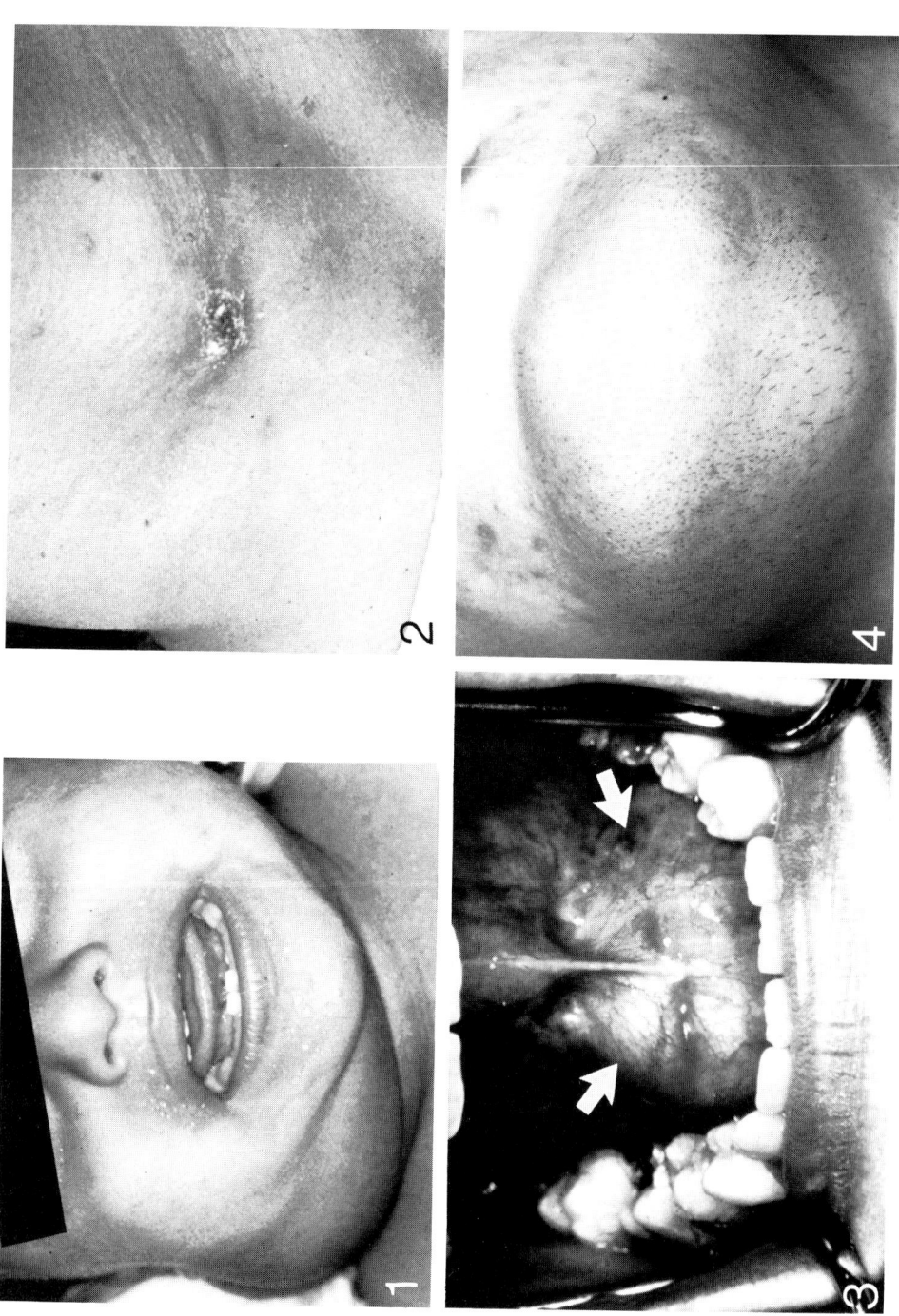

NECK SWELLINGS (continued)

Disease	Clinical Features	Cause	Treatment	Significance
Epidermal cyst	Elevated nodule in skin of neck (or face); usually uninflamed and asymptomatic; up to several centimeters in size; covered by epidermis and near skin surface; common	Epithelial rest proliferation	Excision	Recurrence not expected; more superficially located than other neck lesions discussed
Lymphangioma (Fig. 1) (p. 204–205)	Spongy, diffuse, painless mass in dermis; may become large; lighter than surrounding tissue to red-blue; crepitance; children; rare	Developmental	Excision	May become disfiguring or cause respiratory distress
Thyroglossal tract cyst (Fig. 2) (p. 331–335)	Midline swelling in neck above level of thyroid gland; may develop sinus tract (Fig. 2); most common developmental cyst of neck	Failure of complete descent of thyroid tissue from foramen caecum with subsequent cystification	Excision	Recurrence not uncommon because of tortuous course of cystic space
Thyroid gland tumor	Midline swelling in area of thyroid gland; firm, asymptomatic; uncommon	Unknown	Excision	Prognosis poor to excellent depending upon stage and histologic type of tumor
Dermoid cyst (Figs. 3 and 4) (p. 330–331)	Swelling in floor of mouth or midline of neck; young adults	Unknown	Excision	Recurrence not expected

Chapters 10–15

Jaw Lesions

There are a number of ways to classify jaw lesions. A common way is to separate them according to their general radiographic appearance of lucent, opaque, and mixed pattern. A disadvantage of this method is that an entity may have more than one radiographic pattern. Another is that most lesions in the jaws are radiolucent. The classification chosen for this section is division into the following groups:

Cysts of the oral region
Odontogenic tumors
Benign non-odontogenic tumors
Inflammatory jaw lesions
Malignant non-odontogenic neoplasms of the jaws
Metabolic and genetic jaw diseases

When considering a differential diagnosis, a step-by-step progression through the lesions in these groups provides a convenient and logical sequence of thought. Of considerable clinical importance is the combination of radiographic appearance, patient age, and location of the lesion. These three features taken together are very reliable signs for diagnosis of many jaw lesions and are emphasized in these tables.

Jaw Lesions

Cysts of the Oral Region
Odontogenic Tumors
Benign Non-odontogenic Tumors
Inflammatory Jaw Lesions
Malignant Non-odontogenic Neoplasms of the Jaws
Metabolic and Genetic Jaw Diseases

Chapter 10

Cysts of the Oral Region

ODONTOGENIC CYSTS
Radicular (Periapical) Cyst
Dentigerous Cyst
Lateral Periodontal Cyst
Gingival Cyst of the Newborn
Odontogenic Keratocyst
Calcifying Odontogenic Cyst
NON-ODONTOGENIC CYSTS
"Globulomaxillary" Cyst
Nasolabial Cyst
Median Mandibular Cyst
Nasopalatine Canal Cyst
PSEUDOCYSTS
Aneurysmal Bone Cyst
Traumatic (Simple) Bone Cyst
Static Bone Cyst
Focal Osteoporotic Bone Marrow Defect

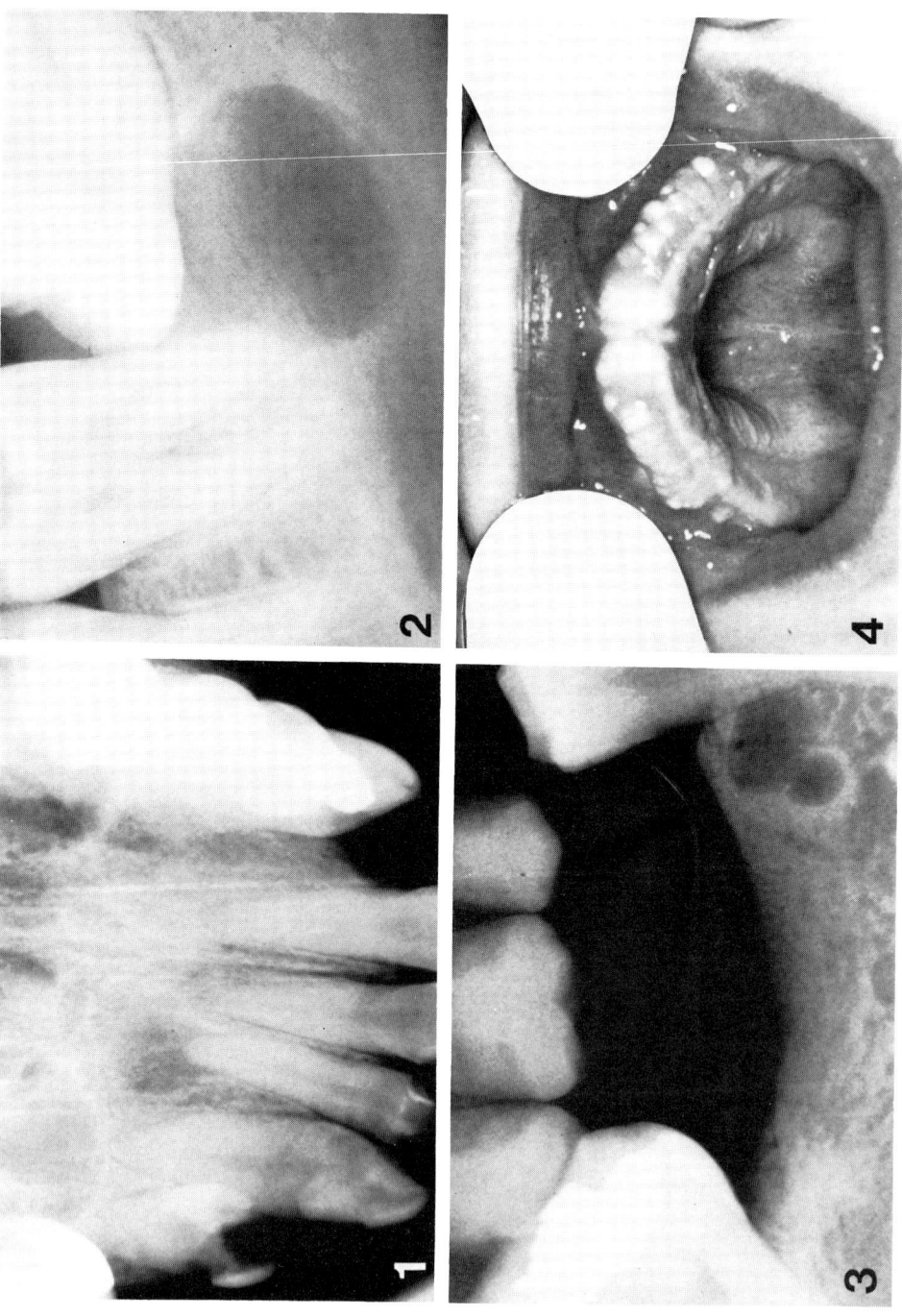

CYSTS OF THE ORAL REGION

Disease	Age	Location	Radiography	Other Features
Radicular (periapical) cyst (Fig. 1) (p. 301–306)	Any age; peaks in third through sixth decades	Apex of any non-vital erupted tooth, especially anterior maxilla	Well-defined lucency at apex of non-vital tooth	Cannot be distinguished radiographically from periapical granuloma; develops from inflammatory stimulation of rests of Malassez; incomplete enucleation results in *residual cyst*; chronic process and usually asymptomatic; common
Dentigerous cyst (Fig. 2) (p. 306–310)	Young adults	Associated most commonly with impacted mandibular third molars and maxillary third molar and cuspids	Well-defined lucency around crown of impacted teeth	Complication of neoplastic transformation of cystic epithelium to ameloblastoma and, rarely, to squamous cell or mucoepidermoid carcinoma; some become very large with rare possibility of pathologic fracture; common; *eruption cyst*—gingival tumescence developing as a dilatation of follicular space over crown of erupting tooth
Lateral periodontal cyst (Fig. 3) (p. 310–313)	Adults	Lateral periodontal membrane, especially mandibular cuspid and premolar area	Well-defined lucency; usually unilocular but may be multilocular	Usually asymptomatic; associated tooth is vital; origin from rests of dental lamina; some keratocytes are found in a lateral root position; gingival cyst of the adult may be soft tissue counterpart
Gingival cyst of the newborn (Fig. 4) (p. 313)	Newborn	Gingival soft tissues	Usually not apparent on radiogram	Newborns—common, multiple, no treatment; adult gingival cyst is rare, solitary, and treated by local excision

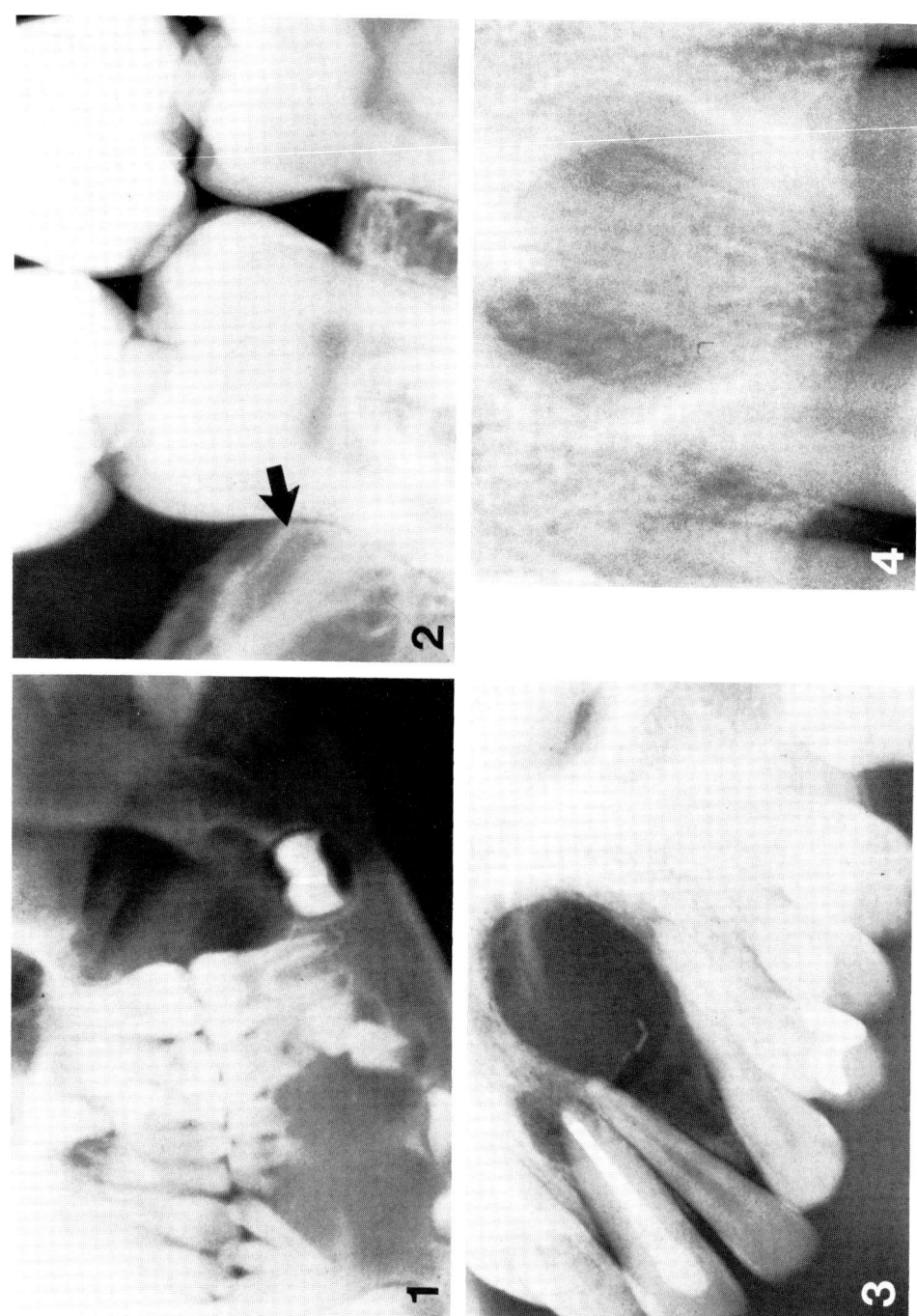

CYSTS OF THE ORAL REGION (continued)

Disease	Age	Location	Radiography	Other Features
Odontogenic keratocyst (Figs. 1 and 2) (p. 313–317)	Any age, especially adults	Mandibular molar-ramus area favored; may be found in position of dentigerous, lateral root, periapical, or primordial cyst	Well-defined lucency; unilocular or multilocular	Recurrence rate of 5 to 62%; may have aggressive behavior; may be part of basal cell nevus syndrome (keratocysts, skeletal anomalies, basal cell carcinomas); follow-up examination necessary; known as *primordial cyst* when found in place of tooth (Fig. 2)
Calcifying odontogenic cyst (p. 317–318)	Any age	Maxilla favored; gingiva second most common site	Well-defined lucency, may have opaque foci	Origin and behavior are in dispute; ghost cell keratinization characteristic; may have aggressive behavior; rare
"Globulomaxillary" cyst (Fig. 3) (p. 319–320)	Any age	Between roots of maxillary cuspid and lateral incisor	Well-defined oval or "pear-shaped" lucency	Teeth are vital; asymptomatic; pathogenesis open to question, may be of odontogenic origin; rare
Nasolabial cyst (p. 320)	Adults	Soft tissue of upper lip, lateral to midline	No change	Origin likely from remnants of nasolacrimal duct; rare
Median mandibular cyst (p. 320–321)	Any age	Midline mandible	Well-defined lucency	Teeth are vital; asymptomatic; pathogenesis open to question; may be of odontogenic origin; rare
Nasopalatine canal cyst (Fig. 4) (p. 321–323)	Any age	Nasopalatine canal or papilla	Well-defined midline maxillary lucency, may be oval or "heart-shaped"	Teeth are vital; may be symptomatic if secondarily infected; may be difficult to differentiate from normal canal; common

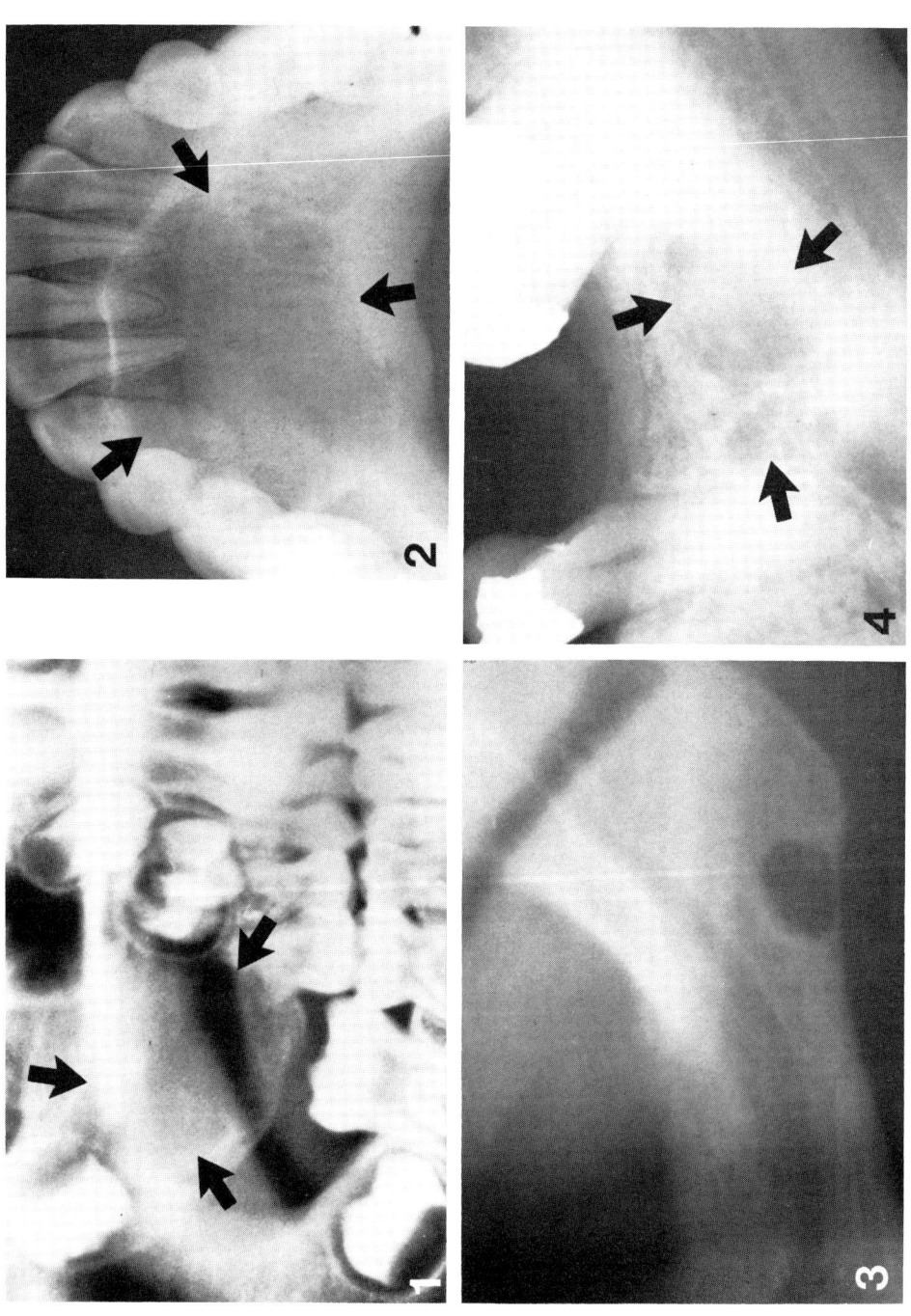

CYSTS OF THE ORAL REGION (continued)

Disease	Age	Location	Radiography	Other Features
Aneurysmal bone cyst (Fig. 1) (p. 323–325)	Second decade favored	Either jaw; also long bones and vertebrae	Lucency, may be poorly defined; may have honeycomb or soap-bubble appearance	Represents vascular anomaly in bone consisting of blood-filled sinusoids; blood wells up when lesion is entered; etiology and pathogenesis unknown; rare; follow-up important
Traumatic (simple) bone cyst (Fig. 2) (p. 325–328)	Second decade favored	Mandible favored	Well-defined lucency often extending between roots of teeth	Represents dead space in bone without epithelial lining; etiology and pathogenesis unknown; uncommon in oral region
Static bone cyst (Fig. 3) (p. 328)	Developmental defect that should be apparent from childhood	Mandibular molar area below alveolar canal	Well-defined oval lucency, does not change with time	Represents lingual depression of mandible; filled with salivary gland or other soft tissue from floor of mouth; asymptomatic; an incidental finding that requires no biopsy or treatment; uncommon
Focal osteoporotic bone marrow defect (Fig. 4) (p. 329)	Adults	Mandible favored	Lucency; often in edentulous areas	Contains normal marrow; must be differentiated from other more significant lesions; uncommon

Jaw Lesions

Cysts of the Oral Region
Odontogenic Tumors
Benign Non-odontogenic Tumors
Inflammatory Jaw Lesions
Malignant Non-odontogenic Neoplasms of the Jaws
Metabolic and Genetic Jaw Diseases

Chapter 11

Odontogenic Tumors

EPITHELIAL TUMORS
Ameloblastoma
Squamous Odontogenic Tumor
Calcifying Epithelial Odontogenic Tumor
Clear Cell Odontogenic Tumor
Adenomatoid Odontogenic Tumor
MESENCHYMAL TUMORS
Odontogenic Myxoma
Central Odontogenic Fibroma
Cementifying Fibroma
Cementoblastoma
Periapical Cemental Dysplasia
MIXED (EPITHELIAL AND MESENCHYMAL) TUMORS
Odontoma
Ameloblastic Fibroma and Ameloblastic Fibro-odontoma

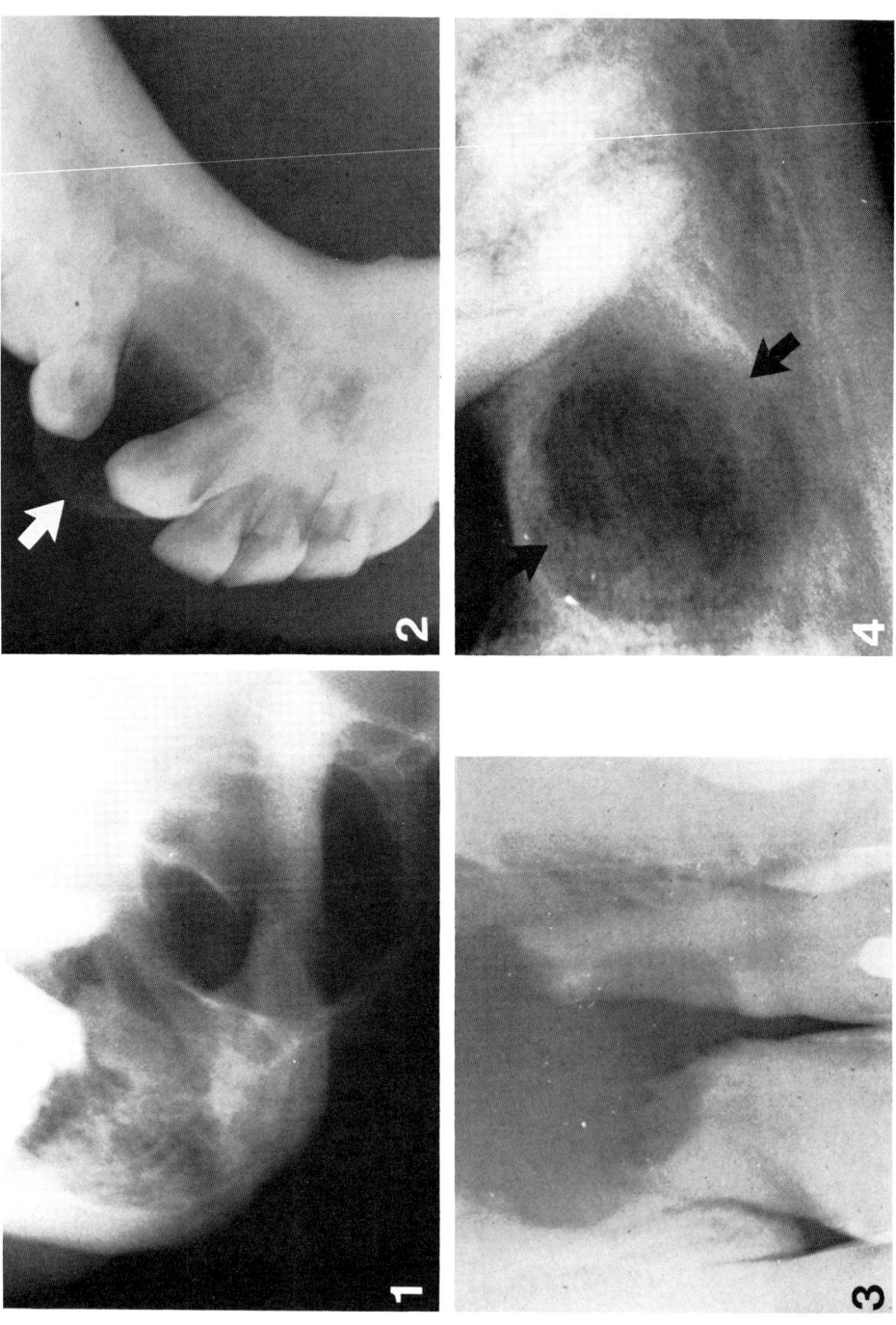

ODONTOGENIC TUMORS

Disease	Age	Location	Radiography	Other Features
Ameloblastoma (Fig. 1) (p. 337–348)	Fourth and fifth decades	Mandibular molar-ramus area favored	Lucent; usually well circumscribed; unilocular or multilocular	May arise in wall of dentigerous cyst; may exhibit aggressive behavior; rarely metastasizes (usually to lung); recurrence rate low for unicystic type; usually asymptomatic; uncommon
Squamous odontogenic tumor (p. 348)	Mean of 40 years; second through seventh decades	Alveolar process; anterior more than posterior	Lucency	Conservative therapy; few recurrences
Calcifying epithelial odontogenic tumor (p. 348–351)	Mean around 40 years; second through tenth decades	Mandibular molar-ramus area favored	Lucent with or without opaque foci; usually well circumscribed; unilocular or multilocular	Behavior and prognosis are similar to ameloblastoma; rare
Clear cell odontogenic tumor (p. 351)	Seventh decade	Mandible, maxilla	Lucency	Rare
Adenomatoid odontogenic tumor (Fig. 2) (p. 351–353)	Second decade	Anterior jaws	Well-defined lucency, may have opaque foci	Usually associated with crown of impacted tooth; no symptoms; does not recur after enucleation; rare
Odontogenic myxoma (Fig. 3) (p. 353–356)	Mean of about 30; ages 10 to 50	Any area of jaws	Lucent lesion, often multilocular or honeycombed; may be poorly defined peripherally	May exhibit aggressive behavior; no symptoms; uncommon; recurrence not uncommon
Central odontogenic fibroma (p. 356–359)	Any	Any area of jaws	Lucency, usually multilocular	Two microscopic subtypes exhibit same benign clinical behavior
Cementifying fibroma (Fig. 4) (p. 359)	Fourth and fifth decades	Posterior mandible	Well-defined, lucent lesion, may have opaque foci	Asymptomatic; grows by local expansion; recurrence unlikely; rare

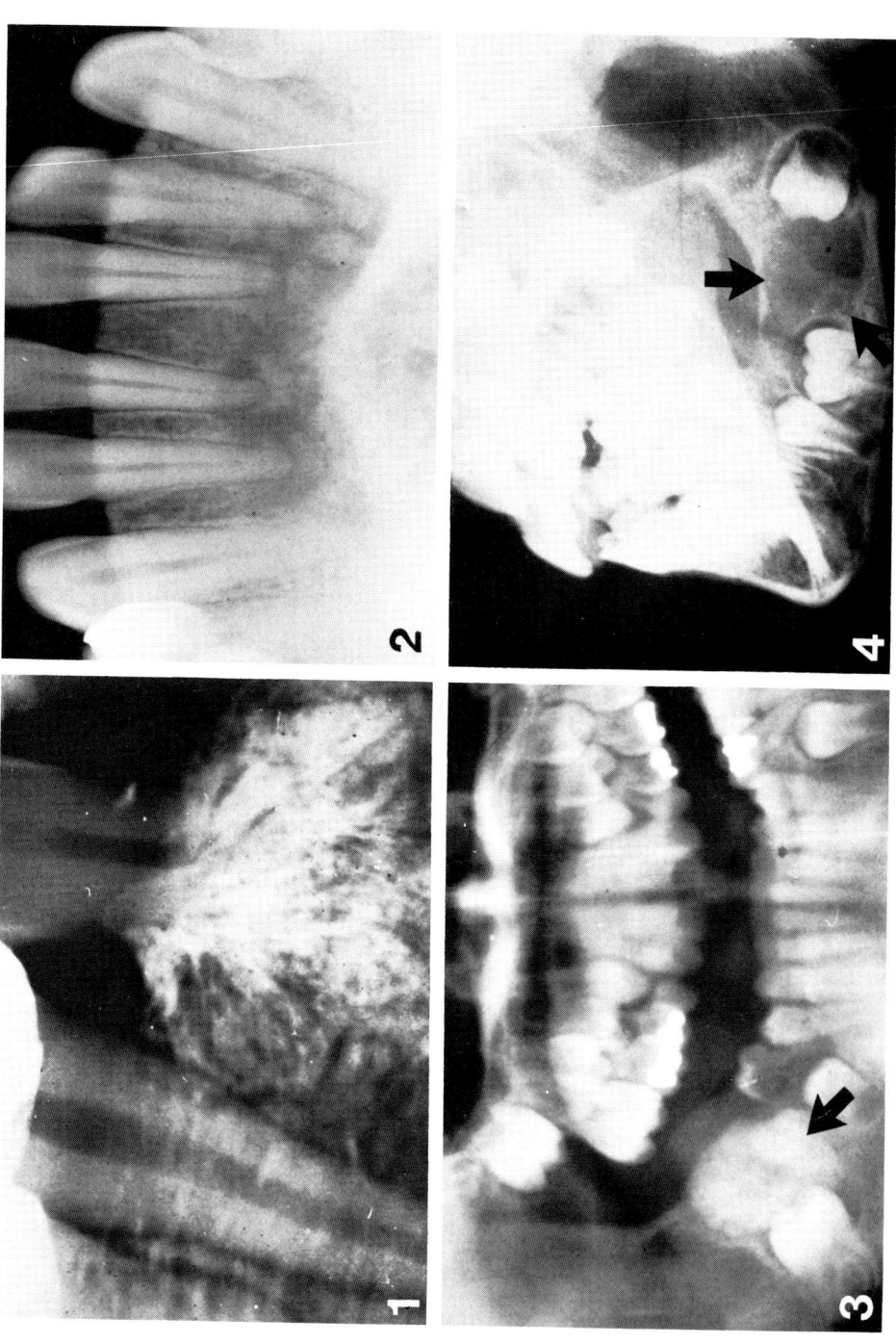

ODONTOGENIC TUMORS (continued)

Disease	Age	Location	Radiography	Other Features
Cementoblastoma (Fig. 1) (p. 359–361)	Second and third decades	Root of posterior teeth; mandible more than maxilla	Opaque lesion; attached to and replaces root; opaque spicules radiate from central area	May cause cortical expansion; tooth and lesion removed together; no symptoms; rare
Periapical cemental dysplasia (Fig. 2) (p. 361–363)	Fifth decade	Mandible, especially apices of anterior teeth; usually more than one tooth affected	Starts as periapical lucencies that eventually become opaque in months to years	Regarded as a reactive lesion; always associated with vital teeth; requires no treatment; asymptomatic; common; rare variant known as *florid osseous dysplasia* represents severe form that may affect one to four quadrants and may have complications of chronic osteomyelitis and traumatic bone cysts
Odontoma (Fig. 3) (p. 363)	Second decade	Anywhere, especially anterior mandible and maxilla	Opaque; *compound type*—tooth shapes apparent; *complex type*—uniform opaque mass	May block eruption of a permanent tooth; *complex type* rarely causes cortical expansion, no recurrence; *compound type* appears as many miniature teeth; *complex type* is conglomeration of enamel and dentin; probably represents hamartoma rather than neoplasm; common
Ameloblastic fibroma and ameloblastic fibro-odontoma (Fig. 4) (p. 364–368)	First and second decades	Mandibular molar-ramus area	Well-defined lucency; may be multilocular and large; fibro-odontoma may have associated opaque mass representing an odontoma	Well encapsulated; recurrence not expected; no symptoms; if odontoma present, the lesion is called ameloblastic fibro-odontoma; rare

Jaw Lesions

Cysts of the Oral Region
Odontogenic Tumors
Benign Non-odontogenic Tumors
Inflammatory Jaw Lesions
Malignant Non-odontogenic Neoplasms of the Jaws
Metabolic and Genetic Jaw Diseases

Chapter 12

Benign Non-odontogenic Tumors*

OSSIFYING FIBROMA
FIBROUS DYSPLASIA
OSTEOBLASTOMA
CHONDROMA
OSTEOMA
CENTRAL GIANT CELL GRANULOMA
HEMANGIOMA OF BONE
IDIOPATHIC HISTIOCYTOSIS (LANGERHANS CELL DISEASE)
TORI AND EXOSTOSES
CORONOID HYPERPLASIA

---

*Because of the similar microscopy presented by a number of benign jaw lesions, they are frequently grouped together as fibro-osseous lesions. They are composed of a benign, fibrous connective tissue stroma with varying amounts of bone or cementum dispersed throughout. Vascularity ranges from slight to prominent in the various lesions. Diagnosis of fibro-osseous lesions is dependent upon the correlation of clinical features, radiographic appearance, and microscopy.

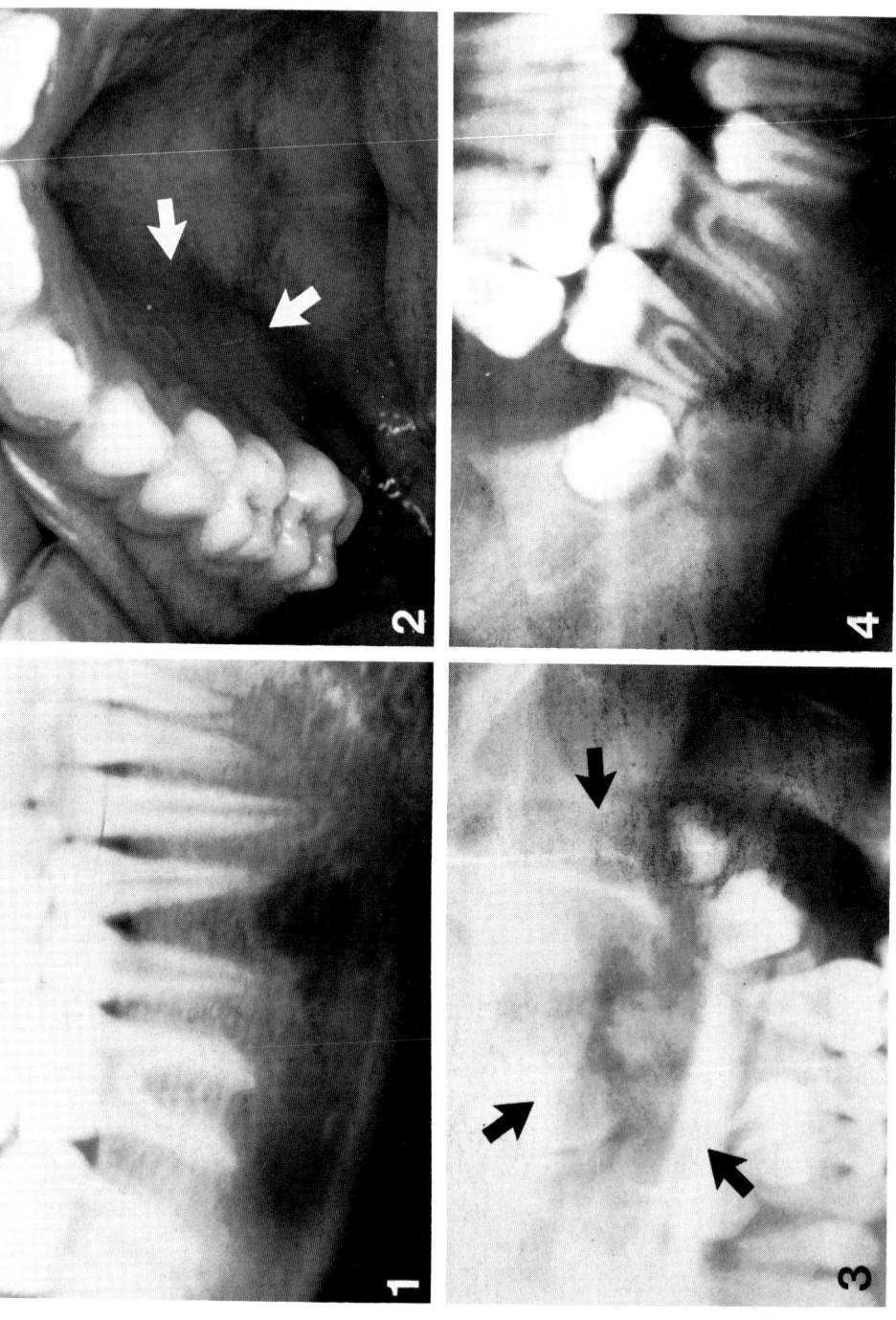

BENIGN NON-ODONTOGENIC TUMORS

Disease	Age	Location	Radiography	Other Features
Ossifying fibroma (Fig. 1) (p. 369–372)	Third and fourth decades	Body of mandible favored	Well-defined lucency, may have opaque foci	Slow growing and asymptomatic; may be indistinguishable from cementifying fibroma; does not recur; microscopy often similar to fibrous dysplasia; uncommon
Fibrous dysplasia (Figs. 2 and 3) (p. 372–375)	First and second decades	Maxilla favored	Poorly defined radiographic mass; diffuse opacification often described as "ground glass"	Slow growing and asymptomatic; causes cortical expansion; may cease growing after puberty; a cosmetic problem treated by recontouring. Variants: *monostotic*—one bone affected; *polyostotic*—more than one bone affected; *Albright's syndrome*—fibrous dysplasia plus café-au-lait macules and endocrine abnormalities (precocious puberty in females); *Jaffe-Lichtenstein syndrome*—multiple bone lesions of fibrous dysplasia and skin pigmentations; rare
Osteoblastoma (Fig. 4) (p. 375–377)	Second decade	Either jaw	Well-defined, lucent to opaque lesion	Diagnostic feature of pain; microscopy often difficult, may be confused with osteosarcoma; recurrence not expected; rare
Chondroma (p. 377–378)	Any age	Any, especially anterior maxilla and posterior mandible	Relative lucency, may have opacities	May be difficult to separate microscopically from chondrosarcoma; rare

BENIGN NON-ODONTOGENIC TUMORS

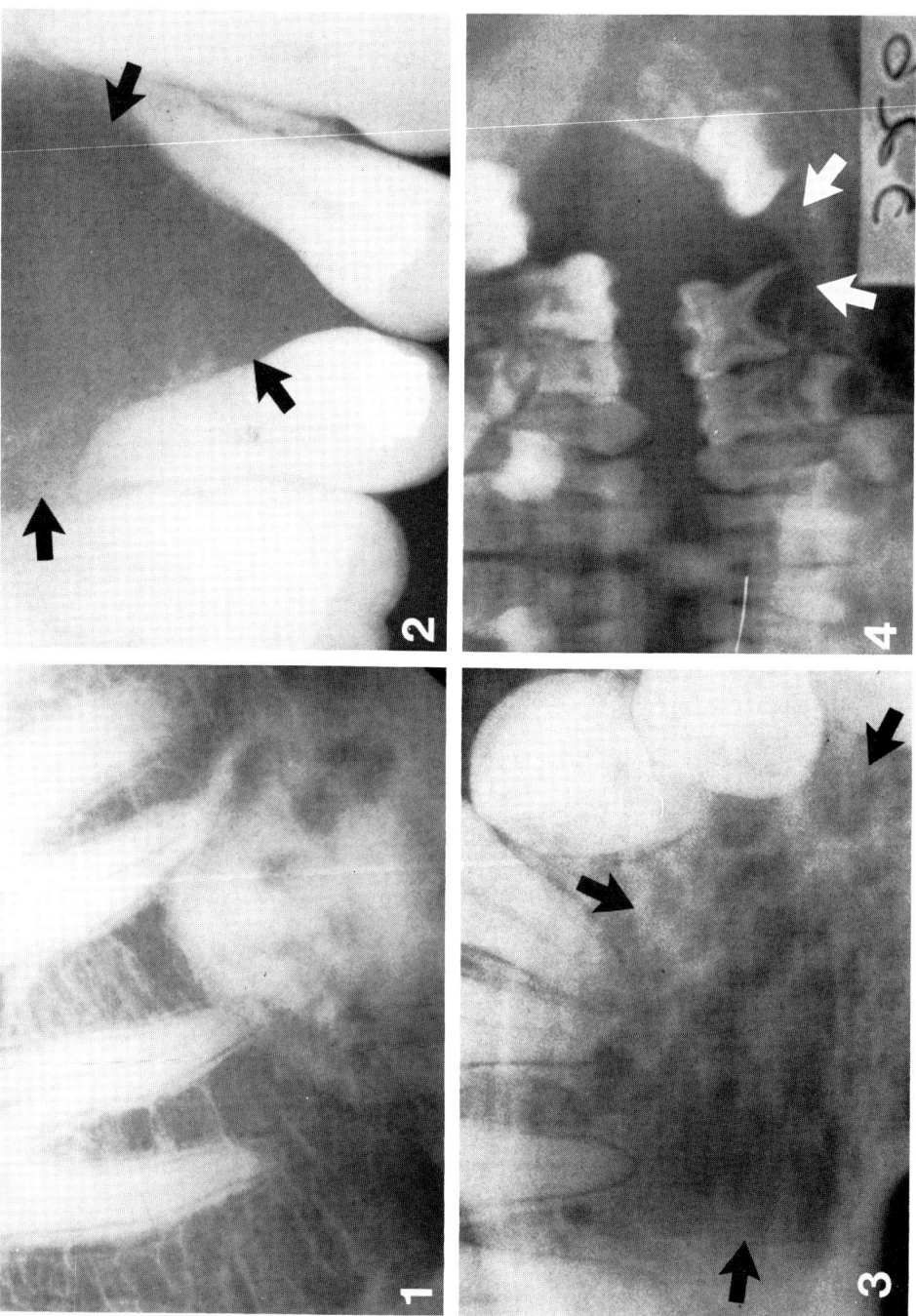

BENIGN NON-ODONTOGENIC TUMORS (continued)

Disease	Age	Location	Radiography	Other Features
Osteoma (Fig. 1) (p. 378–379)	Any age	Either jaw	Well-defined opacity	Asymptomatic; may be part of Gardner's syndrome (osteomas, intestinal polyps, cysts and fibrous lesions of skin, supernumerary teeth); rare
Central giant cell granuloma (Fig. 2) (p. 379–380)	Children and young adults	Either jaw	Usually well-defined lucency; may be multilocular or, less frequently, unilocular	May exhibit aggressive behavior; low recurrence rate; asymptomatic; uncommon
Hemangioma of bone (Fig. 3) (p. 382–383)	Young adults	Either jaw	Lucent lesion; may be "honeycombed" or multilocular	Hemorrhage is significant complication with treatment; asymptomatic; rare
Idiopathic histiocytosis (Langerhans cell disease) (Fig. 4) (p. 383–386)	Children and young adults	Any bone	Single or multiple lucent lesions; some described as "punched out"; "floating teeth" sometimes used to describe lesions around root apices	Three variants: *Letterer-Siwe syndrome* (*acute disseminated*)—organs and bone affected, infants, usually fatal; *Hand-Schüller-Christian syndrome* (*chronic disseminated*)—bone lesions, exophthalmos, diabetes insipidus and organ lesions, children, fair prognosis; *eosinophilic granuloma* (*chronic localized*)—bone lesions only, children and adults, good prognosis; surgery, radiation or chemotherapy; etiology unknown
Tori and exostoses (p. 386–387)	Adults	Palate, lingual mandible, and buccal aspect of alveolar bone	May appear as opacity when large	Torus palatinus in 25% of population, torus mandibularis in 10%; etiology unknown; little significance
Coronoid hyperplasia (p. 387–389)	Young adults	Coronoid process of mandible	Opaque enlargement	Etiology unknown; may affect jaw function

Jaw Lesions

Cysts of the Oral Region
Odontogenic Tumors
Benign Non-odontogenic Tumors
Inflammatory Jaw Lesions
Malignant Non-odontogenic Neoplasms of the Jaws
Metabolic and Genetic Jaw Diseases

Chapter 13

Inflammatory Jaw Lesions

ACUTE OSTEOMYELITIS
CHRONIC OSTEOMYELITIS
Focal Sclerosing Osteomyelitis (Condensing Osteitis)
Diffuse Sclerosing Osteomyelitis
Garrés Osteomyelitis (Chronic Osteomyelitis with Proliferative Periostitis)

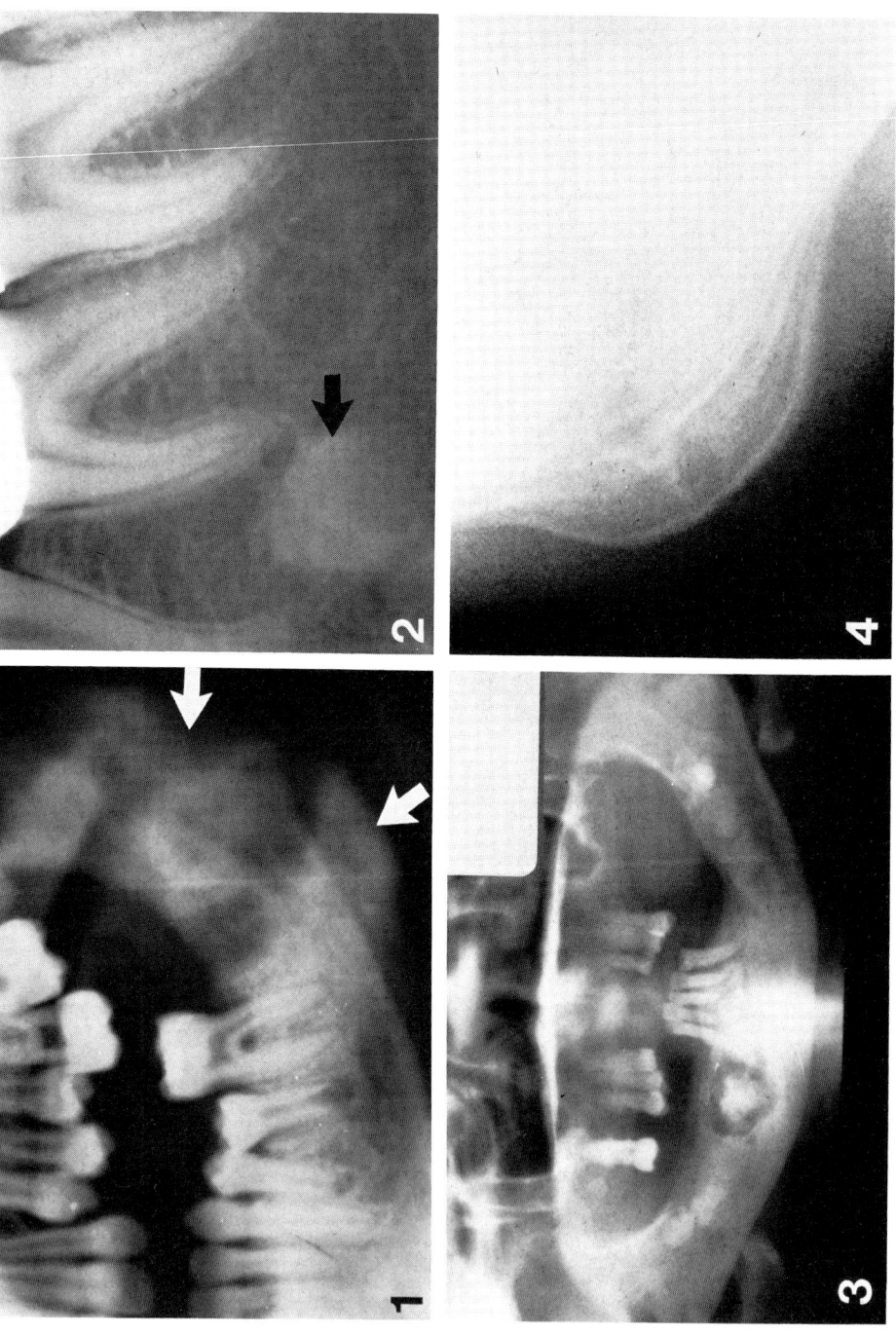

INFLAMMATORY JAW LESIONS

Disease	Age	Location	Radiography	Other Features
Acute osteomyelitis (p. 394–395)	Any age	Mandible favored	Little radiographic change early; after 1 to 2 weeks, a diffuse lucency appears	Pain or paresthesia may be present; pus producing if due to *Staphylococcus* infection; uncommon in severe form; most frequently caused by extension of periapical infection
Chronic osteomyelitis (Figs. 1–4) (p. 395–399)	Any age	Mandible favored	Focal or diffuse; lucent with sclerotic foci described as a "moth-eaten" pattern (Fig. 1); *focal sclerotic type*—well-defined opacification (Fig. 2); *diffuse sclerotic type*—diffuse opacification (Fig. 3); *Garré's type*—"onion-skin" periosteum (Fig. 4)	Usually asymptomatic, but may be painful; most are related to chronic inflammation in bone of dental origin; many are not treated; non-vital teeth should be extracted or root canals filled; common; *Garré's type* is treated by extraction of offending tooth

Jaw Lesions

Cysts of the Oral Region
Odontogenic Tumors
Benign Non-odontogenic Tumors
Inflammatory Jaw Lesions
Malignant Non-odontogenic Neoplasms of the Jaws
Metabolic and Genetic Jaw Diseases

Chapter 14

Malignant Non-odontogenic Neoplasms of the Jaws

OSTEOSARCOMA
Juxtacortical Osteosarcomas
Parosteal Osteosarcoma
Periosteal Osteosarcoma
CHONDROSARCOMA
Mesenchymal Chondrosarcoma
EWING'S SARCOMA
BURKITT'S LYMPHOMA
PLASMA CELL NEOPLASMS
Multiple Myeloma
Solitary Plasmacytoma of Bone
METASTATIC CARCINOMA

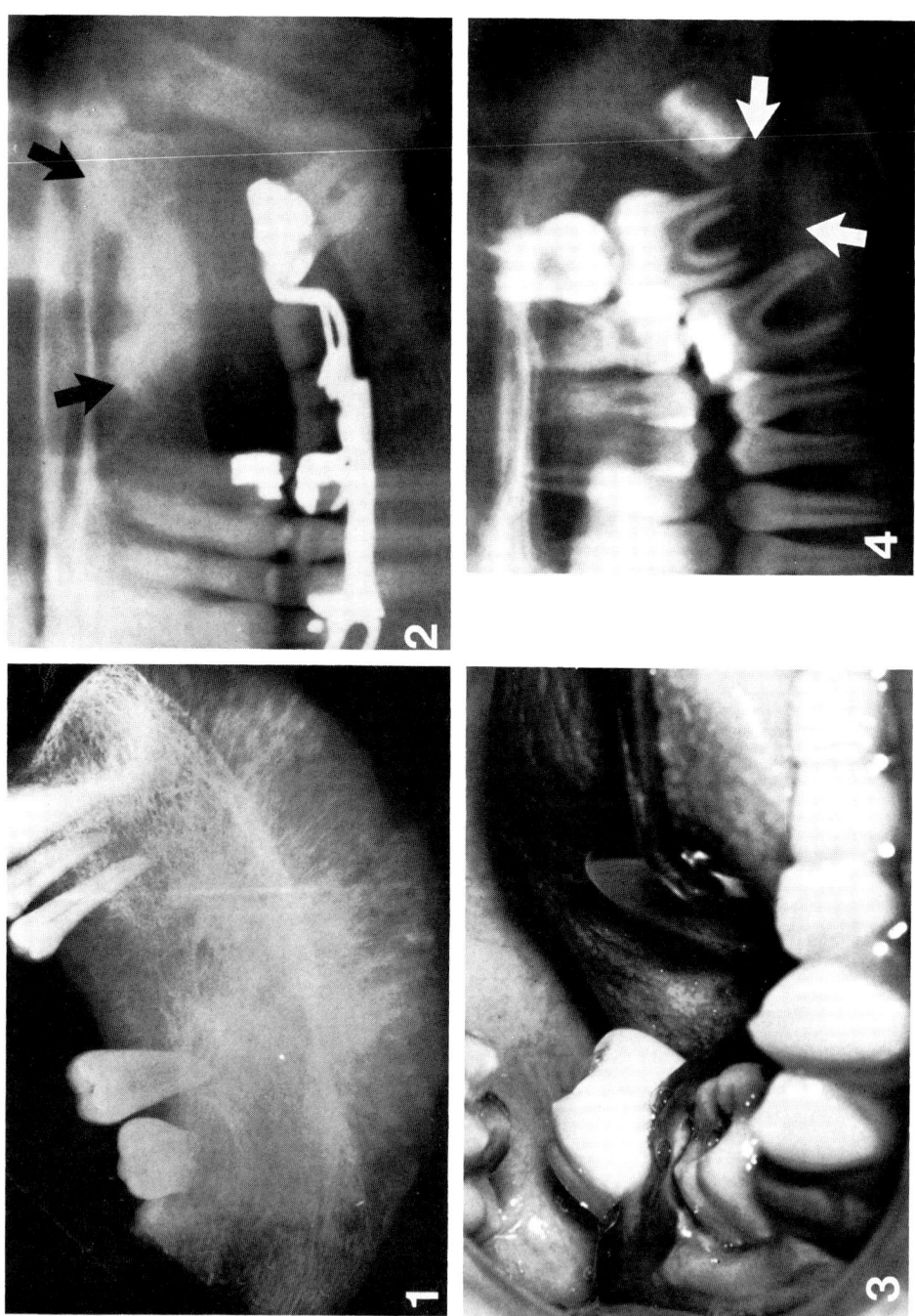

MALIGNANT NON-ODONTOGENIC NEOPLASMS OF THE JAWS

Disease	Age	Location	Radiography	Other Features
Osteosarcoma (Figs. 1 and 2) (p. 405–413)	Third and fourth decades	Mandible or maxilla; juxtacortical subtype (Fig. 2) arises from periosteum	Poorly defined luency with spicules of opaque material; "sunburst" pattern may be seen; juxtacortical lesion appears as radiodense mass on the periosteum	Swelling, pain, or paresthesia are diagnostic features; may have vertical mobility of teeth and uniformly widened periodontal ligament space; prognosis, fair to poor, good prognosis for juxtacortical lesions
Chondrosarcoma (p. 413–416)	Adulthood and old age	Maxilla favored slightly	Poorly defined, lucent to moderately opaque	Swelling, pain, or paresthesia may be present; prognosis fair to poor, better if in mandible; often misdiagnosed as benign cartilage lesion; rare
Ewing's sarcoma (p. 417–419)	Children and young adults	Mandible favored	Diffuse lucency; poorly defined; periosteal reaction, "onionskin," may be present; may be multilocular	Swelling, pain, or paresthesia may be present; prognosis is poor; malignant cell is of unknown origin; rare
Burkitt's lymphoma (Figs. 3 and 4) (p. 419–421)	Children	Mandible or maxilla	Diffuse lucency	Malignancy of B lymphocytes linked to Epstein-Barr virus; pain or paresthesia may be presenting symptoms; prognosis is fair; rare in the U.S.

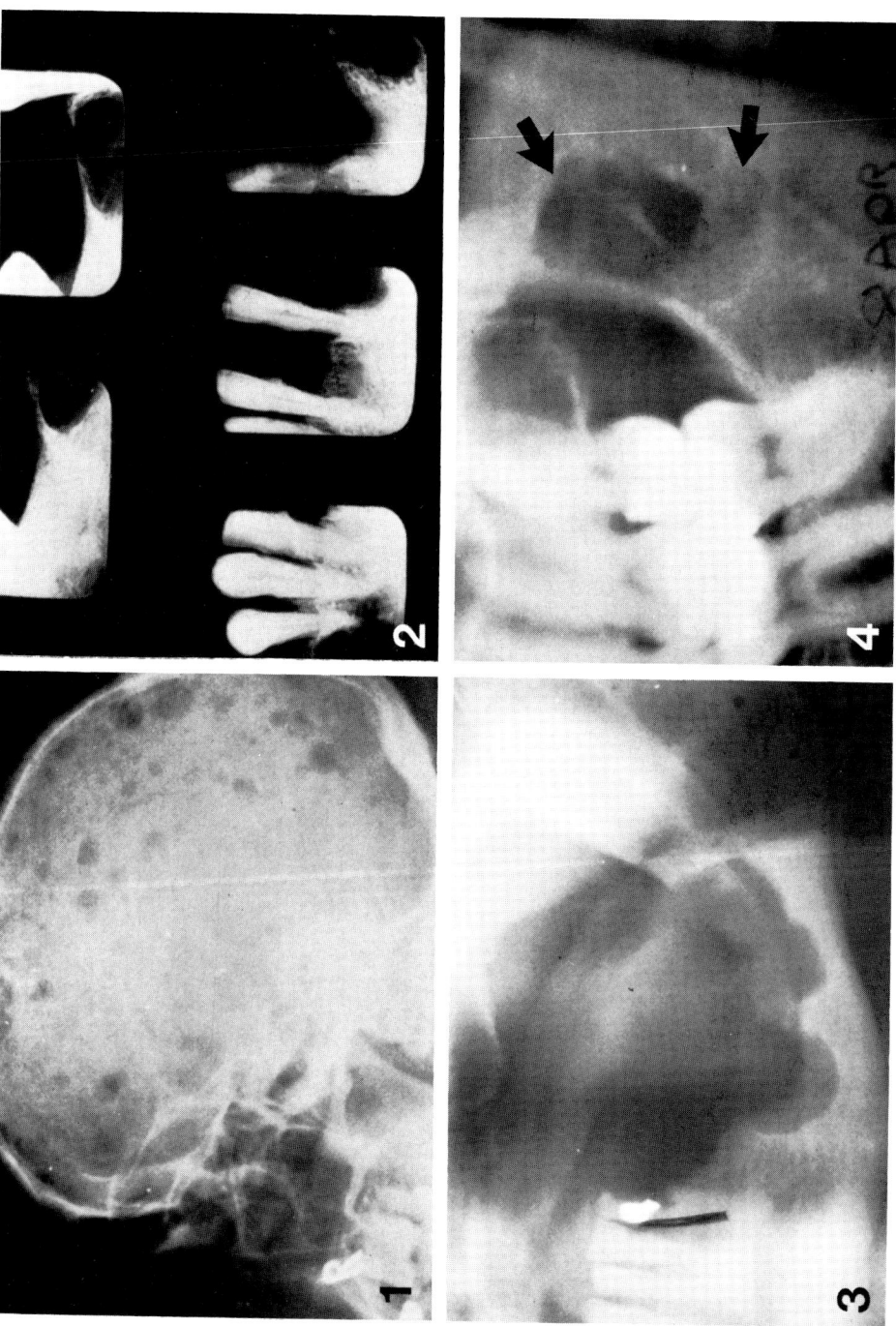

MALIGNANT NON-ODONTOGENIC NEOPLASMS OF THE JAWS (continued)

Disease	Age	Location	Radiography	Other Features
Plasma cell myeloma (Figs. 1 and 2) (p. 421–423)	Adults	Mandible favored	Well-defined lucencies decribed as "punched-out" lesions; some lesions diffuse	Swelling, pain, or numbness may be presenting complaint; Bence Jones protein in urine of a majority of cases; rare to have only jaw lesions; prognosis is poor; solitary lesions eventually become disseminated
Metastatic carcinoma (Figs. 3 and 4) (p. 424–425)	Adults	Mandible favored	Ill-defined, destructive lucency; may be multilocular; some tumors may have opaque foci (e.g., prostate, breast, lung)	Pain or paresthesia often seen; origin is most likely from a malignancy of breast, kidney, lung, colon, prostate, or thyroid; uncommon to rare

Jaw Lesions

Cysts of the Oral Region
Odontogenic Tumors
Benign Non-odontogenic Tumors
Inflammatory Jaw Lesions
Malignant Non-odontogenic Neoplasms of the Jaws
Metabolic and Genetic Jaw Diseases

Chapter 15

Metabolic and Genetic Jaw Diseases

METABOLIC
Paget's Disease
Hyperparathyroidism
Infantile Cortical Hyperostosis
Phantom Bone Disease
Acromegaly
GENETIC
Cherubism
Osteopetrosis
Others (See text)
   Osteogenesis Imperfecta
   Cleidocranial Dysplasia
   Crouzon's Syndrome
   Treacher Collins Syndrome
   Pierre Robin Syndrome
   Marfan's Syndrome
   Ehlers-Danlos Syndrome
   Down's Syndrome
   Hemifacial Atrophy
   Hemifacial Hypertrophy
   Clefts of the Lip and Palate
   Fragile X Syndrome

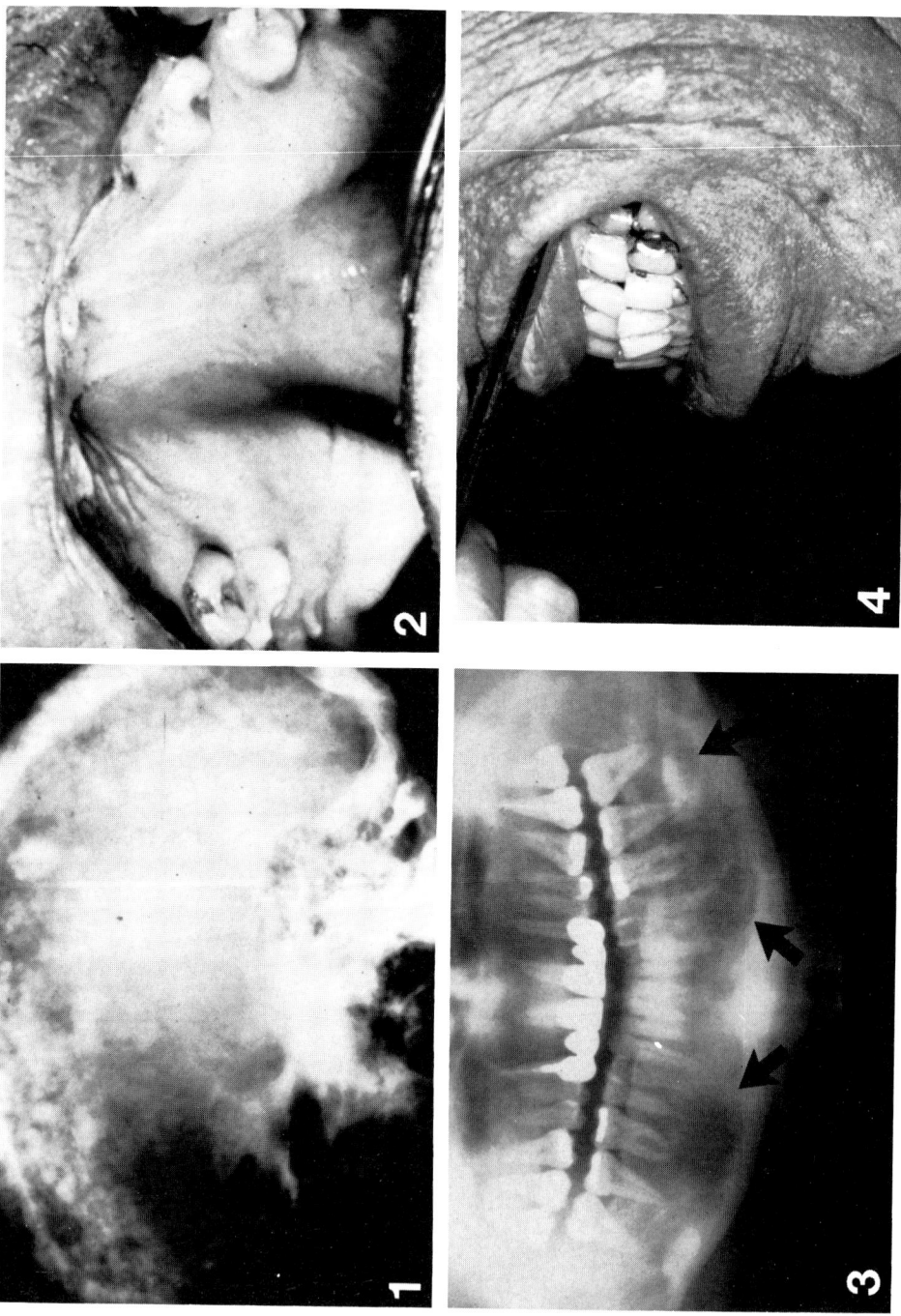

METABOLIC AND GENETIC JAW DISEASES

Disease	Age	Location	Radiography	Other Features
Paget's disease (Figs. 1 and 2) (p. 427–430)	Over 40 years of age	Maxilla favored, bilateral and symmetric	Diffuse lucent to opaque bone changes; opaque lesions described as "cotton wool"; hypercementosis, loss of lamina dura, obliteration of periodontal ligament space, and root resorption may be seen	Patients develop pain, deafness, blindness, and headache because of bone changes; initial complaint may be that denture is too tight; diastemas may develop; complications of hemorrhage early, infection and fracture late; alkaline phosphatase elevated; etiology unknown but affects bone metabolism
Hyperparathyroidism (Fig. 3) (p. 430–432)	Any age	Mandible favored	Usually well-defined lucency(ies); may be multilocular; a minority of patients show loss of lamina dura	Usually asymptomatic; microscopically identical to central giant cell granuloma; serum calcium elevated; most caused by parathyroid adenoma; rare
Infantile cortical hyperostosis (p. 434)	Infants	Mandible and other bones of the skeleton	Cortical thickening/sclerosis	Cause unknown; self-limited; treatment is supportive
Phantom bone disease (p. 434–435)	Young adults	Mandible more than maxilla	Gradual lucency of entire bone	Etiology unknown; no treatment
Acromegaly (Fig. 4) (p. 435–437)	Adults (after closure of epiphyses)	Mandible; uniform, bilateral	Large jaw	Excess production of growth hormone after closure of epiphyses (condyle remains active); prognathism, diastemas may appear; rare

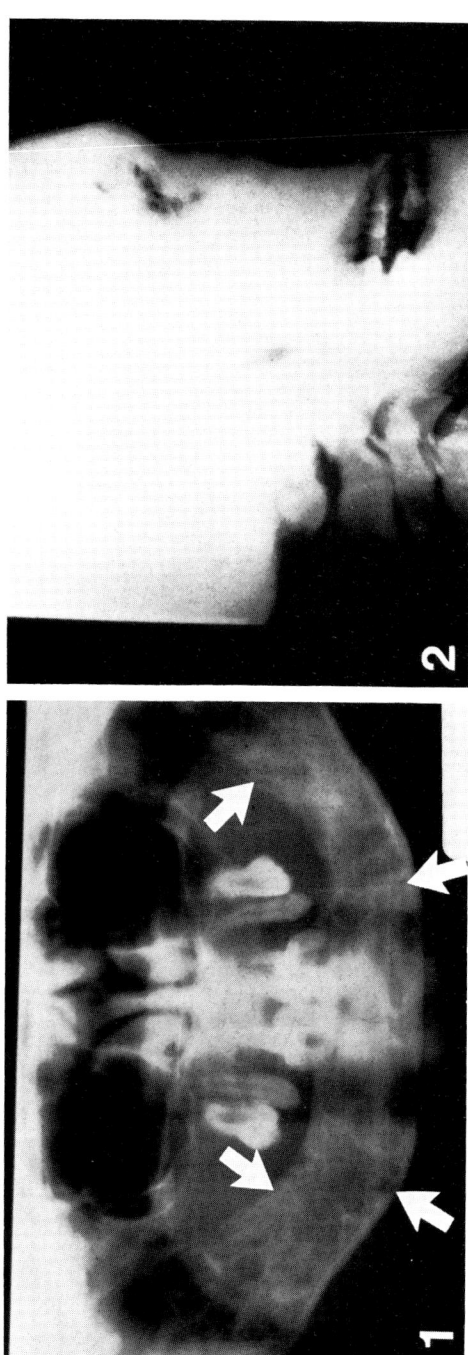

METABOLIC AND GENETIC JAW DISEASES (continued)

Disease	Age	Location	Radiography	Other Features
Cherubism (Fig. 1) (p. 437–439)	Children	Mandible favored; uniform, bilateral	Bilateral multilocular lucencies	Autosomal dominant inheritance pattern; facies is cherub-like; microscopy similar to central giant cell granuloma; process stabilizes after puberty; rare
Osteopetrosis (Fig. 2) (p. 439–441)	Children and adults	Both jaws (and skull)	Diffuse, homogeneous, and symmetric opacification; may cause arrested root development and delayed eruption	Infantile, recessive (severe) and adult, dominant forms; intermediate form also recessive but has mild presentation; results in inhibition of bone resorption; patients develop anemia, blindness, and deafness; dental complications of infection and fracture; rare

The authors make grateful acknowledgment to the following doctors for photographs used in the overview section: S.K. Young (p. O-4, Fig. 4, and p. O-12, Fig. 1), R. Millard (p. O-12, Fig. 1), T. Osborn (p. O-20, Fig. 1), A. Plotzke (p. O-38, Fig. 1), R. Courtney (p. O-38, Fig. 4, and p. O-58, Fig. 2), C. Taylor (p. O-44, Fig. 2), M.M. Ash and H.D. Millard (p. O-64, Fig. 1), and K. Volz (p. O-96, Fig. 2).

Chapter 1

Vesiculo-Bullous Diseases

VIRAL DISEASES
Herpes Simplex Infections
Varicella-Zoster Infections
Hand, Foot, and Mouth Disease
Herpangina
Measles (Rubeola)
CONDITIONS ASSOCIATED WITH
  IMMUNOLOGIC DEFECTS
Pemphigus Vulgaris
Cicatricial Pemphigoid
Bullous Pemphigoid
Dermatitis Herpetiformis
HEREDITARY DISEASES
Epidermolysis Bullosa

VIRAL DISEASES

Oral mucous membranes may be infected by one of several different viruses, each producing a relatively distinct clinical-pathologic picture (Table 1-1). Recognition of accompanying signs and symptoms and utilization of laboratory tests may be important in the separation of oral viral infections from other non-infectious conditions. This distinction may have profound consequences on the patient when treatment is instituted.

Viruses are composed of an inner nucleic acid core (genome) of either DNA or RNA that represents their genetic code. The nucleic acid core is surrounded by a protein coat known as a capsid. With some types of viruses, the capsid is further encased by a lipid envelope. The complete virus particle—consisting of genome and capsid, or genome, capsid, and envelope—is known as the virion and is representative of the infectious and complete viral form outside the cell.

Viruses are infective agents that lack the necessary structures for self-replication. They require the machinery of living cells for maintenance and multiplication. Viruses are, therefore, regarded as intracellular parasites and are usually dependent upon certain cell types in certain hosts. For virus reproduction to occur, the infecting virus must attach to the preferred cell type and penetrate the plasma membrane (Fig. 1-1). Once entry into the cell is accomplished, the capsid (and envelope) are lost, leaving the viral genome to encode the cell for the manufacture of capsid proteins, viral nucleic acid, and enzymes necessary for assembly. Intracellular assembly of new particles is also directed by the infecting virus. Eventually, newly replicated (and enveloped) virus is released, with subsequent infection of other cells. This usually occurs at the expense of the originally infected cell.

In certain types of viral infection, cell death may not occur, allowing the virus to infect dividing host cells in a chronic pattern. Viral latency, in which the infectious agent lies dormant within the host cell, is another non-cytocidal infection. This is common to the herpesviruses, papilloma viruses, and retroviruses. In this latter form of viral infection, overt clinical signs and symptoms of viral replication and infection may follow certain triggering events, such as stress or alterations in the immune state. Another non-cytotoxic type of viral infection is related to tumor-associated viruses that have the ability to become incorporated in the host cell DNA. This newly incorporated viral genetic information results in "transformation" of the host cell into a neoplastic cell.

Table 1–1. VIRUSES AND ASSOCIATED CONDITIONS OF SIGNIFICANCE TO CLINICAL DENTISTRY

Virus Family	Virus	Disease
Herpesvirus	Herpes simplex type 1	Primary herpes gingivostomatitis Secondary herpes (oral and HSL) Herpetic whitlow Occasionally, genital herpes
	Herpes simplex type 2	Genital herpes Occasionally, oral herpes
	Varicella-zoster virus	Varicella, herpes zoster
	Epstein-Barr virus	Mononucleosis Burkitt's lymphoma Nasopharyngeal carcinoma Hairy leukoplakia
	Cytomegalovirus	Salivary gland disease
Papovavirus	Papilloma virus	Oral warts Oral papillomas Condyloma acuminatum Heck's disease ? Carcinoma
Paramyxovirus	Measles virus Mumps virus Parainfluenza virus	Measles Mumps parotitis Respiratory infections
(Orthomyxovirus)	(Influenza virus)	(Influenza)
Picornavirus	Coxsackie virus	Hand, foot, & mouth disease Herpangina
	Rhinovirus	Common cold

Because viruses are integrally associated with host cell biologic function and metabolic pathways and because they utilize similar enzymatic pathways, development of a chemotherapeutic agent that kills the virus and spares the cell has been especially difficult. Drugs directed toward the interruption of viral DNA synthesis or protein synthesis may also interrupt the same processes in the host cell. The thrust of antiviral chemotherapy, therefore, has been directed toward certain enzymes that are virus specific and unique to viral replication.

The herpesviruses are a large family of viruses characterized by a DNA core surrounded by a capsid and an envelope. Five types of herpesviruses are known to be pathogenic for humans, and all have been linked to diseases in the head and neck area. The Epstein-Barr virus has been linked to infectious mononucleosis, Burkitt's lymphoma, nasopharyngeal carcinoma, and oral "hairy" leukoplakia. Cytomegalovirus has been associated with salivary gland disease and systemic disease of immunocompromised patients. Varicella-zoster virus has been shown to cause chickenpox and herpes zoster. Herpes simplex type I (HSV-I) has been shown to be responsible for oral, perioral, and occasionally genital infections. Herpes simplex type II (HSV-II) has been associated with genital infections and occasionally with oral and perioral lesions.

Herpes Simplex Infections

Pathogenesis (Fig. 1–2). Physical contact with an infected individual is the typical route of HSV inoculation for someone (seronegative) who has not been previously exposed to the virus or possibly for someone with a low titer of protective antibody to HSV. Documentation of spread of infection through airborne droplets, through contaminated water, or through contact with inanimate objects is generally lacking. During the primary infection, only a small percentage of individuals show clinical signs and symptoms of infectious systemic disease while a vast majority experience only subclinical disease. This latter group, now seropositive, has been identified through the laboratory evaluation of circulating antibodies to HSV.

The incubation period after exposure ranges

from several days to 2 weeks. A vesiculo-ulcerative eruption typically occurs in the oral and perioral tissues (primary gingivostomatitis). The focus of eruption is expected at the original site of contact.

Following resolution of primary herpetic gingivostomatitis, the virus migrates, through some unknown mechanism, along the periaxon sheath of the trigeminal nerve to the trigeminal ganglion, where it is capable of remaining in a latent or quiescent state. Reactivation of virus may follow exposure to sunlight ("fever blisters"), exposure to cold ("cold sores"), trauma, and stress, causing a secondary or recurrent infection. Viral particles travel by way of the trigeminal nerve to the original epithelial surface, where replication occurs, resulting in a focal vesiculo-ulcerative eruption. Presumably because the humoral and cell-mediated arms of the immune system have been sensitized to HSV antigens, the lesion is limited in extent and systemic symptoms usually do not occur. As the secondary lesion resolves, the virus returns to the trigeminal ganglion and evidence of viral particles can no longer be found within the epithelium. From

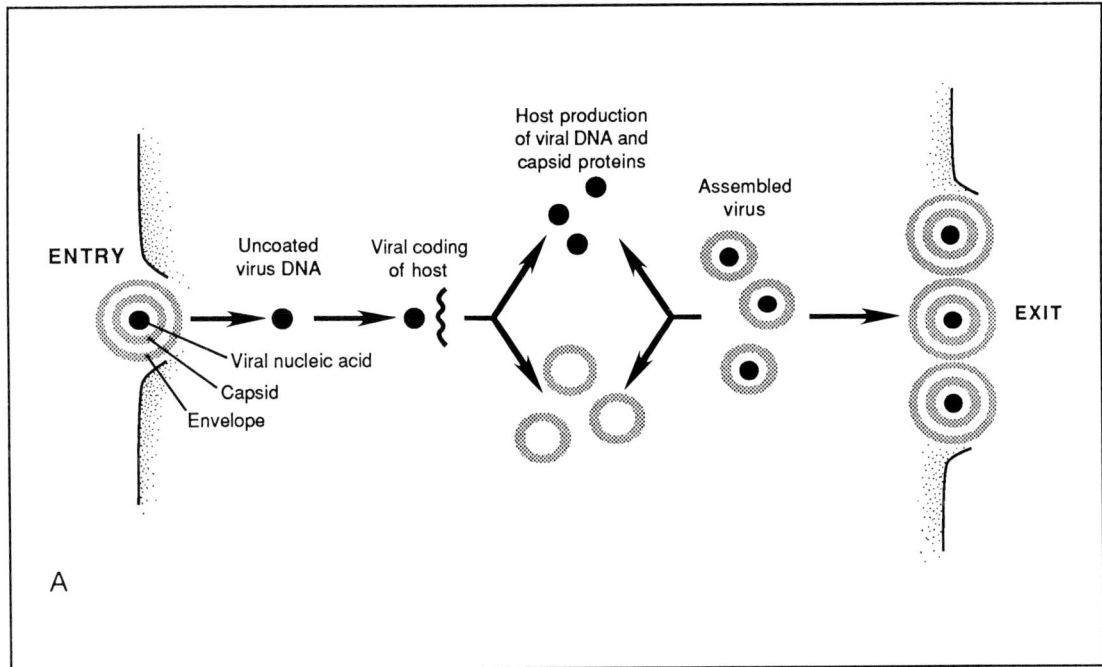

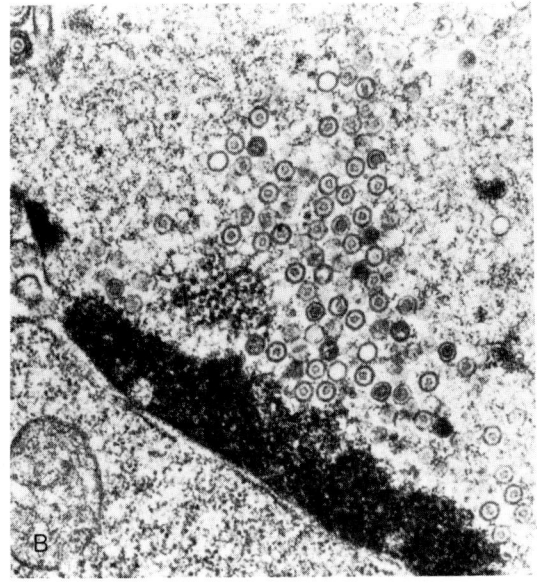

Figure 1–1. *A*, Virus and host cell interaction. *B*, Electron micrograph showing herpes simplex virus in the nucleus of a keratinocyte. Nucleic acid cores are surrounded by electron-dense protein capsid rings. (Courtesy of Dr. S. K. Young.)

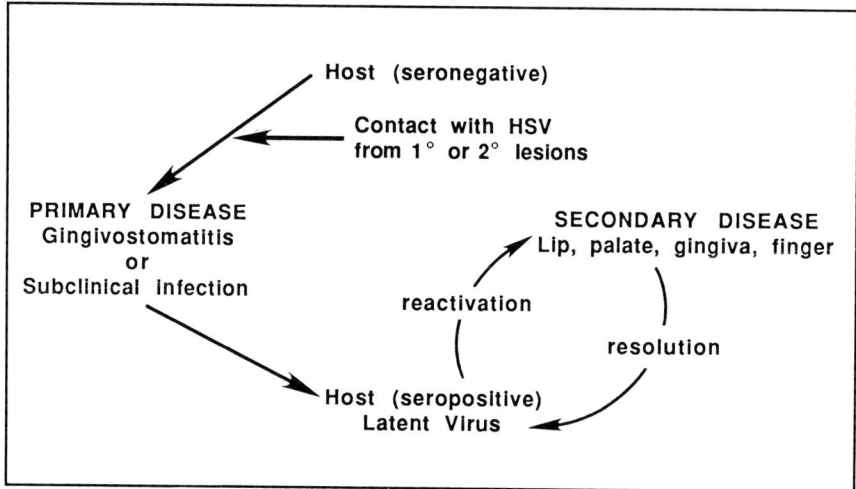

Figure 1–2. Pathogenesis of HSV-I infections.

one third to one half of the United States population experience recurrent herpetic lesions. It is believed that nearly all secondary lesions develop from reactivated latent virus, although reinfection by different strains of the same subtype is considered to be a remote possibility. Also, most of the oral-facial herpetic lesions are due to HSV-I, although a small percentage may be caused by HSV-II secondary to oral-genital contact. Lesions caused by either virus are clinically indistinguishable. HSV-II has a predilection for genital mucosa, with infections having a pathogenesis similiar to HSV-I infections of the head and neck. Latent virus, however, is maintained in the lumbosacral ganglion. Occasional HSV-I infections of the genitalia have also been noted. Previous HSV-I infections may provide some protection against HSV-II infection because of antibody cross-reactivity.

One of the more disconcerting pieces of information to be uncovered about HSV infections is the asymptomatic shedding of intact virus particles in saliva and other secretions of a small percentage of previously infected individuals. The level of risk of infection from such persons has not been measured, although it is probably very low and is certainly much less than the risk of infection from individuals with symptomatic disease. Another problem with herpes infections is their possible carcinogenic potential. Considerable evidence has accumulated linking HSV-II to carcinoma of the cervix. Whether or not HSV-I (or HSV-II) has carcinogenic potential in the head and neck area has yet to be convincingly shown.

Clinical Features

Primary Herpetic Gingivostomatitis. Primary disease is usually seen in children, although adults who have not been previously exposed to HSV or who fail to mount an appropriate response to a previous infection may be affected. The vesicular eruption may appear on the skin, vermilion, or oral mucous membranes (Fig. 1–3). Intraorally, lesions may appear on any mucosal surface. This is in contradistinction to the recurrent form of the disease, in which lesions are confined to hard palate and gingiva. The lesions are accompanied by fever, arthralgia, malaise, headache, and cervical lymphadenopathy.

After the systemic primary infection runs its course of about 1 week to 10 days, the lesions heal without scar. Also, by this time the virus may have migrated to the trigeminal ganglion to reside in a latent form. The number of individuals with primary clinical or subclinical infections in which virus assumes dormancy in nerve tissue is unknown.

Secondary or Recurrent HSV Infections. Secondary herpes represents the reactivation of latent virus. It is believed that only rarely does reinfection from an exogenous source occur in seropositive individuals. A large majority of the population (up to 90%) have antibodies to HSV, and up to 40% of this group may develop secondary herpes. The pathophysiology of recurrence has been related to either a breakdown in focal immunosurveillance or an alteration in local inflammatory mediators that allows the virus to replicate.

There are usually prodromal symptoms of tingling, burning, or pain in the site in which lesions will appear. Within a matter of hours, multiple fragile and short-lived vesicles appear that become ulcerated and coalesce to form a map-like superficial ulcer(s). The lesions heal

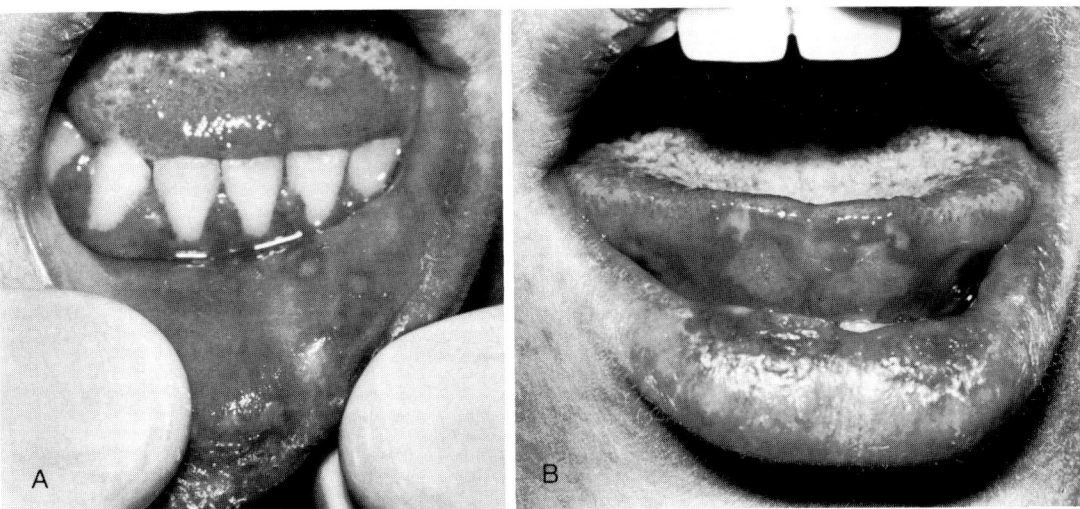

Figure 1–3. *A*, Primary herpes gingivostomatitis in a 14-year-old female. Note lip ulcers and inflamed gingiva. *B*, Same patient with confluent tongue ulcers.

without scarring in 1 to 2 weeks and rarely become secondarily infected (Fig. 1–4). The number of recurrences is variable and ranges from one per year to as many as one per month. Recurrence rate appears to decline with age with each individual. The secondary lesions typically occur at or near the same site with each recurrence. Regionally, most secondary lesions occur on the vermilion and surrounding skin. This type of disease is usually referred to as herpes simplex labialis (HSL) (Fig. 1–5). When recurrences appear intraorally, they are almost always on the hard palate or gingiva (Fig. 1–6).

Herpetic Whitlow. Herpetic whitlow refers to either a primary or a secondary HSV infection involving the fingers (Fig. 1–7). This type of infection typically occurs in dental practitioners who have been in physical contact with infected individuals. In the case of a seronegative clinician, contact may result in a vesiculoulcerative eruption on the digit (rather than in the oral region) along with the signs and symptoms of primary systemic disease. Recurrent lesions, if they occur, would be expected on the fingers. Herpetic whitlow in a seropositive clinician (e.g., one with a history of HSL) is believed to be possible, although less likely because of previous immune stimulation by herpes simplex antigens. The potential occupational hazard of contact with seropositive patients who shed virus in saliva has not been adequately studied. If there is a risk, it is probably very slight.

Pain, redness, and swelling are prominent with herpetic whitlow and can be very pro-

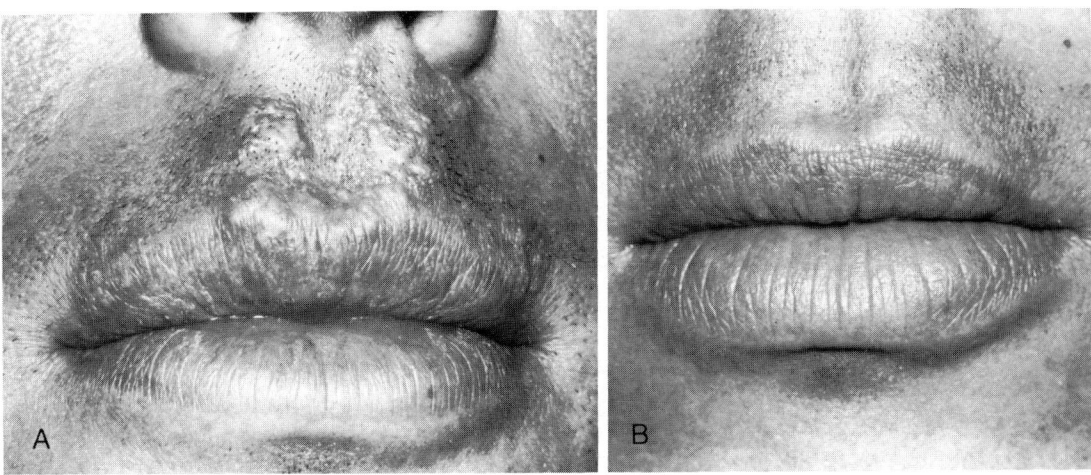

Figure 1–4. *A*, Secondary HSL. *B*, Same patient showing healing without scar 2 weeks later.

6 VESICULO-BULLOUS DISEASES

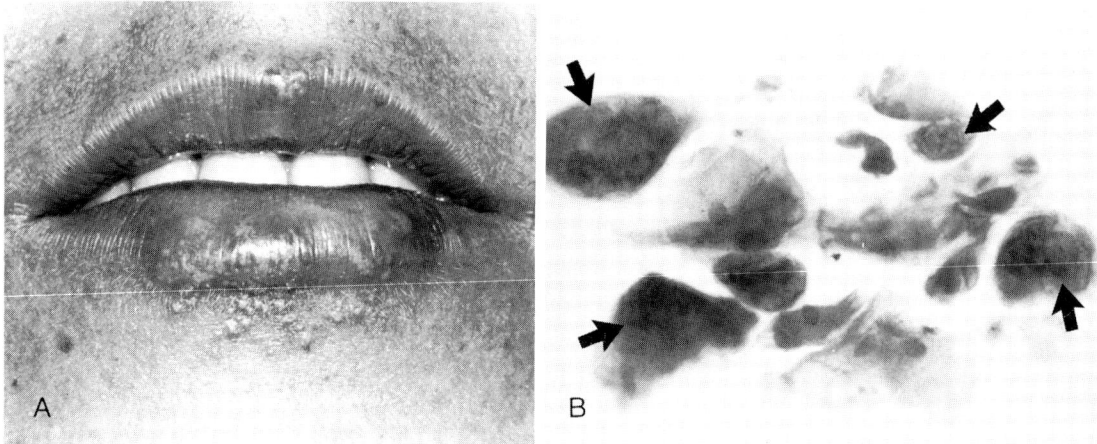

Figure 1–5. *A*, Secondary HSL of the lower and upper lips. *B*, Cytologic preparation from scraping of the base of the vesicles. Note numerous virus-infected multinucleated epithelial cells (arrows). Normal keratinocytes are seen at bottom center.

nounced. Vesicles or pustules eventually break to become ulcers. Axillary or epitrochlear lymphadenopathy may also be present. Duration of herpetic whitlow tends to be more prolonged than in other herpetic infections and may be as long as 4 to 6 weeks. This condition can be especially debilitating for a dental practitioner because of severity of symptoms and duration of lesions. Recurrences may also occur with this form of herpes infection. Lesions would be expected in the same site.

Histopathology. Microscopically, intraepithelial vesicles containing exudate, inflammatory cells, and some virus-infected epithelial cells are seen (Fig. 1–8). Lining the vesicles are highly characteristic epithelial cells that show the effects of HSV infection. Some of these cells contain a single nucleus, and some are multinucleated. The nucleus is homogeneous and glassy, with nuclear material forced to the outer perimeter. These features can also be readily found on cytologic preparations and are indicative of a herpes type infection. On morphologic grounds, however, HSV-I cannot be differentiated from HSV-II or from herpes zoster infections. After several days, herpes-

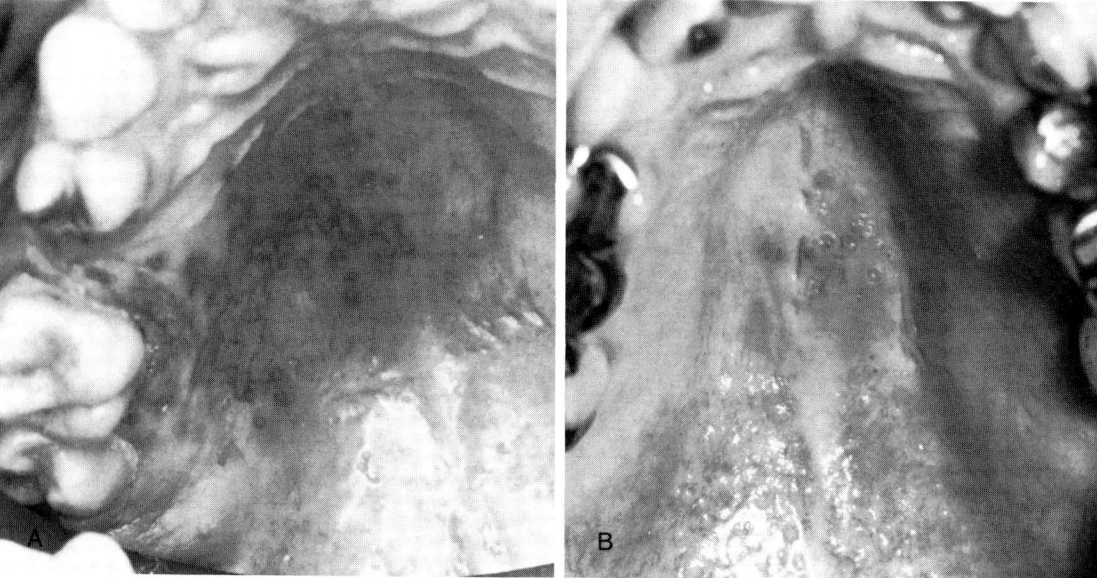

Figure 1–6. *A*, Secondary HSV infection of gingiva and palate. *B*, Secondary HSV infection of palate showing recently ruptured vesicles.

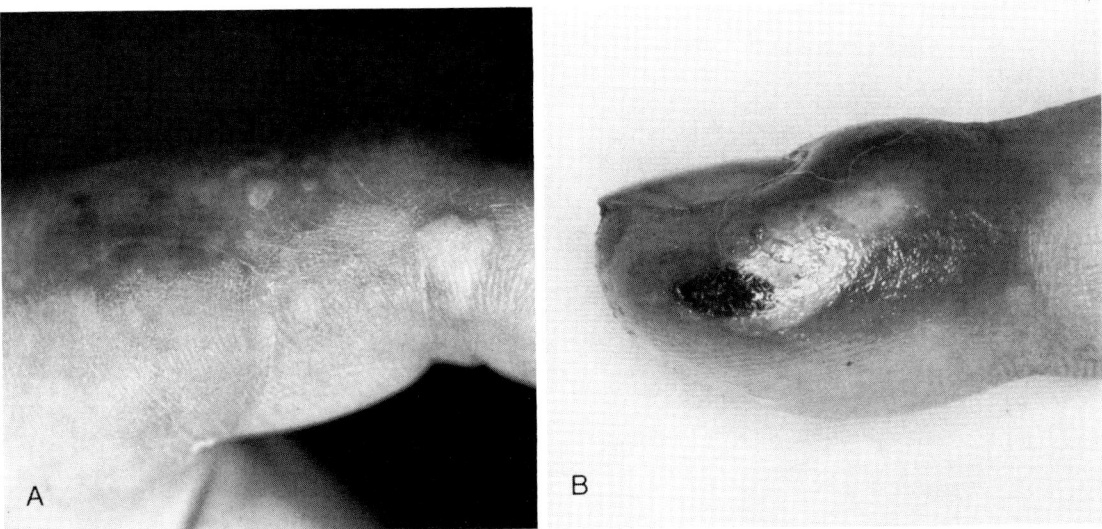

Figure 1–7. *A*, Herpes whitlow showing early vesicular eruption. *B*, Herpes whitlow in later stage showing severe swelling and ulceration. (Courtesy of Dr. S. K. Young.)

infected epithelial cells cannot be demonstrated in either cytologic or biopsy preparations.

Differential Diagnosis. The diagnosis of primary herpetic gingivostomatitis is usually apparent from clinical features. It can be confirmed by a virus culture (which requires 2 to 4 days for positive identification). Immunologic methods utilizing monoclonal antibodies or DNA hybridization techniques have also become useful for specific virus identification.

The systemic signs and symptoms coupled with the oral ulcers may require differentiation from streptococcal pharyngitis, erythema multiforme, and Vincent's infection. Clinically, streptococcal pharyngitis would not involve the lips or perioral tissues, and vesicles would not precede the ulcers. Oral ulcers of erythema multiforme would be larger, usually without a vesicular stage, and would be less likely to affect gingiva. In Vincent's infection (acute necrotizing ulcerative gingivitis) oral lesions would be limited to gingiva, would not be preceded by vesicles, and would demonstrate tissue necrosis. Intraorally, secondary herpes is often confused with aphthous stomatitis but can usually be distinguished from it on the basis of clinical features (Table 1–2). Multiple lesions, vesicles preceding ulcers, and palatal and gingival location are indicative of herpesvirus infection. Other oral conditions that may show clinical features similar to secondary

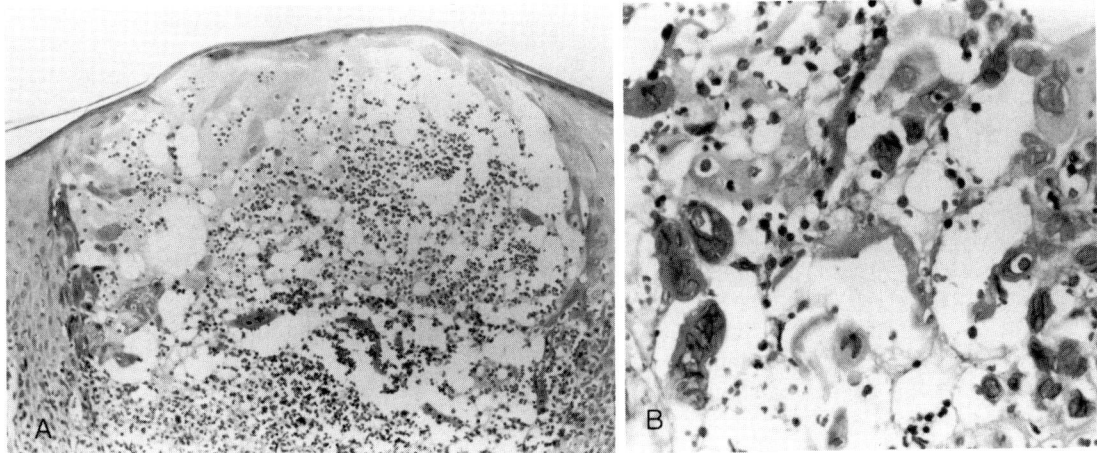

Figure 1–8. *A*, Vesicle of HSV infection. *B*, Syncytium of virus-infected keratinocytes along lateral wall of vesicle. Note multinucleated keratinocytes.

Table 1-2. COMPARISON OF SECONDARY ORAL HERPES SIMPLEX INFECTIONS TO MINOR ORAL APHTHOUS ULCERS

Parameter	Herpes	Minor Aphthae
Cause	HSV-I	Focal immunodysregulation
Precipitating factors	Stress, trauma, UV light, change in immune status	Stress, trauma, hormonal changes, diet, immunologic alterations
Prodromal symptoms	Usually	Occasionally
Cytology	Virus-infected epithelial cells	Non-specific
Vesicular stage	Yes	No
Number of ulcers	Multiple, confluent	Usually one, oval
Pain	Yes	Yes
Location	Vermilion, hard palate, gingiva	All other mucosal sites
Duration	1-2 weeks	1-2 weeks
Scar after healing	No	Major form only
Recurrent	Yes	Yes
Treatment	Antiviral drugs	Steroids

herpes include trauma, chemical burns, and contact allergy. Lip lesions of secondary herpes may need to be distinguished from the pustules of impetigo.

Treatment. One of the most important factors in the treatment of HSV infections is timing. For any drug to be effective, it must be initiated as soon as possible. No later than 48 hours from the onset of symptoms is generally regarded as the ideal time for the start of therapeutic measures. Carriers or vehicles of topical medications are also apparently very important in the chemotherapy of HSV infections. Those agents that facilitate drug absorption are more likely to be successful than those that do not.

A number of virus-specific drugs have been developed, but at present no single therapeutic regimen has proved to be uniformly effective in the treatment of oral and perioral HSV infections. Many remedies and non-specific forms of treatment have been used. All have produced limited or inconsistent results. Development of virus-specific compounds has been slow because of the extreme difficulty in finding a selective viricidal agent that spares the cell but shares metabolic characteristics with the virus.

Limited success has been seen with some herpesvirus-specific drugs. Currently, acyclovir has shown the greatest efficacy in the treatment of mucocutaneous infections. A 5% acyclovir ointment applied five times per day when symptoms first appear reduces slightly the duration of HSL and may abort some lesions. It does not prevent recurrence, however, and may be ineffective in some patients. Oral acyclovir tablets (200 mg, five times per day) are effective in the treatment of primary genital herpes and to a lesser degree in the treatment of recurrent genital disease. Oral acyclovir for the treatment of HSL is probably more effective than the ointment form but at present requires more testing to determine toxicity and long-term effects. The rationale for the use of acyclovir is its ability to interrupt viral replication through inhibition of DNA polymerization. In herpes-infected cells, acyclovir is converted by a virus-induced enzyme, thymidine kinase, and other cellular enzymes to a form that inhibits primarily viral DNA polymerase rather than host cell DNA polymerase. The end result is interruption of viral DNA synthesis and relative sparing of cellular DNA synthesis.

Other virus-specific drugs that have shown some effectiveness in the treatment of herpes infections are vidarabine (ara-A) and idoxuridine. In a 3% ointment, both have been successful in the treatment of ocular herpes infections (herpes keratitis), but neither has shown much ability to alter the course of HSL.

Until new, more effective drugs are developed and tested for mucocutaneous herpetic infections, therapy will necessarily be frustrating and unpredictable. The typically occurring primary herpetic gingivostomatitis is currently best managed with supportive therapy: fluids, rest, oral lavage, and antipyretics. For more severe systemic infections or in the immunosuppressed individual, oral acyclovir may be required.

In conclusion, topical acyclovir, although it is only somewhat effective, is a rational approach to the treatment of problematic cases of secondary oral and perioral herpetic infections. In patients with minor recurrent herpetic lesions, the treatment, at this time, is empirical.

Varicella-Zoster Infections

Etiology and Pathogenesis. Varicella-zoster virus (VZV) is one of the herpesviruses that is pathogenic for humans. The primary infection for the disease in the seronegative individual is known as varicella (chickenpox). The secondary disease or reactivation of latent VZV is known as herpes zoster (shingles). Structurally, VZV is very similar to HSV in that it has a DNA core, a protein capsid, and a lipid envelope. Thus, both have similar light and electron microscopic appearances. There are also some antigenic determinants that are shared by both viruses. Relative to pathogenesis, striking similarities can also be noted. The ability of the virus to remain quiescent in sensory ganglia for indefinite periods following a primary infection is common to both. A cutaneous or mucosal vesiculo-ulcerative eruption following reactivation of latent virus is also typical of VZV and HSV. There are, however, a number of clinical signs and symptoms that appear to be unique to each infection and are discussed next.

Varicella. Transmission of varicella is believed to be predominantly through the inspiration of contaminated droplets. Much less commonly, direct contact is an alternative way of acquiring the disease. During the 2-week incubation period, virus proliferates within macrophages with subsequent viremia and dissemination to skin and other organs. Host defense mechanisms of non-specific interferon production and specific humoral and cell-mediated immune responses are also triggered. Overt clinical disease then appears in most individuals. As the viremia overwhelms body defenses, systemic signs and symptoms develop. Eventually, in the normal host, the immune response is able to limit and halt the replication of virus, allowing recovery in 2 to 3 weeks. During the disease process, the VZV may progress along sensory nerves to the sensory ganglia, where it can reside in a latent, undetectable form.

Herpes Zoster. Reactivation of latent VZV is uncommon but characteristically follows such occurrences as immunosuppressive states from malignancy (especially hematopoietic and lymphoid types) or drug administration, irradiation or surgery on spinal cord, or local trauma. A depressed cellular immune state from whatever cause appears to be a major factor in the development of herpes zoster. Prodromal symptoms of pain or paresthesia develop and persist for several days as the virus infects the sensory nerve of a dermatome (usually of the trunk or head and neck). A vesicular skin eruption that becomes pustular and eventually ulcerated follows. The disease lasts several weeks and may be followed by a troublesome post-herpetic neuralgia (in approximately 10% of patients) that takes several months to resolve. Local cutaneous hyperpigmentation may also be noted on occasion.

Clinical Features

Varicella. A majority of the population experiences a primary infection during childhood. Nearly all adults over age 60 have had VZV infection. Fever, chills, malaise, and headache may accompany a rash that involves primarily the trunk and head and neck. The rash quickly develops into a vesicular eruption that becomes pustular and eventually ulcerates. Successive crops of new lesions appear, owing to repeated waves of viremia. This causes the presence, at any one time, of lesions in all stages of development (Fig. 1–9). The infection is self-limited and lasts several weeks. Oral mucous membranes may be involved in primary disease and usually demonstrate multiple shallow ulcers that are preceded by evanescent vesicles (Fig. 1–10). Because of the intense pruritic nature of the lesions, secondary bacterial infection is not uncommon and may result in healing with scar formation. Complications, including pneumonitis, encephalitis, and inflammation of other organs, may be seen in a very small percentage of cases. If varicella is acquired during pregnancy, fetal abnormalities may occur. When older adults and immunocompromised patients are affected, varicella may be much more severe, protracted, and more likely to produce complications.

Herpes Zoster. Zoster is basically a condition of the older adult population and of individuals who have compromised immune responses. Risk is especially high in those who have lymphoid or hematopoietic malignancies (e.g., Hodgkin's disease, lymphocytic leukemia) and who are also being treated with cytotoxic or immunosuppressive drugs. Other high-risk groups include patients receiving high-dose radiation or steroids, or organ transplants.

The sensory nerves of the trunk and head and neck are commonly affected. Involvement of the various branches of the trigeminal nerve may result in unilateral oral, facial, or ocular lesions (Fig. 1–11). Involvement of facial and

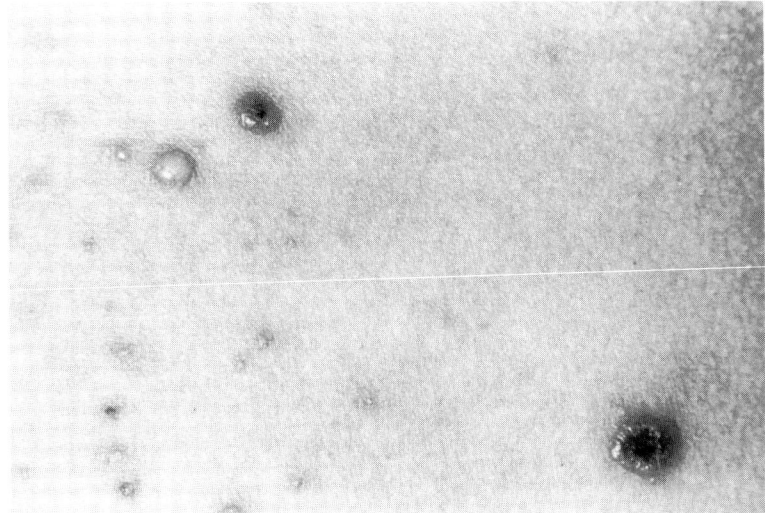

Figure 1–9. Varicella of the trunk showing lesions in all stages of development.

auditory nerves produces the *Ramsay Hunt syndrome,* in which there is facial paralysis accompanied by vesicles of the ipsilateral external ear, tinnitus, deafness, and vertigo.

Following several days of prodromal symptoms of pain or paresthesia in the area of the involved dermatome, a well-delineated unilateral maculopapular rash appears. This may occasionally be accompanied by systemic symptoms as well. The rash quickly becomes vesicular, pustular, and then ulcerative. Remission usually occurs in several weeks. Complications include secondary infection of ulcers, post-herpetic neuralgia (which may be refractory to analgesics), motor paralysis, and ocular inflammation when the ophthalmic division of the trigeminal nerve is involved.

Histopathology. The morphology of the VZV and the inflammatory response to its presence in both varicella and herpes zoster is essentially the same as that seen with HSV. Examination under a light microscope reveals virus-infected epithelial cells showing homogeneous nuclei, representing viral products, with margination of chromatin. Multinucleation of infected cells is also typical. Cytologic smears and histologic specimens both demonstrate these characteristic cellular changes. As infected cells swell, adhesive qualities are lost, resulting in acantholytic vesicles. Inflammatory

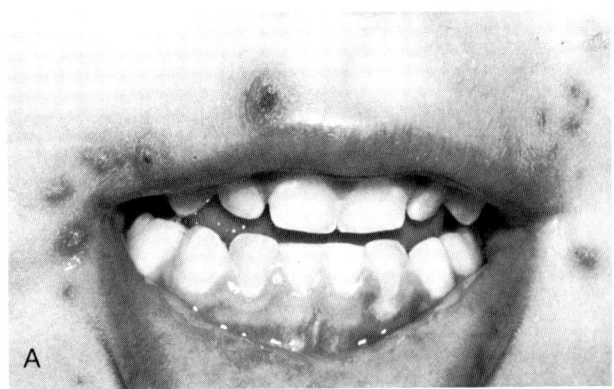
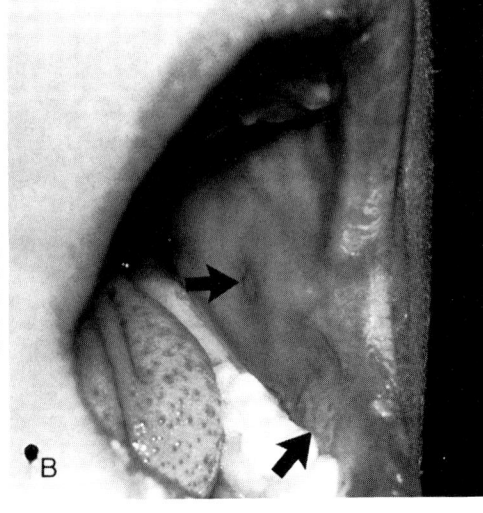

Figure 1–10. *A,* Varicella in a 5-year-old showing perioral and gingival lesions. *B,* Same patient with oral ulcers (arrows).

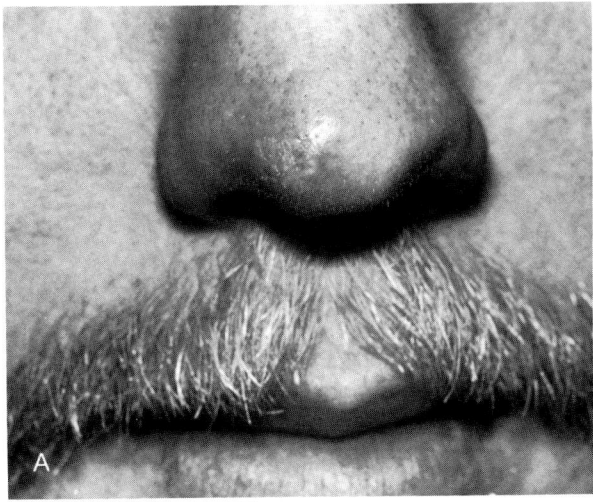
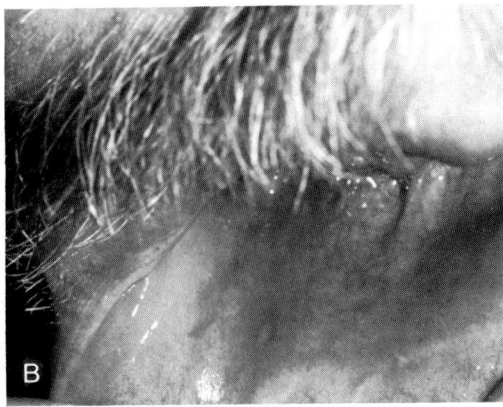

Figure 1-11. Herpes zoster infection in a 24-year-old male. Patient had conjunctivitis, a nose eruption (A), and lip ulcers (B).

cells and exudate add to the vesicle contents, with eventual breakdown and ulceration. In uncomplicated cases, epithelium regenerates from the ulcer margins with little or no scar.

Differential Diagnosis. Varicella is usually clinically diagnosed when history of exposure and type and distribution of lesions are carefully noted. Other primary viral infections that may show some similarities include primary HSV infection and hand, foot, and mouth disease.

Herpes zoster is most commonly confused with recurrent HSV infections and may on clinical grounds be indistinguishable from them. The longer duration, the greater intensity of prodromal symptoms, the unilateral distribution with abrupt ending at the midline, and post-herpetic neuralgia all favor a clinical diagnosis of herpes zoster. Diagnosis of equivocal cases can be definitively made through virus antigen typing using laboratory immunologic tests (e.g., immunoperoxidase or DNA hybridization).

Treatment. For varicella, supportive therapy is generally indicated in normal individuals. However, in the immunocompromised patient, more substantial measures are warranted. Virus-specific drugs that are effective in treating HSV infections have also shown efficacy in the treatment of VZV infections. These include systemically administered acyclovir, vidarabine, and human leukocyte interferon. Corticosteroids are generally contraindicated.

Herpes zoster in patients with intact immune responses is generally treated empirically. Analgesics may be helpful. Topically applied virus-specific drugs may have some benefit if used early. The use of topical or systemic corticosteroids cannot, as yet, be recommended. In patients with compromised immune responses, systemically administered acyclovir, vidarabine, or interferon is indicated although success is variable.

Hand, Foot, and Mouth Disease

Etiology and Pathogenesis. One of the subdivisions of another family of viruses known as picornavirus (literally, small [pico] RNA [rna] virus) is a group known as Coxsackie virus (also known as Coxsackievirus), named after the New York town where the virus was first identified. Certain subtypes of the Coxsackie group of picornaviruses are known to cause oral vesicular eruptions, two of which are hand, foot, and mouth disease (HFM) and herpangina.

HFM is a highly contagious viral infection that is usually caused by Coxsackie type A16, although serologic types A5, A9, A10, B2, B5, and enterovirus 71 (another group of picornaviruses) have been isolated on occasion. The mode of transfer of virus from one individual to another is through either airborne spread or oral-fecal contamination. With subsequent viremia, the virus exhibits a predilection for mucous membranes of the mouth and cutaneous regions of the hands and feet.

Clinical Features. This viral infection typically occurs in epidemic or endemic proportions and affects predominantly children under the age of 5 years. Following a short incubation period, the condition resolves spontaneously in 1 to 2 weeks.

Signs and symptoms are usually mild to

12 VESICULO-BULLOUS DISEASES

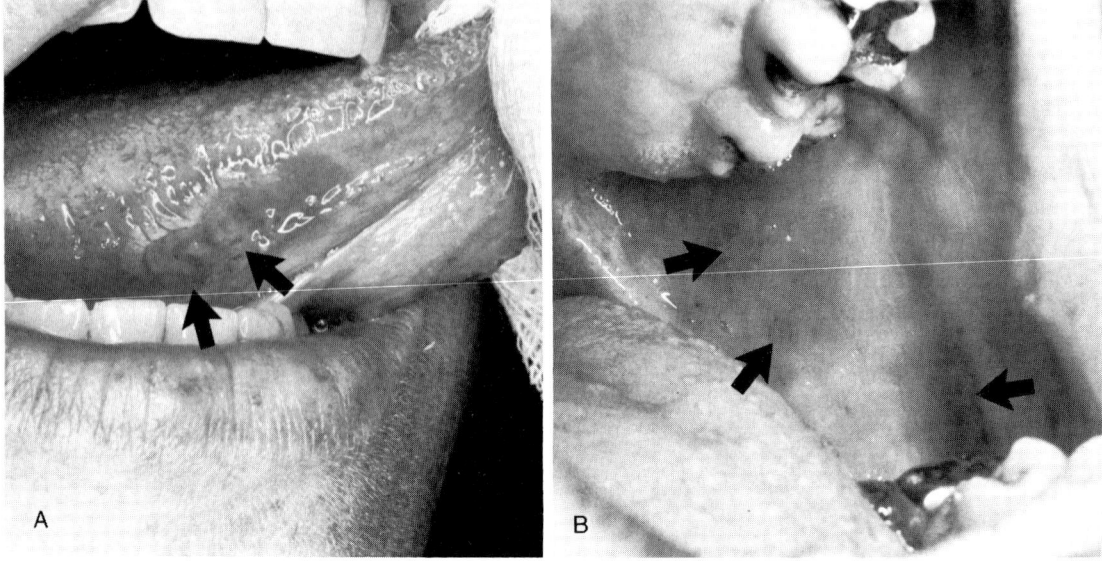

Figure 1–12. *A* and *B*, Hand, foot, and mouth disease—oral ulcers in adult female. (Courtesy of Dr. S. K. Young.)

moderate in intensity and include low-grade fever, malaise, lymphadenopathy, and sore mouth. Pain from oral lesions is often the patient's chief complaint. The oral lesions begin as vesicles that quickly rupture to become ulcers that are covered by a yellow fibrinous membrane surrounded by an erythematous halo (Fig. 1–12). The lesions, which are multiple, can occur anywhere in the mouth, although the palate, tongue, and buccal mucosa are favored sites. Multiple maculopapular lesions, typically on the feet, toes, hands, and fingers, appear concomitant with or shortly after the oral lesions (Fig. 1–13). These lesions progress to a vesicular state and eventually become ulcerated and encrusted.

Histopathology. The vesicles of this condition are found within the epithelium because of obligate viral replication in keratinocytes. Eosinophilic inclusions may be seen within some of the infected epithelial cells. As the keratinocytes are destroyed by virus, the vesicular cavity becomes filled with proteinaceous debris and inflammatory cells.

Differential Diagnosis. Because this disease may express itself primarily within the oral cavity, a differential diagnosis should include primary herpes gingivostomatitis, and possibly

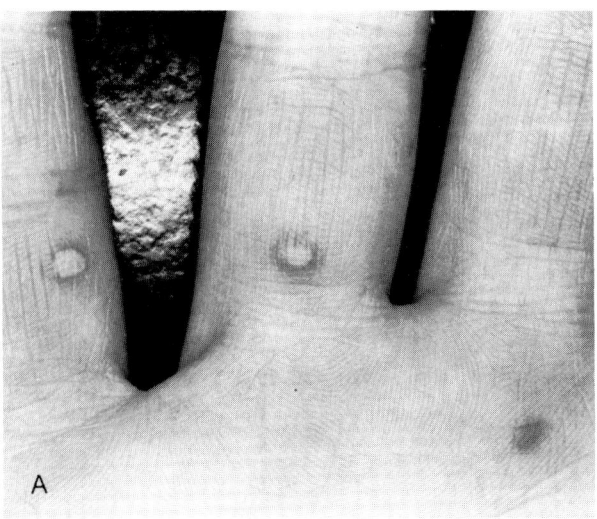
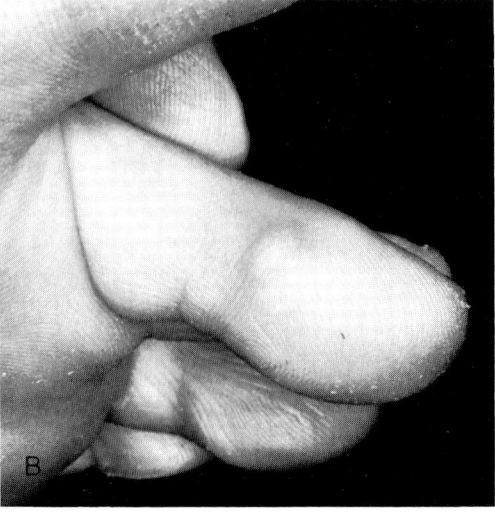

Figure 1–13. *A* and *B*, Hand, foot, and mouth disease—cutaneous expression. (Courtesy of Dr. S. K. Young.)

varicella. The relatively mild symptoms, cutaneous distribution, and epidemic spread should help separate this condition from the others. Virus culture or detection of circulating antibodies may be done to confirm clinical impression.

Treatment. Because of the relatively short duration, the self-limiting nature, and the general lack of virus-specific therapy, treatment for HFM is usually symptomatic. Non-specific mouthwashes may be used to help alleviate oral discomfort.

Herpangina

Etiology and Pathogenesis. This acute viral infection is caused by another Coxsackie type A virus (types A2–6, A8, A10, and possibly others). It is transmitted by contaminated saliva and occasionally through contaminated feces.

Clinical Features. Herpangina is usually endemic, with outbreaks occurring typically in summer or early fall. It occurs more often in children than in adults. They generally complain of malaise, fever, dysphagia, and sore throat following a short incubation period. Intraorally, a vesicular eruption appears on the soft palate, faucial pillars, and tonsils (Fig. 1–14). A diffuse erythematous pharyngitis is also present.

The signs and symptoms are usually mild to moderate and generally last less than a week. On occasion, the Coxsackie virus responsible for typical herpangina may be responsible for subclinical infections or for mild symptoms without evidence of pharyngeal lesions.

Differential Diagnosis. Diagnosis is usually based on historical and clinical information. The characteristic distribution and short duration of herpangina separate it from other primary viral infections such as herpetic gingivostomatitis, HFM, and varicella. The vesicular eruption, mild symptoms, summer presentation, and diffuse pharyngitis also distinguish the condition from streptococcal pharyngitis, and the systemic symptoms distinguish it from aphthous stomatitis. Laboratory confirmation can be made by virus isolation or detection of serum antibodies.

Treatment. Because herpangina is self-limited, is mild and of short duration, and causes few complications, treatment is usually not required.

Measles (Rubeola)

Etiology and Pathogenesis. Measles is a highly contagious viral infection caused by a member of the paramyxovirus family of viruses. The virus, known simply as measles virus, is a DNA virus and is related structurally and biologically to viruses of the orthomyxovirus family, which cause mumps and influenza. The virus is spread by airborne droplets through the respiratory tract.

German measles, or rubella, is a contagious disease that is caused by an unrelated virus of the togavirus family. It shares some clinical features with measles, such as fever, respiratory symptoms, and rash. These features are, however, very mild and short-lived in German measles. Also, Koplik's spots, which are characteristic of measles, do not appear in German

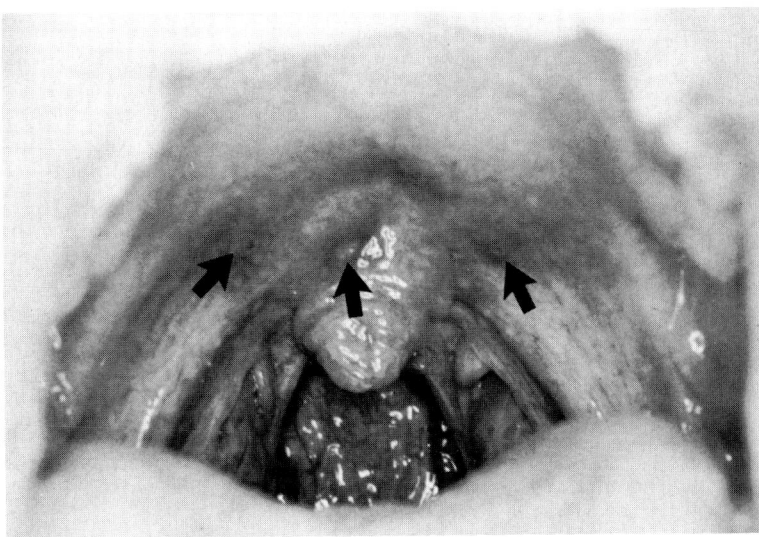

Figure 1–14. Herpangina—multiple oral ulcers with erythematous bases are apparent in the soft palate.

measles. The significance of the German measles virus lies in its ability to cause congenital defects in the developing fetus. The abnormalities produced are varied and may be severe, especially if the intrauterine infection occurs during the first trimester of pregnancy.

Clinical Features. Measles is predominantly a disease of children, often appearing seasonally in winter and spring. Following an incubation period of 7 to 10 days, prodromal symptoms of fever, malaise, coryza, conjunctivitis, photophobia, and cough develop. In 1 to 2 days, pathognomonic, small, erythematous macules with white necrotic centers appear in the buccal mucosa. These herald spots, known as Koplik's spots after the pediatrician who first described them, usher in the characteristic maculopapular skin rash of measles. Koplik's spots generally precede the skin rash by 1 to 2 days. The rash initially affects the head and neck followed by the trunk and then the extremities. Complications associated with the measles virus include encephalitis and thrombocytopenic purpura. Secondary infection may develop as otitis media or pneumonia.

Histopathology. Infected epithelial cells, which eventually become necrotic, overlie an inflamed dermis that contains dilated vascular channels and a focal inflammatory response. Lymphocytes are found in a perivascular distribution. In lymphoid tissues, large characteristic multinucleated macrophages, known as Warthin-Finkeldey giant cells, are seen.

Differential Diagnosis. Diagnosis of measles is usually made on the basis of clinical signs and symptoms. Prodromal symptoms, Koplik's spots, and rash should provide sufficient evidence of measles. If necessary, laboratory confirmation can be made through virus culture or serologic tests for antibodies to measles virus.

Treatment. There is no specific treatment for measles. Supportive therapy of bed rest, fluids, adequate diet, and analgesics generally suffices.

CONDITIONS ASSOCIATED WITH IMMUNOLOGIC DEFECTS

Pemphigus Vulgaris

Etiology and Pathogenesis. Pemphigus is a general term for a group of mucocutaneous diseases characterized by intraepithelial blister formation. This results from a breakdown or loss of intercellular adhesion, thus producing epithelial cell separation known as acantholysis. Pemphigus vulgaris represents the most frequently encountered subset within the pemphigus group of diseases; there are three other recognized forms: pemphigus vegetans (a variant of pemphigus vulgaris), pemphigus foliaceus, and pemphigus erythematosus.

All forms of the disease retain distinctive presentations both clinically and microscopically but share a common autoimmune etiology. Evident are circulating autoantibodies of the IgG type that are reactive against components of epithelial desmosome-tonofilament complexes. The circulating autoantibodies are responsible for the earliest morphologic event: the dissolution or disruption of intercellular junctions and loss of cell-to-cell adhesion. The extent of epithelial cell separation is, generally, directly proportional to the titer of circulating pemphigus antibody. It is believed that the pemphigus antibody, once bound to the target antigen, activates an epithelial intracellular proteolytic enzyme or group of enzymes that act at the desmosome-tonofilament complex.

A less clearly defined concept in etiology is the role of complement. The C3 component of activated complement as well as classical pathway components C1q and C4 has been detected in the intercellular areas. Less frequently, factors of the alternative pathway of complement (properdin and factor B) have been noted. While the exact role of complement in the pathogenesis of pemphigus remains unclear, many believe that it may play an enhancing rather than a primary role in the acantholytic process.

Clinical Features. Patients with pemphigus vulgaris present with the first signs of the disease in the oral mucosa in approximately 60% of cases. Such lesions may precede the onset of cutaneous lesions by periods of up to 1 year. Presentation of the lesions may initially be as fluid-filled bullae (or vesicles) or as shallow ulcers (Fig. 1–15). Bullae rapidly rupture, leaving a collapsed roof. This grayish membrane is easily removed with a gauze sponge, leaving a red, painful ulcerated base. Ulcers range in appearance from small aphthous-like lesions (Fig. 1–16) to large map-like lesions (Fig. 1–17). Gentle traction on clinically unaffected mucosa may produce a stripping of epithelium, the Nikolsky sign. Often a great deal of discomfort occurs with confluence and ulceration of smaller vesicles of the soft palate, buccal mucosa, and floor of the mouth.

The incidence of pemphigus vulgaris is equal in both sexes. There appear to be genetic and

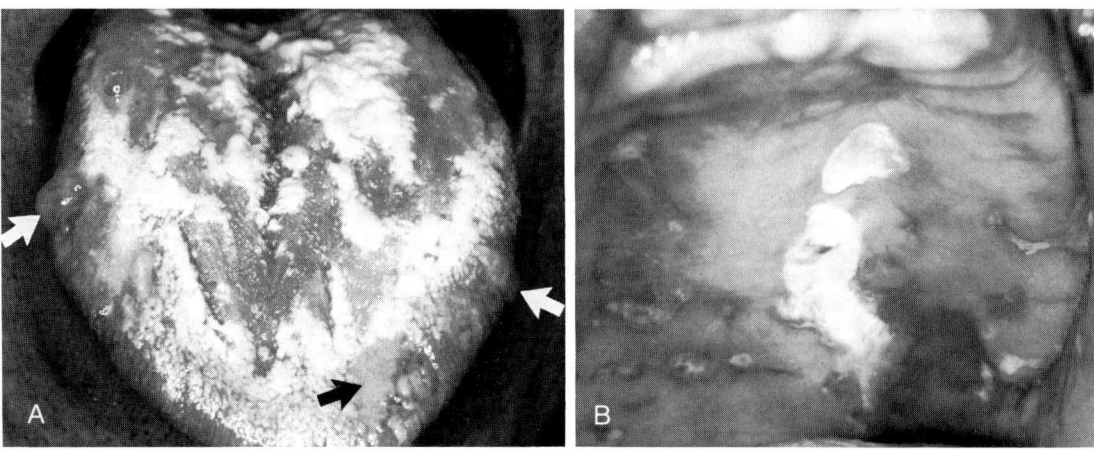

Figure 1–15. *A,* Pemphigus vulgaris of the tongue. Note ulcer (black arrow) and bullae (white arrows). *B,* Pemphigus vulgaris of the palate. Note multiple fibrin-covered ulcers.

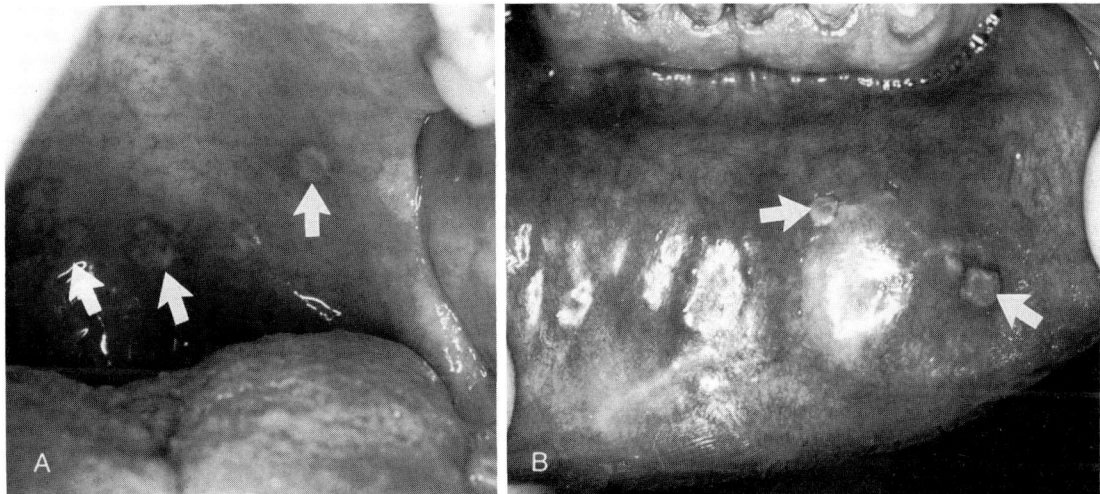

Figure 1–16. *A* and *B,* Pemphigus vulgaris in a 45-year-old man. Multiple aphthous type ulcers are apparent (arrows).

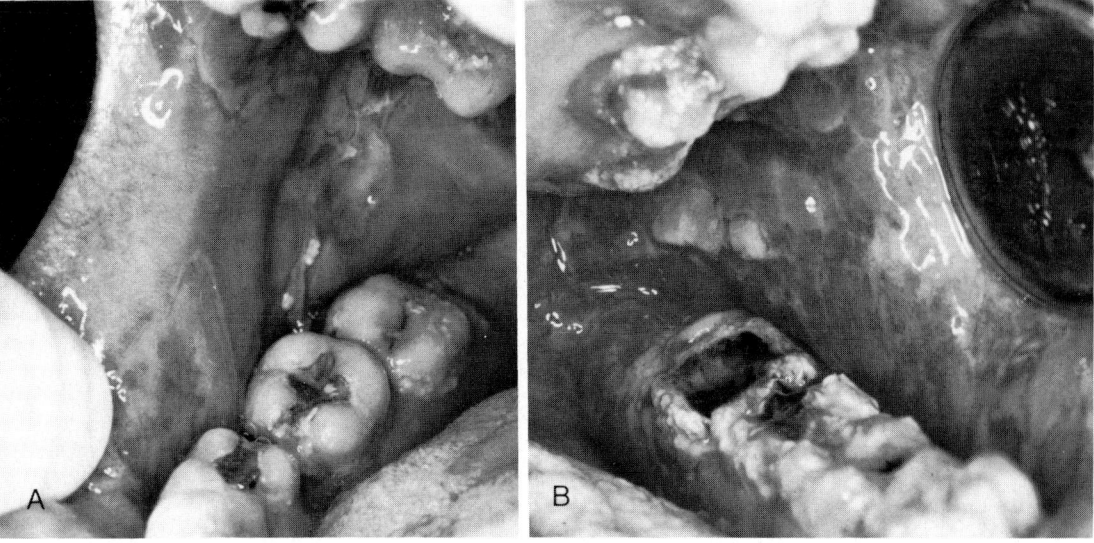

Figure 1–17. *A* and *B,* Pemphigus vulgaris in a 47-year-old male showing widespread ulceration of buccal mucosa.

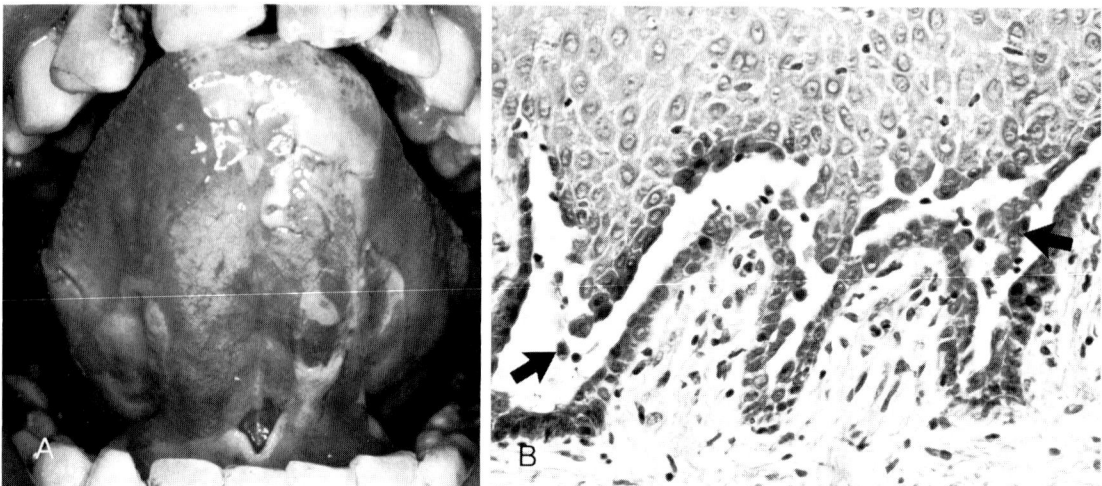

Figure 1–18. *A*, Pemphigus vulgaris of the ventral surface of the tongue. *B*, Biopsy showing intraepithelial separation with free-floating epithelial (Tzanck) cells (arrows).

ethnic factors that predispose to the development of the disease. Pemphigus vulgaris, while generally rare, may be relatively common in some racial and ethnic groups. An increased incidence has been noted in Ashkenazic Jews and in individuals with certain histocompatibility antigen phenotypes (HLA-DRw4, HLA-A10, HLA-Bw3).

Other autoimmune diseases may occur in association with pemphigus vulgaris, such as myasthenia gravis, lupus erythematosus, rheumatoid arthritis, Hashimoto's thyroiditis, thymoma, and Sjögren's syndrome. A wide range has been noted from childhood to the elderly age groups, although most cases are noted within the fourth and fifth decades of life.

Histopathology and Immunopathology. Pemphigus vulgaris represents the prototypical suprabasalar or intraepithelial clefting morphology that generally characterizes all forms of pemphigus. Pathognomonic of pemphigus vulgaris is the acantholytic lesion that features squamous epithelial cells lying free within the bulla of vesicle cavity (Fig. 1–18). Loss of desmosomal attachments and retraction of tonofilaments results in assumption of a more spherical form by the acantholytic epithelial cells (Fig. 1–19). These cells, also known as Tzanck cells, are further characterized by nuclear enlargement and hyperchromasia. Subsequent to formation of the suprabasal cleft, the intact basal layer remains attached to the

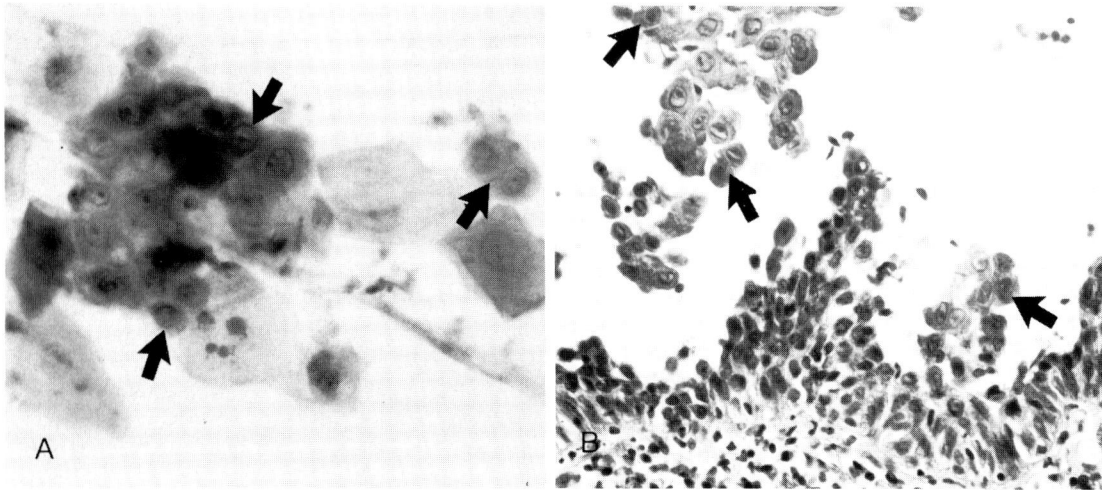

Figure 1–19. *A*, Cytologic smear from pemphigus vulgaris lesion. Note rounded epithelial cells characteristic of this condition (arrows). *B*, Tissue biopsy showing intact basal layer and acantholytic keratinocytes (Tzanck cells) (arrows).

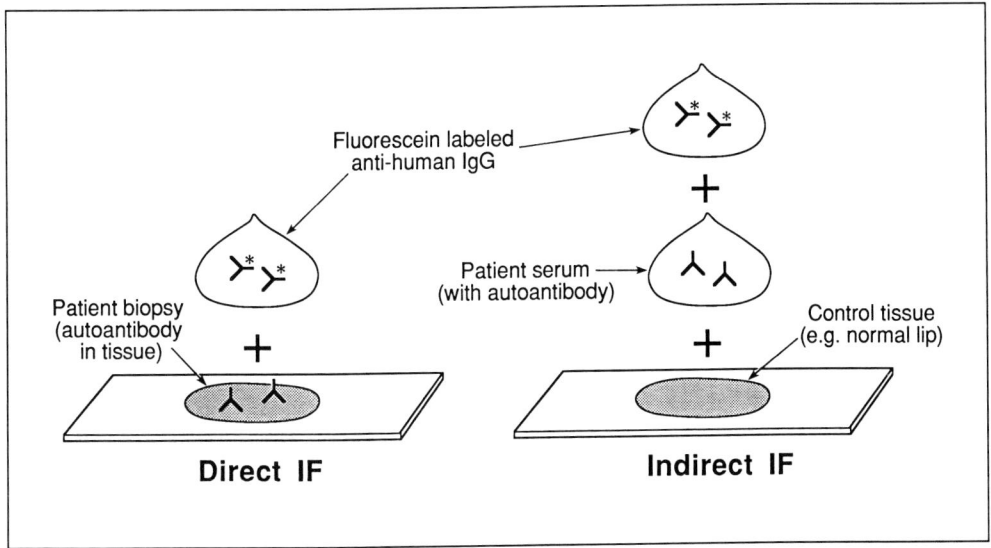

Figure 1–20. Immunofluorescence techniques for demonstrating autoantibodies in either the patient's tissue (direct) or the patient's serum (indirect).

lamina propria, producing a pattern that has been likened to a row of tombstones. In addition to fluid and Tzanck cells, the bulla or vesicle contains variable numbers of neurotophils and occasional eosinophils. When an intact lesion is evident clinically, a cytologic smear, prepared by unroofing the vesicle and gently scraping the base of the lesion, will enable rapid microscopic identification of the acantholytic cells. Initial diagnosis made from a cytologic smear must be confirmed by more definitive procedures.

In addition to a standard biopsy, confirmation of the diagnosis of pemphigus vulgaris can be made with the use of either direct or indirect immunofluorescence testing (Fig. 1–20). Direct immunofluorescence utilizes a patient biopsy in an attempt to demonstrate autoantibody already fixed to the tissue. In pemphigus vulgaris, direct immunofluorescence testing of perilesional tissue will almost always demonstrate intercellular antibodies of the IgG type (Fig. 1–21). The greatest intensity of fluorescence is usually within the parabasal region, with a gradual diminution of fluorescence as the surface is approached. In addition to IgG

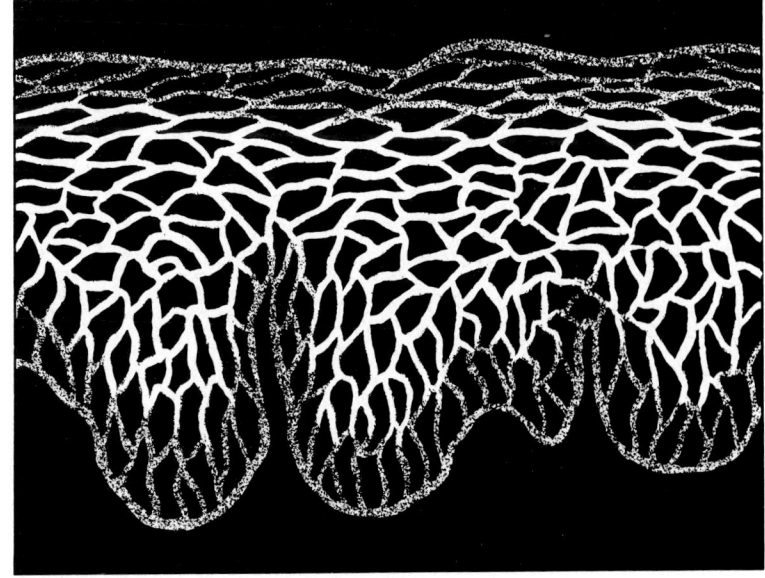

Figure 1–21. Immunofluorescence pattern seen in the epithelium of pemphigus vulgaris. Note that the fluorescence is in the intercellular desmosomal areas, predominantly in the prickle cell zone.

antibodies, C3 and, less commonly, IgA can be detected in the same intercellular fluorescent pattern.

The indirect immunofluorescence technique utilizes the patient's serum reacted with normal control tissue in an effort to demonstrate the presence (and the concentration) of circulating antibody. Such circulating antibodies may be noted in approximately 80% of pemphigus vulgaris patients. This indirect technique allows confirmation of the direct technique and also permits assessment of disease severity, which has been related to titer (or concentration) of circulating antibody. Indirect immunofluorescence titers can then be practically utilized to adjust medication schedules and dosages.

Differential Diagnosis. Clinically the lesions of pemphigus vulgaris must be distinguished from other vesiculo-bullous disease processes such as bullous and cicatricial pemphigoid, erythema multiforme, bullous lichen planus, and dermatitis herpetiformis. When lesions are small, aphthous stomatitis may also be a consideration. Because there is some clinical overlap among these entities, characteristic histologic and immunofluorescence findings must be observed in order to make a definitive diagnosis.

A diagnosis of *pemphigus vegetans,* a variant or closely related form of pemphigus vulgaris, may also be entertained in some situations. Although originally regarded as an infectious disease, subsequent reclassification based upon the presence of acantholysis placed it within the pemphigus group of disorders. It is predominantly a skin disease, but vermilion and intraoral mucosa are frequently involved, often initially (Fig. 1–22). Of importance in distinguishing this rare variant of pemphigus vulgaris from its more common relative is its microscopic appearance. Early acantholytic bullae are followed by epithelial hyperplasia and intraepithelial abscess formation. These pustular "vegetations" contain abundant eosinophils. In general, this form of pemphigus tends to resemble a verrucous or hypertrophic excrescence rather than the blistering of acute pemphigus vulgaris. The course of this disease may parallel the course of pemphigus vulgaris. Pemphigus vegetans–type lesions may also be seen during a lull in the general course of pemphigus vulgaris. Spontaneous remissions may occur in pemphigus vegetans, with complete recovery noted—a phenomenon not characteristic of pemphigus vulgaris.

Treatment and Prognosis. The high morbidity and mortality rate previously associated with pemphigus vulgaris has been radically changed since the introduction of systemic corticosteroids. The reduction in mortality, however, does carry a degree of iatrogenic morbidity associated with chronic corticosteroid use. Indeed the 8 to 10% mortality per 5 years is generally secondary to long-term steroid therapy.

Whether the disease is in an early or stable phase or has progressed to generalized involvement determines the use of one of two treatment alternatives. The former utilizes an intermediate dose of steroid (prednisone), and the latter utilizes an initially high dose of steroid followed by a combined drug approach that includes alternate-day prednisone plus an

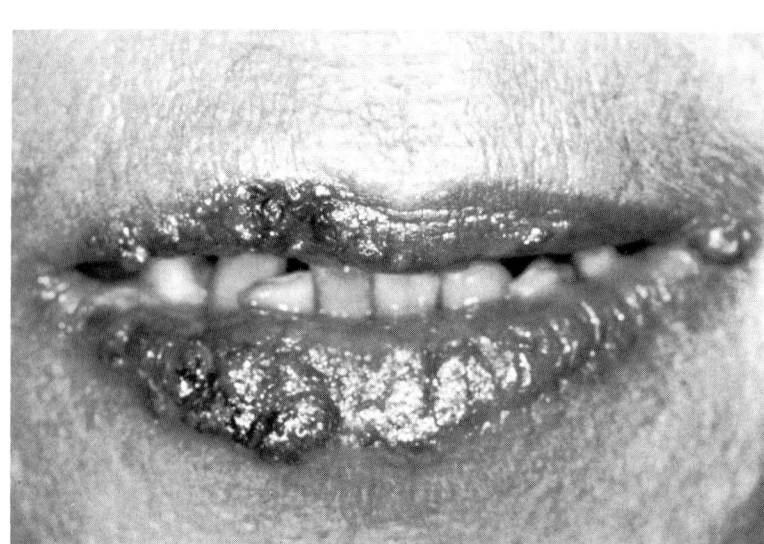

Figure 1–22. Pemphigus vegetans of the lips.

immunosuppressant agent such as azathioprine, methotrexate, or cyclophosphamide. The latter regimen helps reduce both the suppressive effects of steroid on the pituitary-adrenal axis and other complications of high-dose steroid therapy such as immunosuppression, osteoporosis, hyperglycemia, and hypertension. Gold therapy has also been used in the management of patients with pemphigus vulgaris, especially those with steroid-related complications. More recently, the use of plasmapheresis has been suggested as a steroid-sparing alternative.

Overall, a guarded prognosis continues to exist for pemphigus vulgaris patients because of the drugs used and their potential side effects. The major clinical problem, once the disease has been brought under control, is the lifelong treatment commitment required and the potential long-term drug effects.

Cicatricial Pemphigoid

Etiology and Pathogenesis. Cicatricial pemphigoid represents a chronic blistering or vesiculo-bullous disease known by a host of synonymous terms, including benign mucous membrane pemphigoid, ocular pemphigus, and mucosal pemphigoid. When the disorder affects gingiva exclusively, the terms "gingivosis" and "desquamative gingivitis" have been used, although such terms are generally unacceptable because of lack of specificity.

As with its more uncommon relative pemphigus vulgaris, cicatricial pemphigoid is idiopathic and is also considered an autoimmune process (Table 1–3). Autoimmunity is further supported by the almost universal finding of deposits of immunoglobulins and complement components along the basement zone on direct immunofluorescence testing. The role of complement activation in the pathogenesis of this condition is not understood. Unlike its cutaneous counterpart bullous pemphigoid, there are usually no detectable circulating antibodies against basement membrane zone antigens in cicatricial pemphigoid.

The cellular events in lesion production in this disease are less well known in comparison with those in pemphigus vulgaris. More specifically, these events or pathways are more presumed than definitive, since the closely related condition of bullous pemphigoid has served as the source of material in determining actual or likely pathogenetic mechanisms. Such mechanisms will be discussed in a subsequent section dealing with bullous pemphigoid.

Clinical Features. This is a disease of adults and the elderly and tends to affect women more than men. Oral mucosal presentation of cicatricial pemphigoid is quite variable, from incipient erosion or desquamation of attached gingival tissues to large areas of vesiculo-bullous eruptions involving alveolar mucosa, palate, buccal mucosa, tongue, and floor of the mouth (Fig. 1–23). Lesions are chronic and may heal with scarring (cicatrix). Extraoral sites in the order of frequency following oral mucosa are the conjunctiva, larynx, genitalia, esophagus, and skin. Cutaneous lesions are uncommon and usually appear in the head and neck and extremities. Skin lesions follow the appearance of mucosal lesions.

Gingival lesions are the most common form of oral presentation, with manifestations ranging from patchy erythema with mild discomfort to intense generalized erythema and ulceration extending to and beyond the attached alveolar mucosal junction (Fig. 1–24). Severity of surface desquamation generally parallels the level of pain. With chronicity, pain typically diminishes in intensity. Surface areas can often be stripped away with ease, leaving a raw, denuded, bleeding substratum. Often, gentle massage or a shearing force on uninvolved tissue will produce a vesicle or desquamation analogous to that in acantholytic disease (Nikolsky's sign) (Fig. 1–25). Symptoms often preclude performance of routine oral hygiene,

Table 1–3. GENERAL FEATURES OF PEMPHIGUS AND PEMPHIGOID		
Feature	**Pemphigus**	**Pemphigoid**
Detectable circulating Ab	Yes, IgG	No
Tissue-bound autoantibody	Yes, IgG (also complement)	Yes, IgG (also IgA, complement)
Target tissue	Desmosomes	Basement membrane
Vesicles	Intraepithelial	Subepithelial
Sites affected	Oral mucosa, skin	Oral mucosa (esp. gingiva), eye, genitals
Nikolsky's sign	Yes	Yes
Treatment	Systemic steroids	Systemic or topical steroids
Prognosis	Fair to good	Good to excellent

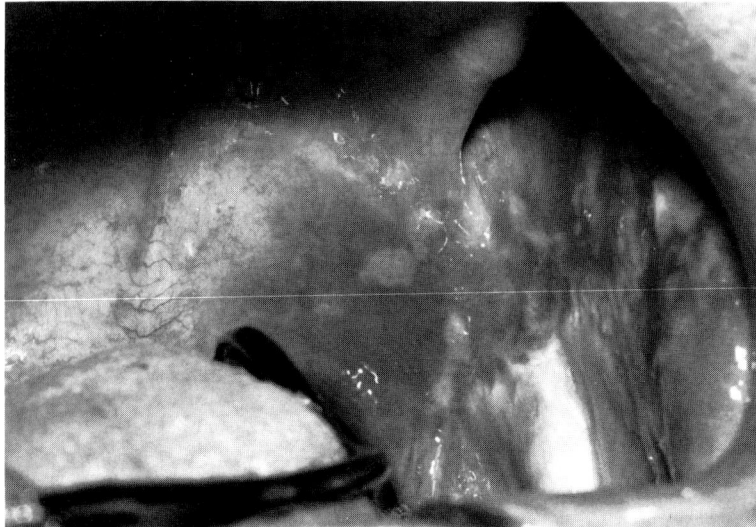

Figure 1–23. Cicatricial pemphigoid showing ulcers and erythema of the soft palate and buccal mucosa.

resulting in considerable plaque accumulation, which in turn further aggravates the gingival tissues. Dietary alterations likewise are often seen, with a shift to soft foods not requiring mastication in an effort to avoid gingival trauma.

Histopathology and Immunopathology. Cicatricial pemphigoid is a subepithelial or subbasal clefting disorder with a clear-cut separation at the basement membrane noted on routine histologic preparations (Fig. 1–26). There is no evidence of acantholysis and no evidence of epithelial degenerative change. The lamina propria is variably infiltrated with lymphocytes and occasional eosinophils and neutrophils. Often a rich adjunct of plasma cells accompanies the lymphocytic infiltrate. Vascular channels often are dilated and prominent in the superficial portion of the lamina propria. Deeper within the submucosa a limited inflammatory cell infiltrate may be seen.

Direct immunofluorescence studies of intact oral mucosa will demonstrate a linear pattern of homogeneous IgG fluorescence (Fig. 1–27). Occasionally IgA may also be detected. Among the complement components commonly found in the same distribution are C3 and occasionally C4 and C1q. Properdin, part of the alternative pathway of complement, is occasionally detected, indicating activation of this system. The frequency of a positive linear continuous pattern in oral disease is over 80%. The pattern is not distinguishable, however, from that seen in bullous pemphigoid or herpes

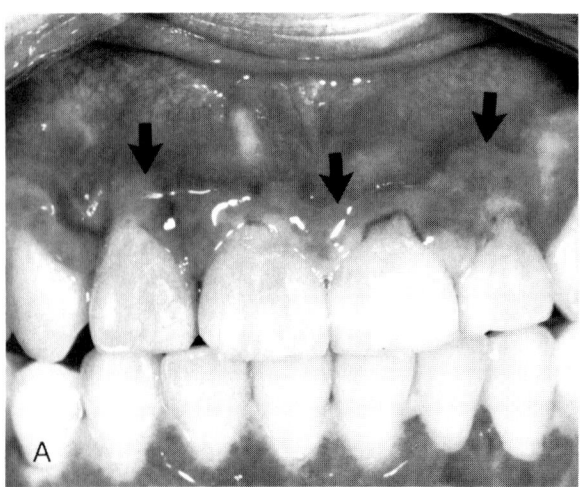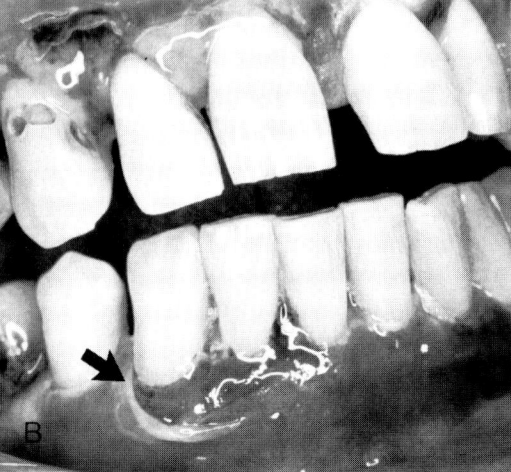

Figure 1–24. *A*, Cicatricial pemphigoid of gingiva showing ulceration of attached gingiva (arrows). *B*, Another pemphigoid patient with maxillary gingival ulcers and traumatic denudation of mandibular gingiva (arrow).

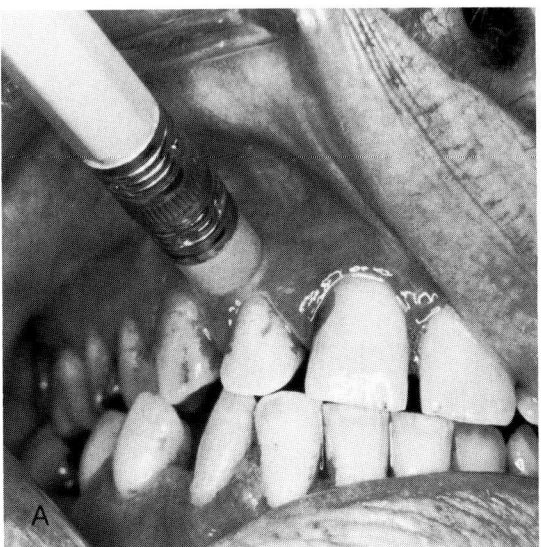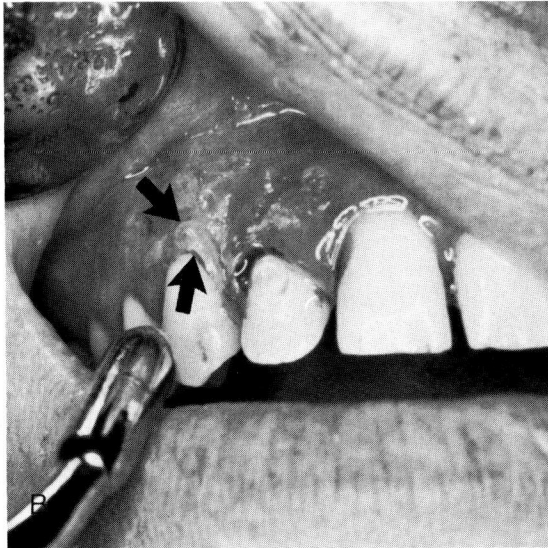

Figure 1–25. *A* and *B*, Pemphigoid patient with induced bulla (Nikolsky's sign) (arrows) produced by gentle twisting of pencil eraser on gingiva.

gestationis. Although indirect immunofluorescence studies are usually negative, IgG and, less commonly, IgA have been occasionally demonstrated in the serum of patients with cicatricial pemphigoid.

Differential Diagnosis. The differential diagnosis of this form of vesiculo-bullous disease must include erosive lichen planus and pemphigus vulgaris. When the attached gingiva is the exclusive site of involvement, discoid lupus erythematosus and contact allergy might also be considered. Separation of diagnoses may be accomplished with histologic or immunologic techniques since each group of lesions demonstrates different histologic or immunopathologic features.

Treatment and Prognosis. Prednisone is frequently used to treat cicatricial pemphigoid, often with disappointing results, however. Response is variable, often requiring high doses to achieve significant results. Since drug side effects may outweigh benefits, especially when lesions are only intraoral, high-potency topical steroids are often used (e.g., betamethasone dipropionate, fluocinonide, desoximetasone). Occlusion of topical corticosteroids often enhances the local response. An occlusive dressing for gingival disease can be adapted from a

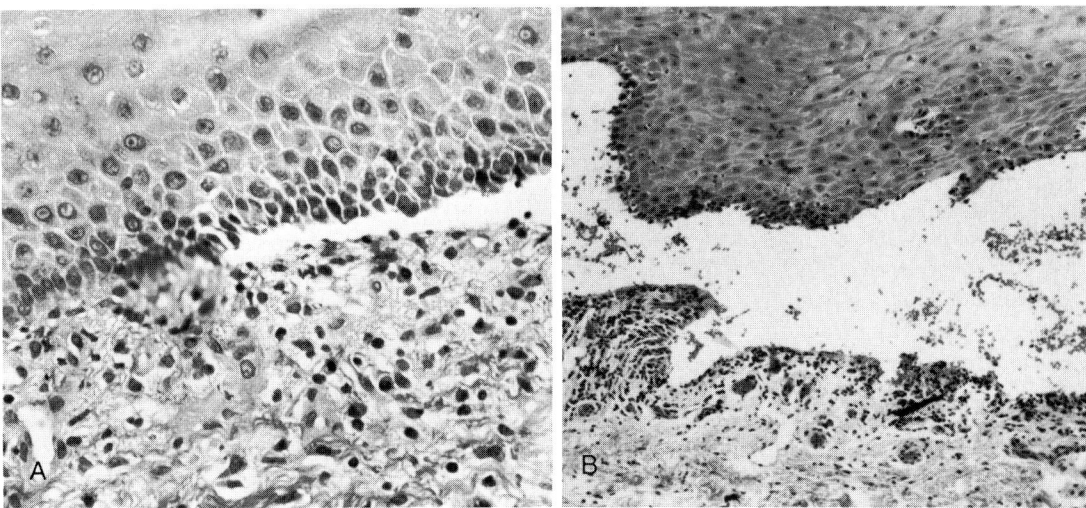

Figure 1–26. *A* and *B*, Cicatricial pemphigoid biopsies showing early *(A)* and later *(B)* separation at the level of the basement membrane.

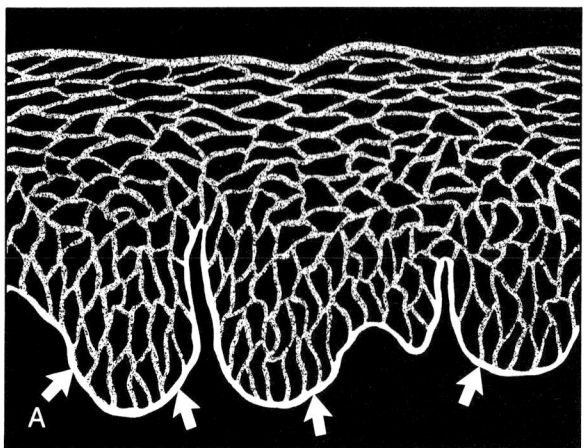 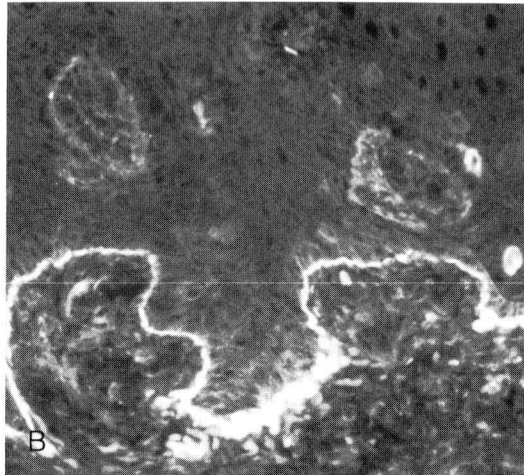

Figure 1-27. *A*, Immunofluorescence pattern of cicatricial pemphigoid. Staining appears along basement membrane (arrows). *B*, Photomicrograph of actual fluorescence stain.

custom-made, flexible mouth guard. Scrupulous oral hygiene further enhances the effectiveness of topical corticosteroids when there is significant gingival involvement.

In cases in which standard therapy has failed, other systemic agents have been utilized with varying success rates. These have included the use of sulfapyridine, sulfones, antibiotics, and nutritional supplementation. Occasionally, in severe cases, the use of immunosuppressive agents (azothioprine, cyclophosphamide) in conjunction with steroids may be justified. This is done to allow reduced steroid dosages and to help avoid steroid complications.

Although cicatricial pemphigoid is benign in terms of not producing mortality, significant debilitation and morbidity can occur. Long-term prognosis is as variable as the short-term response to therapy for this condition. In some cases, a slow but spontaneous improvement may be noted, with complete resolution over a few years. In other cases, however, the course is an extensive one, with some patients exhibiting alternating periods of improvement and exacerbation. Of importance is the occurrence of oral cicatricial pemphigoid with ocular or conjunctival disease. At this latter site, definitive early treatment is critical since corneal damage, conjunctival scarring, and eyelid changes can occur relatively rapidly (Fig. 1-28).

Bullous Pemphigoid

Etiology and Pathogenesis. Bullous pemphigoid and its closely related mucosal counterpart cicatricial pemphigoid (benign mucous membrane pemphigoid) appear to share similar etiologic and pathogenetic factors (Table 1-4). Mechanisms of tissue injury in bullous pemphigoid and, by inference, in cicatricial pemphigoid are evolving. Unlike most cases of cicatricial pemphigoid, there are usually detectable titers of circulating autoantibodies to basement membrane zone antigens in bullous pemphigoid. Such autoantibody titers do not, however, correlate well with the level of disease activity.

Autoantibodies have been demonstrated against distinct components found within the basement membrane zone: namely, laminin, a glycoprotein with a high molecular weight, and so-called bullous pemphigoid antigen, which is found in hemidesmosomes and in the lamina lucida of basement membrane. Subsequent to binding of circulating autoantibodies to tissue antigens, a series of events occur, one of which is complement activation. This attracts neutrophils and eosinophils to the basement membrane zone. These cells then release lysosomal proteases, which in turn participate in degradation of the basement membrane attachment complex. The final event is tissue separation at the epithelial–connective tissue interface. Detailed immunoelectron microscopic studies have demonstrated that the lamina lucida of the basal lamina complex is the actual cleavage plane.

Clinical Features. This bullous disease is found primarily in the elderly, with the peak incidence in the seventh and eighth decades. There is an equal gender distribution, and ethnic predilections are not seen in this condition. A key difference in clinical presentation of this disease compared with cicatricial pem-

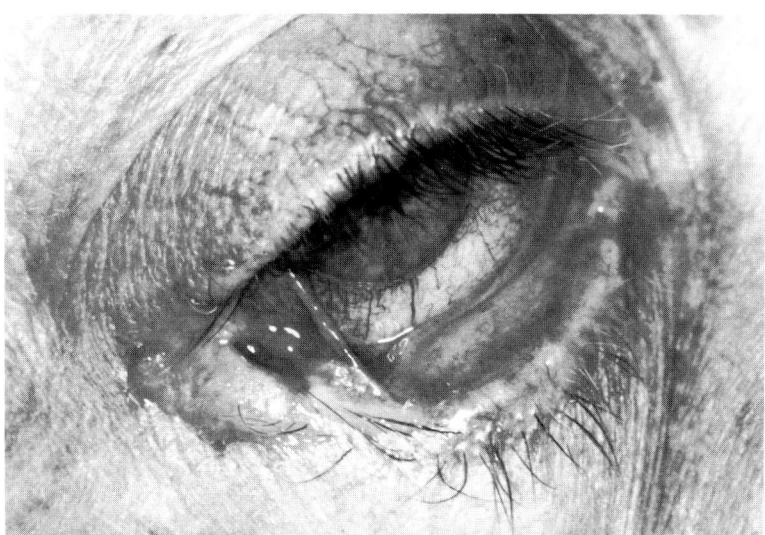

Figure 1-28. Symblepharon, a complication of cicatricial pemphigoid in which there is adhesion between contiguous conjunctival surfaces.

phigoid is the concomitant vesiculo-bullous lesions of skin and oral mucosa (and other mucosal sites) in approximately one third of affected patients. Otherwise, only the skin is affected.

Skin lesions are characterized anatomically by a trunk and limb distribution (Fig. 1-29). While tense vesicles and bullae are typically noted, they are often preceded by or associated with an erythematous papular eruption. Pruritus may be associated with the skin lesions.

Oral mucosal lesions in this form of pemphigoid cannot be distinguished from those of cicatricial pemphigoid. Tense bullae and erosions may be noted, especially on the attached gingiva, a commonly affected site. Other areas of involvement may include the soft palate, buccal mucosa, and floor of the mouth.

Histopathology and Immunopathology. Bullae are subepithelial in bullous pemphigoid and appear similar to those in cicatricial pemphigoid under the light microscope. Ultrastruc-

Table 1-4. COMPARISON AND CONTRAST OF CICATRICIAL AND BULLOUS PEMPHIGOID

Parameter	Cicatricial Pemphigoid	Bullous Pemphigoid
Cause	Autoimmune	Autoimmune
Age	50–80 years	50–80 years
Gender	Females affected more than males	Females & males equally affected
Oral lesions	Oral cavity most common site Gingiva most common intraorally Eye lesions may lead to blindness Ulcers preceded by bullae Ulcers heal with scar	Oral mucosa infrequently affected Oral lesions do not appear before skin lesions Ulcers preceded by bullae Lesions heal without scar
Skin lesions	Uncommon; head, neck, extremities Ulcers preceded by bullae	Trunk & extremities most common sites Ulcers preceded by bullae; rash
Light microscopy	Subepithelial bullae	Subepithelial bullae
Ultrastructure	Separation below basal cells	Separation below basal cells
Immunology	Linear deposits of IgG & C3 No circulating antibody detectable	Linear deposits of IgG & C3 Circulating antibody detectable
Treatment	Corticosteroids, immunosuppressives, dapsone	Corticosteroids, immunosuppressives, dapsone
Course	Chronic, remissions uncommon	Chronic, remissions not uncommon

24 VESICULO-BULLOUS DISEASES

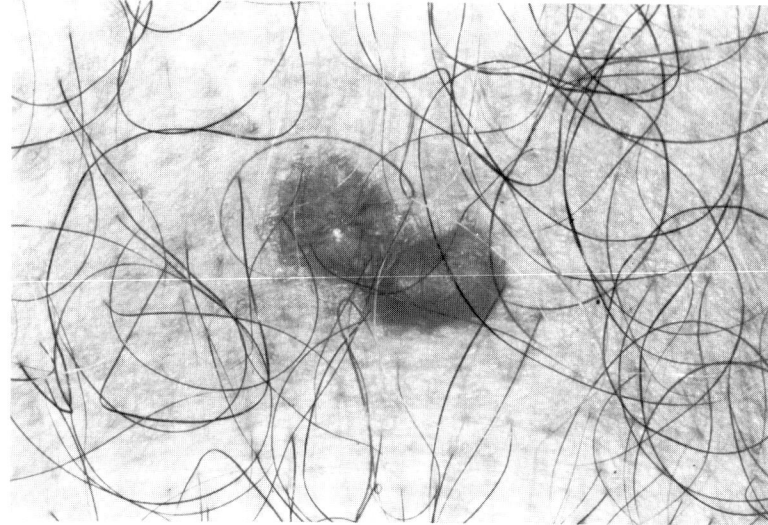

Figure 1–29. Bullous pemphigoid of the skin.

turally, the basement membrane is cleaved at the level of the lamina lucida.

In contrast to cicatricial pemphigoid, bullous pemphigoid demonstrates detectable levels of circulating autoantibodies to basement membrane zone components in approximately 70% of cases. Such antibody titers, however, neither correlate with nor fluctuate with the level of clinical disease, as is the case with pemphigus vulgaris. The direct immunofluorescence findings, corresponding to those in cicatricial pemphigoid, appears as a linear deposition of IgG and C3 along the basement membrane zone in active cases.

Treatment. Periods of clinical remission have been noted with this form of pemphigoid in contrast to the cicatricial form, where remission is less likely. Systemic corticosteroids are generally used to control this disease. Nonsteroidal immunosuppressive agents may also be used to effect control of the disease process as well as to reduce steroid side effects.

Dermatitis Herpetiformis

Etiology and Pathogenesis. The basic cause of dermatitis herpetiformis remains obscure. Although there are no demonstrable circulating autoantibodies noted in the sera of patients, deposits of IgA are evident in the skin and mucosa of patients with this disorder. An often observed association is noted between skin disease and mucosal pathology of the jejunum, in which there is defective fat absorption resembling celiac disease and sensitivity to gluten. Of significance from the patient's vantage is the frequently observed improvement of the malabsorption with a gluten-free diet. Substantiating this relationship is the relapse noted upon reintroduction of gluten-containing foods. The etiologic relationship between cutaneous and intestinal diseases remains obscure, although certain common B lymphocyte–associated antigens are noted in most patients. Additionally, immunogenetic studies have demonstrated an increased incidence of HLA-B8 and HLA-Dw3 histocompatibility antigens in patients with dermatitis herpetiformis and ordinary gluten-sensitive enteropathy.

It must be stressed that, despite its name, there is no relationship to HSV or any member of the herpes family from either an etiologic or a presentation standpoint.

Clinical Features. Dermatitis herpetiformis is a chronic disease typically seen in young and middle-aged adults, with a slight male predilection. It is essentially a cutaneous disease that rarely demonstrates oral mucosal involvement. Periods of exacerbation and remission further characterize this disease. Cutaneous involvement consists of formation of papular, erythematous, and often intensely pruritic lesions that most often are vesicular (Figs. 1–30 and 1–31). Such lesions are usually symmetric in their distribution over the extensor surfaces, especially over the elbows, shoulders, sacrum, and buttocks. Of diagnostic significance is the frequent involvement of the scalp and face. Lesions are usually aggregated (herpetiform) but often are disposed individually. The spectrum of involvement varies from patients with periodic development of lesions to individuals

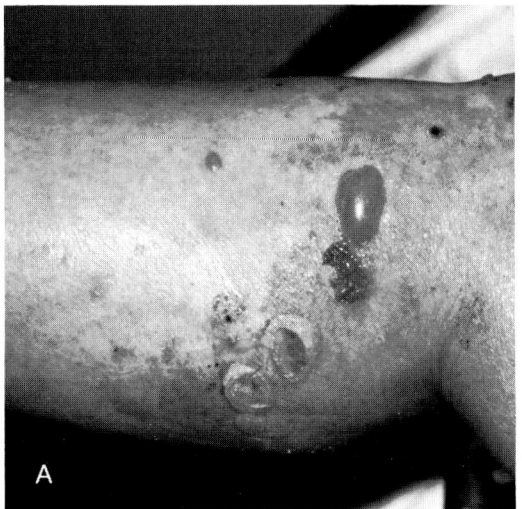 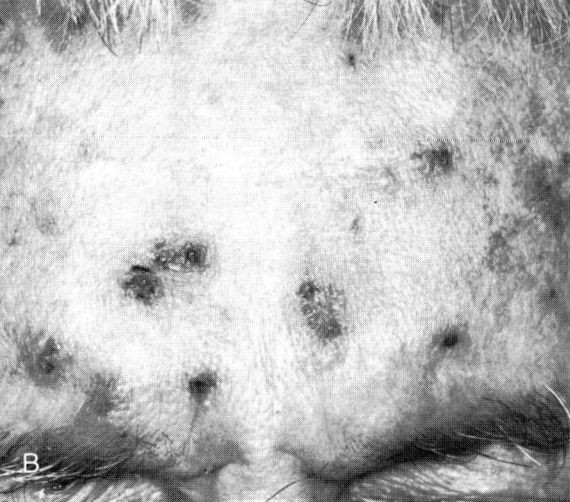

Figure 1–30. *A* and *B*, Dermatitis herpetiformis of the leg and forehead.

with generalized involvement with scores to hundreds of lesions. In time, the healed areas may become hyperpigmented with very slow fading. In some patients, exacerbations may be associated with ingestion of foods or drugs containing iodide compounds. In others, a seasonal (summer months) peak may be seen.

In the oral cavity, vesicles and bullae are evanescent in their presentation and duration. Subsequent to rupture, superficial ulcers with a fibrinous base and surrounding zone of erythema are seen. The ulcers are usually tender and mildly symptomatic in nature and nonspecific in appearance. Lesions may involve both keratinized and non-keratinized mucosa.

Histopathology and Immunopathology. Early lesions of dermatitis herpetiformis, prior to vesiculation, are rather distinctive, especially on the skin. Collections of neutrophils, eosinophils, and fibrin at the papillary tips of the dermis are typical. Subsequent exudation at this location contributes to separation of the overlying epithelium, forming a subepithelial vesicle. Perivascular inflammatory infiltration of a lympho-phagocytic type is present in early lesions.

The immunologic finding of IgA deposits at the tips of the connective tissue papillae is specific for dermatitis herpetiformis. The pattern of IgA deposition at the papillary tips is usually granular to speckled, although linear IgA patterns may be noted. (A linear IgA pattern may also be seen in some other chronic bullous dermatoses.) In addition, it is possible

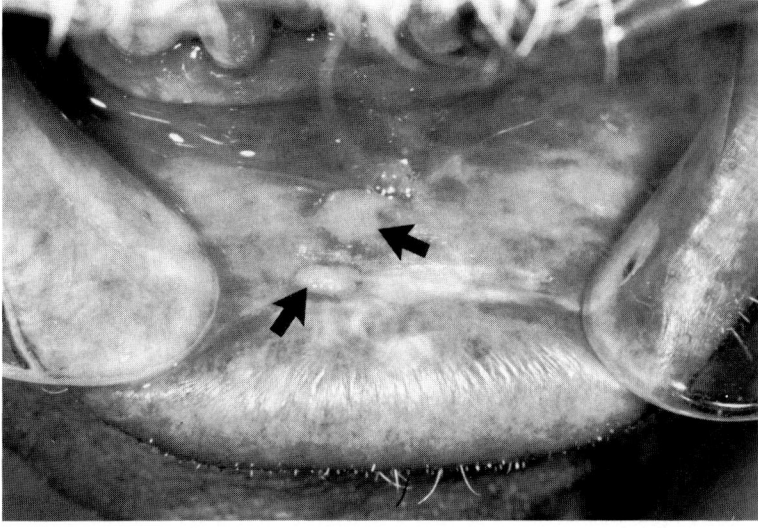

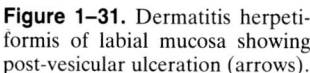

Figure 1–31. Dermatitis herpetiformis of labial mucosa showing post-vesicular ulceration (arrows).

to localize the third component of complement (C3) in lesional and perilesional tissue in a distribution similar to that of IgA.

Diagnosis. Demonstration of specific IgA immunofluorescence enables clear separation of this disease from other mucocutaneous vesiculo-bullous disease. Further supporting the separation of dermatitis herpetiformis from diseases such as bullous pemphigoid is the relationship of dermatitis herpetiformis with gastrointestinal findings, chiefly an asymptomatic gluten-sensitive enteropathy.

Treatment and Prognosis. Dermatitis herpetiformis is generally treated with the drugs dapsone, sulfoxone, and sulfapyridine. Response is usually prompt in the presence of adequate dosage. Since there is usually an associated enteropathy, a gluten-free diet may be also part of the therapeutic regimen. Elimination of gluten from the diet will reduce small bowel pathology and within 2 months produce a return to normal small bowel function. The benefit of dietary changes to skin and oral mucosal disease, however, is less clear-cut and generally not as dramatic.

In most instances, dermatitis herpetiformis is a lifelong condition, often exhibiting long periods of remission. Many patients, however, may be relegated to long-term dietary restrictions or drug treatment or both.

HEREDITARY DISEASES

Epidermolysis Bullosa

Etiology and Pathogenesis. Epidermolysis bullosa is a general term that encompasses one acquired and several genetic varieties of disease that are basically characterized by the formation of blisters at sites of minor trauma. The several genetic types range from autosomal dominant to autosomal recessive in origin and are further distinguished by varying clinical features, histopathology, and ultrastructure. The acquired non-hereditary form known as epidermolysis acquisita is unrelated to the other types, relative to etiologic and pathogenetic aspects. In this acquired type, IgG deposits are frequently found in sub–basement membrane tissue. These antibodies are thought to be a manifestation of the autoimmune nature of this form of the disease.

In the hereditary forms of epidermolysis bullosa, circulating antibodies are not apparently part of the mechanism of disease progression. Pathogenesis appears to be related rather to inherent defects in or degeneration of basal cells, hemidesmosomes, or anchoring connective tissue filaments.

Clinical Features. The feature common to all subtypes of epidermolysis bullosa is bulla formation from minor provocation, usually over areas of stress such as elbows and knees (Fig. 1–32). Onset of disease is during infancy or early childhood for the hereditary forms and during adulthood for the acquired type. Severity is generally greater with the inherited recessive forms. Blisters may be widespread and severe and may result in scarring and atrophy. Nails may be dystrophic in some forms of this disease.

Oral lesions are particularly common and severe in the recessive forms of this group of diseases and uncommon in the acquired form.

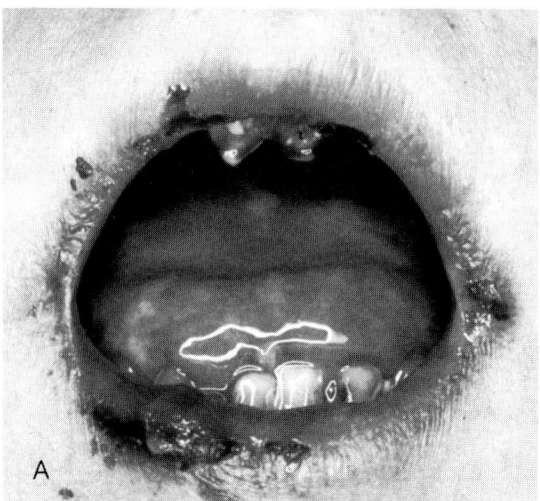
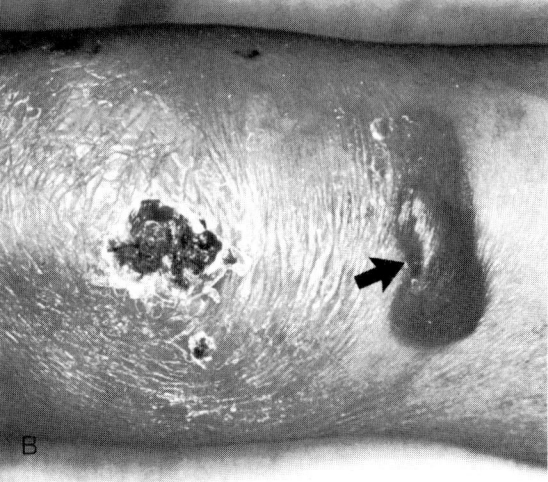

Figure 1–32. *A,* Epidermolysis bullosa in a 9-year-old. The tongue mucosa is atrophic from recurrent lesions, the teeth are hypoplastic, and the oral orifice is restricted because of recurrent lesions. *B,* Knee of same patient showing flaccid bulla (arrow) and other residua of previous lesions.

Oral manifestations include bullae that heal with scar, constricted oral orifice from scar, and hypoplastic teeth (Fig. 1–32). These changes are most pronounced in the type known as recessive dystrophic epidermolysis bullosa.

Treatment and Prognosis. Prognosis is dependent upon the subtype of epidermolysis bullosa. The range varies from life threatening in one of the recessive forms, known as junctional epidermolysis bullosa, to debilitating in most other forms. Therapy includes avoidance of trauma, supportive measures, and chemotherapeutic agents (none of which is consistently effective). Corticosteroids, vitamin E, phenytoin, retinoids, dapsone, and immunosuppressives have all been suggested as possibly producing some benefit to patients.

Bibliography

Viral Diseases

Arvin A, Kushner J, Feldman S, et al. Human leukocyte interferon for the treatment of varicella in children with cancer. N Engl J Med 306:761–765, 1982.

Burke B, Steele R, Beard O, et al. Immune responses to varicella-zoster in the aged. Arch Intern Med 142:291–293, 1982.

Corey L, Spear P. Infections with herpes simplex viruses. N Engl J Med 314:686–691; 749–757, 1986.

Davis B, Dulbecco R, Eisen H, Ginsberg H. Microbiology. 3rd ed. Harper & Row, Philadelphia, 1980, Chaps 55, 57, 59.

Dolin R. Antiviral chemotherapy and chemoprophylaxis. Science 227:1296–1303, 1985.

Douglas J, Critchlow C, Benedetti J, et al. A double-blind study of oral acyclovir for suppression of recurrences of genital herpes simplex virus infection. N Engl J Med 310:1551–1556, 1984.

Fiddian A, Ivanyi L. Topical acyclovir in the management of recurrent herpes labialis. Br J Dermatol 109:321–326, 1983.

Fiddian A, Yeo J, Stubbings R, Dean D. Successful treatment of herpes labialis with topical acyclovir. Br Med J 286:1699–1701, 1983.

Guinan M. Oral acyclovir for treatment and suppression of genital herpes simplex virus infection. JAMA 255:1747–1749, 1986.

Gerson A, Steinberg S, Gelb L. Clinical reinfection with varicella-zoster virus. J Infect Dis 149:137–142, 1984.

Hirsch M, Schooley R. Treatment of herpesvirus infections. N Engl J Med 309:963–970, 1983.

Ishimaru Y, Nakano S, Yamaoka K, Takami S. Outbreaks of hand, foot, and mouth disease by enterovirus 71. Arch Dis Child 55:583–588, 1980.

Jayasuriya A, Nash A. Pathogenesis and immunobiology of herpes simplex virus in mouse and man. Cancer Invest 3:199–207, 1985.

Nicholson K. Antiviral therapy. Lancet 22:677–681, 1984.

Reichman R, Badger G, Mertz G, et al. Treatment of recurrent genital herpes simplex infections with oral acyclovir. JAMA 251:2103–2107, 1984.

Serota F, Starr S, Bryan C, et al. Acyclovir treatment of herpes zoster infections. JAMA 247:2132–2135, 1982.

Spruance S, Overall J Jr, Kern E, et al. The natural history of recurrent herpes simplex labialis. N Engl J Med 297:69–74, 1977.

Spruance S, Schnipper L, Overall J Jr, et al. Treatment of herpes simplex labialis with topical acyclovir in polyethylene glycol. J Infect Dis 146:85–90, 1982.

Straus S, Takiff H, Seidlin M, et al. Suppression of frequently recurring genital herpes—a placebo-controlled double-blind trial of oral acyclovir. N Engl J Med 310:1545–1550, 1984.

Weller T. Varicella and herpes zoster. N Engl J Med 309:1362–1368, 1983.

Whitley R, Soong S, Dolin R, et al. Early vidarabine therapy to control the complications of herpes zoster in immunosuppressed patients. N Engl J Med 307:971–975, 1982.

Immunologic and Hereditary Diseases

Anhalt G, Patel H, Diaz L. Mechanisms of immunologic injury. Arch Dermatol 119:711–713, 1983.

Avalos E, Patel H, Anhalt G, Diaz L. Autoimmune injury of squamous epithelium by pemphigus autoantibodies. Br J Dermatol 111:359–365, 1984.

Brautbar C, Moscovitz M, Livshits T, et al. HLA-DRw4 in pemphigus vulgaris patients in Israel. Tissue Antigens 16:238, 1980.

Daniels T, Quadra-White C. Direct immunofluorescence in oral mucosal disease: a diagnostic analysis of 130 cases. Oral Surg Oral Med Oral Pathol 51:38–46, 1981.

Dubertet L, Bertaux B, Fosse M, et al. Cellular events leading to blister formation in bullous pemphigoid. Br J Dermatol 104:615–624, 1980.

Dvorak A, Mihm M, Osage J, et al. Bullous pemphigoid, an ultrastructural study of the inflammatory response. J Invest Dermatol 78:91–101, 1982.

Economopoulou P, Laskaris G. Dermatitis herpetiformis: oral lesions as an early manifestation. Oral Surg Oral Med Oral Pathol 62:77–80, 1986.

Fine R, Weathers D. Desquamative gingivitis: A form of cicatricial pemphigoid? Br J Dermatol 102:393–399, 1980.

Fitzpatrick T, Eisen A, Wolff K, Freedberg I, Austen K. Dermatology in General Medicine. New York, McGraw-Hill, 1987, Chaps 59 and 64.

Harrison P, Scott D, Cobden I. Buccal mucosa immunofluorescence in coeliac disease and dermatitis herpetiformis. Br J Dermatol 102:687–688, 1980.

Katz S. Dermatitis herpetiformis: clinical, histologic, therapeutic, and laboratory clues. Int J Dermatol 17:529–535, 1978.

Katz S, Strober W. The pathogenesis of dermatitis herpetiformis. J Invest Dermatol 70:63–75, 1978.

Krain L, Landau J, Newcomer V. Cyclophosphamide in the treatment of pemphigus vulgaris and bullous pemphigoid. Arch Dermatol 106:657–661, 1972.

Laskaris G, Angelopoulos A. Cicatricial pemphigoid: direct and indirect immunofluorescent studies. Oral Surg Oral Med Oral Pathol 51:48–54, 1981.

Lever W, Schaumberg-Lever G. Treatment of pemphigus vulgaris. Arch Dermatol 120:44–47, 1984.

Marks J. Dogma and dermatitis herpetiformis. Clin Exp Dermatol 2:189–207, 1977.

Marsden R, McKee P, Boghal B, et al. A study of benign chronic bullous dermatosis of childhood and comparison with dermatitis herpetiformis and bullous pemphigoid occurring in childhood. Clin Exp Dermatol 5:159–172, 1980.

Morioka S, Naito K, Ogaira H. The pathogenic role of pemphigus antibodies and proteinase in epidermal acantholysis. J Invest Dermatol 76:337–341, 1981.

Nisengard R, Chorzelski T, Maciejowska E, et al. Dermatitis herpetiformis: IgA deposits in gingiva, buccal mucosa, and skin. Oral Surg Oral Med Oral Pathol 54:22–25, 1982.

Patel H, Anhalt G, Diaz L. Bullous pemphigoid and pemphigus vulgaris. Ann Allergy 50:144–150, 1983.

Penneys N, Eagelstein W, Frost P. Management of pemphigus with gold compounds: a long-term follow-up report. Arch Dermatol 112:185–187, 1976.

Reginer M, Vaigot P, Michel S, et al. Localization of bullous pemphigoid antigen (BPA) in isolated human keratinocytes. J Invest Dermatol 85:187–190, 1985.

Rogers R, Perry H, Bean S, et al. Immunopathology of cicatricial pemphigoid: Studies of complement deposition. J Invest Dermatol 68:39–43, 1977.

Rogers R, Seehafer J, Perry H. Treatment of cicatricial (benign mucous membrane) pemphigoid with dapsone. J Am Acad Dermatol 6:215–223, 1982.

Singer K, Hashimoto K, Jensen P, et al. Pathogenesis of autoimmunity in pemphigus. Annu Rev Immunol 3:87–108, 1985.

Swanson D, Dahl M. Pemphigus vulgaris and plasma exchange: clinical and serologic studies. J Am Acad Dermatol 4:325–328, 1981.

Wright J. Epidermolysis bullosa: dental and anesthetic management of two cases. Oral Surg Oral Med Oral Pathol 57:155–157, 1984.

Chapter 2

Ulcerative Conditions

REACTIVE LESIONS
BACTERIAL CONDITIONS
Syphilis
Gonorrhea
Tuberculosis
Leprosy
Actinomycosis
Noma
FUNGAL DISEASES
Deep Fungal Diseases
Subcutaneous Fungal Diseases—Sporotrichosis
Opportunistic Fungal Infections—Phycomycosis
CONDITIONS ASSOCIATED WITH
    IMMUNOLOGIC DYSFUNCTION
Aphthous Ulcers
Behçet's Syndrome
Reiter's Syndrome
Erythema Multiforme
Lupus Erythematosus
Drug Reactions
Contact Allergy
Wegener's Granulomatosis
Midline Granuloma
Chronic Granulomatous Disease
NEOPLASMS
Basal Cell Carcinoma
Squamous Cell Carcinoma
Carcinoma of the Maxillary Sinus

An ulcer is defined as a loss of epithelium due to any cause. The term "erosion" generally implies a superficial defect producing some loss of epithelium. For all practical purposes, however, erosion and ulcer are used interchangeably. Ulcers may be preceded by vesicles or bullae that are generally short-lived intraorally. This vesiculo-bullous-ulcerative group of diseases represents a distinct set of oral conditions, which are discussed in Chapter 1. A patient history of "blisters" preceding ulcers is a valuable piece of information that can be used to confine the clinical differential diagnosis to the very specific vesiculo-bullous group of diseases.

Ulcerative lesions are commonly encountered in dental patients. Although many oral ulcers have similar clinical appearances, their etiologies can range from reactive to neoplastic to oral manifestations of dermatologic disease. Diagnosis is important not only for the patient but also for the clinician. Infectious ulcers are potentially communicable to dental personnel and should be approached with caution.

REACTIVE LESIONS

Etiology. The ulcer is probably the most common oral soft tissue lesion. Most ulcers are caused by simple mechanical trauma. A cause and effect relationship is usually obvious, based on historical information or clinical appearance. Most ulcers are the result of accidental trauma and will generally appear in regions that are readily trapped between the teeth, such as the lower lip, tongue, and buccal mucosa (Fig. 2–1). Prostheses, most commonly dentures, are frequently associated with traumatic ulcers, which may be acute or chronic (Fig. 2–2).

In unusual circumstances, lesions may be self-induced because of an abnormal habit that is often associated with some psychologic problem (Fig. 2–3). These so-called factitial injuries are as difficult to decipher as they are to treat. These lesions may prove to be frustrating clinical problems, especially if one has no suspicion of a self-induced etiology. Psychologic counseling may ultimately be required to help resolve the problem.

Traumatic oral ulcers may also be iatrogenic. Respect for the fragility of oral soft tissues is, of course, of paramount importance in the treatment of dental patients. Overzealous tis-

30 ULCERATIVE CONDITIONS

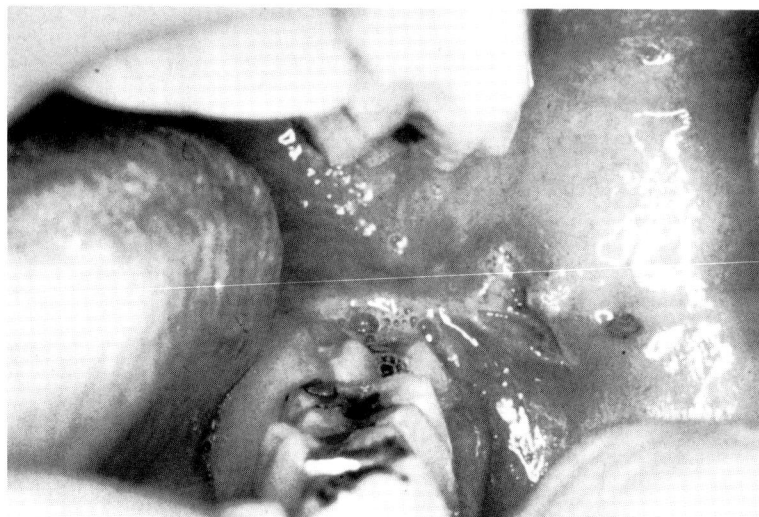

Figure 2–1. Acute traumatic ulcer.

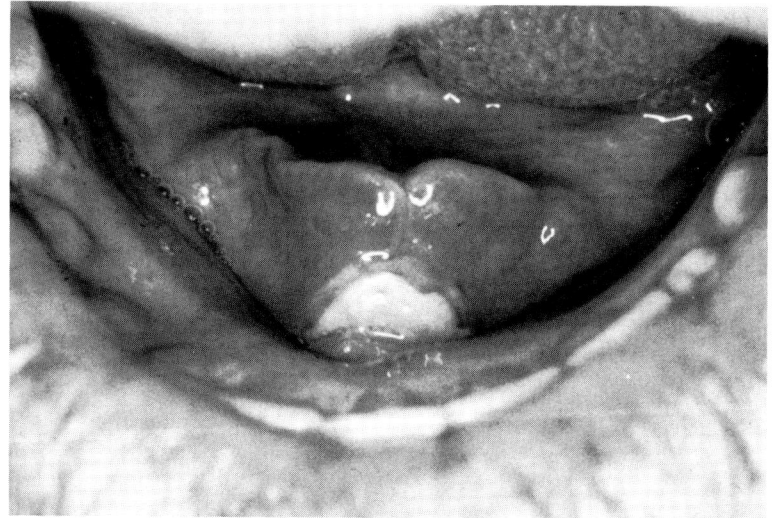

Figure 2–2. Fibrin-covered ulcer in floor of mouth associated with denture flange.

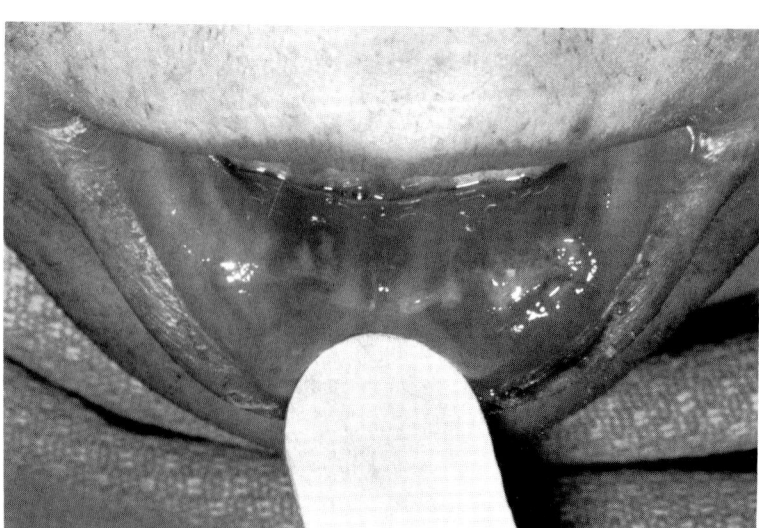

Figure 2–3. Acute self-induced ulcers associated with lip-biting habit.

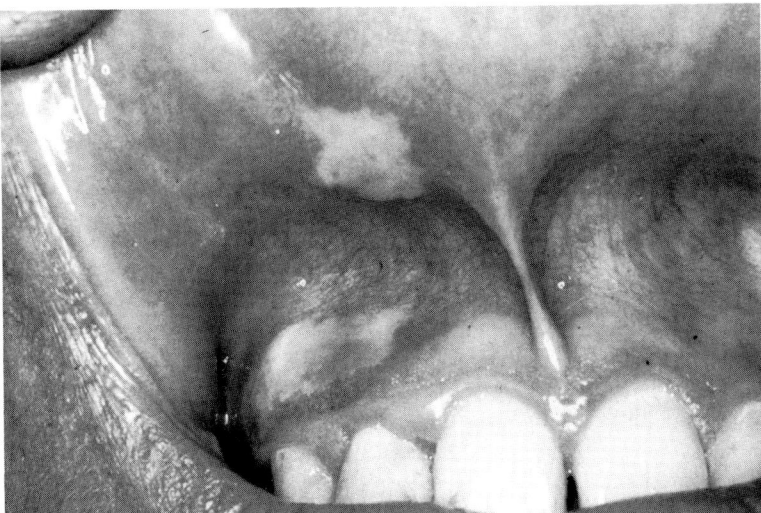

Figure 2-4. Acute iatrogenic "cotton roll" ulcers.

sue manipulation or concentration on treating primarily hard tissues may be responsible for accidental soft tissue injury that can be avoided. Ulcers induced by removal of adherent cotton rolls (Fig. 2-4), by the negative pressure of a saliva ejector, and by accidental striking of mucosa when rotating instruments are not uncommon, but they are preventable.

Chemicals may be the cause of oral ulcers because of their acidic or basic nature or because of their ability to act as irritants or allergens. Lesions may be patient induced or iatrogenic (Fig. 2-5). In spite of a more sophisticated patient population having greater dental awareness, aspirin burns are still seen, although they are much less common than before. When acetylsalicylic acid is placed directly against an area of tooth-related pain, a mucosal burn or coagulative necrosis occurs, the extent being dependent upon the duration and number of aspirin applications. Many over-the-counter medications for toothache, aphthous ulcers, and denture-related injuries have the ability to damage oral mucosa if used injudiciously. Medicines used by dental practitioners can also cause significant soft tissue damage. Cavity medications, especially those containing phenol, may cause iatrogenic oral ulcers. Increasing use of phosphoric acid–etching agents has been associated with mucosal burns of a chemical nature. Endodontic and vital bleaching procedures in which strong oxidizing agents are used (30% hydrogen peroxide), have also produced burns.

Ulcers following heat burns are relatively uncommon intraorally. "Pizza burns," caused by hot cheese, have been noted in the palate. Iatrogenic heat burns may also be seen follow-

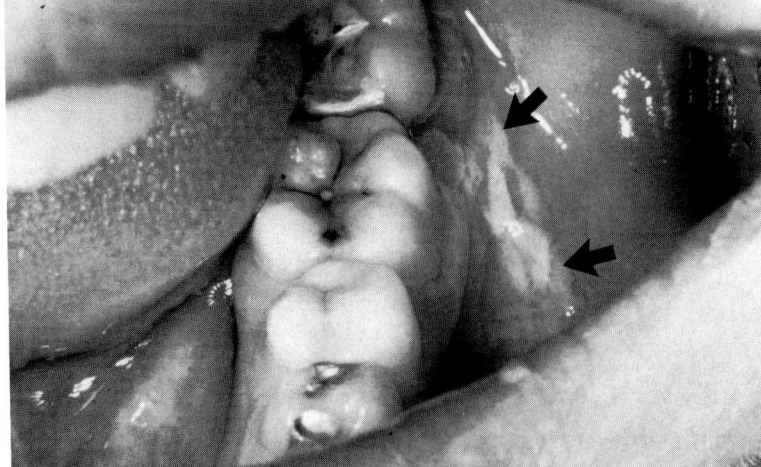

Figure 2-5. Iatrogenic phenol burn (arrows) associated with cavity medication of second molar.

ing the injudicious use of dental impression material, such as wax, hydrocolloid (Fig. 2–6), and compound.

Oral ulcerations are typically seen during the course of therapeutic radiation for head and neck cancers (Fig. 2–7). In those malignancies—namely, squamous cell carcinoma—that require large doses of radiation, in the range of 6000 to 7000 rads, oral ulcers will invariably be seen in tissues within the path of the beam. For malignancies such as lymphoma, in which lower doses of 4000 to 5000 rads are tumoricidal, ulcers are likely but are less severe and of shorter duration. Radiation-induced ulcers persist through the course of therapy and for several weeks after, at which time spontaneous healing occurs without scar.

Clinical Features. Acute reactive ulcers of oral mucous membranes exhibit the clinical signs and symptoms of acute inflammation. The lesions are covered by a yellow-white exudate and are surrounded by an erythematous halo. Varying degrees of pain and tenderness are associated with acute lesions

Chronic reactive ulcers may cause little or no pain. They are covered by a yellow membrane and are surrounded by elevated margins that may show hyperkeratosis (Fig. 2–8). Induration is due to scar and chronic inflammatory cell infiltration.

A particularly ominous-appearing but benign chronic ulcer occasionally may be seen in association with deep soft tissue injury. This crateriform ulcer, known as *traumatic granuloma*, may measure 1 to 2 cm in diameter. It is usually found in the tongue but may occur in the buccal mucosa or lip. Healing may take several weeks. Another ominous-appearing chronic ulcer, characteristically seen in the hard palate, is associated with ischemic necrosis of a minor salivary gland. This lesion, known as necrotizing sialometaplasia, also heals spontaneously in several weeks (see Chapter 8).

Histopathology. Acute ulcers show a loss of surface epithelium that is replaced by a fibrin network containing neutrophils, degenerating cells, and debris. The ulcer base contains dilated capillaries and, with time, granulation tissue. Regeneration of the epithelium begins at the ulcer margins, with proliferating cells coursing over the granulation tissue base and under the fibrin clot.

Chronic ulcers exhibit a granulation tissue base, with scar found deeper in the tissue (Fig. 2–9). Epithelial regeneration may not occur because of continued trauma or because of unfavorable local tissue factors, such as inadequate blood supply. In traumatic granulomas, tissue injury and inflammation extend into subjacent skeletal muscle. A characteristic lush eosinophilic and phagocytic infiltrate dominates the histologic picture.

Diagnosis. With acute reactive ulcers, the cause and effect relationship is usually apparent from the clinical examination and history. When there is a factitial overlay, diagnosis becomes a greater challenge.

The cause of chronic reactive ulcers may not be as readily apparent, making clinical diagnosis more difficult. Under these circumstances, it is important that a differential diagnosis be developed. Conditions to consider are an infectious process (syphilis, tuberculosis, deep fungal infection) or a malignancy. If the lesion is believed most likely to be trau-

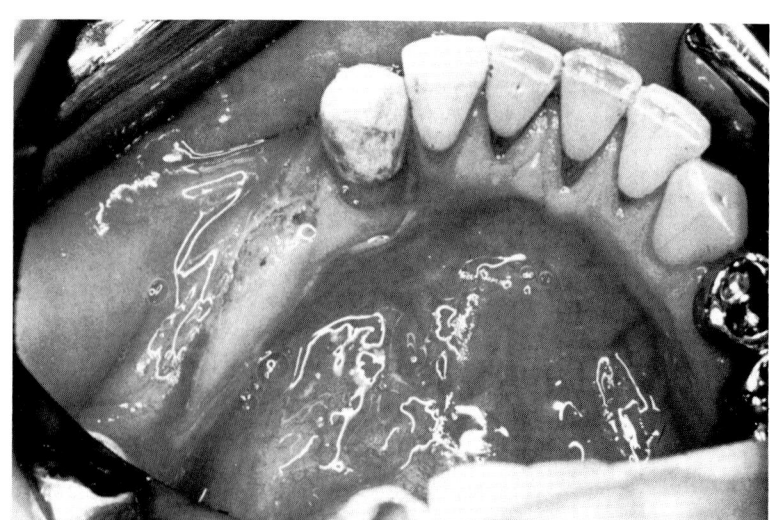

Figure 2–6. Hydrocolloid burn resulting in bone exposure of mandibular ridge.

ULCERATIVE CONDITIONS   33

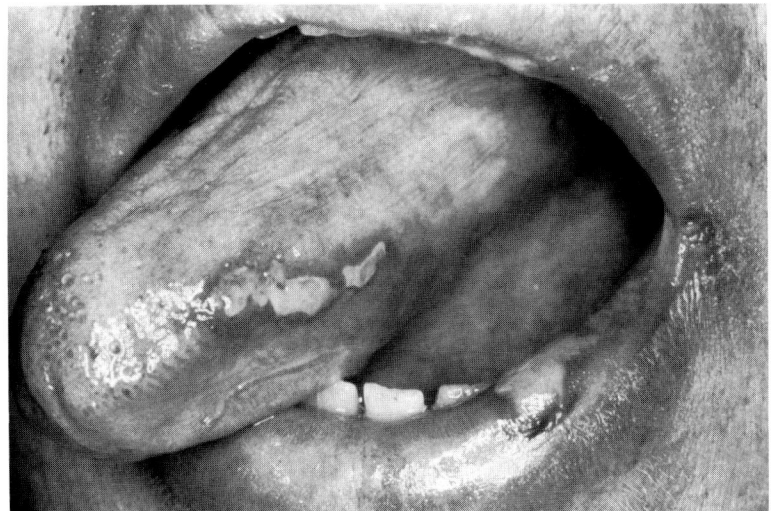

Figure 2–7. Acute radiation ulcers of lip and tongue associated with therapeutic radiation for lymphoma.

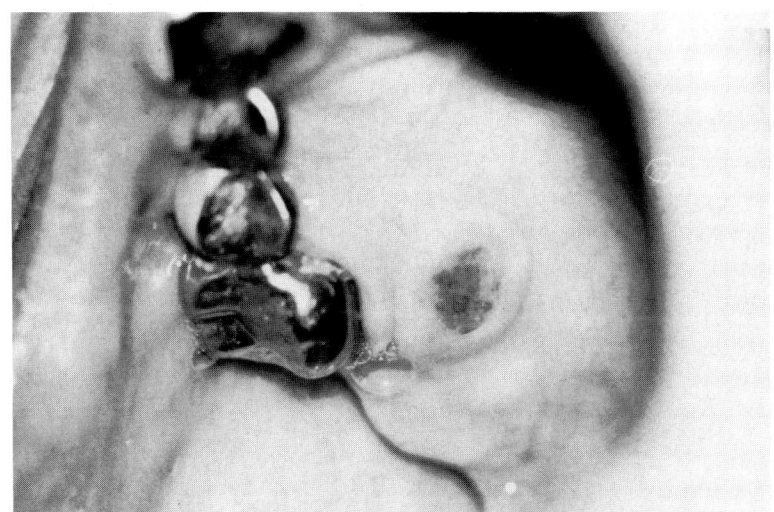

Figure 2–8. Chronic ulcer overlying exostosis of hard palate.

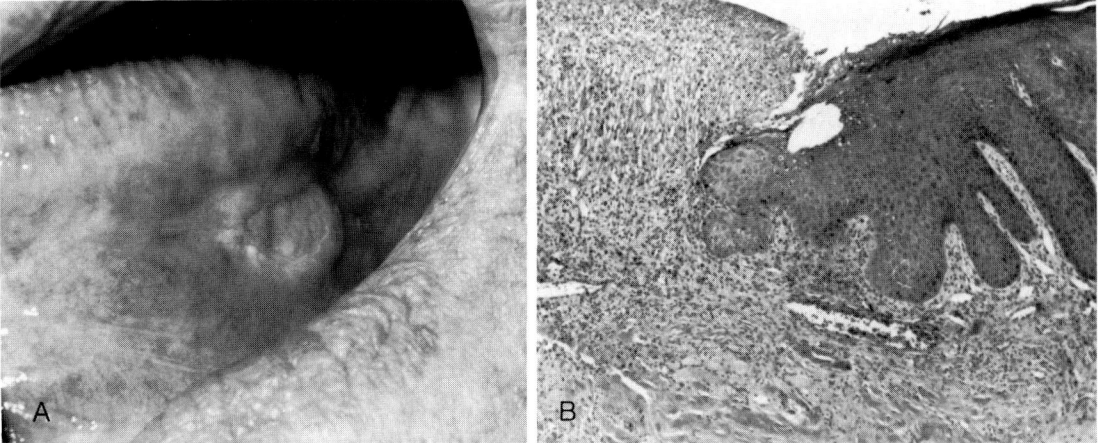

Figure 2–9. *A*, Chronic tongue ulcer. *B*, Ulcer margin showing abrupt transition from epithelium to fibrin membrane.

matic in origin, a 2-week observation period is warranted. If no change is seen or if the lesion increases in size, biopsy should provide a definitive answer.

Treatment. Most reactive ulcers of oral mucous membranes are treated simply with observation. If pain is considerable, symptomatic treatment may be of benefit. This could be in the form of a tetracycline–nystatin–diphenhydramine hydrochloride rinse or topical corticosteroids.

BACTERIAL CONDITIONS

Syphilis

Syphilis is a venereal disease that has been traced as far back as the time of Christopher Columbus, and it has had a profound influence on the history of the world. Whether Columbus's sailors who returned from the Indies were, in fact, responsible for the introduction of syphilis into the Old World is debatable, according to historians. Nonetheless, it was about this time that the virulent pandemic of the "great pox" began. Until Dr. Paul Ehrlich developed his "magic bullet," arsphenamine, around the turn of the century, there was no definitive treatment for syphilis. A stunning change in the control of syphilis followed the introduction of penicillin in the early forties. By 1940, approximately 600,000 new cases were reported in the United States; this decreased over the next 15 years to 6000 cases per year. A slow increase has occurred, to reach the present average of about 28,000 cases per year.

Etiology and Pathogenesis. Syphilis is caused by the spirochete *Treponema pallidum*. It is acquired by sexual contact with a partner with active lesions, by transfusion of infected blood, or by transplacental inoculation from an infected mother.

When spread through contact, the infectious lesion of primary syphilis, known as a chancre, forms at the site of spirochete entry, with the subsequent development of regional lymphadenopathy (Fig. 2–10). The chancre heals spontaneously after several weeks without treatment, leaving the patient with no apparent symptoms. Following a latent period of several weeks, secondary syphilis develops (patients infected via transfusion bypass the primary stage and begin with secondary syphilis). In this stage, there is wide dissemination, with fever, flu-like symptoms, and mucocutaneous lesions appearing with a spirochetemia. Lymphadenopathy is typical, and other organs may also be involved. This stage also resolves spontaneously, and the patient enters another latency period. Relapses to secondary syphilis may occur in some patients. In about one third of those who have entered the latency phase and have not been treated, tertiary or late-stage syphilis develops. These patients may have central nervous system involvement, cardiovascular lesions, or focal necrotic inflammatory lesions, known as gummas, of any organ.

Congenital syphilis occurs during the latter half of pregnancy, when the *T. pallidum* or-

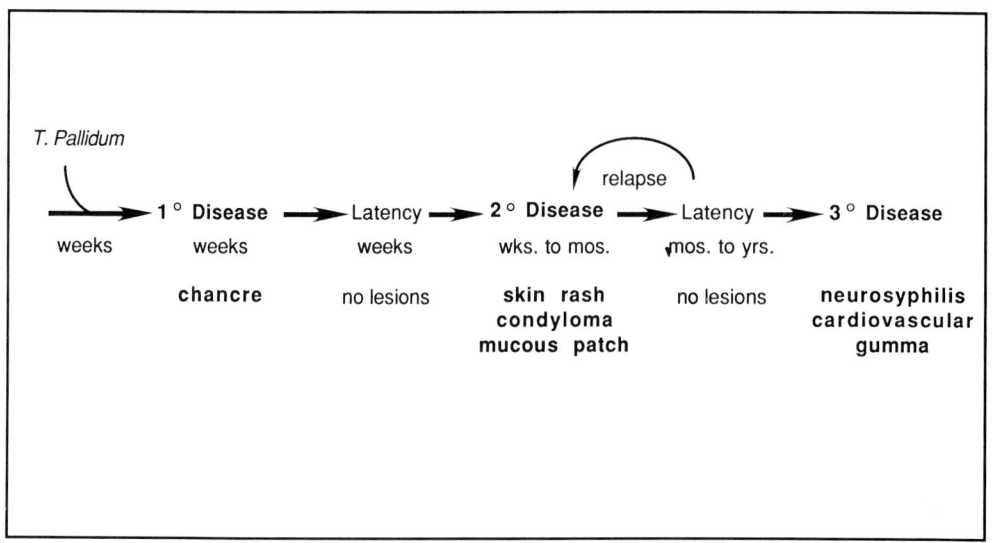

Figure 2–10. Pathogenesis of syphilis.

ganism crosses the placenta from the infected mother. The spirochetemia that develops may result in fetal abortion, or it may produce numerous inflammatory and destructive lesions in various fetal organs.

Clinical Features. Primary syphilis results in a painless indurated ulcer(s) with rolled margins at the site of inoculation (Fig. 2–11). The lesion does not produce an exudate. The location is usually on the genitalia. Lip, oral, and finger lesions do occur occasionally and exhibit similar clinical characteristics. Regional lymphadenopathy, typified by firm, painless swelling, is often part of the clinical picture. The lesion heals without therapy in 3 to 12 weeks, with little or no scarring.

In untreated syphilis, secondary disease begins after about 2 to 10 weeks. The spirochetes are now disseminated widely and are the cause of a reddish-brown maculopapular cutaneous rash (Fig. 2–12) and ulcers covered by a mucoid exudate (mucous patches) on mucous membranes. Elevated broad-based plaques, known as condyloma latum, may also be seen on skin and mucosal surfaces. Inflammatory lesions may potentially occur in any organ during secondary syphilis. These lesions may persist for as long as 8 weeks before spontaneous remission occurs. Patients enter a latency period, during which there may be one or more relapses of disseminated disease.

Tertiary or late-stage disease develops in about one third of latent syphilitics who go untreated. Manifestations take many years to appear and can be profound, since there is a predilection for cardiovascular and central nervous system involvement. Fortunately, this stage of syphilis has become a rarity because of effective antibiotic treatment and possibly because of less virulent organisms. Numerous manifestations of neural syphilis may occur owing to brain, spinal cord, and meningeal involvement. Two of these manifestations are general paresis (paralysis) and tabes dorsalis (locomotor ataxia). Inflammatory involvement of the cardiovascular system, especially the aorta, may result in aneurysms. Focal granulomatous lesions or gummas are also a feature of tertiary syphilis (Fig. 2–13). These are destructive inflammatory lesions that may involve any organ. Intraorally, the palate is typically affected. Development of generalized glossitis with mucosal atrophy has also been well documented in the tertiary stage of this disease. This so-called syphilitic glossitis is known to have a predisposition for the development of squamous cell carcinoma.

The generalized spirochetemia of congenital syphilis may result in numerous clinical manifestations that may affect any organ system in the developing fetus. A mucocutaneous rash may be seen early. When the infectious process involves the vomer, a nasal deformity known as saddle nose develops; or when periostitis of the tibia occurs, excessive anterior bone growth results in a deformity known as saber shin. Other late stigmata of congenital syphilis include three conditions known collectively as Hutchinson's triad: (1) an inflammatory reaction in the cornea, known as interstitial keratitis; (2) eighth nerve deafness; and (3) dental abnormalities consisting of notched or screwdriver-shaped incisors and mulberry molars (Fig. 2–14), presumably occurring because of spirochete infection of the enamel organ of teeth when amelogenesis is active.

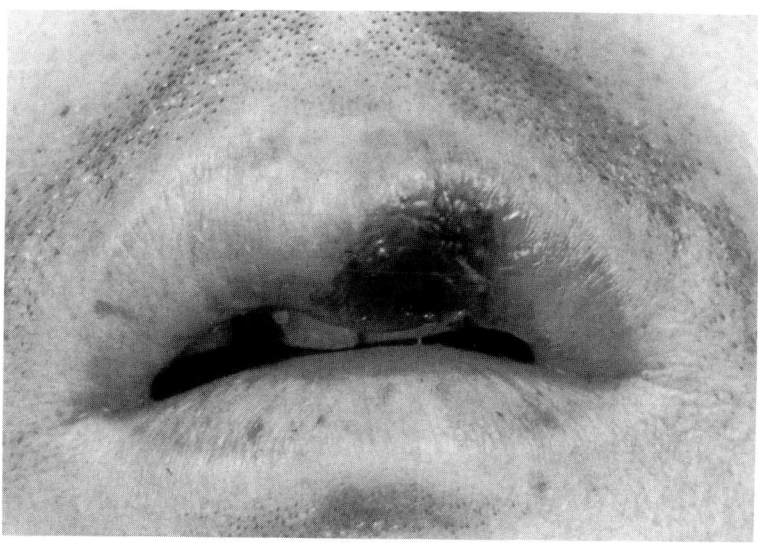

Figure 2–11. Chronic encrusted ulcer (chancre) of primary syphilis. (Reproduced by permission from Kerr, Donald A., Ash, Major M., Jr., and Milliard, H. Dean: Oral Diagnosis, ed. 6, St. Louis, 1983, The C. V. Mosby Co.)

36 ULCERATIVE CONDITIONS

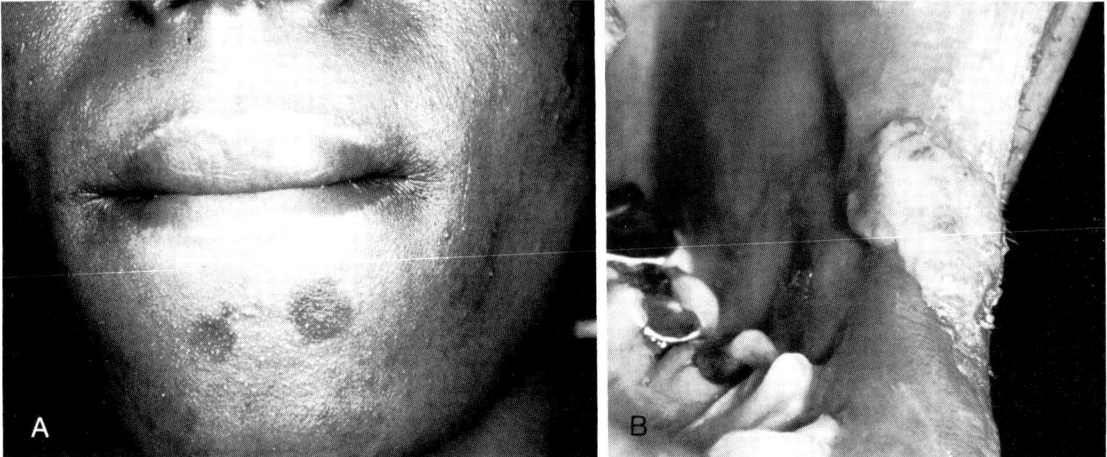

Figure 2–12. Macular lesions *(A)* and condyloma latum *(B)* of secondary syphilis.

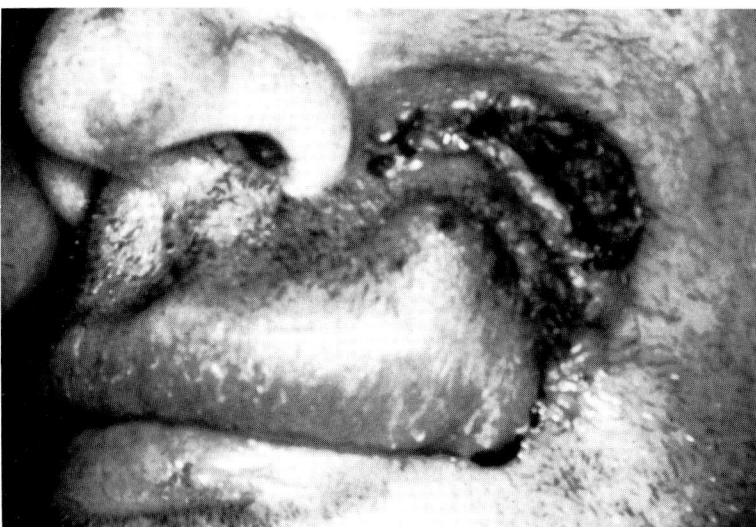

Figure 2–13. Gummatous inflammation of tertiary syphilis.

Figure 2–14. Notched incisors and mulberry molars, part of Hutchinson's triad.

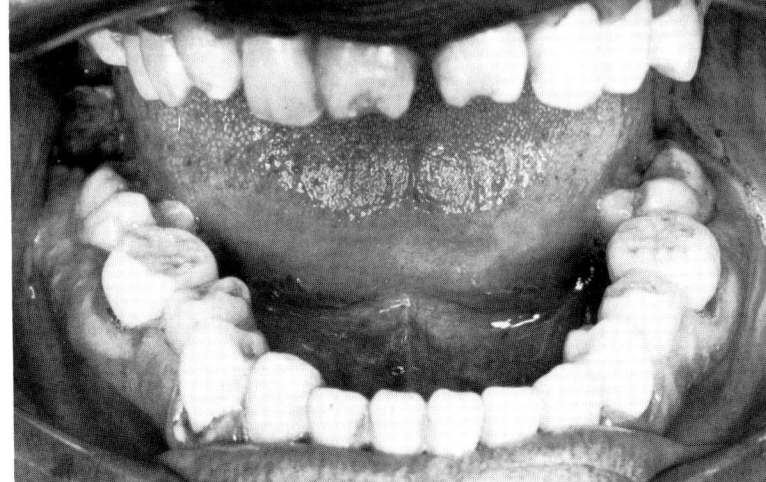

Histopathology. The basic tissue response to *T. pallidum* infections consists of a proliferative endarteritis and a plasma cell infiltrate. Endothelial cells proliferate within small arteries and arterioles, producing a concentric layering of cells that results in a narrowed lumen. Plasma cells, along with lymphocytes and macrophages, are typically found in a perivascular distribution. Using special staining methods, spirochetes can be seen within the various lesions of syphilis, although they may be scant in tertiary lesions. Gummas may additionally show necrosis and greater numbers of macrophages, resulting in a granulomatous lesion that is similar to other conditions, such as tuberculosis.

Differential Diagnosis. Clinically as well as microscopically, syphilis is said to be the great imitator or mimicker because of its resemblance to many other unrelated conditions. When presenting orally, the chancre may be confused with and must be differentiated from squamous cell carcinoma, chronic traumatic lesions, and other infectious diseases, such as tuberculosis and histoplasmosis. The differential diagnosis of secondary syphilis would include many infectious and non-infectious conditions in which there is a mucocutaneous eruption. Oral gummas, though rarely seen, may have a clinical appearance similar to the destructive lesions of midline granuloma.

Definitive diagnosis of syphilis is based upon laboratory test confirmation of clinical impression. Among the several tests available are: (1) darkfield examination of scrapings or exudate from active lesions, (2) special silver stain or immunologic preparation of biopsy tissue, and (3) serologic tests for antibodies to *T. pallidum*.

Treatment. The drug of choice for treating all stages of syphilis is penicillin. Over the years, *T. pallidum* has remained sensitive to penicillin as well as to other antibiotics, such as erythromycin and tetracycline.

Gonorrhea

Etiology. Gonorrhea is one of the most prevalent bacterial diseases in humans. It is caused by the gram-negative diplococcus *Neisseria gonorrhoeae*. Infection is transmitted by direct sexual contact with an infected partner. Containment of the number of infected individuals through the tracing of sexual contacts is enhanced by the short incubation period of less than 7 days but hampered by the absence of symptoms in many individuals, especially females.

Genital infections may be transmitted to the oral or pharyngeal mucous membranes through orogenital contact. Because oral mucosa is more resistant than pharyngeal mucosa, the latter site is much more commonly affected than the former. Risk of developing this form of disease is apparently much more likely with fellatio than with cunnilingus. Individuals may have concomitant genital and oral or pharyngeal infections that result from direct exposure to these areas rather than from spread through blood or lymphatics.

Transmission of gonorrhea from an infected patient to dental personnel is regarded as highly unlikely because the organism is very sensitive to drying and also requires a break in the skin to establish an infection. Gloves, glasses, and a mask should provide adequate protection from accidental infection.

Clinical Features. No specific clinical signs have been consistently associated with the rarely occurring oral gonorrhea. However, multiple ulcerations or generalized erythema have been described. Symptoms range from none to generalized stomatitis.

In the more common pharyngeal gonococcal infections, presenting signs are usually general erythema with associated ulcers and cervical lymphadenopathy. The chief complaint may be sore throat, although many patients are asymptomatic.

Differential Diagnosis. Because of the lack of consistent and distinctive oral lesions, other conditions that cause multiple ulcers or generalized erythema should be included in a differential diagnosis. Aphthous ulcers, herpetic ulcers, erythema multiforme, pemphigus, pemphigoid, drug eruptions, and streptococcal infections should be considered. Diagnosis of gonorrhea is traditionally based upon demonstration of the organism with Gram stains or culture on Thayer-Martin medium. Rapid identification of *N. gonorrhoeae* with immunofluorescent antibody techniques and other laboratory tests may also be used to support clinical impressions.

Treatment. The treatment of choice for gonorrhea is penicillin G. This may be supplemented by oral tetracycline. Ampicillin is apparently ineffective in the treatment of pharyngeal gonorrhea. The clinician should be cognizant of the occurrence of mixed infections and penicillin-resistant gonococcal strains when treating this condition.

Tuberculosis

Etiology and Pathogenesis. Tuberculosis (TB) is caused by the aerobic bacillus *Mycobacterium tuberculosis*. It does not react to Gram stain but appears red with Ziehl-Neelsen stain. With this latter stain, these organisms are not decolorized with acid-alcohol and are therefore also known as acid-fast bacilli.

Although TB has worldwide distribution, it has become much less prevalent than it was before the advent of antibiotics. Significant numbers of patients (e.g., 27,500 United States cases in 1982) continue to develop the active form of this disease. The case rate varies from one region to another and is dependent upon factors that favor spread of communicable diseases, such as poor living conditions, low socioeconomic status, low native resistance, and compromised immunity from debilitating or immunosuppressed conditions. In the United States, a majority of cases can be found in densely populated urban areas, among immigrants from countries with high TB rates (e.g., Southeast Asia and Haiti), and among older individuals with compromised health.

Spread of infection is through small airborne droplets, which carry the organism to pulmonary air spaces. Phagocytosis by alveolar macrophages follows, and the battle between bacterial virulence and host resistance begins. As the immune system is sensitized by the TB antigens, a positive tuberculin reactivity develops. The Mantoux test and the Tine test are skin tests utilizing a tubercular bacillus antigen, called purified protein derivative (PPD), to determine if the individual is hypersensitive to antigen challenge. A positive inflammatory skin reaction indicates that the individual's cell-mediated immune system has been sensitized, and it signifies previous exposure and subclinical infection but does not necessarily imply active disease.

A granulomatous inflammatory response to *M. tuberculosis* follows sensitization. In most cases, the cell-mediated immune response is able to control the infection, allowing subsequent arrest of the disease (Fig. 2–15). Inflammatory foci may eventually undergo dystrophic calcification. Latent organisms in these foci may become reactivated at a later date. In a small number of cases, the disease may progress through airborne, hematogenous, or lymphatic spread, so-called miliary spread.

Oral mucous membranes may become infected through implantation of organisms found in sputum or, less likely, through hematogenous deposition. Similar seeding of the oral cavity may also follow secondary or reactivated TB.

Clinical Features. Unless the primary infection becomes progressive, the infected patient will probably exhibit no symptoms. Skin testing and chest radiograms may provide the only indicators of infection. In reactivated disease, low-grade signs and symptoms of fever, night sweats, malaise, and weight loss may appear. With progression, cough, hemoptysis, and chest pain (pleural involvement) develop. As other organs become involved through spread of organisms, a highly varied clinical picture appears that is dependent upon the organs involved.

Oral manifestations that usually follow im-

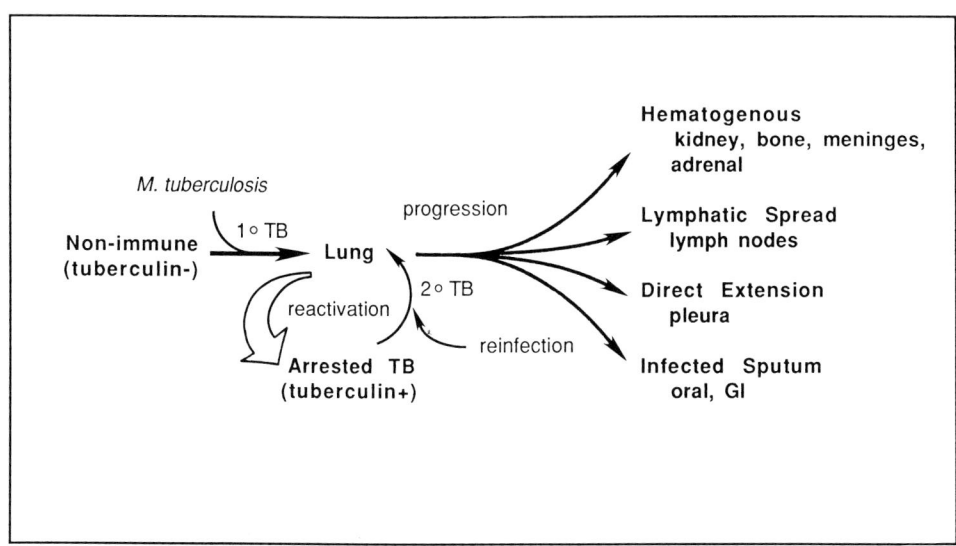

Figure 2–15. Pathogenesis of tuberculosis.

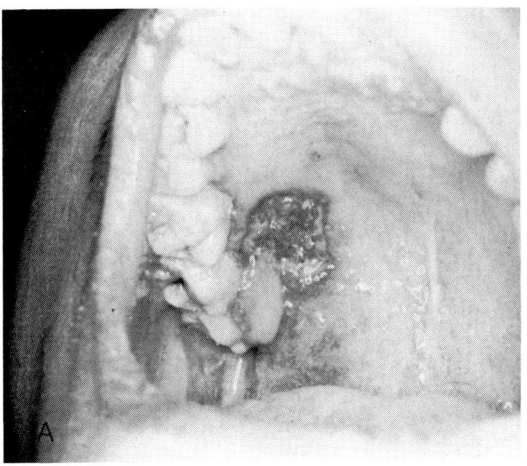 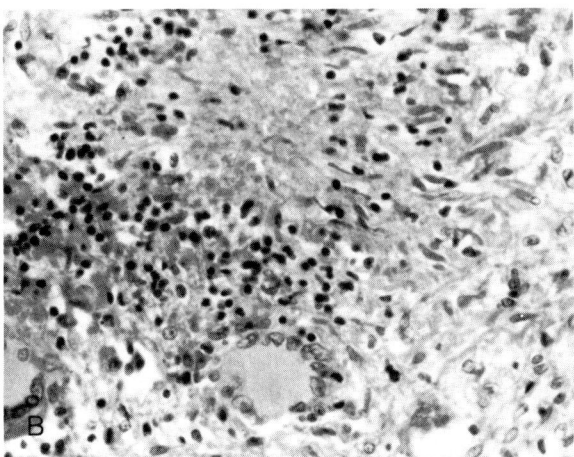

Figure 2–16. *A*, Tuberculous ulcer of the palate in a patient with primary lung disease. *B*, Typical granuloma showing central necrosis (top) and Langhans' giant cells (bottom).

plantation of *M. tuberculosis* from infected sputum may appear on any mucosal surface. The tongue and the palate are favored locations, however (Fig. 2–16). The typical lesion is an indurated, chronic, non-healing ulcer that is usually painful. The causative organism is present in the base of these ulcers, making this a potential infectious hazard to dental personnel, if barrier techniques are not used. Bony involvement of the maxilla and mandible may produce tuberculous osteomyelitis. This most likely follows hematogenous spread of the organism. Pharyngeal involvement results in painful ulcers, and laryngeal lesions may cause dysphagia and voice changes.

Histopathology. The basic microscopic lesion of TB is granulomatous inflammation, in which granulomas show central caseous necrosis. *M. tuberculosis* in tissue incites a characteristic macrophage (histiocyte) response, due, at least in part, to bacterial wall lipids. Focal zones of macrophages become surrounded by lymphocytes and fibroblasts. The macrophages develop abundant eosinophilic cytoplasm, giving them a superficial resemblance to epithelial cells, in which case they are frequently called epithelioid cells. Fusion of macrophages results in the appearance of Langhans' giant cells, in which nuclei are distributed around the periphery of the cytoplasm. As the granulomas age, central necrosis occurs, usually referred to as caseous necrosis because of the gross "cheesy" texture of these zones.

A Ziehl-Neelsen stain must be used to confirm the presence of the organism in the granulomas because several infectious and non-infectious conditions may also produce a similar granulomatous reaction. In the absence of acid-fast bacilli, other microscopic considerations would include syphilis, cat-scratch disease, tularemia, histoplasmosis, blastomycosis, coccidioidomycosis, sarcoidosis, and some foreign body reactions.

Differential Diagnosis. Based on clinical signs and symptoms alone, oral TB cannot be differentiated from several other conditions. A chronic indurated ulcer should prompt the clinician to consider primary syphilis and oral manifestations of deep fungal diseases. Noninfectious processes that should be considered clinically are squamous cell carcinoma and chronic traumatic ulcer. Major aphthae might also be included, although a history of recurrent disease should help separate this condition from the others.

Treatment. Before the advent of effective antibiotics, patients with TB were treated with bed rest and surgery. Chemotherapeutic regimens have now effectively replaced the earlier treatment approaches. Drugs likely to be employed for treatment of TB include isoniazid, rifampin, streptomycin, and ethambutol. Drug combinations are often used, and treatment may be extended as long as 2 years. Oral lesions would be expected to resolve with treatment of the patient's systemic disease.

Patients who convert from a negative to a positive skin test may benefit from prophylactic chemotherapy. This is dependent both upon risk factors involved, such as age and immune status, and upon the opinion of the attending internist.

Leprosy

Etiology and Pathogenesis. Leprosy, also known as Hansen's disease, is a rare infection in the United States but relatively common in other parts of the world, such as southeast Asia, South America, and India. It is caused by an acid-fast bacillus, *Mycobacterium leprae*, that is difficult to grow in culture. Growth has been possible in footpads of mice and in armadillos, both of which exhibit a relatively lower environmental temperature—apparently a requirement for growth of this organism. Leprosy is only moderately contagious, since transmission of the disease requires frequent direct contact with an infected individual over a long period of time. Inoculation through the respiratory tract is also believed to be a potential mode of transmission.

Clinical Features. There is a clinical spectrum of disease that ranges from a limited form (tuberculoid leprosy) to a generalized form (lepromatous leprosy); the latter has a more seriously damaging course. Generally, skin and peripheral nerves are affected. Lesions appear as erythematous plaques or nodules that represent a granulomatous response to the organism. Similar lesions may occur intraorally or intranasally. Damage to peripheral nerves results in anesthesia. In time, severe maxillofacial deformities can appear. Because of nerve dysfunction and anesthesia, the patient's extremities may suffer from trauma, ulceration, and bone resorption.

Histopathology. Microscopically, a granulomatous inflammatory response, in which macrophages and multinucleated giant cells predominate, is usually seen. Infiltration of nerves by mononuclear inflammatory cells is also expected. Acid-fast bacilli can be found within macrophages and are best demonstrated with the Fite stain. Organisms are most numerous in the lepromatous form of leprosy.

Diagnosis. Important for establishing a diagnosis is a history either of contact with a known infected patient or of living in a known endemic area. Signs and symptoms associated with skin and nerves should provide additional clues to the nature of the disease. The appearance of oral lesions without skin lesions seems highly improbable. Biopsy must be done to confirm diagnosis, since there is no laboratory test for leprosy.

Treatment. Current treatment centers around a chemotherapeutic approach in which multiple drugs are used over a period of years. The antileprosy drugs most commonly employed include dapsone, rifampin, and clofazimine.

Actinomycosis

Etiology and Pathogenesis. Actinomycosis is a chronic bacterial disease that, as the name suggests, exhibits some clinical and microscopic features that are fungus-like. It is caused by *Actinomyces israelii*, an anaerobic or microaerophilic, gram-positive bacterium. On rare occasion, other *Actinomyces* species may be involved, or a related aerobic bacterium, *Nocardia asteroides*, may be responsible for a similar clinical picture. *A. israelii* is a normal inhabitant of the oral cavity in a majority of healthy individuals. It is usually found in tonsillar crypts, gingival crevices, carious lesions, and non-vital dental root canals. Actinomycosis is not regarded as a contagious disease, since infection cannot be transmitted from one individual to another. Infections usually appear after trauma, surgery, or previous infection. Tooth extraction, gingival surgery, and oral infections predispose to the development of this condition. Evidence of other important predisposing factors has been slight, although actinomycotic infections have been recorded in osteoradionecrosis of the jaws and in patients with serious systemic illness.

Clinical Features. Most infections by *A. israelii* are seen in the thorax, abdomen, and head and neck and are usually preceded by trauma or direct extension of a contiguous infection. When occurring in the head and neck, the condition is usually designated cervicofacial actinomycosis. It typically presents as a swelling of the mandible that may simulate a pyogenic infection (Fig. 2–17). The lesion may become indurated and eventually form one or more draining sinuses, leading from the medullary spaces of the mandible to the skin of the neck. Less commonly the maxilla may be involved, resulting in an osteomyelitis that may drain through the gingiva. The pus draining from the chronic lesion may contain small yellow granules, known as sulfur granules, that represent aggregates of *A. israelii* organisms. Radiographically, this infection will present as a radiolucency with irregular and ill-defined margins.

Histopathology. A granulomatous inflammatory response with central abscess formation is expected in actinomycosis. In the center of the abscesses, distinctive colonies of organisms (sulfur granules) may be seen. Radiating from the center of the colonies are numerous filaments with clubbed ends.

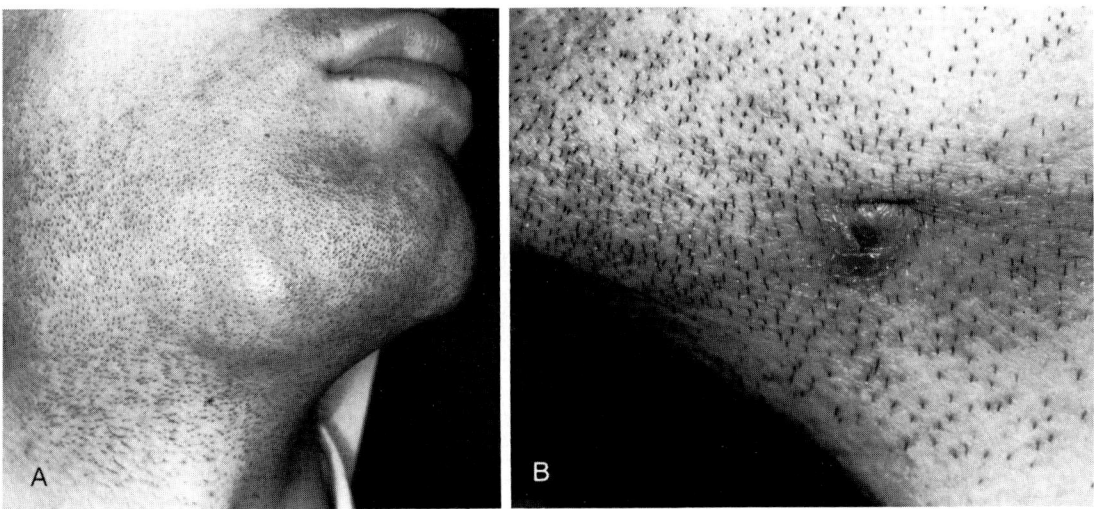

Figure 2-17. *A*, Swelling associated with actinomycosis of the mandible. *B*, Chronic draining sinus tract from mandibular actinomycosis.

Differential Diagnosis. Clinically, actinomycosis may have to be differentiated from osteomyelitis caused by other bacterial or fungal organisms. Infections of the soft tissue of the neck, such as scrofula and *Staphylococcus* infections, may also be considered.

Definitive diagnosis is dependent upon identification of the actinomycotic organism. This may be done through direct examination of exudate, microscopic evaluation of tissue sections, or microbiologic culture of pathologic material.

Treatment. Long-term, high-dose penicillin is the required antibiotic regimen for this disease. Intravenous penicillin (10 to 20 million units per day for 4 to 6 weeks) followed by oral penicillin (4 to 6 gm per day for a period of weeks or months) is a standard regimen for actinomycosis. Tetracycline and erythromycin have also been used to effect cures. Additionally, drainage of abscesses and surgical excision of scar and sinus tracts is recommended to aerate tissue and to enhance penetration of antibiotics.

Noma

Etiology and Pathogenesis. Noma, also known as cancrum oris and gangrenous stomatitis, is a rare disease of childhood that is characterized by a destructive process of orofacial tissues. Necrosis of tissue occurs as a consequence of invasion by anaerobic bacteria (fusiform bacilli and Vincent's spirochetes) in a host whose systemic health is significantly compromised. Malnutrition is the most frequently cited predisposing factor, although debilitation from systemic disease, such as pneumonia or sepsis, has been described. The mechanism by which predisposing factors allow the microorganisms to become virulent pathogens is not understood.

Noma shares many features with the more limited and more benign acute necrotizing ulcerative gingivitis (ANUG or Vincent's infection). Both are caused by the same organisms, both require compromised hosts, and both result in tissue necrosis.

Noma is rarely seen in the United States. It is typically found in relatively underdeveloped countries, especially those in which malnutrition or protein-deficient states are prevalent.

Clinical Features. The initial lesion of noma is a painful ulceration, usually of the gingiva or buccal mucosa, that spreads rapidly and eventually necrotizes (Fig. 2-18). Denudation of the involved bone may follow, eventually leading to necrosis and sequestration. Teeth in the affected area may become loose and may exfoliate. Penetration of organisms into the cheek, lip, or palate may also occur, resulting in fetid necrotic lesions. Before antibiotics were developed, fatalities from this disease were common.

Treatment. Therapy involves treating the underlying predisposing condition as well as the infection itself. Therefore, fluids, electrolytes, and general nutrition are restored, along with the introduction of antibiotics (usually

42   ULCERATIVE CONDITIONS

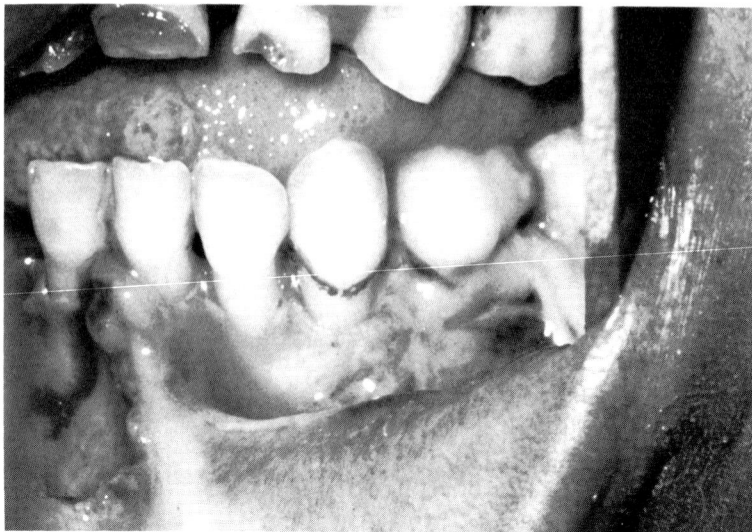

Figure 2–18. Noma involving mandibular gingiva. Tissue is necrotic, resulting in exposure of mandibular bone.

penicillin). Débridement of necrotic tissue may also be beneficial if there is extensive destruction.

FUNGAL DISEASES

Deep Fungal Diseases

Etiology and Pathogenesis. This group of fungal diseases is characterized by primary involvement of the lung. Infections may potentially disseminate from this primary focus to involve other organ systems. Clinically, infections often mimic TB, relative to primary and secondary or reactivated disease.

The deep fungal infections having a significant incidence of oral expression include histoplasmosis, coccidioidomycosis, blastomycosis, and cryptococcosis (Table 2–1). Oral infections will typically follow implantation of oral mucous membranes by infected sputum. Oral infections may also follow hematogenous spread of fungus from a lung focus.

Histoplasmosis is endemic in the midwestern United States, although worldwide in distribution. Inhalation of yeasts from dust of dried pigeon droppings is regarded as a frequent source of infection. Coccidioidomycosis, on the other hand, is endemic in the West, especially in the San Joaquin Valley of California, where it has become known as valley fever. Blastomycosis is usually seen in North America, especially in the Ohio–Mississippi River basin area. *Cryptococcus* infections may be transmitted through inhalation of avian excrement. *Cryptococcus* also may be seen in immunocompromised patients.

Clinical Features. The initial signs and symptoms of deep fungal infections are usually related to lung involvement and include cough, fever, night sweats, weight loss, chest pain, and hemoptysis. Occasionally, a skin eruption of erythema multiforme appears concomitantly with coccidioidomycosis.

Oral lesions are usually preceded by pulmonary infection. Primary involvement of oral mucous membranes is generally regarded as a highly unlikely route of infection. Swallowed infected sputum may potentially cause oral or gastrointestinal lesions. Also, erosion into pulmonary blood vessels by the inflammatory process may result in hematogenous spread to almost any organ. The usual oral lesion is ulcerative in nature (Fig. 2–19). Whether single or multiple, lesions are non-healing, indurated, and frequently painful. Purulence may be an additional feature of blastomycotic lesions.

Histopathology. The basic inflammatory response to deep fungi is granulomatous in nature. In the presence of these microorganisms, macrophages and multinucleated giant cells dominate the histologic picture (Figs. 2–20 and 2–21). Purulence may be a feature of blastomycosis and, less likely, coccidioidomycosis and cryptococcosis. Peculiar to blastomycosis is pseudoepitheliomatous hyperplasia, associated with superficial infections in which ulceration has not yet occurred.

Differential Diagnosis. Clinically, the chronic, non-healing oral ulcers caused by deep fungal infections may be similiar to those of oral squamous cell carcinoma, chronic trauma, oral TB, and primary syphilis. Blastomycosis may also produce a clinical picture

Table 2–1. FEATURES OF DEEP FUNGAL INFECTIONS

	Organism	Pathogenesis	Symptoms	Primary site	Oral lesions	Microscopy	Treatment
Histoplasmosis	*Histoplasma capsulatum*	Inhalation of spores in dust of bird excrement, endemic in midwestern US	Cough, fever, night sweats, weight loss	Lung, may be asymptomatic	Chronic, non-healing ulcer(s), secondary to lung disease	Granulomatous reaction, 2–4 μm yeasts	Amphotericin B, ketoconazole
Coccidioidomycosis	*Coccidioides immitis*	Inhalation of spores, endemic in western US	Cough, fever, weight loss, chest pain, erythema multiforme	Lung, may be asymptomatic	Chronic, non-healing ulcer(s), secondary to lung disease	Granulomatous reaction, 20–60 μm spherules with endospores	Amphotericin B, ketoconazole
Blastomycosis	*Blastomyces dermatitidis*	Inhalation of spores, N. American distribution	Fever, weight loss, night sweats	Lung, some asymptomatic	Chronic, non-healing ulcers, draining sinus, secondary to lung disease	Granulomatous reaction, 5–20 μm budding yeasts	Amphotericin B, ketoconazole
Cryptococcosis	*Cryptococcus neoformans*	Inhalation of spores, pigeons are carriers	Cough, hemoptysis, headache	Lung, some asymptomatic	Chronic, non-healing ulcer(s), secondary to lung disease	Granulomatous reaction, 5–20 μm yeasts	Amphotericin B, flucytosine

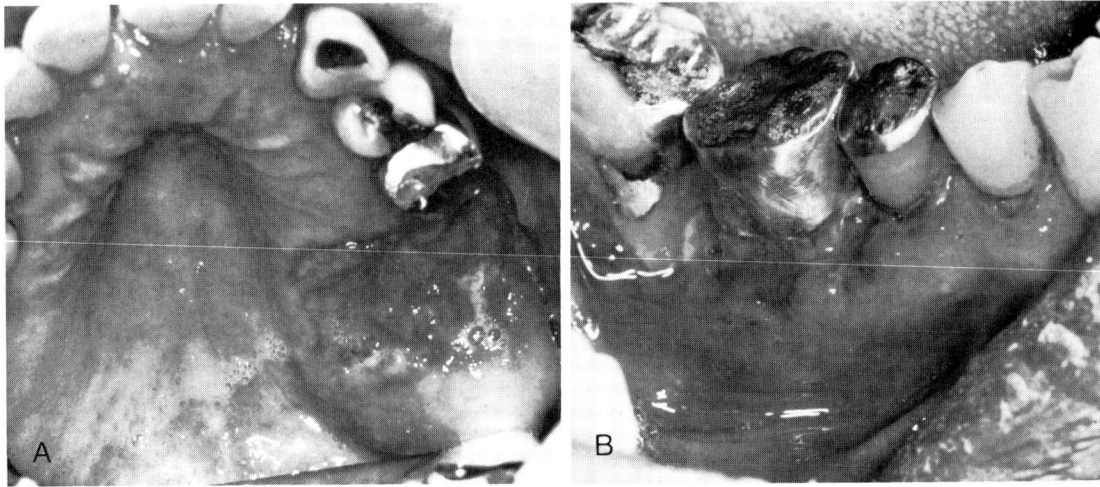

Figure 2–19. *A* and *B*, Palatal and gingival ulcers of oral histoplasmosis.

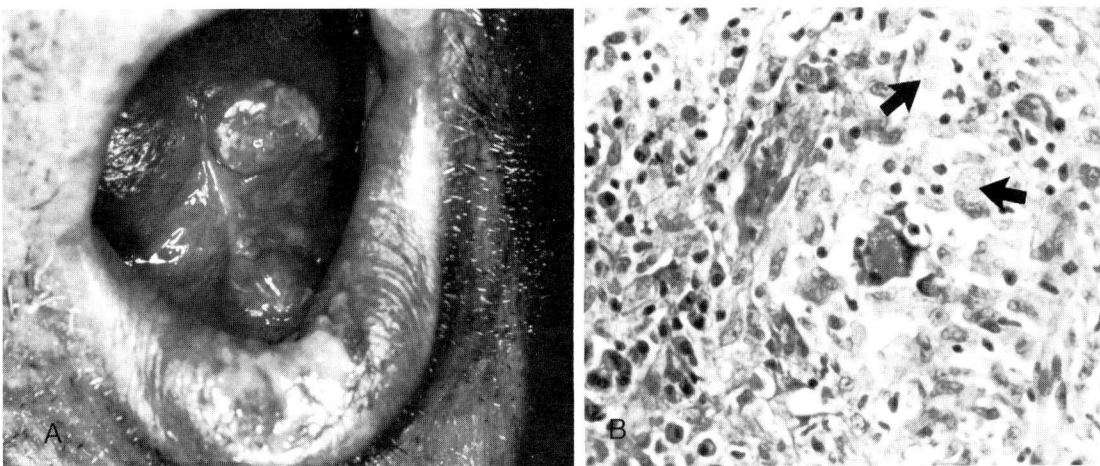

Figure 2–20. *A*, Histoplasmosis of lip and tongue. *B*, Granulomatous inflammation showing tiny *Histoplasma capsulatum* organisms within phagocytic cells (arrows). (Courtesy of Dr. R. Millard.)

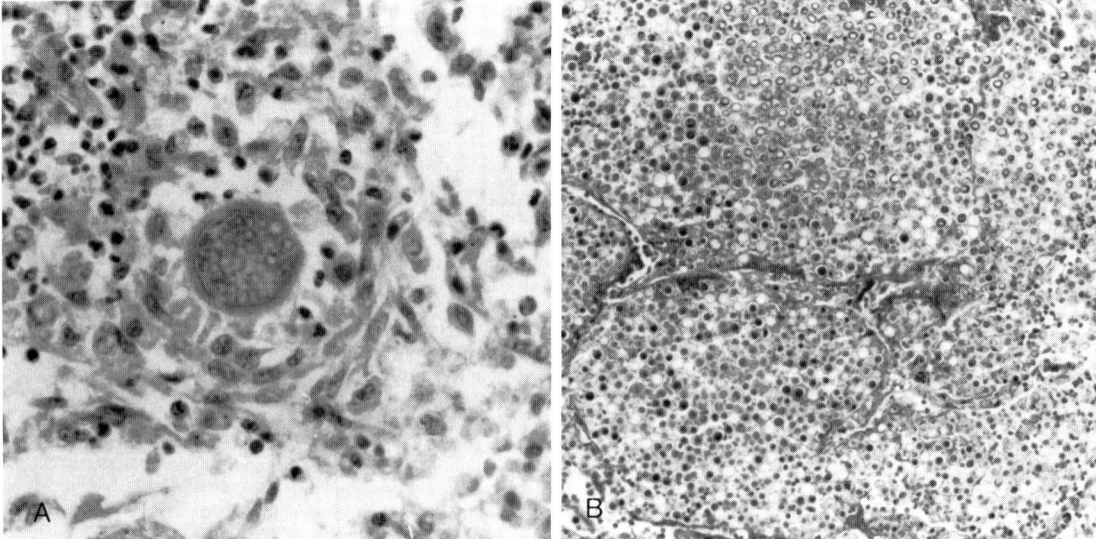

Figure 2–21. *A*, Spherule with endospores of coccidioidomycosis in a granulomatous focus. *B*, Blastomycotic organisms filling lung alveoli.

that simulates cervicofacial actinomycosis. Culture of organisms from lesions or microscopic identification of organisms in biopsy tissue is required to establish definitive diagnosis. Skin tests and serologic tests are generally of little value in the diagnosis of deep fungal infections.

Treatment. Treatment of deep mycotic infections is generally chemotherapeutic. Surgical resection or incision and drainage may occasionally be used to enhance drug effects in treating some necrotic lung infections. Amphotericin B is the drug of choice, although this may be supported or replaced by ketoconazole or flucytosine.

Subcutaneous Fungal Diseases—Sporotrichosis

Etiology and Pathogenesis. Some fungal infections affect primarily subcutaneous tissues. One of these, sporotrichosis, is of significance because it may have oral manifestations. It is caused by *Sporothrix schenckii* and results from inoculation of the skin or mucosa by contaminated soil or thorny plants. After an incubation period of several weeks, subcutaneous nodules that frequently become ulcerated develop. Systemic involvement is rare but may be seen in individuals with defective or suppressed immune responses.

Clinical Features. Lesions appear at the site of inoculation and spread along lymphatic channels. On the skin, red nodules appear with subsequent breakdown, exudate production, and ulceration. Orally, lesions typically present as non-specific chronic ulcers. Lymphadenopathy may also develop.

Histopathology. The inflammatory response to *S. schenckii* is basically granulomatous in nature. Central abscesses may be found in some of the granulomas, and overlying epithelium may exhibit pseudoepitheliomatous hyperplasia. The relatively small, round to oval fungus may be seen in tissue sections.

Diagnosis. Definitive diagnosis is based on culture of infected tissue on Sabouraud's agar. Special silver stains may also be used to identify the organism in tissue biopsies.

Treatment. Sporotrichosis is usually treated with a solution of potassium iodide. In cases of toxicity or allergy to iodides, ketoconazole has been used with limited success. Generally, patients respond well to treatment, with little morbidity developing.

Opportunistic Fungal Infections—Phycomycosis

Etiology and Pathogenesis. "Phycomycosis," also known as mucormycosis, is a generic term that includes fungal infections caused by the genera *Mucor, Rhizopus,* and occasionally others. Organisms of this family of fungi, which normally are found in bread mold or decaying fruit and vegetables, are opportunistic, infecting humans when systemic health is compromised. Infections typically occur in poorly controlled ketoacidotic diabetics, immunosuppressed transplant patients, patients with advanced malignancies, patients being treated with steroids or radiation, or patients who are immunodepressed for any other reason.

Route of infection is through either the gastrointestinal tract or the respiratory tract. Infections may potentially occur anywhere along these routes.

Clinical Features. In the head and neck, lesions are most likely to occur in the nasal cavity, paranasal sinuses, and possibly the oropharynx. Pain and swelling precede ulceration. Tissue necrosis may result in perforation of the palate (Fig. 2–22). Extension into the orbit or brain is a common complication. The fungus has a propensity for arterial walls, where invasion may lead to hematogenous spread, thrombosis, or infarction.

Histopathology. Microscopically, an acute and chronic inflammatory infiltrate is seen in response to the fungus. The organism is usually readily identified in hematoxylin and eosin (H&E) sections in areas of tissue necrosis. Fungus in necrotic vessel walls in which thrombi may be evident is characteristic. Microscopically, the fungus appears as large, pale-staining, non-septate hyphae that tend to branch at right angles.

Differential Diagnosis. It is important for the clinician to recognize that phycomycosis represents one of several opportunistic organisms that may infect an immunocompromised host. Necrotic lesions of the nasal and paranasal sinuses should raise the suspicion of this type of infection. Confirmation must be made by identification of the fungus in biopsy tissue, exudates, or cultures. Because of the severity of underlying disease and the often rapid course that this organism may precipitate, diagnosis of phycomycosis may not be made until after death.

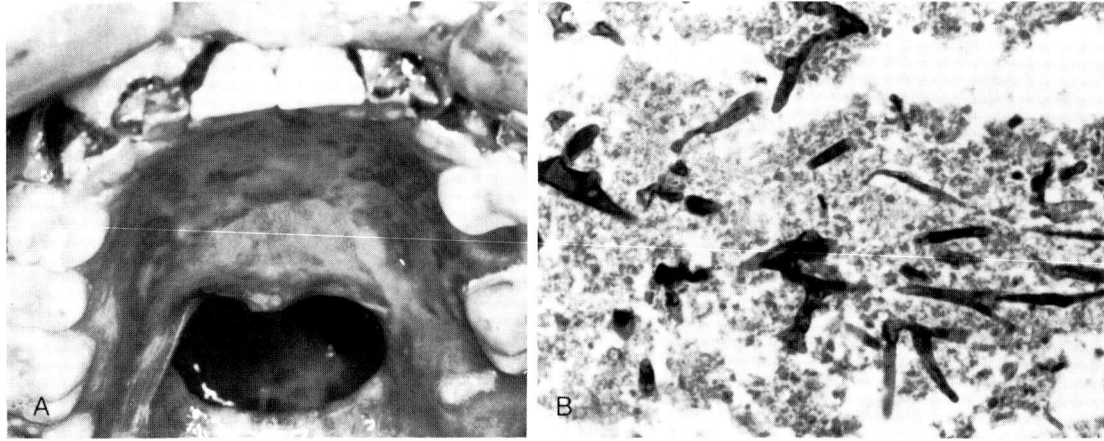

Figure 2–22. *A,* Perforation of palate in diabetic patient with phycomycosis. (Courtesy of Dr. J. Knapp.) *B,* Fungal hyphae in necrotic focus.

Perforating palatal lesions are rather rare but may be seen in association with other diseases. Inflammatory lesions would include gummatous necrosis of tertiary syphilis, midline granuloma, and Wegener's granulomatosis. Rarely, malignancies of nasal and sinus origin (squamous cell carcinoma and salivary gland adenocarcinoma) may present through the palate. Biopsy is required to differentiate these lesions.

Treatment. Amphotericin B is the drug of choice for treatment of phycomycosis. Surgical débridement of the upper respiratory lesions is also often required. Prognosis is generally dependent upon the severity of underlying disease and the institution of appropriate therapy. Death is a relatively frequent consequence of this infection. Generally, lung infections are more likely than upper respiratory infections to be lethal.

CONDITIONS ASSOCIATED WITH IMMUNOLOGIC DYSFUNCTION

Aphthous Ulcers

Of all types of non-traumatic ulceration that affect mucous membranes, aphthous ulcers are probably the most common. Incidence ranges from 20 to 60% depending upon the population studied. Prevalence tends to be higher in professional persons and those in upper socioeconomic groups.

Etiology and Pathogenesis. Although the cause of aphthous ulcerations is unknown, several etiologic factors have been identified.

Immunologic Factors. The most promising avenue of investigation has been in immunology. Although somewhat conflicting, evidence has been presented that implicates a defect in the humoral immune system. Autoantibodies to oral mucous membranes have been demonstrated in patients with aphthous ulcers. These antibodies, however, react with prickle cells rather than with basal cells as would be expected, and they also cross-react with other epithelia where aphthous ulcers do not occur.

Since some investigators believe that circulating immune complexes may be responsible for observed early extravasation of erythrocytes and infiltration of neutrophils in aphthous lesions, an immune-complex vasculitis has been postulated as a cause of this disease. In this theory, neutrophils responding to antigen-antibody complexes and complement in vessel walls release cytoplasmic enzymes, leading to destruction of overlying epithelium. This concept, which is analogous to leukocytoclastic vasculitis, is based on the presence of neutrophils early in this disease, a finding that has not been universally observed.

The most important immunologic findings have indicated that patients with this disease may have a defect in their cell-mediated immune response. Helper/inducer (T4) lymphocytes are seen focally in the very early stages of the disease and, as such, are implicated as mediators. Basal cells in the area also express HLA-DR antigens early, suggesting a role for these cells as well. Since HLA-DR antigens are required for antigen presentation to immunocompetent cells, it could be speculated that these cells are presenting autoantigens to the infiltrating T4 cells, leading to eventual basal cell destruction.

In vitro tests that measure T cell sensitization to antigen have been done in affected patients.

Lymphocyte blast transformation studies have shown that when lymphocytes from affected patients are incubated with mucosal homogenates, blast transformation occurs. Another *in vitro* test, leukocyte migration inhibition, also produces positive results in aphthous patients. T lymphocytes from aphthous patients have also been shown to be cytotoxic to cultured gingival epithelial cells but not to other epithelial cells. Further, patient T lymphocytes show increased antibody-dependent cellular cytotoxicity.

From these studies, even though some of the evidence has been conflicting, it appears likely that aphthous ulcers result from a focal immune dysfunction in which T lymphocytes play a significant role. The nature of the initiating stimulus remains a mystery. The causative agent could be endogenous (autoimmune) antigen or exogenous (hyperimmune) antigen, or it could be a non-specific factor, such as trauma in which chemical mediators may be involved.

Microbiologic Factors. Investigation into other possible causative factors has generally been unproductive. Because of the clinical similarity of oral aphthous ulcers to secondary HSV infections, a viral etiology has been extensively investigated. The only supportive evidence has come from occasional isolation of adenovirus and HSV-I from some lesions, and the detection of part of the herpesvirus genome in peripheral mononuclear cells in some affected patients. Hypersensitivity to bacterial antigens on *Streptococcus sanguis* organisms and others was felt to be a likely cause of aphthous ulcers. This was based on isolation of organisms from ulcers, delayed hypersensitivity reaction with skin testing, and induced leukocyte migration inhibition. However, because the bacteria can be found in normal individuals, and because they do not cause lymphocyte blast transformation, this theory has generally been discarded.

Nutritional Factors. Deficiencies of vitamin B_{12}, folic acid, and iron as measured in serum have been found in a small percentage of patients with aphthous ulcers. Correction of these deficiencies has produced improvement or cures in this small group of patients. However, the etiologic significance of this finding has been questioned because of the absence of uniform serum abnormalities, the absence of malabsorption symptoms, and the general absence of clinical improvement when these items are added to the diet of aphthous patients.

Other Factors. Other causes of aphthous ulcers that have been investigated include hormonal alterations, stress, trauma, and food allergies to substances in nuts, chocolate, and gluten. None of these is seriously regarded as being important in the primary causation of aphthous ulcers, although any of them may have a modifying or triggering role.

Clinical Features. Three forms of aphthous ulcers have been recognized: minor, major, and herpetiform aphthous ulcers (Table 2–2). All are believed to be part of the same disease spectrum, and all are believed to have a common etiology. Differences are essentially clinical and correspond to degree of severity. All forms present as painful recurrent ulcers. Occasionally patients have prodromal symptoms of tingling or burning prior to the appearance of the lesions. The ulcers are not preceded by vesicles and characteristically appear on vestibular and buccal mucosa, tongue, soft palate, fauces, and floor of the mouth. Only rarely do these lesions occur on attached gingiva and hard palate, thus providing an important clinical sign for the separation of aphthous ulcers from secondary herpetic ulcers.

Minor Aphthous Ulcers. This is the most commonly encountered form of aphthous ulcers. It usually appears as a single, painful, oval ulcer, less than 1.0 cm in size, that is covered by a yellow fibrinous membrane and surrounded by an erythematous halo (Fig. 2–23). Multiple oral aphthae may occasionally be seen (Fig. 2–24). When the lateral or ventral surfaces of the tongue are affected, pain tends to be out of proportion to the size of the lesion. The minor aphthous ulcer generally lasts 7 to 10 days and heals without scar formation. Recurrences vary from one individual to another. Periods of freedom from disease may range from a matter of weeks to as long as years.

Major Aphthous Ulcers. This form was previously thought to be a separate entity and was referred to as periadenitis mucosa necrotica recurrens (PMNR), or Sutton's disease. It is now regarded as the most severe expression of aphthous stomatitis. Lesions are larger and more painful and persist longer than minor aphthae. Because of the depth of inflammation, major aphthous ulcers appear crateriform clinically and heal with scar (Fig. 2–25). Lesions may take as long as 6 weeks to heal, and as soon as one ulcer disappears, another one starts. In patients who experience an unremitting course with significant pain and discomfort, systemic health may be compromised

48 ULCERATIVE CONDITIONS

Table 2–2. FEATURES OF THE VARIOUS FORMS OF APHTHOUS ULCERS

Feature	Minor	Major	Herpetiform	Behçet's
Etiology	Immunologic defect	Immunologic defect	Immunologic defect	Immunologic defect, ?vasculitis
Area affected	All areas except gingiva; hard palate, and vermilion	All areas except gingiva, hard palate, and vermilion	Any intraoral area	All areas except gingiva, hard palate, and vermilion
Number of ulcers	Usually one	Several	Multiple (crops)	Few
Clinical appearance	Oval ulcer less than 1 cm	Oval, ragged ulcers, 0.5–2 cm, crateriform, several weeks' duration	Small ulcers in crops	Oval ulcers less than 1 cm
Vesicles preceding ulcers?	No	No	No	No
Extraoral sites	No	No	No	Yes—genitals, eyes
Treatment	None; symptomatic, topical steroids	Topical or systemic steroids	Topical or systemic steroids	Systemic steroids, immunosuppressives

because of difficulty in eating and psychologic stress. The predilection for movable oral mucosa is as typical for major aphthous ulcers as it is for minor aphthae (Fig. 2–26).

Herpetiform Aphthous Ulcers. This form of the disease presents clinically as recurrent crops of small ulcers (Fig. 2–27). Although movable mucosa is predominantly affected, palatal and gingival mucosa may also be involved. Pain may be considerable and healing generally occurs in 1 to 2 weeks. Unlike herpetic infections, herpetiform aphthous ulcers are not preceded by vesicles and exhibit no virus-infected cells. Other than the clinical feature of crops of oral ulcers, there has been no finding that can link this disease to a viral infection.

Histopathology. It is generally accepted that important clues to the etiology and pathogenesis may be found during the early stages in the development of oral aphthous ulcers. Because these ulcers are usually clinically diagnosed, biopsies are unnecessary and rarely done, resulting in the relatively limited availability of histopathologic material. Prospective studies have shown, however, that mononuclear cells are found submucosally and perivascularly in the pre-ulcerative stage. These cells are predominantly T4 lymphocytes that are soon outnumbered by T8 lymphocytes as the ulcerative stage develops. Macrophages and mast cells are also common inhabitants of the ulcer base. Extravasated erythrocytes and neutrophils have been described in the early

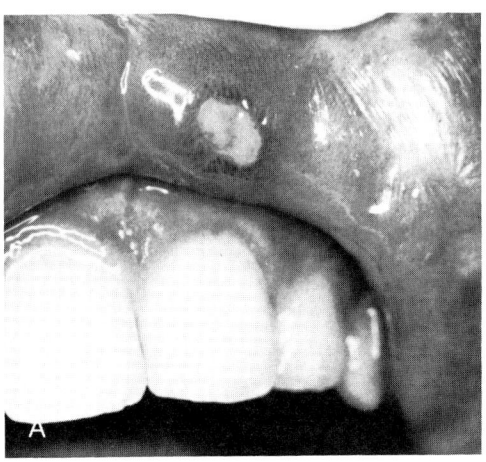 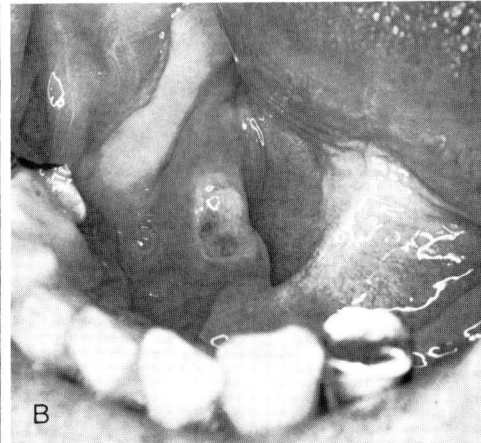

Figure 2–23. *A* and *B*, Minor aphthous ulcers.

ULCERATIVE CONDITIONS   49

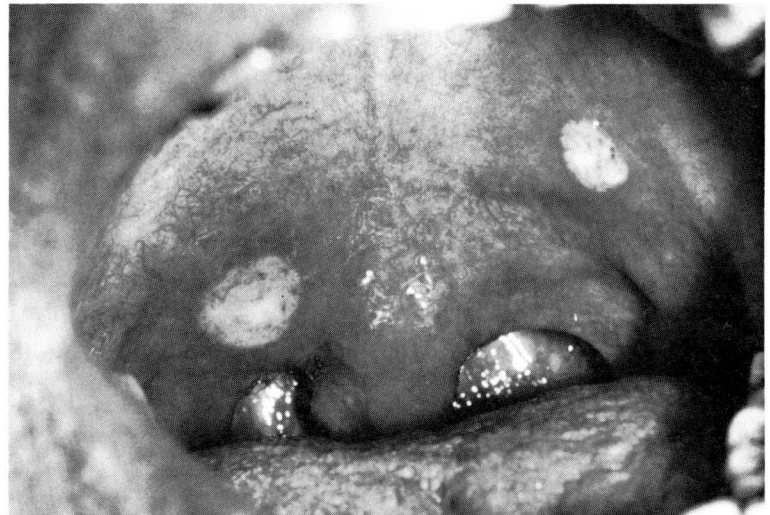

Figure 2–24. Multiple minor aphthae of soft palate.

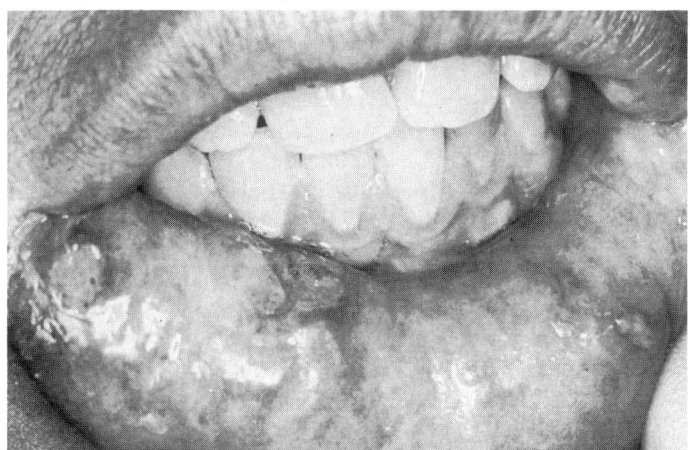

Figure 2–25. Major aphthous ulcers. Residual scars are apparent.

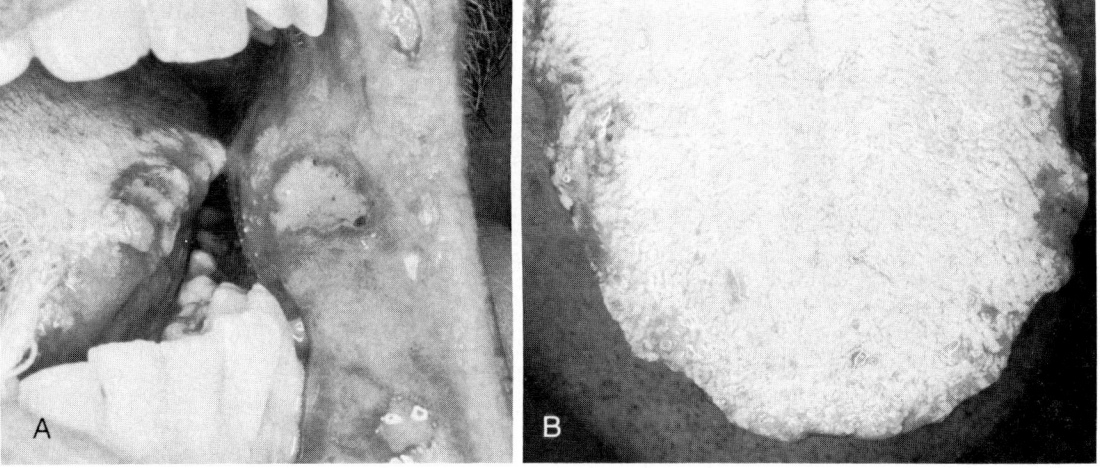

Figure 2–26. *A* and *B*, Major aphthous stomatitis.

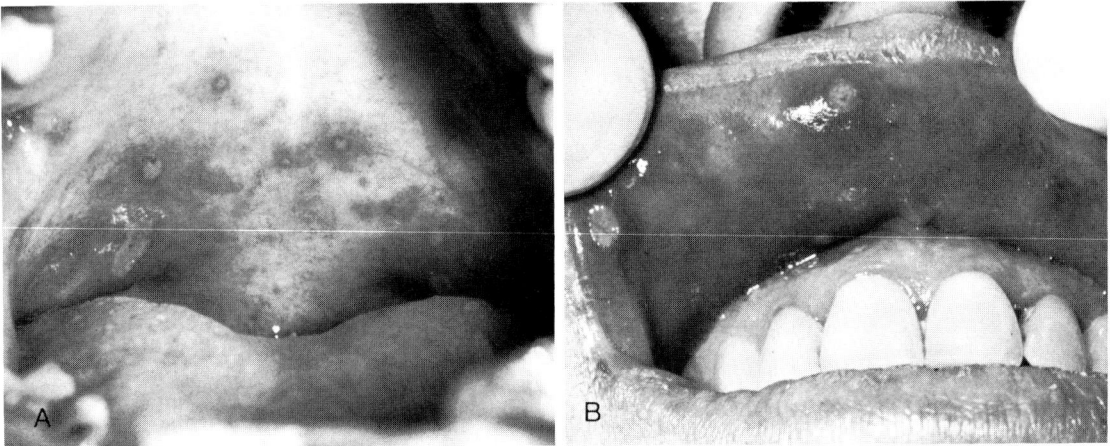

Figure 2–27. *A* and *B*, Herpetiform aphthous stomatitis.

stages of these lesions, lending support for an immune-complex vasculitis etiology.

There are no microscopic diagnostic features of aphthous ulcers. At no time are virus-infected cells evident. Essentially, the same microscopic changes are found in all forms of aphthous ulcers, and all features support an immunologically mediated disease.

Differential Diagnosis. Diagnosis of aphthous ulcers is generally based on history and clinical appearance. Secondary (recurrent) oral herpes is often confused with aphthous ulcers but can usually be distinguished from it. History of vesicles preceding ulcers, location on hard gingiva and hard palate, and crops of lesions indicate herpes rather than aphthous ulcers. Cytologic smears containing virus-infected epithelial cells confirm herpesvirus infection. Cytologic examination of aphthous ulcers results in non-specific findings. Other painful oral ulcerative conditions that may simulate the various forms of aphthous ulcers include trauma, pemphigus vulgaris, cicatricial pemphigoid, and oral expression of a systemic problem, such as Crohn's disease, neutropenia, and sprue.

Treatment. In patients with occasional or few minor aphthous ulcers usually no treatment is needed or sought because of the relatively minor discomfort. Also, a simple, inexpensive, and uniformly effective treatment is not available. However, when patients are more severely affected, some forms of treatment can provide significant control of (but not necessarily cure) this disease. The number of remedies and over-the-counter agents used to treat aphthous ulcers rivals the number used for the treatment of secondary herpetic infections. While some of these are occasionally effective, the rationale for their use is often obscure.

Because aphthous ulcers are most likely related to an immunologic defect, treatment logically includes drugs that can manipulate or regulate immune responses. In this category, corticosteroids currently offer the best chance for disease containment. In severely affected patients, systemic steroids may be used, but in patients with mild to moderate disease, only topical therapy appears justified.

Systemic Steroids. Systemic steroids are appropriate for severe disease but should not be used unless the clinician has experience in this treatment area or is working with a knowledgeable consultant. The systemic effects and complications of glucocorticoids are numerous and can often be profound (Table 2–3).

For immediate control of severe aphthous stomatitis, a low to moderate dose of prednisone over a short period of time is recommended. A typical regimen might be 20 to 40 mg daily for 1 week followed by another week at half the initial dose. Since the adrenals normally secrete most of their daily equivalent of 5 to 7 mg in the morning, all the prednisone should be taken in one bolus early in the morning to simulate the physiologic process and thus minimize interference with the pituitary-adrenal axis and to minimize side effects. It is generally agreed that a slow steroid taper is not necessary if treatment lasts for less than 4 weeks, since adrenal suppression is likely to be minimal.

In patients requiring higher-dose, prolonged, or maintenance steroid therapy, an alternate-day regimen may be used after initial daily therapy. A short-acting steroid (24 to 36 hours), such as prednisone, is desired because

Table 2-3. SYSTEMIC EFFECTS AND SIDE EFFECTS OF GLUCOCORTICOID THERAPY

Effect	Side Effect
Anti-inflammatory by stabilization of biologic membranes and capillaries	Therapeutic
Immunosuppression via lymphocytopenia and monocytopenia	Therapeutic, aggravation of TB and other infections, delayed wound healing
Gluconeogenesis from protein and fat breakdown	Aggravation of diabetes, muscle weakness, osteoporosis
Altered fat metabolism with redistribution in response to protein loss	Buffalo hump, hyperlipidemia
Fluid retention from Na resorption and K excretion	Moon face, weight gain
Potentiation of vasopressors	Blood pressure elevation, aggravation of congestion, heart failure
?Increased gastric secretions	Aggravation of peptic ulcer
Suppression of pituitary-adrenal axis	Adrenal atrophy
CNS effects	Psychologic changes
Ocular effects	Cataracts, glaucoma

it allows recovery or near-normal functioning of the pituitary-adrenal axis on the "off" (no prednisone) days. Additionally, the prednisone tissue effects outlast the ACTH suppression.

Topical Steroids. Topical steroids, if used judiciously, can be relatively efficacious and safe in the treatment of mild to moderate disease. Although nearly all topical compounds have been developed for use on the skin, it appears to be standard practice to prescribe these agents also for use on mucous membranes. The science of topical steroid use in dentistry is relatively primitive when compared with use in dermatology. It has not been established for mucosal diseases whether more potent topical compounds are significantly more effective than less potent topical compounds, or whether more frequent application is more effective than less frequent application. Optimal vehicles for intraoral use of steroids have also not been determined. Currently, empirical judgment is used to decide what type and strength of topical steroid to prescribe.

A number of factors determine the efficacy of a topical steroid. Intrinsic drug potency is significantly enhanced by halogenation of the parent compound, cortisol. Esterification makes it more lipophilic, providing greater penetrability. Increasing drug concentration can improve clinical efficacy, but there are limits beyond which no further gain is noted. For dermatologic use, ointments are probably the most effective because of their occlusive properties. Intraorally, ointments are not very useful because of their inability to adhere to mucous membranes. Creams and gels have received greater acceptance because they are more easily applied. Gels may, however, cause burning upon application in some patients because of the alcohols used in their formulation. It should be noted that there is one vehicle, Orabase (Colgate-Hoyt), that has been developed for oral use. It has, however, received only modest acceptance by clinicians and patients.

Commercially available topical steroids have been ranked in order of potency based on vasoconstriction assay and clinical trials by Cornell and Stoughton (1984). Table 2-4 is a reduced and modified version that should provide a rational basis for choosing an intraoral agent.

Numerous side effects of topical steroids have been recorded following prolonged or intense dermatologic use (Table 2-5). Most important are the suppression of the pituitary-adrenal axis (as indicated by decreasing plasma cortisol) and Cushing's syndrome due to systemic steroid absorption. Other local skin effects include striae, atrophy, hypopigmentation, telangiectasia, induced acne, and folliculitis. Generally, the focal changes are difficult to assess and discern intraorally and are relatively insignificant. Systemic absorption, however, may be a concern if high-potency topical steroids are used liberally for extended periods.

Since only a relatively small amount of topical steroid is needed to cover most oral lesions, it is unlikely that significant systemic effects will occur with judicious intraoral use over short periods of time. Used over a 2- to 4-week period, 15 gm of topical steroid should provide sufficient therapeutic effect for most oral ulcers (especially aphthous ulcers) without risk to the patient.

Antibiotics. Antibiotics (especially tetracycline oral suspension) have been used in the treatment of aphthous ulcers, with fair to good results. The effects are predominantly topical and are most likely related to the elimination

Table 2–4. POTENCY RANKING OF TOPICAL STEROIDS*	
Brand name	Generic name
1. Temovate cream 0.05%	Clobetasol propionate
2. Halog cream 0.1%	Halcinonide
Lidex cream 0.05%	Fluocinonide
Topicort cream 0.25%	Desoximetasone
Lidex gel 0.05%	Fluocinonide
3. Aristocort cream-HP 0.5%	Triamcinolone acetonide
Diprosone cream 0.05%	Betamethasone dipropionate
Florone cream 0.05%	Diflorasone diacetate
Maxiflor cream 0.05%	Diflorasone diacetate
4. Synalar cream-HP 0.2%	Fluocinolone acetonide
Topicort-LP cream 0.05%	Desoximetasone
5. Benisone cream 0.025%	Betamethasone benzoate
Cordran cream 0.025%	Flurandrenolide
Kenalog cream 0.1%	Triamcinolone acetonide
Locoid cream 0.1%	Hydrocortisone butyrate
Synalar cream 0.025%	Fluocinolone acetonide
Valisone cream 0.1%	Betamethasone valerate
Westcort cream 0.2%	
6. Tridesilon cream 0.05%	Desonide
Locorten cream 0.03%	Flumethasone pivalate
7.	Hydrocortisone 1%

*Potency decreases from 1 to 7. Within each group, steroids are of approximately equal potency.
Modified from Cornell R. Stoughton R. The use of topical steroids in psoriasis. Dermatol Clin 2:397–409, 1984.

of secondary bacterial infection of the ulcers. Many clinicians have noted that the combination of tetracycline oral suspension, nystatin oral suspension, and diphenhydramine hydrochloride (Benadryl) elixir often provides more clinical benefit than any of these agents used alone. In this case, the nystatin is probably eliminating secondary *Candida albicans* overgrowth and the diphenhydramine hydrochloride is probably providing a sedative effect. There are numerous variations of this formula that are centered around tetracycline that probably also provide similar good though inconsistent results.

Table 2–5. SIDE EFFECTS OF TOPICAL CORTICOSTEROIDS
Systemic
Suppression of pituitary-adrenal axis
Iatrogenic Cushing's syndrome
Local (skin)
Striae
Atrophy
Hypopigmentation
Telangiectasia
Induced acne
Folliculitis
Candidiasis

The recent introduction of an oral rinse containing chlorhexidine gluconate 0.12% (Peridex [Procter and Gamble]) has been used empirically in this clinical situation with some success. The mechanism allowing for clinical improvement is perhaps related to diminishing the oral bacterial flora load and possibly to the binding to free nerve endings and epithelial cells.

Other Drugs. Two groups of compounds that have immunomodulating effects are the vitamin A derivatives (retinoids). While there is a rational basis for use in aphthous patients, clinical testing has not been done, leaving this, as yet, in the realm of clinical research. Other immunosuppressive drugs, because of their rather profound side effects, are generally not justified for the routine treatment of aphthous ulcers.

Another group of untested drugs include anti-inflammatory agents, such as sulfones and sulfonamides, that alter neutrophil function. If neutrophils are important in the pathogenesis of aphthous ulcers, these drugs may be clinically significant.

In summary, the treatment of aphthous ulcers is somewhat empirical, with no single agent or method being uniformly successful. Current rational treatment centers around the use of steroids or a tetracycline/nystatin–based solution. Although permanent cures are difficult to effect, significant control may be achieved with one of the therapeutic agents discussed here.

Behçet's Syndrome

Etiology. The cause of this condition is basically unknown, although the underlying disease mechanism may be very similar to the one associated with aphthous ulcers. In Behçet's syndrome, there may be a genetic predisposition as well. Also, some indirect evidence has been presented that suggests a viral etiology.

Clinical Features. The lesions of this syndrome typically affect the oral cavity, the eye, and the genitalia (Fig. 2–28). Other regions or systems are less commonly involved. Recurrent arthritis of the wrists, ankles, and knees may be seen. Cardiovascular manifestations are usually of a thrombotic type, and neurologic manifestations are frequently in the form of headaches.

Oral manifestations of this syndrome appear identical to the ulcers of aphthous stomatitis. The ulcers are usually of the minor aphthous type and are found in the typical aphthous distribution.

Ocular changes are found in most Behçet's patients. Uveitis, conjunctivitis, and retinitis are among the more common inflammatory processes.

Genital lesions are ulcerative in nature and may be the cause of significant pain and discomfort. Painful ulcerative lesions may also occur around the anus. Inflammatory bowel disease has been described in some patients.

Histopathology. T lymphocytes are prominent in the ulcerative lesions of Behçet's syndrome. However, neutrophilic infiltrates in which the cells appear within vessel walls have also been described. Some believe that these changes are representative of a leukocytoclastic vasculitis. Immunopathologic support of a vascular target in this condition comes from the demonstration of immunoglobulins and complement in the vessel walls.

Diagnosis. The diagnosis of Behçet's syndrome is based on clinical signs and symptoms from the various regions described above. Biopsy and laboratory tests all produce nonspecific results.

Treatment. Systemic steroids are usually prescribed for the treatment of Behçet's syndrome. Immunosuppressive drugs, such as chlorambucil and azathioprine, may be used instead of or in addition to steroids.

Reiter's Syndrome

Etiology. The underlying cause of this syndrome is unknown, although there appears to be some genetic influence in some cases. An infectious process has been suspected but not substantiated. An abnormal immune response to microbial antigen(s) is now regarded as a likely mechanism for the multiple manifestations of this syndrome.

Clinical Features. The major components of Reiter's syndrome are arthritis, non-gonococcal urethritis, and conjunctivitis or uveitis. The urethritis generally precedes the appearance of the other lesions. Mucocutaneous lesions may be seen in up to half of the patients with Reiter's syndrome. Maculopapular lesions may occur on the genitalia as well as at other sites.

Orally, lesions have been described as relatively painless aphthous type ulcers, occurring almost anywhere in the mouth. Tongue lesions

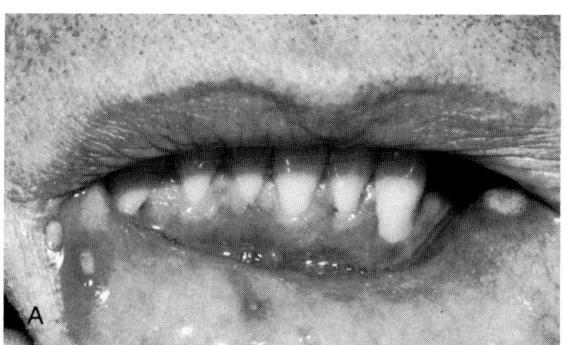
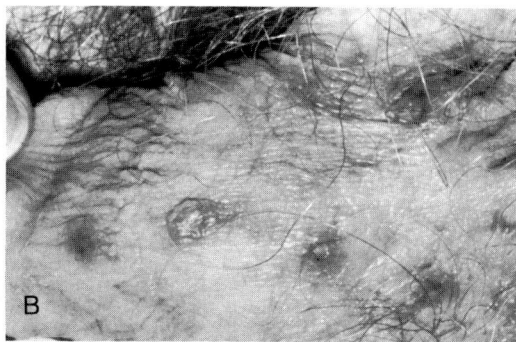

Figure 2–28. *A*, Oral ulcers of Behçet's syndrome. *B*, Penile ulcers in same patient.

have been likened to those of geographic tongue.

Highly characteristic of this syndrome is its occurrence predominantly in white males in their third decade. The duration of the disease varies from weeks to months, and recurrences are not uncommon.

Diagnosis. Diagnosis is dependent upon recognition of the various signs and symptoms associated with this syndrome. There are no specific laboratory tests for Reiter's syndrome.

Treatment. Non-steroidal, anti-inflammatory agents are generally used in the treatment of this disease. Antibiotics have also been added to the treatment regimen, with varied success.

Erythema Multiforme

Etiology and Pathogenesis. The basic cause of erythema multiforme (EM) is unknown, although a hypersensitivity reaction is suspected. There is some evidence that the disease mechanism may be related to antigen-antibody complexes that are targeted for small vessels of the upper dermis or submucosa. In about half the cases, precipitating or triggering factors can be identified. These generally fall into the two large categories of infections and drugs. Other factors, such as malignancy, vaccination, autoimmune disease, and radiotherapy, are occasionally cited as possible triggers. Infections frequently reported include HSV (types I and II), TB, and histoplasmosis. Various types of drugs have precipitated EM, with barbiturates and sulfonamides among the more frequent offenders.

Clinical Features. EM is usually an acute self-limited process that affects the skin or mucous membranes or both. Between 25 and 50% of the patients with cutaneous EM will have oral manifestations of this disease. It may on occasion be chronic, or it may be a recurring, acute problem. In recurrent disease, prodromal symptoms may be experienced prior to any eruption. Young adults are most commonly affected. Individuals will often develop EM in the spring or fall and may have recrudescences seasonally. The term "erythema multiforme" was coined to include the multiple and varied clinical appearances that are associated with the cutaneous manifestations of this disease. The classic skin lesion of EM is the target or iris lesion (Fig. 2–29). It consists of concentric erythematous rings separated by rings of near-normal color. The skin in the center of these lesions may be erythematous or tan, representing resolution. Typically, the extremities are involved, usually in a symmetric distribution. Other types of skin manifestations of EM include macules, papules, vesicles, bullae, and urticarial plaques.

Orally, EM characteristically presents as an ulcerative disease, varying from a few aphthous type lesions to multiple, superficial, widespread ulcers (Figs. 2–30 and 2–31). Short-lived vesicles or bullae are infrequently seen at the initial presentation. Any area of the mouth may be involved, with lips, buccal mucosa, palate, and tongue being most frequently affected. Recurrent oral lesions may appear as multiple painful ulcers similar to the initial episode or as less symptomatic erythematous patches with limited ulceration.

Symptoms range from mild discomfort to severe pain. Considerable apprehension may also be associated with this condition initially because of the occasional explosive onset occurring in some patients. Systemic signs and

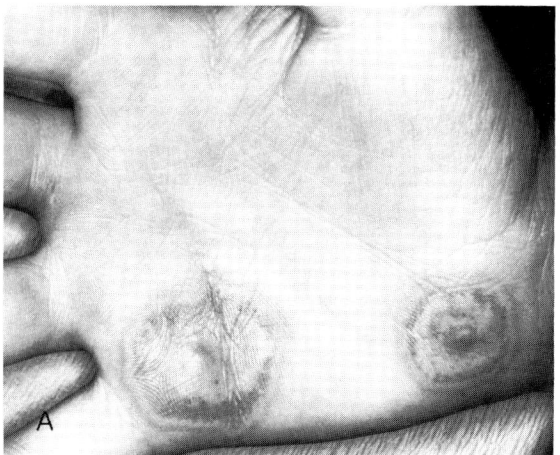
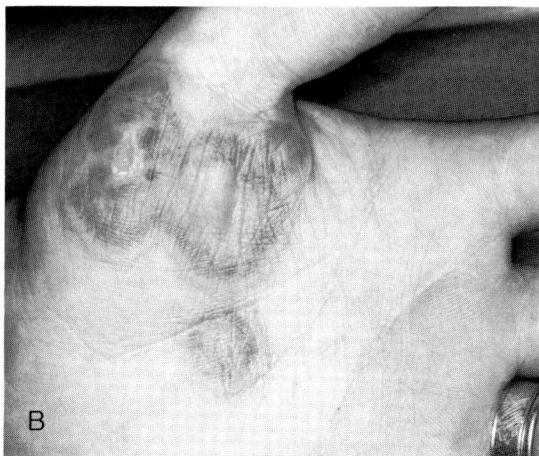

Figure 2–29. *A* and *B*, Target or iris lesions of erythema multiforme.

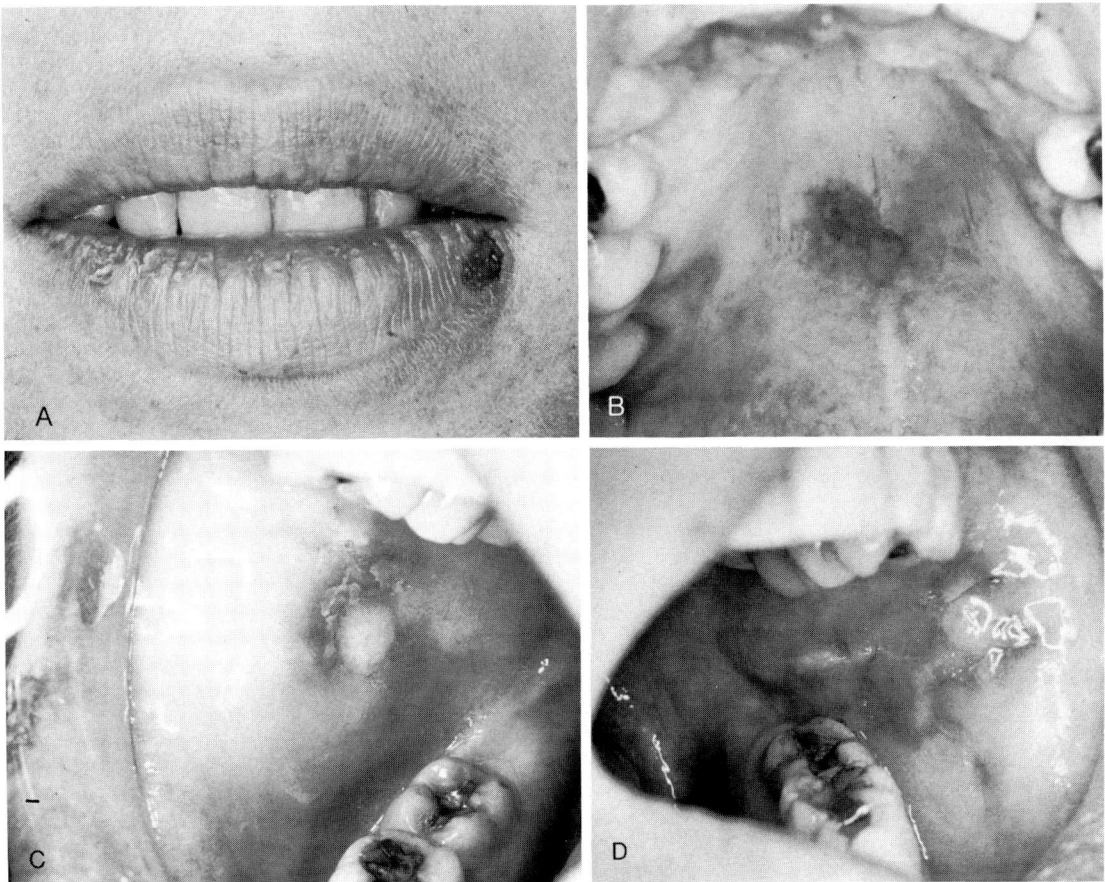

Figure 2–30. *A,* Resolving herpetic lip lesion that triggered oral *(B–D)* and cutaneous (Fig. 2–29) erythema multiforme in a 26-year-old female.

symptoms of headache, slightly elevated temperature, and lymphadenopathy may accompany more intense disease.

At the severe end of the EM spectrum, intense involvement of the mouth, eyes, skin, genitalia, and occasionally the esophagus and respiratory tract may be seen concurrently. This major variant of EM is called *Stevens-Johnson syndrome.* Systemic signs and symptoms in this syndrome may be more pronounced and cutaneous and mucosal lesions may be more extensive than in the usual form of EM. The lips may become encrusted, and oral lesions may cause exquisite pain. Superficial ulceration, often preceded by bullae, is common to all the sites affected. Ocular inflammation (conjunctivitis and uveitis) may lead to scarring and blindness in some patients.

Histopathology. There is no specific or consistent microscopic pattern for EM. A wide range of changes may be seen, affecting both epithelium and supporting connective tissue in the skin and mucous membranes (Fig. 2–32). Intracellular and intercellular (spongiosis) edema, acanthosis, and necrotic keratinocytes may all appear in the epithelium. Vesicles most typically occur at the epithelium–connective tissue interface, although intraepithelial vesiculation has been described in EM. Connective tissue changes usually appear as perivascular infiltrates of lymphocytes and macrophages and edema of the lamina propria or papillary dermis.

Immunopathologic studies are also non-specific for EM. The epithelium shows negative staining for immunoglobulins. Dermal vessels have, however, been shown to have IgM, complement, and fibrin in their walls. This latter finding has been used to support an immune-complex vasculitis cause for EM.

Differential Diagnosis. When target, or iris, skin lesions are present, clinical diagnosis is usually straightforward. However, in the absence of these or any skin lesions, several possibilities should be considered for the oral expression of this disease—included would be primary HSV infections (Table 2–6), aphthous ulcers, pemphigus vulgaris, cicatricial pemphi-

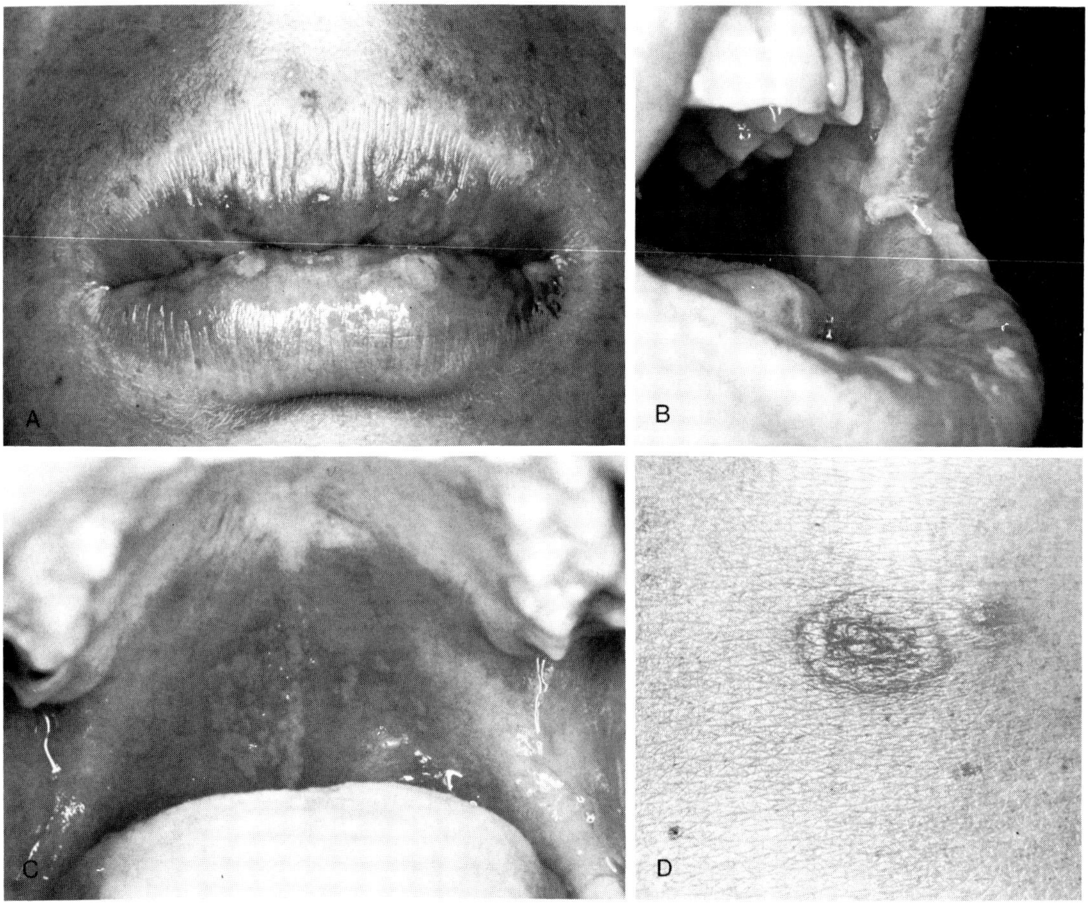

56 ULCERATIVE CONDITIONS

Figure 2–31. *A–D,* Recurrent oral and cutaneous (back) erythema multiforme in a young male.

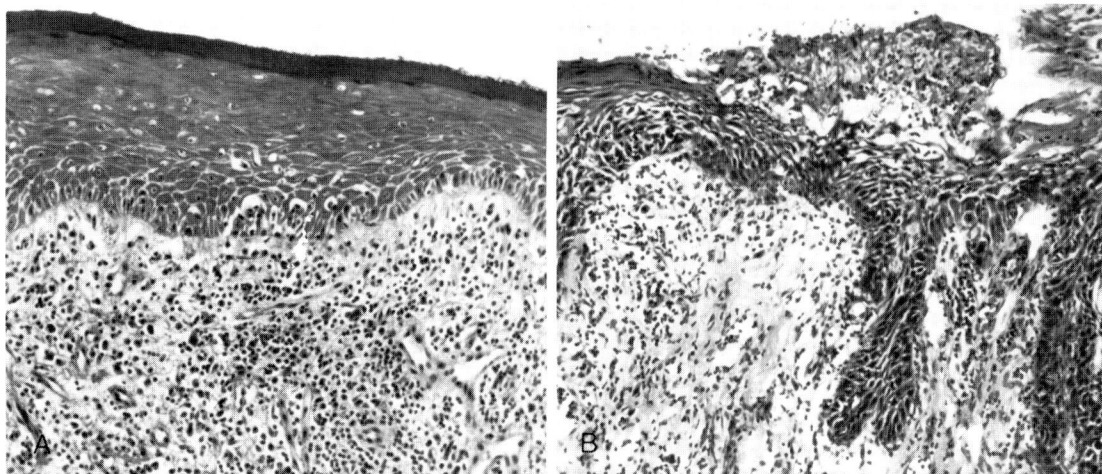

Figure 2–32. *A,* Erythema multiforme showing mononuclear infiltrate, edema, and interface change. *B,* Advanced stage showing intense inflammatory change.

Table 2-6. DIFFERENTIATING FEATURES OF ERYTHEMA MULTIFORME AND PRIMARY HERPES

Feature	Erythema Multiforme	Primary Herpes
Systemic symptoms	None to slight	Pronounced
Typical clinical appearance	Oral—ulcers	Oral—multiple small lesions
	Skin—target lesions	Skin—multiple small ulcers
Areas typically affected	Buccal mucosa, tongue, palate, lips, extremities	Gingiva, lips, perioral skin
Cytology	Non-specific	Virus-infected cells
Age	Young adults	Children
Precipitating factors	Recent drug use or infection (especially HSL)	Exposure to infected patient

goid, and erosive lichen planus. Differentiation from primary herpes is particularly important because of the markedly different treatment required for each, and because of the potential effects of erroneous treatment of herpes with systemic steroids. The general lack of systemic symptoms; the favored oral location of lips, buccal mucosa, tongue, and palate; the larger sized ulcers (usually not preceded by vesicles); the presence of target skin lesions; and a history of recent drug ingestion or infection should favor a diagnosis of EM. Cytologic smears of scrapings of the base of one or two ulcers early in the course of the disease could be diagnostic for a herpetic infection. Sudden onset and limited duration would help separate EM from pemphigus vulgaris, cicatricial pemphigoid, and lichen planus. Although H&E sections and immunopathologic preparations are not specific for EM, they are highly characteristic for pemphigus, pemphigoid, and lichen planus, making the biopsy a good diagnostic tool for EM in an indirect sense. Aphthous ulcers could be ruled out on historical and clinical grounds.

Treatment. Because EM is a self-limited process, only symptomatic treatment is necessary in mild to moderate cases. In severe cases, moderate doses of systemic corticosteroids are used, although this is not universally accepted. Steroids probably shorten the course of the disease and may abort recurrences or reduce their intensity.

Lupus Erythematosus

Lupus erythematosus (LE) encompasses three recognized subsets—systemic (acute) LE, subacute cutaneous LE, and discoid (chronic) LE—all of which may have oral manifestations. In the spectrum of LE, systemic lupus erythematosus (SLE) is of greatest importance because of the profound impact it has on many organ systems. Discoid lupus erythematosus (DLE) is the least aggressive form, affecting predominantly the skin and rarely progressing to a more severe form. It may, however, be of great cosmetic significance because of its predilection for the face. Subacute cutaneous lupus erythematosus (SCLE) lies intermediate between SLE and DLE in that, in addition to skin lesions of mild to moderate severity, there is mild systemic involvement and the appearance of some abnormal autoantibodies.

Etiology and Pathogenesis. LE is generally regarded as an autoimmune process that may be influenced by genetic or viral factors. Both the humoral and the cell-mediated arms of the immune system are involved in the etiology and pathogenesis of this condition.

A large number of autoantibodies directed against various cellular antigens in both the nucleus and the cytoplasm have been identified. These antibodies may be found in the serum or in tissue bound to antigens. Circulating antibodies are responsible for the positive reactions noted in the antinuclear antibody (ANA) and LE cell tests that are done to help confirm the diagnosis of lupus. Also circulating in serum are antigen-antibody complexes that mediate disease in many organ systems.

Indications that the cell-mediated system plays an important role in the pathogenesis of LE are found in the histology of lupus lesions, in which T lymphocytes may appear in prominent numbers, and in the results of abnormal T cell function tests in affected patients. The prevalence of laboratory immunologic abnormalities in LE varies depending upon the disease subtype. Only rarely are serologic alterations demonstrable in DLE. In SCLE, some autoantibodies appear in the serum and tissues of patients. In SLE, the full gamut of immunologic changes may be seen.

Clinical Features

Discoid Lupus Erythematosus. DLE is a disease characteristically seen in middle age, especially in women. Lesions frequently appear solely on the skin, most commonly on the face and scalp. Oral and vermilion lesions are also frequently seen but usually in the company of cutaneous lesions. On the skin, lesions appear as disk-shaped erythematous plaques with hyperpigmented margins (Fig. 2–33). As the lesions expand peripherally, the center heals, with the formation of scar and loss of pigment. Involvement of hair follicles results in permanent hair loss (alopecia).

Mucous membrane lesions appear in about 25% of patients with cutaneous DLE. The buccal mucosa, gingiva, and vermilion are most frequently affected (Figs. 2–34 and 2–35). Lesions may appear as erythematous plaques or erosions. Usually present are delicate, white, keratotic striae radiating from the periphery of the lesions. Keratotic papules may also be seen throughout the lesions. The diagnosis of oral lesions may not be evident on the basis of clinical appearance, but it is often suspected in the presence of skin lesions. Progression of DLE to SLE is very unlikely, although the potential does exist.

Subacute Cutaneous Lupus Erythematosus. In SCLE, a recently recognized subset of LE, skin lesions are annular or papulosquamous in nature. Lesions persist for weeks to months and heal without scar. Oral lesions are similar to those seen in DLE (Fig. 2–36). Mild systemic symptoms in the form of musculoskeletal complaints as well as serologic abnormalities are frequently seen. Circulating antibodies to cytoplasmic components may be found in affected patients. One of these is known as anti-Ro or Sjögren's syndrome A antibody (SS-A), since it may also be found in the serum of patients with Sjögren's syndrome. Another autoantibody less commonly found in both SCLE and Sjögren's syndrome is anti-La (SS-B). Some ANAs may also be demonstrated if a sensitive testing system is used. Overall, clinical and immunologic severity is intermediate between DLE and SLE. Long-term prognosis is believed to be good, with progression to SLE an unlikely event.

Systemic Lupus Erythematosus. In this form of LE, skin and mucosal lesions are relatively mild, and patient complaints are dominated by multiple system involvement. Numerous autoantibodies directed against nuclear and cytoplasmic antigens are found in SLE patients. These antibodies, when complexed to their corresponding antigens either in serum or in the target organ, can cause lesions in nearly any tissue, resulting in a wide variety of clinical signs and symptoms.

Involvement of the skin results in an erythematous rash, classically seen over the malar processes and bridge of the nose. This results in the characteristic "butterfly" distribution usually associated with SLE. Other areas of the face, trunk, and hands may also be involved. The lesions are non-scarring and may flare as systemic involvement progresses. Occasionally, disk-shaped skin lesions, similar to those seen in DLE, appear in SLE.

Oral lesions of SLE are generally similar to those seen in DLE. Ulceration, erythema, and keratosis may be seen (Fig. 2–37). In addition

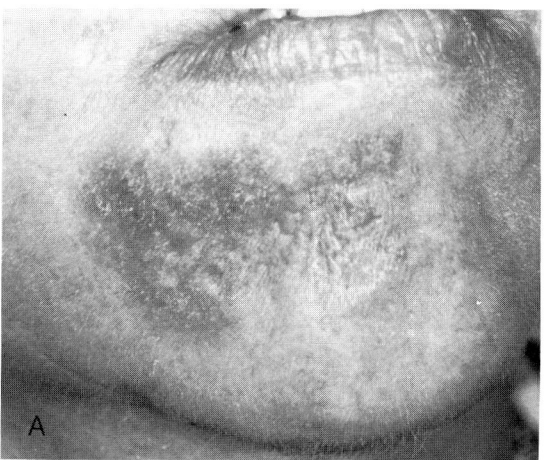
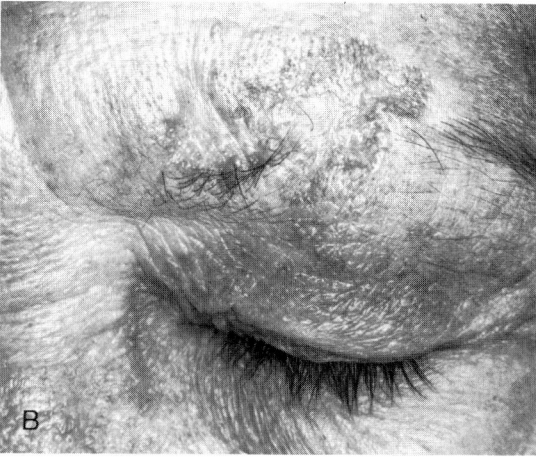

Figure 2–33. *A* and *B*, Cutaneous lesions of DLE. Note loss of eyebrow hair in *B*.

ULCERATIVE CONDITIONS

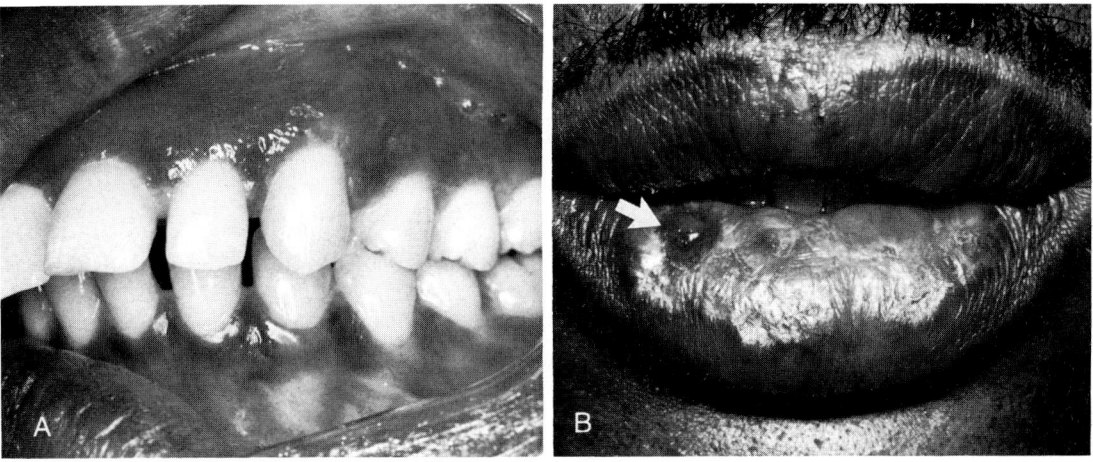

Figure 2–34. DLE of mucous membranes. *A,* The entire maxillary gingiva is erythematous with faint keratic striae. Mandibular gingiva is unaffected. *B,* The lower lip is keratotic with one area of ulceration (arrow).

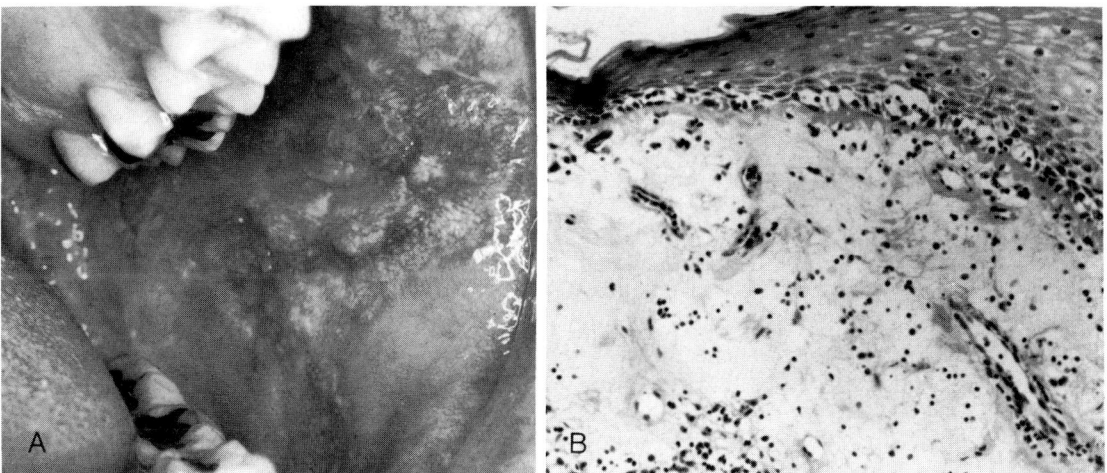

Figure 2–35. *A,* Typical DLE lesion showing erythematous background with speckled keratotic foci. *B,* Microscopic changes include edema, interface change, and epithelial atrophy.

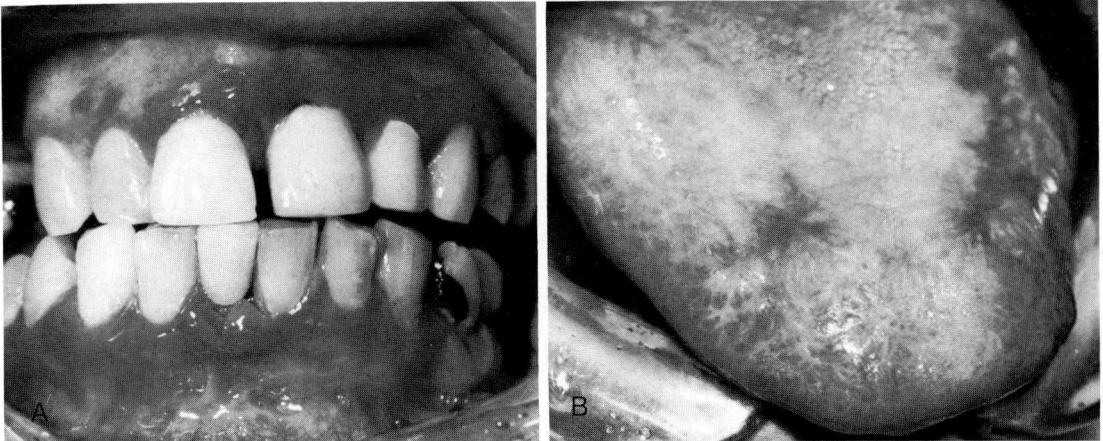

Figure 2–36. Subacute LE. *A,* Most of gingiva is involved by erythematous process. *B,* Tongue is focally reddened (dark areas) with keratotic striae.

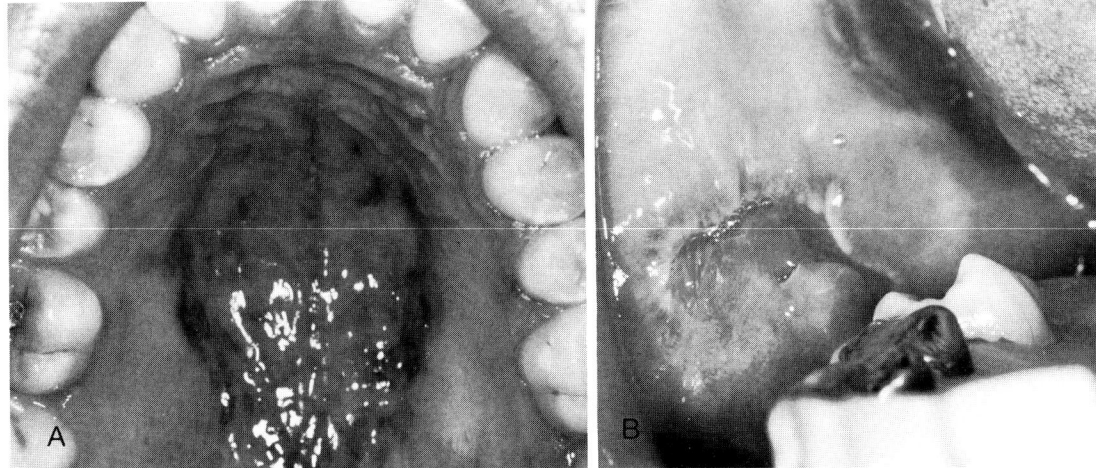

Figure 2-37. Mucosal lesions of SLE. *A*, Predominantly erythematous lesion of palate. *B*, Erythematous and keratotic lesion of buccal mucosa.

to the vermilion, the buccal mucosa, gingiva, and palate are frequently involved.

Systemic expression of SLE may initially be in the form of fever, weight loss, and malaise. Typically, with disease progression many organ systems become involved. Joints, kidneys, heart, and lungs are most frequently affected, although many other organs may express manifestations of this disease. The inflammatory lesions of the variously involved tissues result in a wide array of signs and symptoms. Kidney lesions (glomerulopathy) are, however, the most important, since they are most commonly responsible for the death of SLE patients (Table 2-7).

Serologic tests for autoantibodies are positive in patients with SLE. The ANA test is regarded as the most reliable and is relatively specific for SLE. Among the antibodies that may cause a positive ANA test are anti–single-stranded DNA, anti–double-stranded DNA, and antinuclear ribonuclear protein. Specific tests for these and other autoantibodies of SLE are also available. Another serologic test for SLE is the LE cell test, although it is less sensitive and less specific than the ANA test.

Antibodies to Ro (SS-A) and La (SS-B) cytoplasmic antigens may also be present in SLE.

Histopathology. In DLE, several microscopic changes are seen with relative consistency. Basal cell destruction, hyperkeratosis, epithelial atrophy, lymphocytic infiltration (often in a perivascular distribution), and vascular dilatation with edema of the upper dermis or submucosa are characteristic features. The most important microscopic feature diagnostically is the interface change, since it ap-

Table 2-7. COMPARISON OF DISCOID AND SYSTEMIC LUPUS ERYTHEMATOSUS

Parameter	Discoid Lupus Erythematosus	Systemic Lupus Erythematosus
Organs involved		
Skin	Almost always	Usually
Oral	Frequently	Occasionally
Joints	No	Usually
Kidneys	No	Usually
Heart	No	Usually
Other	No	Often
Symptoms	No	Fever, weight loss, malaise
Serology		
ANA test	Negative	Positive
LE cell test	Negative	Positive
Immunopathology		
Direct immunofluorescence	Positive, granular-linear basement membrane deposits of Ig	Positive, granular-linear basement membrane deposits of Ig

Table 2–8. COMPARISON OF LUPUS ERYTHEMATOSUS AND LICHEN PLANUS

Parameter	Lupus Erythematosus	Lichen Planus
Histopathology		
Basal cell destruction	Yes	Yes
Lymphocytic infiltrate	Yes	Yes
Subepithelial band	No	Yes
Perivascular	Yes	No
Hyperkeratosis	Yes	Yes
Epithelial atrophy	Yes	Occasionally
Submucosal edema	Yes	No
Vasodilatation	Yes	No
Immunopathology (basement membrane)		
Immunoglobulins	Yes	No
Complement	Usually	Often
Fibrinogen	Usually	Usually
Serology		
ANA test	SLE –Positive DLE–Negative	Negative
LE cell test	SLE –Positive DLE–Negative	Negative

pears that the basal cell layer is the primary target in skin and mucous membrane disease. As this is also the case for lichen planus, the two diseases may be difficult to separate microscopically (Table 2–8).

In SLE, oral lesions are microscopically similar to lesions of DLE, although inflammatory cell infiltrates are less evident and more diffuse. Changes in skin lesions will vary from slight to marked, depending on whether lesions are erythematous or "discoid." Interface change, lymphocytic infiltrates, and fibrinoid vascular changes are usually seen.

Other organs, when involved in SLE, show some individual histologic variations. Generally, however, there are basic underlying histologic changes common to all locations. These consist of vasculitis, mononuclear infiltrates, and fibrinoid change.

Direct immunofluorescent testing of skin and mucosal lesions shows granular-linear deposits of immunoglobulins (IgG, IgM, IgA), complement (C3), and fibrinogen along the basement membrane zone in a majority of patients. Since C3 and fibrinogen deposits may appear in several other conditions, immunostaining for these components is felt to be of little value in the diagnosis of LE. Demonstration of immunoglobulin deposits in a granular-linear subepidermal pattern is, however, felt to be relatively specific. This is also the basis of the lupus band test, which utilizes biopsies of involved and uninvolved skin and immunofluorescent staining for immunoglobulins. Positive lupus band staining is seen in lesional skin of most DLE and SLE patients. In uninvolved skin, SLE is usually positive and DLE is negative.

Differential Diagnosis. Clinically, lesions of oral LE most often resemble erosive lichen planus (Fig. 2–38). Oral lupus lesions tend to be less symmetrically distributed than lichen planus. Also, the keratotic striae of LE are much more delicate and subtle than Wickham's striae of lichen planus. When significant ulceration is present, pemphigus vulgaris, cicatricial pemphigoid, EM, and drug reaction might also be considerations. Also, lupus might be confused with erythroplakia, in which there are foci of keratosis (speckled erythroplakia). The presence of characteristic skin lesions or systemic signs and symptoms may help rule in LE. Biopsy and direct immunofluorescent testing should help confirm the clinical impression. Negative serologic tests for autoantibodies (e.g., ANA test) would rule out systemic involvement.

Treatment. DLE is usually treated with topical steroids. High-potency creams can be used intraorally but should be used with caution on facial skin because of secondary cutaneous changes. In refractory cases, antimalarials or sulfones may be used.

Systemic steroids are often utilized in the treatment of SLE (and SCLE). Prednisone dosage is generally dependent upon severity of the disease and may be combined with immunosuppressive agents for their therapeutic and

62 ULCERATIVE CONDITIONS

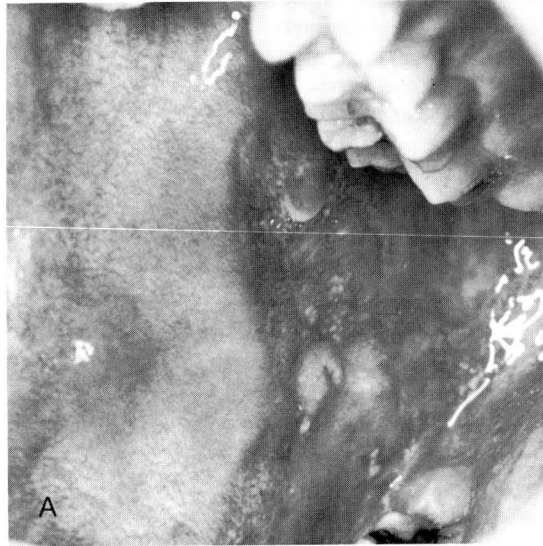 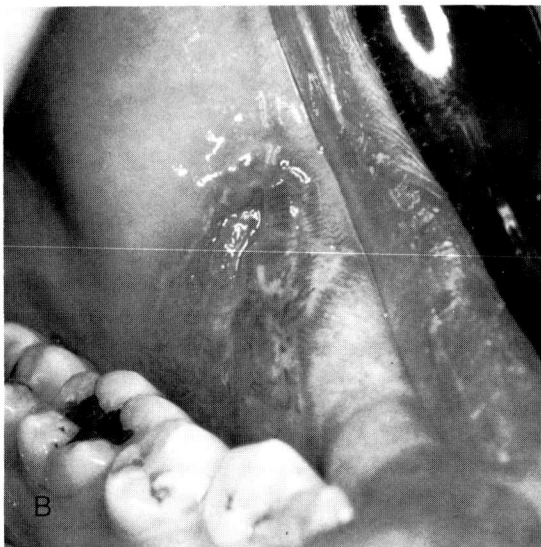

Figure 2–38. *A* and *B*, DLE in a lichenoid distribution. Note dark background with associated delicate white striae.

steroid-sparing effects. Antimalarial and nonsteroidal anti-inflammatory drugs may also be utilized in the control of this disease.

Drug Reactions

Etiology and Pathogenesis. Although the skin is more commonly involved in adverse reactions to drugs, the oral mucosa may occasionally be the target organ. Oral mucous membranes may be the sole site of involvement, or they may be part of a skin reaction to the offending drug. Virtually any drug has the potential to cause an untoward reaction, but some have a greater ability to do so than others. Also, some patients have a greater tendency than others to react to drugs. Some of the drugs that are more commonly cited as being involved in adverse reactions are listed in Table 2–9.

Table 2–9. REPRESENTATIVE DRUGS KNOWN TO CAUSE ADVERSE REACTIONS	
Antimalarials	Meprobamate
Aspirin	Methyldopa
Barbiturates	Oxprenolol
Chlorpromazine	hydrochloride
Cimetidine	Penicillin
Codeine	Phenytoin
Erythromycin	Retinoids
Gold compounds	Streptomycin
Indomethacin	Sulfonamides
Ketoconazole	Tetracycline
Local anesthetics	

Pathogenesis of drug reactions may be related to either immunologic or non-immunologic mechanisms. With the immunologic route, a patient's immune response is triggered by an antigenic component on the drug molecule, resulting in a hyperimmune response or drug allergy. In this type of reaction, the humoral arm of the immune system is predominantly involved. The potential for drug allergy is directly dependent upon the immunogenicity of the drug, the frequency of exposure, the route of administration (topical more likely than oral), and the innate reactivity of the patient's immune system.

One of several mechanisms may be involved in drug allergy. IgE-mediated reactions occur when the drug (allergen) reacts with IgE antibody bound to mast cells. Subsequently, release of chemical mediators from the mast cells produces the clinical disease, which may range from a localized rash to anaphylaxis.

Another pathway for drug reactions involves a cytotoxic reaction in which an antibody binds to a drug (antigen) that is already attached to a cell surface. The target cells may be specific or non-specific and may cause pathologic changes in any organ. If, for example, the red blood cell is the cell involved, the result of this type of reaction would be anemia.

A third pathogenetic mechanism in drug allergy involves circulation of the antigen for extended periods, allowing sensitization of the patient's immune system and the production of new antibody. Subsequent binding of antigen and antibody results in circulating complexes that may be deposited in various sites, producing allergic organopathies, such as nephritis, arthritis, and dermatitis. Disease caused by this mechanism is also known as serum sickness.

Drug reactions that are non-immunologic in nature do not stimulate an immune response in the patient and are not antibody dependent. In this type of response, drugs may directly affect mast cells, causing the release of chemical mediators. The reactions may also be the result of overdose, toxicity, or side effects of the drugs.

Clinical Features. Cutaneous manifestations of drug reactions are widely varied and are dependent upon many factors, some of which include the type of drug, drug dosage, and individual patient differences. Changes may appear rapidly, as in anaphylaxis, angioedema, and urticaria, or, more likely, appear several days after drug use.

Acquired angioedema is an IgE-mediated allergic reaction that is precipitated by drugs or foods such as nuts and shellfish. These substances may act as sensitizing agents (antigens) that elicit IgE production. Upon antigenic rechallenge, mast cells bound with IgE in the skin or mucosa release their contents to cause the clinical picture of angioedema. *Hereditary angioedema* produces similar clinical changes but through a different mechanism. Individuals who inherit this autosomal dominant trait have a qualitative or quantitative deficiency of the inhibitor of the first component of complement, C1 esterase.

Angioedema, by either an acquired or a hereditary pathway, appears as a soft, diffuse, painless swelling, usually of the lips, neck, or face (Fig. 2–39). There is typically no color change. The condition generally subsides after 1 to 2 days and may recur at a later date. Emergency treatment may be required if the process has led to respiratory distress because of glottic or laryngeal involvement. Antihistamines and, in problematic cases, corticosteroids are used to treat this form of allergy.

Other cutaneous manifestations of drug reactions include urticaria, maculopapular rash, erythema, vesicles, ulcers, and target lesions (EM) (Fig. 2–40). An unusual form of drug reaction is known as fixed drug reaction. In patients with this condition, an erythematous lesion appears in the same cutaneous location with each antigenic challenge (Fig. 2–41).

Oral manifestations of drug reactions may be erythematous, vesicular, or ulcerative in nature. They may also mimic erosive lichen planus, in which case they are known as lichenoid drug reactions (Fig. 2–42). The widespread ulcers typical of EM are often representative of a drug reaction.

Histopathology. As with clinical presentation, there is no specific microscopic picture for drug reactions. Although biopsy may not be diagnostic, it may be helpful in ruling out other diagnostic considerations. Nonetheless, many of these microscopic changes may be seen in the various types of drug reactions: mononuclear or polymorphonuclear infiltration in a subepithelial or perivascular distribution, basal cell destruction, edema, and keratinocyte necrosis.

Diagnosis. Because the clinical and histologic features of drug reactions are highly variable and non-specific, the diagnosis of drug reaction requires a high index of suspicion and careful history taking. Recent use of a drug is important, since reaction after several days

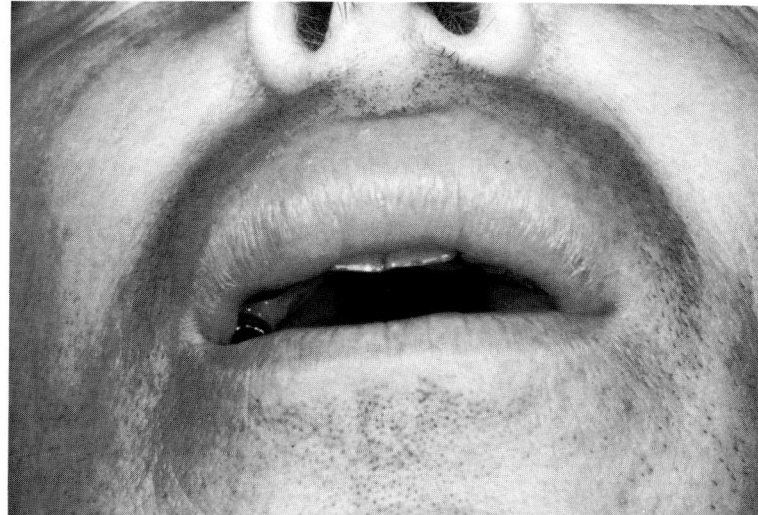

Figure 2–39. Angioedema of the upper lip.

64 ULCERATIVE CONDITIONS

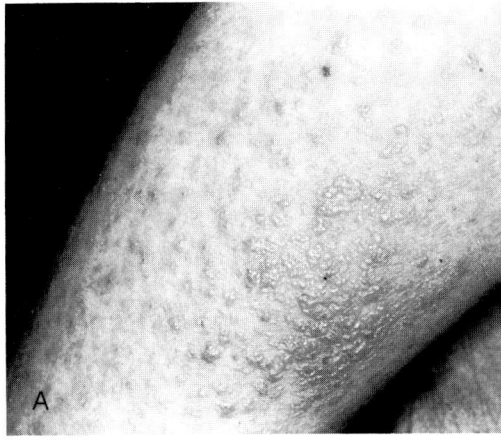
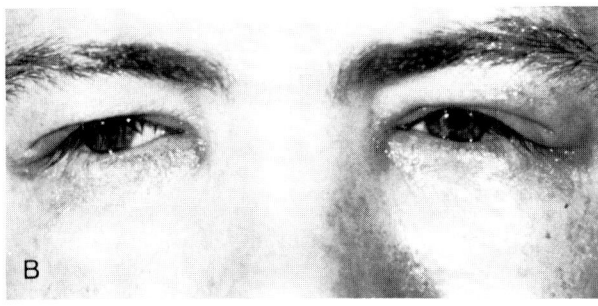

Figure 2–40. Extraoral manifestations of drug reactions. *A,* Vesicular eruption on arm due to phenobarbital. *B,* Conjunctivitis following penicillin ingestion.

tends to rule against drug reaction. An exception is the delayed reaction (up to 2 weeks) noted following the use of ampicillin. Withdrawal of the suspected drug should result in improvement, and reinstitution of the drug (a procedure that is usually ill advised for the patient's safety) should exacerbate the patient's condition. If rechallenge is done, minute amounts of the offending drug or a structurally related drug should cause a reaction. Another consideration that would support a drug reaction is the clinical expression of lesions that are generally regarded as being typically allergic in nature.

Treatment. The most important measure in the management of drug reactions is identification and withdrawal of the causative agent. If this is impossible or undesirable, alternative drugs may have to be substituted or the eruption may have to be dealt with on an empirical basis. Antihistamines and occasionally corticosteroids may be useful in the management of oral and cutaneous eruptions due to drug reactions.

Contact Allergy

Etiology and Pathogenesis. Contact allergic reactions can be caused by antigenic stimulation by a vast array of foreign substances. The immune response is predominantly cell-mediated in nature. In the sensitization phase, the Langerhans cell appears to play a major role in the recognition of foreign antigen. The Langerhans cell differs from its relative the macrophage in that it is widely distributed throughout epidermis and mucosa. It is a dendritic cell found usually midway in the epithelium among keratinocytes; it is responsible for processing antigens that enter the epithelium from the external environment. The Langerhans cell subsequently presents the appropriate antigenic determinants to T lymphocytes. Following antigenic rechallenge, local lymphocytes secrete chemical mediators of inflammation (lymphokines) that produce the clinical

Figure 2–41. Fixed drug reaction induced by tetracycline. (Courtesy of Dr. J. C. B. Stewart.)

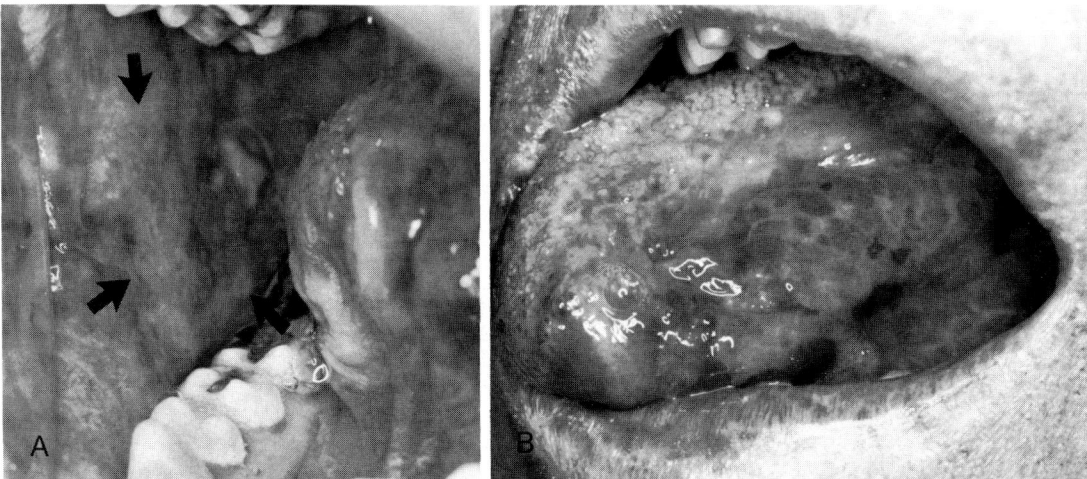

Figure 2–42. Lichenoid drug reaction. *A,* Most of buccal mucosa is ulcerated (arrows). *B,* The tongue shows ulceration and keratotic striae.

and histologic changes characteristic of this process.

Clinical Features. Lesions of contact allergy occur directly adjacent to the causative agent (Fig. 2–43), unless the material is volatile, in which case distant tissue may be affected. Presenting lesions will range from erythematous to vesicular to ulcerative.

Although contact allergy is frequently seen on the skin, it is relatively uncommon intraorally. Some of the many materials containing agents known to cause oral contact allergic reactions are toothpaste, mouthwash, candy, chewing gum, topical antimicrobials, topical steroids, iodine, essential oils, and denture base material (Fig. 2–44). Although denture acrylic is frequently held accountable for allergic contact reactions in the palate, this is probably a misconception. These red lesions are more likely related to chronic candidiasis. If a component of the denture material, especially unpolymerized monomer, were responsible for allergic change, tissue reaction would be seen not only in the palate but also on the alveolar ridge and on the buccal mucosa where contact is made.

Histopathology. Microscopically, the epithelium and connective tissue show inflammatory changes. Spongiosis and vesiculation may be seen within the epithelium. A perivascular lymphophagocytic infiltrate is found in the immediate supporting connective tissue. Blood vessels may be dilated, and occasional eosinophils may be seen.

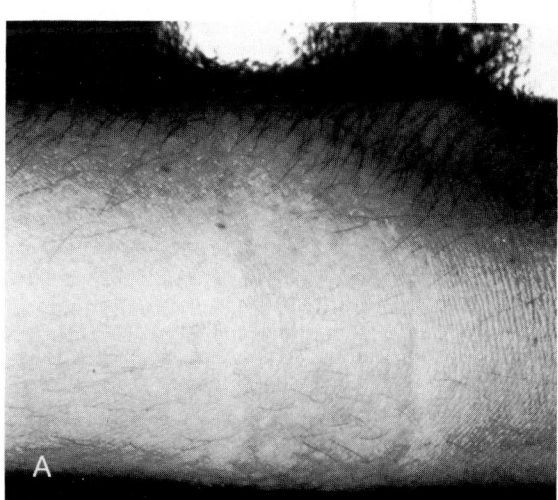
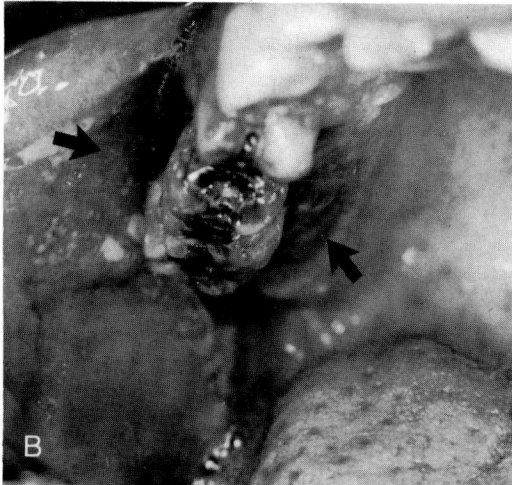

Figure 2–43. *A,* Contact allergic lesion on wrist associated with a watch band. (Courtesy of Dr. S. K. Young.) *B,* Contact allergic reaction of gingiva and buccal mucosa (arrows) caused by periodontal pack.

66 ULCERATIVE CONDITIONS

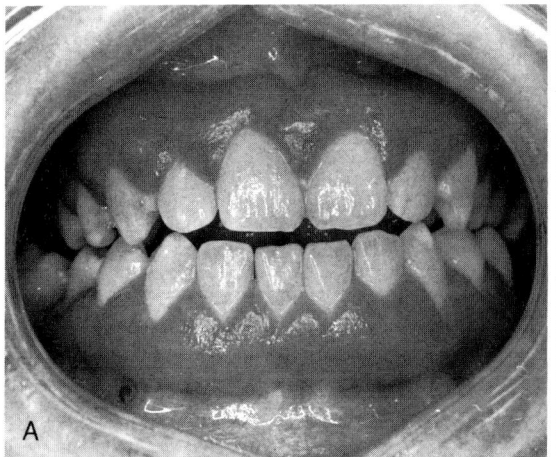 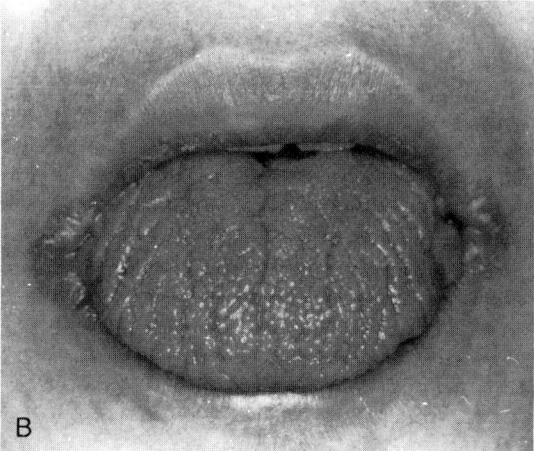

Figure 2–44. *A* and *B*, Oral lesions attributed to an allergen in chewing gum. *A*, Gingiva is intensely erythematous. *B*, Tongue epithelium is atrophic and commissures are fissured.

Diagnosis. Careful history taking is essential. Establishing a cause and effect relationship between offending agent and tissue change may not always be possible. Biopsy may be helpful. Patch testing may be helpful but should be done by an expert in the area because of the possibility of producing false positive results when done on skin and false negative results when attempted on mucosa.

Treatment. Primary treatment should be directed at elimination of the offending material if it can be identified. In uncomplicated cases, lesions should heal in 1 to 2 weeks. Topical steroids may hasten the healing process.

Wegener's Granulomatosis

Etiology. Wegener's granulomatosis is an inflammatory condition of unknown etiology. Efforts to identify a cause have generally focused on infection and immunologic dysfunction but have been unproductive.

Clinical Features. Typically, the triad of upper respiratory tract, lung, and kidney involvement is seen in this condition. Occasionally, only two of the three sites are affected. Lesions may also present in the oral cavity and skin and, potentially, in any other organ system. The basic pathologic process that is common to all foci is necrotizing vasculitis with granuloma formation.

This is a rare disease of middle age. Initial presentation often occurs with head and neck symptoms. Symptoms typical of sinusitis, rhinorrhea, nasal stuffiness, and epistaxis may be seen with or without non-specific complaints of fever, arthralgia, and weight loss. In a majority of cases, nasal or sinus (usually maxillary) involvement is seen and is often present early in the course of the disease. Destructive lesions are typically ulcerated, with necrosis and perforation of nasal septum occasionally seen. Perforation of the hard palate is uncommonly seen in Wegener's granulomatosis. Intraorally, red granular gingival lesions have been reported (Fig. 2–45). The process is generalized and results in relatively uniform enlargement. Most patients have kidney involvement that consists of a focal necrotizing glomerulitis. Renal failure is the final outcome of kidney disease. Inflammatory lung lesions, varying in intensity from slight to severe, may eventually lead to respiratory failure.

Histopathology. The basic pathologic process is granulomatous, with necrotizing vasculitis usually present. Variable numbers of acute and chronic inflammatory cells are seen in the granulomatous zones. Necrosis and multinucleated giant cells may be seen in the granulomatous areas. The affected small vessels show a mononuclear infiltrate within their walls in the presence of fibrinoid necrosis. Definitive diagnosis in the absence of vascular changes is difficult, since the microscopy would be non-specific.

Diagnosis. Diagnosis is generally dependent upon the finding of granulomatous vasculitis in biopsy tissue of upper respiratory tract lesions, evidence of involvement of lung, or kidney lesions. There are no other laboratory tests available that can be used to confirm the diagnosis. On both a clinical and a microscopic level, chronic infectious processes, such as TB, syphilis, histoplasmosis, and blastomycosis, and neoplastic processes, such as lymphoma

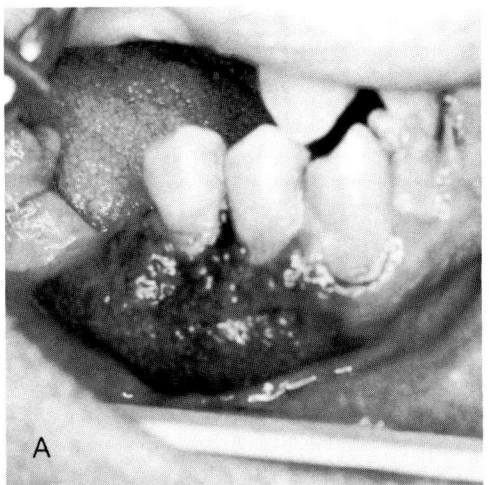
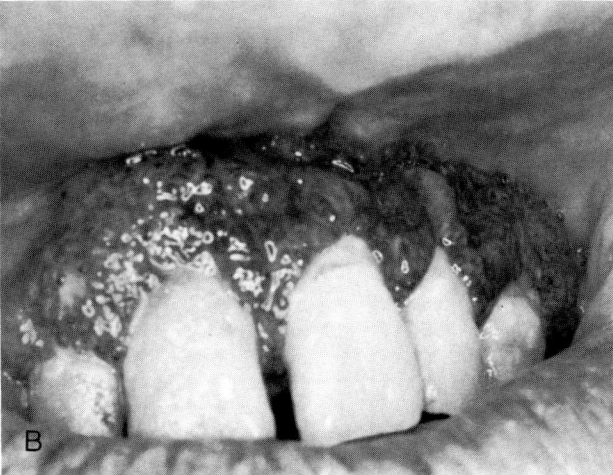

Figure 2–45. *A* and *B*, Granular erosive lesions of Wegener's granulomatosis.

and undifferentiated squamous cell carcinoma, might be serious considerations in a differential diagnosis of this disease. Culture and tissue identification of microorganisms, when negative, would help rule out infectious processes. Immunohistochemical staining or immunofluorescent procedures could be used to help rule out neoplasia, especially on frozen sections.

Treatment. Before the development of chemotherapeutic agents, renal failure and death was a frequent outcome of this disease process. The use of the cytotoxic agent cyclophosphamide and occasionally corticosteroids has provided patients having this disease with a relatively good prognosis.

Midline Granuloma

Etiology. Because midline granuloma has many features that overlap with Wegener's granulomatosis, these two conditions were at one time classified together (Table 2–10). Midline granuloma, like Wegener's granulomatosis, is of unknown etiology, although a hyperimmune response to an as yet unidentified antigen is suspected.

Clinical Features. Midline granuloma is a unifocal destructive process, generally in the midline of the oronasal region, that does not affect other organ systems. Lesions appear clinically as aggressive necrotic ulcers that are progressive and non-healing (Fig. 2–46). Extension through soft tissue, cartilage, and bone is typical. Perforation of the nasal septum and hard palate is characteristic as well. Without treatment, the inflammatory process eventually consumes the patient, and because of continuous erosion into vital structures, especially blood vessels, death has been a typical outcome.

Histopathology. Microscopically, the process is non-specific and typically appears as acute and chronic inflammation in partially necrotic tissue. Because of the almost trivial inflammatory appearance of this condition, several biopsies may be required before one may be confident or comfortable with the diagnosis of midline granuloma.

Differential Diagnosis. Clinically, destructive processes of the midline of the nose or palate would include Wegener's granulomatosis, infectious disease, and neoplasm. Bacterial infection, such as TB and syphilis (gumma),

Table 2–10. COMPARISON OF WEGENER'S GRANULOMATOSIS AND MIDLINE GRANULOMA		
Feature	Wegener's Granulomatosis	Midline Granuloma
Etiology	Unknown	Unknown
Location	Upper respiratory tract, lung, kidney	Upper respiratory tract, oral (may have palate perforation)
Histology	Granulomatous Necrotizing vasculitis	Non-specific Inflammation
Treatment	Cyclophosphamide	Radiation

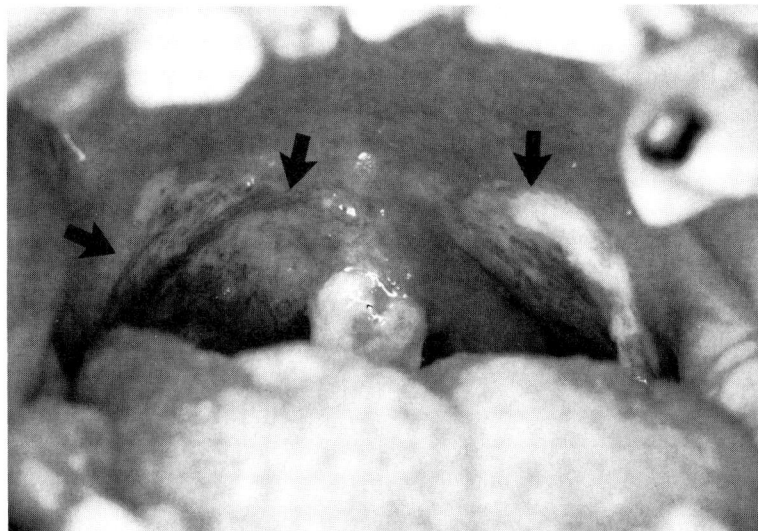

Figure 2–46. Soft palate and uvular ulcers (arrows) of midline granuloma.

may present as a chronic ulcerative process. This is also possible for deep fungal diseases such as histoplasmosis, blastomycosis, and phycomycosis. Neoplasm (poorly differentiated squamous cell carcinoma, sarcomas, and lymphomas) could also present as a destructive midline process.

Treatment. The treatment of choice is high-dose local radiation. It is relatively effective and has produced a reasonably optimistic prognosis. Corticosteroids also have been used with partial success.

Chronic Granulomatous Disease

Etiology and Pathogenesis. This rare systemic disease is inherited in an X-linked manner and occasionally in an autosomal recessive mode. The resulting clinical defect is altered neutrophil and macrophage function. These cells have the capacity to phagocytose microorganisms but lack the ability to kill certain bacteria and fungi owing to insufficient intracellular enzymatic function.

Clinical Features. Manifestations of chronic granulomatous disease appear during childhood and, because of the more frequent X-linked inheritance pattern, occur predominantly in males. The process may affect many organs, including lymph nodes, lung, liver, spleen, bone, and skin, as recurrent or persistent infections. Oral lesions are frequently seen in the form of multiple ulcers that are also recurrent or persistent.

Histopathology. Microscopically, the lesions of chronic granulomatous disease are granular or nodular. Granulomas may exhibit central necrosis.

Diagnosis. The clinical features of recurrent or persistent infections in young patients and the presence in tissue samples of granulomatous inflammation suggest a diagnosis of chronic granulomatous disease. Neutrophil function tests would help confirm the diagnosis. For a differential diagnosis, other granulomatous diseases, such as Crohn's disease, TB, histoplasmosis, blastomycosis, and tularemia, could be included.

Treatment. Treatment is based on the use of specific antimicrobial agents that are directed against the appropriate organism. Those agents that are capable of penetrating mononuclear cell membranes to reach the cytoplasm, where the organisms reside, are especially useful.

NEOPLASMS

Basal Cell Carcinoma

Etiology. This common malignancy, which arises from basal cells of the skin, has a low metastatic potential. Except in very rare instances, it does not occur on mucous membranes, which includes vermilion. Individuals at greater risk for the development of basal cell carcinoma are those with less natural skin pigmentation, those with a long history of chronic sun exposure, those over the age of 40 years, those with a history of cutaneous radiation or burns, and those with one of several predisposing hereditary syndromes. Among the latter is the orally related and important condition of basal cell nevus syndrome, in which individuals may have multiple odontogenic keratocysts, skeletal abnormalities, and multiple basal cell carcinomas. Because of the importance of ultraviolet light in the etiology of this neoplasm, the vast majority of basal cell carcinomas occur on sun-exposed skin. Individuals who have chronic occupational exposure to ultraviolet light or who live in the "Sun Belt" are at greater risk than others to develop basal cell carcinomas.

Clinical Features. This is the most common cancer of the head and neck. The midface is the area in which most basal cell carcinomas are found. The lesion is seen most frequently in older patients, typically between the ages of 50 and 80 years. Men are more commonly affected than women, presumably because of greater cumulative sun exposure. It is believed that this gender difference will equalize in time, as women "catch up" to men relative to their exposure to ultraviolet light.

In early stages, basal cell carcinomas present as indurated, smooth nodules with a pearly appearance and frequent telangiectatic vessels coursing over their surface (Fig. 2–47). With time, the center of the lesion becomes ulcerated and crusted, and as the lesion expands, adjacent vital structures are slowly eroded. Because of their slow but relentless local advancing destructive nature, basal cell carcinomas have earned the name "rodent ulcer" (Fig. 2–48). Other clinical forms may on occasion be seen. These include superficial plaques that grow circumferentially and pigmented lesions that may simulate melanomas or seborrheic keratoses.

Histopathology. Microscopically, most basal cell carcinomas appear as nests and cords of basaloid cells arising from the region of epidermal basal cells. Nuclei have a relatively uniform morphology and tinctorial quality. The neoplastic cells around the periphery of the invading nests and strands are usually palisaded and often columnar.

Several other histologic patterns of basal cell carcinoma have been recognized. The most important is one in which tiny infiltrative nests are found in a fibroblastic stroma. This has been described as an aggressive growth pattern and may portend a more aggressive clinical course. Keratinization in a pattern that resembles that of hair is seen in the uncommon variant, keratotic basal cell carcinomas. The term "adenoid" has been used as a histologic modifier to describe basal cell carcinomas that mimic glandular differentiation. Other histologic types may be described as solid or cystic.

Diagnosis. The diagnosis of basal cell carcinoma is often apparent, based on clinical features. Biopsy usually provides a definitive answer.

Treatment and Prognosis. Several therapeutic modalities are available that can be expected to effect a cure. These include various surgical procedures (standard scalpel surgery, cryosurgery, electrosurgery, Mohs' microscopically guided surgery) and radiation. The type of treatment is dependent upon the experience and training of the therapist and the size and location of the neoplasm.

Since basal cell carcinomas are generally slow growing and rarely metastasize, the prognosis is excellent. Obviously, the smaller the lesion, the better the prognosis, and the better

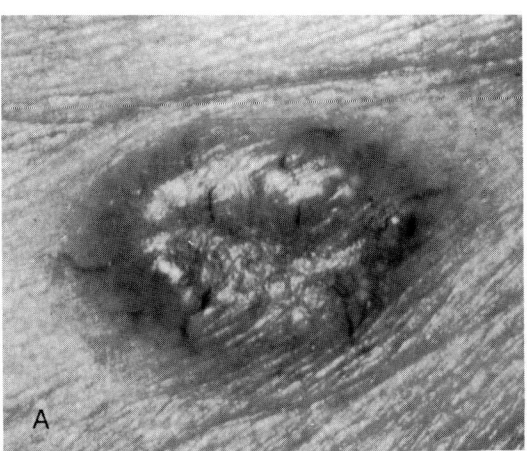
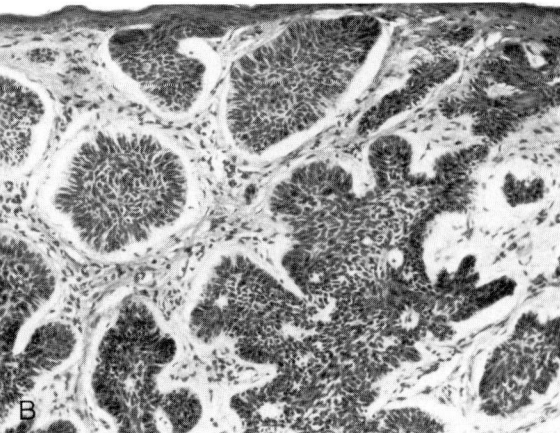

Figure 2–47. *A,* Early basal cell carcinoma of face. (Courtesy of Dr. S. K. Young.) *B,* Nests of basaloid cells invade the dermis in basal cell carcinoma.

70 ULCERATIVE CONDITIONS

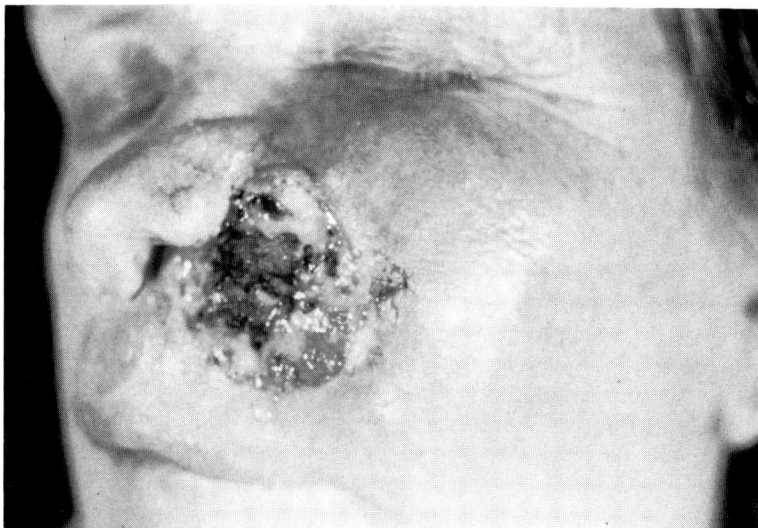

Figure 2–48. Advanced basal cell carcinoma.

the cosmetic result. Death may occasionally occur because of direct tumor extension into vital structures, such as blood vessels or brain.

Squamous Cell Carcinoma

Relative to incidence of all cancers, oral and oropharyngeal squamous cell carcinomas represent about 4% of the total in men (Fig. 2–49) and 2% in women (Fig. 2–50). When stated as numbers, however, the statistics seem more impressive. Annually, about 30,000 new cases of oral (including lip) and oropharyngeal cancer are expected to occur in men and women in the United States. The ratio of men to women is now about 2 to 1. This shift from 3 to 1 has been related to an increase in smoking by women and to their longer life expectancy.

Deaths due to oral and oropharyngeal cancer represent approximately 2% of the total in men and 1% in women. The total number of annual deaths will run as high as 9500.

The trend in survival of patients with this malignancy has been rather disappointing over the past several decades, improving only slightly from 45% to about 50%. The survival rates for blacks were estimated to be significantly and consistently lower. Geographic variations in oral and oropharyngeal carcinoma survival rates exist in the United States and around the world and are most likely connected to habits related to the etiology of this condition.

The survival rate of oral and oropharyngeal cancer has remained disappointingly low and relatively constant, in spite of advances in detection and treatment of many other malignancies. Currently, the greatest hope of improvement of survival rate lies in early detection, an area in which the dental practitioner must play a primary role. The oral cavity is readily accessible for examination and biopsy, making early diagnosis a realistic and achievable goal in oral cancer control.

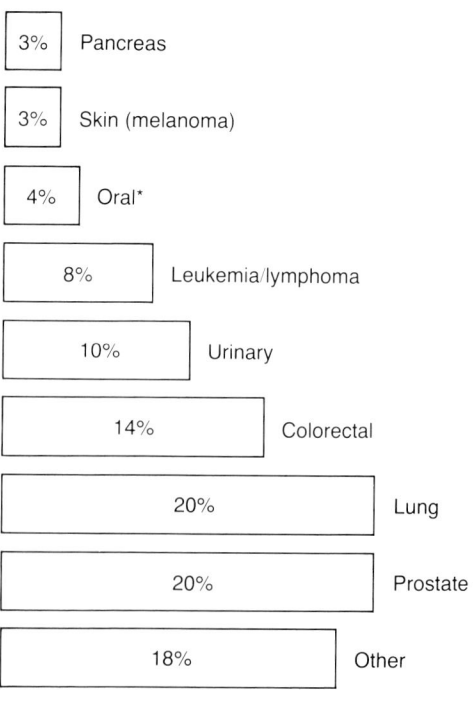

*Represents 20,000 new cases annually.

Figure 2–49. Cancer incidence in men. (Modified from Silverberg E, Lubera J, Cancer statistics, 1988, CA 38:5, 1988.)

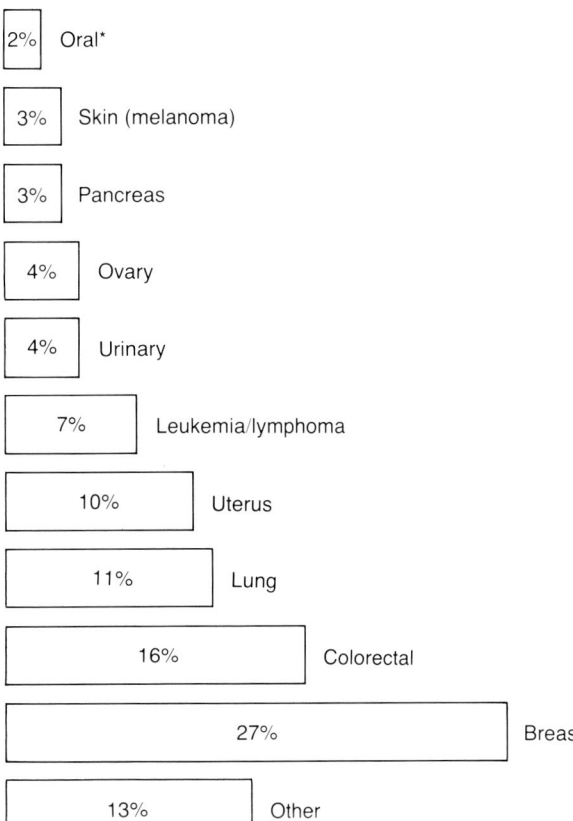

Figure 2–50. Cancer incidence in women. (Modified from Silverberg E, Lubera J, Cancer statistics, 1988, CA 38:5, 1988.)

Etiology. Of all factors believed to contribute to the etiology of oral cancer, tobacco is regarded as the most important. All forms of tobacco smoking as well as the use of smokeless tobacco have been strongly linked to the cause of oral cancer. Cigar and pipe smoking provides greater risk for the development of oral cancer than cigarette smoking, unless "reverse smoking" is done, as may be the habit in India and some South American countries. In this form of smoking, the lighted end of the cigarette is held inside the mouth. The risk then becomes exceedingly high because of the intensity of tobacco combustion adjacent to palatal and lingual tissues. In any event, the time-dose relationship of carcinogens found in tobacco smoke as well as in the tobacco itself is of paramount importance in the cause of oral cancer. The greater the length of time tobacco is used and the greater the amount used, the greater the risk. In addition to an overall increased risk of development of cancer in all regions of the mouth, pipe smokers appear to have a special predilection for squamous cell carcinoma of the lower lip.

With the use of smokeless tobacco, whether in the form of snuff (ground and finely cut tobacco) or chewing tobacco (loose leaf tobacco), the risk of developing oral cancer is significantly increased, especially relative to buccal mucosa and gingiva. A dramatic steady increase in sales and use of smokeless tobacco has been seen over the last decade. Marketing campaigns and peer pressure are generally regarded as primary factors in this rise. Once felt by some to be a relatively safe substitute for cigarettes, the use of smokeless tobacco is now clearly regarded as a significant health hazard. An additional new concern is that young smokeless tobacco users will eventually switch to cigarettes. Not only is there a direct relationship to oral cancer but there is also a direct relationship to elevation of blood pressure, physiologic dependence, and periodontal disease with the use of smokeless tobacco.

The exposure or conditioning period for the appearance of oral cancer from smokeless tobacco is apparently quite long and can be measured in terms of decades. With this in mind, many new oral cancers can be anticipated in the future if smokeless tobacco habits continue at the current rate.

In India and some other Asian countries, oral cancer is the most common type of malignancy and may account for as many as 50% of all cancer cases. This is generally linked to the use of smokeless tobacco mixed with other materials and to the prevalence of its use. The tobacco, typically used with betel nut, slaked lime, and spices, is known as the quid, or pan, and is held in the buccal vestibule for long periods of time. This combination of ingredients, which may vary from one locale to another, is more carcinogenic than tobacco used alone.

Alcohol consumption also appears to add to the risk of oral cancer development. Identification of alcohol alone as a carcinogenic factor has been somewhat difficult because of mixed smoking and drinking habits by most oral cancer patients. Nonetheless, most authorities regard alcohol at least as a promoter if not an initiator of oral cancer. Its effects are simplistically thought to occur through its ability to irritate mucosa and its ability to act as a solvent for carcinogens, especially those in tobacco. Carcinogenic contaminants in alcoholic drinks are also thought to play a role in cancer development.

Some microorganisms have been implicated in oral cancer. The fungus *Candida albicans* has been suggested as a possible causative agent, but this theory has received little support. Historically, the bacterium *T. pallidum* has been implicated because of the occurrence of tongue cancer in tertiary lesions of this organ. This finding has been challenged by the suggestion that the tongue carcinomas are due to the carcinogenic effects of arsenical compounds formerly used to treat syphilis. The link between some viruses and some types of oral cancer has been shown to be relatively strong. Epstein-Barr virus (EBV) has been linked to Burkitt's lymphoma and nasopharyngeal carcinoma. Cytomegalovirus has been linked to Kaposi's sarcoma. It has been suggested that HSV may be related to lip cancer, but support has generally been lacking. Recent studies indicate that members of the papillomavirus group (HPV) may contribute to the etiology of upper aerodigestive tract and laryngeal carcinomas. Verrucous carcinoma in these locations has also been identified as a lesion possibly related to HPV infection.

The only convincing nutritional problem that has been associated with oral cancer is iron deficiency associated with *Plummer-Vinson syndrome,* which typically affects middle-aged females. The syndrome components include a painful red tongue, mucosal atrophy, dysphagia, and a predisposition to the development of oral squamous cell carcinoma.

Ultraviolet light is a known carcinogenic agent that is a significant factor in basal cell carcinomas of the skin and squamous cell carcinomas of the skin and lip. The cumulative dosage of sunlight and the amount of protection by natural pigmentation are of great significance in the development of these cancers. In the ultraviolet light spectrum, radiation with a wavelength of 2900 to 3200 Å (UVB) is more carcinogenic than light of 3200 to 3400 Å (UVA).

Chronic irritation is generally regarded as a modifier rather than an initiator of oral cancer. Mechanical trauma from ill-fitting dentures, broken fillings, and other frictional rubs is unlikely to cause oral cancer. If, however, a cancer is started from another cause, these factors will probably hasten the process. Poor oral hygiene is also regarded as having the same co-carcinogenic effect.

Clinical Features

Carcinoma of the Lips. From a biologic viewpoint, carcinomas of the lower lip should be separated from carcinomas of the upper lip. Carcinomas of the lower lip are far more common than upper lip lesions. Ultraviolet light and pipe smoking are much more important in the cause of lower lip cancer than upper lip cancer. The growth rate is slower for lower lip cancers than for upper lip cancers. The prognosis for lower lip lesions is generally very good, while the prognosis for upper lip lesions is only fair.

Lip carcinomas account for 25 to 30% of all oral cancers. They appear most commonly between 50 and 70 years of age and affect men much more than women. Lesions arise on vermilion and may appear as chronic non-healing ulcers (Fig. 2–51) or as exophytic lesions that are occasionally verrucous in nature (Fig. 2–52). Deep invasion generally appears later in the course of the disease. Metastasis to local submental or submandibular lymph nodes is uncommon but is more likely with larger, more poorly differentiated lesions.

Carcinoma of the Tongue. Squamous cell carcinoma of the tongue is the most common intraoral malignancy. Excluding lip lesions, it accounts for between 25 and 40% of oral carcinomas. There is a definite predilection for males in their sixth, seventh, and eighth decades, although lesions may uncommonly be found in the very young.

Lingual carcinoma is typically asympto-

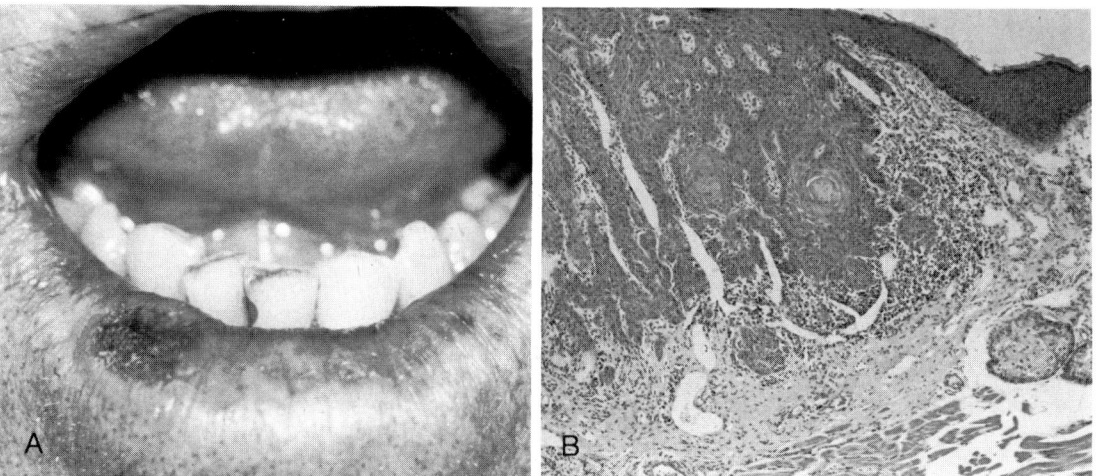

Figure 2–51. *A*, Squamous cell carcinoma of the lower lip. *B*, Elevated margins are due to the presence of neoplasm.

matic. In later stages, as deep invasion occurs, pain or dysphagia may be a prominent patient complaint. The characteristic clinical appearance is one of an indurated, non-healing ulcer with elevated margins (Figs. 2–53 and 2–54). Occasionally, the neoplasm may have a prominent exophytic as well as an endophytic growth pattern. A small percentage of leukoplakias of the tongue represent invasive squamous cell carcinoma or eventually become squamous cell carcinoma. Most erythroplakic patches that appear on the tongue are either *in situ* or invasive squamous cell carcinomas.

The most common location of cancer of the tongue is the posterior lateral border, accounting for up to 45% of tongue lesions. It is particularly uncommon to have lesions develop on the dorsum or in the tip of the tongue. Approximately 25% of tongue cancers occur in the posterior one third or base of the tongue. These lesions are more troublesome than the others because of their silent progression in an area that is difficult to visualize. Accordingly, these lesions are more often metastatic at the time of their discovery, reflecting a significantly poorer prognosis than lesions of the anterior two thirds.

Metastases from tongue cancer are relatively common at the time of primary treatment. In general, metastatic deposits from squamous cell carcinoma of the tongue are found in the lymph nodes of the neck usually on the ipsilateral side. The first nodes to become involved are the submandibular or jugulodigastric nodes at the angle of the mandible. Uncommonly, distant metastatic deposits may be seen in the lung or the liver.

Carcinoma of the Floor of the Mouth. The

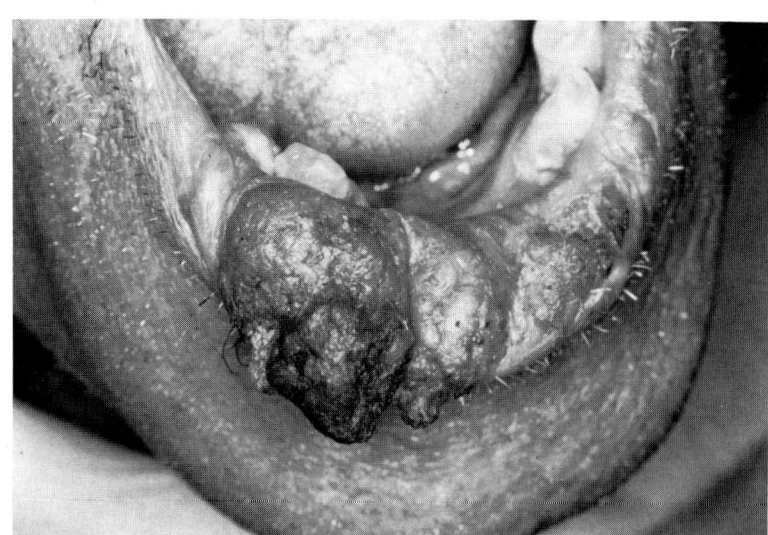

Figure 2–52. Exophytic squamous cell carcinoma of lip.

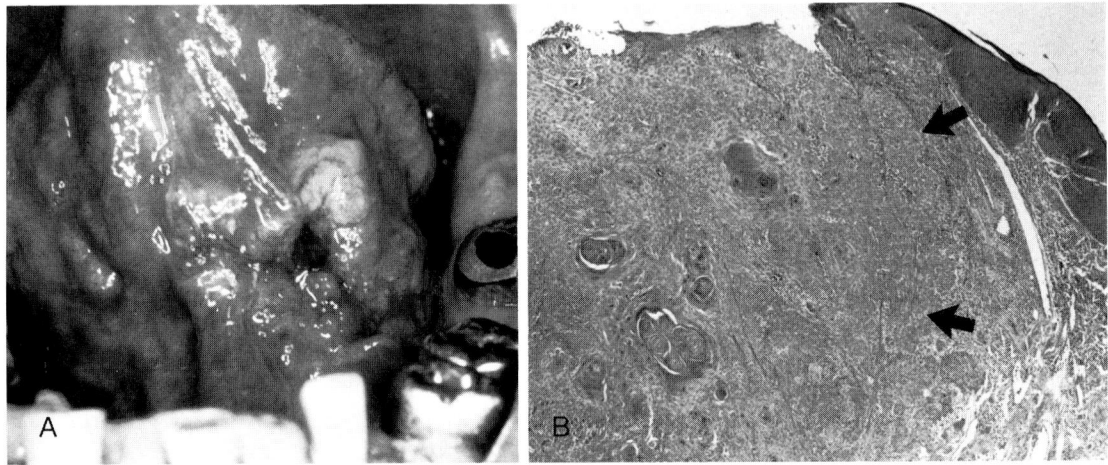

Figure 2–53. *A*, Squamous cell carcinoma of the tongue. *B*, Invasive neoplasm occupies most of submucosa (arrows).

floor of the mouth is the second most common intraoral location of squamous cell carcinomas, accounting for 15 to 20% of cases. Again, carcinomas in this location are seen predominantly in older men, especially those who are chronic alcoholics and smokers. The usual presenting appearance is a painless, non-healing, indurated ulcer (Fig. 2–55). It may also appear as a white or red patch (Fig. 2–56). Occasionally, the lesion may widely infiltrate the soft tissues of the floor of the mouth, causing decreased mobility of the tongue. Metastasis to submandibular lymph nodes is not uncommon for lesions of the floor of the mouth.

Carcinoma of the Buccal Mucosa and Gingiva. Lesions of the buccal mucosa and gingiva each account for approximately 10% of oral squamous cell carcinomas. Men in their seventh decade typify the group affected. Smokeless tobacco is an important etiologic factor in malignant change in these regions. Presenting clinical appearance varies from a white patch to a non-healing ulcer to an exophytic lesion (Fig. 2–57). In the latter group is the clinical pathologic entity *verrucous carcinoma*. This subset of squamous cell carcinoma, most often associated with the use of smokeless tobacco, presents as a broad-based wart-like mass (Fig. 2–58). It is slow growing and very well differentiated, rarely metastasizes, and has a very good prognosis.

Carcinoma of the Palate. There is some justification for the separation of cancers of the hard palate from those of the soft palate. In the soft palate and contiguous faucial tissues, squamous cell carcinoma is a fairly common occurrence, accounting for 10 to 20% of intraoral lesions. In the hard palate, squamous cell carcinomas are relatively uncommon, but adenocarcinomas are relatively common.

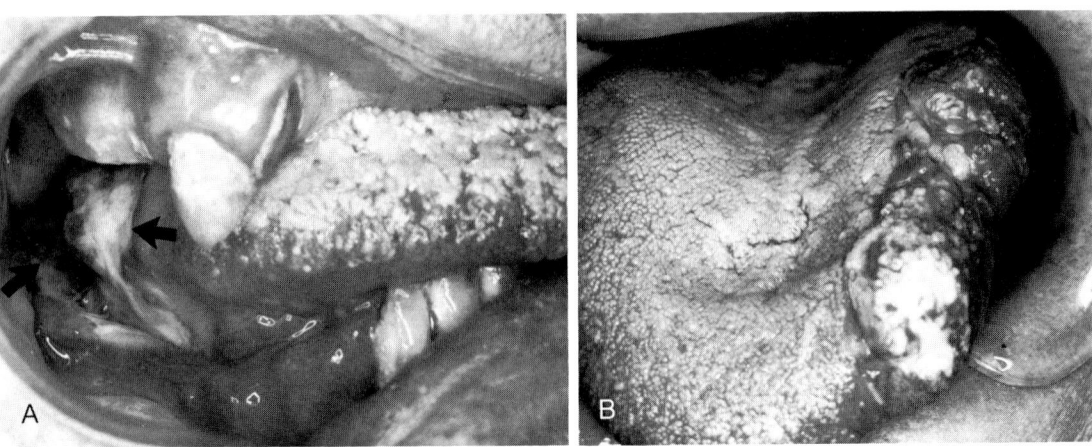

Figure 2–54. *A*, Ulcerative squamous cell carcinoma of posterior lateral tongue (arrows). *B*, Irregular mass representing different clinical pattern of squamous cell carcinoma.

ULCERATIVE CONDITIONS 75

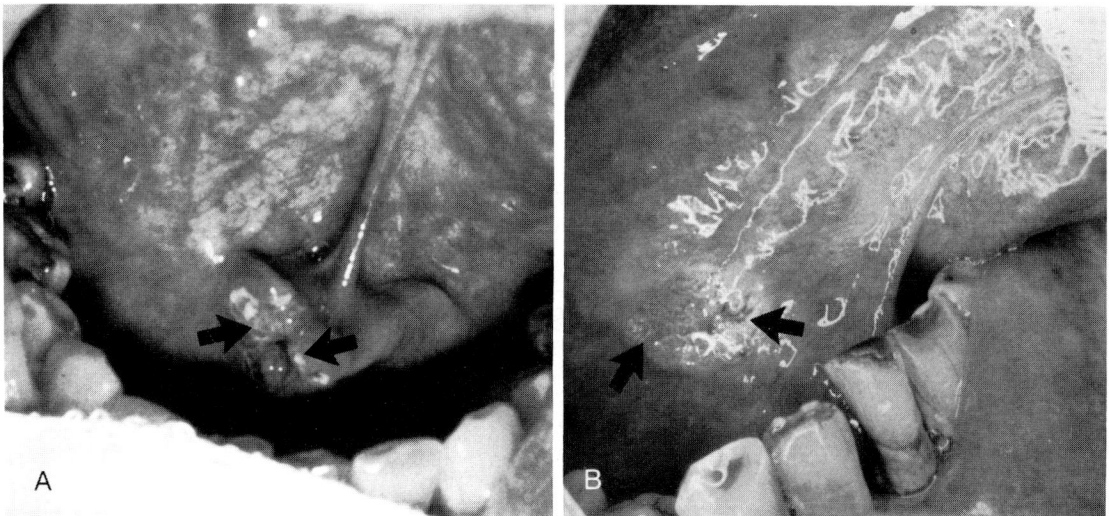

Figure 2–55. *A* and *B*, Early squamous cell carcinomas of the floor of the mouth (arrows). (Courtesy of Dr. E. Ellis.)

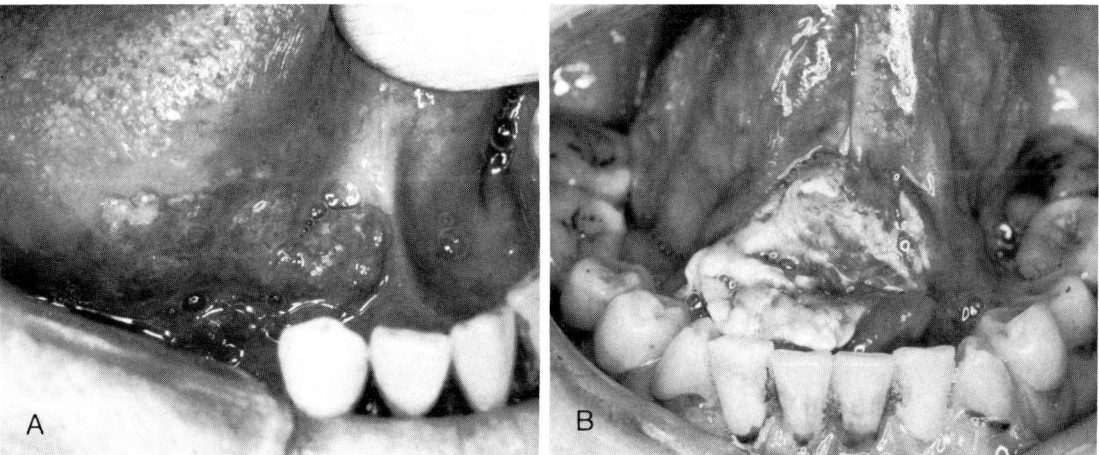

Figure 2–56. *A*, Granular pattern of squamous cell carcinoma in the floor of the mouth. *B*, White (keratotic) mass representing advanced carcinoma.

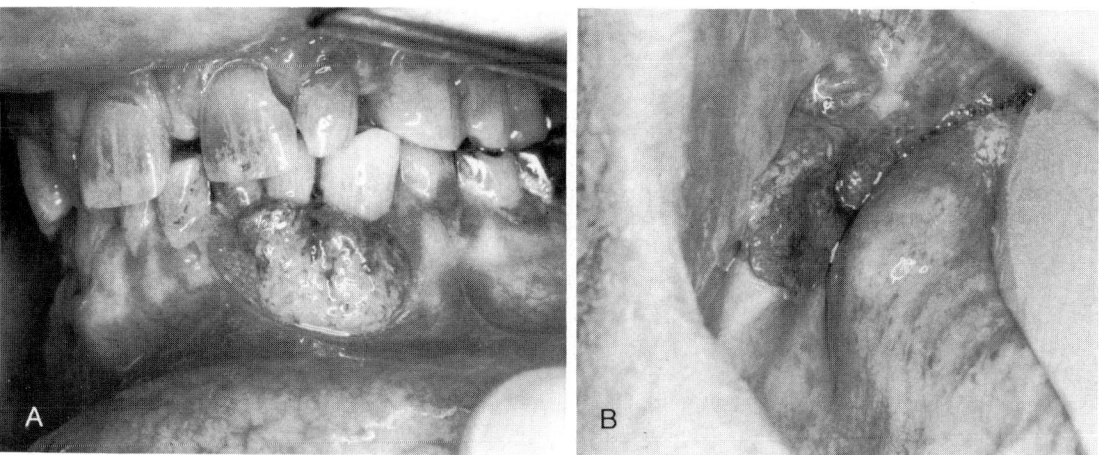

Figure 2–57. *A* and *B*, Squamous cell carcinoma of gingiva and buccal mucosa.

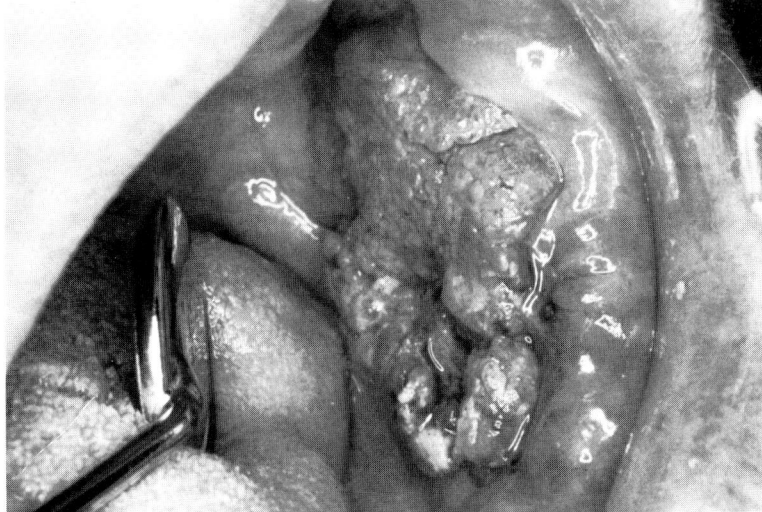

Figure 2–58. Verrucous carcinoma of the buccal mucosa (Courtesy of Dr. J. R. Hayward.)

However, palatal carcinomas are frequently seen in countries such as India where reverse smoking is the custom.

Palatal squamous cell carcinomas generally present as asymptomatic, red or white plaques or as ulcerated masses (adenocarcinomas initially appear as non-ulcerated masses) in older men (Figs. 2–59 and 2–60). Metastasis to cervical nodes or large lesions signifies an ominous course.

Histopathology. Most oral squamous cell carcinomas are moderately or well differentiated lesions. Keratin pearls and individual cell keratinizations are usually evident. Invasion into subjacent structures in the form of small nests of hyperchromatic cells is also typical. Considerable variation between tumors is seen relative to numbers of mitoses, nuclear pleomorphism, and amount of keratinization. In H&E sections of poorly differentiated lesions, keratin is absent or is seen in minute amounts. It can, however, be identified using immunohistochemical techniques for the demonstration of antigenic determinants on otherwise occult keratin intermediate filaments. A significant inflammatory host response is usually found surrounding the nests of invading tumor cells. Lymphocytes, plasma cells and macrophages may all be seen in large numbers.

Rarely, an oral squamous cell carcinoma will appear as a proliferation of spindle cells that may be mistaken for a sarcoma. This type of tumor, known as spindle cell carcinoma, arises from the surface epithelium usually of the lips and occasionally of the tongue. Immunohistochemical staining can be used to identify keratin antigens in this lesion when H&E sections

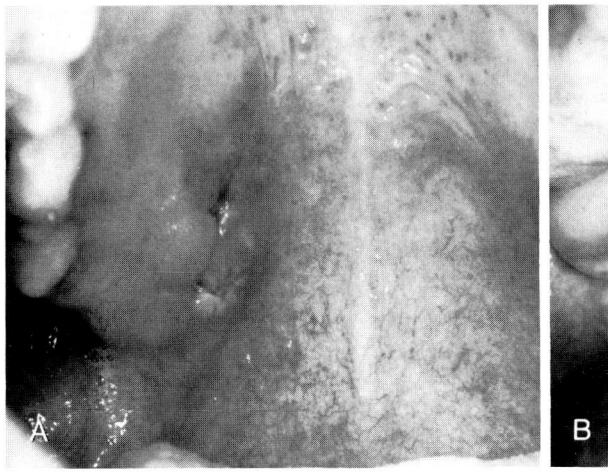
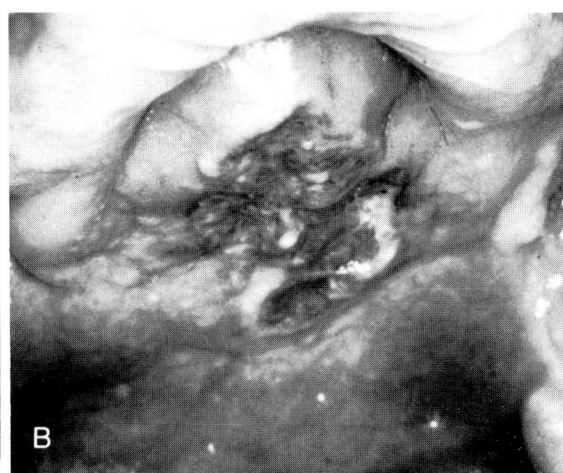

Figure 2–59. *A* and *B*, Squamous cell carcinoma of the palate.

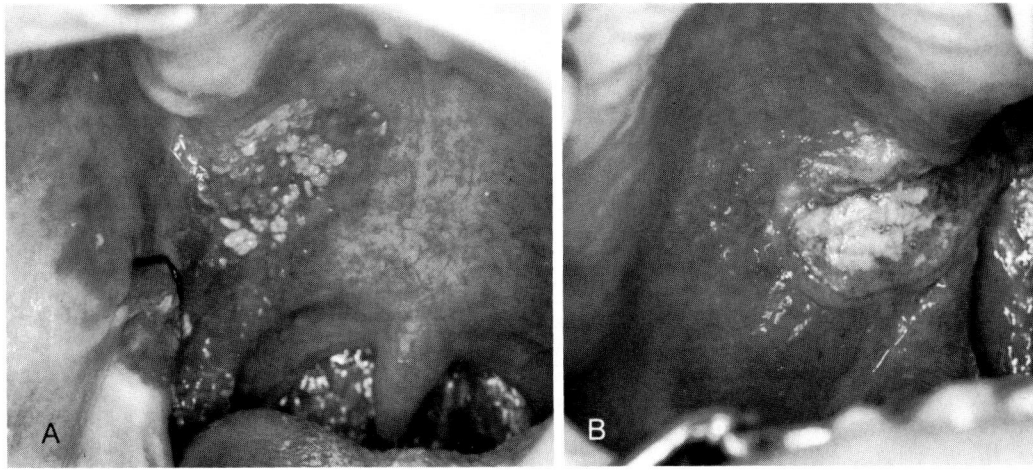

Figure 2–60. Squamous cell carcinoma of soft palate and tonsillar pillar. *A*, Note black silk suture at biopsy site. *B*, Second primary oral cancer in 58-year-old man.

show equivocal findings. Electron microscopy may also be utilized to identify structures such as intracellular tonofilaments and epithelial-type cell junctions desmosomes.

Verrucous carcinoma is characterized by very well differentiated epithelial cells that appear more hyperplastic than neoplastic. A key feature is the invasive nature of the lesion in the form of broad pushing margins. The advancing front is usually surrounded by lymphocytes, plasma cells, and macrophages. Diagnosis based solely on microscopic features is often difficult; it is frequently necessary to consider the lesion in the context of clinical presentation.

Differential Diagnosis. When oral squamous cell carcinomas present in their typical clinical form of chronic non-healing ulcers, other ulcerative conditions should be considered. An undiagnosed chronic ulcer must always be considered potentially infectious until biopsy proves otherwise. It may be impossible on clinical grounds to separate TB, syphilis, and deep fungal infections expressing oral manifestations from oral cancer. Chronic trauma, including factitial injuries, may also mimic squamous cell carcinoma. Careful history taking is especially important, and biopsy will confirm the diagnosis. In the palate and contiguous tissues, midline granuloma and necrotizing sialometaplasia would be serious diagnostic considerations.

Treatment. Generally, oral cancers are best treated with surgery or radiation, or both. Smaller lesions are typically treated with surgery alone, with radiation used as a backup in the event of recurrence. It is not uncommon for radiation to be used alone for smaller lesions. Factors that determine which is to be used include lesion location, histologic type, institution facilities and philosophy, referral patterns, and therapist skills. All things being equal, cure rates are essentially similar. Larger lesions may be treated with either modality or with surgery followed by radiation. Elective or prophylactic neck dissection or radiation is advocated by many in order to eliminate subclinical or occult metastases. Oral squamous cell carcinomas are generally resistant to chemotherapeutic measures. Effects are generally measured in terms of tumor regression rather than elimination. Although anticancer drugs may reduce tumor bulk and delay spread, the profound morbidity associated with this type of treatment may not justify its use. When chemotherapy is employed for oral squamous cell carcinoma, it is usually used as adjunctive therapy in advanced cases.

Therapeutic Radiation Regimens and Complications. In the head and neck, therapeutic radiation is utilized most commonly in the treatment of squamous cell carcinomas and lymphomas. It tends to be more effective on less well differentiated lesions, making its use on verrucous carcinoma questionable. Early reports indicated that verrucous lesions were radioresistant, but recently this concept has been challenged.

The radiation level needed to kill malignant cells ranges from 4000 to 7000 rad. In order to make this tolerable to patients, radiation is fractionated into daily doses of approximately 200 rad. This allows delivery over a 4- to 7-week period of a total tumor dose of 4000 to 5000 rad for lymphomas and 6000 to 7000 rad for squamous cell carcinomas.

Along with the therapeutic effects of radiation are side effects that are dose dependent (Table 2–11). Some of these are reversible, although others are not. Radiation-induced ulcers and the accompanying pain and dysgeusia are known collectively as mucositis (Fig. 2–61). Radiation mucositis is a reversible condition that begins 1 to 2 weeks after the start of therapy and ends several weeks after the termination of therapy. Oral candidiasis often accompanies the mucositis. Permanent damage to salivary gland tissue situated in the beam path may produce significant levels of xerostomia. Some recovery is often seen, especially at lower radiation levels. Xerostomia is frequently the patient's chief complaint during the post-radiation period. Unfortunately, other than the frequent use of water or artificial saliva, there is currently no effective therapeutic measure that can be used to help patients with this problem. With the dryness also comes the potential for the development of cervical or so-called radiation caries (Figs. 2–62 and 2–63). This problem can be minimized with regular patient follow-up dental care and scrupulous oral hygiene (Fig. 2–64).

Skin in the path of the radiation beam will also suffer some damage. Alopecia will be temporary at lower radiation levels but permanent at the higher levels required in the treatment of squamous cell carcinoma. Skin erythema is temporary, but the telangiectasias and atrophy that follow are permanent.

A more insidious and hidden problem lies in the damage that radiation causes to bone, which may result in osteonecrosis. Radiation apparently has deleterious effects on osteocytes, osteoblasts, and endothelial cells, causing reduced capacity of bone to recover from injury. Injury may come in the form of trauma (such as extractions), advancing periodontal disease, and periapical inflammation associated with non-vital teeth (Fig. 2–65). Once osteonecrosis occurs, varying amounts of bone (usually in the mandible) will be lost. This may be an area as small as a few millimeters in size to as large as half the jaw or more (Fig. 2–66). The most important factor responsible for osteonecrosis is the amount of radiation directed through bone on the path to the tumor. Oral health is also of considerable significance. Poor nutrition and chronic alcoholism appear to be influential in the progression of this complication. Because osteonecrosis is a danger that is always present after radiation, tooth extractions should be avoided after therapy. If absolutely necessary, tooth removal should be done as atraumatically as possible, using antibiotic coverage. It is preferable to commit to a treatment plan that schedules tooth removal before radiation therapy begins. Initial soft tissue healing before beginning therapy will

Table 2–11. SIDE EFFECTS OF THERAPEUTIC RADIATION

Temporary Side Effects	Permanent Side Effects
Mucosal ulcers	Xerostomia
Pain	Cervical caries
Dysgeusia/hypogeusia	Osteonecrosis
Candidiasis	Telangiectasia
Dermatitis	Epithelial atrophy
Erythema	Alopecia (higher doses)
Alopecia (lower doses)	

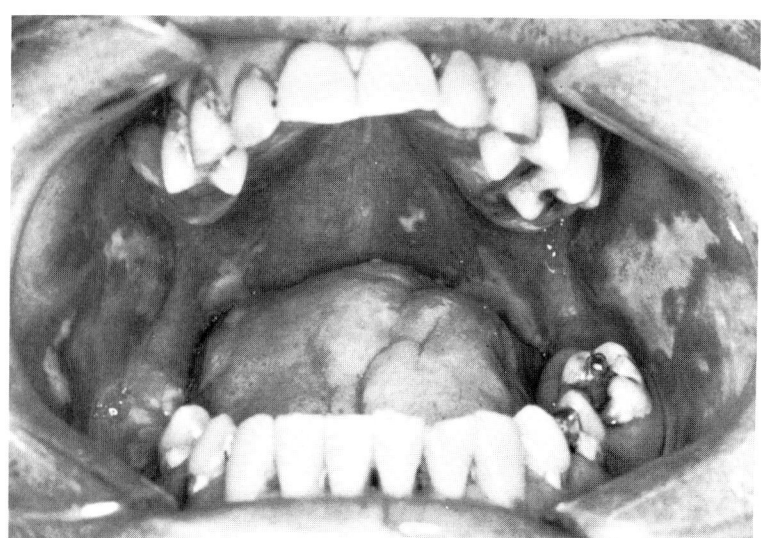

Figure 2–61. Acute radiation-induced ulcers (mucositis).

ULCERATIVE CONDITIONS 79

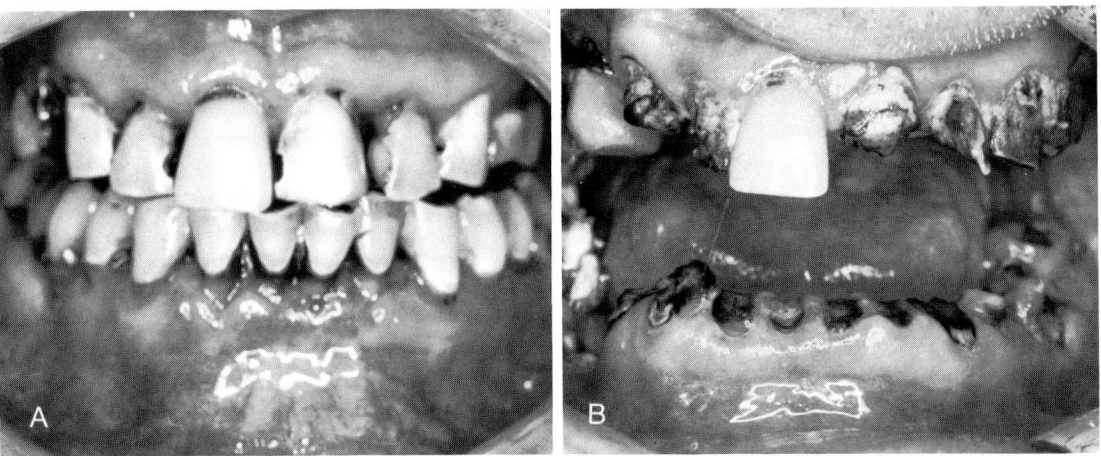

Figure 2–62. *A*, Cervical "radiation" caries resulting from xerostomia and poor oral hygiene. *B*, Same patient 3 years later.

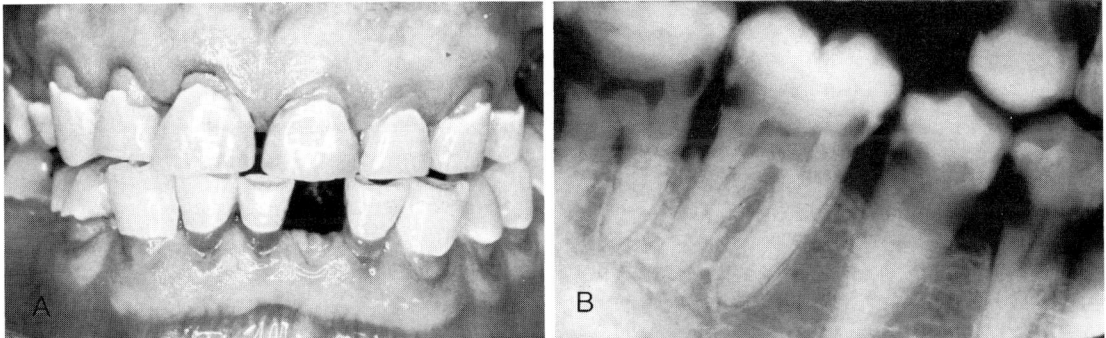

Figure 2–63. *A* and *B*, Radiation-associated cervical caries.

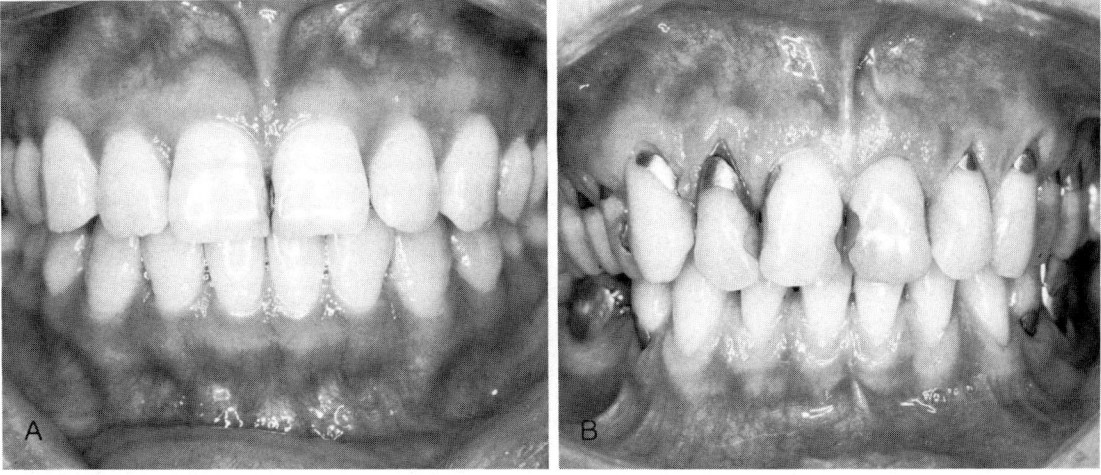

Figure 2–64. *A* and *B*, Post-radiation-status patients with xerostomia but excellent oral hygiene and follow-up care.

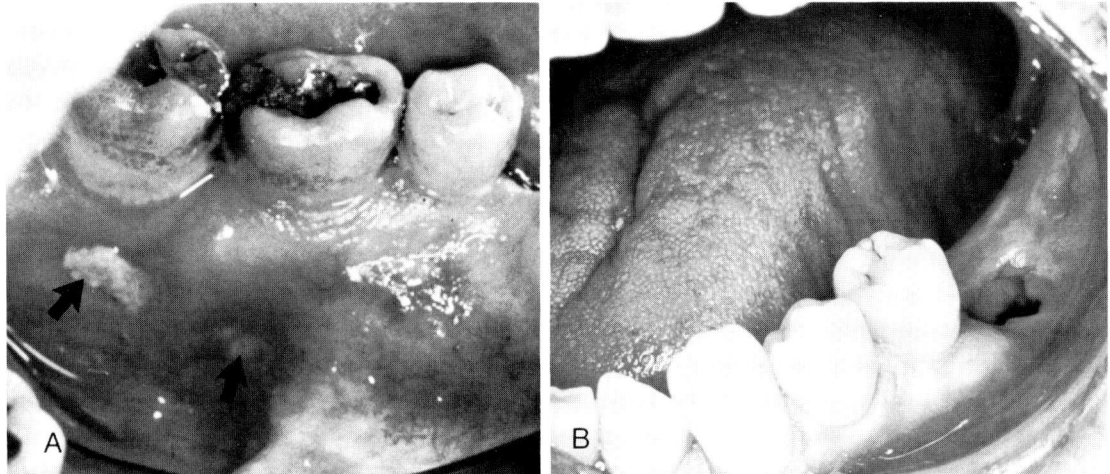

Figure 2–65. *A,* Osteonecrosis of lingual mandible caused by trauma. Note exposed bone (arrows). *B,* Non-healing bone of 2 years' duration in site of post-radiation extraction.

reduce the risk of non-healing of the extraction sites. Prosthetic devices such as dentures and partial dentures, if carefully constructed and monitored, can be worn without difficulty. Xerostomia does not seem to cause difficulty in the wearing of these prostheses. Continued careful surveillance of the patient's oral health, during and after radiation therapy, will help keep complications to an acceptable minimum.

Prognosis. The prognosis for patients with oral squamous cell carcinoma is dependent upon both histologic subtype (grade) and clinical extent (stage) of the tumor. Of the two, clinical stage is more important. Other, more abstract factors that may influence clinical course include age, gender, general health, immune system status, and mental attitude.

The grading of a tumor is the microscopic determination of the differentiation of the tumor cells. Well-differentiated lesions generally have a less aggressive biologic course than poorly differentiated lesions. Of all squamous cell carcinoma histologic subtypes, the most well differentiated, verrucous carcinoma, has the best prognosis. The less-differentiated lesions have a correspondingly poorer prognosis.

The most important indicator of prognosis is the clinical stage of the disease. Once metastasis to cervical nodes has occurred, the 5-year survival rate is reduced by at least half. The overall 5-year survival rate for oral squamous cell carcinoma is around 45 to 50%. If the neoplasm is small and localized, the 5-year cure rate may be as high as 60 to 70% (lower

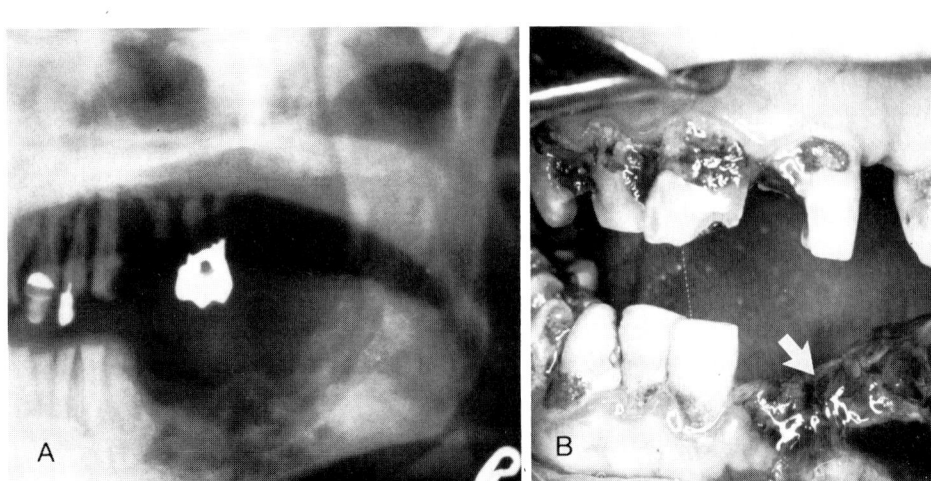

Figure 2–66. *A,* Advanced osteonecrosis of mandible from patient in Figure 2–60. *B,* Advanced cervical caries and necrosis of mandibular bone (arrows).

ULCERATIVE CONDITIONS 81

Table 2-12. TNM STAGING SYSTEM FOR ORAL SQUAMOUS CELL CARCINOMA

T—Tumor
   T_1—Tumor less than 2 cm in diameter
   T_2—Tumor 2–4 cm in diameter
   T_3—Tumor greater than 4 cm in diameter
   T_4—Tumor invades adjacent structures

N—Node
   N_0—No palpable nodes
   N_1—Ipsilateral palpable nodes
   N_2—Contralateral or bilateral nodes
   N_3—Fixed palpable nodes

M—Metastasis
   M_0—No distant metastasis
   M_1—Clinical or radiographic evidence of metastasis

lip lesions may rate as high as 80 to 90%). However, if cervical metastases are present at the time of diagnosis, the survival figures drop precipitously to about 20%.

A numerical system for the clinical staging of oral squamous cell carcinoma has been devised to provide clinical uniformity. It is known as the TNM system—T is a measure of the primary tumor size, N is an estimation of the regional lymph node metastasis, and M is a determination of distant metastases (Table 2–12). Utilization of this system allows more meaningful comparison of data from different institutions and helps guide therapeutic decisions. As the clinical stage advances from I to IV, prognosis worsens (Table 2–13).

Another factor that comes into play in the overall prognosis of oral cancer patients is the increased risk for the development of a second primary lesion. These lesions do not represent recurrence or persistence of the original tumor but new, geographically separate lesions of the upper alimentary tract or even of other organ systems. Approximately 10% of oral cancer patients will develop a second primary lesion, often in the first or second follow-up year. Probably the single most important factor that accounts for this phenomenon is the conditioning by etiologic factors of large areas of mucosa (field effect).

Carcinoma of the Maxillary Sinus

Etiology. Malignancies of the paranasal sinuses occur most commonly in the maxillary sinus. The cause is unknown, although squamous metaplasia of sinus epithelium associated with chronic sinusitis and oral antral fistulas is felt by some investigators to be a predisposing factor.

Clinical Features. This is a disease of older age, affecting predominantly patients over the age of 40. Men are generally afflicted more than women. Past history in these patients frequently includes symptoms of sinusitis. As the neoplasm progresses, a dull ache in the area occurs, with eventual development of overt pain. Specific signs and symptoms referable to oral structures are frequently seen, especially when the neoplasm has its origin in the sinus floor. As the neoplasm extends toward the apices of the maxillary posterior teeth, referred pain may occur. "Toothache," which actually represents neoplastic involvement of the superior alveolar nerve, is a not uncommon symptom in patients with maxillary sinus malignancies. In ruling out dental disease by history and clinical tests, it is imperative that the dental practitioner be aware that sinus neoplasms may present through the alveolus. Without this suspicion, unfortunate delays in definitive treatment may occur. Other clinical signs of invasion of the alveolar process include recently acquired malocclusion, displacement of teeth, and vertical mobility of teeth (teeth undermined by neoplasm). Failure of a socket to heal following an extraction may be indicative of tumor involvement. Paresthesia should always be viewed as an ominous sign and should cause the clinician to consider malignancy within bone. Occasional maxillary sinus cancers may present as a palatal ulcer representing extension through the bone and soft tissue of the palate.

Histopathology. Of the malignancies that originate in the maxillary sinus, squamous cell carcinoma is the most common histologic type. These lesions are generally less differentiated than those occurring in oral mucous membranes. Infrequently, adenocarcinomas arising

Table 2-13. TNM STAGING SYSTEM

Stage I	$T_1 N_0 M_0$
Stage II	$T_2 N_0 M_0$
Stage III	$T_3 N_0 M_0$
	$T_1 N_1 M_0$
	$T_2 N_1 M_0$
	$T_3 N_1 M_0$
Stage IV	$T_1 N_2 M_0$
	$T_2 N_2 M_0$
	$T_3 N_2 M_0$
	$T_1 N_3 M_0$
	$T_2 N_3 M_0$
	$T_3 N_3 M_0$
	$T_4 N_0 M_0$
	Any patients with M_1

presumably from mucous glands in the sinus lining may be seen.

Diagnosis. From a clinical standpoint, when oral signs and symptoms appear to be related to antral carcinoma, dental origin must be ruled out. This is best accomplished by the dental practitioner because of familiarity with normal tooth-jaw relationships and experience in interpretation of vitality tests. Other clinical considerations related to malignancies in the age group in which antral carcinomas occur are metastatic disease and plasma cell myeloma. Osteosarcoma and other less common sarcomas that are usually seen in a younger age group might also be included. Palatal involvement should also cause the clinician to consider adenocarcinoma of minor salivary gland origin, lymphoma, and squamous cell carcinoma.

Treatment and Prognosis. Maxillary sinus carcinomas are generally treated with surgery or radiation, or both. A combination of the two seems to be somewhat more effective than either modality alone. Radiation is often completed first, with surgical resection following. Chemotherapy used in conjunction with radiation has been somewhat successful.

In any event, prognosis is only fair at best. Cure is directly dependent upon the clinical stage of the disease at the time of initial treatment. Compared with oral lesions, sinus lesions are discovered in a more advanced stage because of delays in seeking treatment and delays in making a definitive diagnosis. The anatomy of the area also influences prognosis. Because it is a richly vascular area that is difficult to remove surgically and because it is an area that is difficult to reconstruct, the surgeon may be less aggressive than if the lesion were located elsewhere. The 5-year survival rate is about 25%. If the disease is discovered early, the likelihood of survival increases.

Bibliography

Infectious Diseases

Alfieri N, Fleury R, Opromolla D, et al. Oral lesions in borderline and reactional tuberculoid leprosy. Oral Surg Oral Med Oral Pathol 55:52–57, 1983.

Borssen E, Sundquist G. Actinomyces of infected dental root canals. Oral Surg Oral Med Oral Pathol 51:643–647, 1981.

Fergus H, Savord E. Actinomycosis involving a periapical cyst in the anterior maxilla. Oral Surg Oral Med Oral Pathol 49:390–393, 1980.

Giunta J, Fiumara N. Facts about gonorrhea and dentistry. Oral Surg Oral Med Oral Pathol 62:529–531, 1986.

Griffin J, Bach D, Nespeca J, et al. Noma. Oral Surg Oral Med Oral Pathol 56:605–607, 1983.

Happonen R, Viander M, Pelliriemi L. Actinomyces israelii in osteoradionecrosis of the jaws. 55:580–587, 1983.

Jamsky R, Christen A. Oral gonococcal infections. Oral Surg Oral Med Oral Pathol 53:358–362, 1982.

Mandell G, Douglas R, Bennett J. Principles and Practice of Infectious Diseases. 2nd ed. Wiley & Sons, New York, 1985, Chaps 182, 210, 214, 219.

Mani N. Secondary syphilis initially diagnosed from oral lesions. Oral Surg Oral Med Oral Pathol 58:47–50, 1984.

Michaud M, Blanchette G, Tomich C. Chronic ulceration of the hard palate: first clinical sign of undiagnosed pulmonary tuberculosis. Oral Surg Oral Med Oral Pathol 57:63–67, 1984.

Robbins S, Cotran R, Kumar V. Pathologic Basis of Disease. 3rd ed. W B Saunders, Philadelphia, 1984, pp 351–359.

Rose H, Gingrass D. Localized oral blastomycosis mimicking actinomycosis. Oral Surg Oral Med Oral Pathol 54:12–14, 1982.

Immunologic Diseases

Bangert J, Freeman R, Sontheimer R, et al. Subacute cutaneous lupus erythematosus and discoid lupus erythematosus. Arch Dermatol 120:332–337, 1984.

Batsakis J. Wegener's granulomatosis and midline (nonhealing) granuloma. Head Neck Surg 1:213–222, 1979.

Buchner A, Lozada F, Silverman S. Histopathologic spectrum of oral erythema multiforme. Oral Surg Oral Med Oral Pathol 49:221–228, 1980.

Cornell R, Stoughton R. The use of topical steroids in psoriasis. Dermatol Clin 2:397–409, 1984.

Ford D, da Roza D, Schulzer M. The specificity of synovial mononuclear cell responses to microbiological antigens in Reiter's syndrome. J Rheumatol 9:561–567, 1982.

Fritz K, Weston W. Topical glucocorticosteroids. Ann Allergy 50:68–76, 1983.

Gadol N, Greenspan J, Hoover C, et al. Leukocyte migration inhibition in recurrent aphthous ulceration. J Oral Pathol 14:121–132, 1985.

Gallant C, Kenny P. Oral glucocorticoids and their complications. J Am Acad Dermatol 14:161–177, 1986.

Giunta J, Fiumara N. Ampicillin allergy presenting as secondary syphilis. Oral Surg Oral Med Oral Pathol 57:152–154, 1984.

Glenert U. Drug stomatitis due to gold therapy. Oral Surg Oral Med Oral Pathol 58:52–56, 1984.

Greenspan J, Gadol N, Olson J, et al. Lymphocyte function in recurrent aphthous ulceration. J Oral Pathol 14:592–602, 1985.

Greenspan J, Shillitoe E. Microbial pathogenicity in oral soft tissue diseases. J Dent Res 63:431–434, 1984.

Hansen L, Silverman S, Pons V, et al. Limited Wegener's granulomatosis. Oral Surg Oral Med Oral Pathol 60:524–531, 1985.

Hill C, Rostenberg A. Adverse effects from topical steroids. Cutis 21:624–628, 1978.

Hoover C, Olson J, Greenspan J. Humoral responses and cross-reactivity to viridans streptococci in recurrent aphthous ulceration. J Dent Res 65:1101–1104, 1986.

Jorizzo J. Behçet's disease. Arch Dermatol 122:556–558, 1986.

Kazmierowski J, Wuepper K. Erythema multiforme: immune-complex vasculitis of the superficial cutaneous micro-vasculature. J Invest Dermatol 71:366–369, 1978.

Lindemann R, Riviere G, Sapp P. Oral mucosal antigen reactivity during exacerbation and remission phase of recurrent aphthous ulceration. Oral Surg Oral Med Oral Pathol 60:281–284, 1985.

Lindemann R, Riviere G, Sapp P. Serum antibody responses to indigenous oral mucosal antigens and selected laboratory-maintained bacteria in recurrent aphthous ulceration. Oral Surg Oral Med Oral Pathol 59:585–589, 1985.

Miller M, Ship I, Ram C. A retrospective study of the prevalence and incidence of recurrent aphthous ulcers in a professional population, 1958–1971. Oral Surg Oral Med Oral Pathol 43:532–537, 1977.

Olson J, Feinberg I, Silverman S Jr, et al. Serum vitamin B12, folate, and iron levels in recurrent aphthous ulceration. Oral Surg Oral Med Oral Pathol 54:517–520, 1982.

Savage N, Seymour G, Kruger B. Expression of class I and class II major histocompatibility complex antigens on epithelial cells in recurrent aphthous stomatitis. J Oral Pathol 15:191–195, 1986.

Savage N, Seymour G, Kruger B. T-lymphocyte subset changes in recurrent aphthous stomatitis. Oral Surg Oral Med Oral Pathol 60:175–181, 1985.

Schiodt M. Oral discoid lupus erythematosus. II. Skin lesions and systemic lupus erythematosus in sixty-six patients with six-year follow-up. Oral Surg Oral Med Oral Pathol 57:177–180, 1984.

Schiodt M. Oral discoid lupus erythematosus. III. A histopathologic study of sixty-six patients. Oral Surg Oral Med Oral Pathol 57:281–293, 1984.

Schiodt M, Holmstrup P, Dabelsteen E, Ullman S. Deposits of immunoglobulins, complement, and fibrinogen in oral lupus erythematosus, lichen planus, and leukoplakia. Oral Surg Oral Med Oral Pathol 51:603–608, 1981.

Schroeder H, Muller-Glauser W, Sallay K. Pathomorphologic features of the ulcerative stage of oral aphthous ulcerations. Oral Surg Oral Med Oral Pathol 58:293–305, 1984.

Schroeder H, Muller-Glauser W, Sallay K. Stereologic analysis of leukocyte infiltration in oral ulcers of developing Mikulicz aphthae. Oral Surg Oral Med Oral Pathol 56:629–640, 1983.

Sharquie K. Suppression of Behçet's disease with dapsone. Br J Dermatol 110:493–494, 1984.

Storrs F. Use and abuse of systemic corticosteroid therapy. J Am Acad Dermatol 1:95–105, 1979.

Wermuth D, Geoghegan W, Jordon R. Anti-Ro/SSA antibodies. Arch Dermatol 121:335–338, 1985.

Wiesenfeld D, Scully C, MacFadyed E. Multiple lichenoid drug reactions in a patient with Ferguson-Smith disease. Oral Surg Oral Med Oral Pathol 54:527–529, 1982.

Wray D, Vlagopoulos T, Siraganian R. Food allergens and basophil histamine release in recurrent aphthous stomatitis. Oral Surg Oral Med Oral Path 54:388–400, 1982.

Wysocki G, Brooke R. Oral manifestations of chronic granulomatous disease. Oral Surg Oral Med Oral Pathol 46:815–819, 1978.

Neoplasms

Batsakis J. Tumors of the Head and Neck. 2nd ed. Wiley & Sons, New York, 1979, Chaps 6 and 7.

Beahrs O, Henson D, Hutter R, et al. Manual for Staging of Cancer. 3rd ed. J. B. Lippincott, Philadelphia, 1988, pp 27–30.

Connolly G, Winn D, Hecht S, et al. The reemergence of smokeless tobacco. New Engl J Med 314:1020–1027, 1986.

Rollo J, Rozenbom C, Thawley S, et al. Squamous cell carcinoma of the base of the tongue. Cancer 47:333–342, 1981.

Shibuya H, Amagasa T, Seta K. Leukoplakia-associated multiple carcinomas in patients with tongue carcinoma. Cancer 57:843–846, 1986.

Silverberg E, Lubera J. Cancer statistics, 1988. CA 38:5–22, 1988.

Winn D, Blot W, Shy C, et al. Snuff dipping and oral cancer among women in the southern United States. N Engl J Med 304:745–749, 1981.

Chapter 3

White Lesions

HEREDITARY CONDITIONS
Leukoedema
White Sponge Nevus
Hereditary Benign Intraepithelial Dyskeratosis
Follicular Keratosis
REACTIVE LESIONS
Focal (Frictional) Hyperkeratosis
White Lesions Associated with Smokeless Tobacco
Nicotine Stomatitis
Solar Cheilitis
OTHER WHITE LESIONS
Idiopathic Leukoplakia
Hairy Leukoplakia
Hairy Tongue
Geographic Tongue
Lichen Planus
NON-EPITHELIAL WHITE-YELLOW LESIONS
Candidiasis
Mucosal Burns
Submucous Fibrosis
Fordyce's Granules
Ectopic Lymphoid Tissue
Gingival Cysts
Parulis
Lipoma

White-appearing lesions of the oral mucosa obtain their characteristic appearance from the scattering of light through an altered surface. Such alterations may be the result of a thickened layer of keratin that may form secondary to chronic physical trauma, tobacco use, genetic abnormalities, mucocutaneous diseases, or inflammatory reactions. White-appearing lesions may therefore be divided into classes by etiology or pathogenesis. In many circumstances, a cause may not be identified or known. In others, however, a relationship between an event or a putative agent and the formation of a white lesion may be evident, although an exact mechanism may not be understood or developed. The context of this chapter, therefore, is the clinical white-appearing mucosal lesion with a potentially broad array of etiologic factors and an equally wide spectrum of histologic appearance, from benign reactive to malignant.

When one is confronted in the clinical setting with a white lesion, development of a history can be of considerable significance. Information important to establishing a diagnosis of a white lesion is family history of similar lesions, duration of the process, identification of oral habits such as cheek biting and tobacco use (type and frequency), associated cutaneous or mucosal lesions, current medications, constitutional signs and symptoms, and clinical and laboratory data (including serologic, hematologic, or microbiologic information). A rational treatment plan would then logically follow.

HEREDITARY CONDITIONS

Several hereditary disorders of the oral mucosa are characterized by keratotic or hyperkeratotic disturbances. These disorders share the common clinical finding of a mucosal white lesion. In most instances, hereditary patterns are well established and have been confirmed in numerous studies. In a generic sense, hereditary conditions of the oral mucosa manifesting as white lesions have also been termed "genokeratoses" by some practitioners; others use a more general term, "genodermatosis."

Leukoedema

Etiology and Pathogenesis. To date, no definitive cause or etiology of leukoedema has been established. Attempts to implicate factors such as smoking, alcohol ingestion, bacterial infection, salivary conditions, and electrochemical interactions have been unsuccessful. Some studies, however, indicate a possible relationship between poor oral hygiene and abnormal masticatory patterns. An ethnic or racial clustering of this condition is noted, with blacks the major group affected.

Clinical Features. Leukoedema is usually discovered as an incidental finding. It is asymptomatic, is symmetric in distribution, and occurs on the buccal mucosa (Fig. 3–1). It appears as a gray-white, diffuse, filmy or milky surface. In more exaggerated cases, a whitish cast with surface textural changes, including wrinkling or corrugation, may be seen. With stretching of the buccal mucosa, the opaque changes will dissipate, except in more advanced cases. Gentle stroking with a gauze pad or tongue depressor will not remove leukoedema.

Histopathology. In leukoedema the epithelium is parakeratotic and acanthotic, with marked intracellular edema of spinous cells. The enlarged epithelial cells have small, pyknotic nuclei in optically clear cytoplasm. Alterations in the germinative layer are absent as are inflammatory changes in the lamina propria.

Differential Diagnosis. Leukoplakia, white sponge nevus, hereditary benign intraepithelial dyskeratosis, and the response to chronic cheek biting may show clinical similarities to leukoedema. The overall thickness of these lesions, their persistence upon stretching, and specific microscopic features help separate them from leukoedema.

Treatment and Prognosis. No treatment is necessary since the changes are innocuous. There is no malignant potential, and there is no predisposition to the development of leukoplakia. It is important to recognize this process and avoid unnecessary intervention.

White Sponge Nevus

Clinical Features. White sponge nevus is an autosomal dominant transmitted condition that is often mistaken for leukoplakia. It presents as an asymptomatic, deeply folded, white or gray lesion that may affect several mucosal surfaces. Lesions tend to be somewhat thickened and have a spongy consistency. The presentation intraorally is almost always bilateral and symmetric and usually appears early in life, typically before puberty. The characteristic clinical manifestations of this particular form of keratosis are usually best observed on the buccal mucosa, although other areas such as the tongue, especially along the lateral margins, may also be involved (Fig. 3–2). Although the conjunctival mucosa is often spared, there is a variable degree of involvement of the esophageal, anal, vulval, and vaginal mucosa.

Histopathology. Microscopically, the epithelium is greatly thickened, with marked spongiosis, acanthosis, and parakeratosis. Within the stratum spinosum, marked hydropic or clear cell change may be noted, often beginning in the parabasal region and extending very close to the surface. Nuclei within the acanthotic component tend to be somewhat pyknotic and often eccentric in location. Peri-

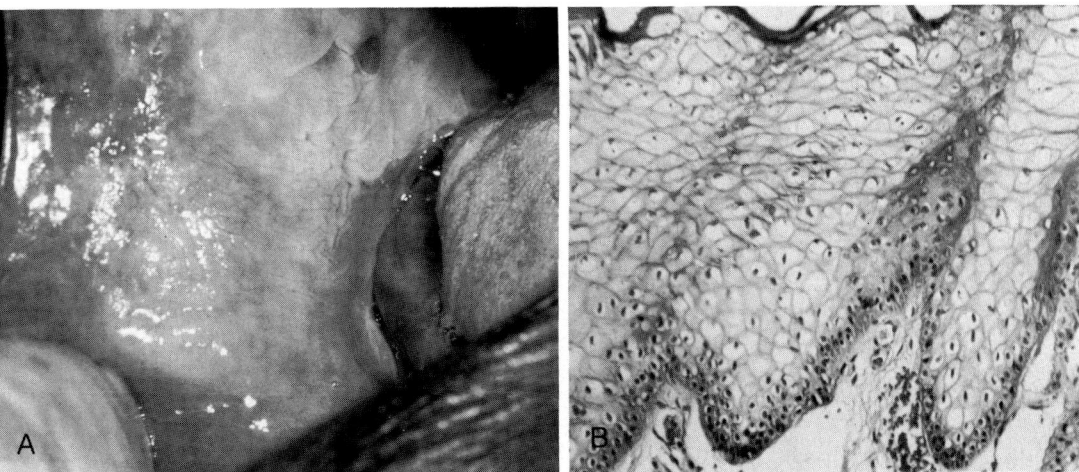

Figure 3–1. *A,* Leukoedema of the buccal mucosa. *B,* Biopsy showing extensive intracellular edema.

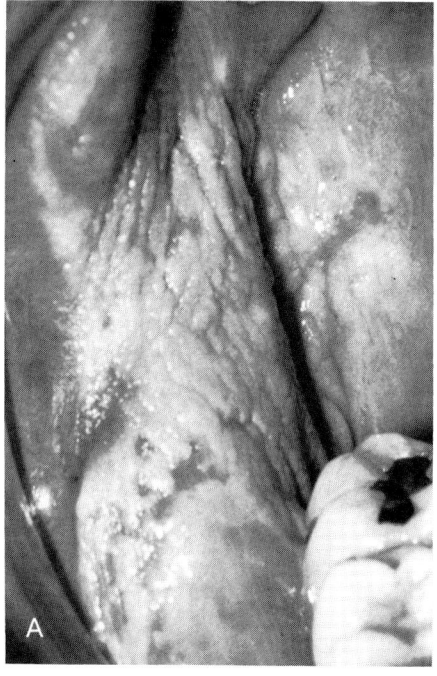
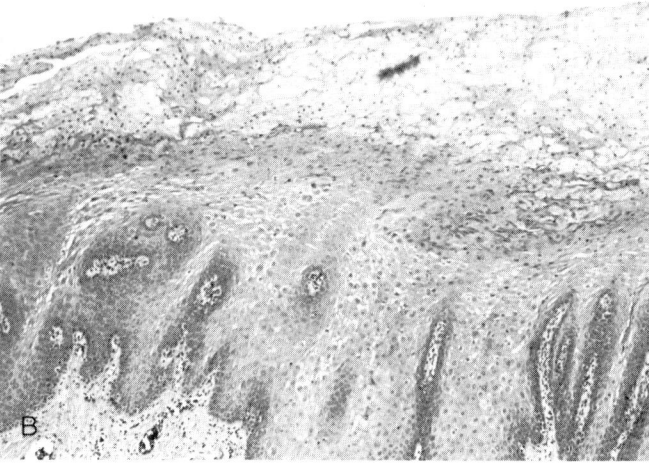

Figure 3–2. *A*, White sponge nevus of buccal mucosa. *B*, Biopsy showing intracellular edema and perinuclear condensation in lower epithelial cells.

nuclear eosinophilic condensation of cytoplasm is characteristic of prickle cells in white sponge nevus. Some limiting membranes are well defined, with occasional individual cells demonstrating premature keratinization within the spinous layer. Generally, it is possible to note the presence of columns of parakeratin extending from the surface into the acanthotic or spinous layer. The lamina propria and submucosa generally are unremarkable.

Several studies attempting to define the ultrastructural characteristics have failed to arrive at a level of consistency and uniformity of findings. This may be due to variations in fixation techniques or laboratory procedures in preparation of tissue for electron microscopy.

Differential Diagnosis. The differential diagnosis would include hereditary benign epithelial dyskeratosis, pachyonychia congenita, and lichen planus of the hypertrophic type. Cheek biting and traumatic or frictional keratosis might also be considered. Once tissue diagnosis is confirmed, no additional biopies are necessary.

Treatment. There is no specific treatment for this particular condition, since it is asymptomatic and benign. Thus far there have been no reports of malignant transformation of white sponge nevus.

Hereditary Benign Intraepithelial Dyskeratosis

Etiology. Hereditary benign intraepithelial dyskeratosis (HBID) is a rare, heritable condition of an autosomal dominant, highly penetrant nature. This condition was noted within a triracial isolate of white, Indian, and black composition in Halifax County, North Carolina. The initial cohort of 75 patients was traced to a single common female ancestor who lived nearly 130 years earlier.

Clinical Features. HBID is actually a syndrome that includes the early onset (usually within the first year of life) of bulbar conjunctivitis and oral lesions. Superimposed upon the bulbar conjunctivitis are foamy gelatinous plaques that tend to be triangular V-shaped, having their base along the limbus and extending medially and temporally.

Oral lesions consist of soft, asymptomatic, white folds and plaques of spongy mucosa. Areas of frequent involvement include the buccal and labial mucosa and labial commissures as well as the floor of the mouth and lateral surfaces of the tongue, gingiva, and palate. The dorsum of the tongue is usually spared. Oral lesions are generally detected within the first year of life, with a gradual increase in intensity until midadolescence. Individual areas of involvement show variable levels of surface alteration, from deeply folded, opaque, white lesions to more delicate, opalescent areas. Frequently, involved areas along the occlusal line will be macerated, further enhancing their shaggy surface texture.

In some patients, ocular lesions may vary seasonally. Some patients may complain of photophobia, especially in early life. Blindness, secondary to corneal vascularization, has been reported. In others, a spontaneous shedding of the conjunctival plaques occurs on a seasonal basis.

Histopathology. Similarities between oral and conjunctival lesions are noted microscopically. Epithelial hyperplasia and acanthosis are present, with significant hydropic degeneration (Fig. 3–3). Enlarged, hyaline, and so-called waxy eosinophilic cells, which are the dyskeratotic elements, are present in the superficial half of the epithelium. Eosinophilic dyskeratotic cells within the middle and superficial spinous regions may become surrounded by adjacent cells, producing a "cell-within-a-cell" pattern. Non-dyskeratotic cells are enlarged and edematous and, in the superficial layers, become elongated. Normal cellular features are noted within the lower spinous and basal layers. Inflammatory cell infiltration within the lamina propria is minimal when present, and the epithelial–connective tissue junction is well defined.

Ultrastructural studies of the dyskeratotic cells show them to be engorged with tonofilaments and vesicular bodies and to contain degenerate nuclei. Cell membrane alterations are also noted in the loss of cellular interdigitations and desmosomes.

Differential Diagnosis. The oral features of HBID are remarkably similar to those of white sponge nevus. Pachyonychia congenita and hypertrophic lichen planus might also be considered, as far as the oral mucosal presentation is concerned. In pachyonychia congenita, however, distinctive fingernail and toenail changes—extreme thickening along the free nail edge—are present. In lichen planus, there is no inheritance pattern evident, although any nail changes present are related to nail fold destruction. Eye changes are not seen in lichen planus, but those in pachyonychia congenita consist of corneal opacities.

Treatment. No treatment is necessary, since this condition is self-limiting. There appears to be no increased risk of malignant transformation.

Follicular Keratosis

Etiology and Pathogenesis. Follicular keratosis (Darier's disease, Darier-White disease) is a genetically transmitted disorder with an autosomal dominant mode of inheritance. In a large series of 200 kindred, there was a 50% chance of an affected offspring developing the disease, with an equal gender distribution. Many cases also appear sporadically or as new mutations. Approximately 50% of cases of follicular keratosis involve the oral cavity. When present, the oral lesions closely follow the onset or the diagnosis of epidermal lesions.

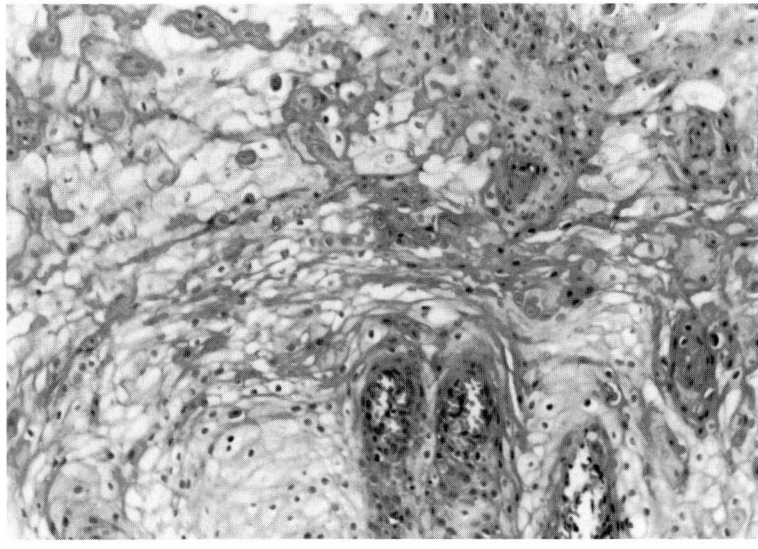

Figure 3–3. Biopsy of hereditary benign intraepithelial dyskeratosis. Dark epithelial cells represent dyskeratosis. Note connective papillae at lower right.

Although the etiology of follicular keratosis is well established, concepts concerning pathogenesis are less well understood and accepted. Four areas of investigation relative to pathogenesis include genetic defects producing abnormalities in the desmosome-tonofilament complex, precocious cell development coupled with altered epidermal cell turnover rates, genetic defects in vitamin A utilization at the epithelial cell level, and possible defects in cell-mediated immunity. The clinical and pathologic end result is an acantholytic process.

Clinical Features. Onset of this disease is usually noted in childhood or adolescence. Skin manifestations are characterized by small, skin-colored papular lesions symmetrically distributed over the face, trunk, and intertriginous areas. Eventually the papules coalesce and become greasy, with a tan to black crust. Subsequently, the coalesced areas form patches of vegetating to verrucous growths that have a tendency to become infected and malodorous. Lesions may also occur unilaterally or in a zosteriform pattern. Thickening of the palms and soles (hyperkeratosis palmaris et plantaris) by excessive keratotic tissue is not uncommon. On the dorsa of the hands, the lesions are similar to flat warts or verruca plana and acrokeratosis verruciformis (Hopf's keratosis). Fingernail changes may include fragility, splintering, and subungual keratosis. Nail changes are often helpful in establishing a diagnosis.

Localized lesions of follicular keratosis may follow sunburn, especially on the legs. Microscopically, these may be reported under the term "warty dyskeratoma."

Oral involvement by this disease is well established (Fig. 3–4). The extent of the oral lesions may parallel the extent of skin involvement. Favored oral mucosal sites include keratinized regions, such as attached gingiva and hard palate, although nearly all oral sites have been reported to be involved. The lesions typically appear as small, whitish papules, producing an overall cobblestone appearance. Papules range from 2 to 3 mm in diameter and may become coalescent. Extension beyond the oral cavity into the oropharynx and pharynx may occur.

Histopathology. Oral lesions closely resemble the cutaneous lesions (Fig. 3–5). Features include (1) suprabasal lacunae (clefts) formation containing acantholytic epithelial cells, (2) basal layer proliferation immediately below and adjacent to the lacunae or clefts, (3) formation of vertical clefts that show a lining of parakeratotic and dyskeratotic cells, and (4) the presence of specific benign dyskeratotic cells—*corps ronds* and *grains*. Corps ronds are large, keratinized squamous cells with round, uniformly basophilic nuclei and intensely eosinophilic cytoplasm. Grains are smaller parakeratotic cells with pyknotic, hyperchromatic nuclei. Ultrastructurally, basal and spinous cells develop into corps ronds as a result of intracellular vacuolization. Grains develop as a result of vacuole compression and premature tonofilament aggregation within the spinous layer cells. Tonofilament separation from attachment plaques with subsequent disappearance of desmosomes has also been observed.

Whether abnormal humoral or cell-mediated immunity exists in patients with this disease is undetermined. Questions relate to the possibility that immunologic dysfunction may be secondary to epidermal disruption. Reported

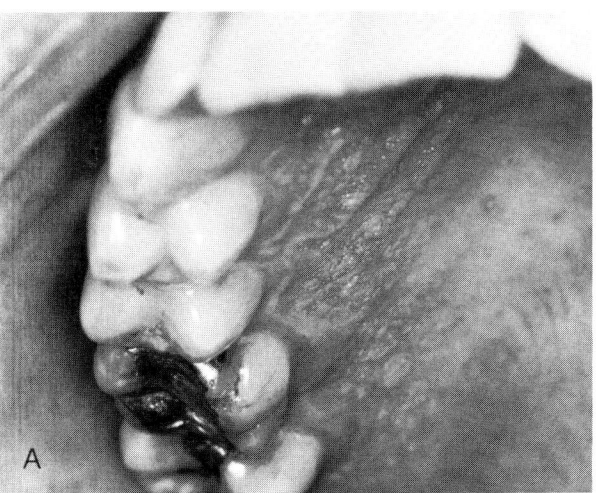
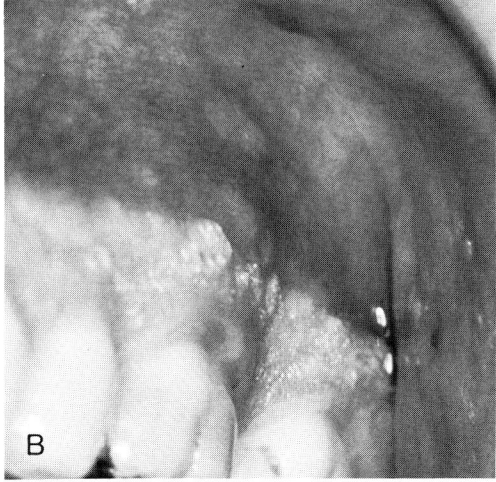

Figure 3–4. *A* and *B*, Follicular keratosis of right hard palate and upper gingiva.

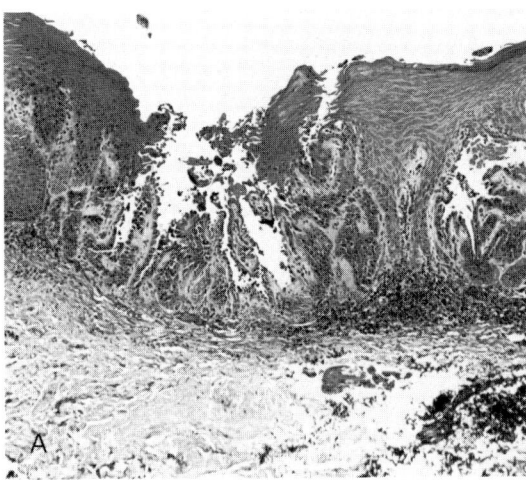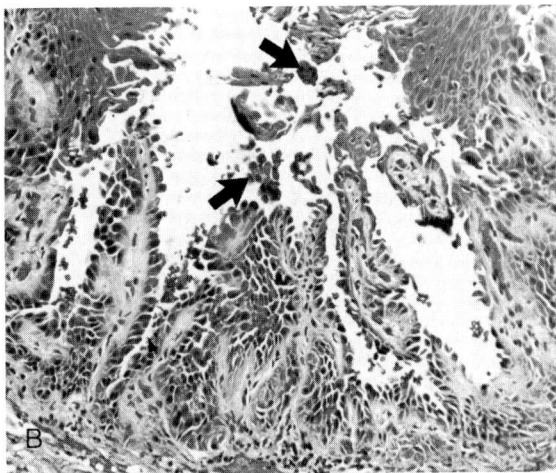

Figure 3–5. *A* and *B*, Microscopy of follicular keratosis showing vertical clefts and acantholytic epithelial cells (arrows).

are alterations in T lymphocyte function as measured by decreased ability to produce migration inhibitory factor, decreased response to *in vitro* mitogens, and cutaneous anergy.

Differential Diagnosis. Follicular keratosis, when affecting the oral mucosa, may bear some clinical resemblance to the rarely occurring conditions dyskeratosis congenita and acanthosis nigricans. Other conditions to be excluded from follicular keratosis are condyloma acuminatum and so-called nicotine stomatitis.

Treatment and Prognosis. In the past, the standard treatment involved the use of large doses of oral vitamin A. However, variable levels of success were reported, and systemic toxicity was also a problem. Recently, vitamin A analogues or retinoids, in the form of etretinate (aromatic retinoid) and isotretinoin (13-cis-retinoic acid), have been used effectively. Side effects, including cheilitis, elevation of serum liver enzymes and triglycerides, and severe dryness of the skin, have also placed some limitations on this treatment method. Discontinuation of treatment usually produces variable periods of remission, with an eventual return to the original level of involvement.

Although the disease is chronic and slowly progressive, remissions may be noted in some patients. Malignant change within oral mucosal lesions has not been reported.

REACTIVE LESIONS

Focal (Frictional) Hyperkeratosis

Etiology. Focal (frictional) hyperkeratosis is a white lesion that is often classified under the general term, "leukoplakia." In this chapter, however, because there may be an obvious cause and effect relationship for this lesion, it is separated from the idiopathic (unknown etiology) leukoplakias.

Chronic rubbing or friction against an oral mucosal surface may result in a hyperkeratotic white lesion that is analogous to a callus on the skin. The tissue response represents a protective action against low-grade long-term trauma.

Clinical Features. Friction-induced hyperkeratoses or leukoplakias occur in areas that are commonly traumatized, such as lips, buccal mucosa along the occlusal line, and edentulous ridges (Figs. 3–6 and 3–7). Chronic cheek or lip chewing may result in opacification (keratinization) of the area affected. Chewing on edentulous alveolar ridges produces the same effect. The etiology of these lesions is self-evident.

Histopathology. As the name indicates, the primary microscopic change is hyperkeratosis. A few chronic inflammatory cells may be seen in the subjacent connective tissue. Dysplastic epithelial changes are not seen in simple frictional hyperkeratotic lesions.

Diagnosis. Careful history taking and examination should indicate the nature of this lesion. If the practitioner is clinically confident of a traumatic cause and keratotic response, no biopsy may be required. The patient should be advised to discontinue the causative habit, however. Then the lesion should resolve with time, confirming the clinical diagnosis. Discontinuing the habit would also allow the unmasking of any underlying lesion that may not be related to trauma.

If the etiology of a white lesion is in doubt, it should be regarded as idiopathic leuko-

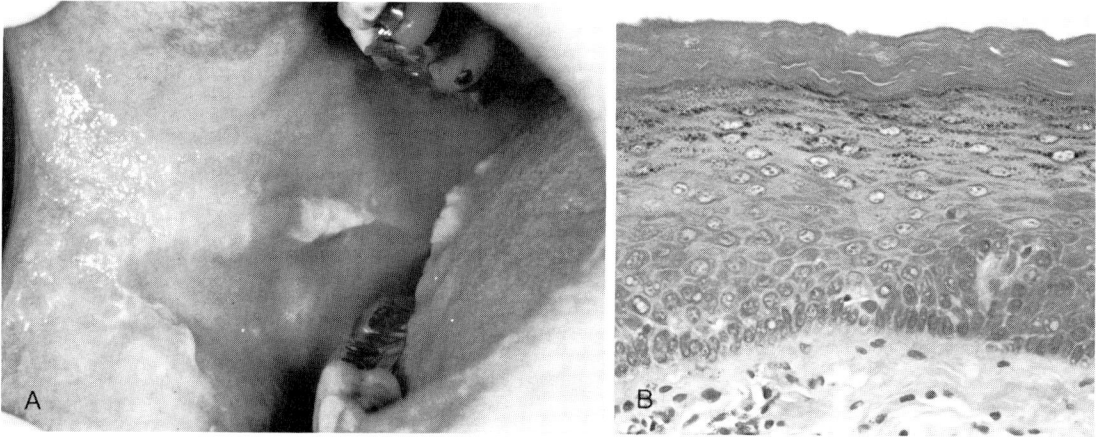

Figure 3–6. *A*, Focal (frictional) hyperkeratosis due to cheek chewing. *B*, Microscopy showing hyperkeratosis.

plakia. Also, if the lesion is not uniformly opaque or has areas of ulceration, induration, or redness, it should be treated as idiopathic leukoplakia.

Treatment. Observation is generally all that is required for simple frictional hyperkeratotic lesions. Control of the habit causing the lesion should result in clinical improvement. Any lesion of questionable etiology should be biopsied.

White Lesions Associated With Smokeless Tobacco

Recently, concern has been expressed within the United States about the steadily increasing use of smokeless tobacco by young people. Geographic differences in tobacco use have also begun to emerge. Numbers of frequent users, which typically have been high in the southern states, are significantly increasing in other areas, especially western states. Current usage by men in New York and Rhode Island is under 1% of the population, but in West Virginia it is over 20%. In a 1986 survey of 25 states and the District of Columbia, 6.5% of men and 0.3% of women were regular users of smokeless tobacco. Earlier literature documenting studies performed in other parts of the world shows many similarities to the more recent American experience.

The general increase in smokeless tobacco consumption has been related to both peer pressure and increased media advertising, which often glamorizes the use of smokeless tobacco or snuff dipping. Additionally, individuals who have been heavy smokers or those who wish to avoid smoking may gravitate to this alternative. The clinical results of long-

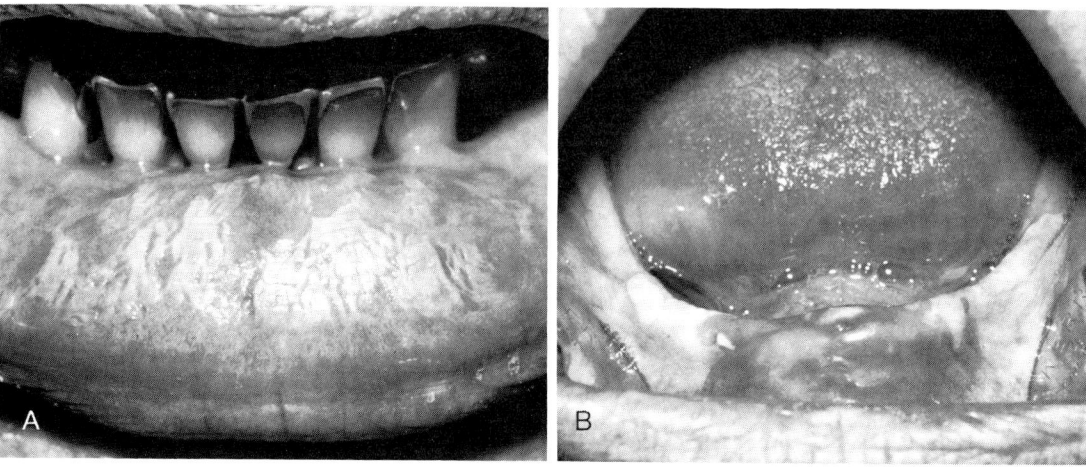

Figure 3–7. Focal (frictional) hyperkeratosis due to habitual rubbing of lip against teeth *(A)*, and the wearing of an ill-fitting denture *(B)*.

term exposure to smokeless tobacco include the development of oral mucosal white patches, dependence, alterations of taste and smell, increased periodontal disease, and significant amounts of dental abrasion.

Etiology. Whether smokeless tobacco is used in the form of chewing tobacco or snuff appears to be insignificant, as all forms may potentially cause alterations in the oral mucosa. The use of this form of tobacco increases the risk of subsequent development of oral mucosal dysplasia. This biologic alteration in tissues is felt to be a response to tobacco constituents and perhaps other agents that are added to tobacco for flavoring or moisture retention. Carcinogens, such as nitrosonornicotine, an organic component of chewing tobacco and snuff, have been identified in the tobacco. The pH of snuff, which ranges between 8.2 and 9.3, may be another factor that relates to the alteration of mucosa, although the buffering capacity of saliva should temper the effect to some degree.

Duration of exposure to smokeless tobacco that is necessary to produce mucosal damage is measured in terms of years. Exposure is believed to result in chemical damage that produces sublethal cell injury within the deeper layers of the oral epithelium. This, in turn, induces a concomitant epithelial hyperplasia. The surface layers of epithelium may be lethally damaged secondary to formation of hydrophobic unsaturated lipids. The observation of variable degrees of sialadenitis suggests that there may be loss of gland function. This, in turn, could relate to decreased protection of the surrounding epithelium against snuff or other exogenous agents.

Clinical Features. The white lesions of the oral mucosa associated with smokeless tobacco use develop in the immediate area where the tobacco is habitually placed (Figs. 3–8 and 3–9). The most common area of involvement is the mucobuccal fold of the mandible, in either the incisor or the molar region. The altered epithelium generally has a granular to wrinkled appearance. In advanced cases, a heavy folded character may be assumed. Less frequently, an erythroplakic or red component may be admixed with the white keratotic component. The lesions are generally painless and asymptomatic, with their discovery often incidental to routine oral examination. Among teenagers, whites are the predominant users of smokeless tobacco, with males making up nearly all of this group.

In other parts of the world, different forms of smokeless tobacco are used. The tobacco preparations are generally of higher (alkaline) pH. In older populations, with a longer exposure to tobacco and other agents, there is often the development of keratinized ridges or spikes of tissue, frequently producing a characteristic pumice-like pattern of keratinization. This pattern has been noted on areas of the oral mucosa that normally do not keratinize.

Histopathology. Slight to moderate parakeratosis is noted over the surface of the affected mucosa. Superficial levels of epithelium may demonstrate vacuolization of the spinous layer. Epithelial hyperplasia is typical, but atrophy and ulceration are unusual. Varying degrees of stromal inflammation may also be seen. Epithelial dysplasia may be noted, with a correspondingly increased inflammatory reaction. In individuals with dysplastic changes, there is generally a longer history of smokeless tobacco use. Salivary gland altera-

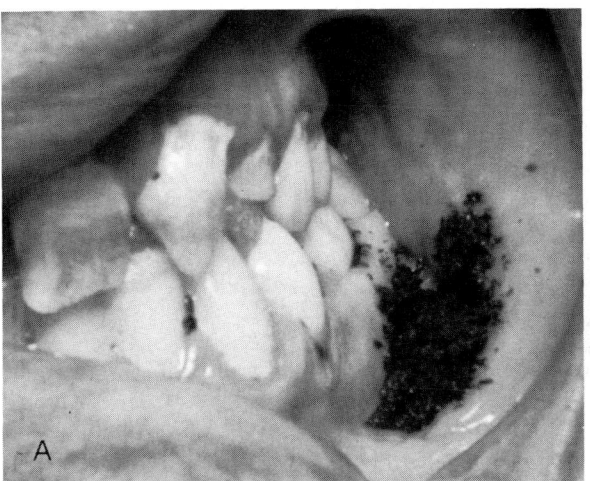
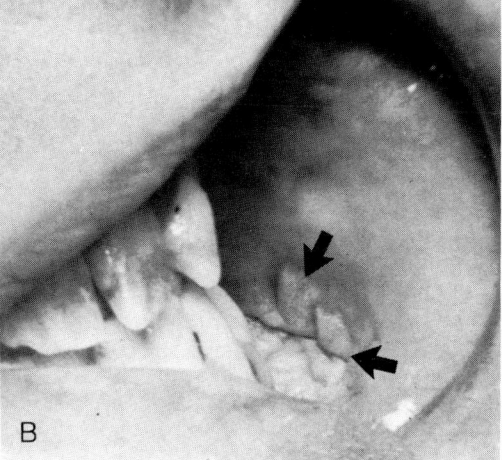

Figure 3–8. Smokeless tobacco user. *A,* Tobacco in place. *B,* Resultant hyperkeratotic pouch (arrows).

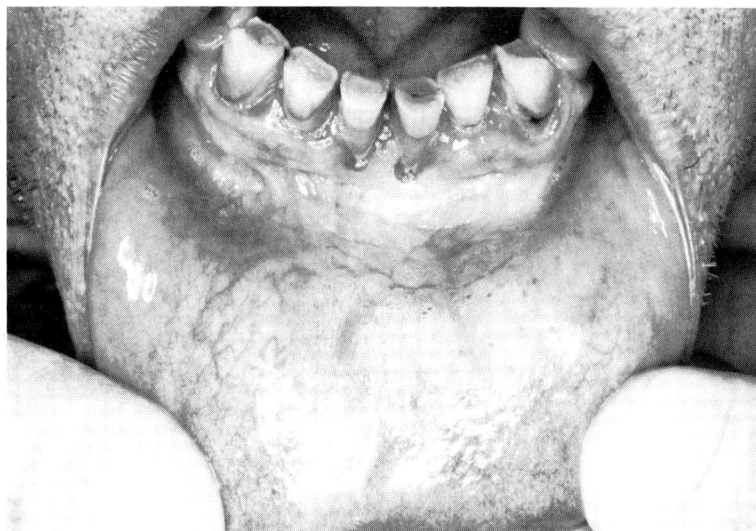

Figure 3–9. Hyperkeratosis caused by smokeless tobacco. Note associated periodontal disease and tooth abrasion.

tions are primarily inflammatory and are seen in approximately 40% of biopsies. As with the oral epithelial changes, increasing degrees of salivary alteration are noted with greater total exposure to smokeless tobacco. Such changes include acinar atrophy, interstitial fibrosis, and dilated excretory ducts. On occasion, a diffuse zone of basophilic stromal alteration may be seen, usually adjacent to minor salivary glands. Stromal mucin pooling may be noted in still fewer cases.

Differential Diagnosis. In the early phases of development, snuff or smokeless tobacco–induced lesions may resemble the diffuse, filmy character of leukoedema, although in leukoedema the change is bilateral and symmetric. The surface alterations in white sponge nevus may approximate the character of lesions related to snuff dipping; however, the bilateral and more general distribution of lesions in white sponge nevus distinguishes the two processes.

Treatment and Prognosis. With elimination of tobacco use, some lesions may disappear after several weeks. Persistent lesions should be removed and examined histologically. Relative to the process of malignant transformation, a long period of exposure to smokeless tobacco appears necessary for such changes to develop. When such changes are evident, the lesions are generally of low-grade malignancy, ranging from verrucous carcinoma to ulcerated squamous cell carcinoma. If there is complete disappearance of a lesion subsequent to discontinuation of a tobacco habit, the prognosis is excellent.

Nicotine Stomatitis

Etiology. This tobacco-related form of keratosis is one of the more common oral forms and is not known to occur in individuals who do not smoke. Nicotine stomatitis is most typically associated with pipe and cigar smoking, with a positive correlation noted between severity of the condition and intensity of smoking. The importance of the direct topical effect of smoke can be appreciated in instances in which the hard palate is covered by a removable prosthesis, resulting in sparing of the mucosa beneath the appliance and hyperkeratosis of exposed areas.

Clinical Features. The palatal mucosa initially responds with an erythematous type reaction and over time with increased levels of keratinization. Subsequent to the opacification or keratinization of the surface, red dots may be noted on the posterior portion of the hard palate (Fig. 3–10). These dots may be surrounded by a white keratotic ring that may be elevated. The dots themselves represent inflammation of the ductal elements of the underlying minor salivary glands. In severe cases a slight furrowed or wrinkled effect may produce an overall roughened appearance.

Histopathology. Biopsy specimens of nicotine stomatitis are generally characterized by a thickened epithelium, with moderate levels of acanthosis and a significant increase in the thickness of the overlying orthokeratin. The minor salivary glands in the area may demonstrate moderate degrees of inflammatory change. Excretory ducts may show squamous

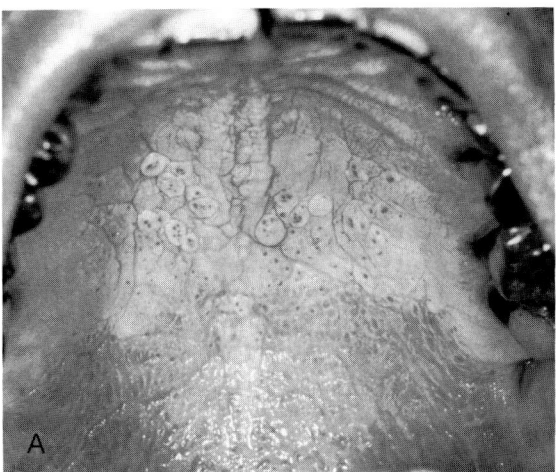 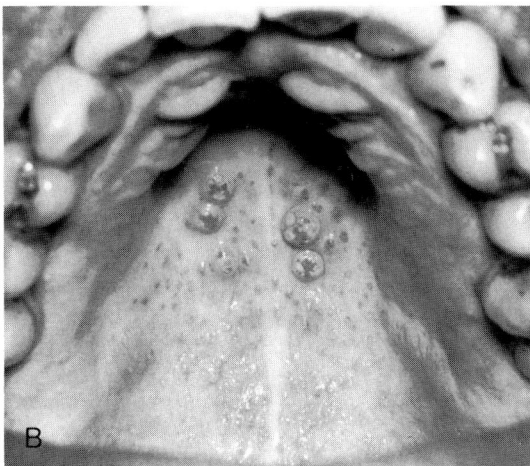

Figure 3–10. *A* and *B*, Nicotine stomatitis.

metaplasia, and glandular tissue will contain chronic inflammatory cells and some scar.

Treatment and Prognosis. The overall significance of nicotine stomatitis in comparison with keratosis in other portions of the oral cavity is minimal. This condition rarely evolves into malignancy except in individuals who "reverse smoke." This habit, which is common in other countries (e.g., India), intensifies the carcinogenic effect of heat and smoke on the palate, resulting in considerable risk of cancer development.

Owing to the overall benign nature of this process, with a minimal risk of carcinoma development in the palate, treatment should be directed toward reduction if not elimination of smoking. When smoking has been discontinued, the condition has been known to revert to normal in some cases.

It should be recognized that the intensity of smoking necessary to produce nicotine stomatitis is likely to have similar effects elsewhere in the oral cavity and the respiratory tract. This significantly increases the overall risk for the development of malignancies in these other regions. Nicotine stomatitis might be viewed as a potential indicator of significant epithelial change at sites other than the hard palate.

Solar Cheilitis

Solar or actinic cheilitis represents accelerated tissue degeneration of the lips, especially the lower lip, secondary to regular and prolonged exposure to sunlight. This particular condition occurs almost exclusively in whites and is especially prevalent in those with fair skin. It is closely correlated to total cumulative exposure to sunlight and amount of skin pigmentation rather than strictly to age of the affected individual.

Etiology and Pathogenesis. The wavelengths of light responsible for actinic cheilitis and, in general, other degenerative actinically related skin conditions are usually considered to be those between 2900 and 3200 Å. Experimental attempts to produce similar lesions with infrared levels of radiation alone have been unsuccessful.

In the past, it has been proposed that subepithelial collagen becomes degraded in time by the effects of ultraviolet light, but subsequent chemical isolation studies have not supported this concept. Rather, it has been shown that the characteristic subepithelial deposits in this condition are elastin and are digested by elastase and not collagenase or trypsin. Additionally, ultrastructural characterization of the filaments is consistent with elastin filaments and not altered collagen. Chemical studies also show decreased concentrations of lysine with concomitant increases in desmosine residues, further substantiating this process as a replacement of collagen by elastin.

Clinical Features. The affected vermilion portion of the lips presents with an atrophic, pale, glossy appearance, often with fissuring and wrinkling at right angles to the cutaneous-vermilion junction (Fig. 3–11). In advanced cases, the junction is irregular or totally effaced, with a degree of epidermization of the vermilion evident. Mottled areas of hyperpigmentation and keratosis are often noted as well as superficial scaling, cracking, and erosion.

Histopathology. The overlying epithelium is generally atrophic and hyperkeratotic. The

WHITE LESIONS

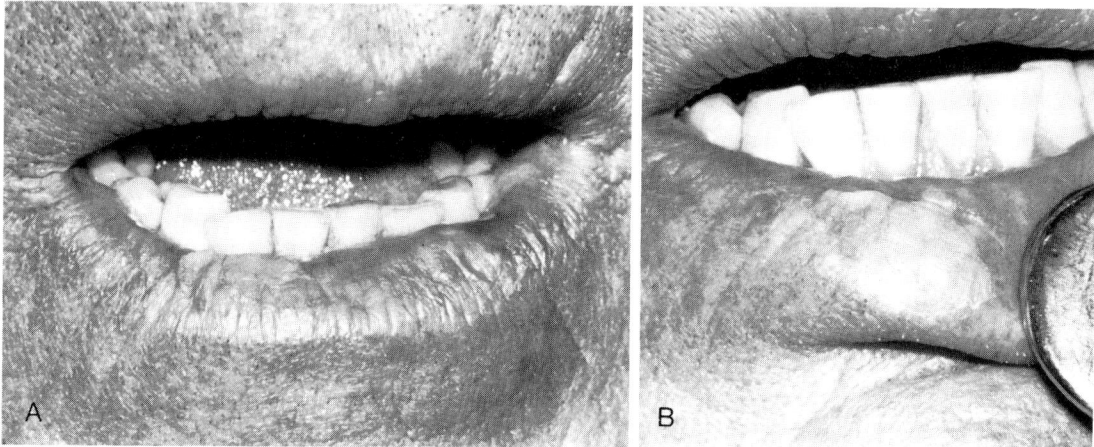

Figure 3–11. *A* and *B*, Solar cheilitis. Note hyperkeratotic plaque in extended lip *(B)*.

basal cells are generally hyperchromatic in nature. Most characteristic is a striking basophilia of the lamina propria and the appearance of telangiectatic vessels (Fig. 3–12). Special stains to highlight elastin show curled or tortuous fibers within an otherwise amorphous mass devoid of a fibrous or collagenous substructure. Digestion with elastase will remove the positive staining material and further confirm the substance's nature as elastin.

Treatment. No specific treatment is indicated. However, there is a very strong relationship to development of carcinoma at this site. Chronic sun damage mandates periodic examination and biopsy if ulceration persists or if induration becomes evident. If atypical changes are noted within the epithelium, a vermilionectomy may be performed in association with a mucosal advancement to replace the excised vermilion area. The use of lip balm containing the sunscreen agent para-aminobenzoic acid (PABA) or its derivatives is indicated during periods of sun exposure in high-risk patients. Sun-blocking opaque agents will also boost the effectiveness of the balm (Table 3–1). Periodic examination is essential once a diagnosis is established.

OTHER WHITE LESIONS

Idiopathic Leukoplakia

"Leukoplakia" is a clinical term indicating a white patch or plaque of oral mucosa that cannot be rubbed off and cannot be characterized clinically as any other disease. This defi-

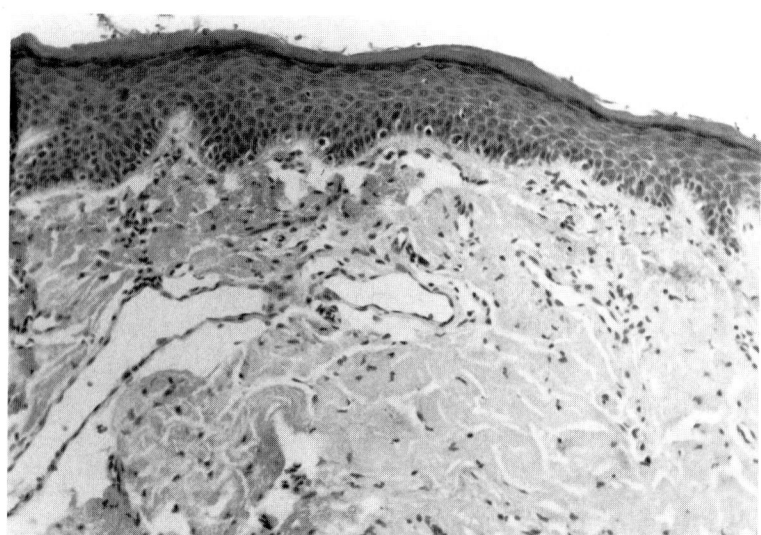

Figure 3–12. Microscopy of solar cheilitis showing hyperkeratosis, epithelial atrophy, telangiectasia, and basophilic change of submucosa.

Table 3–1. AGENTS USED TO PROTECT TISSUE FROM DAMAGING EFFECTS OF UV LIGHT

Sunscreen	Sunblock
Absorbs light	Scatters light
Protects from <3200Å light	Protects from >3200Å light
Reduces burning (erythema)	Reduces tanning (melanogenesis)
e.g., p-aminobenzoate, p-aminobenzoic acid	e.g., zinc oxide, titanium dioxide

nition essentially reflects that of the World Health Organization and seeks to separate lesions that remain after certain diagnostic entities, such as lichen planus, candidiasis, leukoedema, and white sponge nevus, have been eliminated. It is stressed that "leukoplakia" is a clinical term that has no correlation or relation to microscopic features relative to the presence or absence of cellular atypia or dysplasia. Leukoplakias clinically present with similar patterns or appearances but have a considerable degree of microscopic heterogeneity. The absence of any histologic connotation for leukoplakia is an important concept intended to eliminate some of the confusion that formerly existed regarding this term. Because leukoplakias may range microscopically from benign hyperkeratosis to invasive squamous cell carcinomas, biopsy is mandatory to establish a definitive diagnosis. It is important to note that premalignant lesions are not always white and that persistent leukoplakias are usually not premalignant.

Etiology and Pathogenesis. Many cases of leukoplakia are etiologically related to the use of tobacco in smoked or smokeless forms and may regress after discontinuation of tobacco use. The point of irreversibility, however, cannot be defined in terms of duration of tobacco use, forms of tobacco used, or clinical presentation. In addition to use of tobacco, other factors play a role in the etiology of leukoplakia. Lesions due to trauma (focal or frictional hyperkeratosis), such as those produced by an ill-fitting denture, are very common. Nutritional factors within certain populations have also been cited as important, especially relative to iron deficiency anemia and development of sideropenic dysphagia (Plummer-Vinson or Paterson-Kelly syndrome).

There is no doubt that some leukoplakias develop into oral squamous cell carcinoma. Rates of transformation are known to vary considerably from study to study and across cultural habits of tobacco use, in terms of form and combination of tobacco with other agents. Geographic differences in transformation rate as well as prevalence and location of oral leukoplakias are likely related to differences in tobacco habits in various parts of the world. In studies of the United States population, the majority of oral leukoplakias are benign and probably never become malignant. Studies indicate that malignant transformation of leukoplakia occurs over a range from about 1% to as high as 17%.

Clinical Features. Leukoplakia is a condition associated with an older population, with the vast majority of cases occurring over the age of 40 years. Recent trends regarding the use of smokeless tobacco by high-school students may ultimately result in a shift of this age toward a younger population. Over time there has also been a shift in gender predilection, with near parity in incidence of leukoplakia due apparently to the change in smoking habits of young women.

Predominant sites of occurrence have changed over the years. At one time the tongue was the most common site for leukoplakia, although more contemporary studies show the tongue to be one of the least common sites. The mandibular mucosa and the buccal mucosa account for almost half of the leukoplakias (Fig. 3–13). Palate, maxillary ridge, and lower lip are somewhat less frequently involved, and floor of the mouth and retromolar sites are involved comparatively infrequently.

Relative to region affected, the risk of neoplastic transformation is of considerable importance. While the floor of the mouth accounts for a relatively small percentage (10%) of leukoplakias, a large percentage (50%) are dysplastic, carcinoma *in situ,* or invasive lesions when examined microscopically. Leukoplakia of the lips and tongue also exhibits a relatively high percentage (25%) of dysplastic or neoplastic change. In contrast to these sites, the retromolar area exhibits these changes in only about 10% of the cases.

Upon visual examination, leukoplakia may vary from a barely evident, vague whiteness on a base of uninflamed, normal-appearing tissue to a definitive white, thickened, leathery, fissured, verrucous or wart-like lesion. Red zones may also be seen in some leukoplakias, prompting use of the term "speckled leukoplakia." On palpation, the area may be soft, smooth, or finely granular in texture. Other lesions may be roughened, nodular, or indurated.

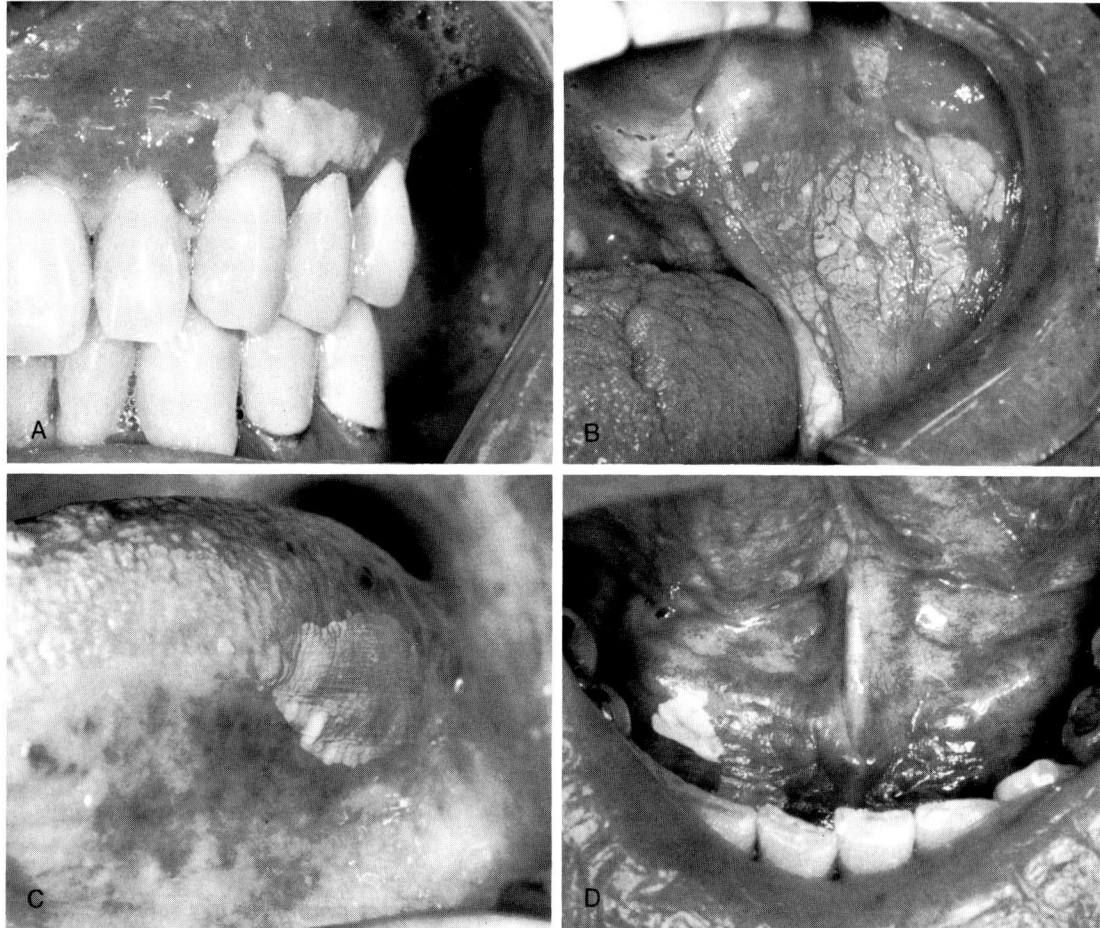

Figure 3–13. *A–D,* Four cases of clinical idiopathic leukoplakia, all of which showed hyperkeratosis microscopically.

An idiopathic form of leukoplakia (so-called leukoplakia simplex) presents with some features that may distinguish it from the leukoplakia of smokers. Presentation is characterized as furrowed, fissured, or wrinkled along the surface, with sharp margins and absence of induration. It has a predilection for middle-aged females who are usually non-smokers.

Proliferative verrucous leukoplakia is a form that has recently been segregated from other leukoplakias. This type of leukoplakia begins as simple keratosis and eventually becomes verrucous in nature. It is persistent, becomes multifocal, and is recurrent. Malignant transformation is not uncommon.

Because there is general consensus that there is no predictable correlation between clinical presentation and histopathology, biopsy is mandatory. This is emphasized by the occasional observation of clinically severe leukoplakia with bland histologic findings contrasted with small, seemingly innocuous leukoplakias with severe histopathologic change.

Histopathology. Epithelial alterations are variable in nature and extent in oral leukoplakias. Histologic changes range from hyperkeratosis, acanthosis, dysplasia, and carcinoma *in situ* to invasive squamous cell carcinoma (Fig. 3–14). By definition the term "dysplasia" refers to disordered growth. Varying degrees of dysplasia may be described in which the epithelial pattern shows mild, moderate, or severe change. This is a subjective determination, and it indicates that the changes do not appear abnormal enough to qualify as neoplastic. The term "atypia" is currently used to indicate abnormal changes of individual cells. (In the past, atypia was used as a synonym for dysplasia.) The diagnosis of epithelial dysplasia may be made when less than the complete thickness of epithelium demonstrates disorderly maturation (Fig. 3–15). Specific characteristics of such dysplasia include (1) drop-shaped epithelial ridges, (2) basal layer hyperplasia, (3) irregular stratification, (4) increased and abnormal mitotic figures, (5) individual or

Normal ⟶ Hyperkeratosis ⟶ Dysplasia ⟶ Carcinoma *in Situ* ⟶ Invasive Carcinoma

◂ - - - - Represents possible reversible process.

Figure 3–14. Microscopic spectrum of idiopathic leukoplakia. Oral lesions may be found anywhere along this spectrum. Some may progress through the various stages over time, whereas others may skip some or all stages to become invasive squamous cell carcinoma.

cell-group keratinization (epithelial pearl formation) within the spinous layer, (6) cellular pleomorphism, (7) nuclear hyperchromatism, (8) altered nuclear-cytoplasmic ratio, (9) enlarged nucleoli, (10) loss of basal cell polarity and "streaming" of spinous layer cells, and (11) loss or diminished intercellular adherence.

When the entire thickness of epithelium is involved with these changes in the so-called top-to-bottom effect, the term "carcinoma *in situ*" may be used (Fig. 3–16). In some cases when cellular atypia is severe, "carcinoma *in situ*" may be used, even though the changes may not be evident from basement membrane to surface. Experience and microscopic judgment is called upon when dealing with this range of epithelial change.

Progression of dysplasia to carcinoma is an assumption that has not been fully documented. It is generally accepted that the more severe the change, the more likely a lesion is to progress to cancer. Also, some lesions can persist for indefinite periods without changing microscopically, and a few others apparently revert to normal. Carcinoma *in situ* is not regarded as a reversible lesion, although it may take many years for invasion to occur.

Invasive squamous cell carcinoma accounts for about 5% of leukoplakias. There is, however, considerable variation in this figure because of variances in study design and population. The overall malignant transformation of benign leukoplakias accounts for approximately another 5% of the lesions.

Differential Diagnosis. The range of lesions that present clinically as a white patch can be reduced significantly simply by scraping the surface of the lesion with an instrument or a gauze pad. If the lesion cannot be removed, many of the processes characterized by the formation of a pseudomembrane can be disregarded. What remains, therefore, is a group of lesions that includes traumatic keratosis or frictional keratosis, galvanic keratosis, verrucous hyperplasia, verrucous carcinoma, lichen planus, discoid lupus erythematosus (DLE), and white sponge nevus.

The element of trauma may be suspected when white lesions involve the lateral margins of the tongue as well as the buccal mucosa. The surface of such lesions is generally eroded and uneven to ragged in surface texture. Areas of erythema or redness that accompany the erosions of traumatically induced lesions are uneven in surface configuration in contrast to erythroplakias, which tend to be more luxuriant or velvety in appearance.

Leukoedema, in contrast to leukoplakia, has

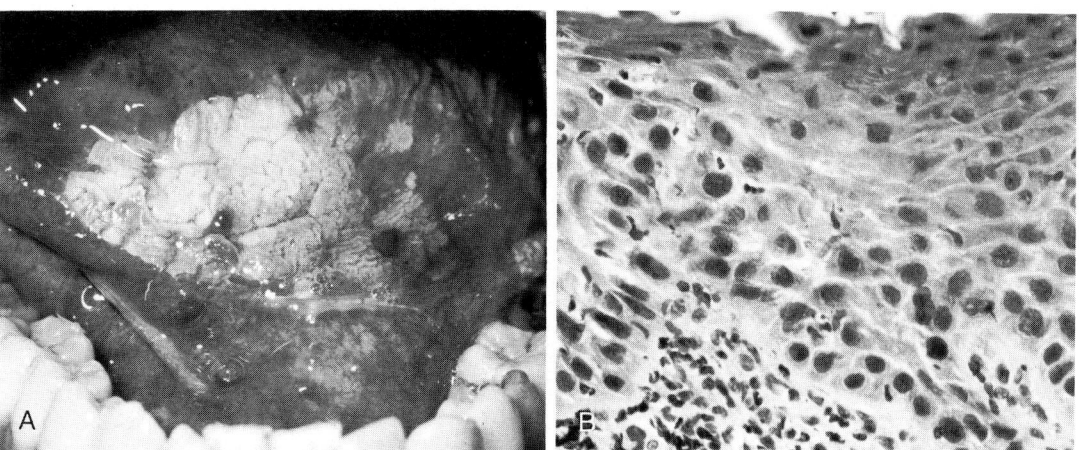

Figure 3–15. *A*, Clinical idiopathic leukoplakia of the left lateral surface of the tongue. *B*, Biopsy showing dysplastic changes of nuclear hyperchromatism and irregular epithelial maturation.

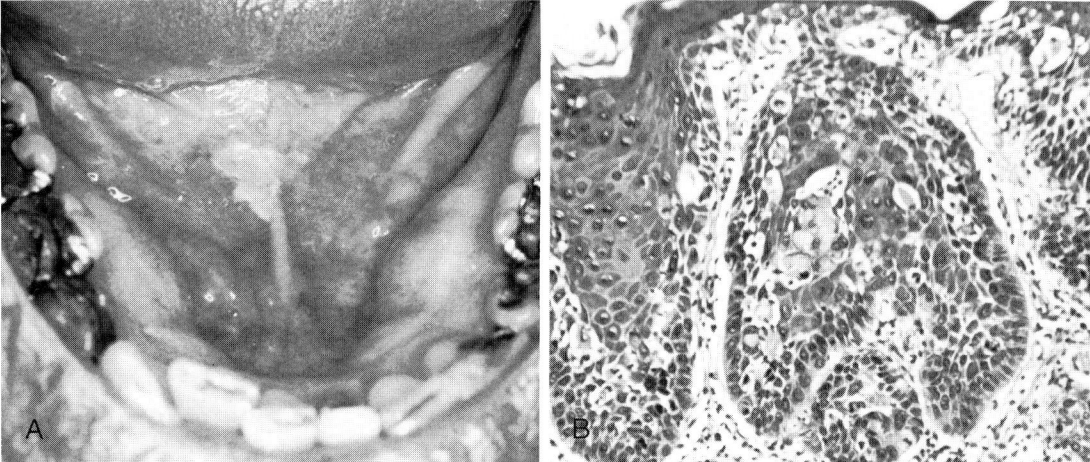

Figure 3–16. *A*, Clinical idiopathic leukoplakia in the floor of the mouth. *B*, Biopsy showing "top-to-bottom" changes of carcinoma *in situ*..

no definitive opaqueness or whiteness but rather presents with an opalescent, milky surface that on occasion may be folded or wrinkled and that disappears upon stretching of the buccal mucosa. This is not the case with leukoplakia, which, in spite of stretching or clinical manipulation, remains opaque and unchanged. Leukoedema is also bilateral and diffuse, and it affects only the buccal mucosa.

Electrogalvanically induced keratosis has increasingly been seen as a cause of white lesions involving the oral mucosa. In general, the appearance of electrogalvanically induced mucosal alteration ranges from definitive plaques to more delicate and diffusely distributed striae with lichen planus–like (lichenoid) forms. The latter presentation will often have associated erythematous areas. In lesions less than a few years old, removal of dissimilar metallic restorations may result in a return to normal.

Verrucous or wart-like keratotic alterations of the oral mucosa may fall into three categories—verrucous carcinoma, proliferative verrucous leukoplakia, and verruca vulgaris. The latter virus-induced lesion, which tends to be discrete, limited, and exophytic, should not be confused with leukoplakic plaques. Verrucous carcinoma, on the other hand, will present as a white, heavily textured, broad-based lesion, with deep folds and fissures intervening between extended fronds of keratotic surface epithelium. Such lesions on the buccal mucosa and attached gingiva may occasionally be considered in a differential diagnosis of white lesions of the same areas. Proliferative verrucous leukoplakia may present as a white patch early in its course and may eventually develop into verrucous carcinoma.

Lichen planus may on occasion be difficult to separate from other white lesions, since many cases of lichen planus lesions tend to be plaque-like in their presentation. However, the lesions will usually be bilateral and affect multiple sites. Leukoplakia generally would not demonstrate the degree of symmetry and bilaterality of lichen planus. Additionally, many patients with lichen planus will have symptomatic complaints. Concomitant with the oral manifestations of lichen planus, many patients will demonstrate lesions of the skin and anogenital regions. Cutaneous lesions tend to be pruritic and papular in their initial presentation and are often distributed in a symmetric pattern along the flexor surfaces of the limbs. Nail changes may also be seen in individuals with oral lichen planus, further helping distinguish this condition from other oral mucosal lesions presenting as white plaques.

A condition often exhibiting a similar clinical presentation to lichen planus is DLE. Overlap relative to site of predilection, clinical appearance, age of patient, and microscopy will often prove problematic in distinguishing DLE from lichen planus and occasionally leukoplakia. It is often necessary to resort to immunofluorescence testing in addition to routine biopsy studies to separate oral DLE from other lesions.

Finally, white sponge nevus may be considered in a differential context in the leukoplakia category. This rare entity is inherited in an autosomal dominant pattern. The symmetry and wide distribution of the lesions also help separate this condition from leukoplakia. The age of onset of lesions before puberty is another valid clinical indicator of this condition in contrast to leukoplakia, which generally tends to develop in the fourth to fifth decade and beyond.

Treatment and Prognosis. The initial step in management of leukoplakia involves identification of etiologic factors. Traumatic influences, such as habit, overextended or inadequate removable appliances, poorly maintained or improperly placed restorations, and displaced teeth, should be rectified. If tobacco or alcohol use is a component of the patient's history, discontinuation is mandatory.

In the management of extensive lesions, multiple biopsies may be required. The clinically most suspicious areas—those that are red, ulcerated, or indurated—should be included. In the absence of dysplastic or atypical epithelial change, periodic and careful follow-up examination is appropriate. If, on the other hand, elements of dysplasia are evident, removal of the lesions by various surgical methods is obligatory. Such procedures may include surgical stripping, cryosurgery, electrodesiccation, or carbon-dioxide laser surgery. In cases of extensive lesions, grafting procedures may be necessary after surgery. Recently, some promise has been seen in the treatment of leukoplakic conditions with systemic and topical retinoid compounds. Patients treated in this manner, however, must be carefully monitored because of undesirable drug side effects and potential for recurrence. Acquisition of more data on this subject appears warranted before it can be recommended for general use.

The issue of reversibility or regression of dysplastic lesions in the oral cavity remains unsettled. Analogous dysplastic lesions of the uterine cervix, when observed over time, are known to regress, persist unchanged, or develop into squamous cell carcinoma. A parallel situation may also exist relative to oral mucosa. In contrast to a progressive sequence of change from hyperplasia to dysplasia to neoplasia, carcinomas may apparently arise without antecedent dysplastic alterations.

Minimal degrees of dysplasia as such do not pose significant risks to the patient. The *site*, however, such as ventral tongue and floor of the mouth, predicates a higher level of significance to dysplastic lesions. As the severity of dysplasia increases, greater caution is in order. Moderately to severely dysplastic lesions should be completely excised.

Hairy Leukoplakia

Etiology and Pathogenesis. An unusual white lesion has been described that occurs along the lateral margins of the tongue, predominantly in male homosexuals. Evidence has suggested that this particular form of leukoplakia, known as hairy leukoplakia, represents an opportunistic infection related to the presence of the Epstein-Barr virus, a herpesvirus. Of importance is the fact that this lesion has been associated with subsequent or concomitant development of the clinical and laboratory features of the acquired immunodeficiency syndrome (AIDS) in up to 80% of cases. Several other oral conditions have also been described as having a greater than expected frequency in AIDS patients (Table 3-2).

The presence of viruses in this lesion has been confirmed, and the specific herpes virus has been identified as the Epstein-Barr virus (EBV). Viral particles have been localized within the nuclei and cytoplasm of the oral epithelial cells of hairy leukoplakia, with DNA Southern blot hybridization studies confirming the presence of the EBV genome. Studies further indicate that this particular virus replicates within the oral hairy leukoplakia lesion. EBV antigens can also be found in epithelial malignancies, such as nasopharyngeal carcinoma, establishing this particular virus as capable of altering epithelial tissues.

It is important to note that replication of EBV within epithelial cells of the tongue has only been reported in individuals reflecting profound immunosuppression. Studies also indicate that both EBV and human papillomavirus (HPV) can simultaneously infect or coexist within the same cell. Speculation has been offered that HPV may facilitate entry, replication, and persistence of EBV in the epithelial cell.

Clinical Features. The clinical appearance of hairy leukoplakia can be quite variable, with unilateral and bilateral presentation reported (Fig. 3-17). An irregular surface contour that is often folded or corrugated is characteristic. Other lesions may be smooth and macular. The vast majority of reported cases

Table 3-2. ORAL MANIFESTATIONS OF AIDS
Hairy leukoplakia
Candidiasis
Kaposi's sarcoma
Squamous cell carcinoma
Lymphoma
Periodontal disease
Xerostomia

100 WHITE LESIONS

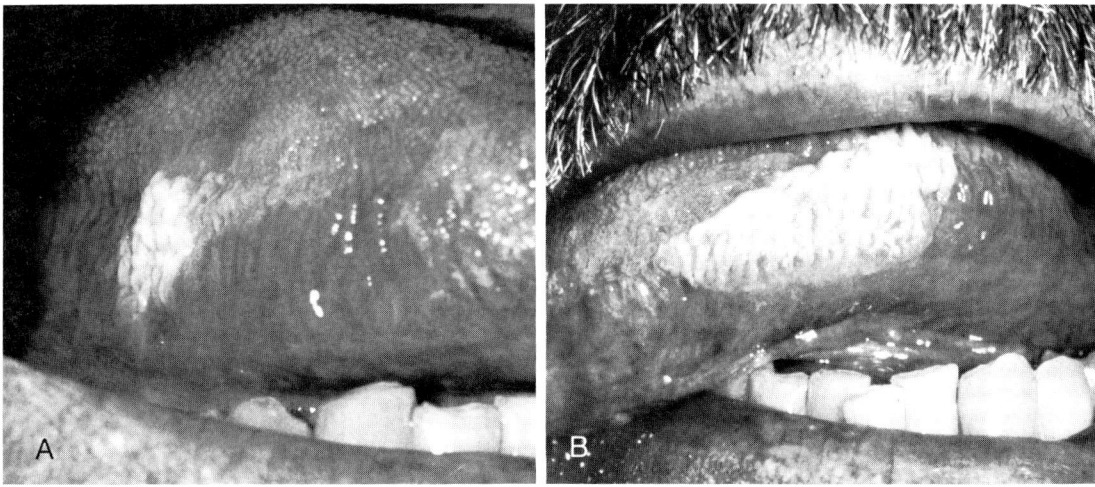

Figure 3–17. *A* and *B*, Bilateral hairy leukoplakia of the tongue. This patient was diagnosed as having AIDS 3 months later. (Courtesy of Dr. J. C. B. Stewart).

have been located along the lateral margins of the tongue. Less commonly, lesions have extended onto the dorsal surface of the tongue and rarely onto the buccal mucosa, the floor of the mouth, or the palate.

In general, there are no associated symptoms, although a suprainfection with *Candida albicans* might call attention to the presence of this condition. In more severe cases, when the entire dorsum of the tongue is involved by the process, the patient may become aware of the lesion and may seek dental consultation.

Histopathology. As with other virus-induced hyperplasias of epithelial tissues, there are several features within hairy leukoplakia that reflect this etiology. The surface layers are markedly hyperparakeratotic, often with the formation of keratotic surface irregularities and ridges (Fig. 3–18). *C. albicans* hyphae are often seen extending into the superficial epithelial cell layers. Beneath the surface, within the spinous cell layer, cells show ballooning degeneration and perinuclear clearing (koilocytosis). Additionally, alterations of nuclear chromatin may be seen in the form of peripheral displacement of chromatin, with a slight central basophilic hue. There is a general paucity of subepithelial inflammatory cells.

Confirmation of the presence of HPV has been made utilizing specific antiviral antibodies in an immunohistochemical staining system. Immunohistochemical and *in vitro* studies have demonstrated the presence of EBV within these cells. Further confirmation has been accomplished by the ultrastructural demonstration of intranuclear virions of EBV (Fig. 3–19). Finally, specific probes for EBV utilizing the Southern blot hybridization procedure

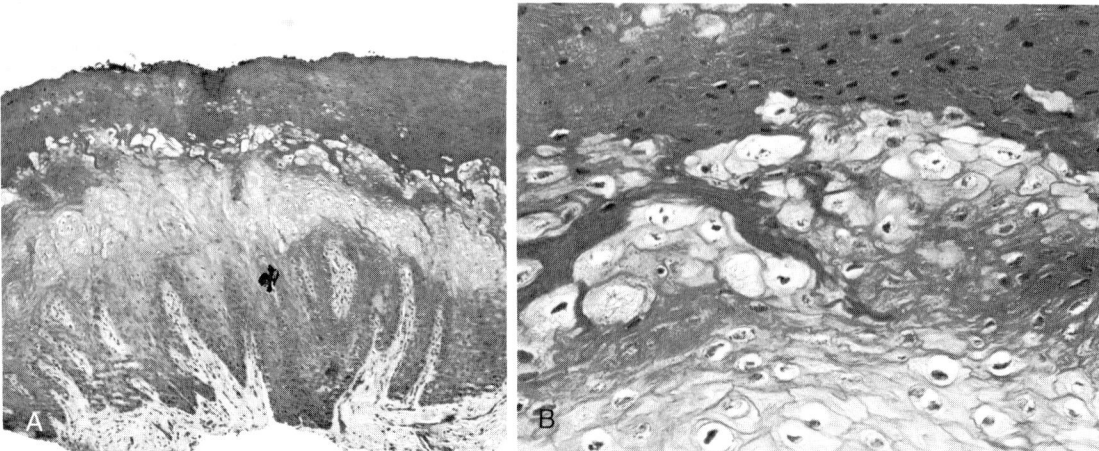

Figure 3–18. *A* and *B*, Biopsy of hairy leukoplakia showing shaggy parakeratosis and koilocytosis.

Figure 3–19. Electron micrographs of Epstein-Barr virus in hairy leukoplakia. *A,* Keratinocyte containing bundles of dark tonofilaments. Chromatin fragments (arrows) are located along the nuclear membrane, and smaller dark viral particles occupy the nucleus (× 8000). *B,* Higher magnification of the nucleus showing detail of viral particles. The outer ring represents the viral capsid (arrow) surrounding a DNA core (× 60,000).

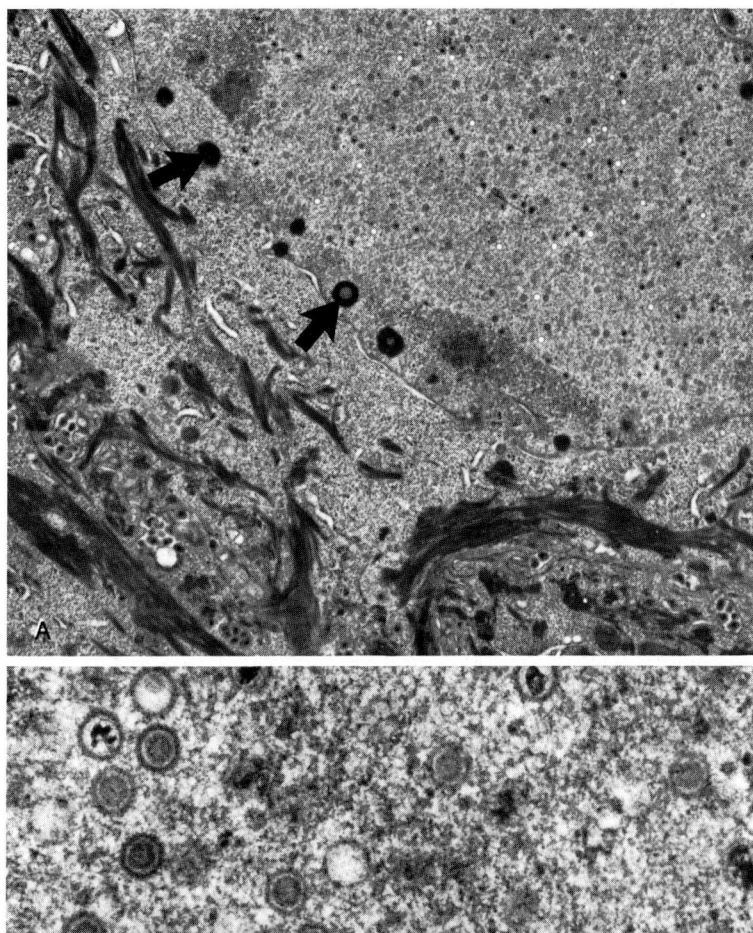

have identified typical EBV patterns, confirming the morphologic studies done previously.

Differential Diagnosis. The clinical differential diagnosis of hairy leukoplakia includes the more common idiopathic leukoplakia and leukoplakia associated with tobacco use. Other entities that might also be considered are lichen planus, chronic hyperplastic candidiasis, and possibly the keratotic reaction associated with electrochemical interactions.

Treatment and Prognosis. There is no specific treatment for hairy leukoplakia, although it is critical for this diagnosis to be confirmed subsequent to its clinical identification. Recent studies indicate that approximately 10% of individuals with diagnosed hairy leukoplakia had AIDS at the time of diagnosis, and an additional 18% developed this disease within 8 months. The probability of AIDS developing in individuals with hairy leukoplakia is nearly 50% at 16 months and up to 80% by 30 months after the diagnosis of hairy leukoplakia is established.

Hairy Tongue

Etiology. The term "white hairy tongue" is a non-specific, clinically descriptive term referring to a condition occurring on the dorsal surface of the tongue. Although hairy tongue is generally idiopathic, there are numerous predisposing factors. Use of broad-spectrum antibiotics, such as penicillin and systemic corticosteroids, is often identified in the clinical history of patients with this condition. Additionally, the use of oxygenating mouth rinses and compounds containing hydrogen peroxide, sodium perborate, and carbamide peroxide has also been cited as a possible contributing factor in this condition. Hairy tongue may also be seen in individuals who are heavy smokers and in individuals who have undergone radiotherapy to the head and neck region for malignant disease. The underlying factor is believed to be related to an alteration in microbial flora, with an attendant overgrowth of fungi and chromogenic bacteria. However, numerous attempts at culture and identification of these organisms have not produced consistent results.

Clinical Features. The clinical alteration relates to hypertrophy of the filiform papillae, with concomitant retardation of the normal rate of desquamation. The result is the production of a thick matted surface, with entrapped bacteria, fungi, cellular debris, and foreign material. Careful examination allows identification of individual filiform papillae that may be as long as several millimeters and that tend to be oriented toward the lateral margins of the tongue.

Symptoms are generally minimal, although when the elongation of the papillae becomes exaggerated, a gagging or a tickling sensation may be felt. Depending upon local conditions and the composition of the bacteria inhabiting the papillary surface, the color may range from white to tan to deep brown or black (Fig. 3–20).

Histopathology. Microscopic examination of a biopsy specimen will confirm the presence of elongated filiform papillae, with surface contamination by clusters of microorganisms and fungi. Keratinization may extend into the mid-portions of the stratum spinosum, with little evidence of basal cell hyperplasia. An orderly sequence of differentiation is noted from the

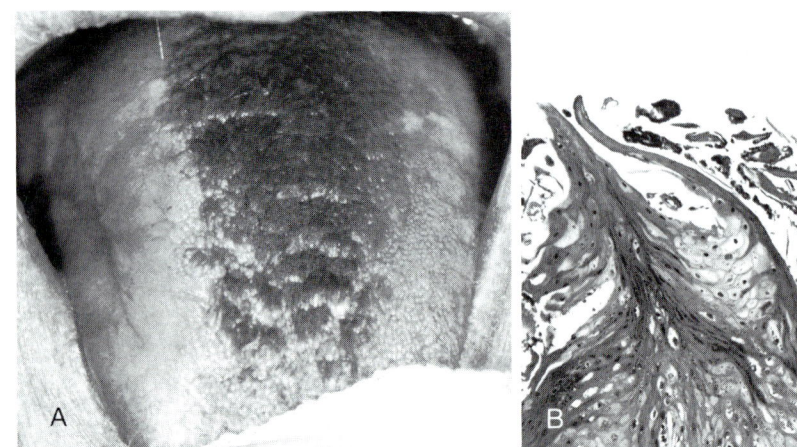

Figure 3–20. *A*, Hairy tongue stained dark by exogenous elements. *B*, Biopsy showing elongation of papillae and trapped bacterial colonies.

basal region through the more superficial elements of the spinous layer. The underlying lamina propria is generally mildly inflamed but otherwise unremarkable.

Diagnosis. Because the clinical features of this lesion are usually quite characteristic, confirmation by biopsy is not necessary. Cytologic or culture studies would not add significantly to the clinical impression.

Treatment and Prognosis. When taking the patient's history, identification of a possible etiologic factor, such as antibiotics or oxygenating mouth rinses, would be helpful. Discontinuing one of these agents should result in the disappearance of the elongated papillae within a few weeks. In cases in which individuals have undergone radiotherapy, with resultant xerostomia and altered bacterial flora, management is more difficult. Brushing of the tongue and fastidious oral hygiene should be of some benefit (application of a 1% solution of podophyllum resin has also been described as a useful treatment). It is important to stress to affected patients that this process is entirely benign and self-limiting, and that, in all likelihood, the tongue will return to normal subsequent to the institution of physical débridement and proper oral hygiene.

Geographic Tongue

Etiology. Geographic tongue, also known as erythema migrans and benign migratory glossitis, is a condition of unknown cause. Numerous theories have attempted to link this disease to emotional stress and fungal and bacterial infections. Geographic tongue has been associated with several different conditions, including psoriasis, seborrheic dermatitis, Reiter's syndrome, and more recently, atopy. In support of the last-named, a significant difference has been noted between prevalence of this condition in atopic patients having intrinsic asthma and rhinitis and its prevalence in patients with negative skin test reactions to various allergens. HLA-B15 antigens may be more commonly associated with an atopic patient and geographic tongue.

Clinical Features. Geographic tongue is seen in approximately 2% of the United States population, affecting women slightly more often than men. Children may occasionally be affected. This condition is characterized initially by the presence of small, round to irregular areas of dekeratinization and desquamation of filiform papillae (Fig. 3–21). The desquamated areas become red and slightly tender, with elevated margins showing a white to slightly yellowish-white rim, often in a circinate pattern. Characteristically, the lesion, when noted over a period of days or weeks, changes in pattern, appearing to move across the dorsum of the tongue. As healing occurs in one area, the process extends to adjacent areas. A positive clinical correlation exists between geographic tongue and plicated or fissured tongue. The significance of this association is unknown, although symptoms may be more common when fissured tongue is present.

Rare cases of similar alterations of mucosa beyond the dorsum of the tongue have been described in which the floor of the mouth, the buccal mucosa, or the gingiva may be involved. The red atrophic lesions with white keratotic margins are similar to lingual counterparts.

Most patients with geographic tongue are asymptomatic. Occasionally, however, patients will complain of irritation or tenderness, especially in relation to consumption of spicy foods and alcoholic beverages as well as smoking. Severity of symptoms varies with time and is often an indicator of the intensity of lesional activity. Lesions may periodically disappear and recur for no apparent reason. In patients with concomitant fissured tongue, symptoms may also be related to secondary *C. albicans* overgrowth within the fissures.

Histopathology. Filiform papillae are often reduced in number and prominence, with the margins of the lesion demonstrating hyperkeratosis and some acanthosis. Closer to the central portion of the lesion, corresponding to the circinate erythematous areas, there is often loss of superficial parakeratin, with significant migration of polymorphic leukocytes and lymphocytes into the epithelium (Fig. 3–22). The leukocytes are often noted within a microabscess near the surface. An inflammatory cell infiltrate within the underlying lamina propria, consisting chiefly of neutrophils, lymphocytes, and plasma cells, can be seen. Also of significance is the fact that this histologic picture is quite reminiscent of psoriasis—indeed it has been considered and described as a psoriasiform type of intraoral eruption. The clinical link, however, between geographic tongue and cutaneous psoriasis has not been substantiated.

Differential Diagnosis. Based on clinical appearance, geographic tongue is usually diagnostic. Only rarely might biopsy be required for a definitive diagnosis. In equivocal cases, clinical differential diagnosis might include candidiasis, leukoplakia, lichen planus, and lupus erythematosus (LE).

Treatment and Prognosis. Because of the

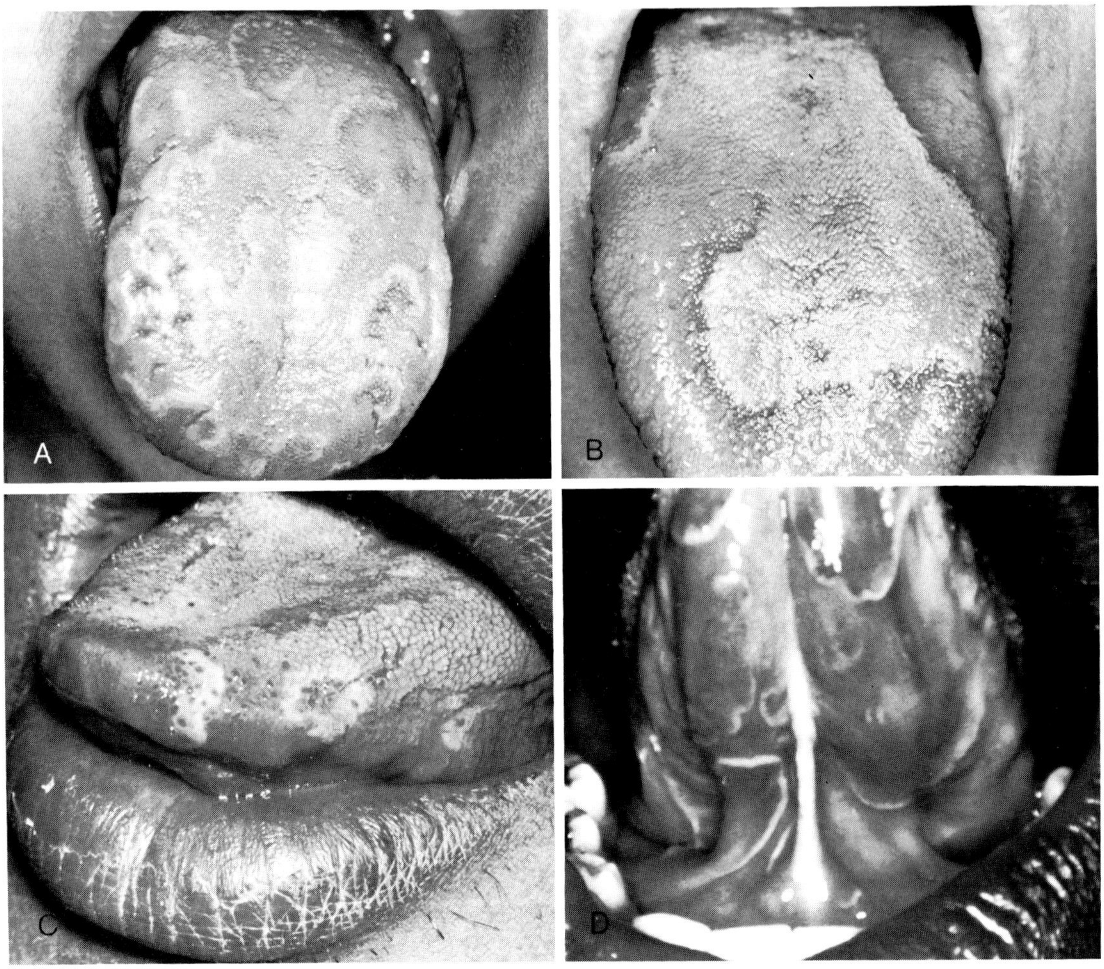

104 WHITE LESIONS

Figure 3–21. *A–D*, Various patterns of geographic tongue.

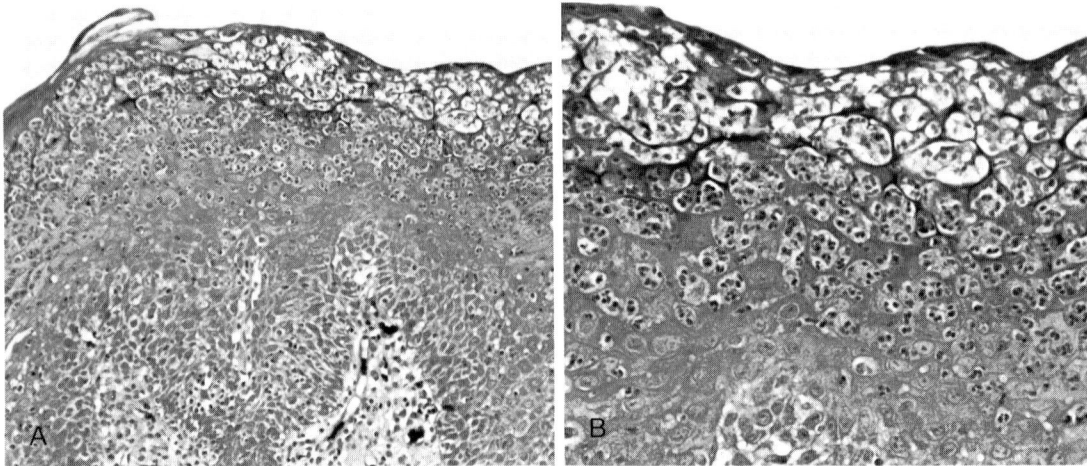

Figure 3–22. *A* and *B*, Biopsy of erythematous zone of geographic tongue showing relative keratin loss and intense neutrophilic infiltration.

self-limiting and usually asymptomatic nature of this condition, treatment is not required. However, when symptoms occur, treatment tends to be empirical and symptomatic. Topical steroids, especially ones containing an antifungal agent, may be helpful. Reassuring patients that this condition is totally benign and does not portend more serious disease in the future will help relieve anxiety.

Lichen Planus

Lichen planus is a rather common, chronic inflammatory mucocutaneous disease. It was first described clinically by Wilson in 1869 and histologically by Dubreuilh in 1906. Since the turn of the century, numerous theories concerning etiology and clinical interrelationships with other diseases have been postulated, and they will be described here. The importance of this disease relates to its degree of frequency within the general population, its frequency of misdiagnosis, its multiplicity of presentations, and its possible connection to malignancy.

Etiology and Pathogenesis. Epithelial basal cells are the primary target in lichen planus. The mechanism of basal cell damage appears to be related to a cell-mediated immune process involving Langerhans cells, T lymphocytes, and macrophages. Theoretically, Langerhans cells (and macrophages) in the epithelium process antigens and present the antigenic information to T lymphocytes. After a proliferative period, T8 lymphocytes become cytotoxic for basal keratinocytes. Similar immunologic mechanisms have also been reported for other conditions such as graft versus host disease and allergic contact dermatitis.

It is hypothesized that in this series of events Langerhans cells contact and "recognize" an antigen, possibly of microbiologic, pharmacologic, or allogeneic origin. The Langerhans cells then process and present appropriate antigenic determinants to T lymphocytes that have been attracted to the area by a Langerhans/macrophage lymphokine known as interleukin-1. The interleukin-1 stimulates the T lymphocytes to produce interleukin-2, which causes T cell proliferation. Activated lymphocytes are subsequently cytotoxic for basal cells. They also secrete gamma-interferon, which induces keratinocytes to express the class II histocompatibility antigens HLA-DR and increase their rate of differentiation, with formation of a thickened surface. This latter feature is seen clinically as a white lesion. The HLA-DR expression may also help explain the lymphocytic "attraction" to the epithelium. It is known that antigenic information is transferred from Langerhans cells (and macrophages) to lymphocytes when there is mutual expression of HLA-DR antigens. If keratinocytes are induced to produce HLA-DR antigens, lymphocytes normally expressing HLA-DR antigens may contact the epithelial cells. During this contact, inappropriate epithelial antigenic information may be passed to lymphocytes because of the HLA-DR linkage. With this mechanism, self-antigens may be recognized as foreign, resulting in an autoimmune response. The destruction of the basal cell layer may also be explained in terms of keratinocytes demonstrating antigens on their surface that are structurally similar to foreign antigens and are recognized erroneously by host T lymphocytes. These cells may then become cytotoxic for the epithelial cells in a hyperimmune reaction.

Clinical Features. Lichen planus is a disease of middle age that affects men and women in nearly equal numbers. Children are rarely affected. Frequently, the severity of the disease parallels the patient's level of stress.

The oral manifestations of lichen planus demonstrate considerable variation in appearance and presentation. Several types of lichen planus within the oral cavity have been described. The most common type is the *reticular form,* which is characterized by the presence of numerous interlacing keratotic lines or striae (so-called Wickham's striae) that produce an annular or lacy pattern (Figs. 3–23 and 3–24). The buccal mucosa is the site most commonly involved. The striae, while occurring typically in a symmetric fashion on the buccal mucosa, may also be noted on the tongue and less frequently on the gingiva and the lips (Fig. 3–25). Almost any mucosal tissue may demonstrate manifestations of lichen planus. This form generally presents with minimal clinical symptoms and is often an incidental discovery.

The *plaque form* of lichen planus tends to resemble leukoplakia clinically, with a multifocal distribution. Such plaques generally range from slightly elevated and smooth to slightly irregular (Fig. 3–26). The primary sites for this variant are over the dorsum of the tongue and on the buccal mucosa.

The *atrophic form* of lichen planus may be seen in conjunction with reticular or erosive variants. The proportion of keratinized to atrophic areas varies from one area to another within this same anatomic region and will also vary over time within the region. The attached gingiva is frequently involved in this form of

106　WHITE LESIONS

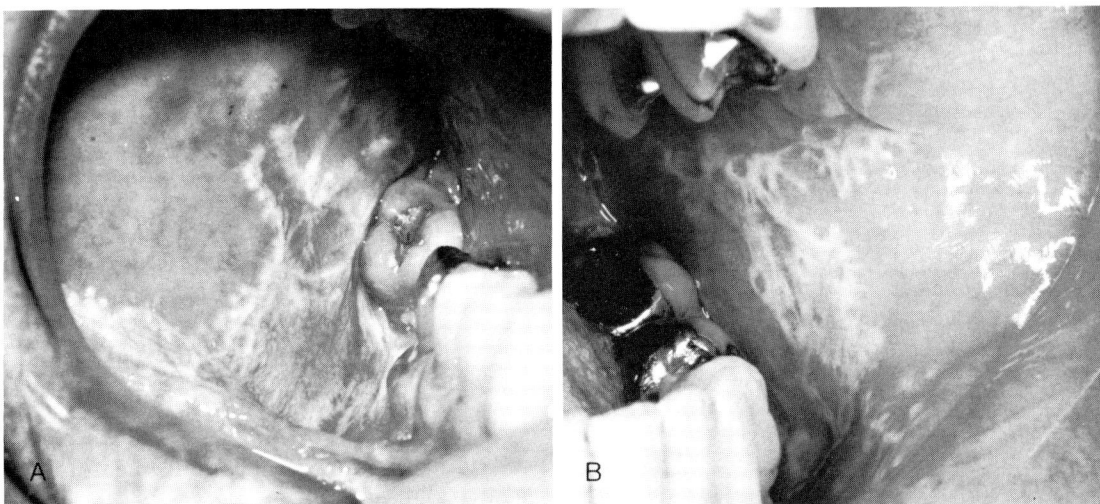

Figure 3–23. *A* and *B*, Typical reticular pattern of lichen planus in two different patients.

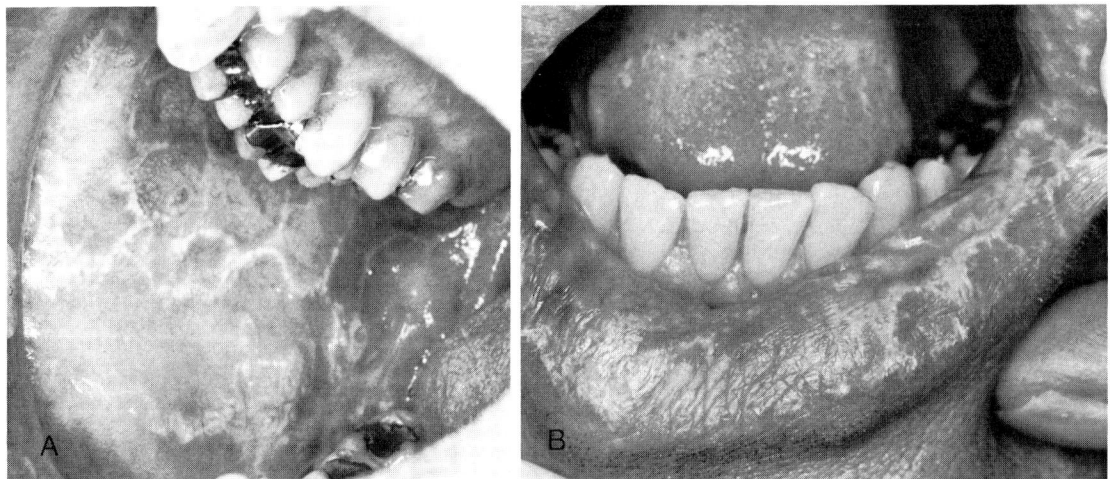

Figure 3–24. *A* and *B*, Lichen planus. Reticular pattern in two different patients.

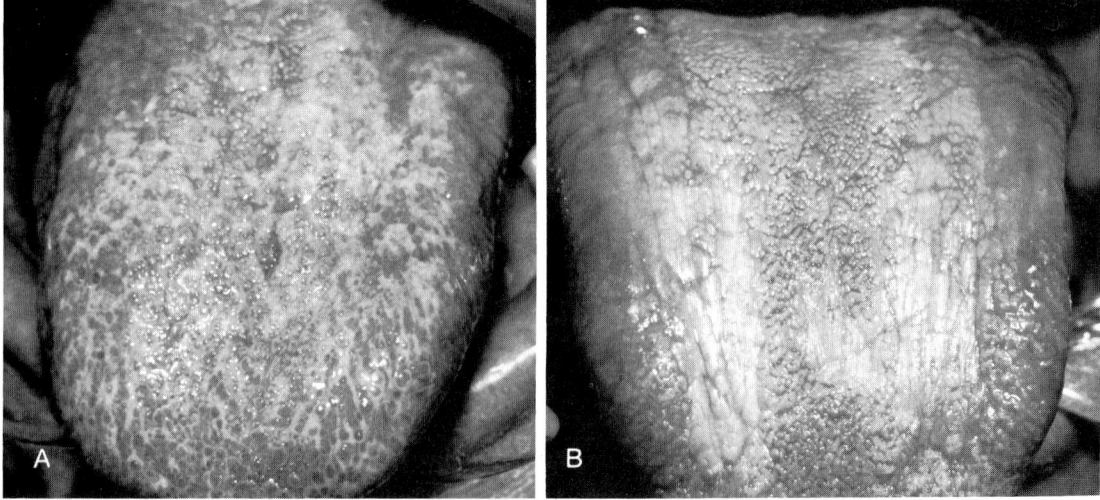

Figure 3–25. Lichen planus of the tongue. *A*, Reticular pattern. *B*, Plaque pattern with atrophy of tongue papillae.

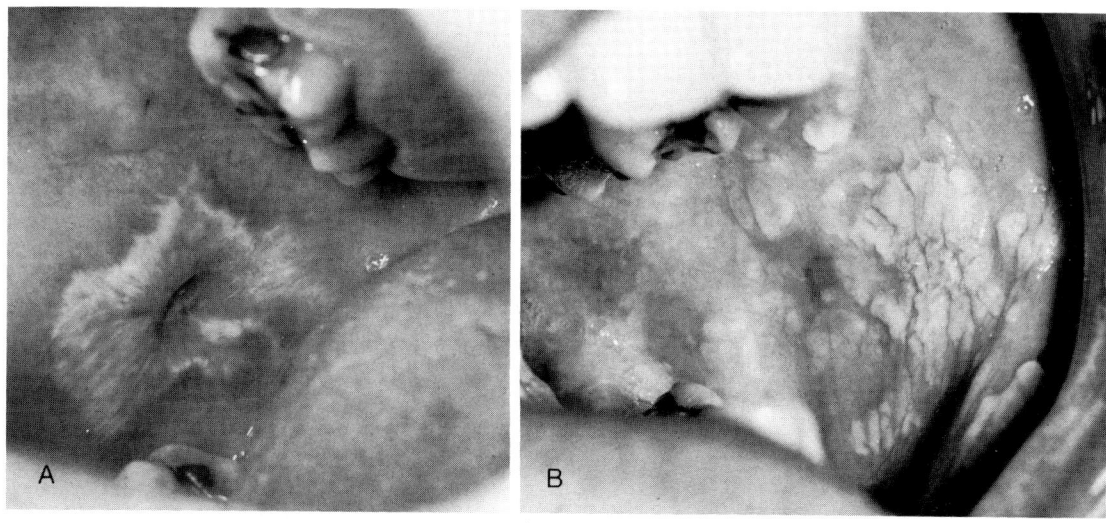

Figure 3-26. *A* and *B,* Lichen planus. Plaque-type lesions in two different patients.

lichen planus, in a so-called desquamative gingivitis pattern (Fig. 3-27). The latter term is non-specific and may represent a variety of disturbances affecting the attached gingiva. At the margins of the atrophic zones, whitish keratotic striae are usually evident, radiating peripherally and blending into surrounding mucosa. When the gingiva is involved, it tends to have a patchy distribution over all four quadrants in a relatively symmetric fashion. Lingual gingiva is usually spared or is less severely involved. The atrophic form of lichen planus will almost always be symptomatic, with patients complaining of burning or pain in the area of involvement.

In the *erosive form* of lichen planus, the surface is generally granular and brightly erythematous, and it may bleed upon slight provocation or manipulation. A fibrinous plaque or pseudomembrane covers areas where erosion is significant. The process is a rather dynamic one, with changing patterns of presentation and involvement noted from week to week. Careful examination usually demonstrates a keratotic component, generally peripheral to the site of erosion, with either reticular or finely radiating keratotic striae.

The most unusual form of lichen planus is the *bullous variant.* The bullae or vesicles range from a few millimeters to several centimeters in diameter. Such bullae are generally short-lived and, upon rupturing, leave an ulcerated, extremely uncomfortable surface. Commonly, the lesions are seen on the buccal

Figure 3-27. Atrophic lichen planus of the gingiva. Note atrophic dark areas (arrows) from which keratotic striae radiate.

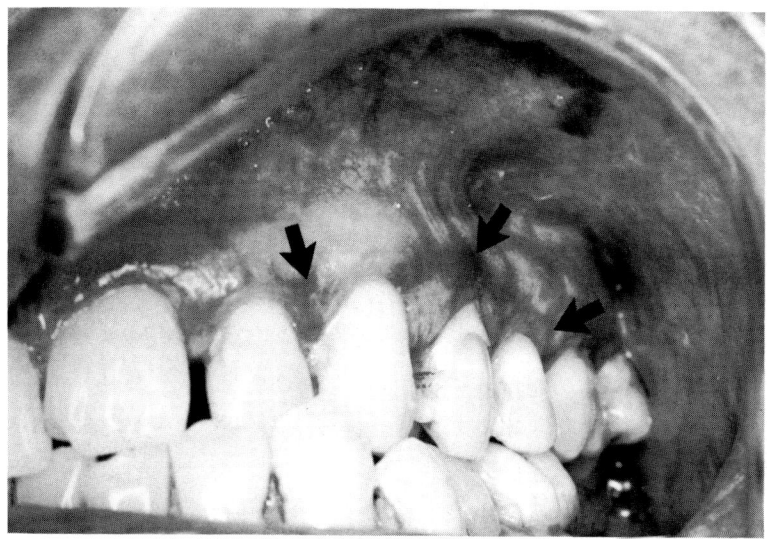

mucosa, especially in the posterior and inferior regions adjacent to the second and third molars. Another common site is the lateral margin of the tongue. Rarely, such lesions may be found on the gingiva and along the inner aspect of the lips. The latter site seems to be more characteristic of drug-induced lichen planus or lichenoid reactions, however. With this variant of the disease, careful examination will often demonstrate the presence of reticular or striated keratotic components.

Recent studies have emphasized the prevalence of secondary oral candidiasis in patients with oral lichen planus, with rates approximating 50%. The data suggest that an altered status of cellular immunity in such lesions may be responsible.

On the skin, lichen planus is characterized by the presence of small, violaceous, polygonal, flat-topped papules with a predilection for the flexor surfaces (Fig. 3–28). Other clinical varieties include hypertrophic, atrophic, bullous, follicular, and linear forms. Cutaneous lesions are noted in approximately 20 to 60% of patients presenting with oral lichen planus. Although the oral changes are more constant over time, it has been noted that the corresponding skin lesions will wax and wane periodically.

Histopathology. The microscopic criteria for the more common variants of lichen planus include the presence of hyperorthokeratosis or hyperparakeratosis. Variable degrees of acanthosis may be seen. The basal layer will characteristically demonstrate liquefaction to the extent of a near-total absence of basal cells (Fig. 3–29). A general effacement or destruction of the epithelial–connective tissue interface is noted, with an intense infiltration of lymphocytes in a band pattern found within the lamina propria parallel to the surface. Within the epithelium, there are increased numbers of Langerhans cells (as demonstrated with immunohistochemistry), presumably processing and presenting antigens to the subjacent T lymphocytes (Fig. 3–30). Discrete eosinophilic ovoid bodies representing necrotic keratinocytes are occasionally noted at the basal cell level or within the surrounding inflammatory cell infiltrate. Although not specific for lichen planus, these colloid or so-called Civatte bodies are suggestive of it. Also noted in a significant number of cases is the presence of a narrow eosinophilic band adjacent to the basement membrane zone, often between the lymphocytic infiltrate and the epithelial cells.

Direct immunofluorescence study demonstrates the presence of fibrinogen along the basement membrane zone in 90 to 100% of cases. While immunoglobulins and complement factors may be found as well, they are far less common than fibrinogen deposition. The immunofluorescence pattern in this disease is not specific or diagnostic, since such patterns may also be seen in LE and erythema multiforme (EM).

Differential Diagnosis. Clinically, other diseases with a white or keratotic component should be considered in a differential diagnosis. Such entities include atrophic candidiasis, leukoplakia, squamous cell carcinoma, drug eruption, and DLE.

Erosive or atrophic lichen planus affecting the attached gingiva must be differentiated from cicatricial pemphigoid, since both may

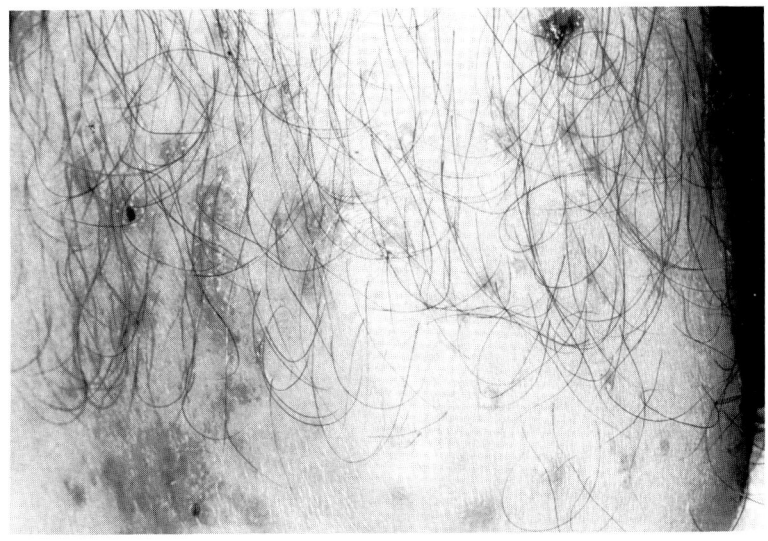

Figure 3–28. Lichen planus of the skin of the ankle presenting as an excoriated papular eruption.

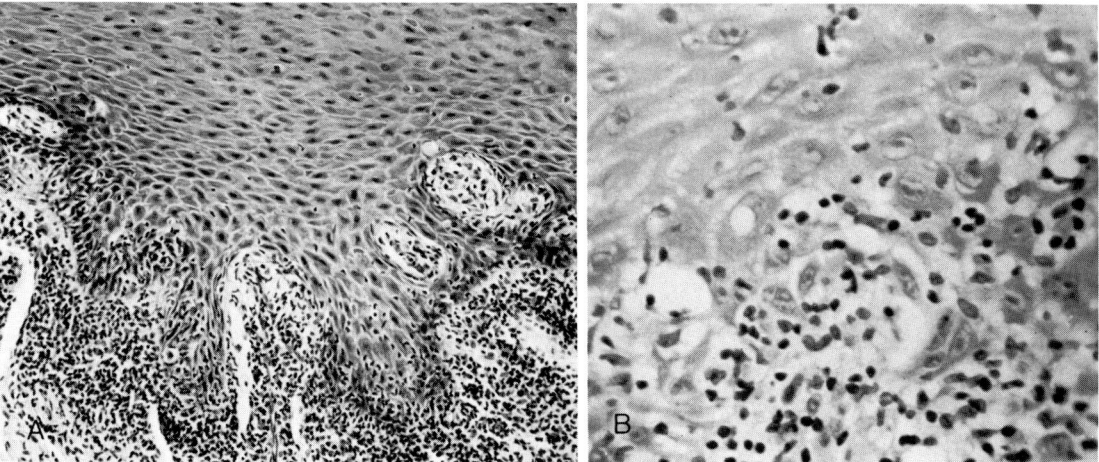

Figure 3–29. *A*, Microscopy of lichen planus showing interface changes of lymphocyte infiltration and basal cell loss. *B*, High magnification of epithelial–connective tissue interface.

present with a desquamative clinical appearance. The differential diagnosis in this case can be aided by direct immunofluorescence studies, since cicatricial pemphigoid has a diagnostic pattern. Colloid or civatte bodies mentioned earlier will often contain immunoglobulin deposits and are rather characteristic for lichen planus; linear immunoglobulin deposits along the basement membrane zone would indicate cicatricial pemphigoid.

Treatment and Prognosis. No specific systemic or local therapy is uniformly successful in the management of lichen planus, although many therapeutic methods have been attempted in an effort to control or eliminate the disease. Corticosteroids are the single most useful group of drugs in the treatment of lichen planus. The rationale for their use is their ability to modulate inflammation and the immune response. Topical application as well as local injection of steroids has been successfully used in controlling but not curing the disease. In circumstances in which symptoms are severe, systemic steroids may be used for management of oral lichen planus, although this is not a routine practice. Recently, because of their antikeratinizing and immunomodulating effects, systemic and topical vitamin A analogues (retinoids) have been utilized in the management of the keratinized reticular and plaque variants of lichen planus (Fig. 3–31). Reversal of white striae can be achieved with topical retinoids, although the effects may be only temporary. Systemic retinoids have been used in cases of severe lichen planus with varying degrees of success. The benefits of

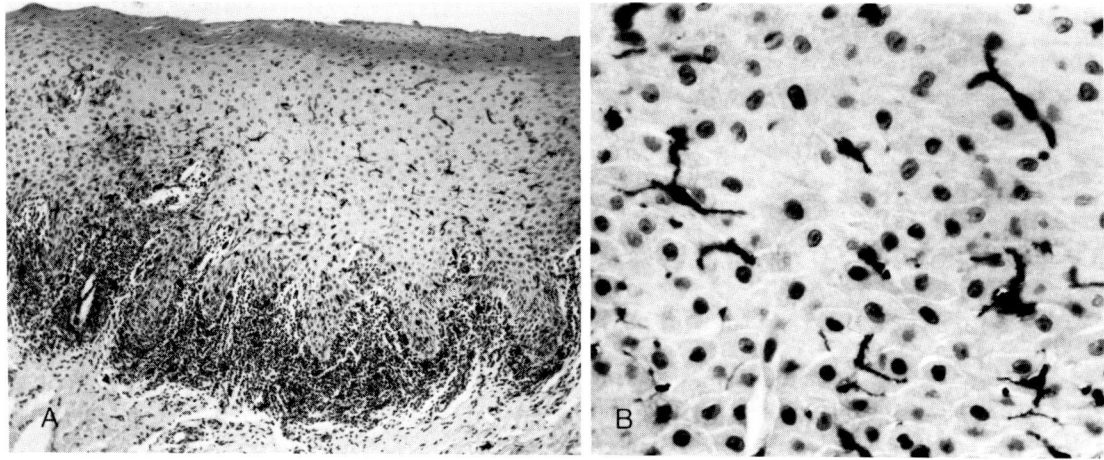

Figure 3–30. *A*, Immunohistochemical stain (S-100 protein) of Langerhans cells in oral lichen planus. *B*, High-magnification detail of dendritic Langerhans cells in the mid-epithelial zone.

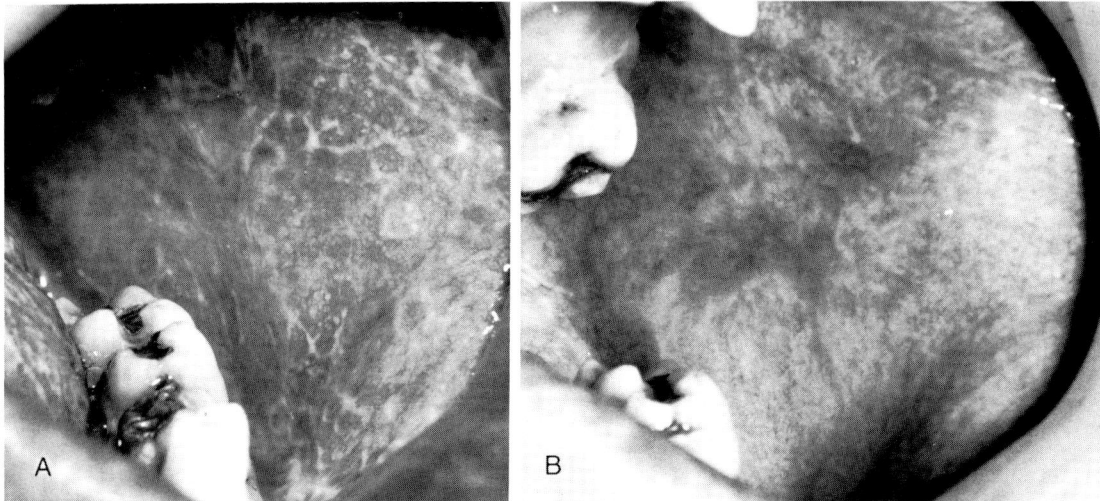

Figure 3–31. *A*, Oral lichen planus before treatment. *B*, Same patient at the end of treatment with topical 13-cis-retinoic acid.

systemic therapy must be carefully weighed against the rather significant side effects—cheilitis, elevation of serum liver enzymes and triglycerides, and teratogenicity.

In cases with significant tissue involvement, more than one drug may be indicated. Various combinations of systemic steroids, topical steroids, and retinoids may be used with some success. However, these methods should be attempted only by experienced clinicians or through consultation with an expert with these drugs.

Finally, control of severe forms of erosive lichen planus has been reported with the use of dapsone (diaminodiphenylsulfone). It is postulated that this particular agent may help control the lymphocyte-mediated process of lichen planus by modulating the release of inflammatory or chemotactic factors from mast cells or neutrophils.

Although there is some debate about the malignant potential of oral lichen planus, it appears that a slightly higher rate of oral squamous cell carcinoma is seen in lichen planus patients as compared with the general population. The actual frequency of malignant transformation appears to be rather low overall and is more commonly noted in the erosive and the atrophic forms of the disease. Since lichen planus is a chronic condition, patients should be observed periodically. This is particularly important for those with the erosive or the atrophic form of the disease and for those with a history of tobacco or alcohol abuse.

NON-EPITHELIAL WHITE-YELLOW LESIONS

Candidiasis

"Candidiasis" is a term that encompasses a group of mucosal and cutaneous conditions with a common etiologic agent from the *Candida* genus of fungi. It is the most common oral mycotic infection, although frequency rates are difficult to determine because of the prevalence of the causative organism in a large proportion of the population. The relationship between the commensal state and pathogenicity is a complex one, based on local factors alone in some cases and local plus systemic factors in others. Oral manifestations may be acute or chronic with variable degrees of severity. Numerous systems of classification have been formulated, indicating the complexity of this condition, the many modes of clinical presentation, and the interrelationship with local and systemic factors. In addition, a relationship has been reported between a subset known as candidal leukoplakia and squamous cell carcinoma.

Etiology and Pathogenesis. Candidiasis is caused by *C. albicans* and the related but far less common species *C. parapsilosis, C. tropicalis, C. glabrata, C. krusei, C. pseudotropicalis,* and *C. guilliermondi. C. albicans* is a commensal organism residing in the oral cavity in a majority of healthy persons. Transformation or escape from a state of commensalism to pathogen by this organism relates to local and systemic factors that are extremely difficult to create experimentally. The organism is a unicellular yeast of the Cryptococcaceae family and may exist in three distinct biologic and morphologic forms: the vegetative or yeast form of oval cells (blastospores), measuring 1.5 to 5 μm in diameter; the elongated cellular form (pseudohyphae); and the chlamydospore form, which consists of cell bodies measuring 7 to 17 μm in diameter, with a thick, refractile, enclosing wall. In the commensal state, the pseudohyphal form is present. The persistence of this organism in its vegetative state is noted intraorally (and intravaginally) and is stated to be related in part to its symbiotic partnership with *Lactobacillus acidophilus*. As evidenced by its frequency in the general population, *C. albicans* is of weak pathogenicity, thereby reflecting the necessity for local or systemic predisposing factors (Table 3–3).

Infection with this organism is usually superficial, affecting the outer aspects of the involved oral mucosa or skin. In severely debilitated and immunocompromised patients, such as AIDS patients, infection may extend into the alimentary tract (candidal esophagitis), bronchopulmonary tract, or other organ systems. The opportunistic nature of this organism is observed in the frequency of mild forms of the disease secondary to the short-term use of systemic antibiotic therapy for minor bacterial infections.

Clinical Features. Oral manifestations of this disease are variable, with numerous forms noted (Table 3–4). The most common form is the acute pseudomembranous form known as thrush (Fig. 3–32). Extremes of infancy and advanced age characterize two groups frequently affected. Estimates of disease frequency range up to 5% of neonates, 5% of cancer patients, and 10% of institutionalized, debilitated elderly patients. This infection is common in patients being treated with radiation or chemotherapy for leukemia and solid tumors, with up to half of those in the former group and 70% in the latter group affected. Candidiasis has also been recognized in patients who suffer from AIDS and those who are in other high-risk groups.

Oral lesions are characteristically white, soft to gelatinous plaques or nodules that grow centrifugally and merge. Plaques are composed of fungal organisms, keratotic debris, inflammatory cells, desquamated epithelial cells, bacteria, and fibrin. Wiping away the plaques or pseudomembranes with a gauze sponge or cotton-tipped applicator will leave an erythematous, eroded, or ulcerated surface that is often tender. Although lesions of thrush may develop at any location, favored sites include the buccal mucosa and mucobuccal folds, the oropharynx, and the lateral aspects of the dorsal tongue. In most instances in which the pseudomembrane has not been disturbed, the associated symptoms are minimal. In severe examples, patients may complain of tenderness, burning, and dysphagia.

Persistence of acute pseudomembranous candidiasis may eventually result in loss of the pseudomembrane, with presentation as a more generalized red lesion, known as acute atrophic candidiasis (Fig. 3–33). Along the dorsum of the tongue, patches of depapillation and dekeratinization may be noted. In the past, this particular form of candidiasis was known as antibiotic stomatitis or antibiotic glossitis, because of its frequent relationship to antibiotic treatment of acute infections. Of interest is that broad-spectrum antibiotics or concurrent administration of multiple narrow-spectrum antibiotics may produce this secondary infection to a much greater degree than do single narrow-spectrum antibiotics. Withdrawal of the offending antibiotic and institu-

Table 3–3. PREDISPOSING FACTORS FOR *CANDIDA* INFECTION

Immunologic immaturity of infancy
Endocrine disturbances
    Diabetes mellitus
    Hypoparathyroidism
    Pregnancy
    Systemic steroid therapy/hypoadrenalism
Advanced malignancy
Malabsorption and malnutrition
Systemic antibiotic therapy
Cancer chemotherapy
Other forms of immunosuppression (e.g., AIDS)

Table 3–4. ORAL CANDIDIASIS CLASSIFICATION

Acute candidiasis
    Pseudomembranous
    Atrophic
Chronic candidiasis
    Atrophic
    Hypertrophic/hyperplastic
Mucocutaneous forms
    Localized (oral, face, scalp, nails)
    Familial
    Syndrome associated

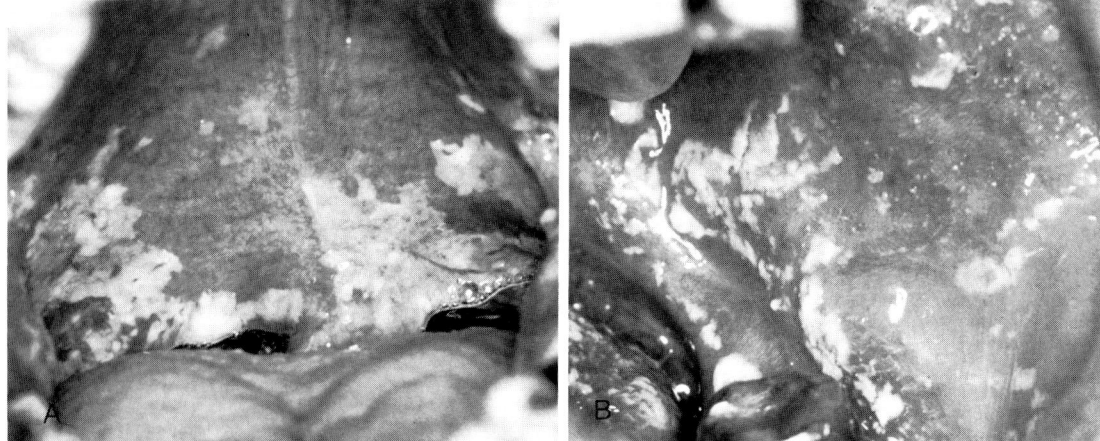

Figure 3–32. *A* and *B,* Acute (pseudomembranous) candidiasis.

tion of appropriate oral hygiene will lead to improvement. In contrast to the acute pseudomembranous form, oral symptoms of the acute atrophic form are quite marked, because of numerous erosions and intense inflammation.

Chronic candidiasis, often called denture sore mouth, is a commonly seen atrophic subset (Fig. 3–34). This particular form of candidiasis occurs in up to 65% of geriatric individuals who wear complete maxillary dentures. Expression of this form of candidiasis depends upon the oral mucosa being conditioned by a covering prosthesis. There is a distinct predilection for the palatal mucosa as compared with the mandibular alveolar arch. Women show a greater propensity for developing this form of the disease than men. Chronic, low-grade trauma secondary to poor prosthesis fit, less than ideal occlusal relationships, and failure to remove the appliance at night all contribute to the development of this condition. The clinical appearance is that of a bright red, somewhat velvety to pebbly surface, with relatively little keratinization. In severe examples, small confluent vesicles and erosions may be seen.

Also seen in individuals with denture-related chronic atrophic candidiasis is angular cheilitis (Fig. 3–34). This condition is especially prevalent in individuals who demonstrate deep folds at the commissures secondary to overclosure. In such circumstances, small accumulations of saliva gather in the skin folds at the commissural angles and are subsequently colonized by yeast organisms. Clinically, the lesions are moderately painful, fissured, eroded, and encrusted. Angular cheilitis may also be

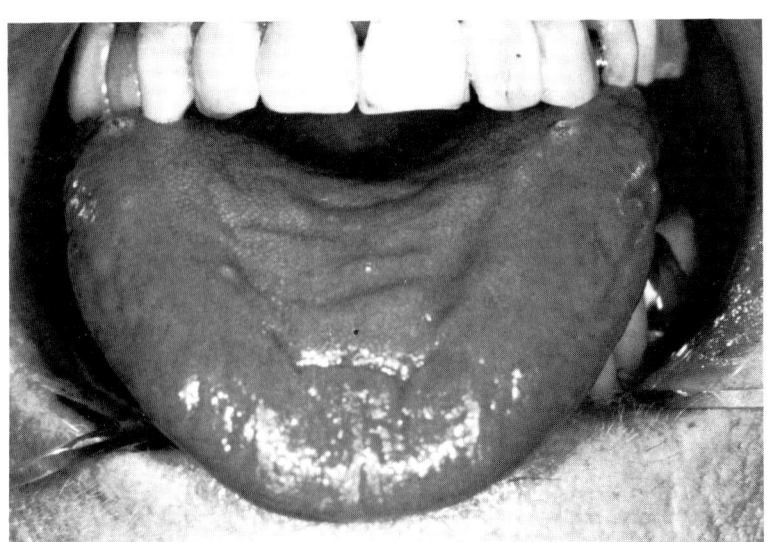

Figure 3–33. Acute atrophic candidiasis.

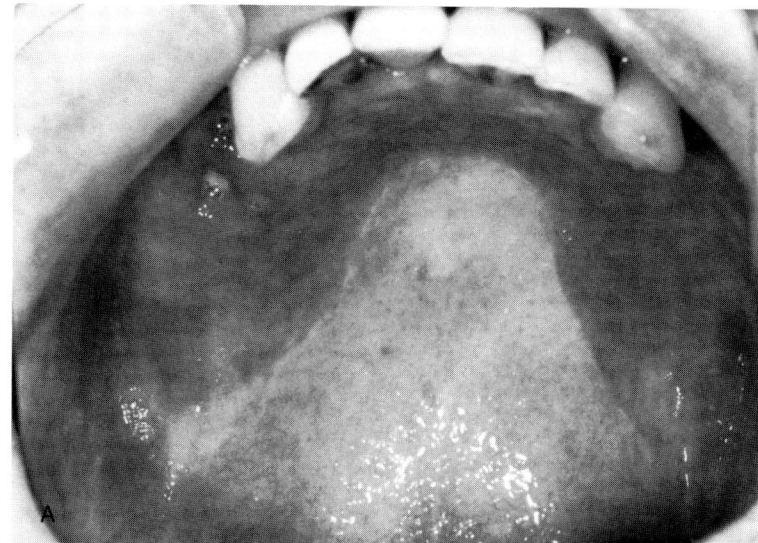
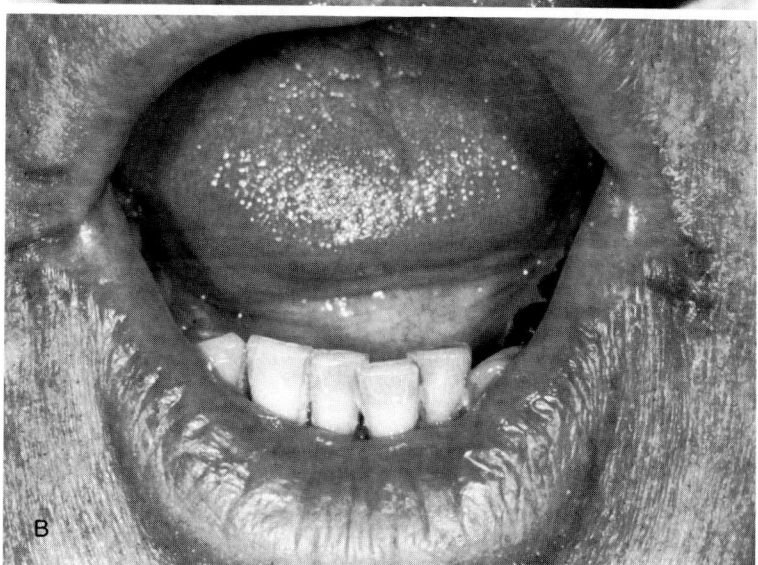

Figure 3–34. Chronic atrophic candidiasis. *A*, Denture "sore mouth" type. *B*, Angular cheilitis or perlèche type.

seen in individuals who habitually lick their lips and deposit small amounts of saliva in the commissural angles. The pathogenesis of the condition, however, is identical to that in denture wearers.

A circumoral type of atrophic candidiasis may be seen in those with severe lip-licking habits with extension of the process onto the surrounding skin. The skin is fissured and demonstrates a degree of brown coloration on a slightly erythematous base. This condition is to be separated from perioral dermatitis, which characteristically shows less crusting and a zone of uninvolved skin immediately adjacent to the cutaneous-vermilion junction.

Chronic candidal infections are also capable of producing a hyperplastic tissue response. When occurring in the retrocommissural area, the lesion resembles speckled leukoplakia and, in some classifications, is known as candidal leukoplakia. It occurs in adults with no apparent predisposition to infection by *C. albicans,* and it is felt by some clinicians to represent a premalignant lesion.

Hyperplastic candidiasis may involve the dorsum of the tongue in a pattern referred to as median rhomboid glossitis (Fig. 3–35). It is usually asymptomatic and is generally discovered on routine oral examination. The lesion is found anterior to the circumvallate papillae and has a rhomboid outline. It may have a smooth, nodular, or fissured surface. It may be slightly indurated and may range in color from white to a more characteristic red. In the past, this particular condition was felt to be a developmental anomaly, thought to have oc-

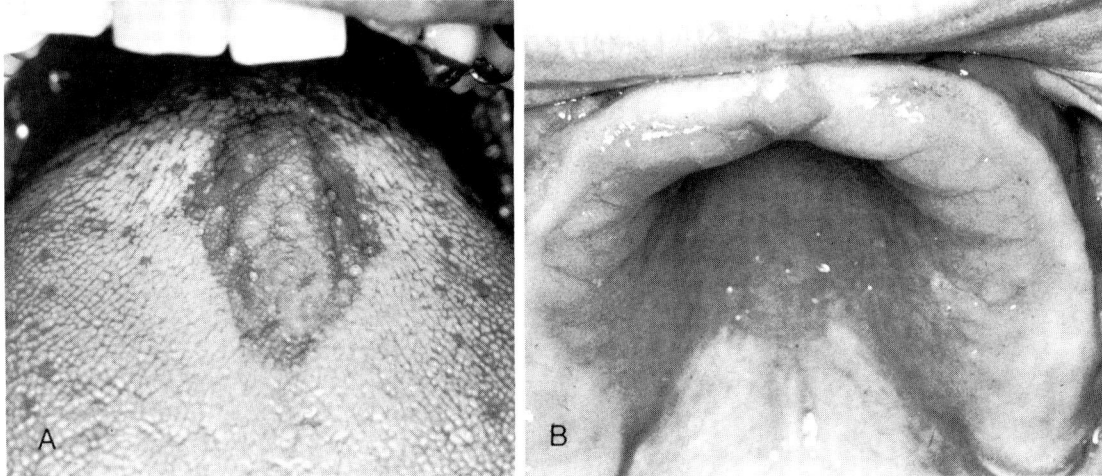

Figure 3–35. Chronic hypertrophic/hyperplastic candidiasis. *A*, Median rhomboid glossitis type. *B*, Palatal papillary type.

curred secondary to persistence of the tuberculum impar of the developing tongue. Recent evidence indicates, however, that this is more likely a hypertrophic form of candidiasis.

Nodular papillary lesions of the hard palatal mucosa predominantly seen beneath maxillary complete dentures are felt to represent, at least in part, a response to chronic yeast infection (Fig. 3–35). The papillary hyperplasia is composed of individual nodules that are ovoid to spherical and form excrescences measuring 2 to 3 mm in diameter on an erythematous background.

The mucocutaneous forms of candidiasis are rather diverse in their presentation and in the groups of patients affected. The localized form of mucocutaneous candidiasis is characterized by long-standing and persistent candidiasis of the oral mucosa, nails, skin, and vaginal mucosa (Fig. 3–36). This form of candidiasis is often resistant to treatment, with only temporary remission following the use of standard antifungal therapy. As with all forms of chronic mucocutaneous candidiasis, this form begins early in life, usually within the first 2 decades. The disease begins as a pseudomembranous type of candidiasis and is soon followed by nail and cutaneous involvement. Nail changes range from slight involvement of a single nail to severe disfigurement of all nails. Secondary granulomatous changes occur in the nail bed as well as in the associated skin lesions.

A familial non-syndrome form of candidiasis may be seen in approximately 20% of cases with mucocutaneous presentation. This form of the disease is felt to be transmitted in an autosomal recessive fashion, with nearly 50% of such patients demonstrating an associated endocrinopathy. This endocrinopathy usually consists of hypoparathyroidism, Addison's dis-

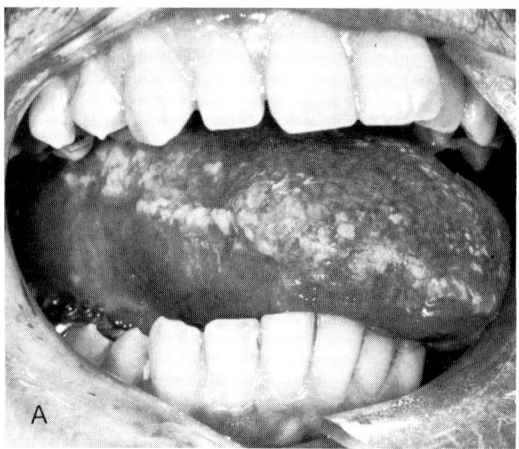
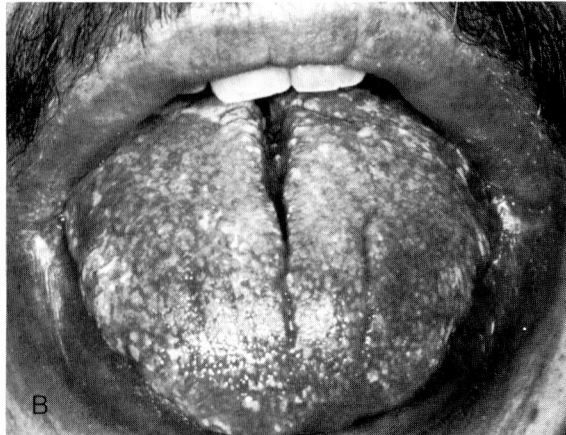

Figure 3–36. *A* and *B*, Mucocutaneous candidiasis.

ease, and occasionally hypothyroidism or diabetes mellitus. In other forms of familial chronic mucocutaneous candidiasis, there is an associated iron deficiency, often without clinical signs of anemia. Patients absorb iron normally, although there is a chronic depletion of iron stores believed to be due to a genetically determined abnormality of iron metabolism. Subsequently, there may be a secondary deficiency of the cellular immune system, which favors infection by the fungal organism.

There are other forms of familial mucocutaneous candidiasis that have in common abnormalities of iron metabolism and alterations of cell-mediated immunity. One form is characterized by late onset of the candidiasis, is generally limited to the oral cavity, and is seen beyond 35 years of age. A second subset of patients will, in addition to demonstrating susceptibility to candidiasis as well as other forms of infection, demonstrate an excessive epithelial and connective tissue reaction to the proliferating organisms.

The triad of chronic mucocutaneous candidiasis, myositis, and thymoma was initially reported in 1968. Several cases have been reported since then. Usually myositis is the initial manifestation, followed by mucocutaneous expression of the disease. Muscle biopsies in this disorder demonstrate sharply demarcated, intense lymphocytic infiltration between bundles of striated muscle. The role of the thymus relates to a deficiency in T cell–mediated immunologic function, hence providing an opportunity for yeast proliferation. It is theorized that appropriately armed T lymphocytes may control *Candida* infections by manufacturing and releasing a lymphokine-like substance that is reported to be toxic for the organism.

A final form of candidiasis is becoming increasingly evident within the immunosuppressed population of patients, in particular those infected with the human immunodeficiency virus (HIV) and with other manifestations of AIDS. This form of candidiasis was originally described in 1981 and is now well recognized as being one of the more important opportunistic infections that afflicts this group of patients. The significantly depleted cell-mediated arm of the immune mechanism is felt to be responsible for allowing the development of the severe candidiasis.

Laboratory Findings. Clinical laboratory tests for this organism involve removal of a portion of the candidal plaque, which is then smeared on a microscope slide and macerated with 20% potassium hydroxide. The slide is subsequently examined for typical hyphae. Culture identification and quantification of organisms may be performed with a variety of media, including Sabouraud's broth, blood agar, and cornmeal agar. Immunofluorescent identification may be necessary in forms of the disease in which no colonies are clinically evident, especially in the chronic atrophic form of the disease. Traditional methods of laboratory characterization of *C. albicans* and other species relate to viable carbohydrate fermentation and assimilation studies as well as microscopic characteristics.

Histopathology. Microscopic examination of the pseudomembranous lesions of candidiasis will show a localized superficial inflammatory reaction with erosion or ulceration of the surface. Ulcers are covered with a thick layer of cellular debris, fibrin, inflammatory exudate, and large numbers of yeast hyphae. In superficial infections, the fungi are limited to the surface layers of the epithelium; in more severe examples hyphae will extend deeper into the epithelium (Fig. 3–37). Neutrophilic infiltration of the epithelium with superficial microabscess formation is typically seen. Yeast elements may be morphologically enhanced by staining with methenamine silver or periodic acid–Schiff (PAS) reagent. The predominant fungal forms growing in this particular form of the disease are pseudohyphae. These pseudohyphae penetrate the epithelium and may actually enter keratinocytes to become intracellular parasites. The chronic varieties of candidiasis have epithelial hyperplasia in common. Epithelial hyperplasia is a rather characteristic feature of this form of the disease and has been shown to be induced by the presence of the yeast organism. Since experimental evidence indicates that such an infection is capable of producing epithelial hyperplasia and since chronic candidiasis may give rise to oral leukoplakia, the importance of this infection becomes apparent. This must be tempered with the fact that there is no clear evidence that chronic candidiasis is in and of itself a precancerous state. It is possible, however, that epithelial invasion by this organism and subsequent proliferation may contribute to neoplastic change.

Differential Diagnosis. Candidal infections must be differentiated from several entities, including the slough associated with chemical burns, superficial bacterial infections and colonization, gangrenous stomatitis, traumatic ulcerations, and mucous patches of syphilis. When isolated red lesions of the acute atrophic form of candidiasis are present, they must be

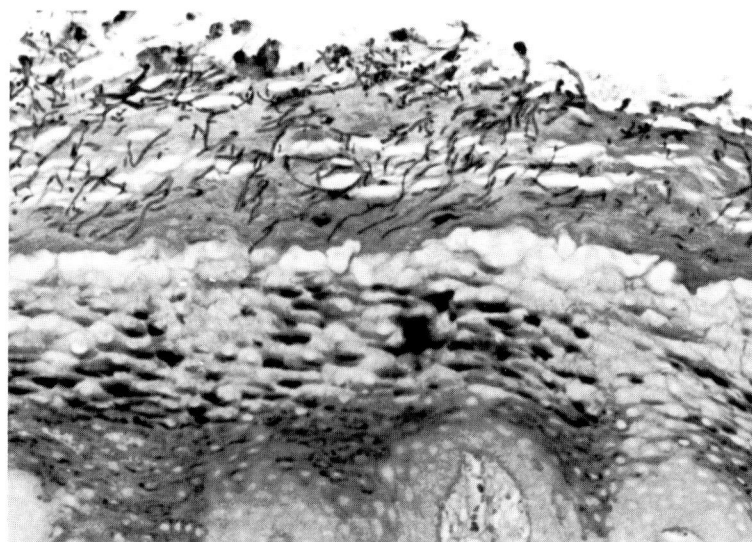

Figure 3–37. Microscopic section (PAS stain) of acute candidiasis. Numerous dark-stained hyphae and spore forms of *C. albicans* are present in the parakeratotic layer.

differentiated from drug reactions and thermal burns. In addition, these red lesions may resemble erosive lichen planus, DLE, and early or mild cases of EM.

Treatment and Prognosis. The majority of *C. albicans* infections may be simply treated with topical applications of nystatin suspension. In the case of denture-related disease, nystatin cream may be used on the affected tissue and in the denture itself to provide prolonged contact and eliminate organisms in the denture material. Withdrawal of broad-spectrum antibiotics will usually produce resolution of the oral yeast infection. If oxygenating agents, such as hydrogen peroxide, have been used chronically, withdrawal of these particular substances should allow for reestablishment of normal oral bacterial flora and relief of symptoms. Clotrimazole can be conveniently administered in lozenge or troche form. Topical applications of either nystatin or clotrimazole should be continued for approximately 1 week beyond the disappearance of clinical manifestations of the disease. In cases of chronic mucocutaneous candidiasis or oral candidiasis associated with immunosuppression, topical agents may not be effective. In such instances, systemic administration of medications such as amphotericin B, ketoconazole, and flucytosine may be necessary. Caution must be exercised, however, since flucytosine and ketoconazole may be hepatotoxic and can also depress hematopoiesis.

The prognosis for acute and most other forms of chronic candidiasis is excellent. The underlying defect in most types of mucocutaneous candidiasis, however, militates against cure, although intermittent improvement may be noted following the use of systemic antifungal agents.

Mucosal Burns

Etiology. The most common form of superficial "burn" of the oral mucosa is associated with topical applications of chemicals, such as aspirin or caustic agents, to the mucosa. Placement of recreational drugs, accidental placement of phosphoric acid–etching solutions or gel by a dentist, or overly fastidious use of alcohol-containing mouthwashes may produce similar effects.

Clinical Features. In cases of short-term exposure to agents capable of inducing tissue necrosis, a localized mild erythema may be evident. As the concentration of the offending agent increases and as the contact time increases, surface coagulative necrosis is more likely to occur, resulting in a white slough or membrane (Fig. 3–38). Beneath the membrane will be a friable, painful surface that will bleed easily upon manipulation. With gentle traction, the surface slough will peel from the denuded connective tissue, producing considerable tenderness and pain.

Thermal burns are commonly noted on the hard palatal mucosa and are generally associated with sticky foods that adhere to the palate. Hot liquids are more likely to burn the tongue or the soft palate. Such lesions are generally erythematous rather than white (necrosis), as is seen with chemical burns.

Another form of burn that is potentially quite serious is the electrical burn. In particular, children who chew through electrical cords receive rather characteristic initial burns that are often symmetric. The result of such accidents is significant tissue damage, frequently followed by scarring and reduction in the size of the oral opening. The surface of such lesions tends to be characterized by a thickened slough that extends deep into the surrounding connective tissue and muscles.

Histopathology. In cases of chemical and thermal burns in which an obvious clinical slough has developed, the epithelial component will show coagulative necrosis through its entire thickness. A fibrinous exudate is also evident. The underlying connective tissue will be intensely inflamed. Electrical burns will be more destructive, showing deep extension of necrosis, often into muscle.

Differential Diagnosis. The fundamental element in establishing the diagnosis of a mucosal burn relates to obtaining an accurate history, with the identification of an agent that may produce tissue damage. Among the most frequent agents involved with localized mucosal sloughs traditionally has been aspirin used as topical treatment for toothache.

In the absence of a history of use of a chemical likely to produce a burn or a history of ingestion of excessively hot food, accumulated materia alba over the soft tissues secondary to poor oral hygiene might be considered. A fibrinous exudate over an ulcerated pyogenic granuloma or a pseudomembrane associated with acute necrotizing ulcerative gingivitis (ANUG) might also be included in a differential diagnosis.

Treatment. Management of chemical, thermal, or electrical burns is quite variable. For the thermal or chemical burn patient, local symptomatic therapy with or without the use of systemic analgesics is appropriate. Topical therapy utilizing hydrocortisone acetate with or without benzocaine may be helpful. Application of dilute solutions of topical anesthetic such as 1% dyclonine hydrochloride (Dyclone) will also reduce symptoms. For the electrical burn patient, management may be much more difficult. The services of the pediatric dentist, the oral and maxillofacial surgeon, and, on occasion, the plastic surgeon may be necessary in more severe cases. Pressure stents may be required over the damaged areas to prevent early contracture of the wounds. Subsequent to healing, further definitive surgical or reconstructive treatment may be necessary because of extensive scar formation or loss of significant amounts of tissue.

Submucous Fibrosis

Etiology. The postulated etiology of this condition is hypersensitivity to dietary constituents such as spicy foods, especially chili. Habits such as betel nut chewing and the use of tobacco in betel nut quids are also believed to have etiologic importance. In addition, general nutritional or vitamin deficiencies have been mentioned as potential etiologic factors. Experimental models for the study of submucous fibrosis have been developed; *in vitro* studies have demonstrated that components of the betel nut *(Areca catecha)* increase collagen synthesis by 170% as compared with controls.

Clinical Features. This disease is rarely seen in North America. It is generally noted in individuals who have emigrated from southeast

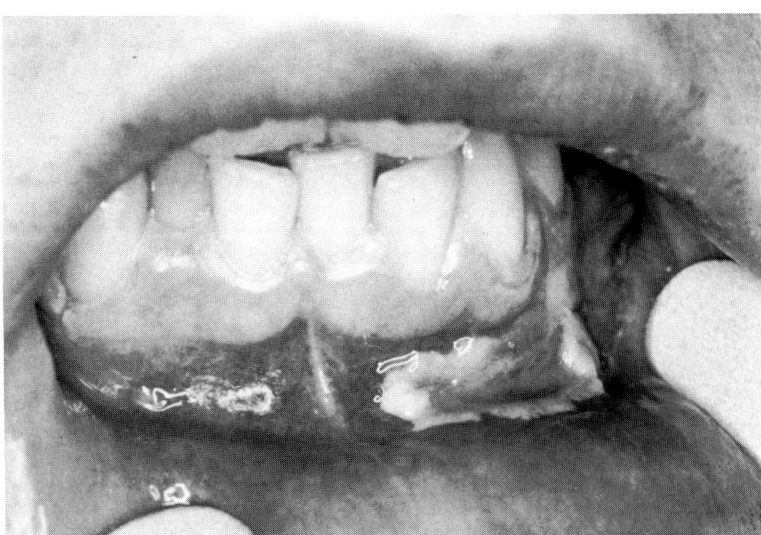

Figure 3–38. Chemical burn of the vestibular mucosa.

Asia or India. Other ethnic clustering may be noted within Pakistanis and Burmese, with sporadic cases observed in South Vietnamese, Thais, Chinese, and Nepalese. Those affected are typically between the ages of 20 and 40, although the condition may be seen in younger and older individuals as well.

Oral submucous fibrosis presents as a whitish-yellow lesion that has a chronic insidious biologic behavior. It is typically seen within the oral cavity but on occasion may extend into the pharynx and the esophagus. Submucous fibrosis may occasionally be preceded by or be associated with vesicle formation. In time the affected mucosa, especially the soft palate and the buccal mucosa, loses its resilience and elasticity, with resultant trismus and considerable difficulty in eating. The process progresses from the lamina propria initially to the underlying musculature.

Histopathology. Microscopically, the principal features include extreme thinning and atrophy of the epithelium, with variable degrees of dysplastic change. The superficial portions of the lamina propria are poorly vascularized and hyalinized (Fig. 3–39). Fibroblasts are few in number, with a variable chronic inflammatory infiltrate ranging from minimal to moderate.

Differential Diagnosis. The clinical differential diagnosis of submucous fibrosis includes a relatively small number of entities. Radiation-related subepithelial fibrosis may produce a degree of trismus and mucosal atrophy, although not to the same degree as submucous fibrosis. Mucosal scarring secondary to thermal or chemical burns may produce associated trismus, although the actual pattern of the scars in relation to these circumstances is probably more demonstrative than those associated with submucous fibrosis.

Treatment and Prognosis. Treatment has included stretching exercises and intralesional injections of corticosteroids. Surgical releasing procedures likewise have been attempted. All methods of treatment, however, have proved to be of little help in this essentially irreversible condition.

The primary importance of submucous fibrosis relates to its reported premalignant nature. The development of squamous cell carcinoma has been noted in up to one third of patients with submucous fibrosis. It has been speculated that the fibroblastic degeneration and epithelial atrophy form the physical basis for carcinogen penetration through the epithelium. The restriction or elimination of tobacco use should be attempted, and etiologic dietary agents should be withdrawn.

Fordyce's Granules

Etiology. Fordyce's granules represent ectopic sebaceous glands or sebaceous choristomas (normal tissue in an abnormal location). The origin of such granules is felt to be developmental.

Clinical Features. Fordyce's granules are multiple, often seen in aggregates or in confluent arrangements (Fig. 3–40). The sites of predilection include the buccal mucosa and the vermilion of the upper lip. The lesions generally are symmetrically distributed. Males show larger numbers of lesions per unit area than do women. The age of appearance generally

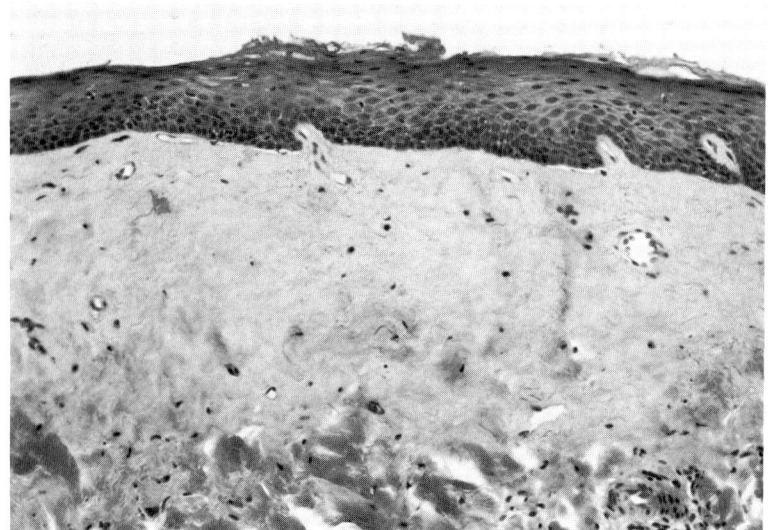

Figure 3–39. Biopsy of oral submucous fibrosis showing hyalinization of connective tissue and epithelial atrophy.

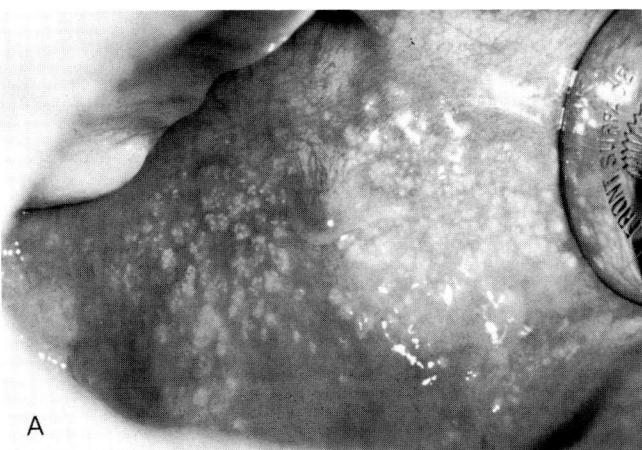
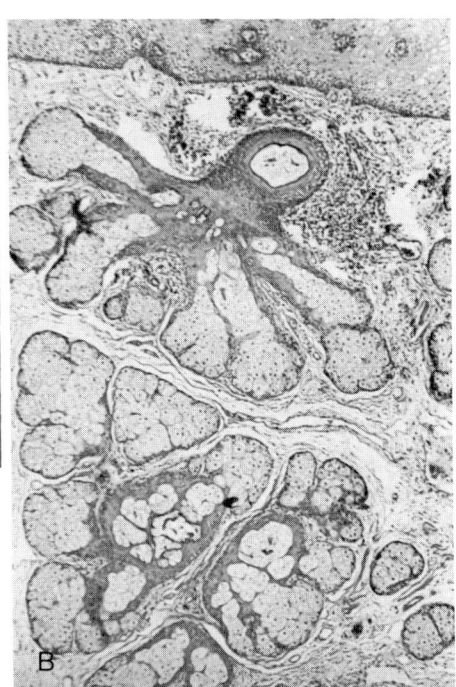

Figure 3–40. *A*, Fordyce's granules of the buccal mucosa. *B*, Biopsy showing numerous lobules of sebaceous glands.

is post-pubertal, with numbers of lesions reaching a peak between 20 and 30 years of age, although areas of involvement increase up to the sixth decade. The lesions are asymptomatic and are often discovered incidentally by the patient or by the practitioner during a routine oral examination. A large proportion of the population is affected by this particular condition; it is seen in approximately 80% of individuals.

Histopathology. Superficially located lobules of sebaceous glands are seen aggregated around or adjacent to excretory ducts. The ducts themselves contain sebaceous and keratinous debris. The heterotopic glands are well formed and appear functional. Individual cells demonstrate a granular, relatively clear cytoplasm with basally placed nuclei that are slightly pyknotic in nature. Except for the relationship of sebaceous glands to hair in the skin, there is virtual identity of the oral glands with those of the skin.

Differential Diagnosis. The appearance and distribution of the glands may on occasion be mistaken for small clusters of *C. albicans* organisms. Simple wiping of the surface of the Fordyce granules, however, would not result in their disappearance as would be the case with candidal colonies. Very few other conditions could be mistaken for this particular entity.

Treatment and Prognosis. No treatment is indicated for this particular condition, since the glands are normal in character and do not cause any untoward effects.

Ectopic Lymphoid Tissue

Ectopic lymphoid tissue may be found in numerous oral locations. It is normally found in the posterolateral aspect of the tongue, where it is known as the lingual tonsil. Aggregates of lymphoid tissue may commonly be seen in the soft palate, the floor of the mouth, and the tonsillar pillars, although they may occur in other sites as well.

Lymphoid tissue has a yellow or yellow-white color clinically and typically produces small, dome-shaped elevations (Fig. 3–41). The tissue appears uninflamed, and the patient is unaware of its presence. Crypts in the lymphoid tissue may on occasion become obstructed, causing "cystic" dilatation of the area. These lesions may then be called lymphoepithelial cysts. In a strict sense, however, lymphoepithelial cysts are believed to be derived from cystic change of embryonically entrapped epithelium within lymphoid tissue.

Generally, lymphoid tissue can be diagnosed on clinical features alone. Since this is basically normal tissue, no biopsy is necessary.

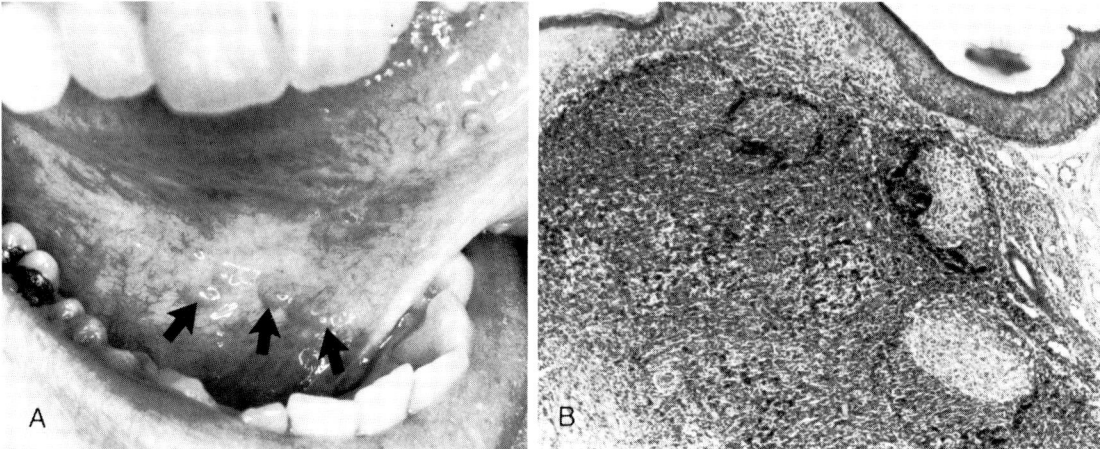

Figure 3–41. *A*, Ectopic lymphoid tissue (arrows). *B*, Microscopy showing lymphoid tissue covered by intact epithelium.

Gingival Cysts

Gingival cysts of odontogenic origin occur in adults as well as in infants. In infants, the relative frequency is highest in the neonatal phase, and by 3 months the cysts are rarely noted. Observations of such cysts from the neonatal period forward indicate that the vast majority involute spontaneously or rupture and exfoliate. Two eponyms have been commonly used as synonyms for gingival cysts, although these eponyms were originally intended to designate different neonatal cysts. The term "Epstein's pearls" was used to designate cysts noted along the palatal midline that had no relationship to the tooth-forming apparatus. The term "Bohn's nodules" referred to cysts noted along the alveolar ridges that were believed to be related to salivary gland remnants.

Etiology and Pathogenesis. Neonatal gingival cysts are thought to arise from the dental lamina remnants. Fetal tissues between 10 and 12 weeks of age show small amounts of keratin within elements of the dental lamina. Toward the end of the twelfth week of gestation, disruption of the dental lamina is evident, with many fragments demonstrating central cystification and keratin accumulation. Gingival cysts are generally numerous in the fetus and infant, increasing in number to the twenty-second week of gestation.

Midline palatal cysts, or Epstein's pearls, are thought to result from epithelial entrapment within the midline of palatal fusion. Small epithelial inclusions within the line of fusion produce microcysts that contain keratin and usually rupture early in life. Detailed developmental studies have shown that fewer than 20 midline palatal keratinizing cysts are noted in any fetus by the fourteenth week of gestation, with no increased tendency to exceed that number with time.

The origin of the gingival cyst of the adult is probably from remnants of the dental lamina (rests of Serres). Cystic change of these rests may occasionally result in a multilocular lesion. An alternative theory of pathogenesis relates to the traumatic implantation of surface epithelium into gingival connective tissue.

Clinical Features. The gingival cyst in the neonate will present as a white or off-white, broad-based nodule approximately 2 mm in diameter, with one to many cysts being evident along the alveolar crests (Fig. 3–42). The midline palatal cysts, on the other hand, present along the midpalatal raphe toward the junction of the hard and soft palate. The overall incidence has been estimated at 76%.

The gingival cyst of the adult occurs chiefly within the fifth and sixth decades. It appears more frequently in the mandible than in the maxilla (Fig. 3–43). There is a great deal of similarity between the gingival cyst in the adult and the lateral periodontal cyst, including site of predilection, age of occurrence, clinical behavior, and overall morphology.

The gingival cyst of the adult is painless, well circumscribed, and slow growing. The lesions generally occur in the attached gingiva, often within the interdental papilla. Only rarely are such lesions found along the lingual gingiva. Premolar and bicuspid regions of the mandible are favored locations. The overlying epithelium is intact and smooth. The lesion may appear white-yellow to blue. In cases of long duration and large size (approaching 1 cm in diameter), there may be slight sauceri-

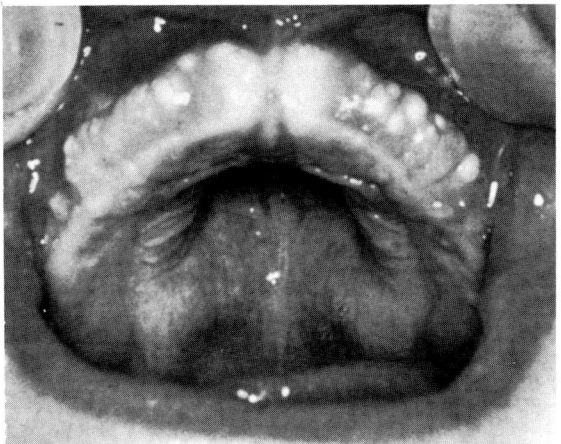

Figure 3–42. Gingival cysts of the newborn.

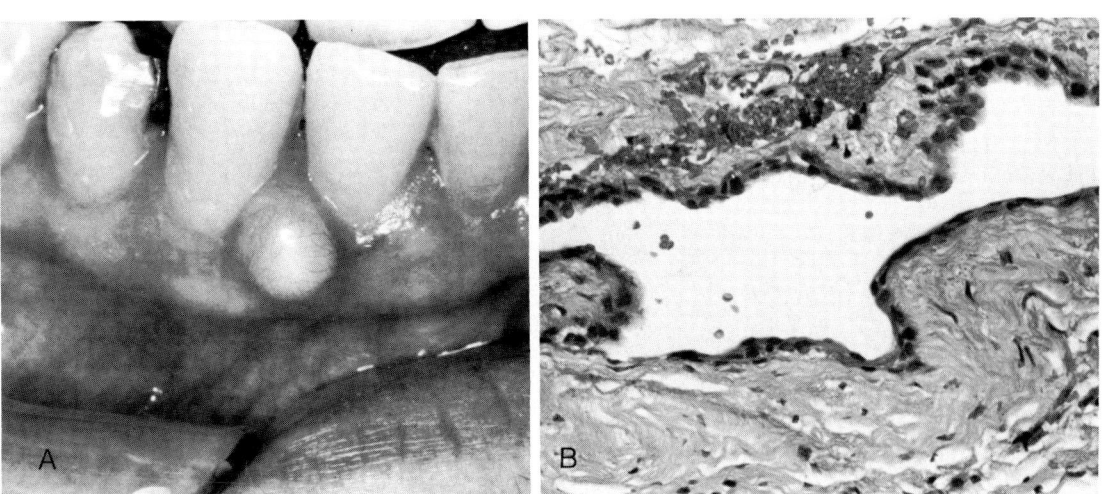

Figure 3–43. *A*, Gingival cyst of the adult. *B*, A thin, non-keratinized epithelium lines the cyst.

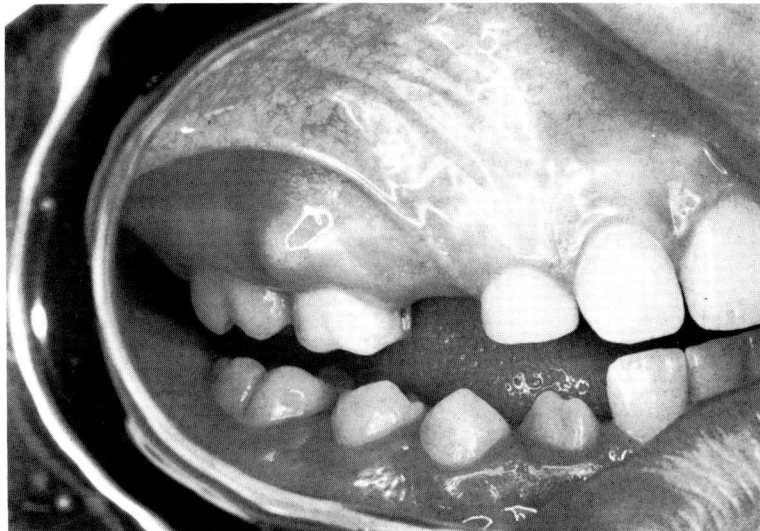

Figure 3–44. Parulis adjacent to upper molar.

zation of the underlying alveolar crestal bone, especially in the interdental region. In these cases, a subtle semilunar shadow or lucency, indicating erosion of the superior aspect of the alveolar crest, may be seen.

Histopathology. In the neonatal gingival cyst, subepithelial cystic structures demonstrate an epithelial lining that is often thin and attenuated. The basal layer is characteristically flattened, but the surface parakeratinized squames fill the lumen. Dystrophic mineralization is occasionally noted within the cyst cavity as well as within the cyst wall.

A thin layer of cuboidal or flattened epithelial cells lines the gingival cyst of the adult. Nuclei tend to be hyperchromatic but uniform from one cell to another. The epithelial–connective tissue junction is flattened, with some cysts demonstrating plaques or focal epithelial thickenings, often with clear cell changes. Infrequently, the cyst lining will keratinize. Small, solid clusters of epithelium may also be seen within the connective tissue wall of the cyst, apart and separate from the epithelial lining.

Treatment. No treatment is indicated for gingival or palatal cysts of the newborn, since they spontaneously rupture early in life or at the time of tooth eruption. Treatment of gingival cysts of the adult is surgical excision, with inclusion of the overlying epithelium recommended. Recurrence is unlikely.

Parulis

The parulis or "gum boil" represents a focus of pus in the gingival connective tissue. It is

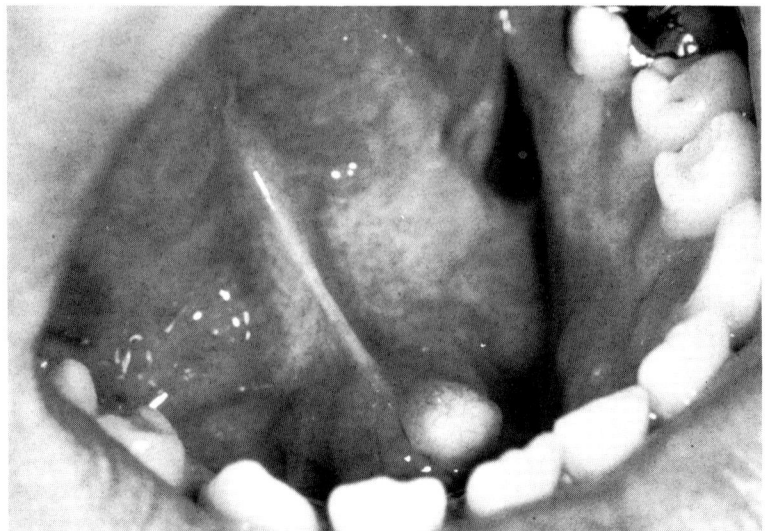

Figure 3–45. Lipoma on the floor of the mouth.

derived from an acute infection, either at the base of an occluded periodontal pocket or at the apex of a non-vital tooth. If the path of least resistance leads to gingival submucosa, a soft tissue abscess or parulis results. The lesion presents as a yellow-white gingival tumescence with variable amounts of erythema (Fig. 3–44). Pain is typical, and once the pus escapes to the surface, symptoms are temporarily relieved. Treatment of the underlying condition (periodontal pocket or non-vital tooth) is required to achieve resolution of the gingival abscess.

Lipoma

Lipoma presents as a yellow or yellow-white uninflamed submucosal mass (Fig. 3–45) and is included in this section for completeness. Detailed discussion of this lesion is found in Chapter 7.

Bibliography

Hereditary Conditions

Burge SM, Wilkinson JD, Miller AJ, et al. The efficacy of an aromatic retinoid, Tigason (etretinate), in the treatment of Darier's disease. Br J Dermatol 104:675–679, 1981.

Dicken CH, Bauer EA, Hazen PG, et al. Isotretinoin treatment of Darier's disease. J Am Acad Dermatol 118:278–279, 1982.

Jegasothy BV, Hameniuk JM. Darier's disease: a partially immunodeficient state. J Invest Dermatol 76:126–132, 1981.

Miller RL, Bernstein ML, Arm RN. Darier's disease of the oral mucosa: clinical case report with ultrastructural evaluation. J Oral Pathol 11:79–89, 1982.

Sadeghi EM, Witkop CJ; Ultrastructural study of hereditary benign intraepithelial dyskeratosis. Oral Surg Oral Med Oral Pathol 44:567–577, 1977.

Witkop CJ, Gorlin RJ. Four hereditary mucosal syndromes. Arch Dermatol 84:762–771, 1961.

Reactive Lesions

Centers for Disease Control. Smokeless tobacco use in the United States–behavioral risk factor surveillance system, 1986. MMWR 36:337–340, 1987.

Christen AG. The case against smokeless tobacco: five facts for the professional to consider. J Am Dent Assoc 101:464–469, 1980.

Connolly G, Winn D, Hecht S, et al. The recmergence of smokeless tobacco. N Engl J Med 314:1020–1027, 1986.

Greer RO, Poulsion TC. Oral tissue alterations associated with the use of smokeless tobacco by teenagers. Oral Surg Oral Med Oral Pathol 56:275–284, 1983.

Hirsch JM, Heyden G, Thilander H. A clinical, histomorphological and histochemical study of snuff-induced lesions of varying severity. J Oral Pathol 11:337–348, 1982.

Koop C. The campaign against smokeless tobacco. N Engl J Med 314:1042–1044, 1986.

Sundstrom B, Mornstad H, Axell T. Oral carcinoma associated with snuff dipping. J Oral Pathol 11:245–251, 1982.

Tipton J. The selection of sun blocking topical agents to protect the skin. Plast Reconstr Surg 62:223–228, 1978.

Other White Lesions

Axell T, Holmstrup P, Kramer IRH, et al. International seminar on oral leukoplakia and associated lesions related to tobacco habits. Community Dent Oral Epidemiol 12:145–158, 1982.

Basham T, Nickoloff B, Merigan T, et al. Recombinant gamma interferon induces HLA-DR expression on cultured human keratinocytes. J Invest Dermatol 83:88–90, 1984.

Belton CM, Eversole LR. Oral hairy leukoplakia: ultrastructural studies. J Oral Pathol 15:493–499, 1986.

Eversole LR, Jacobsen P, Stone CE, et al. Oral condyloma planus (hairy leukoplakia) among homosexual men: a clinicopathologic study of thirty-six cases. Oral Surg Oral Med Oral Pathol 61:249–255, 1986.

Falk DK, Latour DL, King LE. Dapsone in the treatment of erosive lichen planus. J Am Acad Dermatol 12:567–570, 1985.

Giustina TA, Stewart JCB, Ellis CN, et al. Topical application of isotretinoin gel improves oral lichen planus. Arch Dermatol 122:534–536, 1986.

Greenspan D, Greenspan J, Conant M, et al. Oral "hairy" leukoplakia in male homosexuals: evidence of association with both papillomavirus and a herpes-group virus. Lancet 2:831–834, 1984.

Greenspan D, Greenspan J, Hearst N, et al. Relation of oral hairy leukoplakia to infection with the human immunodeficiency virus and the risk of developing AIDS. J Infect Dis 155:475–481, 1987.

Greenspan D, Pindborg JJ, Greenspan JS, Schiodt M. Hairy Leukoplakia in AIDS and the Dental Team. Munksgaard, Copenhagen, 1986.

Greenspan J, Greenspan D, Lennette ET, et al. Replication of Epstein-Barr virus within the epithelial cells of oral "hairy" leukoplakia, an AIDS-associated lesion. N Engl J Med 313:1564–1571, 1986.

Hansen L, Olson J, Silverman S. Proliferative verrucous leukoplakia. Oral Surg Oral Med Oral Pathol 60:285–298, 1985.

Hong WK, Endicott J, Itri LM, et al. 13-cis-retinoic acid in the treatment of oral leukoplakia. N Engl J Med 315:1501–1505, 1986.

Hunter J. The Langerhans cell: from gold to glitter. Clin Exp Dermatol 8:569–592, 1983.

Krogh P, Homstrup P, Thorn J. Yeast species and biotypes associated with oral leukoplakia and lichen planus. Oral Surg Oral Med Oral Pathol 63:48–54, 1987.

Krutchkoff DJ, Cutler L, Laskowski S. Oral lichen planus: the evidence regarding potential malignant transformation. J Oral Pathol 7:1–7, 1978.

Krutchkoff DJ, Eisenberg E. Lichenoid dysplasia: a distinct histopathologic entity. Oral Surg Oral Med Oral Pathol 60:308–315, 1985.

Loning T, Schmitt D, Becker W, et al. Application of the biotin-avidin system for ultrastructural identification of suppressor/cytotoxic lymphocytes in oral lichen planus. Arch Dermatol Res 272:177–180, 1982.

Lundstrom LMC. Allergy and corrosion of dental materials in a patient with oral lichen planus. Int Oral Surg 13:16–24, 1984.

Mahrle G, Meyer-Hamme S, Ippen H. Oral treatment of keratinizing disorders of skin and mucous membranes with etretinate. Arch Dermatol 118:97–100, 1982.

Marx R. HLA antigen in geographic tongue. Tissue Antigens 15:60–62, 1980.

Milestone LM. Prescribing retinoids: the art and science. Arch Dermatol 122:761–763, 1986 (editorial).

Morhenn VB. The etiology of lichen planus: a hypothesis. Am J Dermatopathol 8:154–156, 1986.

Pindborg JJ, Barnes D, Roed-Peterson B. Epidemiology and histology of oral leukoplakia and leukoedema among Papuans and New Guineans. Cancer 22:379–384, 1968.

Ralls AS. Stomatitis areata migrans affecting the gingiva. Oral Surg Oral Med Oral Pathol 60:197–200, 1985.

Ruzicka T, Wasserman SI, Soter NA, et al. Inhibition of rat mast cell arachidonic acid cyclo-oxygenase by dapsone. J Allergy Clin Immunol 72:365–370, 1983.

Schubert MM, Sullivan KM, Morton TH, et al. Oral manifestations of chronic graft vs host disease. Arch Intern Med 144:1591–1595, 1984.

Shear M, Pindborg JJ. Verrucous hyperplasia of the oral mucosa. Cancer 46:1855–1862, 1980.

Silverman S Jr, Gorsky M, Lozada F. Oral leukoplakia and malignant transformation. Cancer 53:563–568, 1984.

Silverman S Jr, Gorsky M, Lozada-Nur F. A prospective follow-up study of 570 patients with oral lichen planus: persistence, remission, and malignant association. Oral Surg Oral Med Oral Pathol 60:30–34, 1985.

Silverman S, Migliorati C, Lozada-Nur F, et al. Oral findings in people with or at high risk for AIDS: a study of 375 homosexual males. J Am Dent Assoc 112:187–192, 1986.

Simon M, Hornstein OP. Prevalence rate of candida in the oral cavity of patients with oral lichen planus. Arch Dermatol Res 267:317–318, 1980.

Simon M, Reimer G, Schardt M, et al. Lymphocytotoxicity for oral mucosa in lichen planus. Dermatologica 167:11–15, 1983.

Slobert K, Jonsson R, Jontell M. Assessment of Langerhans' cells in oral lichen planus. J Oral Pathol 13:516–529, 1984.

Standish SM, Moorman WC. Treatment of hairy tongue with podophyllin resin. J Am Dent Assoc 68:535–540, 1964.

Waldron CA, Shafer WG. Leukoplakia revisited. Cancer 36:1386–1392, 1975.

Zegarelli DJ. Ulcerative and erosive lichen planus: treated by modified topical steroid and injection steroid therapy. NY State Dent J 53(3):23–25, 1987.

Non-epithelial White-Yellow Lesions

Buchner A, Hansen L. The histomorphologic spectrum of the gingival cyst in the adult. Oral Surg Oral Med Oral Pathol 48:531–539, 1979.

Canniff JP, Harvey W. The aetiology of oral submucous fibrosis: the stimulation of collagen synthesis by extracts of areca nut. Int J Oral Surg 10:163–167, 1981.

Dreizen S. Oral candidiasis. Am J Med 77:28–33, 1984.

Fromm A. Epstein's pearls, Bohn's nodules and inclusion-cysts of the oral cavity. J Dent Child 34:275–281, 1967.

Gottlieb MS, Schroff R, Schantez HM, et al. Pneumocystis carinii and mucosal candidiasis in previously healthy homosexual men: evidence of a new acquired cellular immunodeficiency. N Engl J Med 305:1425–1431, 1981.

Klein R, Harris C, Small C, et al. Oral candidiasis in high-risk patients as the initial manifestation of the acquired immunodeficiency syndrome. N Engl J Med 311:354–358, 1984.

Montes L, Ceballos R, Cooper MD, et al. Chronic mucocutaneous candidiasis, myositis, and thymoma: a new triad. JAMA 222:1619–1623, 1972.

Moreillon MC, Schroeder HE. Numerical frequency of epithelial abnormalities, particularly microcysts, in the developing human oral mucosa. Oral Surg Oral Med Oral Pathol 53:44–55, 1982.

Pindborg JJ. Lesions of the oral mucosa to be considered premalignant and their epidemiology. *In* Mackenzie IC, Dabelsteen E, Squier CA (eds). Oral Premalignancy. University of Iowa Press, Iowa City, 1980, pp 2–14.

Pindborg JJ, Bhonsle RB, Murti PR, et al. Incidence and early forms of submucous fibrosis. Oral Surg Oral Med Oral Pathol 50:40–44, 1980.

Small CB, Klein RS, Friedland GH, et al. Community-acquired opportunistic infections and defective cellular immunity in heterosexual drug abusers. Am J Med 74:433–441, 1983.

Smith CB. Candidiasis: pathogenesis, host resistance and predisposing factors. *In* Bodey G, Fainstein V (eds). Candidiasis. Raven Press, New York, 1985, pp 53–64.

Wysocki GP, Brannon RB, Gardner DG, et al. Histogenesis of the lateral periodontal cyst and the gingival cyst of the adult. Oral Surg Oral Med Oral Pathol 50:327–334, 1980.

Chapter 4

Red-Blue Lesions

INTRAVASCULAR, FOCAL
Developmental Lesions
   Hemangioma
Reactive Lesions
   Pyogenic Granuloma
   Peripheral Giant Cell Granuloma
   Median Rhomboid Glossitis
Neoplasms
   Erythroplakia
   Kaposi's Sarcoma
Unknown Etiology
   Geographic Tongue
   Psoriasis
INTRAVASCULAR, DIFFUSE
Metabolic-Endocrine Conditions
   Vitamin B Deficiencies
   Pernicious Anemia
   Iron Deficiency Anemia
   Burning Mouth Syndrome
Infectious Conditions
   Scarlet Fever
   Atrophic Candidiasis
Immunologic Abnormalities
   Plasma Cell Gingivitis
   Drug Reactions and Contact Allergies
EXTRAVASCULAR—PETECHIAE AND ECCHYMOSES

INTRAVASCULAR, FOCAL

Developmental Lesions

Hemangioma

Etiology. The term "hemangioma" is used here in the generic sense to encompass a variety of vascular neoplasms, hamartomas, and malformations that appear predominantly at or around birth. Because of the confusion surrounding the basic origin of many of these lesions, classification of clinical and microscopic varieties has been difficult. None of the numerous proposed classifications has had uniform acceptance, although there is merit in separating benign neoplasms from vascular malformations because of different clinical and behavioral characteristics. Using this approach, the term "congenital hemangioma" is used in a more restricted sense to identify benign congenital neoplasms of proliferating endothelial cells. Vascular malformations include lesions resulting from abnormal vessel morphogenesis (Table 4–1). Separation of vascular lesions into one of these two groups can be of considerable significance relative to the treatment of patients. Unfortunately, in actual practice, some difficulty may be encountered in classifying lesions in this way because of overlapping clinical and histologic features.

In any event, congenital hemangiomas have traditionally been subdivided into two microscopic types—capillary and cavernous—that essentially reflect differences in vessel diameter. Vascular malformations may exhibit similar features but may also show vascular channels that represent arteries and veins.

Clinical Features. The congenital hemangioma, also known as strawberry nevus, usually presents around the time of birth but may not be apparent until childhood (Fig. 4–1). This lesion may exhibit a rapid growth phase followed several years later by an involution phase. In contrast, vascular malformations are generally persistent lesions that grow with the individual and do not involute (Figs. 4–2 and 4–3). Both types of lesions may range in color from red to blue, depending upon the degree of congestion and their depth in tissue. When they are compressed, blanching occurs. This simple clinical test can be used to separate these lesions from hemorrhagic lesions in soft tissue (ecchymoses). Congenital hemangiomas and vascular malformations may be flat, nodular, or bosselated. Other clinical signs include

Table 4–1. FEATURES OF HEMANGIOMAS	
Congenital Hemangioma	**Vascular Malformation**
Abnormality of endothelial cell proliferation	Abnormality of vessel morphogenesis
Results from increased number of capillaries	Results from dilatation of arteries, veins, or capillaries
Appears weeks after birth	Usually present at birth
Rapid growth	Progressive enlargement—grows with the patient
Spontaneous involution	Persistent
Rarely affects bone	Frequently affects bone
Resectable	Difficult to resect
Surgical bleeding controllable	Surgical hemorrhage a potential problem
Often circumscribed	Poorly circumscribed
Recurrence uncommon	Recurrence common
No bruit or thrill	May produce bruit or thrill

the presence of a bruit or a thrill, features associated predominantly with vascular malformations. Lesions are most commonly found in lips, tongue, and buccal mucosa. Lesions that affect bone are probably vascular malformations rather than congenital hemangiomas.

Sturge-Weber syndrome, or *encephalotrigeminal angiomatosis,* is a condition that includes vascular malformations. In this syndrome, venous malformations involve the leptomeninges of the cerebral cortex, usually with similar vascular malformations of the face. The associated facial lesion, also known as *port-wine stain* or *nevus flammeus,* involves the skin innervated by one or more branches of the trigeminal nerve (Fig. 4–4). Port-wine stains may also occur as isolated lesions of the skin without the other stigmata of Sturge-Weber syndrome. The vascular defect of Sturge-Weber syndrome may extend intraorally to involve the buccal mucosa and the gingiva. Ocular lesions may also appear.

Neurologic defects of Sturge-Weber syndrome may include mental retardation, hemiparesis, and seizure disorders. The patient may be taking phenytoin (Dilantin) for control of the latter problem, with possible secondary development of drug-induced generalized gingival hyperplasia. Calcification of the intracranial vascular lesion may provide radiologic evidence of the process in the leptomeninges.

Differential diagnosis would include *angio-osteohypertrophy syndrome,* which is characterized by vascular malformations of the face

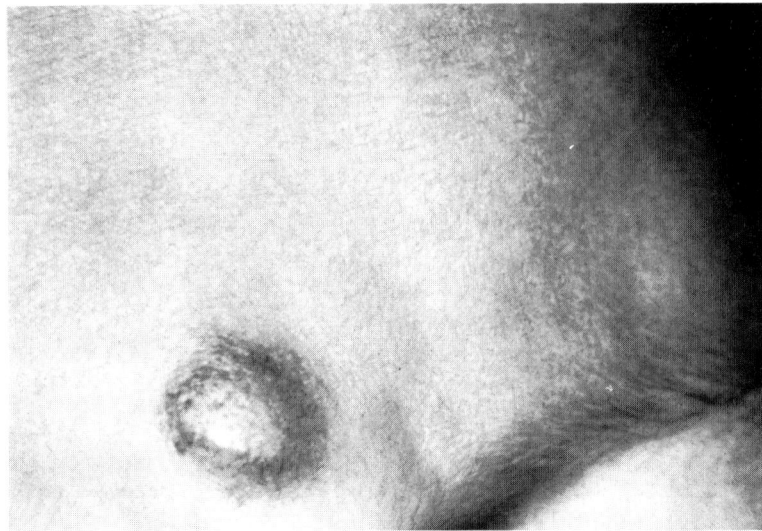

Figure 4–1. Congenital hemangioma on forehead of infant.

Figure 4–2. Vascular malformations (hemangiomas) of buccal mucosa *(A)* and maxillary gingiva *(B)* (arrows).

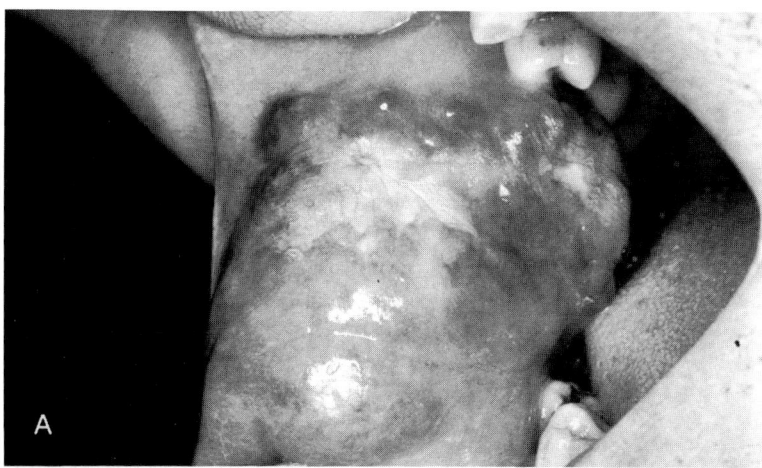
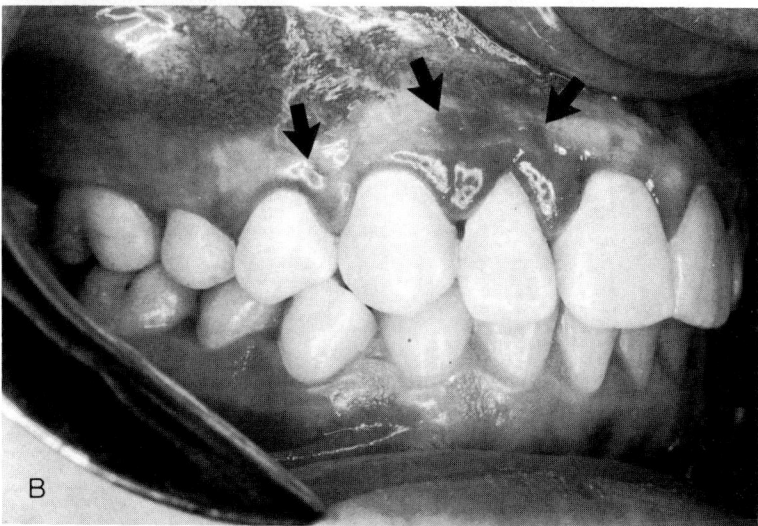

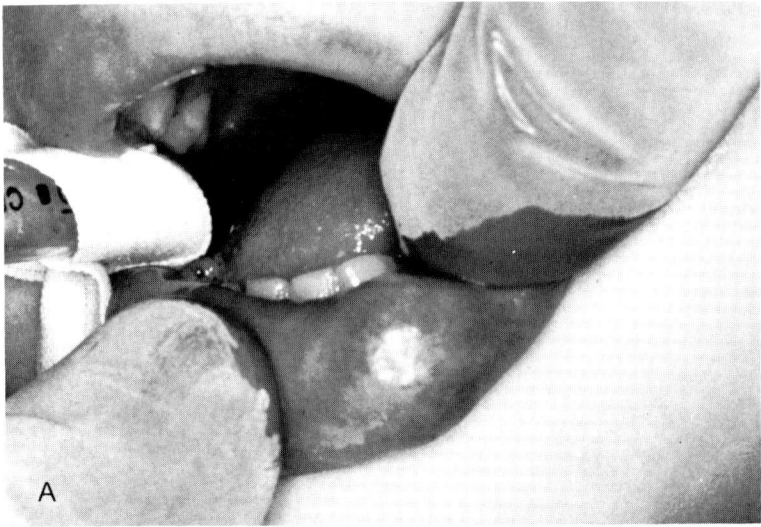
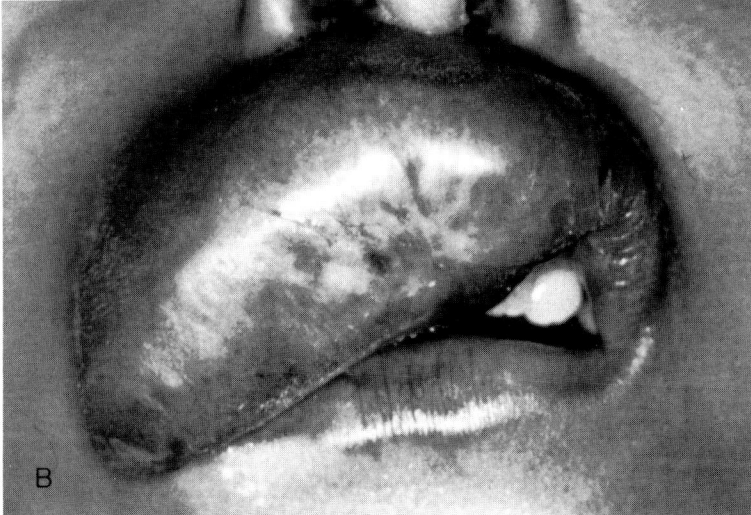

Figure 4–3. *A* and *B*, Vascular malformations (hemangiomas) of the lips. (Courtesy of Dr. W. Wade).

Figure 4–4. Vascular malformation (hemangioma) or port-wine stain of the type associated with Sturge-Weber syndrome.

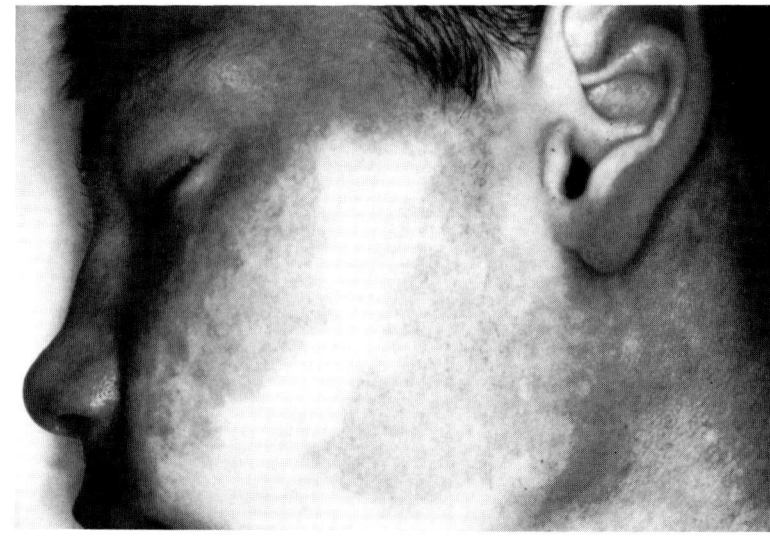

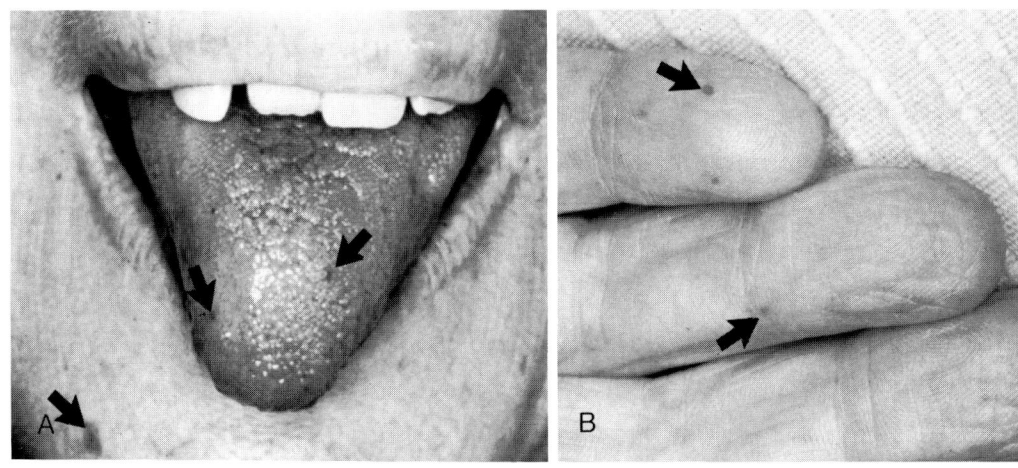

Figure 4–5. *A* and *B,* Hereditary hemorrhagic telangiectasias (Rendu-Osler-Weber syndrome) of tongue, face, and fingers (arrows).

(port-wine stains), varices, and hypertrophy of bone. The bony abnormality usually affects long bones but may also involve the mandible or maxilla, resulting in asymmetry, malocclusion, and altered eruption pattern.

Rendu-Osler-Weber syndrome, or *hereditary hemorrhagic telangiectasia,* is a rare condition featuring abnormal vascular dilatations of terminal vessels in skin, mucous membranes, and occasionally viscera (Fig. 4–5). The telangiectatic vessels in this autosomal dominant condition appear clinically as red macules or papules, typically on the face, chest, and oral mucosa. Lesions appear early in life and persist throughout adulthood.

Intranasal lesions are responsible for epistaxis, the most common presenting sign of Rendu-Osler-Weber syndrome. Bleeding from oral lesions is also a frequent occurrence in affected patients. Control of bleeding may on occasion be a difficult problem. Chronic bleeding may also result in anemia.

Diagnosis of Rendu-Osler-Weber syndrome is based on clinical findings, hemorrhagic history, and family history. Another condition that might be considered in a differential diagnosis is the *CREST syndrome.* This includes calcinosis cutis, Raynaud's disease, esophageal dysfunction, sclerodactyly, and telangiectasia.

The *venous varix* or varicosity is an abnormal vascular dilatation. It is a relatively trivial vascular malformation when it appears in the oral mucosa (Fig. 4–6). Varices in the ventral aspect of the tongue are common developmental abnormalities. Varices are also common on the lower lip in older adults, especially those with chronic sun exposure. Varices are typically blue and blanch with compression. Oc-

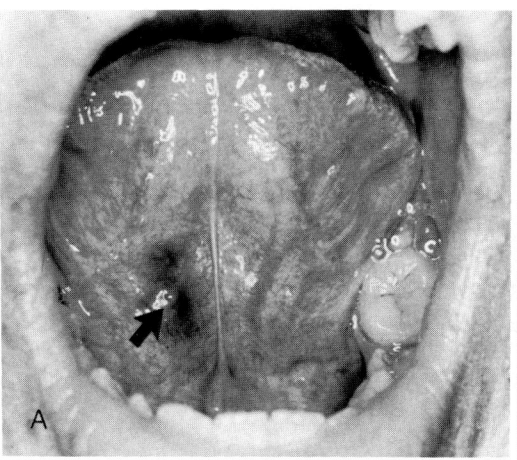
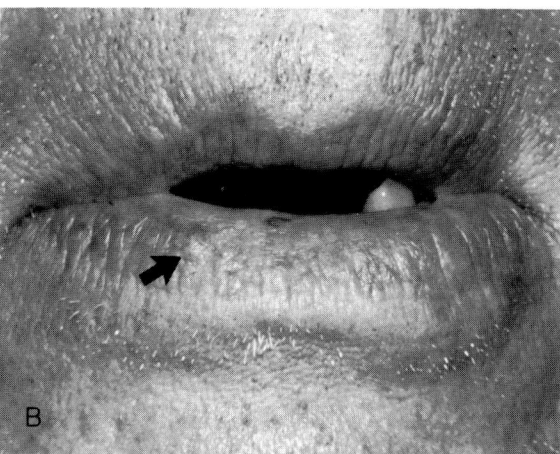

Figure 4–6. Venous varix of ventral tongue *(A)* and lip *(B)* (arrows).

casionally thrombosis, insignificant in these lesions, occurs, giving them a firm texture. No treatment is required for venous varix.

Histopathology. Congenital hemangiomas have been classified microscopically as capillary or cavernous, depending upon the size of the vascular spaces (Fig. 4–7). Spaces are lined by endothelium without muscular support. Clinically, there appears to be no significant difference between capillary and cavernous hemangiomas.

Vascular malformations may consist not only of capillaries but also of venous, arteriolar, and lymphatic channels. Lesions may be of purely one type of vessel, or they may be combinations of two or more.

Diagnosis. As a generic group, hemangiomas are usually self-evident on clinical examination. When they affect the mandible or the maxilla, a radiolucent lesion with a "honeycombed" pattern is expected. Differentiation between congenital hemangiomas and vascular malformations can be difficult and occasionally impossible. A complete history, a clinical examination, and angiography should be definitive.

Treatment. Spontaneous involution during early childhood is likely for congenital hemangiomas. If these lesions persist into the later years of childhood, involution is improbable and definitive treatment may be required. Vascular malformations generally do not involute and require intervention if eradication is the goal. Because the margins of these lesions are frequently ill defined, total elimination may not be practical or possible.

Treatment of vascular lesions continues to center around a careful surgical approach. Adjuncts include selective arteriole embolization and sclerosant therapy.

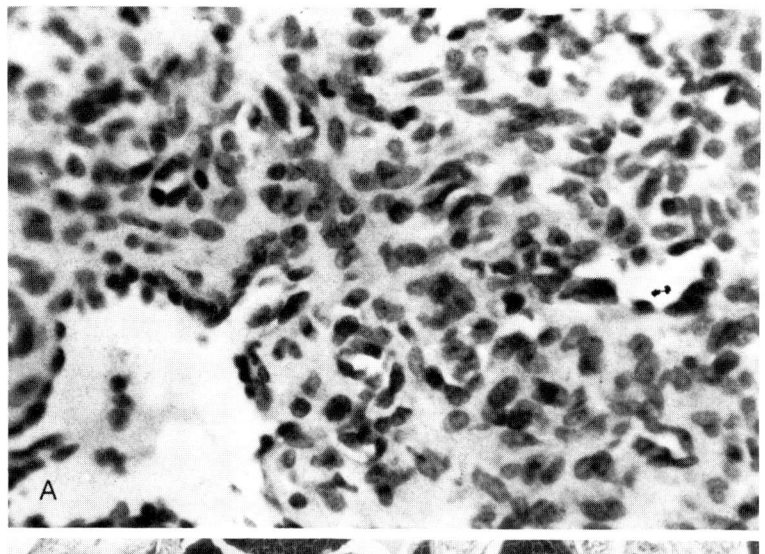
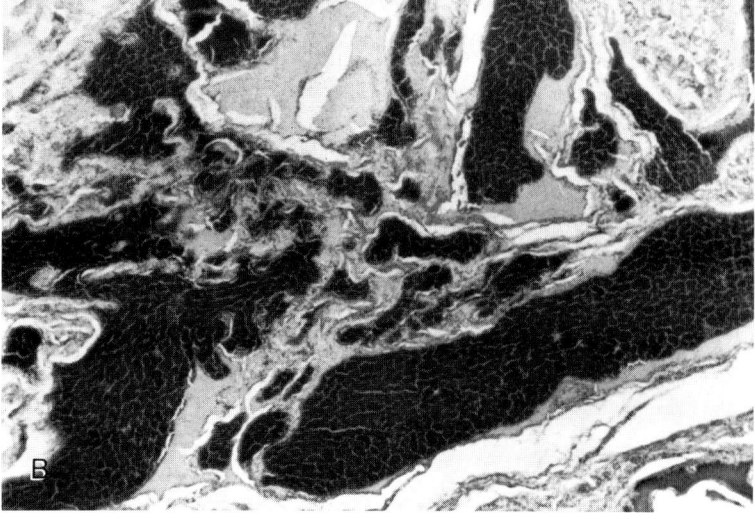

Figure 4–7. Microscopy of capillary *(A)* and cavernous *(B)* hemangiomas.

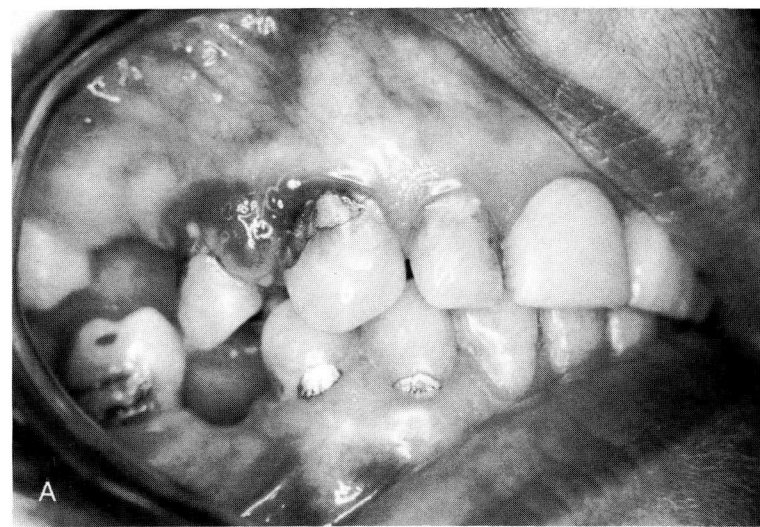
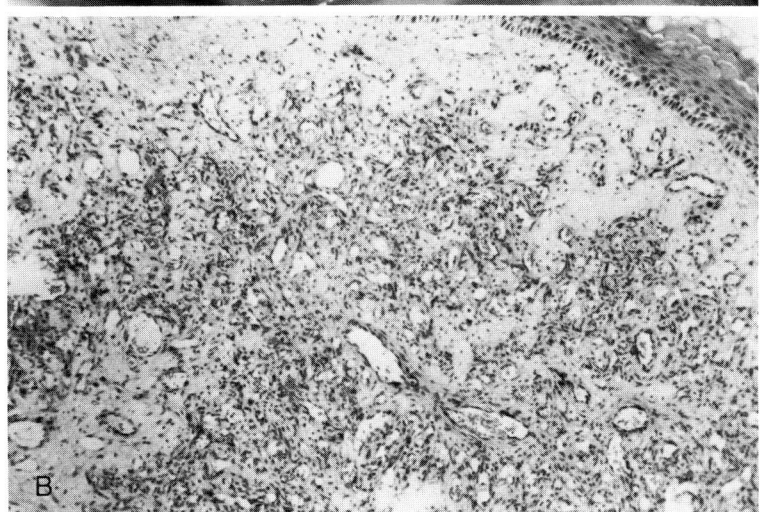

Figure 4–8. *A*, Pyogenic granuloma of gingiva. *B*, Microscopy showing numerous capillaries responsible clinically for the dark color.

Reactive Lesions

Pyogenic Granuloma

Etiology. This lesion represents an overexuberant connective tissue reaction to a known stimulus or injury. It appears as a red mass, because it is composed predominantly of hyperplastic granulation tissue in which capillaries are very prominent. The term "pyogenic granuloma" is somewhat of a misnomer in that it is not pus producing, as "pyogenic" implies. It is, however, a "tumor" of granulation tissue, as "granuloma" implies.

Clinical Features. The pyogenic granuloma is commonly seen on the gingiva, where it is presumably caused by calculus or foreign material within the gingival crevice (Figs. 4–8 and 4–9). Hormonal changes of puberty and pregnancy may modify the gingival reparative response to injury. Under these circumstances, multiple gingival lesions or generalized gingival hyperplasia may be seen. Pyogenic granulomas are uncommonly seen elsewhere in the mouth but may appear in areas of frequent trauma, such as the lower lip, the buccal mucosa, and the tongue.

Pyogenic granulomas are typically red. Occasionally, they may become ulcerated because of secondary trauma. The ulcerated lesion may then become covered by a yellow, fibrinous membrane. They may be pedunculated or broad based and may range in size from a few millimeters to several centimeters. These lesions may be seen at any age and tend to occur in females more frequently than in males.

Histopathology. Microscopically, these lesions are composed of lobular masses of hyperplastic granulation tissue. Some scarring may be noted in some of these lesions, suggesting that there occasionally may be maturation of the connective tissue repair process.

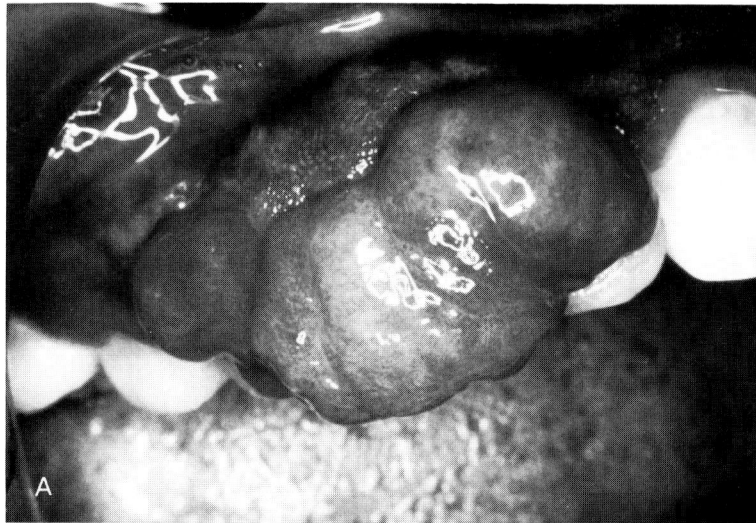
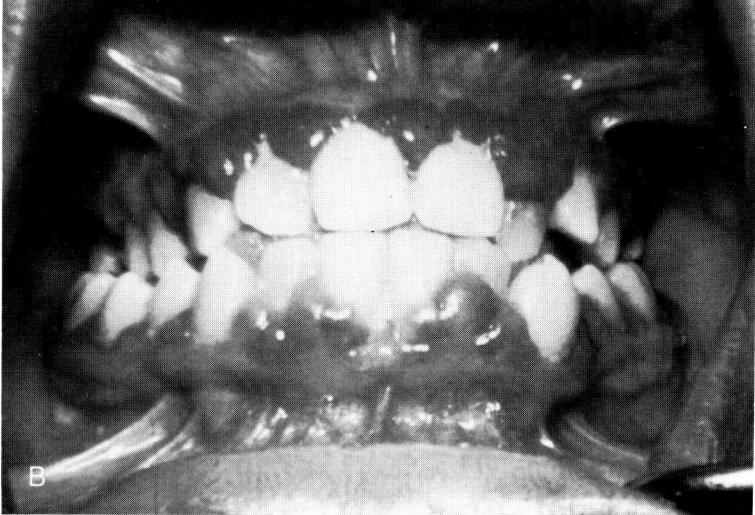

Figure 4–9. *A*, Large pyogenic granuloma of gingiva. *B*, Generalized gingival hyperplasia (multiple pyogenic granulomas) associated with pregnancy.

Variable numbers of chronic inflammatory cells may be seen. Neutrophils will be present in the superficial zone of ulcerated pyogenic granulomas.

Differential Diagnosis. Clinically, this lesion must be differentiated from the peripheral giant cell granuloma, which also occurs as a red gingival mass. A peripheral fibroma may be another consideration, although these tend to be much lighter in color. Biopsy is definitive.

Treatment. Pyogenic granulomas should be surgically excised. When gingival lesions are being removed, the excisional process should include removal of the connective tissue from which the lesion arises as well as removal of any local etiologic factors, such as calculus.

Recurrence is occasionally seen and is believed to be due to incomplete excision, failure to remove etiologic factors, or reinjury to the area.

Peripheral Giant Cell Granuloma

Etiology. The peripheral giant cell granuloma represents a relatively uncommon and unusual hyperplastic connective tissue response to injury of gingival tissues. It is one of the "reactive hyperplasias" commonly seen in oral mucous membranes, representing an exuberant reparative response. The feature that sets this lesion apart from the others is the appearance of multinucleated giant cells. The reason for their presence remains a mystery.

Clinical Features. Peripheral giant cell granulomas are seen exclusively in gingiva, usually in the area between the first permanent molars and the incisors (Fig. 4–10). They presumably arise from periodontal ligament or periosteum and cause, on occasion, resorption of alveolar bone. When this process occurs on the edentulous ridge, a superficial, cup-shaped radiolucency may be seen (Fig. 4–11). Peripheral giant cell granulomas typically present as red to blue broad-based masses. Secondary ulceration due to trauma may give the lesions a focal yellow zone caused by the formation of a fibrin clot over the ulcer. These lesions, most of which are about 1 cm in diameter, may occur at any age and tend to be seen more frequently in females than in males.

Histopathology. Hyperplastic granulation tissue is a basic element of the peripheral giant cell granuloma. Scattered throughout the lobulated granulation tissue mass are abundant multinucleated giant cells. Ultrastructural and immunologic studies have shown that the giant cells are derived from macrophages. Ultrastructurally, fusion of plasma membranes of adjacent macrophages has been demonstrated. Immunohistochemically, macrophages and giant cells share similar antigenic markers, such as muramidase and alpha-1-antichymotrypsin. Nonetheless, the giant cells appear to be nonfunctional in the usual sense of phagocytosis and bone resorption.

Islands of metaplastic bone occasionally may be seen in these lesions. This finding has no clinical significance. Variable numbers of chronic inflammatory cells will be present, and neutrophils will be found in ulcer bases.

Differential Diagnosis. Generally, this lesion is clinically indistinguishable from a pyogenic granuloma. Although the peripheral giant cell granuloma is more likely to cause bone resorption than is the pyogenic granuloma, the differences are otherwise slight. Biopsy will provide definitive results. Microscopically, the peripheral giant cell granuloma is identical to its central or intraosseous counterpart the central giant cell granuloma, which is derived from

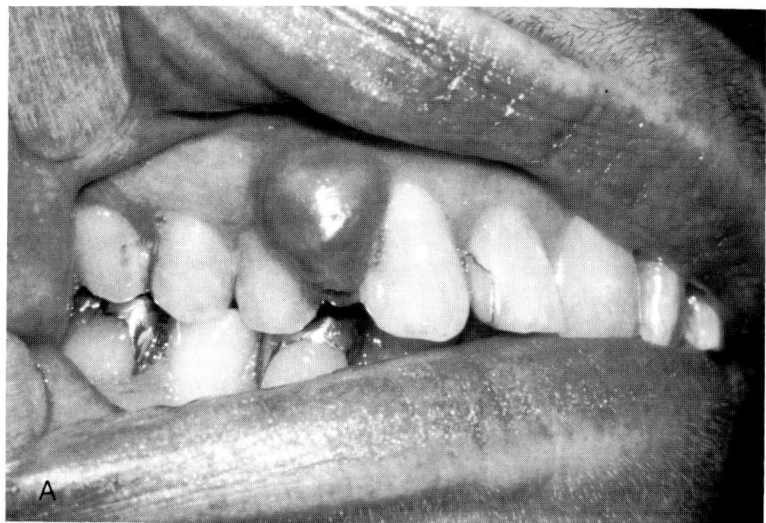
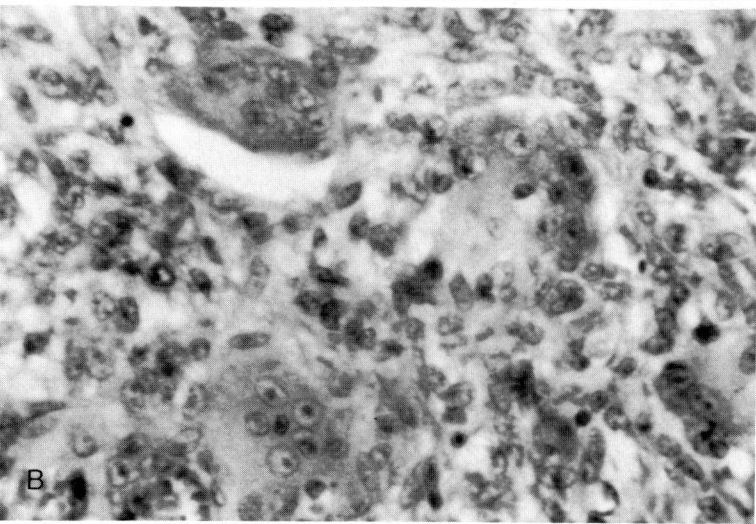

Figure 4–10. *A,* Peripheral giant cell granuloma. *B,* Microscopy showing young fibroblasts, capillaries, and giant cells.

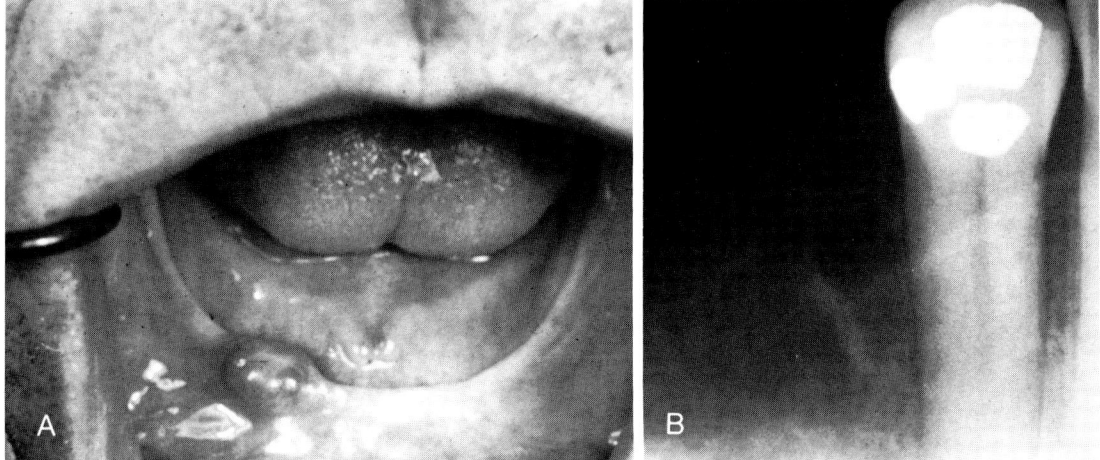

Figure 4–11. *A*, Peripheral giant cell granuloma of an edentulous ridge. *B*, Superficial erosion of mandibular cortex caused by peripheral giant cell granuloma.

the medullary tissue of the mandible and the maxilla. Clinical features adequately separate these two microscopically identical lesions.

Treatment. Surgical excision is the preferred treatment for peripheral giant cell granulomas. Removal of local factors or irritants is also required. Recurrence is uncommon.

Median Rhomboid Glossitis

Etiology. This entity was once thought to be a congenital abnormality related to the persistence of an embryonic midline tongue structure known as the tuberculum impar. This lesion is now believed to be related to a chronic infection by *Candida albicans*. The exact role of this fungus in the pathogenesis of the lesion is yet to be established.

Clinical Features. This lesion usually presents as a red elevated rhomboid or oval lesion in the dorsal midline of the tongue, just anterior to the circumvallate papillae (Fig. 4–12). The lesion may occasionally be mildly painful, although most are asymptomatic.

Histopathology. Microscopically, epithelial hyperplasia is evident in the form of bulbous rete ridges (Fig. 4–13). *C. albicans* hyphae can usually be found in the upper levels of the epithelium. A thick band of hyalinized connective tissue separates the epithelium from deeper structures.

Diagnosis. The diagnosis of median rhomboid glossitis is generally evident from clinical appearance. Since oral cancer rarely occurs at this location, squamous cell carcinoma is usually not a serious clinical consideration.

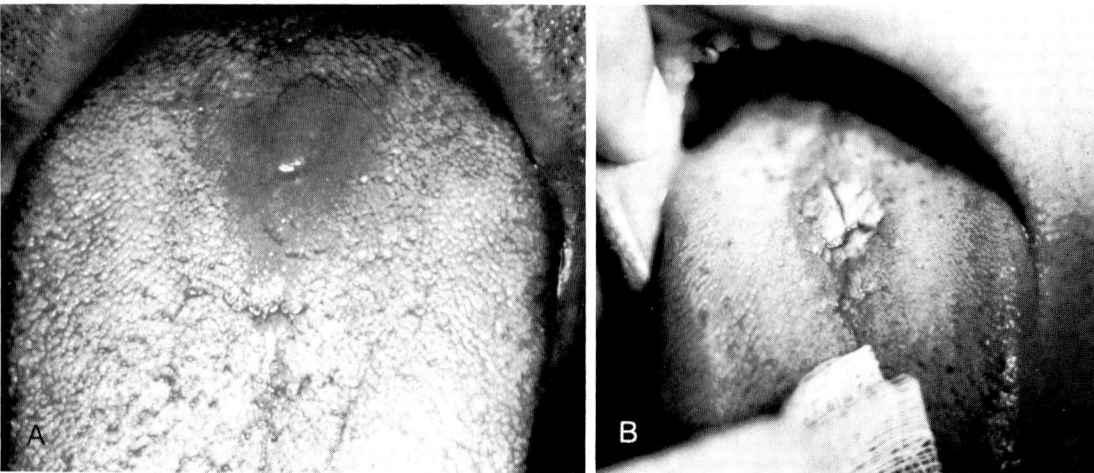

Figure 4–12. *A* and *B*, Median rhomboid glossitis. The central area of *B* is white because of secondary candidiasis.

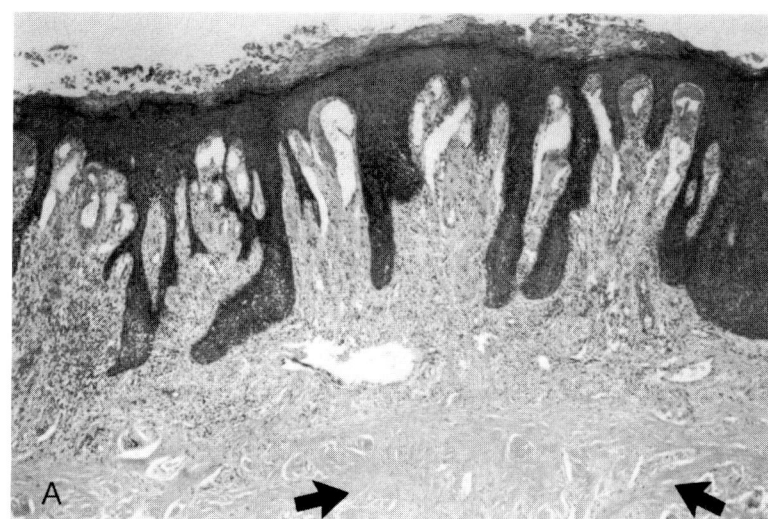
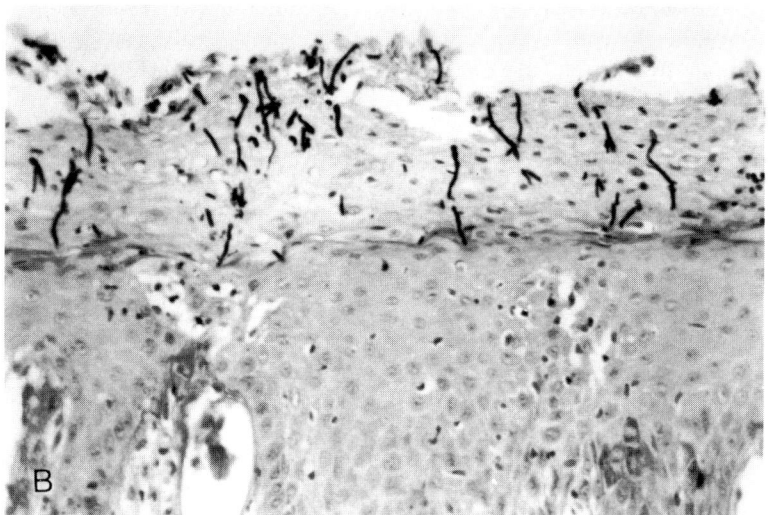

Figure 4–13. *A,* Microscopy of median rhomboid glossitis showing epithelial hyperplasia, prominent capillaries, and a band of hyalinized connective tissue at the base (arrows). *B,* PAS stain showing hyphae of *C. albicans* in the parakeratotic layer.

Treatment. Generally no treatment is necessary for median rhomboid glossitis. If the lesion is painful, symptomatic treatment may be necessary. If malignancy is part of a clinical differential diagnosis, biopsy should be done. Median rhomboid glossitis itself is generally regarded as having no malignant potential.

Neoplasms

Erythroplakia

Etiology. "Erythroplakia" is a clinical term that refers to a red patch on oral mucous membranes. It does not indicate a particular microscopic diagnosis, although after biopsy most will be found to be severe dysplasia or carcinoma. The cause of this lesion is unknown. It is generally assumed, however, that the etiologic factors for erythroplakia are similar to those responsible for oral cancer. Therefore, tobacco probably plays a significant role in the induction of many of these lesions. Alcohol, nutritional defects, chronic irritation, and other factors may also play contributing or modifying roles.

Clinical Features. Erythroplakia is seen much less frequently than its leukoplakia counterpart. It should, however, be viewed as a more serious lesion, because of the significantly higher percentage of malignancies associated with it. The lesion appears as a red patch with fairly well defined margins (Fig. 4–14). It may be seen in any oral region, although it is most commonly found in the floor of the mouth; the next most frequent site is the retromolar area. Individuals between 50 and 70 years of age are usually affected, and there appears to be no gender predilection. Focal white areas representing keratosis may also be seen in some lesions. Erythroplakia is usually

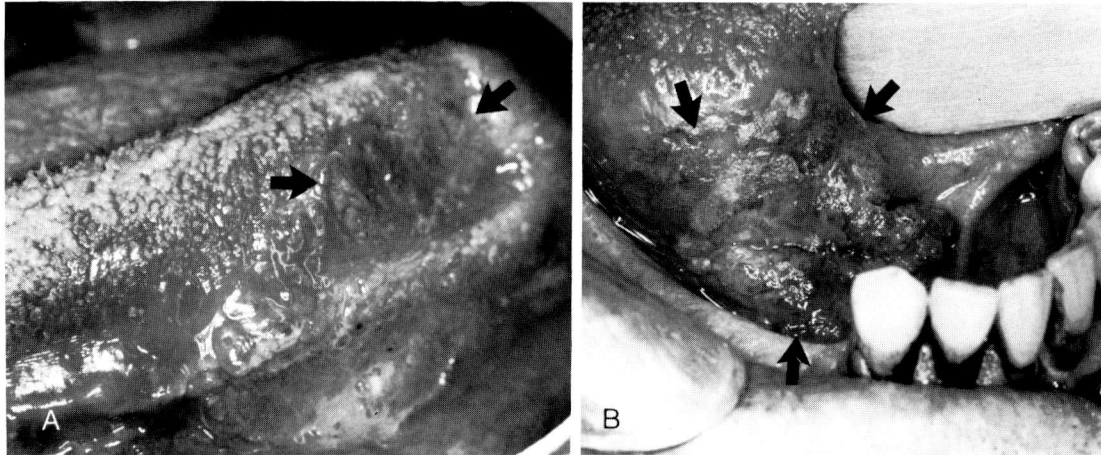

Figure 4–14. Erythroplakia of the posterolateral tongue *(A)* (arrows) and the floor of the mouth *(B)* (arrows).

supple to the touch, although some induration may be noted in invasive lesions.

Histopathology. On biopsy, approximately 90% of erythroplakias show at least severe dysplastic change—about half are invasive squamous cell carcinomas, and 40% are severe dysplasias or *in situ* carcinomas (Fig. 4–15). The remainder are mild to moderate dysplasias. A relative reduction in keratin production and a relative increase in vascularity accounts for the clinical color of these lesions. Products of keratinocyte terminal differentiation, such as keratin, involucrin, and filaggrin, are found in reduced or negligible amounts in these lesions when stained immunohistochemically.

A rare histologic subtype of carcinoma *in situ*, known as *Bowen's disease*, may be seen as a red (or white) patch in the oral mucosa. When this process occurs on the glans penis, it is known as *erythroplasia of Queyrat*. Microscopic features that separate this lesion from the usual carcinoma *in situ* include marked disordered growth, multinucleated keratinocytes, large hyperchromatic keratinocyte nuclei, and atypical individual cell keratinization.

Differential Diagnosis. The clinical features of erythroplakia may occasionally be shared by several other red lesions. Atrophic candidiasis results in a red mucosal lesion, but symptoms are usually present. A macular form of Kaposi's sarcoma, an ecchymotic patch, a contact allergic reaction, a vascular malformation, and psoriasis might also be considered in an expanded differential diagnosis. A careful clinical history and examination should separate most of these lesions. Biopsy provides a definitive answer.

Treatment. The treatment of choice for erythroplakia is surgical excision. It is generally more important to excise widely than deeply in dysplastic and *in situ* lesions, because of their superficial nature. However, because the epithelial changes may extend down the salivary gland excretory ducts in the area, the

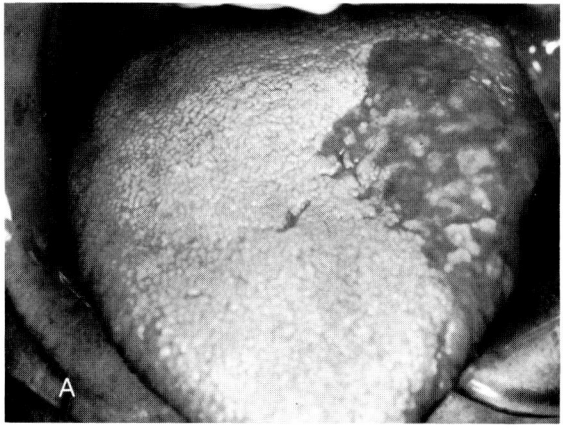
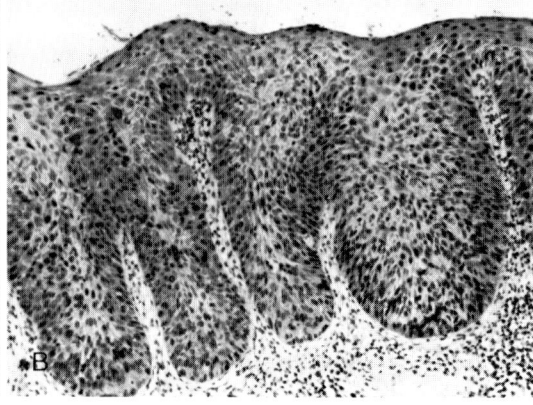

Figure 4–15. *A* and *B*, Erythroplakia of the tongue. Biopsy *(B)* was diagnosed as carcinoma *in situ*.

Table 4-2. FEATURES OF KAPOSI'S SARCOMA

Parameter	Classic Type	African Type	Immunodeficiency Type
Geography	Mediterranean basin	Africa	Metropolitan areas
Prevalence	Rare	Endemic	Relatively common
Age	Older men	Children and adults	Adults
Skin lesions	Lower extremities	Extremities	Any site
Oral lesions	Rare	Rare	Common
Other organs	Occasionally	Occasionally	Frequently
Course	Indolent	Prolonged	Aggressive
Prognosis	Fair	Fair	Poor

deep surgical margin should not be too shallow. Multiple histologic sections may be necessary to adequately assess the involvement of ducts.

It is generally accepted that severely dysplastic and *in situ* lesions eventually become invasive. The time required for this event can range from months to years. Follow-up examinations are critical for patients with these lesions, because of the potential field effect caused by etiologic agents.

Kaposi's Sarcoma

Etiology. Kaposi's sarcoma is a malignant neoplasm of endothelial cell origin. The various etiologic factors cited as possibly having significance include genetic predisposition, infection (especially viral), environmental influences of various geographic regions, and immune disregulation, such as reduced immunosurveillance.

Clinical Features. Three different clinical patterns of Kaposi's sarcoma have emerged since it was first described by Kaposi in 1872 (Table 4–2). It was initially seen as a rare skin lesion, predominantly in older men living in the Mediterranean basin. In this classic form, it appears as multifocal reddish-brown nodules primarily in the skin of the lower extremities, although any organ may be affected. Oral lesions are rare in this type. This classic form has a rather long indolent course and a fair to good prognosis.

The second pattern of Kaposi's sarcoma was identified in Africa, where it is now considered to be endemic. It is seen typically in the extremities of blacks. The most commonly affected organ is skin. Oral lesions are rarely seen. The clinical course is prolonged, and the overall prognosis is fair.

The third pattern of Kaposi's sarcoma has been seen in patients with AIDS and other conditions associated with immunodeficiency. This type differs from the other two forms in several ways. Skin lesions are not limited to the extremities but may be seen anywhere. A younger age group is affected. Oral and lymph node lesions are relatively common (Fig. 4–16). The clinical course is relatively rapid and aggressive, and the prognosis is correspondingly poor.

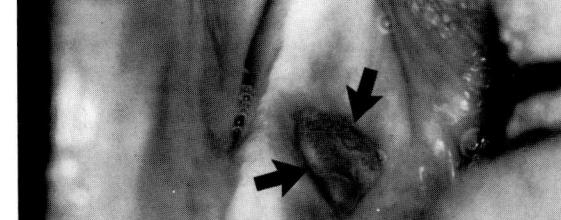

Figure 4–16. Kaposi's sarcoma of the lingual side of the mandible (arrows).

Kaposi's sarcoma occurs in about one third of AIDS patients, with about half of these developing oral lesions. It has been described in most oral regions, although the palate is by far the most common location. Oral Kaposi's sarcoma ranges from a rather trivial-appearing, flat lesion to a rather ominous, nodular exophytic lesion. It may be single or multifocal. The color is usually red to blue.

Histopathology. Early lesions of Kaposi's sarcoma may be of considerable diagnostic challenge, because of their similarity to capillary hemangiomas and pyogenic granulomas (Fig. 4–17). Atypical vascular channels, extravasated red blood cells (RBCs), hemosiderin, and inflammatory cells are characteristic of Kaposi's sarcoma. However, with the exception of atypical vascular channels, these histologic features may also be seen with other vascular lesions. In late stages of Kaposi's sarcoma, the appearance of a prominent spindle cell component and mitotic figures aids in the microscopic interpretation of this condition.

Differential Diagnosis. Other clinical considerations would include hemangioma, erythroplakia, melanoma, and pyogenic granuloma. Microscopically, reactive (pyogenic granuloma), congenital (hemangioma), and neoplastic (pericytoma, angiosarcoma) lesions might deserve consideration.

Treatment. Various forms of treatment have been used for Kaposi's sarcoma, but none has been uniformly successful. Surgery has been useful on localized lesions, and low-dose radiation and chemotherapy have been used for larger and multifocal lesions. Chemotherapeutic regimens that include several anticancer

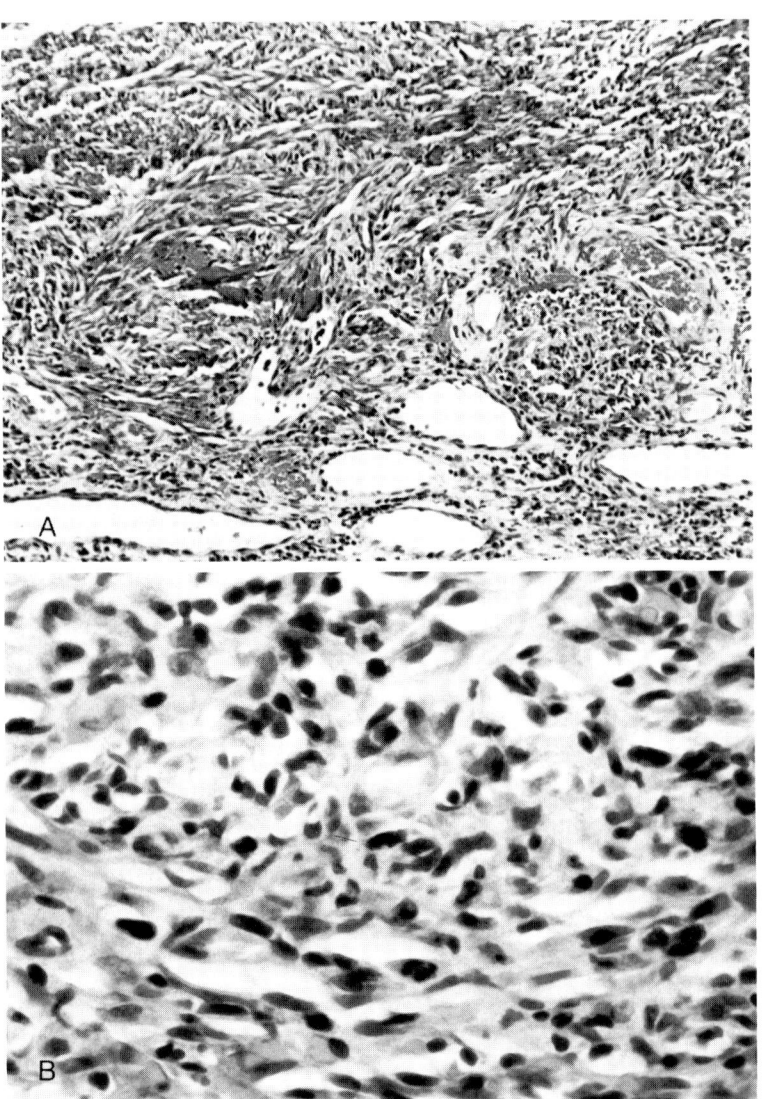

Figure 4–17. Kaposi's sarcoma. *A*, Low magnification showing atypical vascular channels and spindle cells. *B*, High magnification showing numerous slit-like vascular channels and atypical spindle cells.

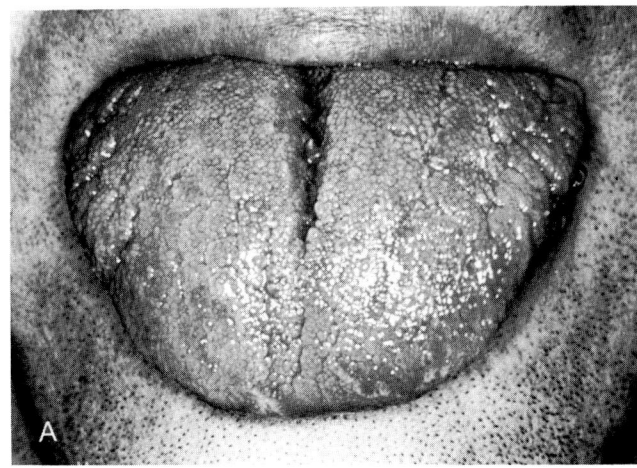
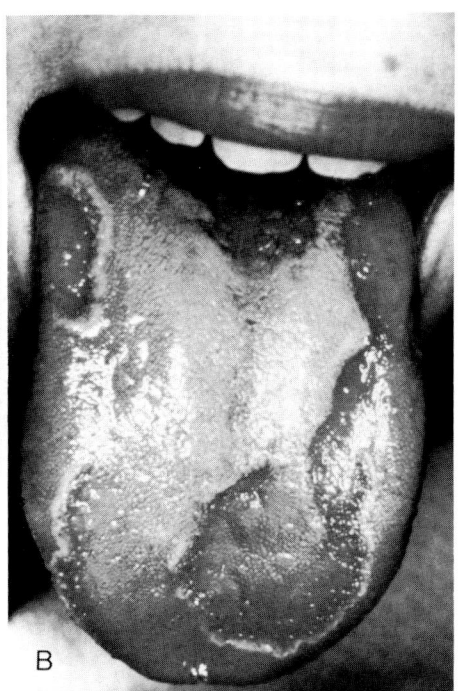

Figure 4–18. *A* and *B*, Geographic tongue. Note dark patches surrounded partially by subtle white keratotic rings *(A)*.

drugs seem to be gaining favor in treating more aggressive tumors.

Unknown Etiology

Geographic Tongue

Geographic tongue, or benign migratory glossitis, is described in Chapter 3, but it is mentioned here because it can on occasion appear as a predominantly red tongue lesion (Fig. 4–18). When the zones of papillary atrophy are relatively prominent and the keratotic margins are relatively subdued, geographic tongue presents as a red lesion. Careful clinical examination should reveal the nature of the lesion. Although this entity should be included in a differential diagnosis of red tongue lesions, it has the same significance as its more typical form.

Psoriasis

Etiology. Psoriasis is a common (1% of the United States population) skin disease that rarely affects the oral mucous membranes. It is of unknown etiology but has a strong hereditary influence. The epidermal changes appear to be related to a defect in the control of keratinocyte proliferation. The hyperproliferative state of the affected epidermis produces a turnover rate that is up to eight times greater than normal.

Clinical Features. Psoriasis occurs at any age but most commonly appears during young adult life. It is a chronic disease that may persist throughout life, with periods of exacerbation and remission. Various triggers, such as trauma, infection, and stress, may precipitate new episodes. The development of psoriatic lesions following trauma of normal-appearing skin is known as Koebner's reaction or phenomenon.

Several clinical patterns of psoriasis may be seen. The basic skin lesion of psoriasis is well defined and covered by silvery scales (Fig. 4–19). When the scales are removed, small pinpoint bleeding is seen, because of increased vascularity under focal areas of epidermal thinning. This feature of psoriasis is known as the Auspitz sign.

Oral lesions of psoriasis are apparently rare clinical observations. No consistent pattern has been described, with lesions ranging in type from red plaques to white plaques to ulcers. Geographic tongue has also been listed as an oral manifestation of psoriasis, but this is most likely a coincidental finding.

In a small percentage of psoriatics, a seronegative polyarthritis may be seen. The temporomandibular joint may occasionally be one of the joints involved in this process. Pain and

140 RED-BLUE LESIONS

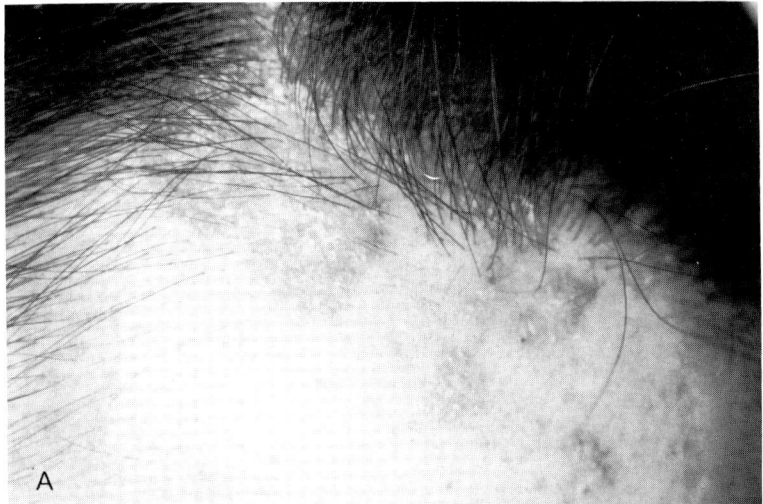
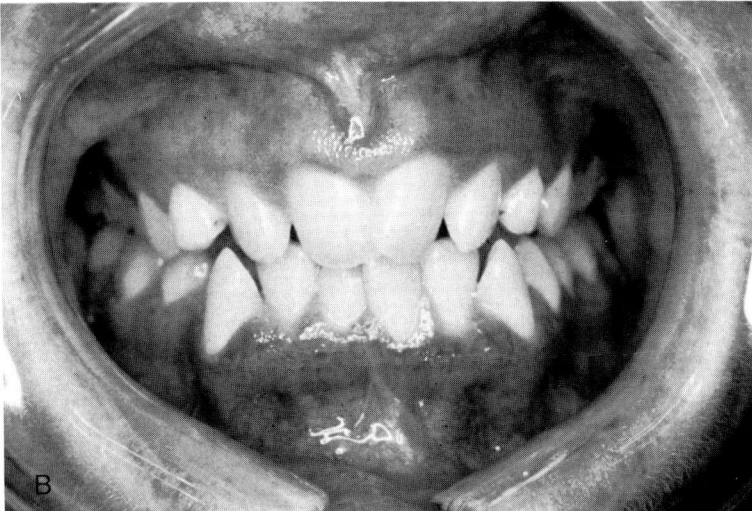

Figure 4–19. *A*, Dark, scaly psoriatic lesions of forehead. *B*, Lesions of attached gingiva that were diagnosed microscopically as being consistent with psoriasis (dark areas).

restricted motion are seen with erosion of the condyle.

Histopathology. Because of the hyperproliferative nature of psoriasis, epithelial hyperplasia due to acanthosis and parakeratosis is seen (Fig. 4–20). Connective tissue papillae contain lymphocytes and prominent capillaries that are covered by thinned epithelium. Bleeding from these foci provides the clinical Auspitz sign. Neutrophils are usually found in the epithelium, often in aggregates between epithelial cells producing Munro microabscesses.

Diagnosis. The diagnosis of cutaneous psoriasis is based on clinical history, clinical examination, and biopsy. Diagnosis of oral lesions is dependent upon confirmation of concurrent cutaneous disease. It is highly doubtful that oral lesions exist without skin lesions. Because psoriasiform microscopic changes are occasionally seen in many oral inflammatory conditions, biopsy of a solitary oral lesion should not be relied upon to provide conclusive evidence of oral psoriasis. The presence of cutaneous disease and the waxing and waning of oral lesions with skin lesions would also be necessary.

Treatment. A wide variety of drugs are available for the treatment of cutaneous psoriasis. The drug or combination of drugs used is dependent upon the clinician's training and experience and the patient's response. Topical preparations (tars, anthralin, and corticosteroids), systemic agents (methotrexate and retinoids), and photochemotherapy (psoralens plus UVA light) all have their advantages and proponents. Patients are best managed by the dermatologic expert.

INTRAVASCULAR, DIFFUSE

Metabolic-Endocrine Conditions

Vitamin B Deficiencies

Etiology. In various areas of the world, especially those with poor socioeconomic conditions, vitamin B deficiencies may be relatively common because of inadequate dietary intake. In the United States, deficiencies of the B vitamins are relatively uncommon.

Vitamin B deficiencies may involve one or several of the water-soluble B complex vitamins. Decreased intake through malnutrition associated with alcoholism, starvation, or fad diets may lead to clinically apparent disease. Decreased absorption because of gastrointestinal disease (e.g., malabsorption syndromes) or increased utilization because of increased demand (e.g., hyperparathyroidism) may also account for deficiencies.

Most of the vitamins classified under the B complex (biotin, nicotinamide, pantothenic acid, and thiamine) are involved in intracellular metabolism of carbohydrates, fats, and proteins. Others (vitamin B_{12} and folic acid) are involved in RBC development. Deficiencies of individual vitamins may produce dis-

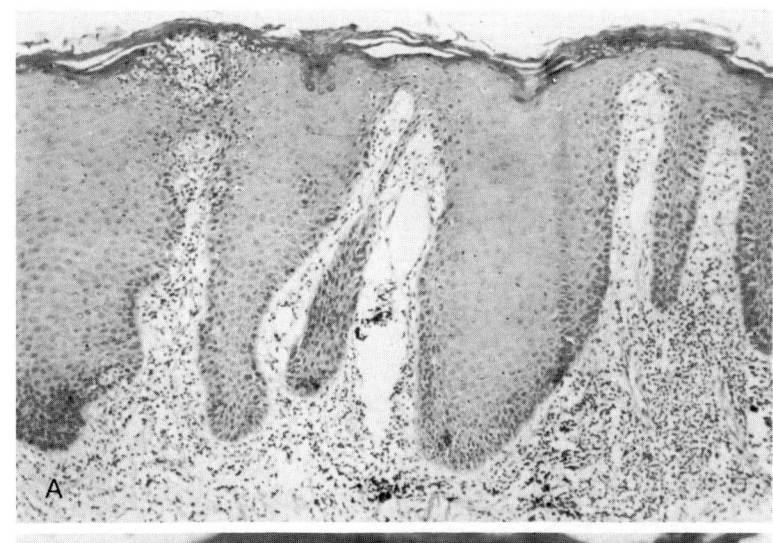
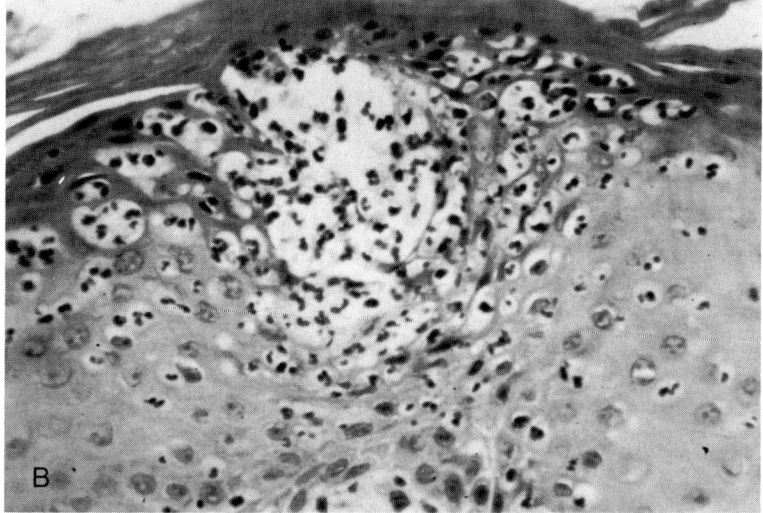

Figure 4–20. *A* and *B,* Psoriasis of the skin featuring epithelial hyperplasia, intermittent epithelial thinning, prominent capillaries, and microabscesses of Munro *(B)*.

tinctive clinical pictures. Significant oral changes have been well documented in deficiencies of riboflavin (ariboflavinosis), niacin (pellagra), folic acid (one of the megaloblastic anemias), and vitamin B_{12} (pernicious anemia).

Clinical Features. In general, the oral changes associated with vitamin B deficiencies consist of cheilitis and glossitis (Fig. 4–21). The lips may exhibit cracking and fissuring that is exaggerated at the corners of the mouth, in which case it is called angular cheilitis. The tongue becomes reddened with atrophy of papillae, and the patient complains of pain and burning.

In addition to these oral changes, riboflavin deficiency results in keratitis of the eyes and a scaly dermatitis focused on the nasolabial area and genitalia. Niacin deficiency is associated with extraoral problems as well. The four Ds of niacin deficiency are dermatitis, diarrhea, dementia, and death. The most striking and consistent feature is a symmetrically distributed dermatitis that eventually shows marked thickening and pigmentary changes. Dementia is in the form of disorientation and forgetfulness. The glossitis in this deficiency may be severe and may extend to other mucosal surfaces.

Folic acid deficiency results in a megaloblastic (enlarged RBC precursors) bone marrow, a macrocytic (enlarged circulating RBCs) anemia, and gastrointestinal abnormalities, including diarrhea and the general oral lesions described previously. Vitamin B_{12} deficiency shares many of the signs and symptoms of folic acid deficiency. These are detailed in the following section on anemias.

Diagnosis and Treatment. Diagnosis of B complex deficiencies is based upon history, clinical findings, and laboratory data. Replacement therapy should be curative.

Pernicious Anemia

Etiology. This is essentially a deficiency of vitamin B_{12} (erythrocyte maturing factor or extrinsic factor), which is necessary for DNA synthesis, especially in rapidly dividing cells, such as those found in bone marrow and the gastrointestinal tract. Pernicious anemia results from the inability to transport vitamin B_{12} across intestinal mucosa because of a relative lack of a gastric substance (intrinsic factor). This intrinsic factor is normally complexed to vitamin B_{12}, making the vitamin available to mucosal cells for absorption. An autoimmune

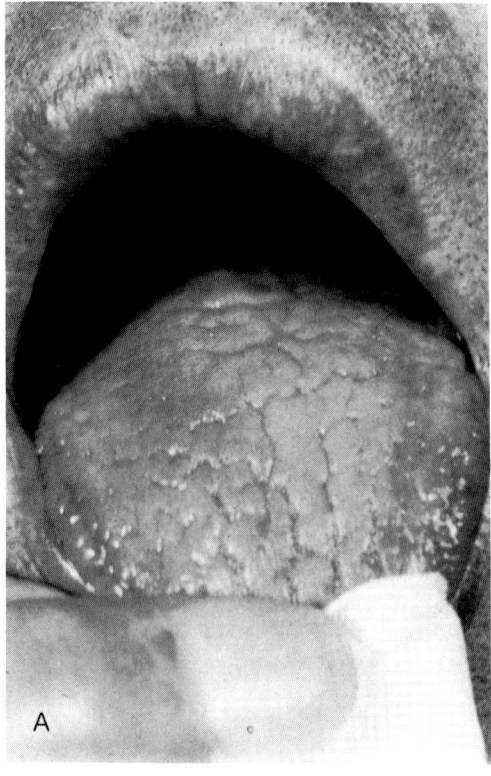
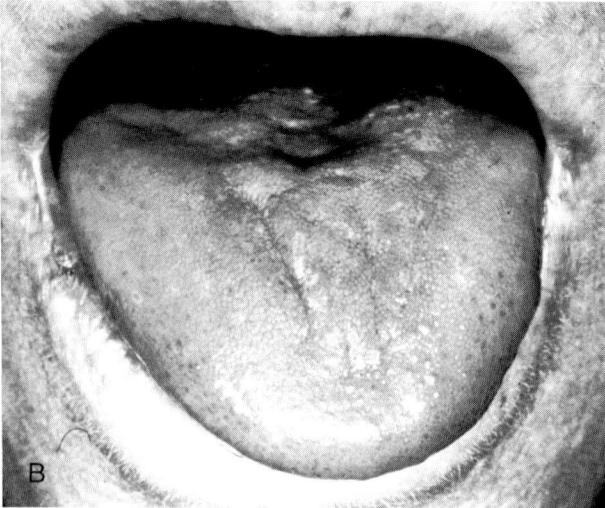

Figure 4–21. Atrophic tongues associated with pernicious anemia *(A)* and vitamin B deficiency *(B)*.

response directed against the intrinsic factor or the gastric mucosa is believed to be a probable mechanism responsible for pernicious anemia. The end result is atrophic gastritis, achlorhydria, neurologic changes, megaloblastic bone marrow, and macrocytic anemia. Additionally, significant oral manifestations may be seen.

Clinical Features. Pernicious anemia affects adults of either gender. The clinical signs of anemia—weakness, pallor, shortness of breath, difficulty in breathing, and increased fatigue on exertion—may be present. Also, in more severe cases, central nervous system manifestations (headache, dizziness, and tinnitus) and gastrointestinal manifestations (nausea, diarrhea, and stomatitis) may be present.

Specific oral complaints center around the tongue. Pain and burning are typical symptoms. The tongue appears more red because of atrophy of the papillae. The resultant smooth, red appearance has been referred to as Hunter's glossitis or Moeller's glossitis.

Diagnosis. The clinical picture of pernicious anemia can be only presumptive of this disease. Diagnosis is based upon laboratory demonstration of a megaloblastic, macrocytic anemia.

Treatment. Parenteral administration of vitamin B_{12} is curative for this condition. An increased risk of the development of gastric carcinoma is associated with the chronic atrophic gastritis that may be seen in pernicious anemia.

Iron Deficiency Anemia

Etiology. Iron deficiency is the cause of this rather common anemia. The deficiency may be due to inadequate dietary intake, impaired absorption due to a gastrointestinal malady, chronic blood loss due to such problems as excessive menstrual flow, gastrointestinal bleeding, and aspirin ingestion, and increased demand as experienced during childhood and pregnancy.

Clinical Features. This is a relatively prevalent form of anemia that affects predominantly women. In addition to the clinical signs and symptoms associated with anemias in general, iron deficiency anemia may also result in brittle nails and hair and koilonychia (spoon-shaped nails). The tongue may become red, painful, and smooth. Angular cheilitis may also be seen.

In addition to iron deficiency, the Plummer-Vinson syndrome includes dysphagia, atrophy of the upper alimentary tract, and a predisposition to the development of oral cancer.

Diagnosis. Laboratory blood studies show a slight to moderately reduced hematocrit and reduced hemoglobin level. The RBCs are microcytic and hypochromic. Serum iron is also low.

Treatment. Recognition of the underlying cause of iron deficiency anemia is necessary to effectively treat this condition. Dietary iron supplements are required to elevate hemoglobin levels and replenish iron stores.

Burning Mouth Syndrome

Burning mouth or burning tongue syndrome usually exhibits no clinically detectable lesions, although symptoms of pain and burning can be intense. This relatively common, "non-lesion" clinical problem is included in this section because the symptoms associated with burning mouth also appear in vitamin B deficiency, pernicious anemia, iron deficiency anemia, and chronic atrophic candidiasis. This is a particularly frustrating problem for both patient and clinician, because there is usually no clear-cut cause and no uniformly successful treatment.

Etiology. The etiology of burning mouth syndrome is varied and often difficult to decipher clinically. The symptoms of pain and burning appear to be the result of one of many possible causes. Factors cited as having possible etiologic significance include

1. Microorganisms—especially fungi *(C. albicans)* and possibly bacteria (staphylococci, streptococci, anaerobes).

2. Xerostomia associated with Sjögren's syndrome, age changes, or drugs such as antihypertensives, antihypoglycemics, beta-blockers, and non-steroidal anti-inflammatories.

3. Nutritional defects associated primarily with B vitamin complex or iron.

4. Anemias, namely pernicious anemia and iron deficiency anemia.

5. Hormone imbalance, especially hypoestrinism associated with post-menopausal changes.

6. Neurologic abnormalities, such as depression, cancer phobia, and other psychogenic problems.

7. Diabetes mellitus.

8. Mechanical trauma, such as an oral habit or chronic denture irritation.

9. Idiopathic causes.

In some patients, more than one of these

may be contributing to the problem of burning mouth syndrome.

Other potential etiologic factors that might be explored are those related to dysgeusia (altered taste), an occasional clinical feature of burning mouth syndrome. Dysgeusia is associated with an equally long list of factors that include zinc deficiency, drugs (especially antibiotics), endocrine abnormalities, Vincent's infection, heavy-metal intoxication, chorda tympani injury, and psychogenic and idiopathic causes.

The mechanism by which such a varied group of factors causes symptoms of burning mouth syndrome is completely enigmatic. There seems to be no common thread or underlying defect that can tie these factors together. It is apparent that burning mouth syndrome represents a diverse, complex group of patients. Determination of etiology is a difficult and challenging clinical problem that requires careful extensive history taking and, frequently, laboratory support.

Clinical Features. This is a condition that typically affects middle-age females. Men are affected but generally at a later age than females. Burning mouth syndrome is rare in children and teenagers, very uncommon in young adults, but relatively common in adults over the age of 40.

Symptoms of pain and burning may be accompanied by altered taste and xerostomia. Occasionally, a patient may attribute the initiation of the malady to recent dental work, such as placement of a new bridge or extraction of a tooth. Symptoms are frequently described as severe and ever-present or worsening late in the day and evening. Any and all mucosal regions may be affected, although the tongue is by far the most commonly involved site.

Highly characteristic of the complaint of intense burning mouth or tongue is a completely normal-appearing oral mucosa. Tissue is intact and has the same color as the surrounding tissue, with normal distribution of tongue papillae.

Some laboratory studies that may prove useful are cultures for *C. albicans,* serum tests for Sjögren's syndrome antibodies (SS-A, SS-B), complete blood count, serum iron, total iron-binding capacity, and serum B_{12} and folic acid levels. Whether any or all of these tests should be performed is a consideration to be made on an individual basis, dependent upon clinical history and clinical suspicion of chronic candidiasis, Sjögren's syndrome, vitamin deficiency, or anemia.

Histopathology. Since there is typically no clinical lesion associated with burning mouth syndrome and since symptoms are more generalized than focal, biopsy is generally not indicated. When an occasional arbitrary site in the area of chief complaint is chosen for biopsy, tissue appears within normal limits in hematoxylin and eosin (H&E) sections. Special stains may reveal the presence of a few *C. albicans* hyphae.

Diagnosis. Diagnosis is based on detailed history, negative clinical examination, laboratory studies, and exclusion of all other possible oral problems. Making the clinical diagnosis of burning mouth syndrome is generally not the difficult aspect of these cases. Rather, it is determining the subtle factor(s) that led to the symptoms that is difficult if not impossible.

Treatment. If a nutritional deficit is the cause, replacement therapy will be curative. If a patient wears a prosthetic device, careful inspection of its fit and tissue base should be done. Relining or remaking it may help eliminate chronic irritation. If fungal cultures are positive, topical nystatin or clotrimazole therapy should produce satisfactory clinical results. If drugs may be involved, consultation with the patient's physician for an alternative drug may prove beneficial.

Since most patients will not fall neatly into one of these categories in which an identified problem can be rectified, treatment becomes difficult. Hormonal changes, neurologic problems, and idiopathic disease are as difficult to identify as they are to treat. A sensitive empathetic approach should be used when treating patients with this problem. The clinician should be supportive and offer an explanation of the various facets and frustrations of burning mouth syndrome. No great optimism or easy solution should be offered, since a patient may ultimately have to accept the disease and learn to live with the problem.

Other referrals may be useful, if only to exhaust all possibilities and reassure the patient. The need for psychologic counseling is often difficult to broach with these patients, but it may be necessary after all logical avenues of investigation have been explored.

Empirical treatment is frequently the approach most clinicians are forced to use for patients with burning mouth syndrome. Even though there may be no evidence of candidiasis, nystatin or clotrimazole may cause a lessening of symptoms. A solution of tetracycline–nystatin–diphenhydramine hydrochloride (Benadryl) or similar remedy may likewise make the patient more comfortable. Topical steroids, such as betamethasone (with or without antifungal agent), applied to the area of chief complaint may also be of some benefit. Generally, viscous lidocaine provides only temporary relief of pain, and saliva substitutes are of minimal value in patients suffering from an associated xerostomia.

Infectious Conditions

Scarlet Fever

Etiology. The characteristic effects of this systemic bacterial infection are the result of an erythrogenic toxin produced by some strains of group A streptococci that causes capillary damage. Other strains of group A streptococci that are unable to elaborate the toxin can cause pharyngitis and all the attendant features of infection but without the red skin rash and oral signs of scarlet fever. Spread of all group A streptococcal infections is generally via droplets from contact with an infected individual and, less likely, a carrier. Crowded living conditions promote the spread of streptococcal infections.

Clinical Features. Children are typically affected, following an incubation period of several days. In addition to the usual symptoms of all group A streptococcal infections—pharyngitis, tonsillitis, fever, lymphadenopathy, malaise, and headache—the child also exhibits a red skin rash that starts on the chest and spreads to other surfaces. The face is flushed except for a zone of circumoral pallor. The palate may show inflammatory changes, and the tongue may become covered with a white coat in which fungiform papillae are enlarged and reddened (strawberry tongue). Later, the coat is lost, leaving a beefy red tongue (red strawberry tongue or raspberry tongue). In untreated, uncomplicated cases, the disease subsides in a matter of days.

Complications of pharyngeal suppuration (abscesses), direct extension to adjacent structures, and metastatic infection may occasionally be seen. Non-suppurative hypersensitivity complications of rheumatic fever and glomerulonephritis are also important potential problems.

Differential Diagnosis. *Staphylococcus aureus* infections, viral infections, and drug eruptions might also be viable considerations in clinical evaluation of children with pharyngitis and an exanthematous skin eruption. Definitive diagnosis is based on history, clinical presentation, and throat culture.

Treatment. Penicillin is the drug of choice for the treatment of group A streptococcal infections. Erythromycin should be used in patients allergic to penicillin. The rationale for antibiotic treatment of this short-lived, self-limited disease is the prevention of complications, especially rheumatic fever and glomerulonephritis.

Atrophic Candidiasis

Caused by the fungus *C. albicans*, this form of the disease appears as a red lesion rather than the traditional white lesion usually associated with candidiasis. The fungus is a prevalent intraoral microorganism that can be cultured from the mouths of most normal individuals. When local or systemic conditions change in favor of fungus growth (see Chapter 3), *C. albicans* takes an opportunistic role and causes overt infection.

Acute atrophic candidiasis follows the loss of the white fungal colonies from the surface of the mucosa. The lesion is red and painful. Chronic atrophic candidiasis also appears as a red, painful lesion, typically under a maxillary denture (denture sore mouth) or at the commissurae of the mouth (angular cheilitis or perlèche). Detailed discussion of atrophic candidiasis can be found in Chapter 3.

Immunologic Abnormalities

Plasma Cell Gingivitis

Etiology. This highly characteristic condition was first given the name "plasma cell gingivostomatitis," because of the prominent plasma cell infiltrate in the tissues affected and because of the undetermined origin. This condition was subsequently named allergic gingivostomatitis because many cases were linked to chewing gum that was believed to be eliciting an allergic reaction. When gum was removed from the diet of affected patients, tissues reverted to normal in a matter of weeks. Similar clinical lesions, however, were noted in patients who did not chew gum, thereby opening to question the original hypothesis. Clinical and microscopic evidence still supports an allergic or hypersensitive reaction. A possible explanation of the appearance of disease in non–gum chewers might be that it represents a reaction to an ingredient in chewing gum, such as mint or cinnamon flavorings, that might be found in other foods.

This peculiar condition is of historical interest because it was relatively prevalent at one time but is rarely seen today. In the early 1970s, numerous cases, all nearly identical, were seen throughout the United States. Within a few years, the phenomenon all but disappeared. Clinicians speculated that formulas or sources of the offending ingredient(s) were changed, making the product non-allergenic.

Clinical Features. This condition affects adults and occasionally children of either gender. Burning mouth, tongue, or lips is the usual complaint of patients with plasma cell gingivitis. The onset is rather sudden, and the discomfort can wax and wane. This condition should not be classified with burning mouth syndrome, because distinctive clinical changes are present. The attached gingiva is fiery red but not ulcerated; the tongue mucosa is atrophic and red; and the commissures are reddened, cracked, and fissured (Fig. 4–22). There is no cervical lymphadenopathy, and there are no systemic complaints.

Histopathology. The affected epithelium is spongiotic and is infiltrated by various types of inflammatory cells (Fig. 4–23). Langerhans cells are also prominent, and occasionally necrotic keratinocytes may be seen. The lamina propria displays prominent capillaries and is infiltrated by plasma cells of normal morphology.

Differential Diagnosis. The triad of gingivitis, glossitis, and angular cheilitis differentiates this from other oral conditions. If tongue and commissure changes are particularly prominent, vitamin B deficiency or anemia might be included in a differential diagnosis. If gingival changes are particularly prominent, discoid lupus erythematosus, atrophic lichen planus, psoriasis, cicatricial pemphigoid, and contact allergic reaction might be considerations.

Treatment. Most patients respond rather quickly to the cessation of gum chewing. In non–gum chewers and those gum chewers who do not respond to the elimination of gum, careful dietary history taking is indicated in an attempt to identify an allergic source.

Drug Reactions and Contact Allergies

Allergic reactions to drugs taken systemically or used topically frequently affect the skin but may also affect oral mucous membranes. A wide variety of agents are known to have this capacity, especially in patients who have a predisposition to the development of allergies.

The clinical appearance of allergic response in the skin ranges from red erythematous lesions to an urticarial rash to a vesiculo-ulcerative eruption. The same types of changes may appear in oral mucosa. In the less intense and less destructive injuries, the mucosa exhibits a generalized redness. When the tongue is the primary target, the pattern may be similar to the changes of vitamin B deficiency and anemia. (A detailed discussion on this subject can be found in Chapter 2.)

EXTRAVASCULAR—PETECHIAE AND ECCHYMOSES

Etiology. Soft tissue hemorrhages in the form of petechiae (pinpoint size) or ecchy-

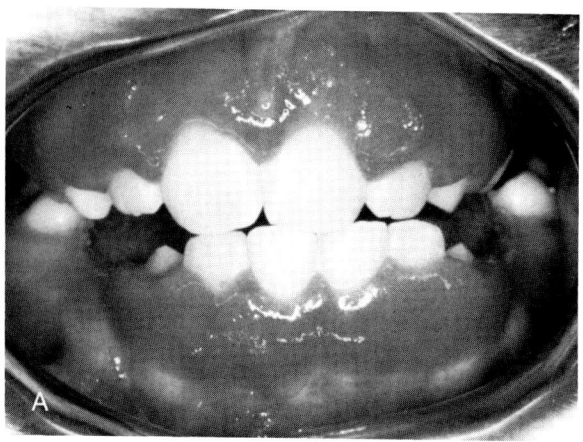
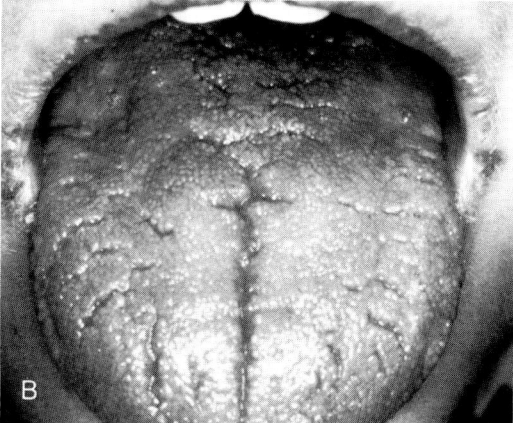

Figure 4–22. *A* and *B*, Plasma cell gingivitis of attached gingiva, tongue, and commissures.

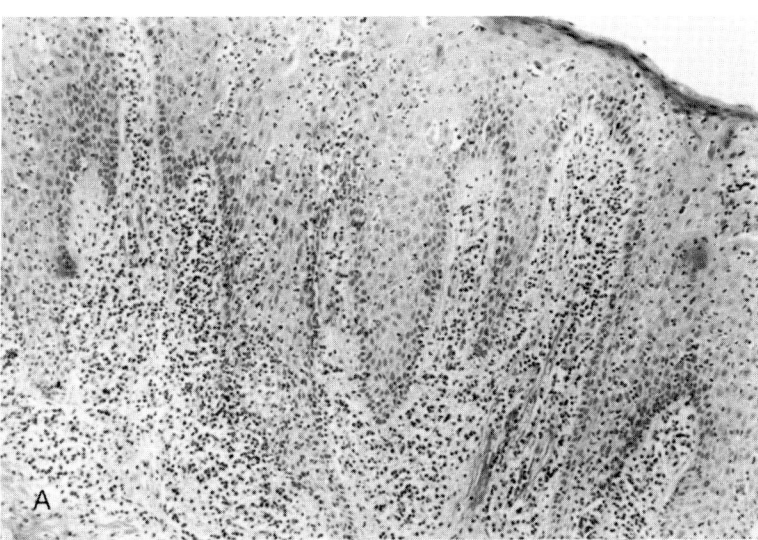
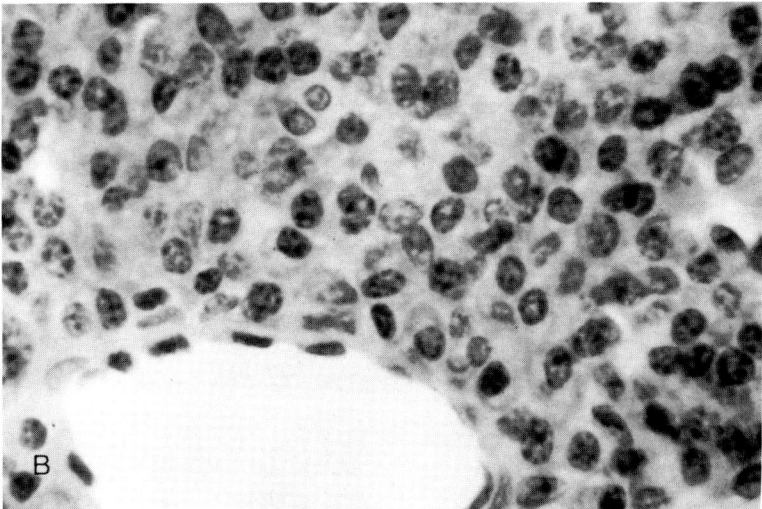

Figure 4–23. Plasma cell gingivitis showing spongiosis and inflammatory cell response *(A)*. Most cells in the connective tissue infiltrate are plasma cells *(B)*.

Table 4–3. BLOOD DYSCRASIAS THAT FREQUENTLY HAVE ORAL MANIFESTATIONS
Leukemia
Monocytic > myelocytic > lymphocytic
Acute > chronic
Agranulocytosis
Cyclic neutropenia
Infectious mononucleosis
Idiopathic thrombocytopenic purpura
Secondary thrombocytopenic purpura
Hemophilias
Macroglobulinemia

Table 4–4. ORAL MANIFESTATIONS OF BLOOD DYSCRASIAS
Petechiae, ecchymoses
Gingival enlargement
"Spontaneous" gingival hemorrhage
Prolonged bleeding following oral surgery
Gingivitis refractory to treatment
Loose teeth
Mucosal ulcers

moses (larger than pinpoint size) appear intraorally, generally because of trauma or blood disease (dyscrasia) (Table 4–3). Traumatic injury, if blood vessels are significantly damaged, can result in leakage of blood into surrounding connective tissue, producing red to purple lesions. The types of injury are many and, among other things, related to cheek biting, coughing, fellatio, trauma from prosthetic appliances, injudicious hygiene procedures, and iatrogenic dental injuries.

In patients with blood dyscrasia, the presenting sign of minor trauma may be oral red to purple macules (Table 4–4). The dental practitioner can therefore play a significant role in the recognition of this abnormality. After ruling out a traumatic etiology, the practitioner should refer the patient to an internist or hematologist.

All the various types of leukemia have the potential to produce intraoral lesions. In actual practice, monocytic leukemia (monocyte series) is most often associated with oral manifestations, myelocytic leukemia (granulocyte series) is next, and lymphocytic leukemia (lymphocytes) is least likely to be associated with oral signs. Acute forms of the leukemias are also more likely than chronic forms to be associated with oral lesions.

Platelet and clotting defects make up another large group of blood dyscrasias that may be responsible for petechiae, ecchymoses, and other intraoral manifestations. Platelet problems may be qualitative or quantitative in nature. They may also be of unknown origin (idiopathic thrombocytopenic purpura), or they may appear secondary to a wide variety of systemic factors, such as drug ingestion, infection, and immunologic disease. Hemophilia and related disorders in which clotting factors are deficient or defective are predominantly hereditary and are characteristically associated with prolonged bleeding and occasional ecchymoses.

Clinical Features. The color of these lesions varies from red to blue to purple, depending upon the age of the lesion and the degree of degradation of the extravasated blood (Fig. 4–24). Soft tissue hemorrhagic lesions usually appear in areas accessible to trauma, such as buccal mucosa, lateral tongue, lips, and junc-

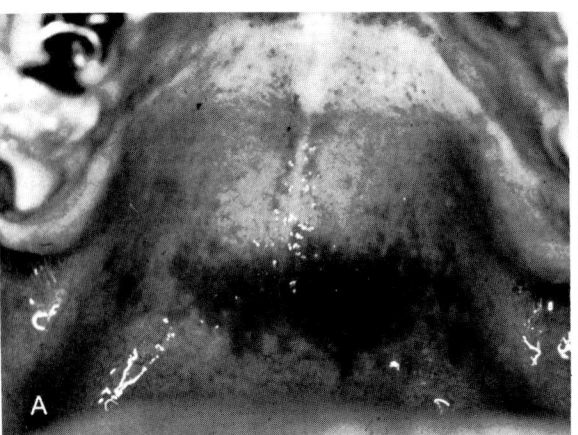
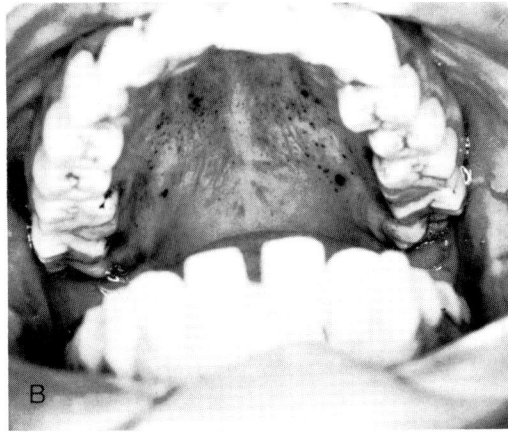

Figure 4–24. *A*, Palatal ecchymosis associated with trauma. (From Ash MM Jr. Kerr and Ash's Oral Pathology, 5th ed. Lea & Febiger, Philadelphia, 1986. Reprinted by permission.) *B*, Petechiae of the palate associated with a blood dyscrasia.

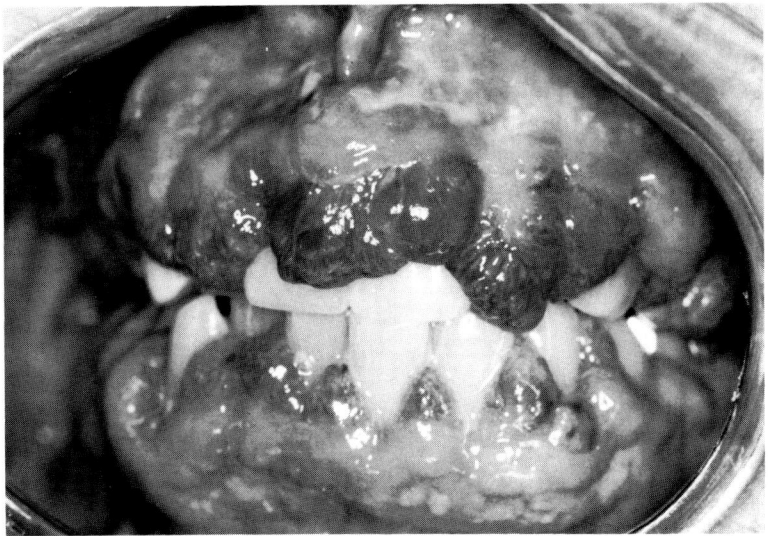

Figure 4–25. Enlargement of the gingiva associated with acute monocytic leukemia.

tion of hard and soft palate. In those injuries that are related to uncomplicated trauma, a cause and effect relationship can usually be established after a history has been taken.

The lesions that develop secondary to blood dyscrasias may follow trivial or otherwise insignificant trauma. In addition to petechiae and ecchymoses, other clinical oral signs of blood dyscrasias include gingival enlargement (especially with monocytic leukemia [Fig. 4–25]), gingivitis, "spontaneous" gingival hemorrhage, prolonged bleeding after oral surgery, loose teeth, and mucosal ulcers.

Diagnosis. The inability to otherwise explain the appearance of any of these clinical signs should cause the clinician to suspect one of the blood dyscrasias. Gingivitis that is refractory to standard therapy should be viewed as a potential dyscrasia. The concomitant presence of lymphadenopathy, weight loss, weakness, fever, joint pain, and headache should add to the suspicion of serious systemic disease. The dentist in this situation should see that the patient is evaluated by an internist or hematologist.

Bibliography

Intravascular, Focal

Bluminfeld W, Egbert B, Sagebiel R. Differential diagnosis of Kaposi's sarcoma. Arch Pathol Lab Med 109:123–127, 1985.

Brauer M, Gates P, Doyle J. Visceral Kaposi's sarcoma presenting with gingival lesions. Oral Surg Oral Med Oral Pathol 50:151–155, 1980.

Green T, Beckstead J, Lozada-Nur F, et al. Histopathologic spectrum of oral Kaposi's sarcoma. Oral Surg Oral Med Oral Pathol 58:306–314, 1984.

Itoiz M, Conti C, Lanfranchi H, et al. Immunohistochemical detection of filaggrin in preneoplastic and neoplastic lesions of the human oral mucsoa. Am J Pathol 119:456–161, 1985.

Kaban L, Mulliken J. Vascular anomalies of the maxillofacial region. J Oral Maxillofac Surg 44:203–213, 1986.

Littner M, Dayan D, Gorsky M, et al. Migratory stomatitis. Oral Surg Oral Med Oral Pathol 63:555–559, 1987.

Lozada F, Silverman S, Migliorati C, et al. Oral manifestations of tumor and opportunistic infections in the acquired immunodeficiency syndrome (AIDS): findings in 53 homosexual men with Kaposi's sarcoma. Oral Surg Oral Med Oral Pathol 56:491–494, 1983.

Rasmussen O, Bakke M. Psoriatic arthritis of the temporomandibular joint. Oral Surg Oral Med Oral Pathol 53:351–357, 1982.

Regezi J, Zarbo R, Lloyd R. HLA-DR antigen detection in giant cell lesions. J Oral Pathol 15:434–438, 1986.

Regezi J, Zarbo R, Lloyd R. Muramidase, α-1 antitrypsin, α-1 antichymotrypsin, and S-100 protein immunoreactivity in giant cell lesions. Cancer 59:64–68, 1987.

Sassoon A, Said J, Nash G, et al. Involucrin in intraepithelial and invasive squamous cell carcinoma. Hum Pathol 16:467–470, 1985.

Shafer W, Waldron C. Erythroplakia of the oral cavity. Cancer 36:1021–1028, 1975.

van der Waal I, Beemster G, van der Kwast W. Median rhomboid glossitis caused by Candida? Oral Surg Oral Med Oral Pathol 47:31–35, 1979.

Weiss R, Guillet G, Freedberg I, et al. The use of monoclonal antibody to keratin in human epidermal disease: alterations in immunohistochemical staining pattern. J Invest Dermatol 81:224–230, 1983.

Intravascular, Diffuse

Dreizen S, McCredie K, Keating M, et al. Malignant gingival and skin "infiltrates" in adult leukemia. Oral Surg Oral Med Oral Pathol 55:572–579, 1983.

Grushka M. Clinical features of burning mouth syndrome. Oral Surg Oral Med Oral Pathol 63:30–36, 1987.

Katz J, Benoliel R, Leviner E. Burning mouth sensation associated with fusospirochetal infection in edentulous patients. Oral Surg Oral Med Oral Pathol 62:152–154, 1986.

Kerr D, McClatchey K, Regezi J. Idiopathic gingivostomatitis. Oral Surg Oral Med Oral Pathol 32:402–423, 1971.

Lamey P, Hammond A, Allam B, et al. Vitamin status of patients with burning mouth syndrome and the response to replacement therapy. Br Dent J 160:81–84, 1986.

Lowental U, Pisanti S. The syndrome of oral complaints: etiology and therapy. Oral Surg Oral Med Oral Pathol 46:2–6, 1978.

vander Ploeg H, vander Wal N, Eijkman M, et al. Psychological aspects of patients with burning mouth syndrome. Oral Surg Oral Med Oral Pathol 63:664–668, 1987.

Zegarelli D. Burning mouth: an analysis of 57 patients. Oral Surg Oral Med Oral Pathol 58:34–38, 1984.

Chapter 5

Pigmentations of Oral and Perioral Tissues

BENIGN LESIONS OF MELANOCYTE ORIGIN
Physiologic Pigmentation
Smoking-Associated Melanosis
Ephelis
Lentigo
Café-au-lait Macules
Oral Melanotic Macule
Vitiligo
NEOPLASMS
Nevi
Melanoma
Neuroectodermal Tumor of Infancy
PIGMENTATIONS CAUSED BY EXOGENOUS DEPOSITS
Amalgam Tattoo/Focal Argyrosis
Heavy-Metal Pigmentations
Minocycline Pigmentation

BENIGN LESIONS OF MELANOCYTE ORIGIN

Melanin-producing cells (melanocytes) have their embryologic origin in the neural crest. These cells find their way to epithelial surfaces and reside among basal cells. They exhibit numerous dendritic processes that extend to adjacent keratinocytes, where transfer of pigment occurs (Fig. 5–1). The packaged pigment granules (melanosomes) produced by these melanocytes are ordinarily not retained within the cell itself but rather are delivered to the surrounding keratinocytes and occasionally to the subjacent macrophages. Light, hormones, and genetic constitution influence the amount of pigment produced.

Melanocytes are found throughout the oral mucosa but go unnoticed because of their relatively low level of pigment production and because of their clear, non-staining cytoplasm on routine preparation. When focally or generally active in pigment production or proliferation, they may be responsible for several different recognized entities in the oral mucous membranes, ranging from physiologic pigmentation to malignant neoplasia.

A physiologic relative of the melanocyte, the nevus cell, is also responsible for other benign (nevi) and malignant (melanomas) neoplastic lesions. Although they exhibit morphologic differences from melanocytes, including an oval shape and a tendency to nest with other similar cells, nevus cells possess the same enzyme, tyrosinase, as melanocytes. This enzyme is responsible for conversion of tyrosine to melanin in the melanosome organelle.

Oral melanin pigmentations range from brown to black to blue, depending upon amount of melanin produced and depth or location of the pigment. Generally, superficial pigmentation is brown, whereas deeper pigmentation is black to blue. Darkening of a pre-existing lesion that has not been stimulated by known factors suggests that pigment cells are producing more melanin or invading deeper tissue.

Physiologic Pigmentation

Clinical Features. This type of pigmentation is symmetric and persistent and does not alter normal architecture, such as gingival stippling (Fig. 5–2). This pigmentation may be seen in patients at any age and is without gender

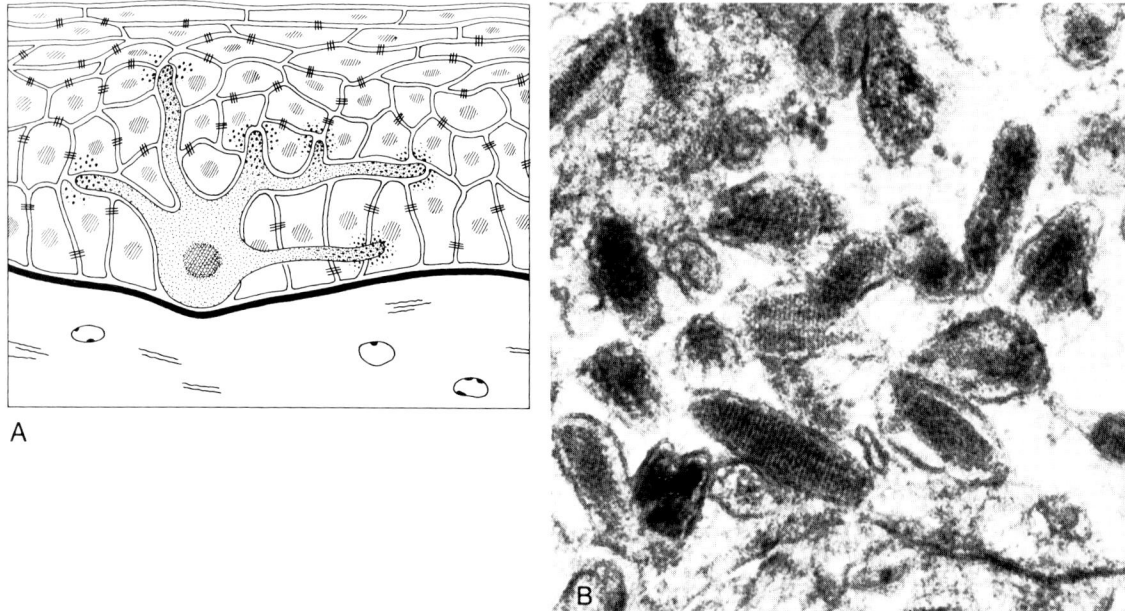

Figure 5–1. *A*, Typical melanocyte showing dendritic morphology and relationship to keratinocytes. Maturing melanosomes are evident in dendritic processes of the melanocyte. Mature granules can be found in the keratinocytes. *B*, Electron micrograph of maturing melanosomes (premelanosomes) in dendritic process of a melanocyte. Note internal lattice structure of the ovoid premelanosomes.

predilection. Physiologic pigmentation may be found in any location, although the gingiva is the most commonly affected intraoral tissue. A related type of pigmentation, called post-inflammatory pigmentation, is occasionally seen following mucosal reaction to injury. In occasional cases of lichen planus of the buccal mucosa, areas surrounding active disease may eventually show mucosal pigmentation (Fig. 5–3).

Histopathology. Physiologic pigmentation is due not to increased numbers of melanocytes but rather to increased melanocyte activity. The melanin is found in surrounding basal keratinocytes and subjacent macrophages (melanophages).

Differential Diagnosis. Clinical differential diagnosis would include smoking-associated melanosis, the syndromes associated with oral melanosis—Peutz-Jeghers syndrome and Addison's disease (Table 5–1)—and melanoma. Although physiologic pigmentation is usually clinically diagnostic, biopsy may be justified if clinical features are atypical.

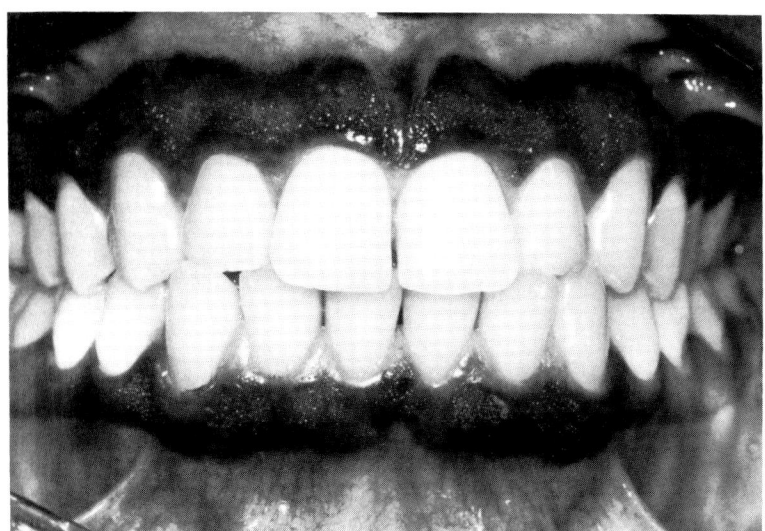

Figure 5–2. Physiologic pigmentation in young adult male. Note symmetry and normal gingival stippling. (Courtesy of Dr. A. Plotzke.)

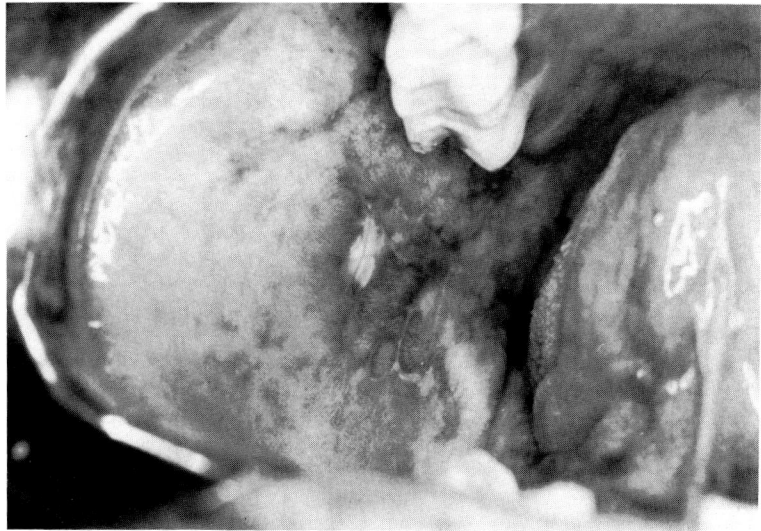

Figure 5–3. Post-inflammatory pigmentation in patient with oral lichen planus.

Smoking-Associated Melanosis

Etiology and Pathogenesis. Abnormal melanin pigmentation of oral mucosa has been linked to cigarette smoking and may be designated smoking-associated melanosis or smoker's melanosis. The pathogenesis is believed to be related to a component in tobacco smoke that stimulates melanocytes. Female sex hormones are also believed to be modifiers in this type of pigmentation, since females (especially those on birth control pills) are more commonly affected than males.

Clinical Features. Anterior labial gingiva is the region most typically affected (Fig. 5–4). Palate and buccal mucosa pigmentation has been associated with pipe smoking. The use of smokeless tobacco has not been linked to oral melanosis. In smoking-associated melanosis, the intensity of pigmentation appears to be time and dose related.

Histopathology. Melanocytes show increased melanin production as evidenced by pigmentation of adjacent basal keratinocytes (Fig. 5–4). The microscopic appearance is essentially similiar to that seen in physiologic pigmentation and melanotic macule.

Differential Diagnosis. Other entities to consider before definitive diagnosis is established are physiologic pigmentation, melanosis related to Peutz-Jeghers syndrome and Addison's disease, and melanoma.

Treatment. With cessation of smoking, improvement is expected over the course of months to years. Smoker's melanosis, per se, appears to be of little significance. It may, however, potentially mask other lesions or may be cosmetically objectionable.

Ephelis

Clinical Features. Ephelides, or freckles, are common, small (less than 5 mm in diameter), tan or brown macules. On the skin, they appear during childhood and are found on sun-exposed areas of the skin. These lesions will darken with exposure to ultraviolet light and lighten during periods of non-exposure.

Table 5–1. SYNDROMES ASSOCIATED WITH ORAL AND CUTANEOUS MACULAR PIGMENTATION

Syndrome	Features
Peutz-Jeghers syndrome	Perioral ephelides, intestinal polyposis (not premalignant), autosomal dominant
Addison's disease	Diffuse cutaneous pigmentation, oral ephelides, adrenal cortical insufficiency
Albright's syndrome	Café-au-lait macules, polyostotic fibrous dysplasia, precocious puberty
Neurofibromatosis	Café-au-lait macules, oral and cutaneous neurofibromas (malignant potential); some inherited as autosomal dominant

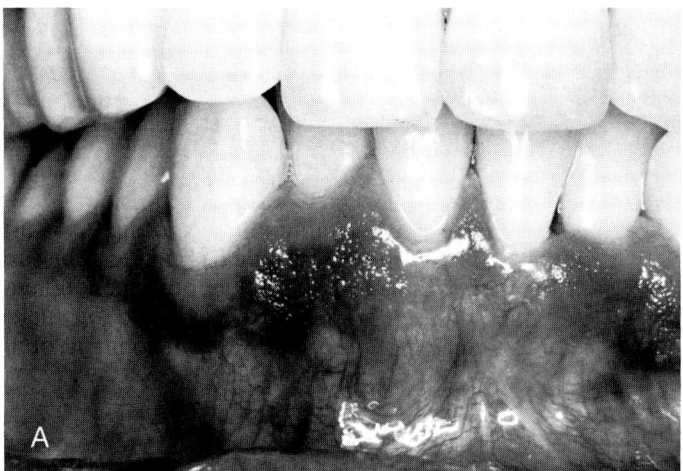
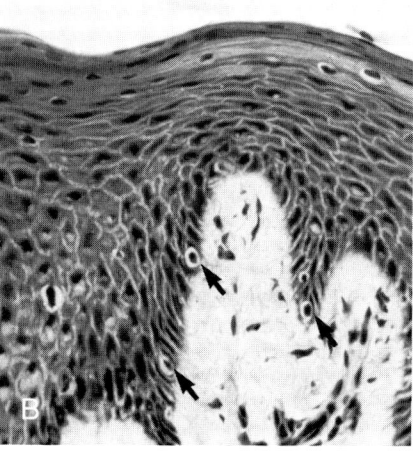

Figure 5–4. *A*, Smoker's melanosis in young adult female. Pigmentation faded slowly after cessation of cigarette smoking. (Courtesy of Dr. P. Chiravalli.) *B*, Biopsy showing normal melanocytes in basal cell layer (arrows).

When freckles as well as larger pigmented macules that may be termed melanotic macules are seen in excess in an oral and perioral distribution, *Peutz-Jeghers syndrome* (Fig. 5–5) and *Addison's disease* (Fig. 5–6) should be considered. Peutz-Jeghers syndrome is a condition that is inherited in an autosomal dominant pattern. In addition to ephelides and other melanotic macules, intestinal polyposis is seen. These polyps are regarded as being hamartomatous without, or with very limited, neoplastic potential. They are usually found in the small intestine (jejunum) and may produce signs and symptoms of abdominal pain, rectal bleeding, and diarrhea.

Addison's disease, primary adrenal cortical insufficiency, may result from adrenal gland infection (tuberculosis), autoimmune disease, or idiopathic causes. With reduced cortisol production by the adrenals, pituitary adrenocorticotropic hormone (ACTH) and melanocyte-stimulating hormone (MSH) increase as part of a negative feedback mechanism. Overproduction of both ACTH and MSH results in stimulation of melanocytes, leading to diffuse pigmentation of the skin. Oral freckles and larger melanotic macules occur with the generalized pigmentation. Other presenting signs and symptoms of this syndrome include weakness, weight loss, nausea, vomiting, and hypotension.

Histopathology. Ephelides result from increased melanocyte function or melanin production rather than from increased numbers of melanocytes. Increased amounts of melanin are found in the basal cell layer because of

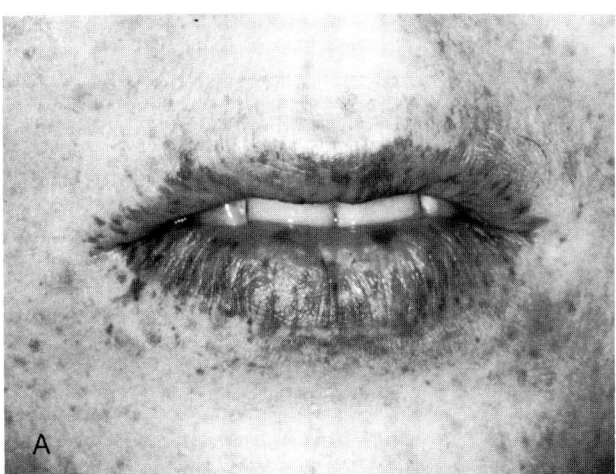
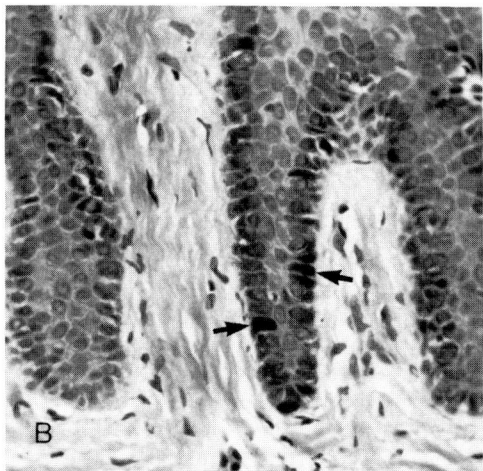

Figure 5–5. *A*, Perioral ephelides (freckles) associated with Peutz-Jeghers syndrome. *B*, Photomicrograph of an ephelis showing melanin deposits in basal keratinocytes (arrows).

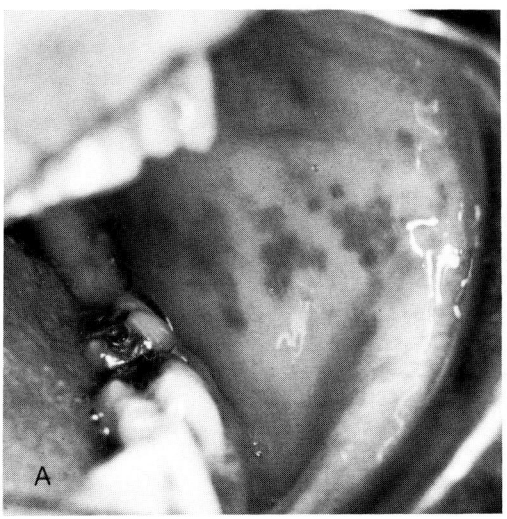 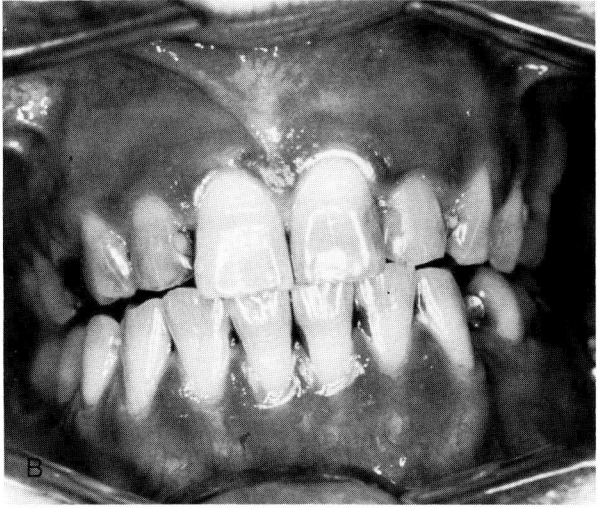

Figure 5–6. Pigmented macules of Addison's disease on the buccal mucosa *(A)* and gingiva *(B)*.

focal melanocyte hyperactivity and melanosome transfer to the basal keratinocytes.

Treatment. There is no treatment indicated for this lesion. Its significance is negligible, unless associated with one of the two syndromes mentioned.

Lentigo

Clinical Features. Lentigines are brown macules of the skin that are larger than freckles and are usually associated with solar exposure and aging ("age spots," "liver spots") (Fig. 5–7). Common in middle-aged and older individuals, these skin lesions are persistent and do not require ultraviolet stimulation to become apparent, as may be the case with freckles. This is a rare lesion intraorally and would be better classified under a generic term, "melanotic macule."

Histopathology. Microscopically, these lesions show increased numbers of melanocytes as well as increased pigment production. Basal keratinocytes subsequently exhibit increased amounts of melanin. Elongation of rete ridges is also noted.

Treatment. Lentigines are believed to have no malignant potential and are of only cosmetic significance. This lesion should not be confused with the low-grade malignancy known as lentigo maligna melanoma.

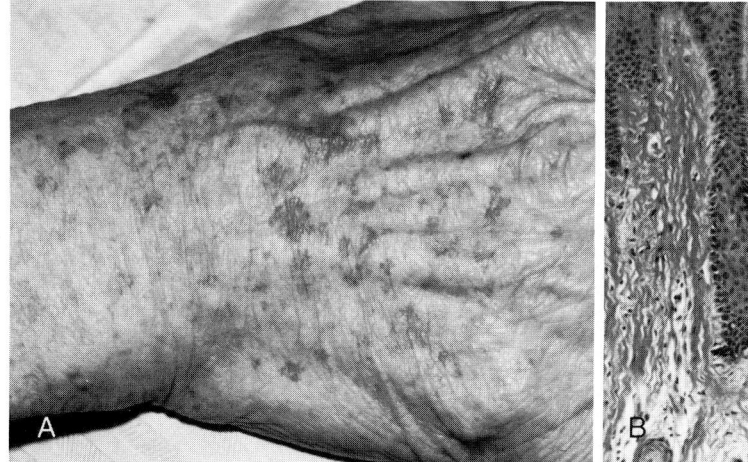 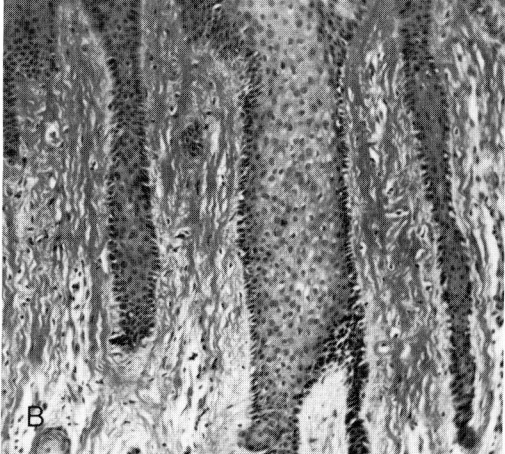

Figure 5–7. *A*, Lentigines on the back of the hand of a 70-year-old female. *B*, Melanin pigmentation of basal cells in elongated rete ridges of a lentigo.

Café-au-lait Macules

Clinical Features. Café-au-lait macules are large (greater than 2 cm), brown skin macules that may occur as independent (sporadic) events or as part of Albright's syndrome or neurofibromatosis (Fig. 5–8 and Table 5–1). These lesions appear during childhood and have a uniform brown appearance with irregular margins. They darken with ultraviolet light exposure and do not disappear with shading (as is the case with freckles) or with age. In Albright's syndrome, patients manifest polyostotic fibrous dysplasia plus precocious puberty and various endocrinopathies. The finding of six or more café-au-lait macules in any individual is generally regarded as being a highly suspicious sign for neurofibromatosis (von Recklinghausen's disease of skin). Patients with neurofibromatosis develop multiple neurofibromas that may have malignant potential. Ephelides are also common in this condition, especially in the axillae (Crowe's sign).

Histopathology. Microscopically, melanocytes are increased in number as well as in activity level. Giant melanosomes have also been described as being characteristic of this lesion.

Treatment. These lesions require no treatment, unless they are cosmetically objectionable. They are of little significance, unless associated with one of the aforementioned syndromes, in which case treatment of the underlying disease is necessary.

Oral Melanotic Macule

Clinical Features. "Oral melanotic macule" is a term used clinically to describe a focal pigmented lesion that may represent one of several conditions. Microscopically, the synonym "oral focal melanosis" may be used to describe this lesion. Either designation may refer to (1) an idiopathic pigmented spot, (2) an intraoral freckle or lentigo, (3) post-inflammatory pigmentation, or (4) the macules associated with Peutz-Jeghers syndrome or Addison's disease.

Melanotic macules have been described as occurring predominantly on the vermilion of the lips and gingiva, although they may appear on any mucosal surface (Fig. 5–9). They are asymptomatic and apparently have no malignant potential.

Histopathology. Microscopically, these lesions are characterized by normal numbers of melanocytes that show increased melanin production and increased basal cell pigmentation (Fig. 5–9). Melanophagocytosis may also been seen.

Differential Diagnosis. These oral pigmentations must be differentiated from early superficial melanomas (Table 5–2). They may be confused with blue nevi or amalgam tattoo, especially when occurring on gingiva. If they are multiple, Peutz-Jeghers syndrome and Addison's disease may be possible clinical considerations.

Treatment. Biopsy may be required to establish definitive diagnosis of this lesion. Otherwise, no treatment is indicated.

Vitiligo

Etiology. Unlike the conditions discussed earlier, vitiligo is a depigmentary process in which melanocytes disappear from affected tissues. The cause is unknown, although au-

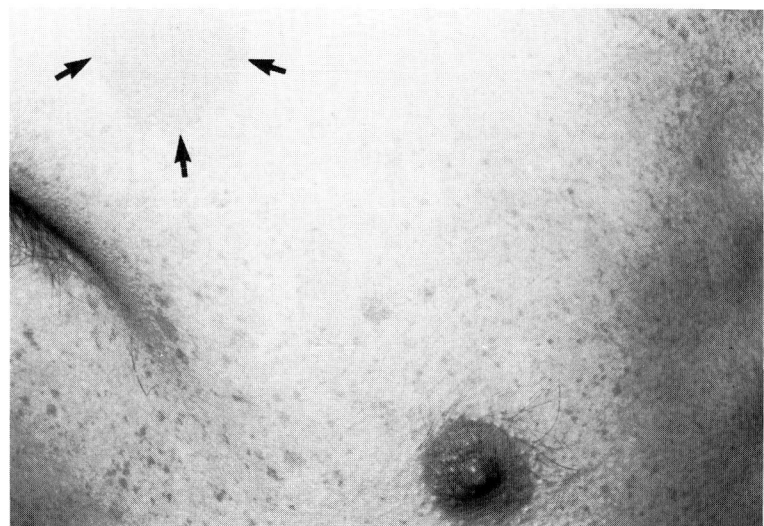

Figure 5–8. Café-au-lait macule seen as part of neurofibromatosis. Note axillary ephelides (lower left).

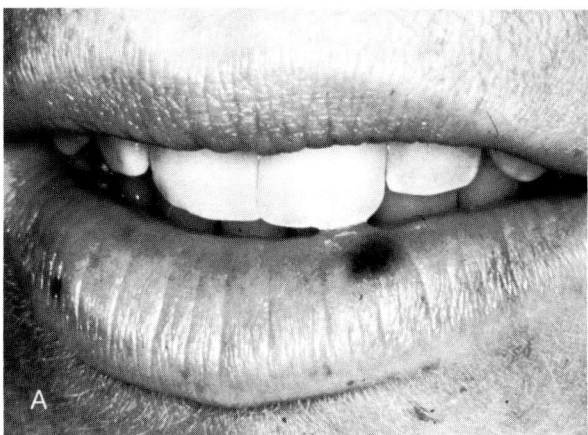 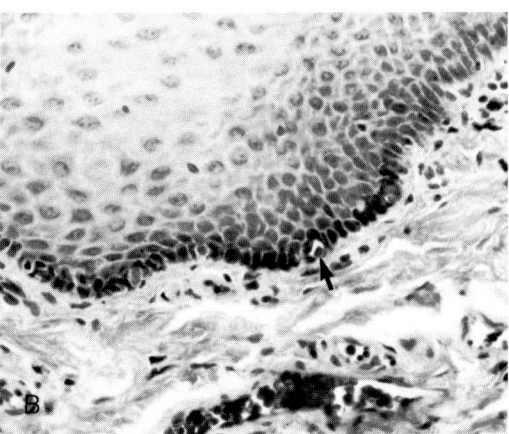

Figure 5–9. *A*, Melanotic macules on the vermilion of the lips. *B*, Microscopy of melanotic macule showing basal keratinocyte pigmentation. Note melanocyte (arrow).

toimmune reaction directed against melanocytes and toxic destruction of melanocytes by some unknown mediator have been proposed. Stress, trauma, chemicals, hormonal changes, and ultraviolet light have all been cited as possible precipitating factors.

Clinical Features. Vitiligo is a condition that affects predominantly the skin but may involve oral and perioral tissues (Fig. 5–10). Clinically, the depigmented vitiliginous macules range from several millimeters to several centimeters in size. The lesions are white and have relatively distinct, and possibly hyperpigmented, margins. The lesions may occur at any age and in either sex. On the face, perioral and periocular tissues are commonly affected. Other zones where lesions occur are the nape of the neck and areas of repeated trauma, such as knees, elbows, and hands.

Treatment. The clinical course of this condition is protracted and unpredictable. Spontaneous repigmentation may occur in a small number of patients, although most exhibit an abatement or a progression of the process. Treatment is difficult and may center around the use of tanning creams (e.g., psoralens), the use of depigmentation creams (e.g., hydroquinones) on normal adjacent skin, or the use of cosmetic cover-ups.

NEOPLASMS

Nevi

Etiology. "Nevus" is a general term that may refer to any congenital lesion of various cell types or tissue types, such as epidermis, vessels, and pigment cells. In the usual context, however, "nevus," used without a modifier, refers to the pigmented lesion composed of nevus cells. It is sometimes called, more specifically, nevocellular nevus or melanocytic nevus.

Nevi (moles) are collections of nevus cells that, except for the tendency to "nest" and their lack of dendrites, are cytologically identical to melanocytes. They may be found in epithelium or supporting connective tissue, or both. The origin of nevus cells is not completely known. It has been postulated that they are derived from pigment cells that migrate

Table 5–2. CLINICAL DIFFERENTIATION OF ORAL PIGMENTATIONS FROM EARLY MELANOMA	
Lesion	**Differentiating Features**
Focal argyrosis	Uniform slate-gray color, history of dental trauma, macular, no change with time
Physiologic pigment	Symmetric, not recently acquired, uniform color, no obstruction of normal landmarks
Melanotic macule	Uniform color, macular, relatively uniform contour
Melanoma	Recently acquired, variable color, irregular margins, satellite lesions, may be ulcerated or papular

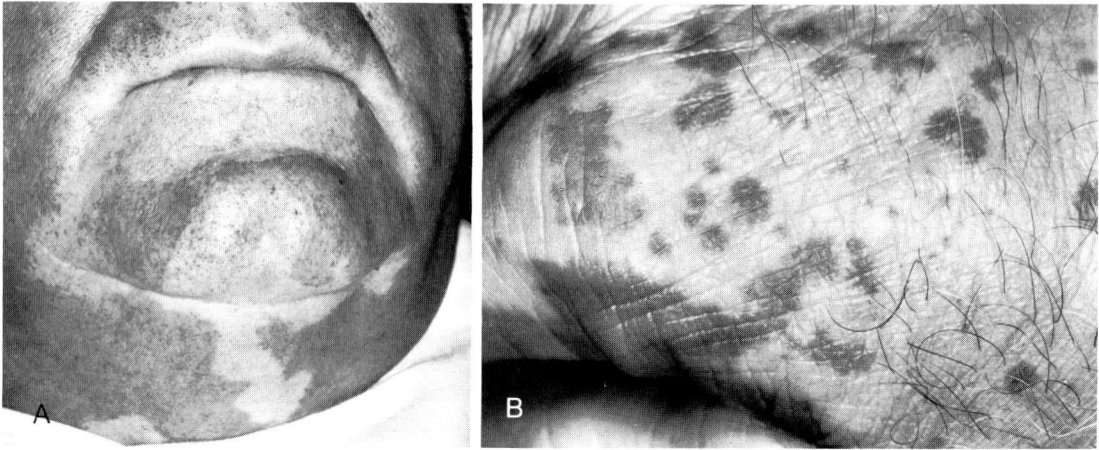

Figure 5-10. *A*, Vitiligo of lips, chin, and neck. *B*, Same patient with vitiligo on back of hand; dark areas represent normal pigmented areas.

from the neural crest to the epithelium and dermis (submucosa) or that they develop from altered resident melanocytes.

Clinical Features. Nevi of the skin are common acquired papular lesions seen in a large majority of the population (Fig. 5-11). They usually appear shortly after birth and throughout childhood. They may appear in any site. Intraoral nevi are uncommon, if not rare, lesions that may occur at any age. Most oral lesions present as elevated papules, occasionally non-pigmented, usually on the hard palate (Fig. 5-12). Less frequent sites are buccal mucosa, labial mucosa, gingiva, alveolar ridge, and vermilion.

Histopathology. Microscopically, several subtypes are recognized. Classification is dependent upon whether nevus cells are located in the epithelium at the connective tissue junction (junctional nevus), in the dermis (intradermal nevus), or in the submucosa (intramucosal nevus), or in a combination of zones (compound nevus) (Fig. 5-13). A fourth type of nevus, in which cells are spindle shaped and found deep in the connective tissue, is known as the blue nevus. Skin lesions that exhibit junctional proliferation of nevus cells or melanocytes are usually viewed as having malignant potential. Although this relationship is believed to be generally applicable to oral lesions, conclusive evidence is not available, because of the small numbers reported and limited knowledge of natural history. Probably more important than the junctional nevus is the reported pre-existing melanosis associated with some oral melanomas, a phenomenon that most likely represents a radial growth phase of the melanoma. Because junctional

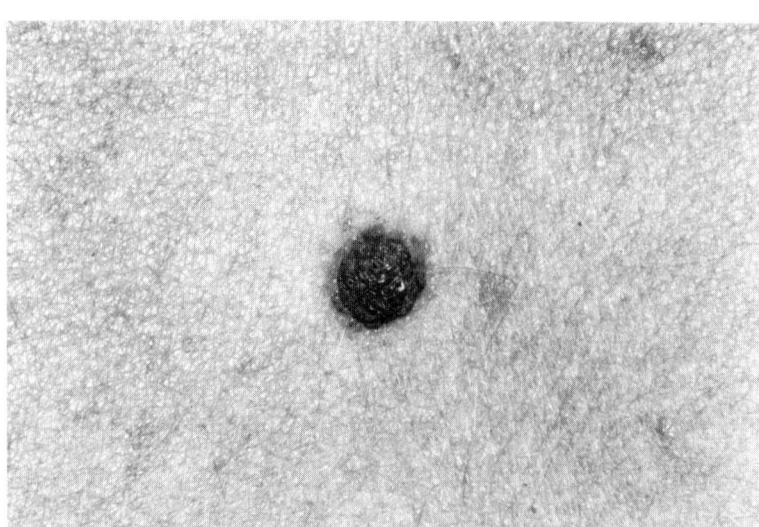

Figure 5-11. Pigmented nevus on skin of the back. The lesion is symmetric, evenly colored, and elevated.

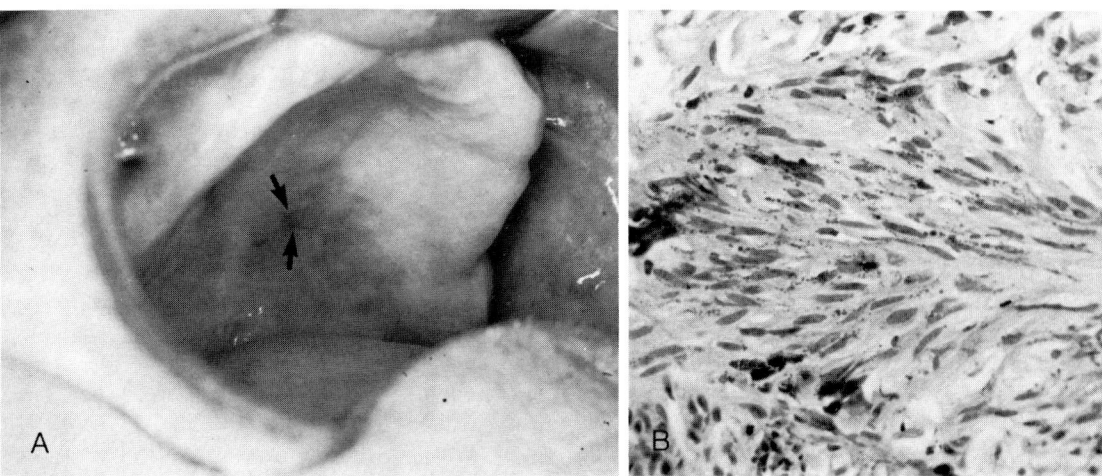

Figure 5–12. *A*, Blue nevus of hard palate. *B*, Microscopy of blue nevus showing pigment granules in spindle-shaped melanocytes deep in the submucosa.

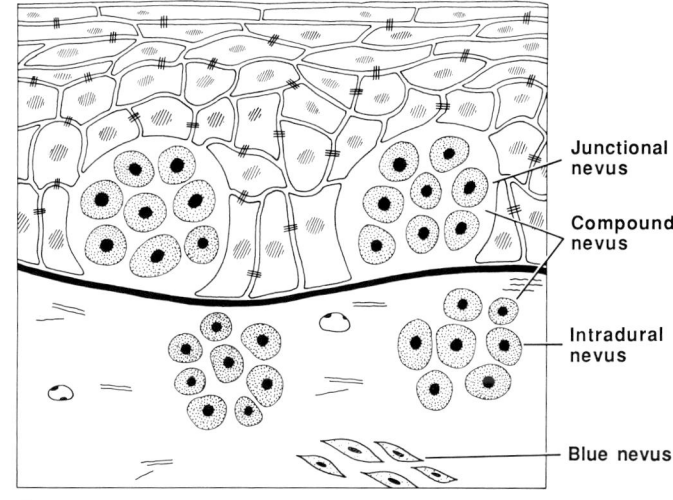

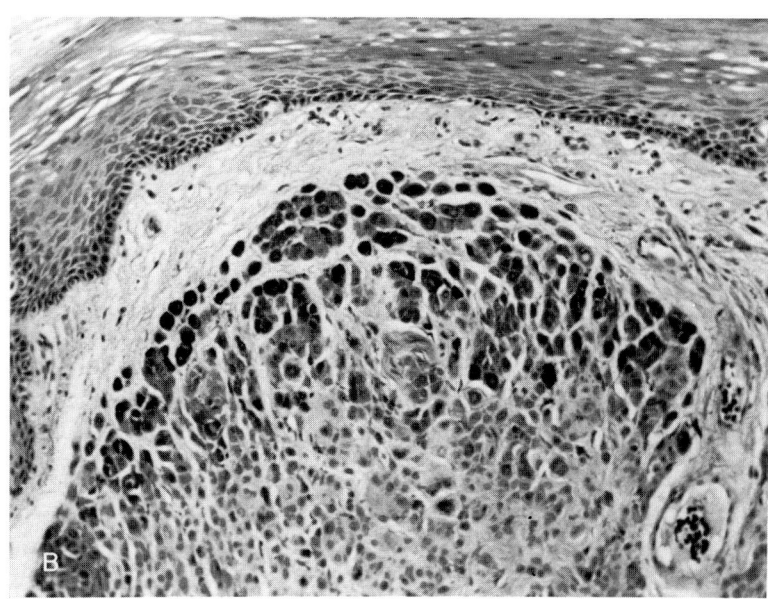

Figure 5–13. *A*, Nevus cells showing location of cells in the various types of nevi. *B*, Biopsy of intramucosal nevus. Pigmentation is most intense near surface.

changes cannot be appreciated in the clinical setting, biopsy of any oral pigment-producing lesion is mandatory in order to identify any of those with malignant potential.

In the oral cavity, intramucosal nevi are the most common variety seen, and blue nevi are the second most common. Compound and junctional nevi occur relatively rarely in the oral mucosa.

Differential Diagnosis. Other clinical considerations that should be included along with any type of oral nevus are melanotic macule, amalgam tattoo, and melanoma. Lesions of vascular origin might also be considered. These include hematoma, varix, and hemangioma. Diascopy (compression) could be used to rule out the last two lesions, in which the blood is contained within a vascular system.

Treatment. The significance of these lesions lies in the potential for malignant transformation of lesions with junctional change. This relationship is less well supported intraorally than in the skin, because of the relative infrequency of junctional nevi in the oral mucosa. The role of irritation in malignant transformation of nevi is not established. By and of itself, it is probably not a carcinogenic factor, although it may be responsible for inflammatory changes that make microscopic diagnosis difficult.

Because of the infrequency with which oral nevi occur, because of the inability to clinically judge the presence of junctional change, and because of the possible confusion with early melanoma, all oral nevi should be excised. Since their size is generally under 1 cm, excisional biopsy would usually be indicated.

Melanoma

Etiology. Melanomas of the skin have been increasing in frequency over the past several years and now represent approximately 2% of all cancers (excluding carcinomas of the skin). Overall, the cancer-related death rate due to melanoma of the skin is about 1 to 2%. Cutaneous melanoma is more common in southern climates than in northern climates and is much more common in whites than in blacks and Asians. In the oral mucous membranes, there are no geographic differences, and the racial predilection seen with skin melanomas does not occur. In fact, blacks and Asians appear to be proportionately more frequently affected with this neoplasm in the oral mucosa than are whites.

Melanomas may arise from neoplastic transformation of either melanocytes or nevus cells. Predisposing factors for skin lesions include amount of sun exposure (increased risk), degree of natural pigmentation (reduced risk), and precursor lesions, such as junctional nevi. Intraorally, pre-existing melanosis has been thought to appear prior to melanoma development. This pigmentary process, however, very likely represents an early growth phase of these lesions. It is now well recognized that some types of melanomas in skin and mucosa may exhibit a prolonged superficial or radial growth phase occurring at the junction of epithelium and connective tissue before they enter an invasive vertical growth phase.

Clinical-Pathologic Features. Melanomas of oral mucosa are much less common than their cutaneous counterparts. Cutaneous melanomas generally occur in a younger population than do mucosal lesions (which usually appear over the age of 50). There is no sex predilection. Cutaneous melanomas occurring in the head and neck region are most often seen in sun-exposed areas. Oral lesions occur predominantly on the hard palate and gingiva, followed by the lips and the buccal mucosa. Pigmentation patterns that suggest melanoma include different mixtures of color—such as brown, black, blue, and red—asymmetry, and irregular margins.

Recognition of radial and vertical growth phases in melanomas has led to the subclassification of these lesions into several clinical-pathologic entities. Subtypes occurring in the skin are known as nodular melanoma, superficial spreading melanoma, lentigo maligna melanoma, and acral-lentiginous melanoma. Each of these is now known to exhibit distinctive microscopic and clinical features and natural histories. Comparable lesions have been identified intraorally for nodular melanoma and superficial spreading melanoma. There is no direct oral counterpart to the sun-induced lentigo maligna melanoma. Oral acral-lentiginous melanomas have been reported.

Nodular melanoma appears clinically as darkly pigmented elevations in skin or mucous membrane (Fig. 5–14). It is composed of malignant cells whose growth pattern is described as vertical. Cells may penetrate the overlying epithelium as well as the subjacent connective tissue. This form of melanoma is invasive from the beginning and metastasizes early. Consequently it has a relatively poor prognosis.

Superficial spreading melanoma is the most common form of melanoma. It develops over several years into a well-defined, slightly elevated, pigmented patch (Fig. 5–15). During its

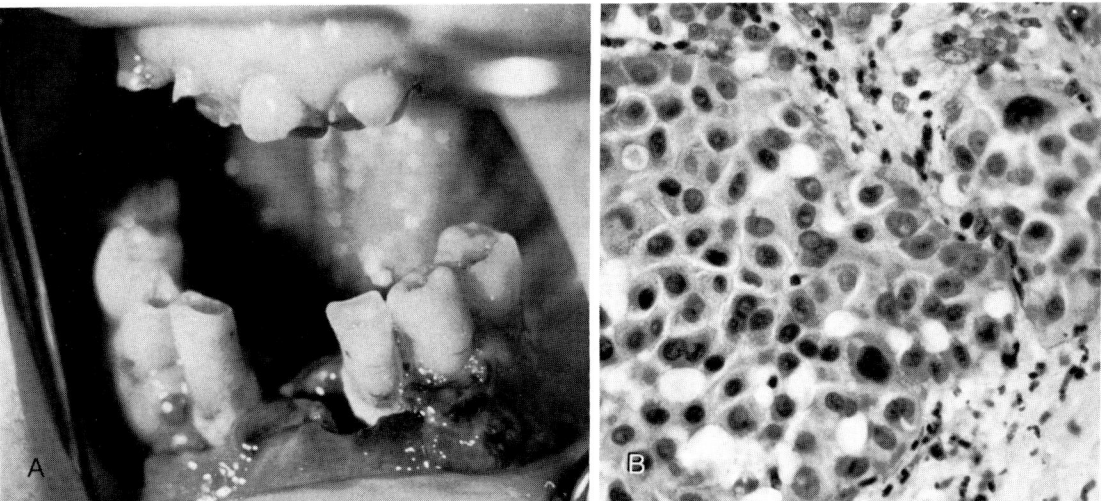

Figure 5–14. *A*, Nodular melanoma of mandibular gingiva. *B*, Microscopy shows tumor cells with hyperchromatic and pleomorphic nuclei.

radial growth phase, the neoplastic cells are found at the junction of epithelium and connective tissue. Invasion of the epidermis by malignant cells has produced what has been described as a pagetoid appearance, after Paget's disease of the breast. After several years of centrifugal growth, the neoplasm enters into a vertical growth phase that subsequently gives the lesion metastatic potential. Because of the prolonged radial growth phase of this lesion, its prognosis is better than that for nodular melanoma.

Lentigo maligna melanoma occurs predominantly on sun-exposed skin of the elderly. It also has a radial growth phase that, in this case, may last up to 25 or 30 years. Clinically, this lesion appears as a flat, irregularly pigmented patch with ill-defined margins. Prognosis is generally considered excellent for this lesion until it enters its vertical growth phase, at which time the prognosis worsens.

Acral-lentiginous melanomas are a small group of oral melanomas that share microscopic and behavioral features with melanomas occurring around the nail bed (Figs. 5–16 and 5–17). At present, distinction from superficial spreading melanomas is academic, since it has not been shown that these two subtypes exhibit significantly different behavioral characteristics when occurring intraorally.

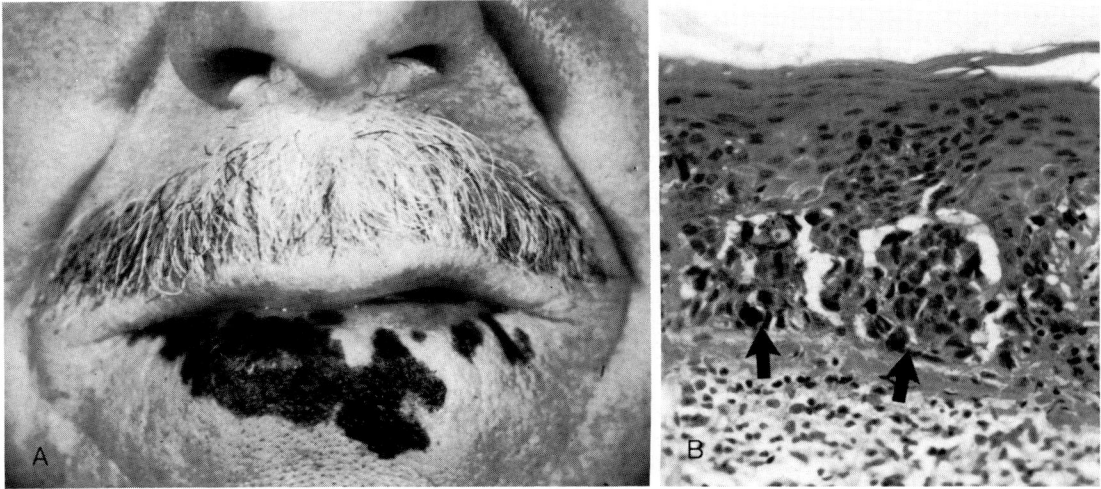

Figure 5–15. *A*, Superficial spreading melanoma of 8 years' duration. *B*, Microscopy showing nests of malignant melanocytes at the junction of epithelium and connective tissue (arrows).

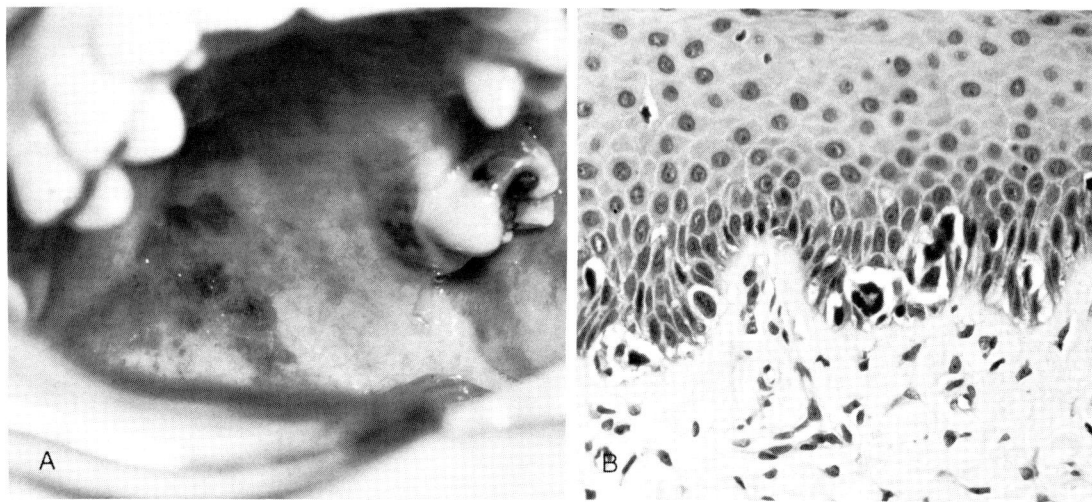

Figure 5–16. *A*, Acral-lentiginous melanoma. *B*, Malignant cells are found along basement membrane during radial growth phase.

Differential Diagnosis. Intraorally, differential considerations would most often include amalgam tattoo, physiologic pigmentation, and melanotic macule. History, symmetry, and uniformity and evenness of pigmentation would all be of significant value in differentiating these lesions. Because melanomas may initially have a relatively innocuous appearance, biopsy should be done on any questionable acquired pigmentations.

Treatment and Prognosis. Surgery remains the primary mode of treatment for melanomas. Chemotherapy is often employed, and occasionally immunotherapy is used as an adjunct. Radiotherapy has not been fully explored as a primary treatment method, but it may play a supportive role in disease management. Treatment failures of mucosal melanomas are most commonly linked to incomplete excision, resulting in local recurrence and distant metastasis. Regional lymph node metastasis seems to be a less important reason for persistence of disease. The necessity of wide surgical excision of melanomas with a radial growth pattern is apparent from the microscopy of this phenomenon.

Prognosis is based on both histologic subtype and depth of tumor invasion. The latter feature is a well-established prognosticator for skin lesions that has only recently been applied to oral melanomas. Oral lesions have been found to be of considerably greater thickness (and

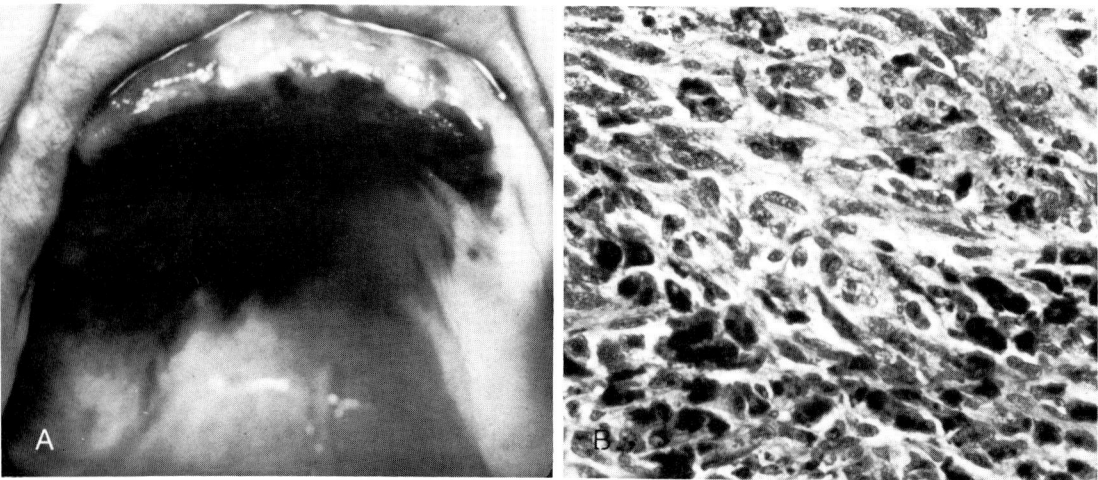

Figure 5–17. *A*, Advanced acral-lentiginous melanoma. *B*, Malignant cells in vertical growth phase are spindle shaped, a feature typical of this type of melanoma.

consequently to be more advanced) than skin lesions at the time of biopsy. The overall poor prognosis of oral lesions as compared with skin lesions may be related therefore to late recognition of the oral lesions. Another factor is probably the more confining and difficult treatment area of the oral cavity. Oral lesions may also be inherently biologically more aggressive than skin lesions. Until more lesions are subclassified and measured for depth of invasion, these questions will go unanswered. After 5 years, the survival rate of cutaneous melanomas is about 65% and the prognosis for oral lesions is about 20%. Unfortunately, the survival rate for the oral lesions continues to fall after the traditional measure of 5 years.

Neuroectodermal Tumor of Infancy

Etiology. This rare, benign neoplasm is composed of relatively primitive pigment-producing cells. Like melanocytes and nevus cells, these cells have their origin in the neural crest.

Clinical Features. This lesion is found in infants usually under the age of 6 months and occurs typically in the maxilla, although the mandible and the skull have been involved. This lesion usually presents as a non-ulcerated and occasionally darkly pigmented mass (Fig. 5–18). The latter feature is due to melanin production by tumor cells. Radiographs show an ill-defined lucency that may contain developing teeth.

Histopathology. This neoplasm exhibits an alveolar pattern, i.e., nests of tumor cells with small amounts of intervening connective tissue (Fig. 5–19). The variably sized nests of round to oval cells are found within a well-defined connective tissue margin. Cells located centrally within the neoplastic nests are dense and compact; peripheral cells are larger and often contain melanin.

Differential Diagnosis. Few other lesions would present in this age group and in this characteristic location. Malignancies of early childhood, such as neuroblastomas, sarcomas, or "histiocytic" tumors, might be considered. Odontogenic cysts and tumors would not be seriously entertained in a differential diagnosis.

Treatment and Prognosis. This lesion has been treated with surgical excision with good results. A few cases of local recurrence have been recorded, and at least one case has been documented in which metastasis has followed local excision.

PIGMENTATIONS CAUSED BY EXOGENOUS DEPOSITS

Amalgam Tattoo/Focal Argyrosis

Etiology. Amalgam tattoo or focal argyrosis is an iatrogenic lesion that follows traumatic soft tissue implantation of amalgam particles. This usually follows tooth extraction or preparation of teeth having old amalgam fillings for gold-casting restorations.

Clinical Features. This is the most common pigmentation of oral mucous membranes.

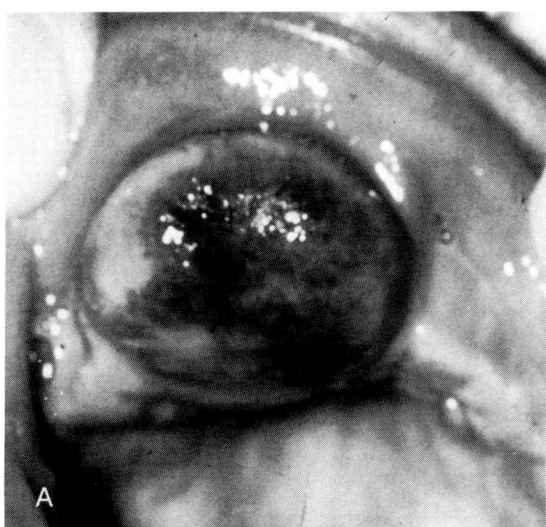 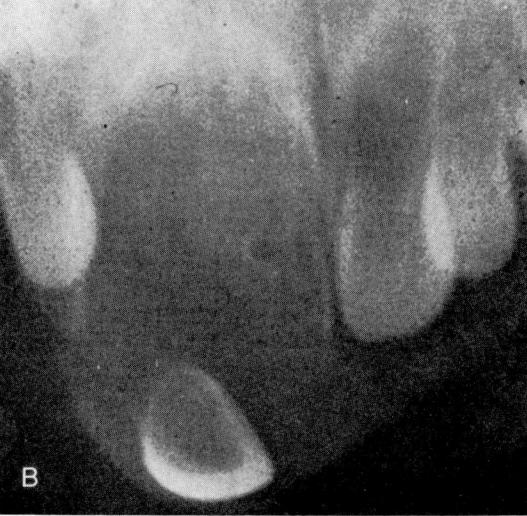

Figure 5–18. *A*, Neuroectodermal tumor of infancy in the maxilla. *B*, Radiograph showing a poorly defined lucency.

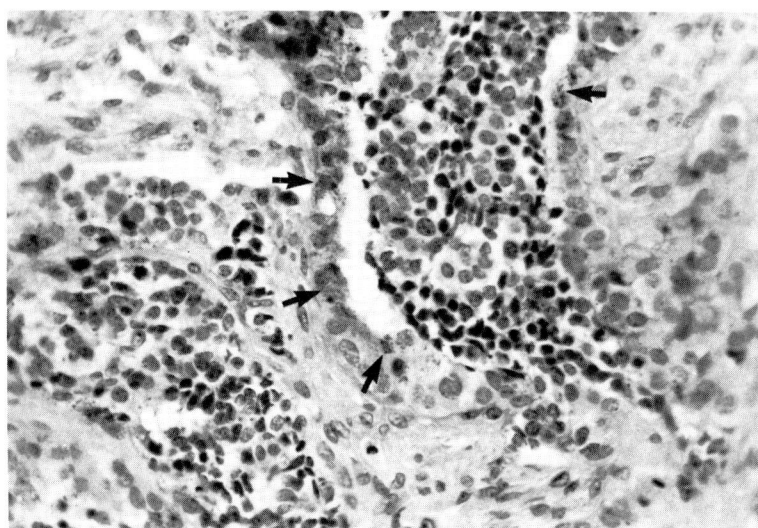

Figure 5-19. Microscopy of neuroectodermal tumor showing nests of round tumor cells. Pigment granules can be seen in peripheral layer of cells (arrows).

These lesions would be expected in the soft tissues contiguous with teeth restored with amalgam alloy (Fig. 5–20A). Therefore, the most frequently affected sites are gingiva, buccal mucosa, palate, and tongue. Because amalgam is relatively well tolerated by soft tissues, clinical signs of inflammation are rarely seen. The lesions are macular and gray and do not change appreciably with time. If the amalgam particles are of sufficient size, they may be detected on soft tissue radiographs (Fig. 5–20B).

Histopathology. Microscopically, amalgam particles are typically aligned along collagen fibers and around blood vessels (Fig. 5–21). Few lymphocytes and macrophages are found, except in cases in which particles are relatively large. Multinucleated, foreign-body giant cells may also be seen.

Differential Diagnosis. The significance of the amalgam tattoo lies in its clinical similarity to melanin-producing lesions. In a gingival or a palatal location, separation from nevi and, more important, early melanoma is mandatory, since these are the most common areas for the latter lesions as well. Radiographs, history, and an even, persistent gray appearance would all help separate amalgam tattoo from melanoma. Any questionable lesions should be biopsied.

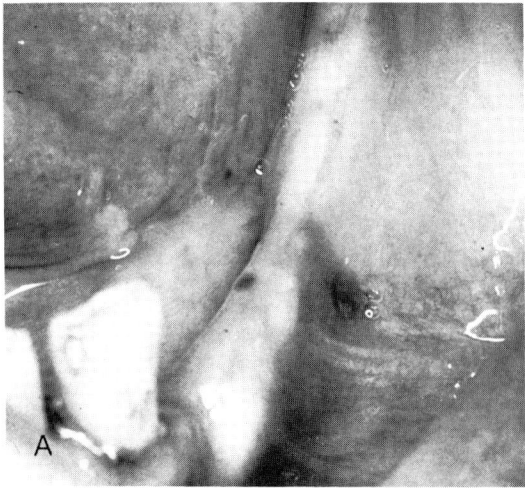
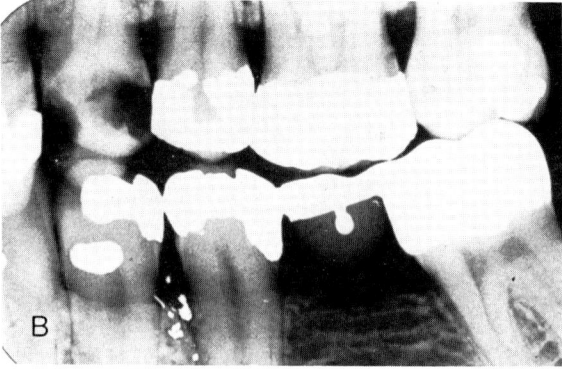

Figure 5-20. *A*, Focal argyrosis of alveolar ridge and vestibule. *B*, Focal argyrosis with large particles that can be seen in a radiograph.

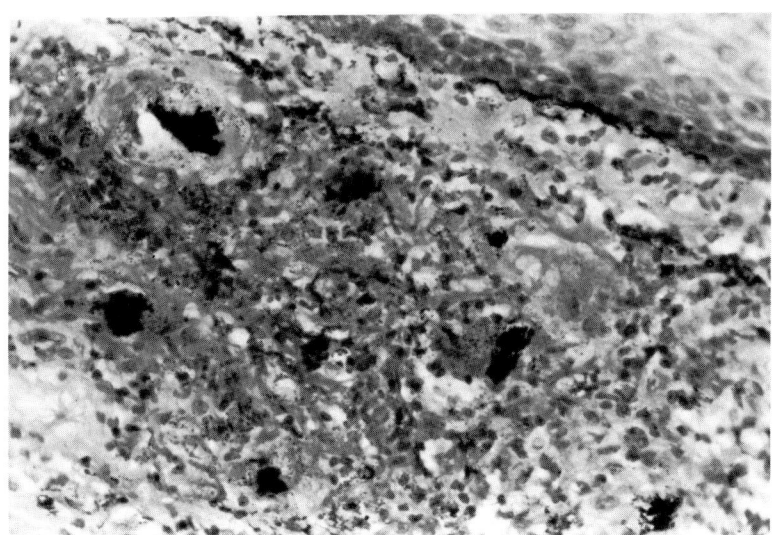

Figure 5–21. Focal argyrosis showing connective tissue deposits of various-sized amalgam particles. Note deposition along basement membrane (top right).

Heavy-Metal Pigmentations

Etiology. Some heavy metals (arsenic, bismuth, lead, mercury) may be responsible for oral pigmentation. This phenomenon occurs predominantly following occupational exposure to vapors of these metals. Historically, arsenic and bismuth compounds were used to treat diseases such as syphilis, lichen planus, and other dermatoses, providing another method for oral heavy-metal deposition.

Clinical Features. These heavy metals may be deposited in both skin and oral mucosa (especially in gingiva). The characteristic color is gray to black, and the distribution is linear when found along the gingival margin. Bismuth and lead staining of gingival tissues are known as bismuth line and lead line (Fig. 5–22), respectively. This is proportional to the amount of gingival inflammation and appears to be the result of the reaction product of the heavy metal with hydrogen sulfide in the inflammatory zones.

Significance. The metallic deposits in oral mucosa, per se, are relatively insignificant. The underlying cause must be investigated because of detrimental effects of systemic toxicity. For dental personnel, chronic mercury vapor exposure is now recognized as a significant occupational hazard, if dental amalgam is handled carelessly and without proper precautions. Dental patients, however, are apparently at no risk, because of the relatively short exposure periods that they experience with routine office

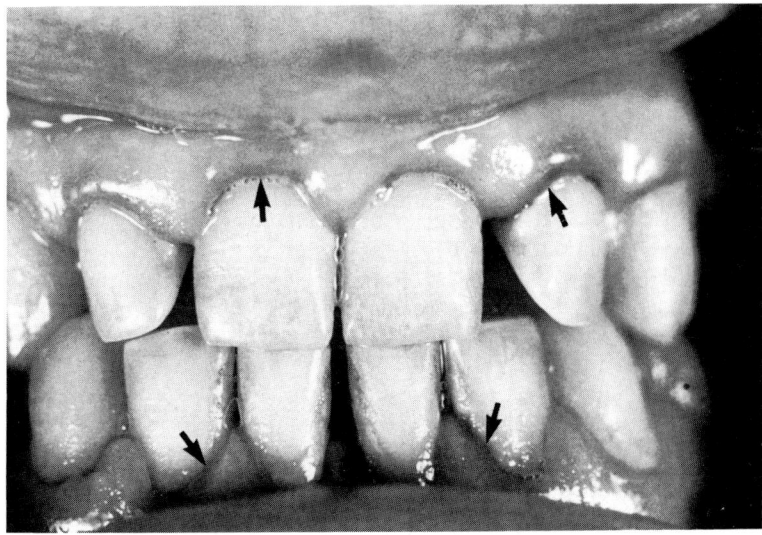

Figure 5–22. Gingival pigmentation (lead line) associated with lead intoxication (arrows).

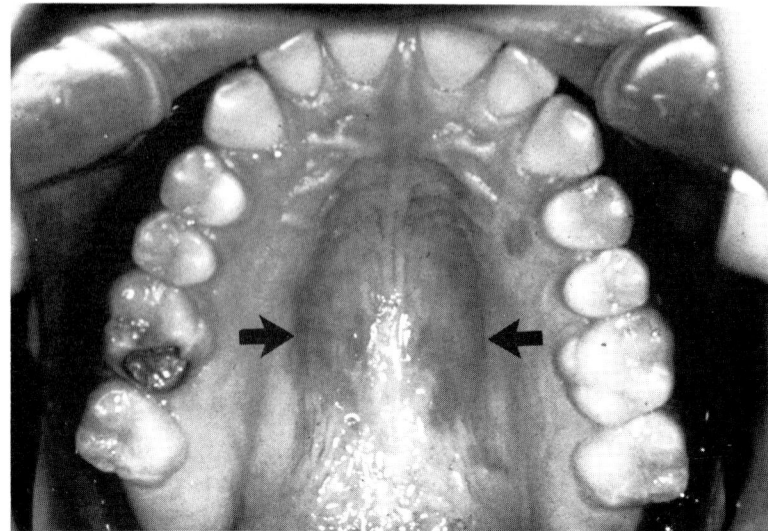

Figure 5–23. Minocycline pigmentation of palate (arrows). (Courtesy of Dr. C. Witkop.)

visits. Toxicity from the restorations themselves is also apparently negligible.

If, in the dental office, the atmospheric air has elevated mercury vapor levels, dental personnel may show elevated body levels of mercury as measured in hair, nails, saliva, and urine. *Chronic mercury intoxication* may produce symptoms of tremors, loss of appetite, nausea, depression, headache, fatigue, weakness, and insomnia. Hazard due to mercury can be eliminated in the dental office if precautions are observed. The most common recommendations include (1) storage of mercury in sealed containers, (2) coverage of mercury spills with sulfur dust to prevent vaporization, (3) utilization of hard, seamless floor surfaces instead of carpeting, (4) working in well-ventilated spaces with frequent air filter changes, (5) storage of amalgam scraps under water in a sealed container, (6) use of well-sealed amalgamation capsules, and (7) utilization of water spray and suction when grinding amalgam.

Minocycline Pigmentation

This type of pigmentation may be found after the treatment of acne with prolonged high doses of minocycline. There may be either diffuse skin pigmentation in sun-exposed areas or pigment deposits in scars, in isolated patches of the legs and feet, in the periorbital skin, in the palate (Fig. 5–23), and on the roots of teeth. In the diffuse form, microscopic changes are found in melanocytes that are more active in pigment production. In the patchy form, macrophages containing iron that is presumably complexed to minocycline in some form are seen.

Other exogenous drugs that may produce pigmentation of oral tissues include aminoquinolines (e.g., chloroquine), cis-platinum, and cyclophosphamide.

Bibliography

Axell T, Hedin C. Epidemiologic study of excessive oral melanin pigmentation with special reference to the influence of tobacco habits. Scand J Dent Res 90:432–442, 1982.

Batsakis J, Regezi J, Solomon A, Rice D. The pathology of head and neck tumors: mucosal melanomas. Head Neck Surg 4:404–418, 1982.

Berthelsen A, Andersen A, Jensen T, Hansen H. Melanomas of the mucosa in the oral cavity and the upper respiratory passages. Cancer 54:907–912, 1984.

Buchner A, Hansen L. Melanotic macule of the oral mucosa: a clinicopathologic study of 105 cases. Oral Surg Oral Med Oral Pathol 48:244–249, 1979.

Buchner A, Hansen L. Pigmented nevi of the oral mucosa: a clinicopathologic study of 36 new cases and review of 155 cases from the literature. Part I: a clinicopathologic study of 36 new cases. Oral Surg Oral Med Oral Pathol 63:566–572, 1987.

Buchner A, Hansen L. Pigmented nevi of the oral mucosa: a clinicopathologic study of 36 new cases and review of 155 cases from the literature. Part II: analysis of 191 cases. Oral Surg Oral Med Oral Pathol 63:676–682, 1987.

Dehner L, Sibley R, Sauk J Jr, et al. Malignant melanotic neuroectodermal tumor of infancy. Cancer 43:1389–1410, 1979.

Fitzpatrick T, Eisen A, Wolff K, Freedberg I, Austen K. Dermatology in General Medicine. McGraw-Hill, New York, 1987, Chaps 79–81.

Regezi J, Hayward J, Pickens T. Superficial melanomas of oral mucous membranes. Oral Surg Oral Med Oral Pathol 45:730–740, 1978.

Rupp N, Paffenbarger G. Significance to health of mercury used in dental practice: a review. J Am Dent Assoc 82:1404–1406, 1971.

Snow G, van der Esch E, van Slooten E. Mucosal melanomas of the head and neck. Head Neck Surg 1:24–30, 1978.

Chapter 6

Verrucal-Papillary Lesions

REACTIVE LESIONS
Papillary Hyperplasia
Condyloma Latum
Squamous Papilloma/Oral Verruca Vulgaris
Condyloma Acuminatum
Focal Epithelial Hyperplasia
NEOPLASMS
Keratoacanthoma
Verrucous Carcinoma
UNKNOWN ETIOLOGY
Pyostomatitis Vegetans
Verruciform Xanthoma

The oral mucosa may be the site of a class of lesions that may be designated verrucal-papillary. The majority of verrucal-papillary lesions are benign exophytic growths capable of arising from any portion of the oral mucosa in both keratinized and non-keratinized areas. A wide range of etiologic factors, including viral, bacterial, fungal, traumatic, and neoplastic, may be implicated in this class of lesions. These lesions range from relatively trivial to potentially life threatening. Clinical differential diagnosis can be rather wide, encompassing many etiologically unrelated conditions.

REACTIVE LESIONS

Papillary Hyperplasia

Etiology. Papillary hyperplasia or palatal papillomatosis appears almost exclusively on the hard palate and almost always in association with a removable prosthesis. A definitive physical relationship with the mucosa covered by a removable denture base is seen; this may be noted in 1 in 10 people who wear appliances that cover the hard palatal mucosa.

The precise cause of papillary hyperplasia arising in the context described is not well understood, although it appears to be associated with ill-fitting or loose dentures that may predispose to or potentiate growth of *Candida albicans* organisms beneath or at the interface of the denture base material and the mucosa. The hyperplastic phenomenon has been related to the presence of the fungal organism in the setting of low-grade chronic trauma.

Clinical Features. The area of mucosa over the palate that tends to be most frequently involved is the vault. Less commonly the alveolar ridge or the palatal incline is affected.

Presentation is characterized by multiple erythematous and edematous papillary projections that are tightly aggregated, producing an overall verrucous granular or "cobblestone" appearance (Fig. 6–1). The projections may be slender and almost villous, although, in a majority of cases, each projection tends to be rounded and blunted, with narrow spaces on either side. Ulceration is rare, although at times intense erythema may provide an overall appearance of erosion. Focal telangiectatic sites may also be noted on occasion.

Histopathology. On perpendicular cross section, the lesion appears as numerous small fronds or papillary projections covered with intact parakeratotic stratified squamous epithelium (Fig. 6–1). The epithelium is supported by hyperplastic central cores of well-vascularized stromal tissue. The epithelium is hyperplastic and often demonstrates pseudoepitheliomatous features, occasionally severe enough

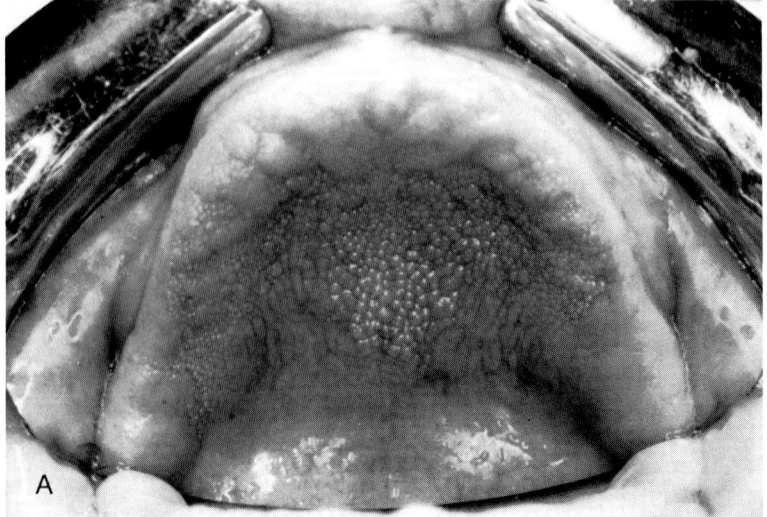
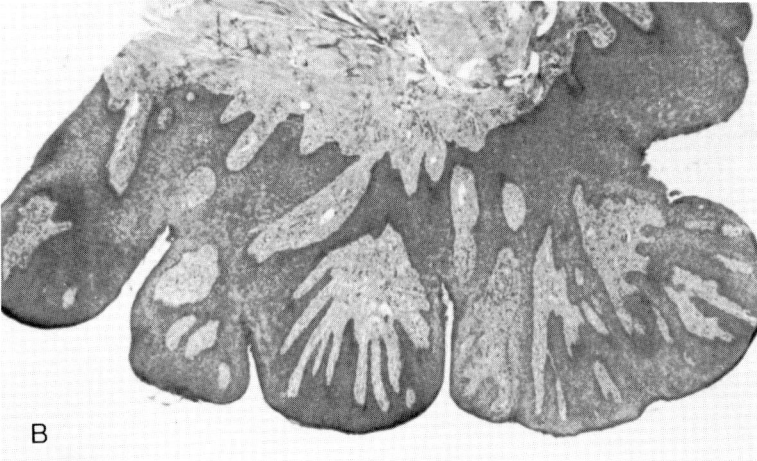

Figure 6–1. *A* and *B*, Papillary hyperplasia of the hard palate.

to mimic squamous cell carcinoma. There is no evidence of dysplasia in association with this lesion, and there is no tendency for malignant transformation.

Differential Diagnosis. The differential diagnosis of papillary hyperplasia of the palate is rather narrow, since this particular entity is seldom confused with other forms of pathology. The chief lesion to be separated from papillary hyperplasia is nicotine stomatitis involving the hard palate; however, nicotine stomatitis does not occur on the hard palate of pipe smokers who wear complete maxillary removable appliances. Also, nicotine stomatitis tends to be more keratinized and usually demonstrates the presence of a small dot or punctum in the center of each nodular excrescence, which represents the orifice of the subjacent minor salivary gland duct. Rarely, in Darier's disease, the mucosa of the palate may demonstrate numerous papules. Multiple squamous papillomas may occur on the palate; however, these lesions tend to be more keratinized with more delicate projections. Finally, in the multiple hamartoma syndrome (Cowden's syndrome), the oral mucosa may exhibit multiple papillary mucosal nodules.

Treatment and Prognosis. Surgical removal is indicated, prior to reconstructing a denture for the patient. The actual surgical method is often a matter of individual preference and may include curettage, cryosurgery, electrosurgery, mucoabrasion, and laser ablation.

Removal of appliances at bedtime and maintenance of good oral hygiene coupled with antifungal therapy may significantly reduce intensity of lesions. In mild cases, utilization of soft tissue conditioning agents and liners, with frequent changing of lining material, can produce sufficient resolution to preclude surgery.

Condyloma Latum

Condyloma latum is one of the many and variable expressions of secondary syphilis. As with all forms of syphilis, cutaneous, mucosal, and systemic lesions that mimic other conditions or diseases can be seen. Characteristic of condyloma latum is the presence of exophytic, sometimes friable, papillary to polypoid lesions within the oral cavity. Condyloma latum contains abundant microorganisms *(Treponema pallidum)*, making it a potential source of infection.

Condyloma latum usually appears on the skin, especially around the anal and the genital areas. Lesions may also be noted within the oral cavity—the tissue involved is formed into a soft, red, often mushroom-like mass with a generally smooth, lobulated surface (Fig. 6–2). It is unlike condyloma acuminatum, which is not covered by a hyperkeratotic or a digitate surface. Within the oral cavity, condyloma latum may be noted at any location.

Microscopically, the overlying epithelium demonstrates significant acanthosis, along with intracellular and intercellular edema and transmigration of neutrophils. A perivascular plasma cell infiltrate is common within the lamina propria in the absence of a true vasculitis.

The patient requires systemic administration of antibiotics to eliminate the underlying bacteremia. The oral lesions will generally regress as the systemic disease is brought under control.

Squamous Papilloma/Oral Verruca Vulgaris

"Oral squamous papilloma" is used as a generic term to include papillary and verrucal growths composed of benign epithelium and minor amounts of supporting connective tissue.

Oral squamous papilloma (including vermilion) is the most common papillary lesion of the oral mucosa, making up approximately 2.5% of all oral lesions. Whether all intraoral squamous papillomas are related etiologically to classic cutaneous verruca vulgaris is unknown. However, at least some oral squamous papillomas have been shown to be associated with the same human papillomavirus (HPV) subtype that causes cutaneous warts (Table 6–1). Other oral papillomas have been associated with different HPV subtypes. Whether all oral papillomas are of viral etiology is open to question. It has recently been shown that the class of human papillomaviruses is very large (over 50 subtypes) and that individually these viruses are associated with many conditions of squamous epithelium. For example, HPV subtypes 2 and 4 have been isolated and demonstrated within cutaneous warts; flat warts of the skin have been identified with HPV subtypes 3 and 10. HPV subtype 11 has been found within papillomas of the sinonasal tract and the oral cavity. HPV subtypes 16 and 18 have been related to neoplastic changes of squamous epithelium.

Etiology. A putative etiologic agent of papillomas of the upper aerodigestive tract is a member of the papovavirus group, currently designated human papillomavirus. This is a DNA virus containing a single molecule of double-stranded DNA. The viruses themselves are non-enveloped icosahedral particles rang-

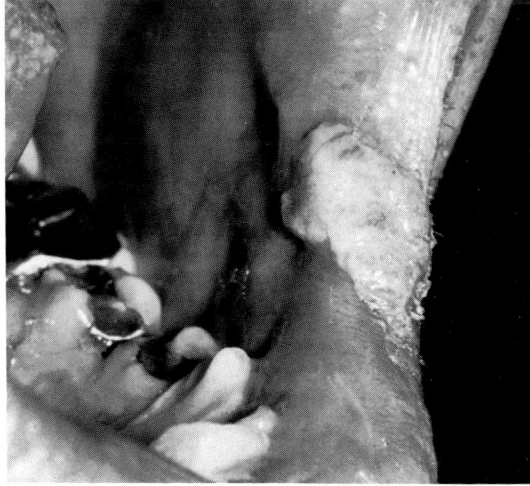

Figure 6–2. Condyloma latum of the commissure. (Courtesy of Dr. C. G. Taylor.)

Table 6–1. LESIONS ASSOCIATED WITH HUMAN PAPILLOMAVIRUS	
Location/Diagnosis	**HPV Subtype**
Oral squamous papilloma (including oral verruca vulgaris)	2, 6, 11
Cutaneous verruca vulgaris	2, 4
Flat warts	3, 10
Condyloma acuminatum	6, 11
Laryngeal papillomas	11
Conjunctival papillomas	11
Focal epithelial hyperplasia	13
Squamous dysplasia/neoplasia	16, 18

ing from 45 to 55 nm in diameter with 72 capsomeres in a skewed arrangement. Various species are antigenically distinct, with some common antigenic determinants shared by many such species. The phases of cell infection are initiated by attachment of the virus to the plasma membrane of the cell prior to its penetration into the cytoplasm by either pinocytosis or fusion with the plasma membrane. Subsequently, the virus is released into the cytoplasm and uncovered. Actual synthesis or replication of HPV occurs within the nuclei of epithelial cells as a result of stimulation of cellular DNA synthesis (Fig. 6–3). The viral genome is expressed in both early and late stages with the host histone proteins being incorporated into the virions. If progeny production is blocked, persistent infection may result. However, if intact viruses in the complete form are produced, new infective viruses can be released with or without cell death.

It has yet to be shown that HPV DNA exists in basal keratinocytes of papillomas. This is probably due to the fact that the number of copies of viral DNA is below the threshold level of detection with current laboratory methods. In studies of cultured keratinocytes from laryngeal papillomas, only about 10 copies of HPV-16 DNA were noted per cell, a level considerably lower than that detectable by autoradiographic techniques.

Infections caused by HPV that are associ-

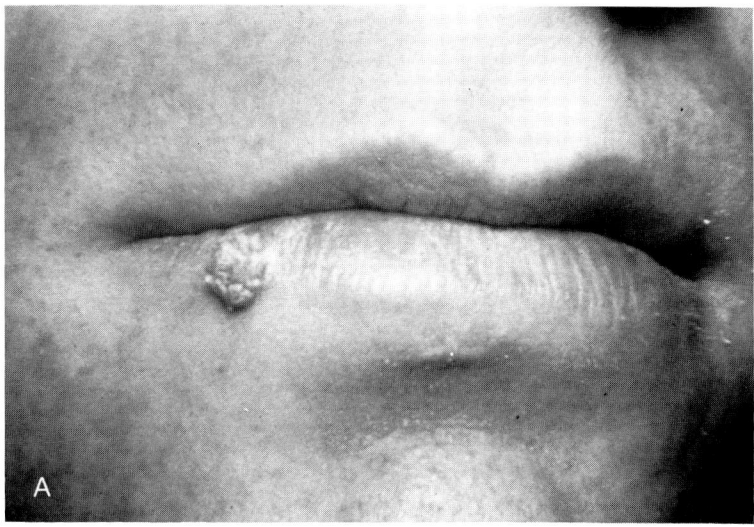
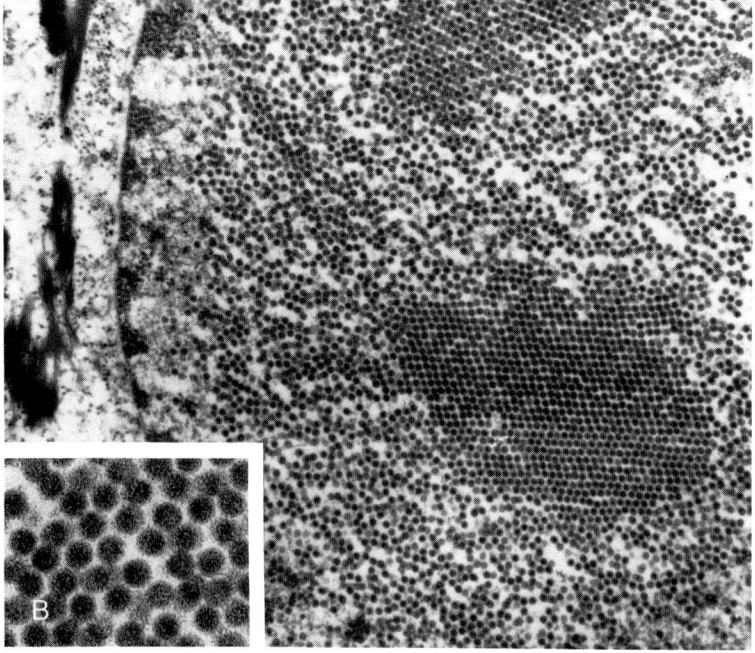

Figure 6–3. *A,* Squamous papillomas (verruca vulgaris) of vermilion. *B,* Electron micrograph of human papillomavirus in nucleus of epithelial cell ($\times$ 33,000; inset, $\times$ 100,000).

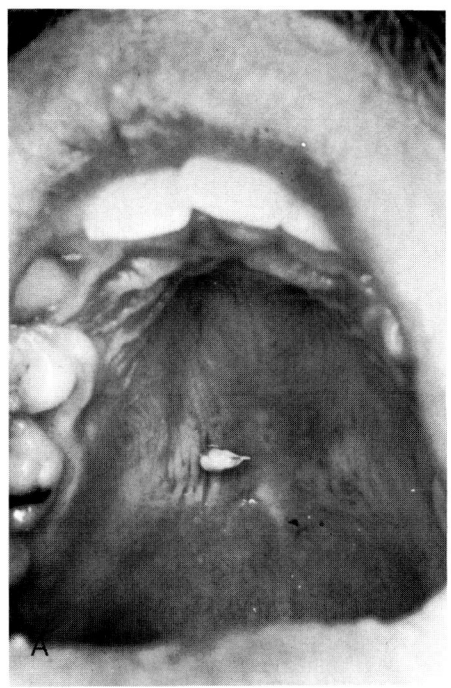
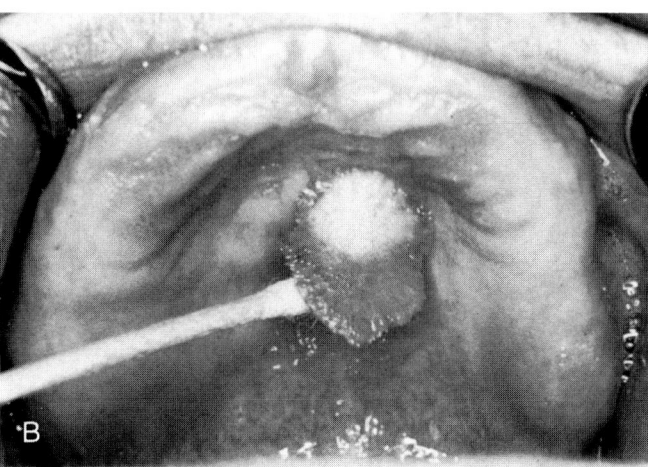

Figure 6–4. *A* and *B*, Squamous papillomas of the palate.

ated with only small quantities of progeny virus show signs of viral growth in the upper layers of the lesion, especially those in the larynx and the oral cavity as well as condyloma acuminatum in the oral and genital regions. The reasons for reduced production of HPV at these sites are unclear.

Clinical Features. Oral squamous papillomas may be found on the vermilion portion of the lips and any intraoral mucosal site, with predilection for the hard and the soft palates and the uvula (Fig. 6–4). The latter three sites account for approximately one third of the lesions found. The soft palate appears to be most commonly affected, with the tongue the site of one fourth of the lesions found, and the lips accounting for approximately 15% of oral squamous papillomas. The lesions themselves generally measure less than 1 cm and appear as exophytic granular to cauliflower-like surface alterations. The lesions generally are solitary in their presentation, although on occasion multiple lesions may be noted. The lesions are generally asymptomatic.

Histopathology. Oral squamous papillomas represent an exaggerated growth of normal squamous epithelial cell components. Extensions of surface epithelium, supported by a well-vascularized connective tissue stroma, project from the free surface of the epithelium (Fig. 6–5). Secondary and tertiary branchings that are covered by orthokeratin or parakeratin, or both, may be seen in approximately 80% of cases. The histologic architecture may on occasion mimic the pattern of the cutaneous wart (Fig. 6–6). Koilocytosis of upper-level epithelial cells may be found. A distinct maturational sequence may be noted from the basal layer through the most superficial cell layers. A variable level of inflammatory cell response or presence may be noted within the lamina propria and the submucosa.

Many oral squamous papillomas demonstrate variable levels of cellular atypia, especially those involving the soft palate and the more posterior areas of the oral cavity. When atypia is present, it seems to be of little importance and in all probability represents an expression of rapid cellular turnover.

Differential Diagnosis. The differential diagnosis of the oral squamous cell papilloma, when solitary, includes verruciform xanthoma, warty dyskeratoma, and condyloma acuminatum. The verruciform xanthoma may resemble the squamous papilloma, although this lesion has a distinct predilection for the gingiva and the alveolar ridge. The warty dyskeratoma, or so-called localized Darier's disease, also resembles the squamous papilloma but generally tends to be multiple in its presentation. The condyloma would be larger than the papilloma and would have a broader base.

Treatment and Prognosis. Although many oral squamous papillomas appear to be virally induced, the infectivity of the HPV must be of a very low order. Route of transmission of the

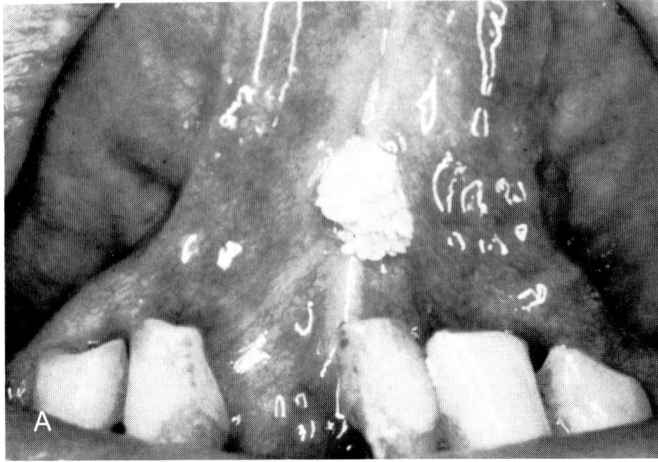
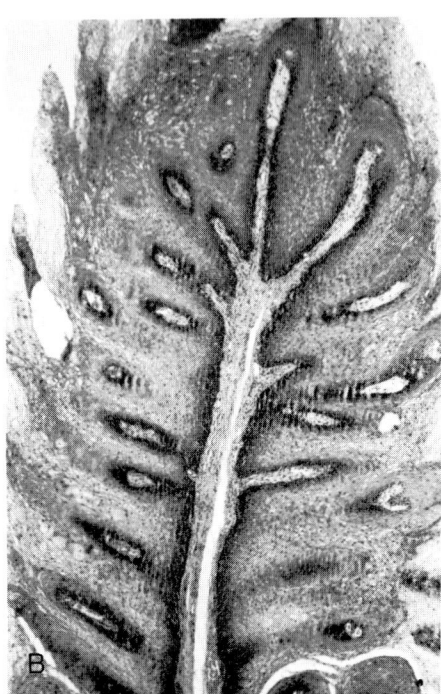

Figure 6–5. *A*, Squamous papilloma of lingual frenum. *B*, Microscopy showing benign epithelium supported by fibrovascular cores.

virus is unknown for oral lesions, although direct contact would be favored.

Surgical removal is the treatment of choice by either routine excision or laser ablation. Recurrence is rare, except for lesions involving the larynx.

Condyloma Acuminatum

Condyloma acuminatum is an infectious lesion that is characteristically located in the anogenital region but may also involve the oral mucosa. Common to these sites is a warm, moist squamous epithelial surface. An increasing frequency of this lesion has been noted within the AIDS group of patients, reflecting an aspect of opportunistic infection.

Etiology and Pathogenesis. Condyloma acuminatum is a verrucous or a papillary growth that has been etiologically related to HPV subtypes 6 and 11. The maturation of the various subtypes of HPV within oral and genital mucosal cells is essentially the same. The keratinized cells act as the natural hosts for the virus, with the replication closely linked to the process of keratinization and altered keratinocyte differentiation.

Clinical Features. Characteristic of early condyloma acuminatum formation is a group of multiple pink nodules that grow and ultimately coalesce. The result is a soft, pedunculated to sessile, exophytic papillary growth that may be keratinized or non-keratinized.

One to three months after viral implantation—presumably as a result of orogenital contact with an infected partner—the disease becomes apparent. The lesions at times may be rather extensive, but they are generally self-limiting. The risk of autoinoculation is a distinct possibility, thus offering a rationale for complete elimination of the lesions.

Histopathology. Papillary projections extending from the base of each lesion are covered by stratified squamous epithelium that is often parakeratotic but at times may be non-keratinized (Fig. 6–7). Upper-level epithelial cells demonstrate nuclei that are pyknotic and crenated, often surrounded by an edematous or optically clear zone forming the so-called koilocytic cell. This cell is felt to be indicative of a virally altered state. The epithelial layer itself is hyperplastic without evidence of premalignancy or dysplastic change. The underlying stroma is well vascularized and may contain a trace of chronic inflammatory cells.

Ultrastructurally, it is often impossible to demonstrate intact virions within the nucleus or the cytoplasm of the presumably infected cells. Numerous degenerative changes are noted, however, including the presence of intranuclear fibrillar or filamentous deposits and significant intranuclear and intracytoplasmic vacuolization.

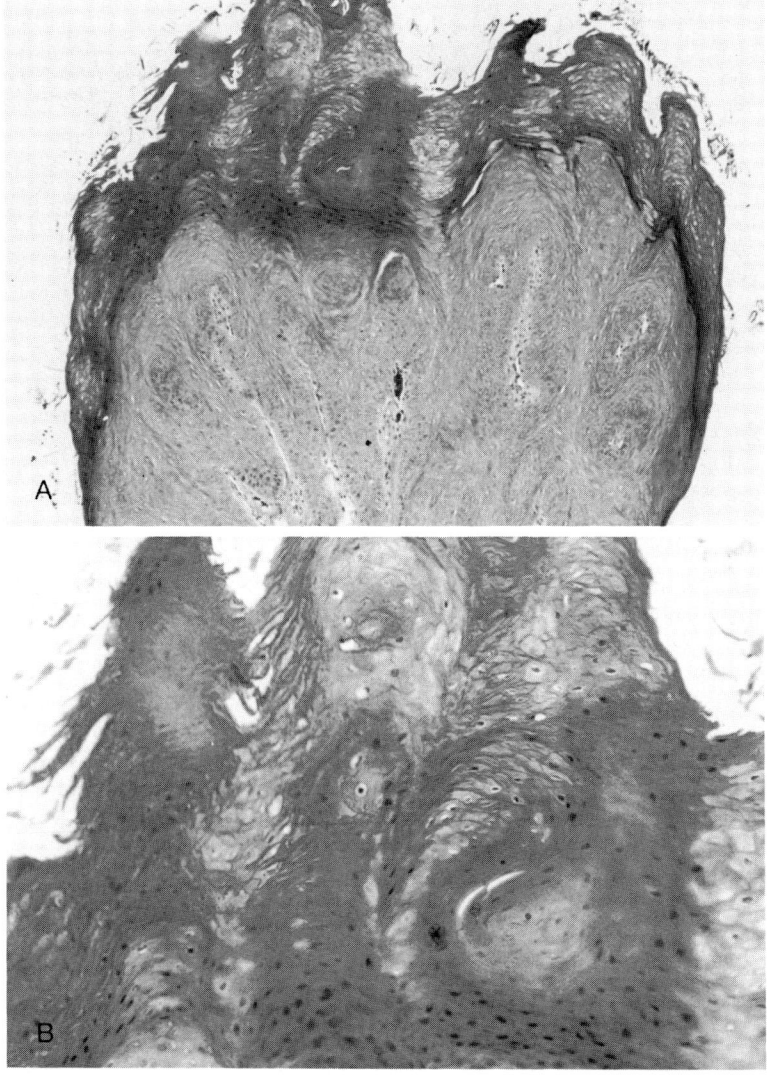

Figure 6–6. *A* and *B*, Oral verruca vulgaris. Note columns of keratin and occasional clear cells (koilocytes).

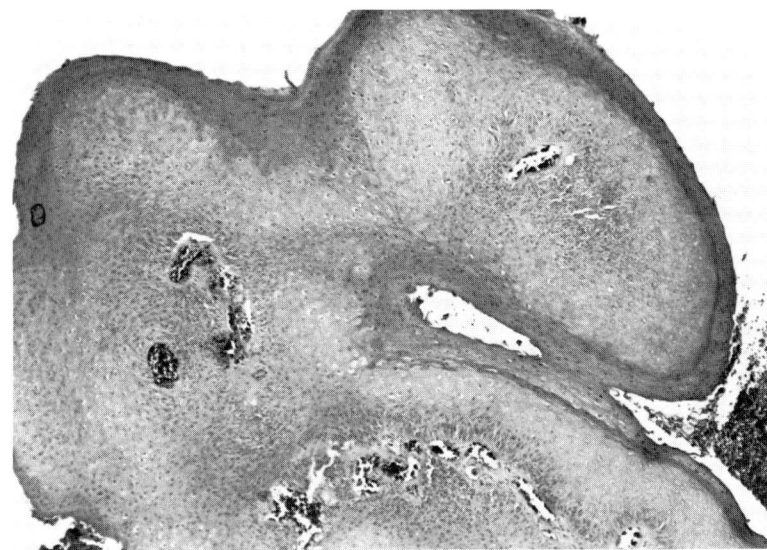

Figure 6–7. Broad papillary fold of condyloma acuminatum.

Differential Diagnosis. Condyloma acuminatum may resemble focal epithelial hyperplasia in some cases. Multiple intraoral verruca vulgaris may be a consideration, indeed representing the same type of infection. There are no universally accepted microscopic features that are capable of delineating condyloma acuminatum from verruca vulgaris. *In situ* DNA hybridization studies may be required to accurately classify these lesions.

Treatment and Prognosis. Treatment for these lesions is generally simple surgical excision, including cryosurgery, scalpel excision, electrodesiccation, and carbon dioxide laser ablation. Recurrences are common, perhaps reflective of the infectious nature of this process in which the surrounding normal-appearing tissue may be harboring the infectious agent. Use of interferon holds promise as an effective new treatment.

Focal Epithelial Hyperplasia

Focal epithelial hyperplasia (Heck's disease) was identified as a distinct entity in 1965, eliminating much confusion about this condition. Former designations for this particular entity included multiple polypous hyperplasias, verruca, and papillomata. Most early studies described lesions in American Indians, in both the United States and Brazil, and in Eskimos. More recent studies have also identified other populations and ethnic groups including South Africans, Mexicans, and Central Americans, as developing this rare disorder.

Etiology and Pathogenesis. The definitive cause of this condition is unknown. Theories ranging from local low-grade irritation to vitamin deficiencies have been proposed. More recently, however, convincing evidence has indicated that HPV subtype 13 plays an important etiologic role. Suggestions that genetic factors are involved have been made but not substantiated.

Clinical Features. This condition is characterized by the presence of multiple nodular soft tissue masses distributed over the mucosal surfaces, especially the buccal mucosa, the labial mucosa, and the tongue. Lesions may appear as discrete papules or as clusters of papules, often similar in color to the surrounding mucosa. If found in areas of occlusal trauma, they may appear whitish. The lesions are asymptomatic and are often discovered incidentally. Initially described in children, this condition is now known to affect a wide age range. An equal gender distribution has also been noted.

Histopathology. Acanthosis and parakeratosis are consistent findings (Fig. 6–8). Prominent clubbing and anastomosis of epithelial ridges with basal orientation is also seen. Enlarged ballooning cells with abnormal nuclear chromatin patterns are often seen within the spinous layer. More superficial elements demonstrate cytoplasmic granular changes and nuclear fragmentation. Cells immediately beneath the surface often show pyknotic nuclei with a surrounding zone of cytoplasmic vacuolization.

Ultrastructurally, crystalline arrangements of virus-like particles may be noted. Such particles measure approximately 50 mm in

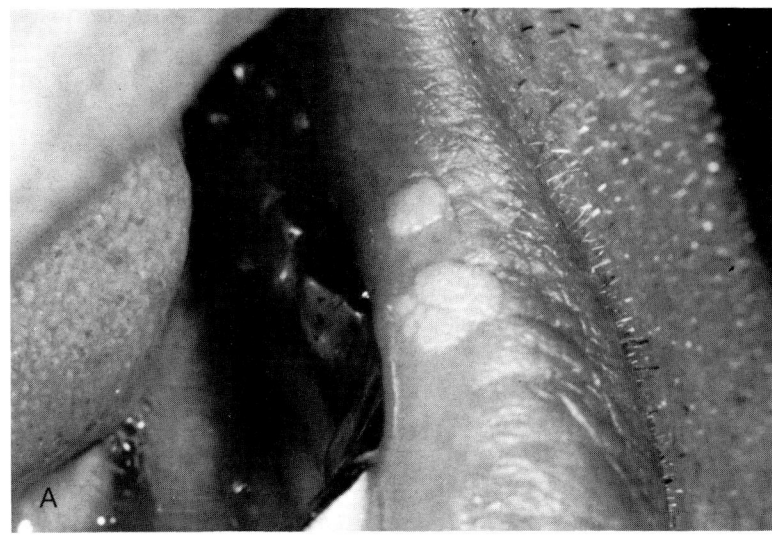

Figure 6–8. *A*, Focal epithelial hyperplasia of the lip. Note acanthosis and parakeratosis in biopsy specimen *(B)*.

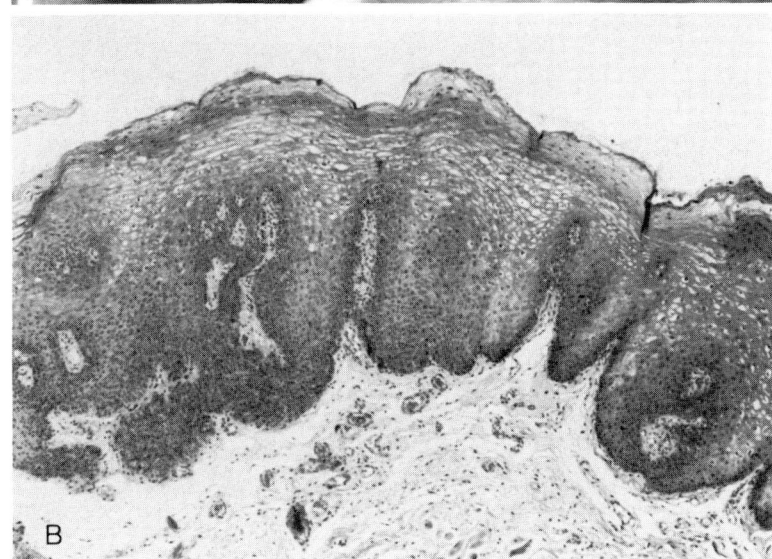

diameter, within the superficial spinous cells. Viruses may be found within the nucleus as well as the cytoplasm of spinous layer cells.

Differential Diagnosis. A differential diagnosis would include verruca vulgaris and multiple squamous papillomas. The oral mucosal lesions of the Cowden or multiple hamartoma syndrome may present similarly and should be ruled out. Additionally, lesions of Darier's disease, oral manifestations of Crohn's disease, and pyostomatitis vegetans might also be considered.

Treatment. No particular treatment is indicated, especially with widespread involvement. Surgical removal may be used if few lesions are present. Of significance is the fact that spontaneous regression has been noted in many cases, perhaps an expression of viral recognition and cell-mediated immunity.

NEOPLASMS

Keratoacanthoma

Etiology. The keratoacanthoma is a benign lesion of unknown cause that occurs chiefly on sun-exposed skin and, far less commonly, at the mucocutaneous junction. Rarely has this lesion been reported to arise on mucous membranes. In skin, the keratoacanthoma originates within the pilosebaceous apparatus, which explains its predominance in skin. The rare intraoral examples suggest that ectopic sebaceous glands may represent the tissue of origin. Virus-like intranuclear inclusions have been described in keratoacanthoma. However, attempts to produce such lesions in experimental animals by inoculation of tumor tissue have been unsuccessful. In addition to sunlight and viruses, suspected etiologic agents include chemical carcinogens, trauma, and genetic factors.

Clinical Features. Keratoacanthomas may be solitary or multiple (Fig. 6–9). The lesion usually begins as a small red macule that soon becomes a firm papule with a fine scale over its highest point. Rapid enlargement of the papule occurs over approximately 4 to 8 weeks, resulting ultimately in a hemispheric, firm, elevated, asymptomatic nodule that contains a central plug of keratin. When fully developed, the keratoacanthoma contains a core of keratin surrounded by a concentric collar of raised skin or mucosa. A peripheral rim of erythema at the lesion base may parallel the raised margin. Generally, there is no evidence of induration and fixation to the underlying structures.

If the lesion is not removed, spontaneous regression occurs. The central keratin mass is exfoliated, leaving a saucer-shaped lesion that heals with scar formation.

Histopathology. Keratoacanthoma is characterized by a central keratin plug with an overhanging lip or a marginal buttress of epithelium (Fig. 6–10). Marked pseudoepitheliomatous hyperplasia is evident, along with an intense mixed inflammatory infiltrate.

Of great importance is the histologic similarity between the keratoacanthoma and a well-differentiated squamous cell carcinoma. Numerous histologic criteria such as high level of differentiation, formation of keratin masses, smooth symmetric infiltration, and abrupt epithelial changes at lateral margins have been used to distinguish keratoacanthoma from carcinoma, but these have proved somewhat inconsistent. Analysis of intraepithelial elastic fibers has been helpful in distinguishing between these two lesions when they occur on sun-exposed skin. Recently, special immuno-

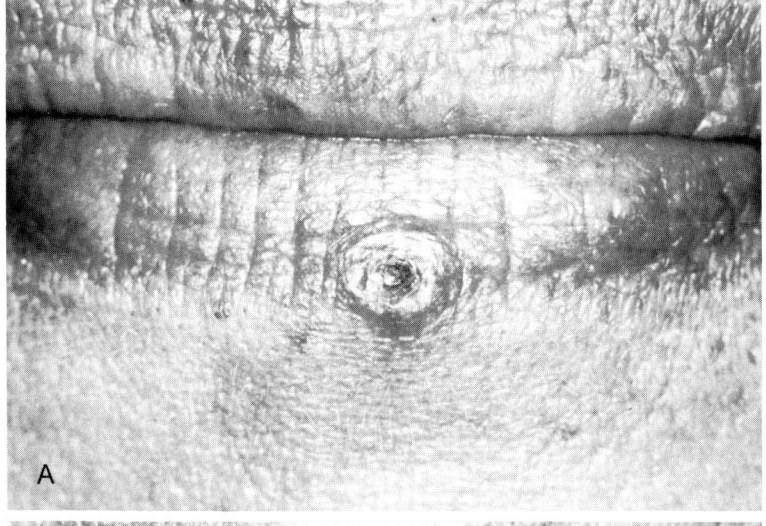
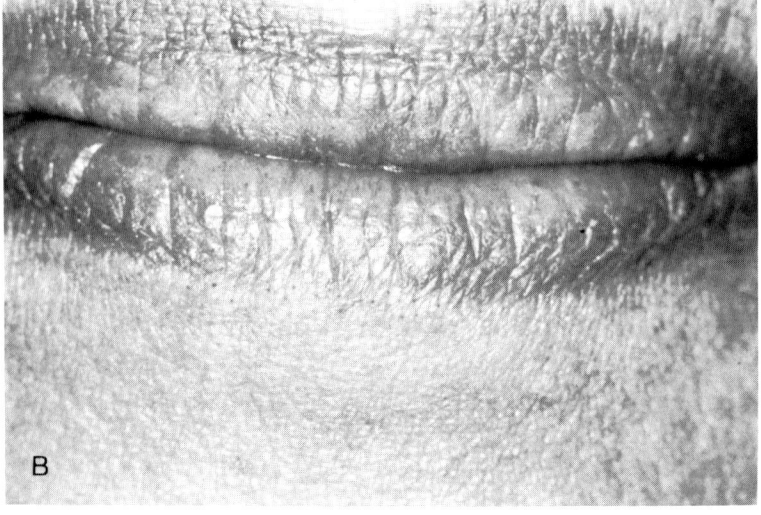

Figure 6–9. *A*, Keratoacanthoma of the lower lip. *B*, Same patient several weeks later showing spontaneous regression of the lesion.

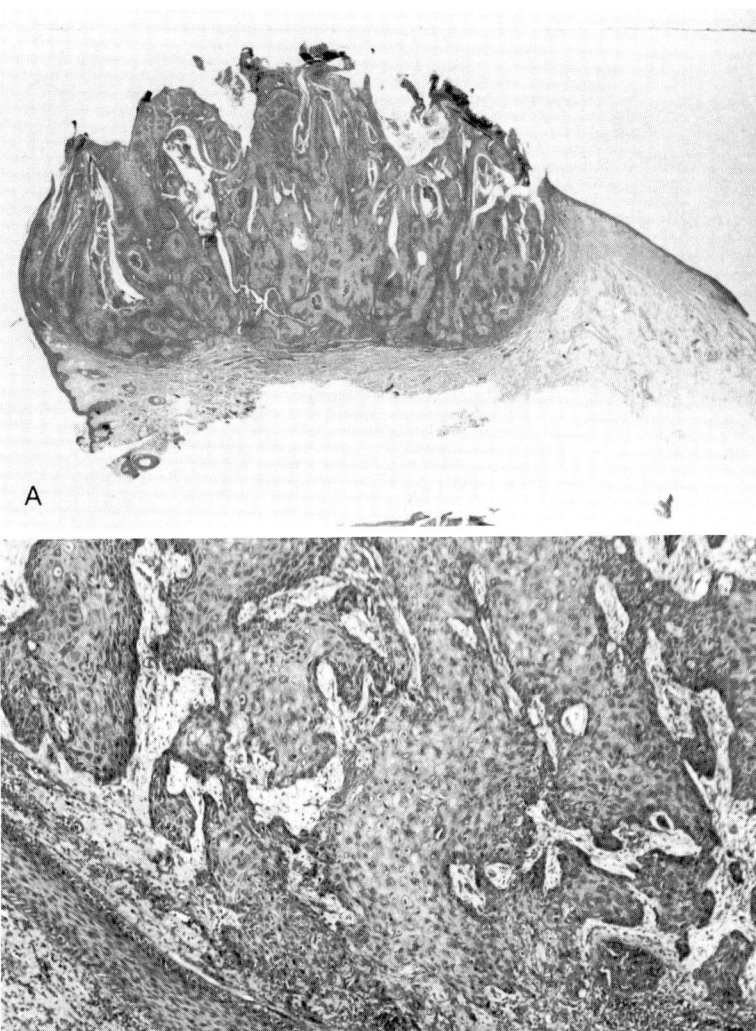

Figure 6–10. *A,* Low magnification of a keratoacanthoma showing its cup-shaped outline and central keratin plug. *B,* The base of a keratoacanthoma exhibiting epithelial proliferation similar to squamous cell carcinoma.

histochemical studies suggest that antigens (e.g., involucrin) that are markers of various levels of differentiation may be useful in microscopic diagnosis of these lesions.

Differential Diagnosis. The primary entity to be distinguished from the solitary keratoacanthoma is the squamous cell carcinoma, from both a clinical and a microscopic perspective. Squamous cell carcinomas have a relatively slow growth rate, are of irregular shape, and generally begin later in life. On the lip, other conditions to be differentiated include molluscum contagiosum, solar keratosis, verruca vulgaris, and warty dyskeratoma. Most of these entities, however, can be easily excluded on the basis of histologic examination of the biopsy specimen.

Treatment and Prognosis. At the least, a very careful follow-up is required in all cases because of the difficulties in diagnosis and distinction from squamous cell carcinoma. Any dubious lesion should be treated, since there are no absolutely reliable diagnostic, clinical, or histologic criteria to differentiate these two lesions. Additionally, during the early phase of this lesion, prediction of its ultimate size may be impossible.

The solitary keratoacanthoma may be removed by surgical excision or by thorough curettage of the base; both methods are equally effective. No recurrence is expected. In cases in which no treatment is accomplished, spontaneous involution is the rule, often with a superficial scar or surface alteration evident.

Verrucous Carcinoma

Since the original description of verrucous carcinoma in 1948, significant confusion has developed regarding assessment and interpretation of the proper diagnostic criteria. As a result, much confusion remains relative to its morphologic, behavioral, and therapeutic characteristics. Recently, a lesion designated as verrucous hyperplasia has been defined in the oral mucosa, adding to the confusion surrounding these verrucal growths. Currently, many believe that on both histologic and clinical grounds verrucous hyperplasia may represent an early biologic form of verrucous carcinoma.

Etiology. Depending upon the site of origin, etiologic factors involved in the initiation of verrucous carcinoma vary. When it appears in the oral cavity, verrucous carcinoma is most closely associated with use of tobacco in various forms, including chewing tobacco and snuff. The possible role of HPV in either a primary or an ancillary relationship awaits elucidation.

Clinical Features. This form of carcinoma accounts for 5% of all intraoral squamous cell carcinomas. The sites of predilection for verrucous carcinoma are highest in the oral cavity and the larynx. Within the oral cavity, the buccal mucosa accounts for over half of all cases, and the gingiva is the location for nearly one third (Table 6–2). The mandibular gingiva shows a slight predominance over the maxillary gingiva. There is a distinct male predominance, and most individuals are over 50 years of age.

Early lesions, which in all probability are represented by the term "verrucous hyperplasia," are relatively superficial by palpation and tend to be white, representing hyperkeratosis. These lesions often arise in clinical leukoplakia with well-demarcated margins. In time, the borders become irregular and more indurated. As fully developed verrucous carcinoma develops, the lesion tends to become exophytic with a whitish to gray shaggy surface (Fig. 6–11). Although not highly infiltrative, the lesion extends into surrounding tissues, and when it involves the gingival tissues, it becomes fixed to the underlying periosteum. If it is untreated, gradual invasion of periosteum and destruction of bone occurs (Fig. 6–12).

Histopathology. At low levels of magnification, surface papillary fronds are seen to be covered by a markedly acanthotic and highly keratinized epithelial surface (Fig. 6–13). Bulbous, well-differentiated epithelial masses extend into the submucosa, with margins that are blunted and pushing rather than narrow and infiltrative. The level of differentiation of

Table 6–2. INTRAORAL SITES OF VERRUCOUS CARCINOMA

Site	Number
Buccal mucosa	101
Gingiva	49
Tongue	12
Floor of mouth	7
Palate	7

From Batsakis JG, Hybels R, Crissman JD, Rice DH, The pathology of head and neck tumors, part 15. Verrucous carcinoma. Head Neck Surg 5:29–38, 1982.

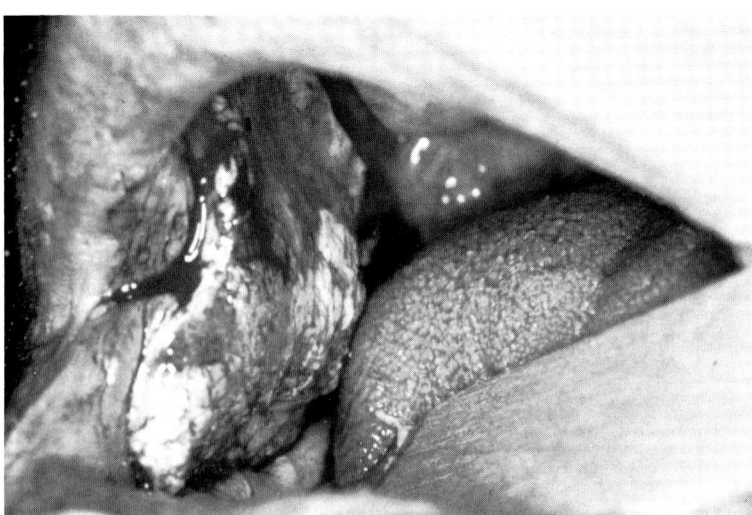

Figure 6–11. Verrucous carcinoma of the buccal mucosa.

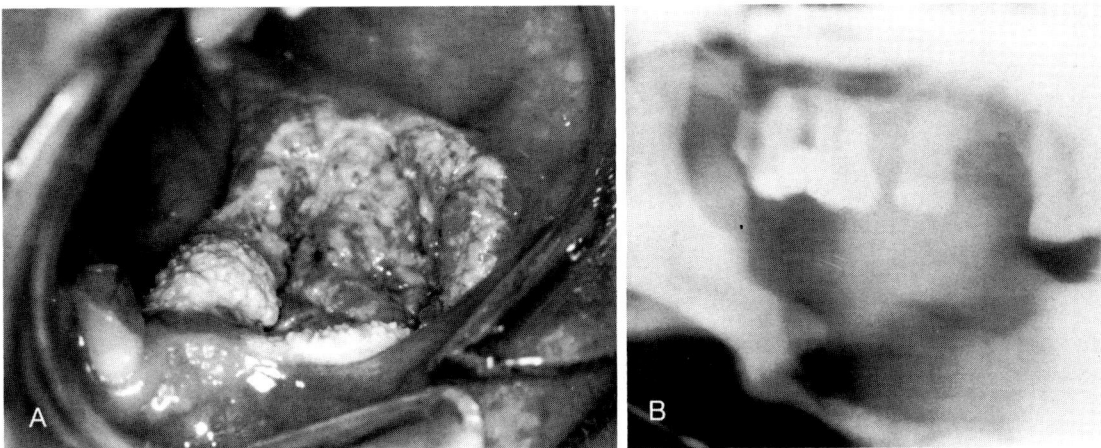

Figure 6-12. *A*, Verrucous carcinoma of alveolar ridge and vestibule. *B*, Invasion of mandible by neoplasm in the same patient.

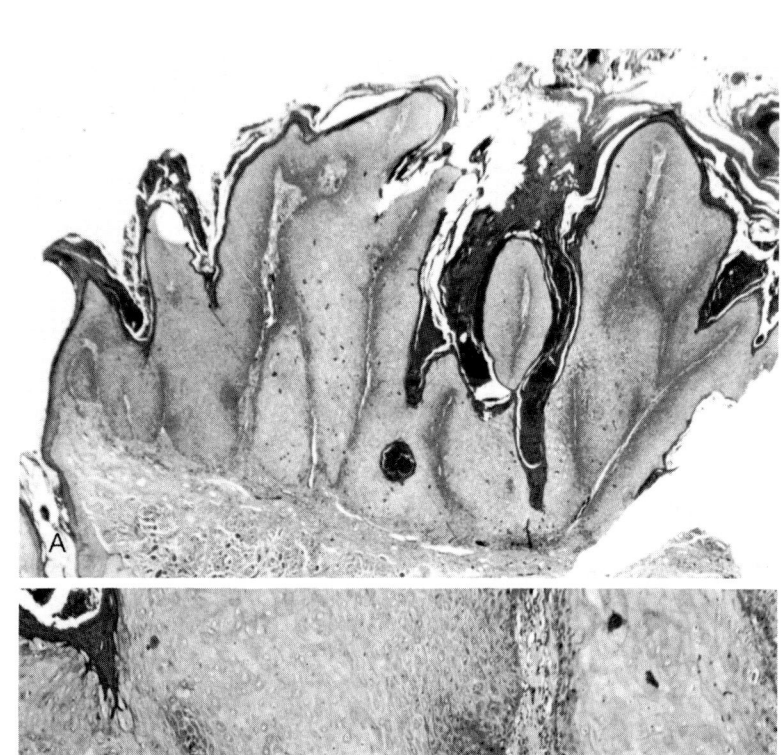

Figure 6-13. *A*, Verrucous carcinoma. *B*, Base of lesion showing well-differentiated blunt margins.

the squamous elements is high. There is an absence of cytologic alteration and significant dysplasia characteristic of other forms of malignancy. Adjacent to the pushing margins of the carcinoma, a rich lymphocytic infiltrate, which at times may show focal areas of acute inflammation surrounding foci of well-formed keratin, is usually found.

Of importance is the absence of anaplasia and a deceptively benign appearance. An acceptable diagnosis can be assured only by providing a biopsy of sufficient depth to evaluate the full thickness of the epithelial component as well as the stromal interface.

Differential Diagnosis. In well-developed cases of verrucous carcinoma, the clinical-pathologic diagnosis is straightforward. However, in less than obvious situations, leukoplakia would be a consideration. Also to be included would be papillary squamous carcinoma, which may be distinguished from verrucous carcinoma by its more infiltrative nature and its more rapid growth. An entity recently described as proliferative verrucous leukoplakia, although at this point not extensively documented, must be included.

Treatment and Prognosis. Surgical methods are generally used as the primary form of therapy in most cases of verrucous carcinoma. This is chiefly due to early reports of frequent anaplastic transformation occurring in verrucous carcinoma following radiotherapy. Recent literature, however, suggests that transformation to an anaplastic state occurs far less frequently than had been reported. Aggressive radiotherapy employed early or in combination with surgery may offer a significant chance of cure.

Regardless of therapeutic method, it is well documented that verrucous carcinoma rarely metastasizes but is locally destructive. In advanced cases in which the maxilla or the mandible exhibits significant destruction, resection is mandated.

The prognosis for verrucous carcinoma is excellent, primarily because of its high level of differentiation and the general rarity of metastatic spread. Local recurrence, however, remains a distinct possibility if inadequate treatment is rendered.

UNKNOWN ETIOLOGY

Pyostomatitis Vegetans

Originally described in 1949, this benign chronic and pustular form of mucocutaneous disease is most often seen in association with inflammatory bowel disease. In two of the three original patients with oral lesions, the lesions were confined to the oral mucosa. The etiology of pyostomatitis vegetans is unknown, although it may be seen in association with ulcerative colitis, spastic colitis, chronic diarrhea, and Crohn's disease.

Clinical Features. Early in the evolution of pyostomatitis vegetans, the oral mucosa appears erythematous and edematous, often thrown into deep folds, especially in the buccal mucosal region. Multiple pustules, ranging from 2 to 3 mm in diameter, and small vegetating papillary projections may be seen. Oral mucosal involvement may include gingiva, hard and soft palates, buccal and labial mucosa, lateral and ventral tongue, and floor of the mouth. Males are affected nearly twice as often as females, and the age range is generally between the third and sixth decades, with an average age of 34 years. Laboratory values are generally within normal limits, although in many patients peripheral eosinophilia or anemia may be noted.

Histopathology. The oral mucosa demonstrates hyperkeratosis and pronounced acanthosis, often in a papillary surface configuration or with attending pseudoepitheliomatous hyperplasia. A pronounced inflammatory infiltrate composed of neutrophils and eosinophils is a constant finding. Superficial abscesses may be seen within the lamina propria, with extension into the parabasal regions of the overlying epithelium. Ulceration and superficial epithelial necrosis may also be noted.

Treatment and Prognosis. The management of this entity relates to controlling the associated bowel disease. Topical agents, such as corticosteroids, may be used intraorally. Additionally, antibiotics, multivitamins, and nutritional supplements may be employed; however, all are associated with variable and ultimately dismal results. Remission of oral lesions reflects control of the underlying bowel disease and serves as a specific mucosal marker for the process.

Verruciform Xanthoma

The verruciform xanthoma is an uncommon oral mucosal lesion that is benign and that occasionally may be found on the skin as well. The etiology is obscure, although it has recently been suggested that this entity belongs in a category of immunologic disorders characterized by the presence of large numbers of Langerhans cells.

Clinical Features. Clinically, the verruciform xanthoma of the oral cavity is well circumscribed, with a granular to papillary surface. A wide range in size from 2 mm to over 2 cm has been reported. Either an exophytic or a depressed surface is present, and occasionally the lesion may be ulcerated. The level of keratinization of the surface will influence its color, which ranges from white to red.

The majority of cases have been reported in whites; there is no gender predilection. The average age is 45 years, with a few cases reported within the first and second decades. The lesions are usually discovered incidentally, although occasional cases have been reported in which a long history is noted, often years in duration.

Histopathology. Lesions may be flat or slightly raised with a papillomatous or verrucous surface composed of parakeratinized epithelial cells (Fig. 6–14). Uniformly invaginated crypts alternate with papillary extensions. Elongated epithelial ridges extend into the lamina propria at a uniform level or depth. The epithelial component is normal with no evidence of dysplasia or atypia.

The most characteristic feature is the presence of numerous foam or xanthoma cells within the lamina propria or connective tissue papillae. Characteristic of the foam cells is a granular to flocculent cytoplasm that may contain periodic acid–Schiff (PAS) positive, diastase-resistant granules or lipid droplets, or both. Ultrastructurally, the foam cells are best characterized as macrophages. Occasionally, the foam cells may extend deeper into the lamina propria, intermingling with the inflammatory cells that are usually present. Recent

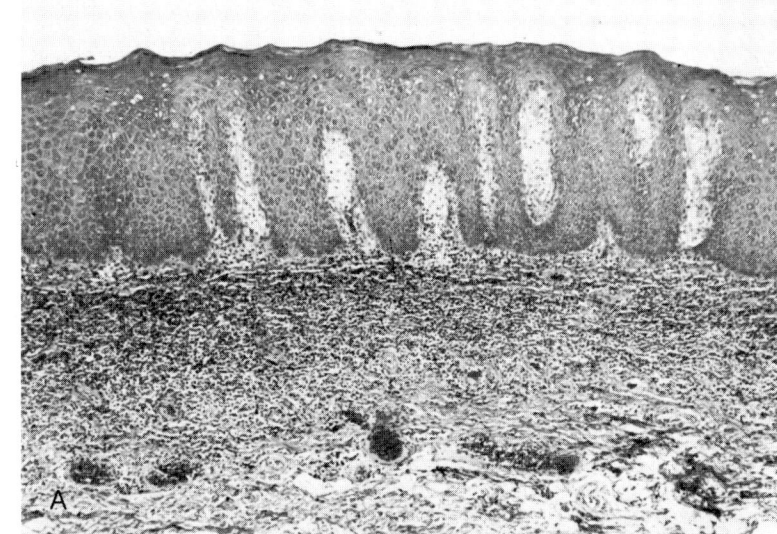

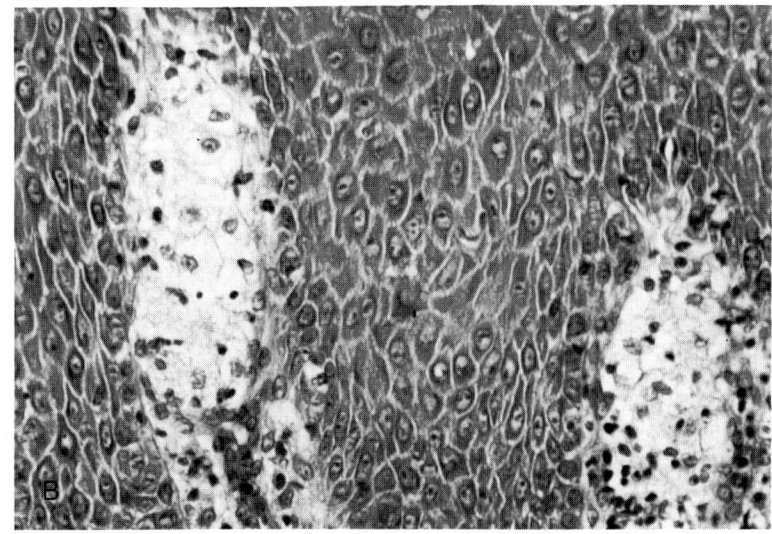

Figure 6–14. *A* and *B*, Verruciform xanthoma. Note pale xanthoma cells in the lamina propria.

immunohistochemical studies have demonstrated the presence of Langerhans cells, suggesting an immunologic participation in histogenesis.

Differential Diagnosis. A differential diagnosis for this entity includes squamous papilloma, papillary squamous carcinoma, and condyloma acuminatum. When multiple lesions are noted, focal epithelial hyperplasia may be considered.

Treatment. The treatment is conservative excision. No recurrences have been reported.

Bibliography

Papillary Hyperplasia

Gorlin RJ, Peterson WC. Warty dyskeratoma: a note concerning its occurrence on the oral mucosa. Arch Dermatol 95:292–293, 1967.

Swart JGN, Lekkas C, Allard RHB. Oral manifestations in Cowden syndrome. Oral Surg Oral Med Oral Pathol 59:264–268, 1985.

Condyloma Latum

De Swaan B, Tjiam KH, Vuzevski VD, et al. Solitary oral condyloma lata in a patient with secondary syphilis. Sex Transm Dis 12:238–240, 1985.

Manton SL, Egglestone SI, Alexander I, et al. Oral presentation of secondary syphilis. Br Dent J 160:237–238, 1986.

Squamous Papilloma/Oral Verruca Vulgaris

Batsakis JG, Raymond AK, Rice DH. The pathology of head neck tumors: papillomas of the upper aerodigestive tract, part 18. Head Neck Surg 5:332–344, 1983.

Brandsma J, Abramson A, Sciubba JJ, et al. Papillomavirus infection of the nose. In Steinberg B, Brandsma J, Taichman LB (eds). Papillomaviruses. Cold Spring Harbor Laboratory, Cold Spring Harbor, New York, 1987, pp 301–308.

Eversole LR, Laipis PJ, Green TL. Human papillomavirus type 2 DNA in oral and labial verruca vulgaris. J Cutan Pathol 14:319–325, 1987.

Green TL, Eversole LR, Leider AS. Oral and labial verruca vulgaris: clinical, histological, and immunohistochemical evaluation. Oral Surg Oral Med Oral Pathol 62:410–416, 1986.

Lutzner M, Kuffer R, Blanchet-Bardon C, et al. Different papillomaviruses as causes of oral warts. Arch Dermatol 118:393–397, 1982.

McNab J, Walkinshaw S, Cordiner J, et al. Human papillomavirus in clinically and histologically normal tissue of patients with genital cancer. N Engl J Med 315:1052–1058, 1986.

Scully C, Prime S, Maitland N. Papillomaviruses: their possible role in oral disease. Oral Surg Oral Med Oral Pathol 60:166–174, 1985.

Syrjanen S, Syrjanen K, Lamberg M. Detection of human papillomavirus DNA in oral mucosal lesions using in situ DNA-hybridization applied on paraffin sections. Oral Surg Oral Med Oral Pathol 62:660–667, 1986.

Taichman LB, LaPorta RF. The expression of papillomaviruses in epithelial cells. In Salzman NP, Howley PM (eds). The Papovaviridae, vol 2. Plenum, New York, 1987, pp 109–139.

Condyloma Acuminatum

Eron L, Judson F, Tucker S, et al. Interferon therapy for condyloma acuminata. N Engl J Med 315:1059–1064, 1986.

Marquard JV, Racey GL. Combined medical and surgical management of intraoral condyloma acuminatum. J Oral Surg 39:459–461, 1981.

Silverman S Jr, Migliorati CA, Lazada-Nur F, et al. Oral findings in people with or at high-risk for AIDS: a study of 375 homosexual males. J Am Dent Assoc 112:187–192, 1986.

Steinberg BM, Topp WC, Schneider PS, et al. Laryngeal papillomavirus infection during clinical remission. N Engl J Med 308:1261–1264, 1983.

Summers L, Booth DR. Intraoral condyloma acuminatum. Oral Surg 38:273–278, 1974.

Focal Epithelial Hyperplasia

Pfister H, Hettich I, Runne V, et al. Characterization of human papilloma virus type 14 from focal epithelial hyperplasia (Heck) lesions. J Virol 47:363–366, 1983.

Praetorius-Clausen F. Rare oral viral disorders molluscum contagiosum, localized keratoacanthoma, verrucae, condyloma acuminatum, and focal epithelial hyperplasia. Oral Surg 34:604–618, 1972.

Van Wyck CW, Staz J, Farman AG. Focal epithelial hyperplasia in a group of South Africans: its ultrastructural features. J Oral Pathol 6:14–24, 1977.

Keratoacanthoma

Ellis GL. Differentiating keratoacanthoma from squamous cell carcinoma of the lower lip: an analysis of intraepithelial elastic fibers and intracytoplasmic glycogen. Oral Surg Oral Med Oral Pathol 56:527–532, 1983.

Rook A, Whimster I. Keratoacanthoma: a 30-year retrospect. J Am Acad Dermatol 100:41–47, 1979.

Smoller BR, Kwan TH, Said JW, et al. Keratoacanthoma and squamous cell carcinoma of the skin: immunohistochemical localization of involucrin and keratin proteins. J Am Acad Dermatol 14:226–234, 1986.

Sumitomo S, Kumasa S, Iwai Y, et al. Involucrin expression in epithelial tumors of oral and pharyngeal mucosa and skin. Oral Surg Oral Med Oral Pathol 62:155–163, 1986.

Svirsky JA, Freedman PD, Lumerman H. Solitary intraoral keratoacanthoma. Oral Surg 43:116–122, 1977.

Verrucous Carcinoma

Ackerman LV. Verrucous carcinoma of the oral cavity. Surgery 23:670–678, 1948.

Batsakis JG, Hybels R, Crissman JD, et al. The pathology of head and neck tumors, part 15. Verrucous carcinoma. Head Neck Surg 5:29–38, 1982.

Burns HP, van Nostrand AWP, Palmer JA. Verrucous carcinoma of the oral cavity: management by radiotherapy and surgery. Can J Surg 23:19–25, 1980.

Hansen LS, Olson JA, Silverman S Jr. Proliferative verrucous leukoplakia. A long-term study of 30 patients. Oral Surg Oral Med Oral Pathol 60:285–298, 1985.

McDonald JS, Crissman JD, Gluckman JL. Verrucous carcinoma of the oral cavity. Head Neck Surg 5:22–28, 1982.

Perez CA, Kraus FT, Evans JC, et al. Anaplastic transformation of verrucous carcinoma of the oral cavity after radiation therapy. Radiology 86:108–115, 1966.

Schwade JG, Wara WM, Dedo HH, et al. Radiotherapy for verrucous carcinoma. Radiology 120:677–679, 1976.

Shear M, Pindborg JJ. Verrucous hyperplasia of the oral mucosa. Cancer 46:1855–1861, 1980.

Pyostomatitis Vegetans

Cataldo E, Covino MC, Tesone PE. Pyostomatitis vegetans. Oral Surg 52:172–177, 1981.

Hansen LS, Silverman S Jr, Daniels TE. The differential diagnosis of pyostomatitis vegetans and its relations to bowel disease. Oral Surg Oral Med Oral Pathol 55:363–373, 1983.

Neville BW, Laden SA, Smith SE, et al. Pyostomatitis vegetans. Am J Dermatopathol 7:69–77, 1985.

Van Hale HM, Rogers RS III, Zone JJ, et al. Pyostomatitis vegetans. A marker for inflammatory disease of the gut. Arch Dermatol 121:94–98, 1985.

Verruciform Xanthoma

Neville B. The verruciform xanthoma. A review and report of eight new cases. Am J Dermatopathol 8:247–253, 1986.

Nowparast B, Howell FV, Rick GM. Verruciform xanthoma. A clinicopathologic review and report of 54 cases. Oral Surg 51:619–625, 1981.

Rowden D, Lovas G, Shafer W, et al. Langerhans cells in verruciform xanthomas: an immunoperoxidase study of ten oral cases. J Oral Pathol 15:48–53, 1986.

Santa Cruz DJ, Martin SA. Verruciform xanthoma of the vulva. Report of two cases. Am J Clin Pathol 71:224–228, 1979.

Van der Waal I, Kerstens HCJ, Hens CJJ. Verruciform xanthoma of the oral mucosa. J Oral Maxillofac Surg 43:623–626, 1985.

Chapter 7

Connective Tissue Lesions

FIBROUS CONNECTIVE TISSUE LESIONS
Reactive Hyperplasias
   Pyogenic Granuloma and Peripheral Giant Cell Granuloma
   Peripheral Fibroma
   Generalized Gingival Hyperplasia
   Traumatic Fibroma
   Denture-Induced Fibrous Hyperplasia
Neoplasms
   Myxoma
   Juvenile Nasopharyngeal Angiofibroma
   Nodular Fasciitis
   Fibromatosis
   Fibrosarcoma
   Benign Fibrous Histiocytoma
   Malignant Fibrous Histiocytoma
VASCULAR LESIONS
Reactive Lesions
   Venous Varix
Congenital Lesions
   Hemangioma
   Lymphangioma
Neoplasms
   Hemangiopericytoma
   Angiosarcoma
   Kaposi's Sarcoma
NEURAL LESIONS
Reactive Lesions
   Traumatic Neuroma
Neoplasms
   Granular Cell Tumors
   Schwannoma
   Neurofibroma
   Mucosal Neuromas of Multiple Endocrine Neoplasia Syndrome, Type III
   Neurogenic Sarcoma
   Esthesioneuroblastoma
LESIONS OF MUSCLE AND FAT
Reactive Lesions
   Myositis Ossificans
Neoplasms
   Leiomyoma and Leiomyosarcoma
   Rhabdomyoma and Rhabdomyosarcoma
   Lipoma and Liposarcoma

FIBROUS CONNECTIVE TISSUE LESIONS

Reactive Hyperplasias

This is a group of fibrous connective tissue lesions that commonly occur in oral mucosa secondary to injury. The group represents a chronic process in which there is overexuberant repair (granulation tissue and scar) following, occasionally, a single causative event such as trauma or, more likely, following continued low-grade injury. As a group, these lesions present as submucosal masses that may become secondarily ulcerated when traumatized during mastication. Their color ranges from lighter than the surrounding tissue (because of a relative increase in collagen) to red (because of an abundance of well vascularized granulation tissue). Because nerve does not proliferate with the reactive hyperplastic tissue, these lesions are painless. The reason for the overexuberant repair is unknown. Treatment is generally surgical excision and removal or modification of the irritating factor.

Although these are all pathogenically related lesions, different names or subdivisions have been devised because of variations in anatomic site, clinical appearance, or microscopic picture. Those lesions that present as prominent red masses are discussed in Chapter 4.

Pyogenic Granuloma and Peripheral Giant Cell Granuloma

These conditions are discussed in detail in Chapter 4.

Peripheral Fibroma

Clinical Features. By definition, this reactive hyperplastic mass occurs in the gingiva and may be derived from connective tissue of the submucosa or the periodontal ligament (Fig. 7–1). Some lesions may represent a "mature" pyogenic granuloma in which the granulation tissue has been largely replaced by collagen. It may occur at any age, although it does have a predilection for young adults. Females develop these lesions more commonly than do males, and the gingiva anterior to the permanent molars is most frequently affected.

The peripheral fibroma presents clinically as either a pedunculated or a sessile mass that is similar in color to the surrounding connective tissue. Ulceration may be noted over the summit of the lesion. It rarely causes erosion of subjacent alveolar bone.

Histopathology. The peripheral fibroma is a focal fibrous hyperplasia that may also be called hyperplastic scar. It is highly collagenous and relatively avascular and may contain a mild to moderate chronic inflammatory cell infiltrate. This is basically the gingival counterpart to the traumatic fibroma occurring in other mucosal regions.

Microscopically, several subtypes of this lesion have been identified. These are essentially of academic interest, since biologic behavior and treatment of these microscopic variants are the same.

The *peripheral ossifying fibroma* is a gingival mass in which calcified islands, presumed to be bone, are seen (Fig. 7–2). The bone is

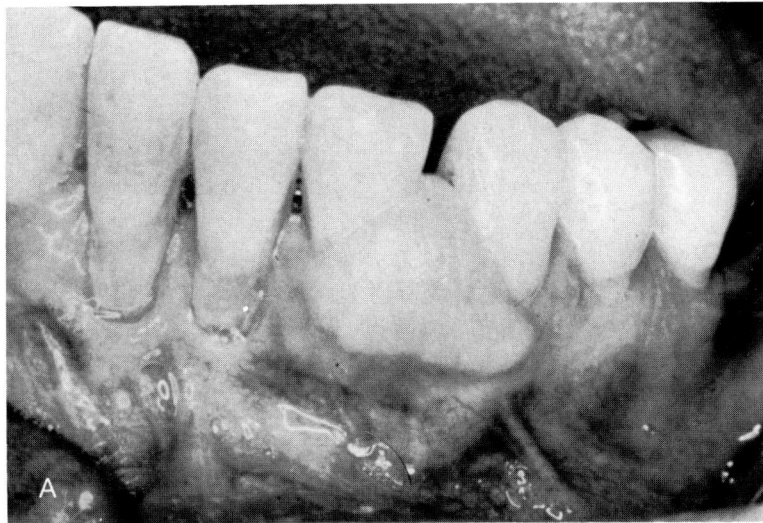
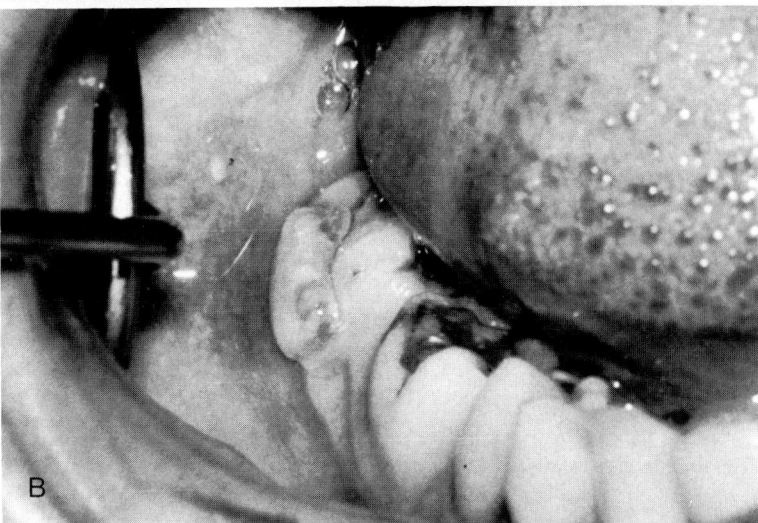

Figure 7–1. *A*, Peripheral fibroma. *B*, Peripheral fibroma with ossification.

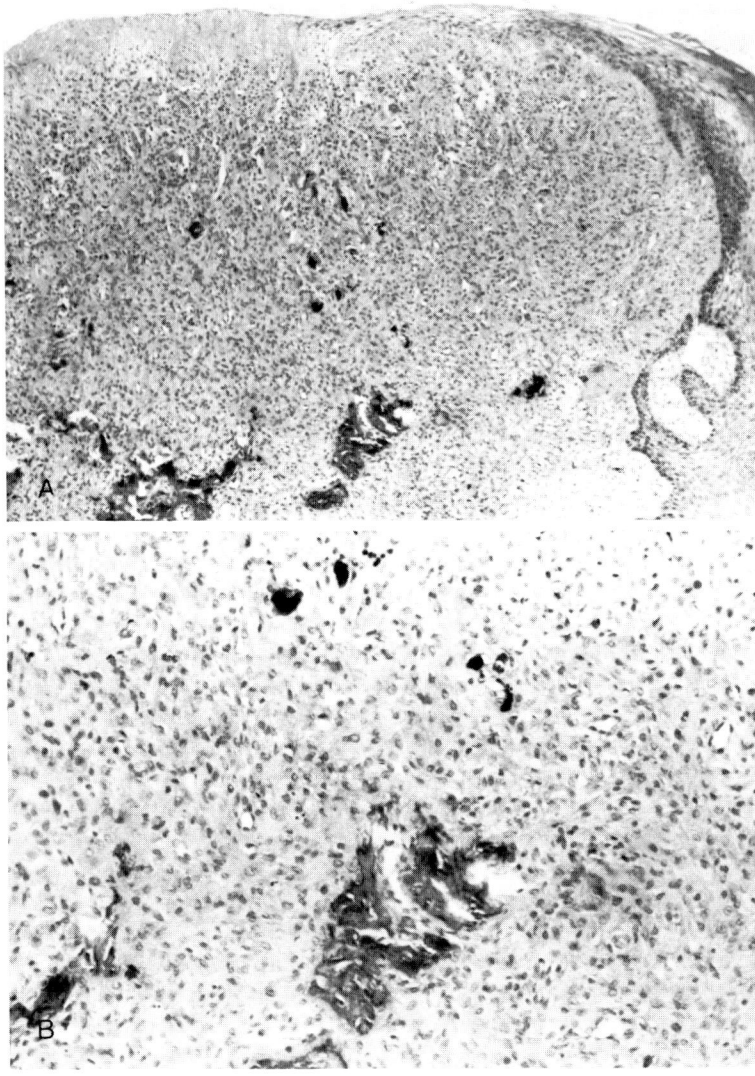

Figure 7-2. Peripheral fibroma with ossification. Low magnification *(A)* showing surface ulceration. High magnification *(B)* of ossification area showing benign fibroblasts.

found within a non-encapsulated proliferation of plump benign fibroblasts. Chronic inflammatory cells tend to be seen around the periphery of the lesion. The surface is often ulcerated.

The *peripheral odontogenic fibroma* is a gingival mass composed of well-vascularized fibrous connective tissue. The distinguishing feature of this variant is the presence of strands of odontogenic epithelium, often abundant, throughout the connective tissue (Fig. 7-3). The lesion is usually non-ulcerated.

The so-called *giant cell fibroma* is a focal fibrous hyperplasia in which fibroblasts, many of which are multinucleated, assume a stellate shape (Figs. 7-4 and 7-5). These same peculiar fibroblasts can also be found in focal fibrous hyperplastic lesions throughout the oral mucosa and occasionally on the skin (fibrous papule).

Differential Diagnosis. Clinically, these lesions are usually not confused with anything else. There may, however, be some overlap with pyogenic granuloma and, rarely, peripheral giant cell granuloma, when these two lesions do not have a prominent vascular component.

Treatment. Peripheral fibroma should be treated by local excision that should include the periodontal ligament, if involved. Also, any identifiable etiologic agent, such as calculus or other foreign material, should be removed. Recurrence may occasionally be associated with the microscopic subtype peripheral ossifying fibroma, but this is usually not a significant problem.

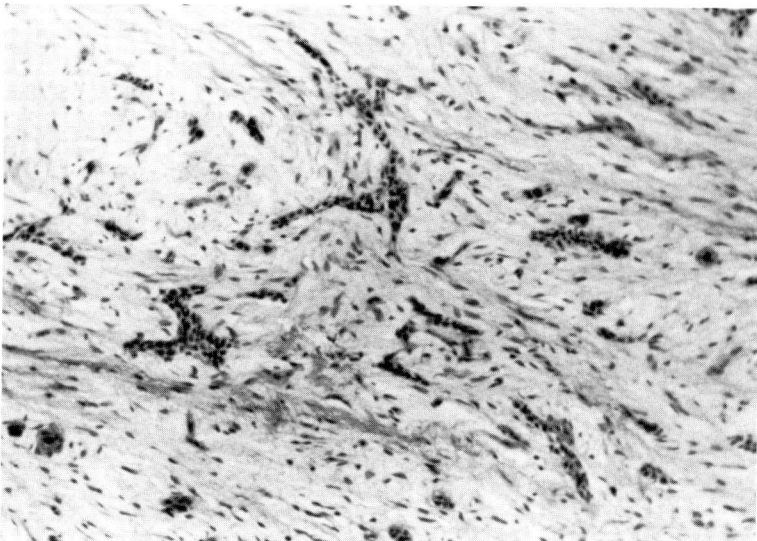

Figure 7–3. Peripheral odontogenic fibroma. Note numerous strands of odontogenic epithelium.

Generalized Gingival Hyperplasia

Etiology. In this form of gingival enlargement, overgrowth may vary from mild enlargement of interdental papillae to such severe uniform enlargement that the crowns of the teeth may be covered by hyperplastic tissue. Uniform or generalized gingival fibrous connective tissue hyperplasia may be due to one of several etiologic factors. Most cases are nonspecific and are a result of an unusual hyperplastic tissue response to chronic inflammation associated with local factors such as plaque, calculus, or bacteria (Fig. 7–6). Why only some patients have a propensity for the development of connective tissue hyperplasia in response to local factors is unknown.

Other conditions such as hormonal changes and drugs can significantly potentiate or exaggerate the effects of local factors on gingival connective tissue. Hormonal changes occurring during pregnancy and puberty have long been known to be associated with generalized gingival hyperplasia. The hyperresponsiveness during pregnancy has led to the infrequently used and inappropriate term "pregnancy gingivitis." Altered hormonal conditions act in concert with local irritants to produce the hyperplastic response. It is questionable whether significant gingival enlargement during periods of hormonal imbalance would be seen in individuals with scrupulous oral hygiene.

Phenytoin (Dilantin), the drug used in the

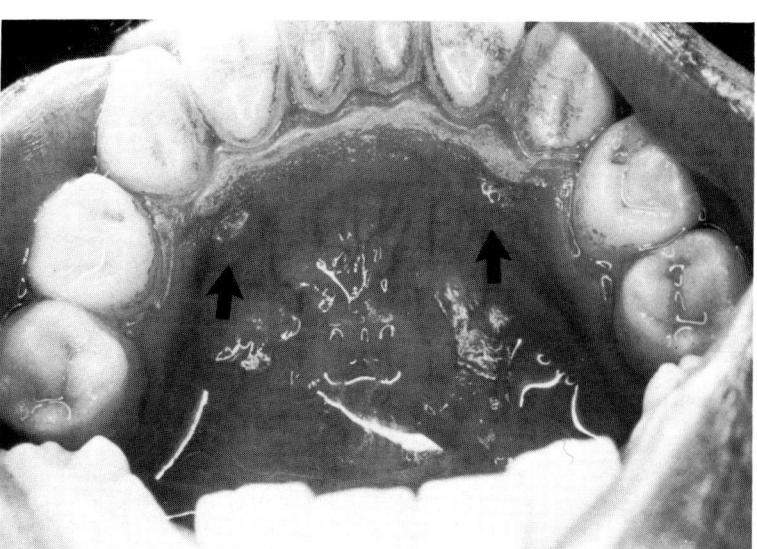

Figure 7–4. Peripheral fibroma (arrows), "giant cell" type.

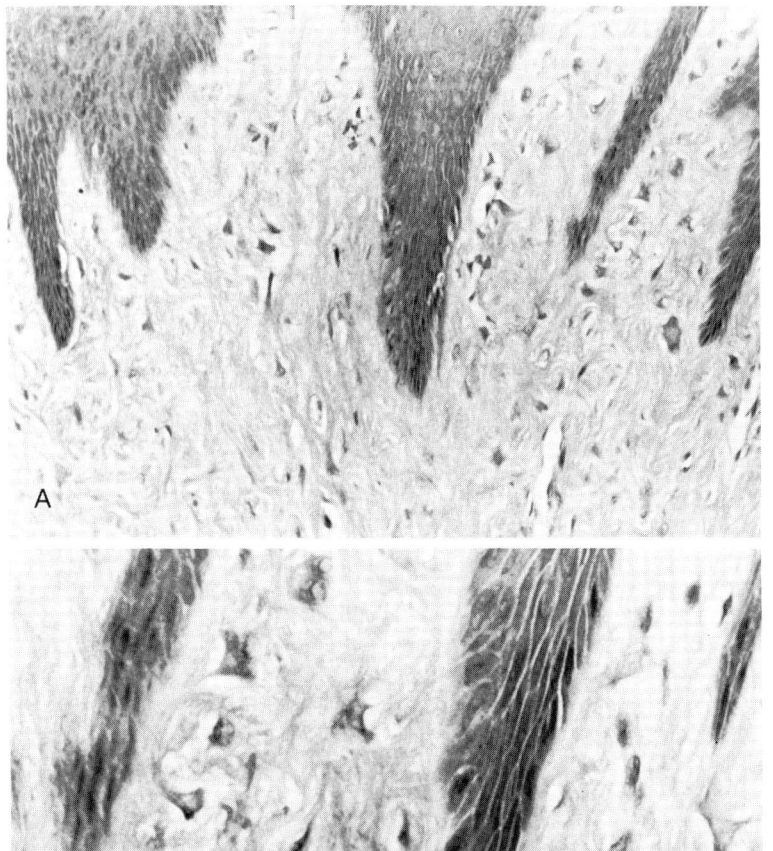
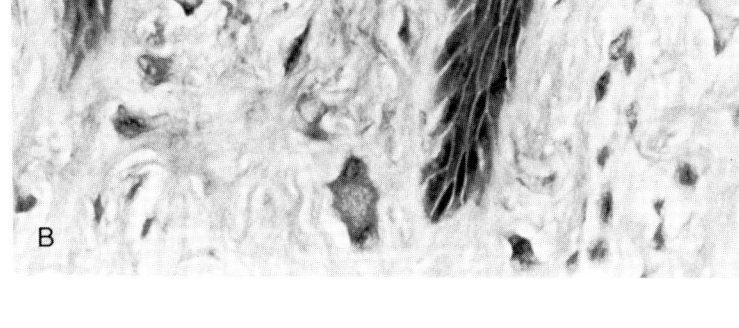

Figure 7–5. *A* and *B*, Peripheral fibroma, "giant cell" type. Note stellate and multinucleated fibroblasts.

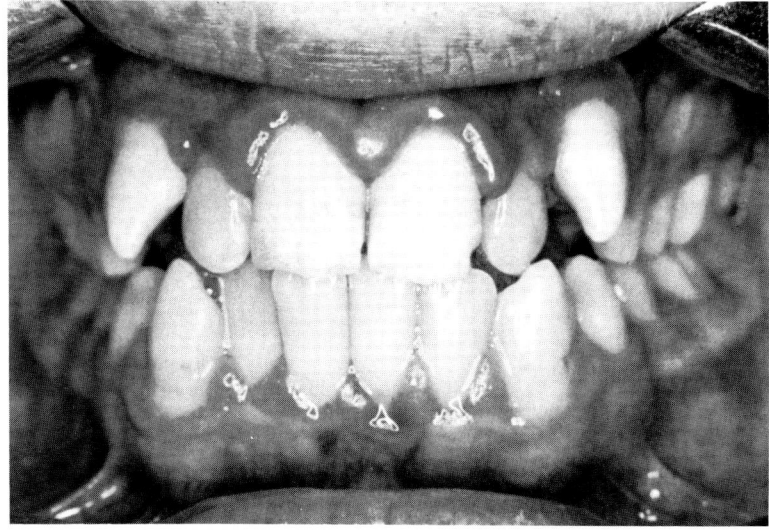

Figure 7–6. Generalized gingival hyperplasia due to reaction to local factors.

control of seizure disorders, is a well-known etiologic factor in generalized gingival enlargement (Fig. 7–7). The extent or severity of so-called *Dilantin hyperplasia* is dependent upon the presence of local factors. The effect of time and dosage of drug on gingival tissue is not clear. The reported prevalence of this condition has ranged from 0 to 80%, depending upon the investigator's clinical criteria and the number of patients observed. A 50% figure is generally accepted as the probable level of prevalence. In any event, the fact that not all patients taking Dilantin develop gingival hyperplasia indicates that some patients are predisposed to the development of this condition. It has only rarely been described in edentulous patients and children prior to tooth eruption. The mechanism by which the drug causes fibrous hyperplasia is unclear, although the drug appears to have a regulating effect on fibroblast enzymes or growth rate. All fibroblasts are thought to be susceptible to the drug to some degree. The exaggerated response of gingival fibroblasts is probably related to the influence of concomitant inflammation.

A side effect of another drug, *cyclosporine*, has more recently been linked to fibrous hyperplasia of the gingiva. Cyclosporine is an immunosuppressive drug that is used to suppress T lymphocyte function in transplant patients and in patients with various autoimmune diseases. It may also find use in the treatment of alopecia because of another of its side effects, hirsutism. Although the drug is chemically unrelated to phenytoin (Dilantin), there are many clinical gingival parallels. Not all patients are affected (10 to 70%), local factors play a synergistic role, and clinical appearance

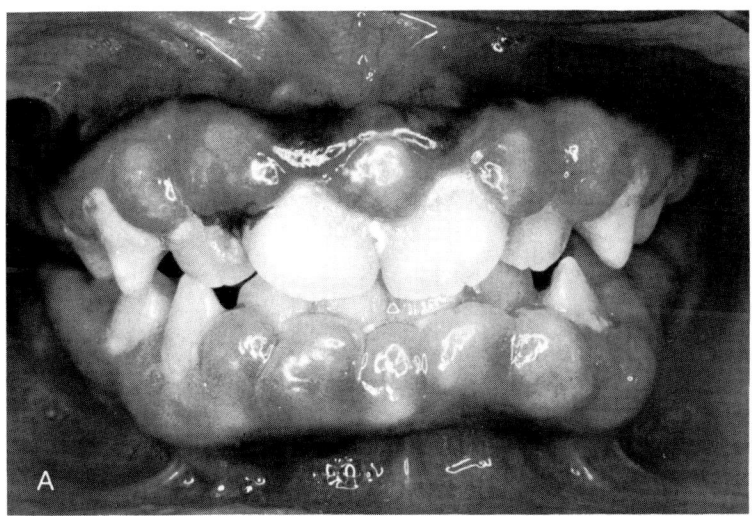

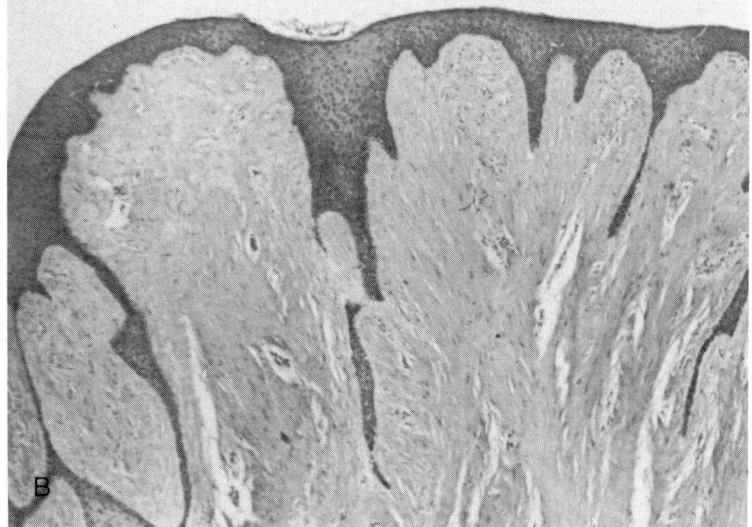

Figure 7–7. *A* and *B*, Generalized gingival hyperplasia, phenytoin (Dilantin) induced. Note dense collagen making up bulk of the enlargement.

is similar. Unlike Dilantin hyperplasia, cyclosporine-induced hyperplasia is a reversible process following cessation of drug use.

Gingival enlargement is also known to occur in patients with leukemia, especially those with the monocytic type. This is believed to be the result of infiltration of the gingival soft tissues by malignant white blood cells (WBCs). This may also be due, totally or in part, to reactive fibrous hyperplasia caused by local factors (Fig. 7–8). Because of the bleeding tendency associated with leukemia, patients may be reluctant to practice good oral hygiene, resulting in accumulation of plaque and debris. This accumulation may provide the inflammatory stimulus for connective tissue hyperplasia.

Another form of gingival enlargement, appearing early in childhood, is known as *idiopathic hyperplasia* or *hereditary gingival fibromatosis* (Fig. 7–9). In this rarely seen condition, some patients have a hereditary predisposition, whereas others have no apparent genetic link.

Clinical Features. The clinical feature common to the variously caused gingival hyperplasias is an increase in the bulk of the free and attached gingiva, especially the interdental papillae. Stippling is lost, and gingival margins become rolled and blunted. Consistency will range from soft and spongy to firm and dense, depending directly upon the degree of fibroplasia. A range of color from red-blue to lighter than surrounding tissue is also seen; this depends upon the severity of the inflammatory response as well. Generally, the hyperplasias associated with non-specific local factors and hormonal changes will appear more inflamed clinically than the drug-induced and

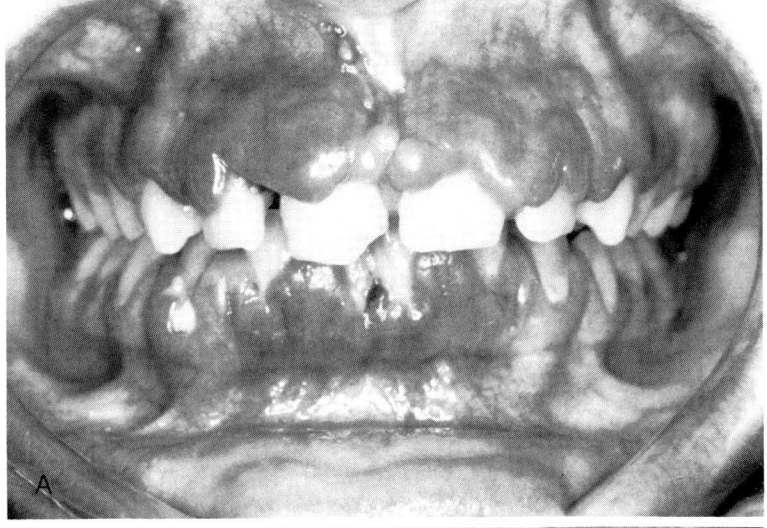
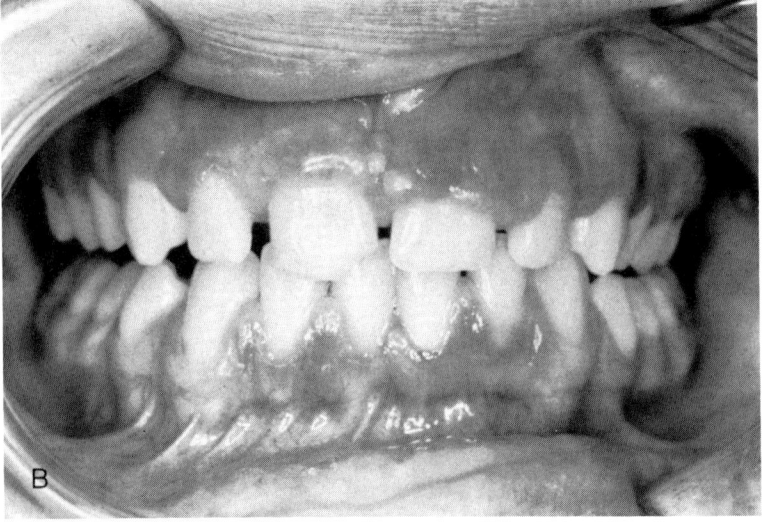

Figure 7–8. *A*, Generalized gingival hyperplasia in a leukemic patient. *B*, Same patient after prophylaxis and improved home care.

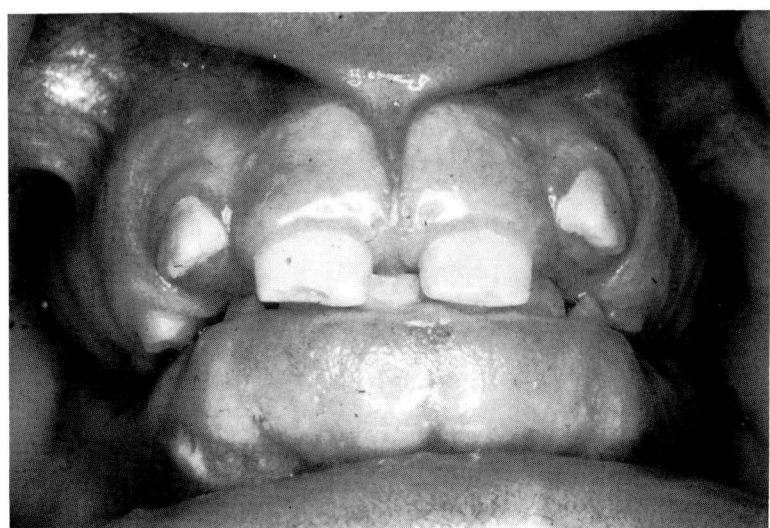

Figure 7–9. Generalized gingival hyperplasia, idiopathic type.

the idiopathic forms. The idiopathic type is particularly dense and fibrous, with relatively little inflammatory change.

Histopathology. The microscopic picture of gingival hyperplasia is one in which abundant collagen deposition dominates. Fibroblasts are increased in number, and varying degrees of chronic inflammation are seen. In some cases, especially those in which hormonal changes are important, capillaries may be increased and prominent. The overlying epithelium will usually exhibit some hyperplasia. In leukemic enlargements, atypical and immature WBCs, representing a malignant infiltrate, may be seen.

Treatment. In all forms of generalized gingival hyperplasia, good oral hygiene is necessary to minimize the effects of inflammation on fibrous proliferation and the effects of systemic factors. Gingivoplasty or gingivectomy may be required but should be done in combination with prophylaxis and oral hygiene instruction.

Traumatic Fibroma

Etiology. Traumatic fibroma, also known as irritation fibroma, focal fibrous hyperplasia, and hyperplastic scar, is a reactive lesion caused usually by chronic trauma to oral mucous membranes. Overexuberant fibrous connective tissue repair results in a clinically evident submucosal mass.

Clinical Features. There is no gender or racial predilection for the development of this intraoral lesion. It is a very common reactive hyperplasia that is typically found in frequently traumatized areas, such as buccal mucosa, lateral border of the tongue, and lower lip (Fig. 7–10). It is a painless, broad-based swelling that is lighter than the surrounding tissue, because of its relative lack of vascular channels. The surface may occasionally be traumatically ulcerated, particularly in larger lesions. Traumatic fibromas have limited growth potential, usually not exceeding 1 cm in diameter and rarely greater than 2 cm.

Histopathology. Collagen overproduction is the basic process that dominates the microscopy of this lesion (Fig. 7–11). Fibroblasts are mature and widely scattered in a dense collagen matrix. Sparse chronic inflammatory cells may be seen, usually in a perivascular distribution. Overlying epithelium is often thinned and hyperkeratotic, because of chronic low-grade friction.

Differential Diagnosis. This is a relatively trivial lesion that should be removed to rule out other pathologic processes. Depending upon location, several other entities might be included in a clinical differential diagnosis of small, asymptomatic submucosal masses. Neurofibroma, neurilemoma, and granular cell tumor would be possibilities for masses in the tongue. In the lower lip and buccal mucosa, lipoma, mucocele, and salivary gland tumors might be considered. Although rare, benign neoplasms of mesenchymal origin could present as submucosal masses not unlike the traumatic fibroma.

Treatment. Simple surgical excision is usually effective. Infrequently, recurrences may be caused by continued trauma to the involved area. These lesions have no malignant potential.

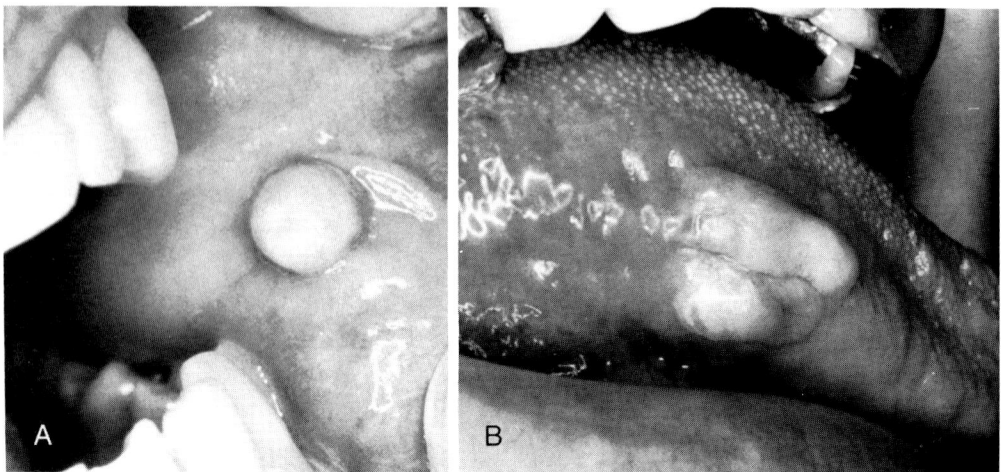

Figure 7–10. *A* and *B*, Traumatic fibromas.

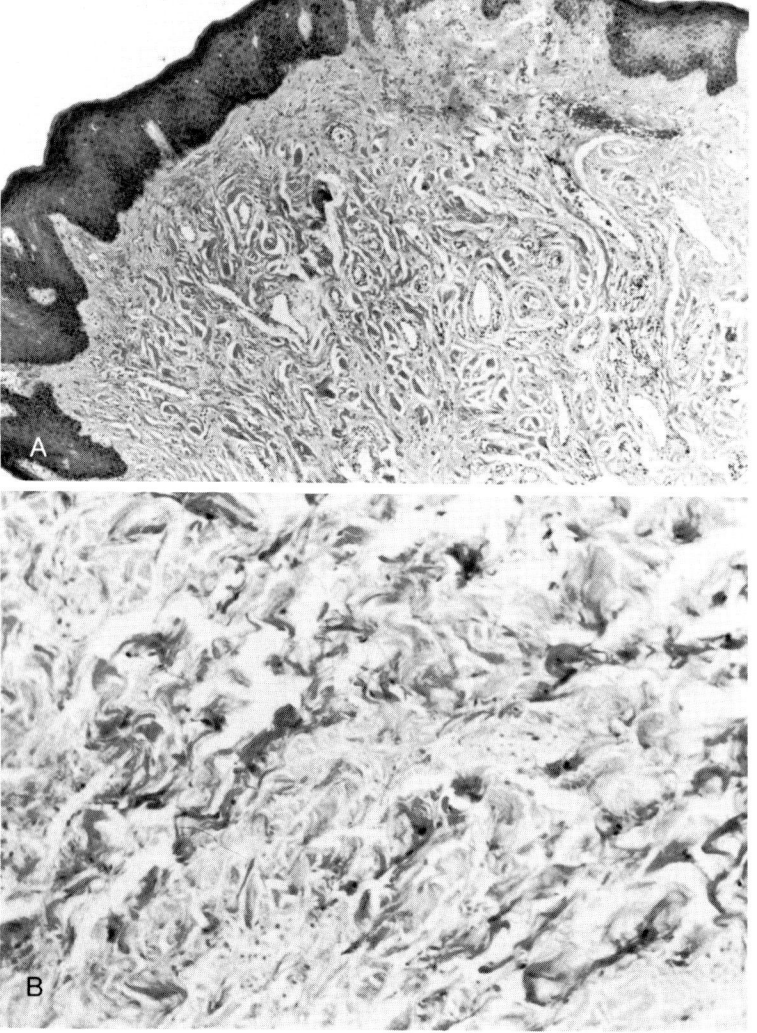

Figure 7–11. *A* and *B*, Traumatic fibroma. Lesion is composed of dense collagen.

Denture-Induced Fibrous Hyperplasia

Etiology. This fibrous hyperplasia of oral mucosa is related to the chronic trauma produced by an ill-fitting denture. It is essentially the same process that leads to the traumatic fibroma, except that a denture is specifically identified as the causative agent. This lesion has also been designated by the outdated synonyms "inflammatory hyperplasia," "denture hyperplasia," and "epulis fissuratum."

Clinical Features. Denture-induced fibrous hyperplasia is a common lesion that occurs in the vestibular mucosa where the denture flange contacts tissue (Figs. 7–12 and 7–13). As the bony ridges of the mandible and the maxilla resorb with long-term denture use, the flanges gradually extend farther into the vestibule. There, chronic irritation and trauma may incite an overexuberant fibrous connective tissue reparative response. The result is the appearance of painless folds of fibrous tissue surrounding the overextended denture flange.

Treatment. Some reduction in size of the lesion may follow prolonged removal of the denture. However, because the hyperplastic scar is relatively permanent, surgical excision is usually required. Construction of a new denture or relining of the old one is also required to prevent recurrences.

Neoplasms

Myxoma

Clinical Features. The oral soft tissue myxoma is a rare lesion that presents as a slow-growing, asymptomatic submucosal mass. There appears to be no gender predilection, and the lesion may occur at any age. Myxomas have been reported in all oral locations, although the palate is most frequently affected.

Oral myxomas have been reported in an autosomal dominantly inherited syndrome consisting of myxomas, spotty mucocutaneous pigmentation (similar to Peutz-Jeghers syndrome), and endocrine abnormalities. Of greatest significance is the occurrence of cardiac myxoma, which may be life threatening because of its growth potential in this vital organ. Young patients with a diagnosed oral myxoma should be considered at risk for the syndrome if they have multiple or recurrent lesions and perioral pigmentation.

Histopathology. Oral myxomas are not encapsulated and may exhibit infiltration of surrounding soft tissue. Dispersed stellate and spindle-shaped fibroblasts are found in a loose myxoid stroma (Fig. 7–14). With the use of special stains, collagen fibers appear relatively sparse, and reticulin fibers are apparent. Inflammatory cells are generally not seen within the tumor mass.

Differential Diagnosis. As an asymptomatic uninflamed mass in mucous membrane, myxomas are usually regarded clinically as mucoceles or traumatic fibromas. Ordinarily, myxomas would not be included in a differential diagnosis of soft submucosal masses, because of their rarity.

Microscopically, soft tissue myxomas may be confused with several other myxoid lesions. Included in a microscopic differential diagnosis would be nerve sheath myxoma and oral focal mucinosis (Table 7–1). Secondary considerations might also be given to myxoid lipoma,

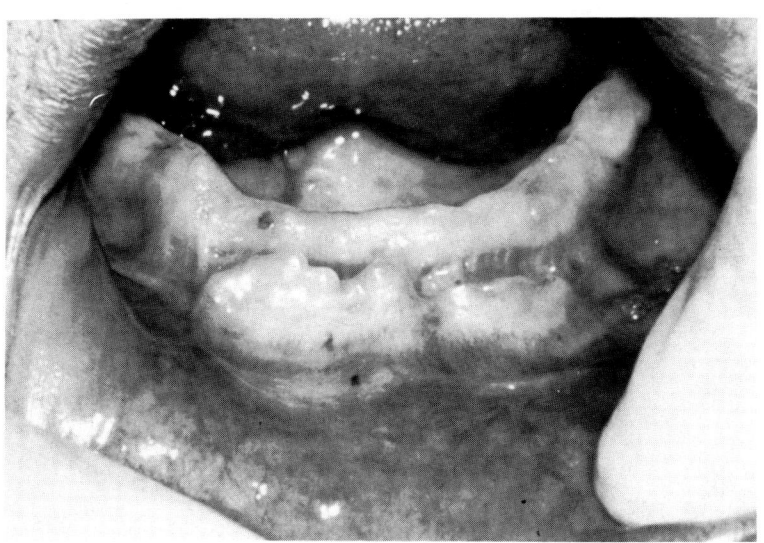

Figure 7–12. Denture-induced fibrous hyperplasia of anterior vestibule.

194 CONNECTIVE TISSUE LESIONS

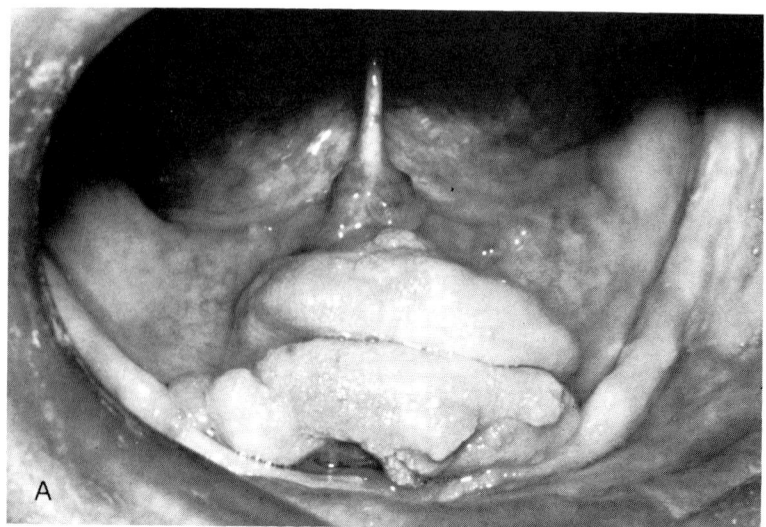

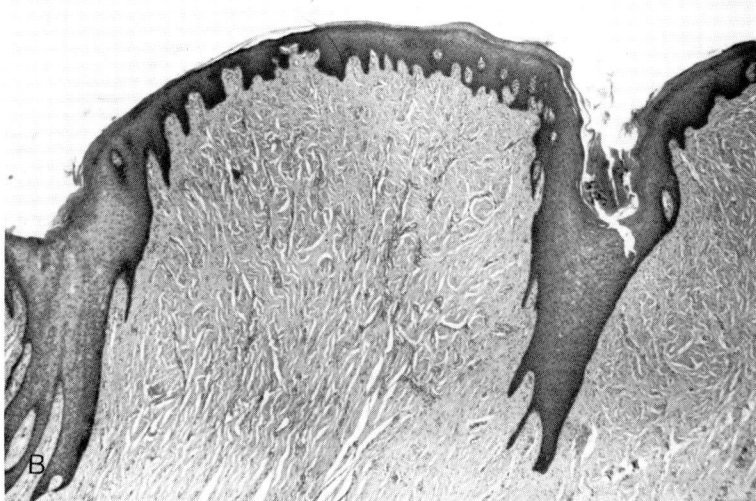

Figure 7–13. *A*, Denture-induced fibrous hyperplasia. *B*, Microscopy showing folds of dense collagen.

Figure 7–14. Soft tissue myxoma.

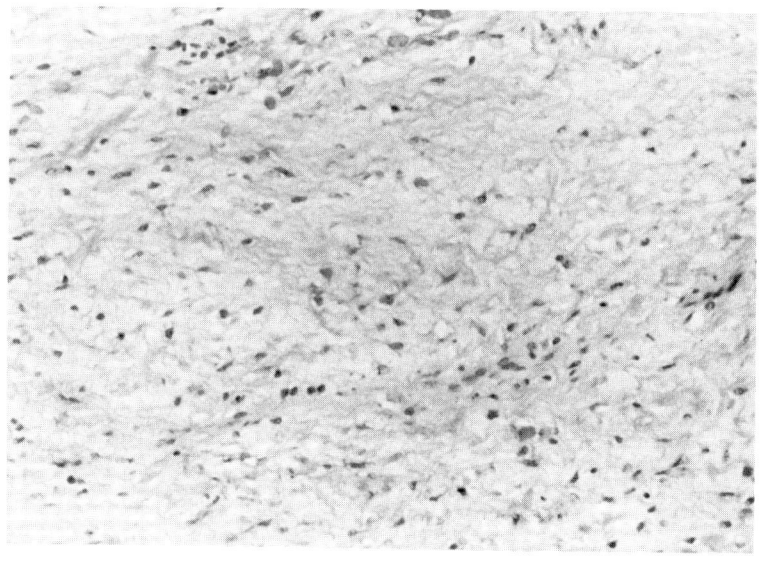

Table 7-1. MICROSCOPIC DIFFERENTIATION OF ORAL MYXOID LESIONS				
Lesion	Mast Cells	Reticulin Fibers	Pattern	Periphery
Soft tissue myxoma	No	Yes	Diffuse, uniform	Blending, infiltration
Nerve sheath myxoma	Yes	Yes	Lobular	Condensed fibrous tissue
Focal mucinosis	No	No	Uniform	Well circumscribed

mucocele, and myxomatous change in a fibrous lesion or neurofibroma.

Nerve sheath myxoma arises from the endoneurium of a peripheral nerve. It typically exhibits lobulated mucoid tissue containing stellate and spindle-shaped cells. Condensed connective tissue, representing perineurium, surrounds the lesion. A fine reticulin network is seen throughout, with special stains. Mast cells are characteristically present in this lesion.

Oral focal mucinosis represents the mucosal counterpart of cutaneous focal mucinosis. The lesion appears as a well-circumscribed area of myxomatous connective tissue in the submucosa or the dermis. It contains no mast cells and no reticulin network except that which surrounds supporting blood vessels.

Treatment. The treatment of choice for oral soft tissue myxoma as well as other myxoid lesions is surgical excision. Recurrence is not uncommon for myxomas but is unexpected for nerve sheath myxoma and focal mucinosis. All are benign processes and require conservative therapy only.

Juvenile Nasopharyngeal Angiofibroma

Clinical Features. Nasopharyngeal angiofibroma is also known as juvenile nasopharyngeal angiofibroma, because of its almost exclusive occurrence in the second decade of life. It is an uncommon to rare neoplasm that nearly always affects males. It characteristically produces a mass in the nasopharynx that leads to obstruction or epistaxis that may, on occasion, be severe. Rarely, this lesion may present intraorally, causing palatal expansion in which there is a blue color owing to the intense vascularity of the lesion. This lesion can generally be described as benign and slow growing but unencapsulated and locally invasive. On occasion, it may exhibit aggressive clinical behavior in which there is direct extension into the bones of the midface and the skull base.

Histopathology. Microscopically, nasopharyngeal angiofibroma has the appearance of a mature, well-collagenized lesion containing cleft-like vascular channels (Fig. 7-15). The fibroblasts have a uniform benign appearance. The vascular channels vary in size and are lined by endothelium that may occasionally be rimmed by smooth muscle cells.

Differential Diagnosis. The presentation of a submucosal bluish mass in the palate should suggest several clinical possibilities. Hemangioma, lymphoma, salivary gland tumor, and mucus extravasation phenomenon would be likely candidates in a differential diagnosis. Nasopharyngeal angiofibroma should be included if the patient also has symptoms involv-

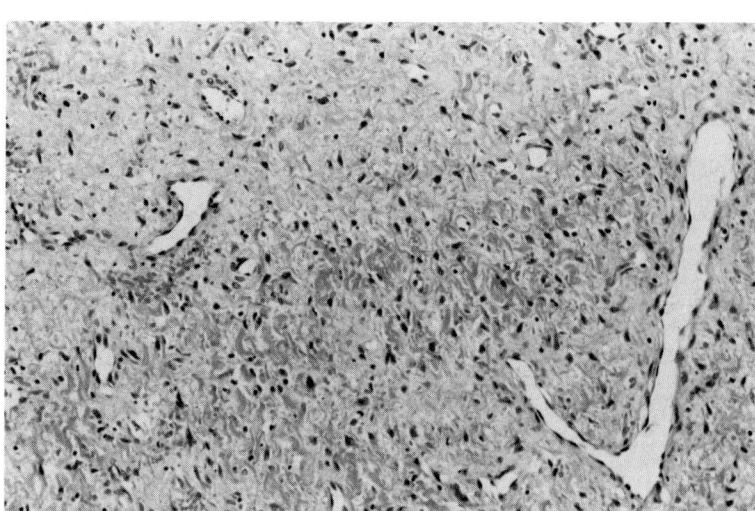

Figure 7-15. Nasopharyngeal angiofibroma.

ing the nasal cavity. Otherwise, the clinician may generally exclude this lesion from a diagnostic list, since there is a very low probability of a nasopharyngeal angiofibroma presenting orally. Biopsy of a lesion that is felt to be an angiofibroma should be done with caution and in a hospital setting, because of the potential for excessive bleeding. Radiographic and angiographic studies would be especially helpful in establishing a definitive diagnosis.

Treatment. Although numerous forms of treatment, such as radiation, exogenous hormone administration, sclerosant therapy, and embolization, have been used for nasopharyngeal angiofibroma, surgery remains the preferred form of therapy. Recurrences are common (up to 50% of cases) and are due to incomplete excision, because of the invasive nature of the lesion and the surgically difficult anatomic location.

Nodular Fasciitis

Clinical Features. Nodular fasciitis, also known as pseudosarcomatous fasciitis, is a well-recognized entity representing a reactive fibrous connective tissue growth (Table 7–2). The cause of this proliferation is unknown, although trauma is believed to be important in many cases because of the location of lesions over bony prominences such as the angle of the mandible and zygoma. The lesion typically presents as a firm mass in the dermis or the submucosa. It exhibits such rapid growth clinically that malignancy may be suspected. Pain or tenderness often accompanies the process. There is no gender predilection, and young adults and adults are usually affected. The trunk and extremities are the areas most commonly involved, with about 10% of cases appearing in the head and neck, usually in the skin of the face and the parotid sheath.

Histopathology. As the name implies, this lesion exhibits a nodular growth pattern (Fig. 7–16). It is often well circumscribed but may show some infiltrative tendency. Plump fibroblasts with vesicular nuclei are seen in a haphazard to a storiform or a cartwheel arrangement. Myxoid areas are often found. Multinucleated giant cells are occasionally present and may originate from adjacent muscle or from fusion of macrophage-histiocytes (tumor giant cells). Mitotic figures may be frequent but are morphologically normal in appearance. Capillaries in the tumor are immature, with prominent endothelial cells, and are arranged in a radial or a parallel fashion. Inflammatory cells and extravasated red blood cells (RBCs) are also microscopic features of nodular fasciitis.

Several subtypes of nodular fasciitis have been reported that represent variations on the typical microscopic picture. These include proliferative fasciitis, parosteal fasciitis, and intravascular fasciitis. The terms "myxoid," "cellular," and "fibrous" have also been used to describe these lesions when one of these characteristics is present.

An analogous lesion occurring within muscle is known as *proliferative myositis*. This reactive lesion, which usually occurs in the trunk and rarely in the head and the neck (sternocleidomastoid muscle), parallels the clinical course of nodular fasciitis. It does, however, appear in an older age group.

Differential Diagnosis. Diagnostic problems relative to nodular fasciitis occur because many of its microscopic features are shared by other fibrous proliferations, such as fibromatosis, fibrous histiocytoma, and fibrosarcoma (Table 7–3). Fibromatosis is more infiltrative than nodular fasciitis, and it exhibits a fascicular growth pattern. It also produces more collagen and has fewer mitotic figures. Fibrous histiocytoma has a dual population of fibroblasts and macrophage-histiocytes, and it may not be as well circumscribed as nodular fasciitis. Fibrosarcoma is infiltrative and exhibits a "her-

Table 7–2. COMPARATIVE CLINICAL FEATURES OF NODULAR FASCIITIS AND FIBROMATOSIS

Feature	Nodular Fasciitis	Fibromatosis
Tumor type	Reactive	Benign aggressive
Age affected	Young adults, adults	Children, young adults
Symptoms	Often	Infrequently
Areas affected	Trunk and extremities (head and neck 10%)	Shoulder and trunk (head and neck 10%)
Growth rate	Rapid	Moderate
Periphery	Often circumscribed	Infiltrative
Recurrence	Rarely	Frequently
Treatment	Conservative surgery	Aggressive surgery

CONNECTIVE TISSUE LESIONS   197

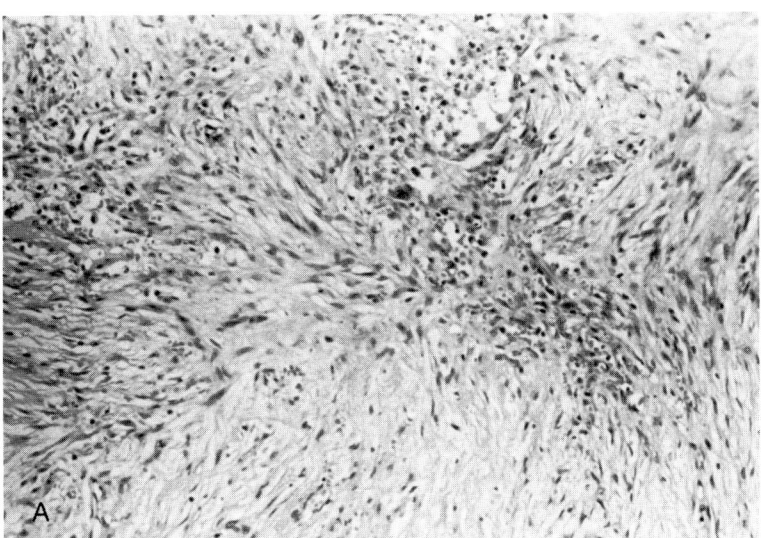

Figure 7–16. A and B, Nodular fasciitis. Note inflammatory cells and giant cell (arrow).

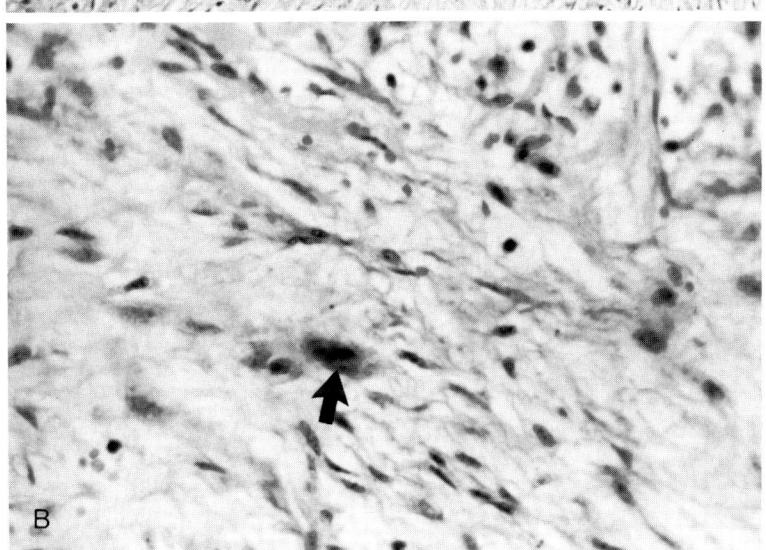

Table 7–3. COMPARATIVE MICROSCOPIC FEATURES OF FIBROUS PROLIFERATIONS

Feature	Nodular Fasciitis	Fibromatosis	Benign Fibrous Histiocytoma	Fibrosarcoma
Periphery	Often circumscribed	Infiltrative	Occasionally circumscribed	Infiltrative
Growth pattern	Nodular, haphazard to storiform	Fascicular	Storiform	"Herringbone"
Mitoses	Frequent, normal	Few, normal	Few, normal	Few to many, abnormal
Cellular atypia	No	No	No	No
Inflammatory cells	Yes	No	No	No
Extravasated RBCs	Yes	No	No	No
Tumor giant cells	Occasionally	No	Frequently	Infrequently
Macrophage-histiocytes	No	No	Yes	No

ringbone" pattern. Nuclei are pleomorphic and hyperchromatic, and mitoses are more abundant and atypical.

Treatment. Conservative surgical excision is the treatment of choice for nodular fasciitis. Recurrences are rarely seen.

Fibromatosis

Clinical Features. Fibromatosis, also known as extra-abdominal fibromatosis, is a benign fibrous proliferation that may be a troublesome clinical problem, because of often aggressive behavior and its tendency for recurrence (Table 7–2). It is seen in children and young adults, with approximately equal gender distribution. This lesion is most commonly found in the shoulder area and trunk, with about 10% of cases appearing in the soft tissues of the head and neck. It is slower growing than nodular fasciitis and less likely to be symptomatic.

Histopathology. Fibromatosis is a non-encapsulated infiltrative lesion with a fascicular growth pattern (Fig. 7–17). The lesion is composed of highly differentiated connective tissue containing uniform compact fibroblasts, often surrounded by abundant collagen. Nuclei are not atypical, and mitotic figures are infrequent. When muscle invasion occurs, giant cells of muscle origin may be seen. Slit-like vascular spaces are usually seen as well. Overall, the bland microscopic appearance of this lesion belies its locally aggressive growth (Table 7–3).

Treatment. Recurrence rates in the range of 20 to 60% have been reported. Because of this and because of the locally destructive nature of fibromatosis, an aggressive surgical approach is recommended.

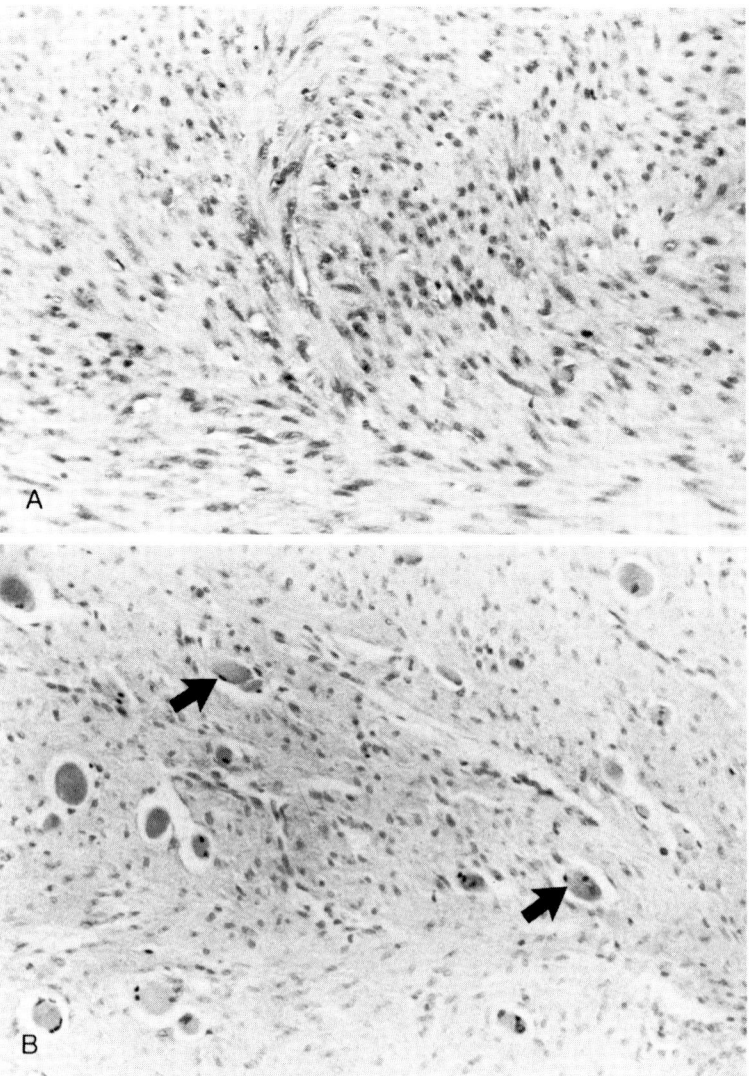

Figure 7–17. *A* and *B*, Two cases of fibromatosis showing the range of cellularity in this lesion. Note residual muscle in *B* (arrows).

Fibrosarcoma

Clinical Features. Fibrosarcoma is a rare soft tissue and bony malignancy of the head and neck. When occurring in bone, the lesion may theoretically arise from periosteum, endosteum, or periodontal ligament.

A tumescence resulting from proliferation of malignant fibroblasts appears at the site of origin (Fig. 7–18). Secondary ulceration may be seen as the lesion enlarges. Young adults are most commonly affected. This is an infiltrative neoplasm that is more of a locally destructive problem than a metastatic problem.

Histopathology. Microscopically, fibrosarcoma exhibits malignant-appearing fibroblasts, typically in a "herringbone" or interlacing fascicular pattern (Fig. 7–19). Collagen may be sparse and mitotic figures frequent. Cell differentiation from one tumor to another may be quite variable. The periphery of this lesion is ill defined, since the neoplasm freely invades surrounding tissue.

Treatment. Wide surgical excision is generally advocated for fibrosarcoma, because of the difficulty in controlling local growth. Although recurrence is not uncommon, metastasis is infrequently seen. Bone lesions are more likely to metastasize via the blood stream than are soft tissue lesions. The overall 5-year survival rate ranges between 30 and 50%. Generally, patients with soft tissue lesions fare better than patients with primary lesions of bone. Also, those with well-differentiated lesions have a better prognosis than do those with poorly differentiated lesions.

Benign Fibrous Histiocytoma

"Fibrous histiocytoma" is a generic term that encompasses benign neoplasms consisting of a dual population of fibroblasts and macrophage-histiocytes (Table 7–4). Although the precise histogenesis remains in dispute, immunohistochemical evidence has favored a fibroblast cell of origin over a macrophage-histiocyte origin.

Clinical Features. Benign fibrous histiocytoma is a rare oral neoplasm that may affect either soft tissue or bone. It is a lesion of adults, typically seen in the fifth decade. It presents as a mass that may be ulcerated and is usually painless (Fig. 7–20). Intrabone lesions present as radiolucencies, often with ill-defined margins. They are often initially interpreted as osteomyelitis on radiographic examination.

Histopathology. The dual population of fibroblasts and macrophage-histiocytes must be present before a diagnosis of benign fibrous histiocytoma can be considered (Fig. 7–21). The cellular proliferation is typically in a storiform pattern that is often circumscribed peripherally. Tumor giant cells may be seen. There is no cellular atypia, and mitotic figures are infrequent and normal (see Table 7–3).

Treatment. Surgical excision is the treatment of choice for benign fibrous histiocytoma. Recurrence is usually not seen.

Malignant Fibrous Histiocytoma

Clinical Features. Malignant fibrous histiocytoma is an infrequently reported lesion in

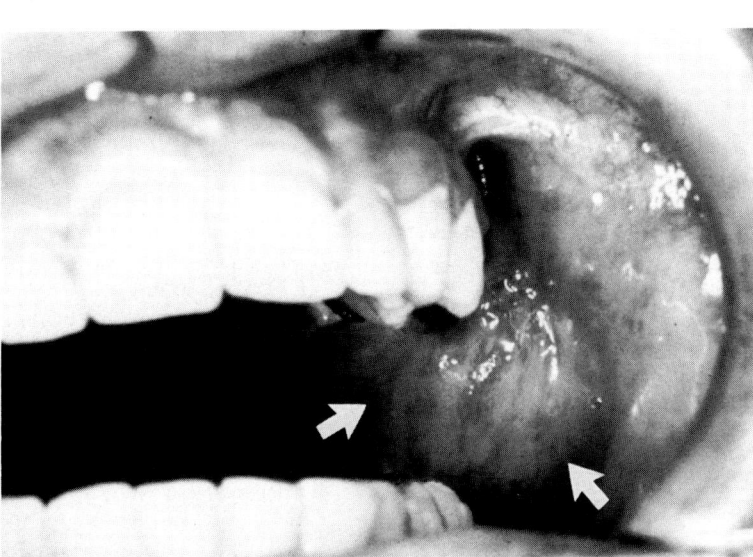

Figure 7–18. Fibrosarcoma of the buccal mucosa (arrows).

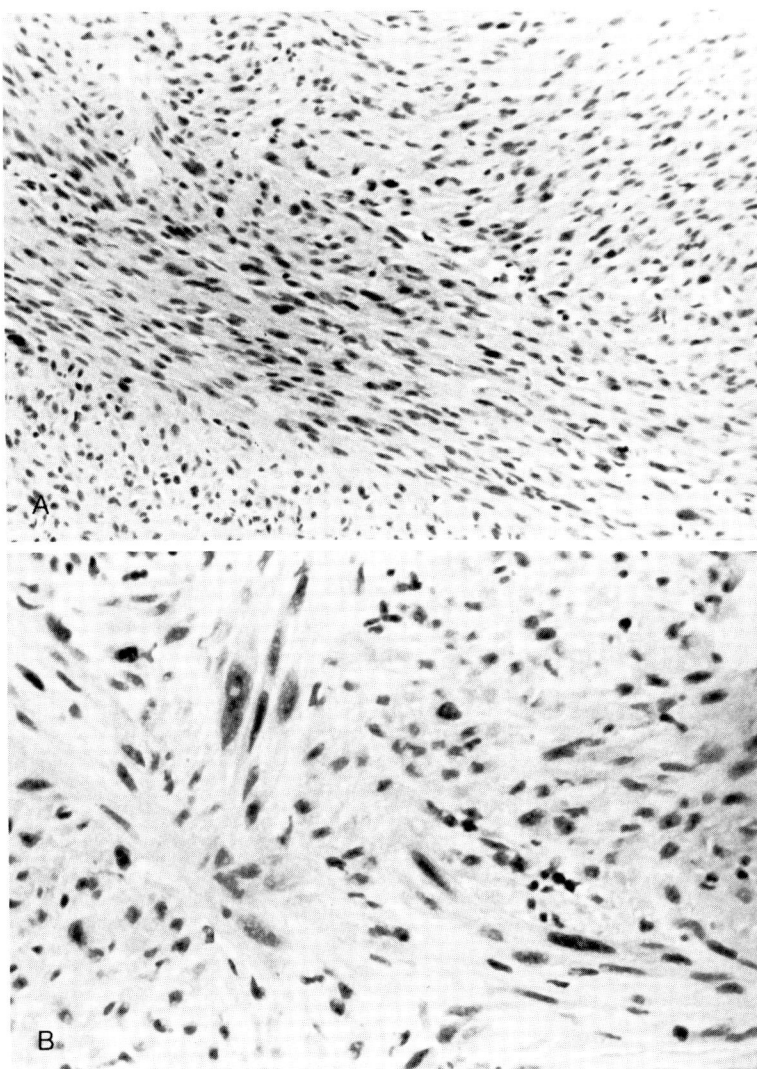

Figure 7-19. *A* and *B*, Fibrosarcoma of oral soft tissues. Moderate nuclear pleomorphism is evident in *B*.

Table 7-4. CLASSIFICATION OF FIBROUS HISTIOCYTOMAS
Benign
Benign fibrous histiocytoma (oral)
Dermatofibroma (skin)
Giant cell tumor of tendon sheath
Xanthogranuloma
Atypical fibroxanthoma (skin)
?Peripheral ossifying fibroma
?"Giant cell" fibroma
Malignant
Dermatofibrosarcoma protuberans (skin)
Malignant fibrous histiocytoma
Storiform-pleomorphic
Myxoid
Giant cell
Inflammatory
Angiomatoid

the head and neck, although it is the most common adult soft tissue sarcoma in the rest of the body. It may also occur in bone, where it follows a more aggressive course than in soft tissue. Biologically, it has significant recurrence and metastatic potential that is dependent, in part, upon clinical factors such as anatomic site, superficial or deep location, and size.

Overall, malignant fibrous histiocytomas occur in late adult life and are rare in children. Males are affected more frequently than females. The extremities and retroperitoneum are favored sites.

In the extremities, these tumors typically present as painless masses. In the retroperitoneum, signs and symptoms of malaise, anorexia, weight loss, and hyperpyrexia may ac-

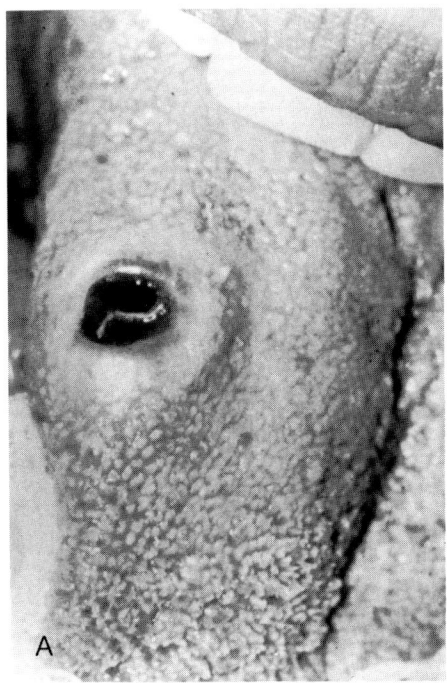
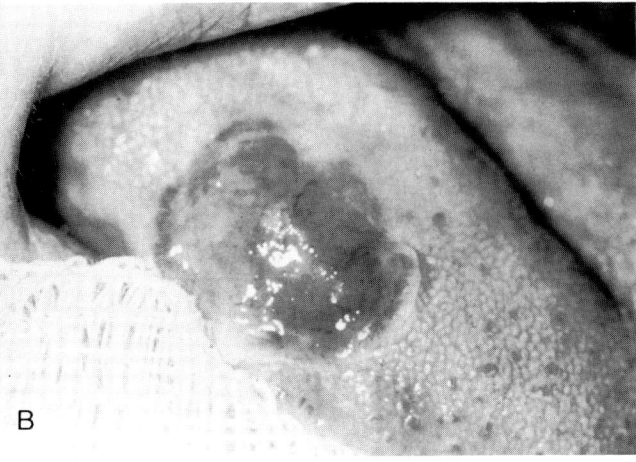

Figure 7-20. *A* and *B*, Benign fibrous histiocytoma of the tongue. *B* shows the appearance of the same lesion after a 2-week observation period.

company tumor growth. In the head and neck, these neoplasms present usually as a mass. Other accompanying signs and symptoms are dependent upon specific location in the head and neck. Pain, facial paralysis, epistaxis, rhinorrhea, hemoptysis, and dysphagia may be seen.

Malignant fibrous histiocytomas have been reported in the mandible and the maxilla. These lesions cause radiolucencies with poorly defined margins and may have a "moth-eaten" appearance. Cortical expansion may be seen, and pathologic fracture may occur with larger lesions.

Intraoral soft tissue lesions appear to have no site predilection. Although only a small number have been reported, almost all regions have been affected.

Histopathology. Basic to all malignant fibrous histiocytomas is the proliferation of fibroblasts, macrophage-histiocytes, and giant cells (Fig. 7-22). Abnormal and frequent mitotic figures, necrosis, and extensive cellular atypia may be seen. In some lesions, a storiform pattern may dominate the microscopic picture; in others, myxoid zones, giant cells, acute inflammatory cells, xanthoma cells, or blood vessels may be prominent (Table 7-4). The recognition of these different microscopic features has led to subclassification into storiform-pleomorphic (most common), myxoid, giant cell, inflammatory, and angiomatoid types. There are conflicting data relative to prediction of behavior from each histologic subtype.

Treatment. Wide surgical excision is the usual treatment. Radiation or chemotherapy apparently offers limited additional benefit, although these methods have not been fully explored.

Location of the neoplasm is an important factor for prognosis. Lesions located in deeper soft tissues generally have exhibited a more aggressive clinical course. Intraosseous neoplasms exhibit a worse prognosis than soft tissue lesions. As the size of the lesion increases, the metastatic potential increases. The presence of an inflammatory cell host response improves the prognosis. Survival is variable and is dependent in large part upon the factors discussed here.

The 5-year survival rate ranges from 20 to 60%. Patients with oral lesions generally do somewhat worse than others. Recurrence and metastatic rates are about 40%.

VASCULAR LESIONS

Reactive Lesions

Venous Varix

This condition is discussed in detail in Chapter 4.

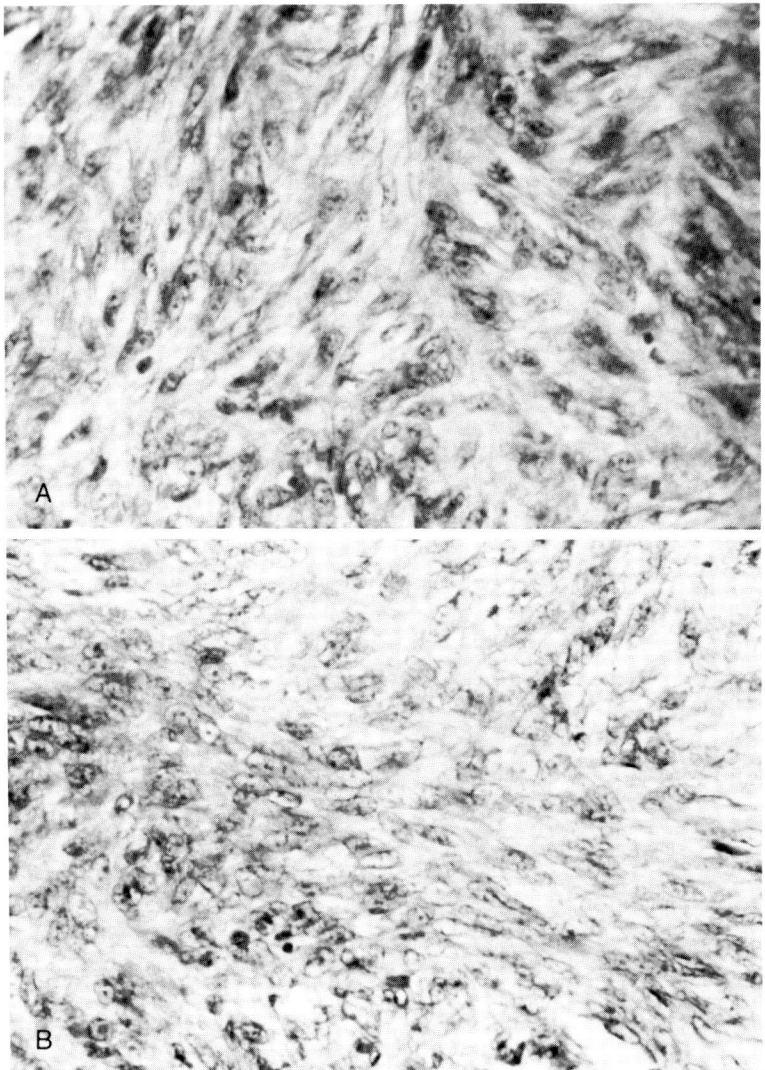

Figure 7–21. *A* and *B,* Benign fibrous histiocytomas.

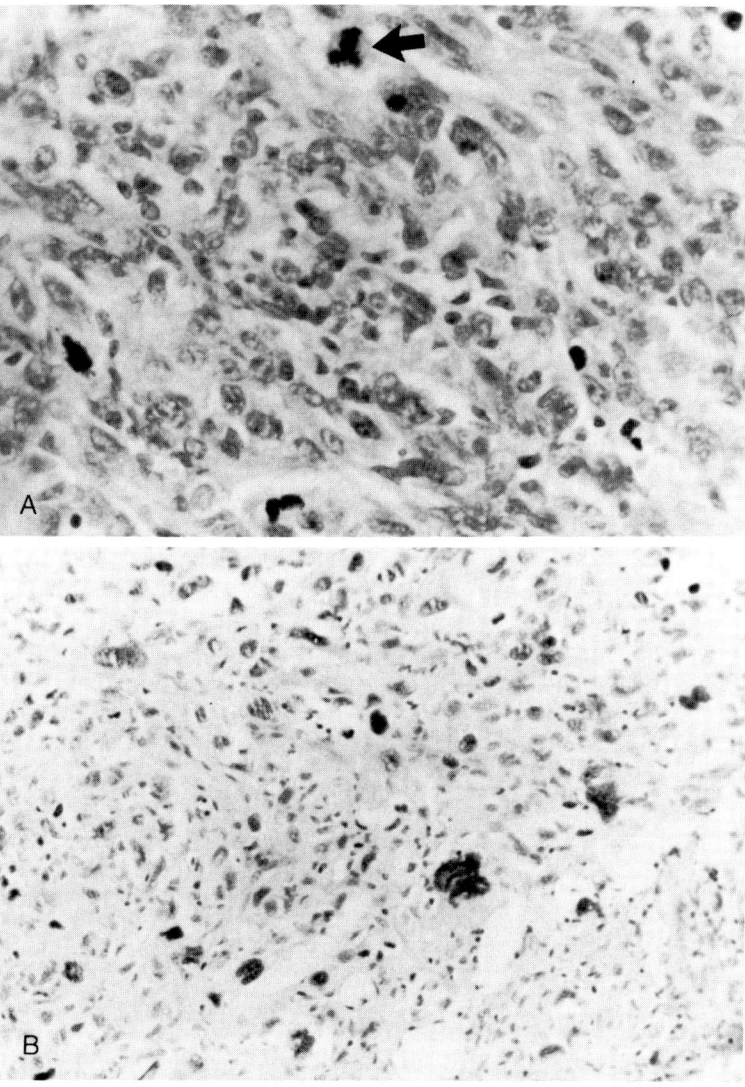

Figure 7–22. *A* and *B*, Malignant fibrous histiocytomas. Note tripolar mitotic figure in *A* (arrow) and nuclear pleomorphism of macrophage histiocytes in *B*.

Congenital Lesions

Hemangioma

This condition is discussed in detail in Chapter 4.

Lymphangioma

Etiology. Lymphangiomas are generally regarded as congenital lesions rather than as neoplasms. Often present at or around the time of birth, they usually appear within the first 2 decades of life. Involution over time is usually not seen with these lesions, in contrast to congenital hemangiomas.

Clinical Features. Lymphangiomas present as painless, nodular, vesicle-like swellings when superficial, or as a submucosal mass if located deeper (Fig. 7–23). The color ranges from lighter than the surrounding tissue to red-blue when capillaries are part of the congenital malformation. On palpation, the lesions may produce a crepitant sound as lymphatic fluid is pushed from one area to another.

The tongue is the most common intraoral site, and the lesions may be responsible for macroglossia when diffusely distributed throughout the submucosa. Lymphangioma of the lip may cause a macrocheilia. Lymphangioma of the neck is known as *cystic hygroma*, hygroma colli, or cavernous lymphangioma. This diffuse soft tissue swelling may be life threatening, because it involves vital structures of the neck. Respiratory distress, intralesional

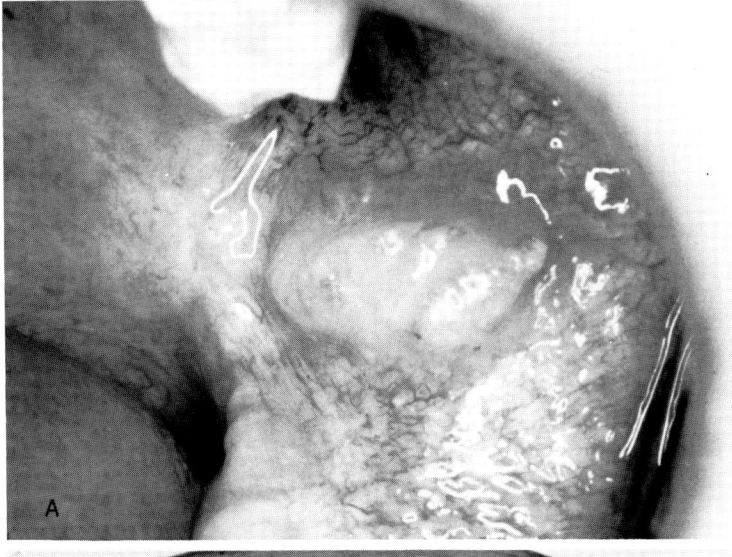
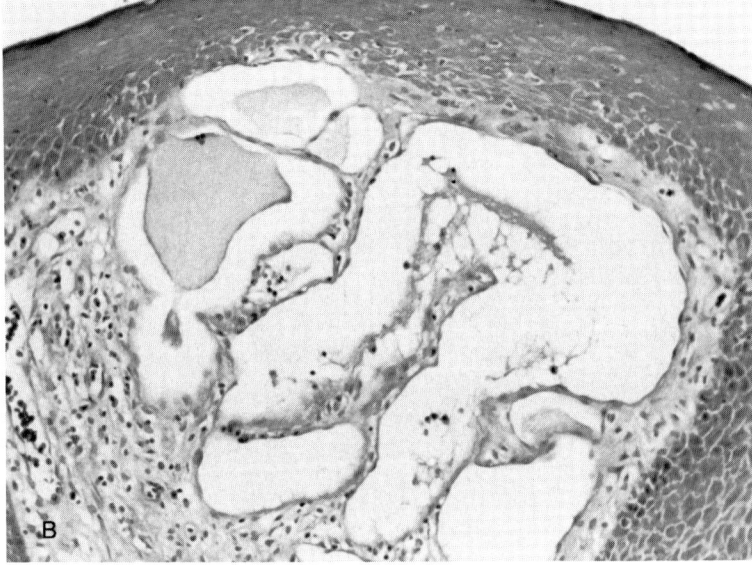

Figure 7–23. *A* and *B*, Lymphangioma of the buccal mucosa. Note endothelium-lined spaces in *B*.

hemorrhage, and disfigurement are all potential sequelae to cystic hygroma.

Histopathology. Endothelium-lined lymphatic channels are diffusely distributed in the submucosa. The channels contain eosinophilic lymph that occasionally includes RBCs, especially in mixed lymphatic and capillary proliferations. There is no capsule. A characteristic feature is the location of lymphatic channels directly adjacent to overlying epithelium, without any apparent intervening connective tissue.

Differential Diagnosis. Clinically, the lymphangioma may occasionally appear similar to hemangioma when there is a significant capillary component. When small, the lesions may be confused with mucoceles. Superficial lesions should not be confused with vesiculo-bullous eruptions, since lesions associated with the latter are short-lived and often painful and inflamed.

Treatment. Lymphangiomas are usually surgically removed, but, because of their lack of encapsulation, recurrences are common. Large lymphangiomas, such as cystic hygromas, may require staged surgical procedures to gain control of the lesion. Sclerosant therapy and radiation have been used with limited success, and they are not generally recommended as standard therapy.

Neoplasms

Hemangiopericytoma

The hemangiopericytoma is a rare neoplasm that is derived from the pericyte. This cell is normally found in capillaries and venules, between the basement membrane and endothelium. The cell probably has a contractile property and serves as an endothelial reserve cell. The neoplasm that arises from this cell may appear as a mass in any location of the body across a wide age spectrum. There are no distinguishing clinical signs that would suggest a diagnosis of hemangiopericytoma (Fig. 7–24).

Microscopically, the neoplasm is characterized by proliferation of well-differentiated, oval to spindle-shaped mesenchymal cells separated by small, slit-like vascular channels (Fig. 7–25). The vessels are thin walled and may exhibit "staghorn" profiles.

The biologic behavior of the hemangiopericytoma is unpredictable, exhibiting on occasion a benign course and on other occasions an aggressive metastatic course. Unfortunately, there are no reliable histologic criteria that can be used to predict clinical course, although necrosis, numerous mitotic figures, and hypercellularity may be suggestive of a more aggressive lesion. The treatment of choice is wide surgical excision. Recurrence and metastases are not uncommon.

Angiosarcoma

Angiosarcoma is a rare neoplasm of endothelial cell origin. A distinct clinical pathologic variant of angiosarcoma is Kaposi's sarcoma.

The scalp is the usual location for angiosarcomas, although occasional lesions have been reported in the maxillary sinus and the oral cavity (Fig. 7–26). The lesion consists of an unencapsulated proliferation of anaplastic endothelial cells enclosing irregular luminal

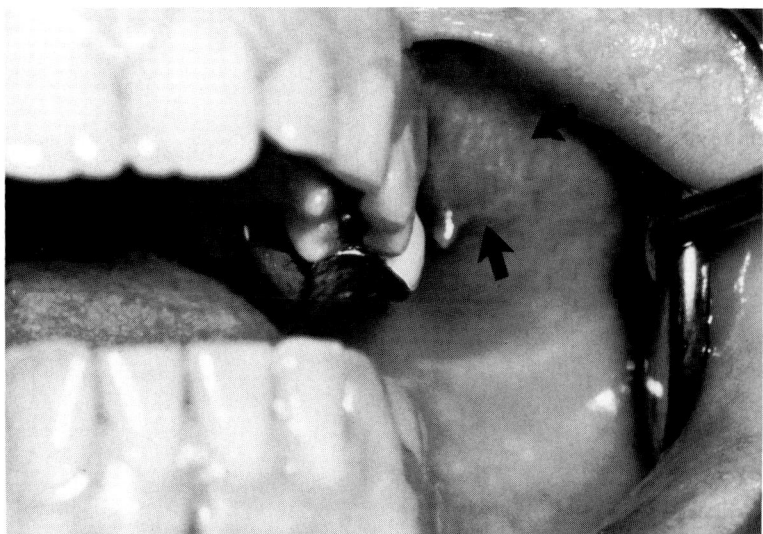

Figure 7–24. Hemangiopericytoma of the buccal mucosa (arrows).

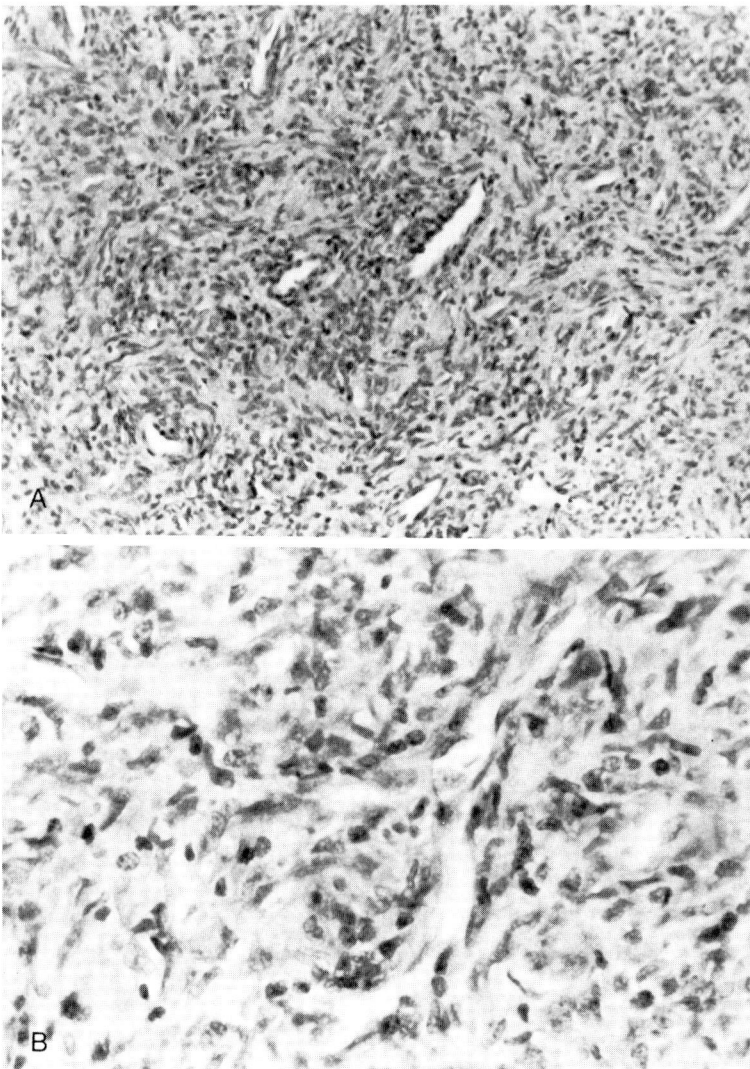

Figure 7-25. *A* and *B*, Hemangiopericytoma showing numerous capillary spaces.

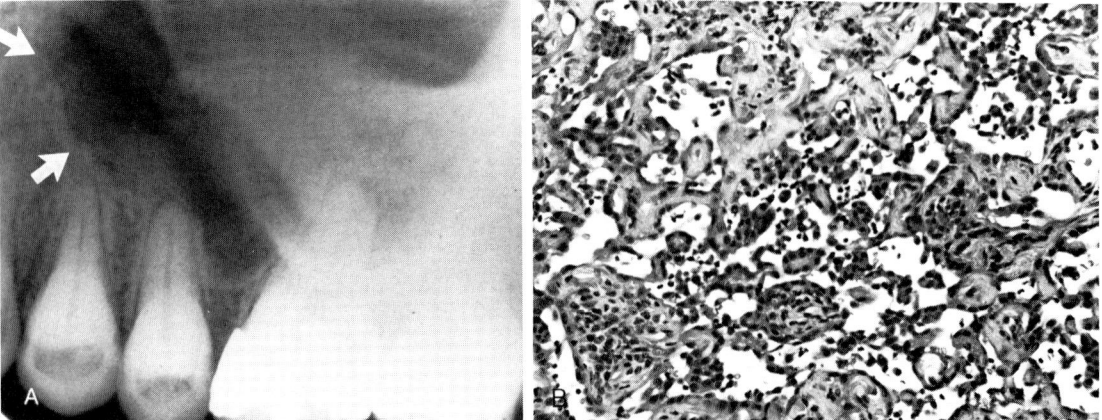

Figure 7-26. *A*, Angiosarcoma of the maxillary sinus. Note erosion of sinus wall (arrows). *B*, Angiosarcoma showing anaplastic endothelial cells lining irregular vascular spaces.

spaces. It has an aggressive clinical course and a poor prognosis.

Kaposi's Sarcoma

This condition is discussed in detail in Chapter 4.

NEURAL LESIONS

Reactive Lesions

Traumatic Neuroma

Etiology. As the name suggests, this lesion is caused by trauma to a peripheral nerve. In the oral cavity, the injury may be in the form of trauma from a surgical procedure such as a tooth extraction, from a local anesthetic injection, or from an accident. Transection of a sensory nerve can result in inflammation and scarring in the area of injury. As the proximal nerve segment proliferates in an attempt to regenerate into the distal segment, it becomes entangled and trapped in the developing scar, resulting in a composite mass of fibrous tissue, Schwann cells, and axons. This may be regarded as another type of reactive hyperplasia.

Clinical Features. About half the patients with oral traumatic neuromas have associated pain. The type of pain varies from one patient to another and ranges from occasional tenderness to constant severe pain. Radiating facial pain may occasionally be caused by a traumatic neuroma. Injection of local anesthesia into the area of tumescence relieves the pain.

There is a wide age range in which the lesions occur, although most are seen in adults. The mental foramen is the most common location, followed by extraction sites in the anterior maxilla and the posterior mandible (Fig. 7–27). Lower lip, tongue, buccal mucosa, and palate are also relatively common locations.

Histopathology. Microscopically, bundles of nerves are found admixed with dense, collagenous fibrous tissue. A chronic inflammatory cell infiltrate may be seen in a minority of cases, particularly those that are symptomatic.

Diagnosis. Clinical diagnosis may be difficult, if patients present with atypical facial pain. Excisional biopsy of a suspected mass or radiolucency will ultimately be required to prove the clinical impression. Traumatic neuroma should be included in a clinical differential diagnosis of any small mass that is spontaneously painful or painful when compressed. Acute infection may cause similar symptoms, but other clinical signs of inflammation should separate this process from traumatic neuroma.

Treatment. Even though surgical transection of a peripheral nerve may have caused the lesion, surgical excision is the treatment of choice. Recurrence is infrequently seen. Nerve sectioning or alcohol injection is much less effective and is generally not used for this condition.

Neoplasms

Granular Cell Tumors

Etiology and Histogenesis. The granular cell tumor, formerly known as granular cell myoblastoma, is an uncommon neoplasm of unknown etiology. The unique granular cells that make up the lesion are readily identified microscopically, but they do not have a known normal cell counterpart. This has led to considerable speculation over the histogenesis of this lesion. The controversy of its origin has persisted since it was originally described in 1926. Because of the intimate relationship of granular cells to skeletal muscle, the myoblast was originally thought to be the progenitor cell. The light microscopic appearance also suggested a macrophage origin. Results of ultrastructural studies suggested, instead, origin from the pericyte, the undifferentiated mesenchymal cell, or the Schwann cell. Immunohistochemistry has facilitated demonstration of a protein (S-100 protein) in the granular cells that is usually found predominantly in the nervous system. This has been the strongest evidence in support of origin from Schwann cells. Subsequently, antigens associated with peripheral nerve myelin protein have been found in granular cells. Striated muscle proteins have not been identified in these cells with immunohistochemical techniques.

A related lesion known as *congenital gingival granular cell tumor* (congenital epulis) is composed of cells that are identical, seen under a light microscope to those of the granular cell tumor that occurs in older patients. Slight differences have been noted ultrastructurally and immunohistochemically, however. In the cells making up the congenital gingival granular cell tumor, so-called angulate bodies are not found ultrastructurally, and S-100 protein is absent immunohistochemically. These findings suggest that the congenital gingival tumor has a different histogenesis than the granular cell tumor. It has been suggested that, rather than having a neural origin, the congenital

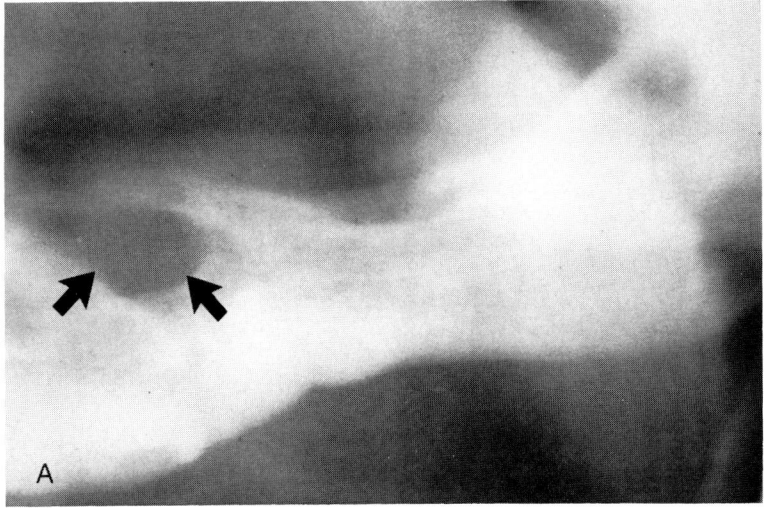

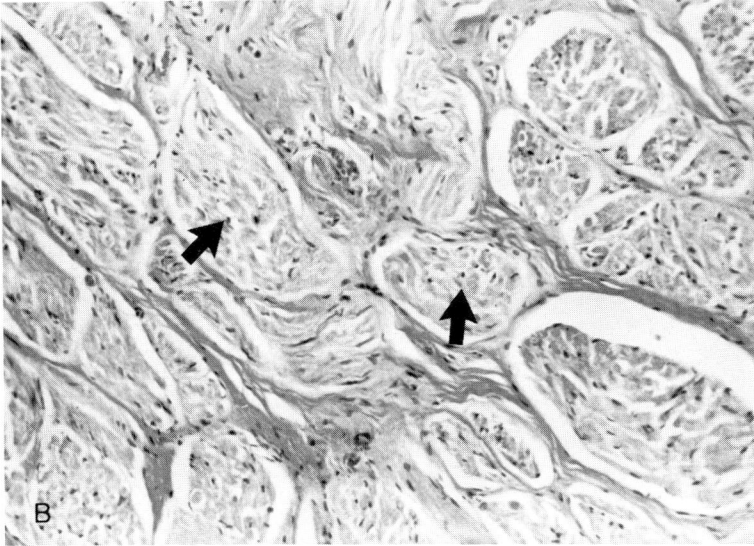

Figure 7-27. *A*, Traumatic neuroma in mental nerve area (arrows). *B*, Microscopy showing proliferating nerve (arrows) and scar.

gingival tumor may be derived from the pericyte or a related cell with potential smooth muscle differentiation.

Granular cell lesions may also be found in other tissues and diverse sites such as the jaw (e.g., granular cell ameloblastoma), skin, gastrointestinal tract, and respiratory tract. Because histologic and ultrastructural similarities are seen in the granular cells of all these lesions, it is suggested that granular cells represent a common morphologic expression of an unusual degenerative process from several different origins.

Clinical Features. Granular cell tumors appear in a range of patients from children to the elderly, with the mean usually in middle adult life (Table 7-5). Some studies have shown a predilection for females; others have shown near-equal gender distribution. In the head and neck, the tongue is by far the most common location for granular cell tumors (Fig. 7-28). However, any oral location may be affected.

Presentation is typically as an uninflamed asymptomatic mass less than 2 cm in diameter. The overlying epithelium is intact. Multiple lesions have occasionally been described.

The congenital gingival granular cell tumor appears on the gingiva (usually anterior) of newborns (Fig. 7-29). It presents as a noninflamed, pedunculated or broad-based mass. The maxillary gingiva is more often involved than the mandibular gingiva, and females are affected more than males. The lesion does not recur, and spontaneous regressions have been reported.

Histopathology. The clinical tumescence of granular cell tumors is due to the presence of

Table 7-5. COMPARATIVE FEATURES OF ORAL GRANULAR CELL LESIONS

Feature	Granular Cell Tumor	Congenital Gingival Granular Cell Tumor
Age	All	Infants
Gender	Females ≧ males	Females > males
Location	Oral, mucosa, skin, other	Gingiva only
Light microscopy		
Granular cells	Yes	Yes
Pseudoepitheliomatous hyperplasia	Yes, frequently	No
Ultrastructure		
Autophagic vacuoles	Yes	Yes
Angulate bodies	Yes	No
Smooth muscle features	No	Yes
Immunohistochemical		
S-100	Positive	Negative
Carcinoembryonic antigen	Positive	Positive
HLA-DR	Positive	Positive
Antichymotrypsin	Negative	Negative
Muscle actin	Negative	Negative

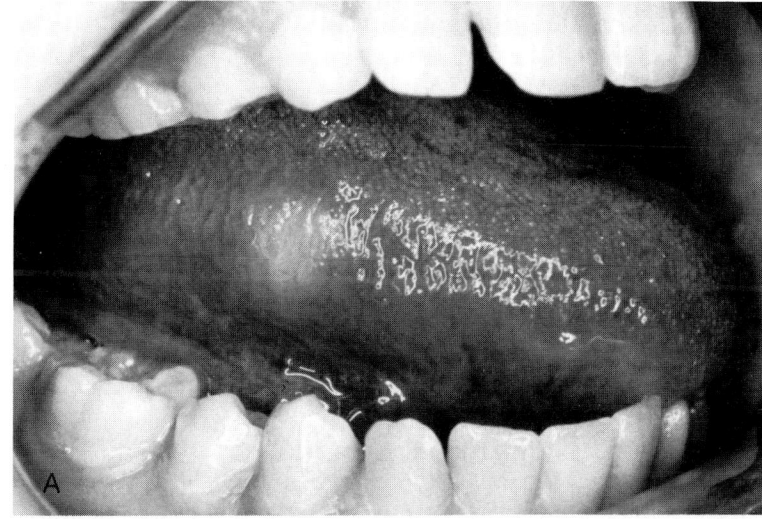
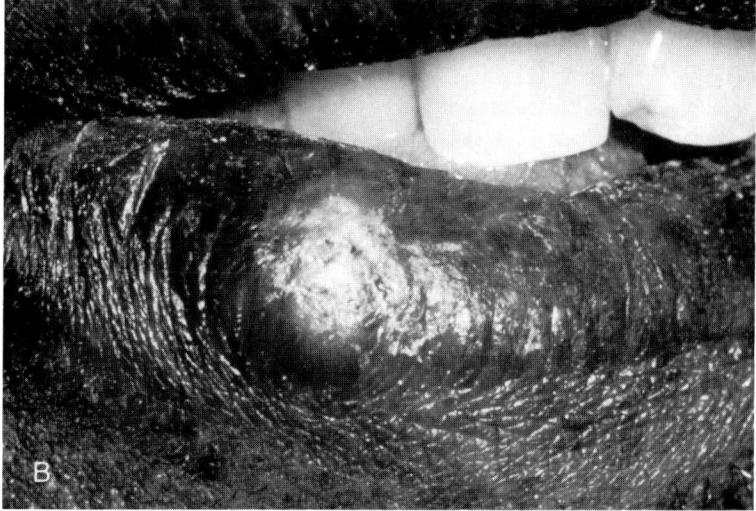

Figure 7-28. *A* and *B*, Granular cell tumors of tongue and lip. (Courtesy of Dr. W. Jerome.)

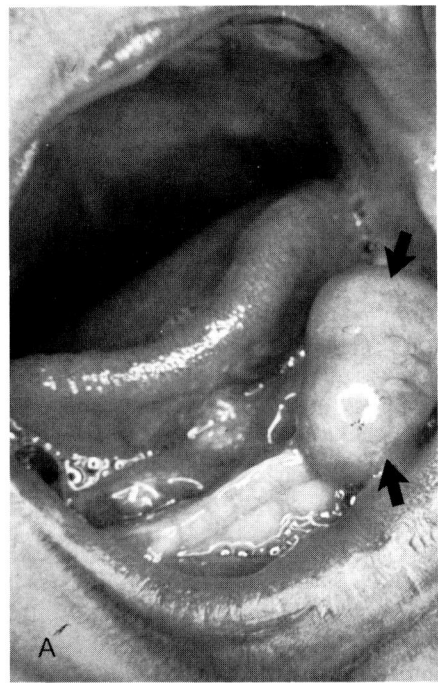
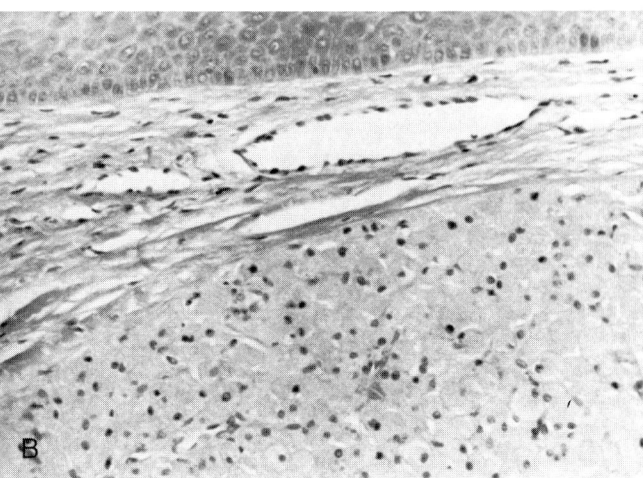

Figure 7–29. *A*, Congenital gingival granular cell tumor (arrows). *B*, Microscopy showing granular cells below and non-papillated epithelium above.

unencapsulated sheets of large polygonal cells with pale, granular or grainy cytoplasm (Figs. 7–30 and 7–31). The nuclei are small, compact, and morphologically benign. Mitotic figures are rare. Pseudoepitheliomatous hyperplasia of the overlying oral epithelium is seen in about half the cases. This may be such a prominent feature that subjacent granular cells are overlooked, resulting in an overdiagnosis of squamous cell carcinoma. The pseudoepitheliomatous hyperplasia of granular cell tumor represents a completely benign process; it is not known to have malignant potential. The absence of a chronic inflammatory cell infiltrate, which would be typically seen in well-differentiated squamous cell carcinomas, indicates that the epithelial changes are hyperplastic rather than neoplastic.

The cells of the congenital gingival granular cell tumor appear identical to those of the granular cell tumor. Seen with the light microscope, the only difference between the two lesions is that the former does not exhibit overlying pseudoepitheliomatous hyperplasia.

Ultrastructurally, granular cells of both the granular cell tumor and the congenital gingival counterpart contain autophagic vacuoles (Fig. 7–32). One of the consistent differences noted has been the absence of angulate bodies in the gingival lesion. Also, in some gingival lesions, the presence of microfilaments with fusiform dense bodies, pinocytotic vesicles, and basement membrane has been noted.

Immunohistochemically, both lesions contain carcinoembryonic and HLA-DR antigens. However, only the granular cell tumor contains S-100 protein. Both tumors are negative for α-1 antichymotrypsin and muscle actin.

Differential Diagnosis. Clinically, the granular cell tumor might be confused with other connective tissue lesions. Neurofibroma and schwannoma would be prime considerations for tongue lesions. Salivary gland tumors, lipoma, and other benign mesenchymal neoplasms may present intraorally as asymptomatic lumps similar to granular cell tumor. Traumatic fibroma is a common reactive lesion that should be included in a differential diagnosis. Biopsy is the only way to achieve a definitive diagnosis.

The congenital gingival granular cell tumor is clinically distinctive because of the age of the patient and the location in which the mass is seen. Other submucosal lumps that occur in the gingiva of infants, such as gingival cyst and neuroectodermal tumor of infancy, are more deeply seated and broad based.

Treatment. Granular cell tumors are surgically excised, and recurrence is not expected. Spontaneous regression has been noted but is apparently a rare event.

Schwannoma

Etiology. The schwannoma or neurilemoma is a benign neoplasm with no known cause or

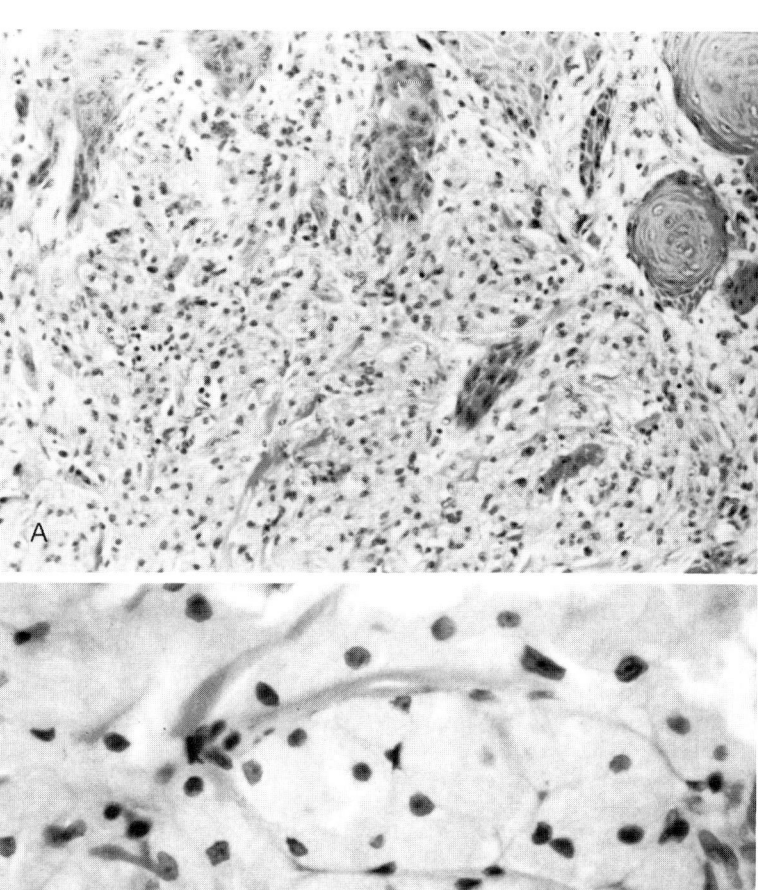

Figure 7–30. *A,* Granular cell tumor cells with overlying pseudoepitheliomatous hyperplasia. *B,* High magnification of granular cells.

stimulus. It is derived from proliferation of Schwann cells (neural crest origin) of the neurilemma that surrounds peripheral nerves. As the lesion grows, the nerve is pushed aside and does not become enmeshed within the tumor.

Clinical Features. This is an encapsulated submucosal mass that presents typically as an asymptomatic lump in patients of any age (Table 7–6). The tongue is the favored location, although lesions have been described in the palate, floor of the mouth, buccal mucosa, gingiva, lips, vestibule, and jaws. Bony lesions produce a radiolucent pattern and may also cause pain or paresthesia. The schwannoma is usually slow growing but may undergo a sudden increase in size, thought in some cases to be due to intralesional hemorrhage. Of considerable clinical significance is the fact that solitary schwannomas are not seen in the syndrome neurofibromatosis. If multiple, however, they may rarely be part of this syndrome. Another important clinical feature is the extremely low rate of malignant transformation associated with schwannoma as compared with the relatively high rate associated with neurofibroma in neurofibromatosis.

Histopathology. The microscopic features of schwannoma are usually highly characteristic, making diagnosis relatively easy (Fig. 7–33). Spindle cells that assume two different patterns are surrounded by a capsule. In one pattern, so-called Antoni A areas consist of spindle cells organized in palisaded whorls and waves. These cells frequently surround an acellular eosinophilic zone (Verocay body). Ultrastructurally, the acellular zone has been shown to

212 CONNECTIVE TISSUE LESIONS

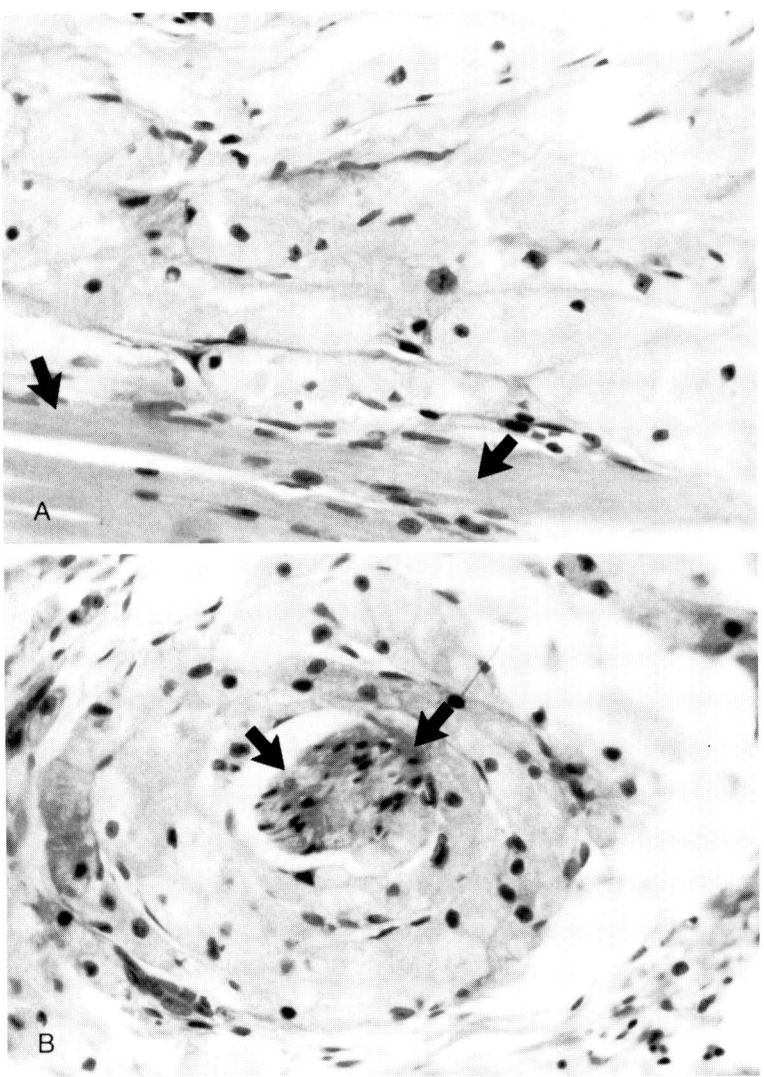

Figure 7-31. Granular cell tumor cells intimately associated with muscle *(A* arrows) and nerve *(B* arrows).

Table 7-6. COMPARATIVE FEATURES OF NEURAL TUMORS			
Feature	**Schwannoma**	**Neurofibroma**	**Mucosal Neuroma**
Cell of origin	Schwann cell	Schwann cell or perineural fibroblast	Nerve tissue ?Hamartoma
Age	Any	Any	Children, young adults
Location	Any, especially tongue	Any, tongue, buccal mucosa, vestibule	Tongue, lip, buccal mucosa
Number	Usually solitary	Solitary to multiple	Multiple
Bone lesions?	Occasionally	Frequently	No
Part of neurofibromastosis?	Rarely	Typical	No
Malignant change?	Rarely	Frequently	No
Part of MEN III?	No	No	Typical

Figure 7–32. Electron micrographs of autophagic vacuoles *(A)* and angulate bodies *(B)* found in granular cells of the granular cell tumor.

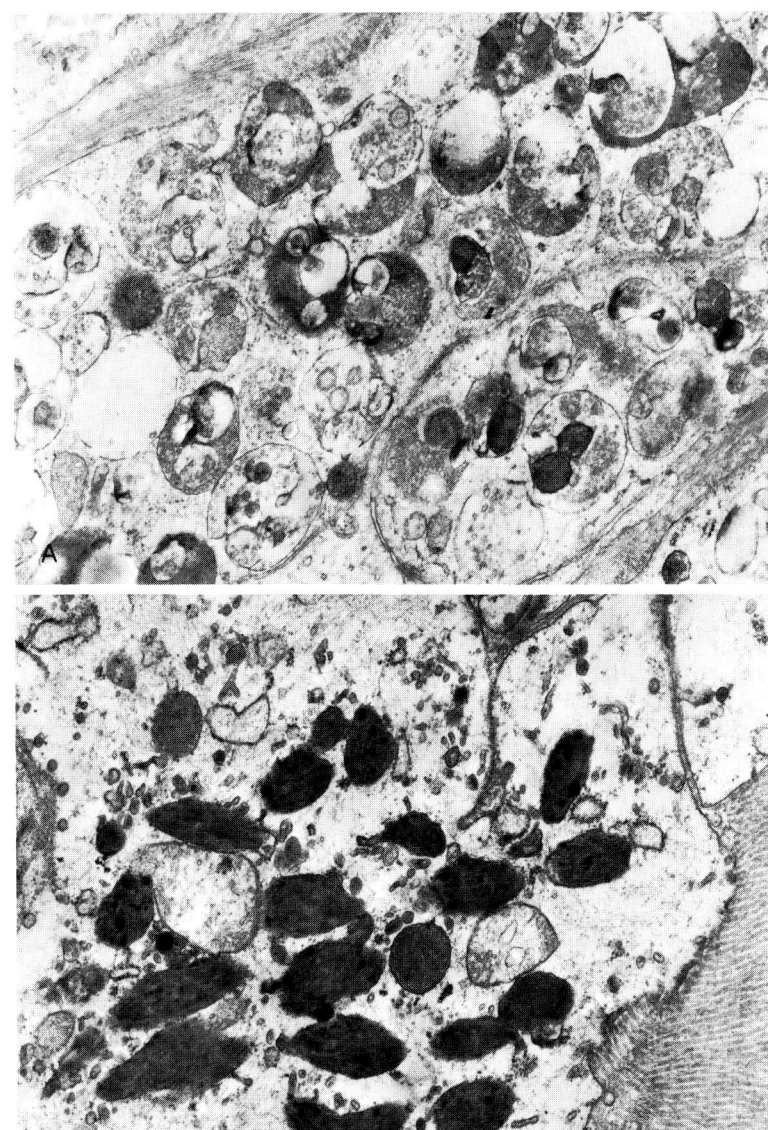

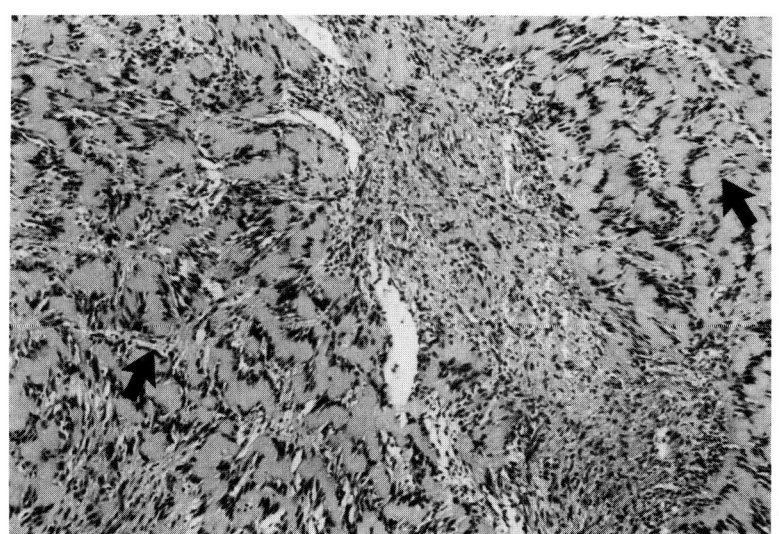

Figure 7–33. Micrograph of schwannoma showing areas of so-called Antoni A tissue (arrows) and so-called Antoni B tissue between (center). Note acellular foci in the Antoni A tissue.

be composed of interdigitated cytoplasmic processes and reduplicated basement membrane. The other pattern is the so-called Antoni B tissue, consisting of spindle cells haphazardly distributed in a light fibrillar matrix.

A microscopic variant known as *ancient schwannoma* has been described. This unusual designation was coined to reflect what was believed to be degenerative changes in a longstanding schwannoma. In this variant, fibrosis, inflammatory cells, and hemorrhage may be seen. Some nuclear atypia may also be present. The clinical and behavioral characteristics are believed to be the same as those for schwannoma.

Differential Diagnosis. There are no distinctive features of schwannoma that allow identification of this lesion on clinical grounds. Intraorally, differential diagnosis would include other benign mesenchymal neoplasms, salivary gland tumors, and traumatic fibroma.

Treatment. Schwannomas are surgically excised, and recurrence is unlikely. Prognosis is excellent.

Neurofibroma

Etiology. Neurofibromas may appear as solitary lesions or as multiple lesions as part of the syndrome neurofibromatosis (von Recklinghausen's disease of skin). The etiology of solitary neurofibroma is unknown. Neurofibromatosis, on the other hand, is inherited as an autosomal dominant trait. It has variable expressivity and often (50% of cases) appears following spontaneous mutation.

The cell of origin of the neurofibroma is not clearly established. Most investigators believe it is the Schwann cell; others believe that the perineural fibroblast is responsible.

Clinical Features. The solitary neurofibroma presents at any age as an uninflamed, asymptomatic, submucosal mass (Table 7–6). The tongue, buccal mucosa, and vestibule are the oral regions most commonly affected.

Neurofibromatosis is a relatively common syndrome (one in 3000 births) that includes multiple neurofibromas, cutaneous café-au-lait macules, bone abnormalities, central nervous system changes, and other stigmata. The neurofibromas range clinically from discrete superficial nodules to deep diffuse masses (Fig. 7–34). Lesions may be so numerous and prominent that they become cosmetically significant. Intraoral neurofibromas may be seen in up to 25% of patients with neurofibromatosis. When other oral stigmata such as enlarged fungiform papillae and bone abnormalities are included, oral manifestations may be seen in as many as 70% of neurofibromatosis patients. Malignant degeneration of neurofibromas into neurogenic sarcoma is seen in between 5 and 15% of patients with this syndrome.

The presence of six or more café-au-lait macules greater than 1.5 cm in diameter is generally regarded as being indicative of neu-

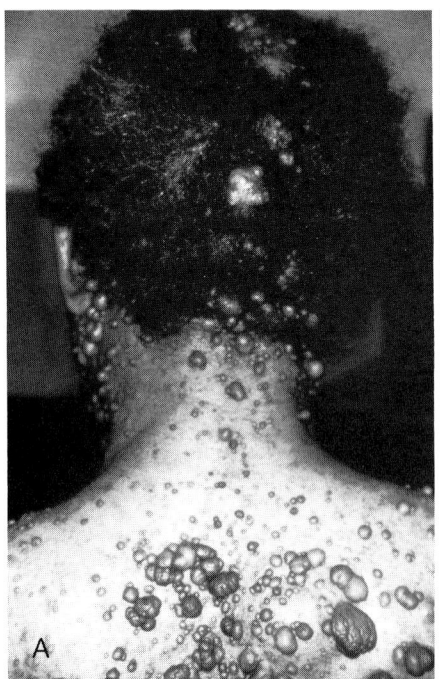
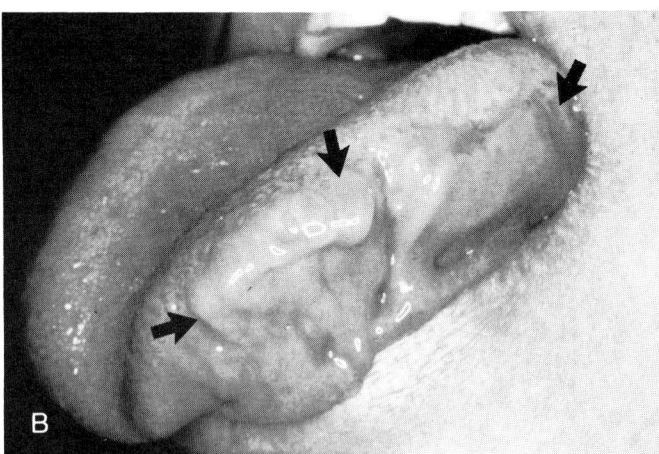

Figure 7–34. *A*, Neurofibromatosis. (Courtesy of Dr. R. Wesley.) *B*, Neurofibroma of the tongue (arrows).

rofibromatosis until proved otherwise. Axillary freckling (Crowe's sign) and iris freckling (Lisch spots) are also commonly seen pigmentary abnormalities.

Bone changes may be seen in half or more of patients with neurofibromatosis. The changes may be in the form of cortical erosion from adjacent soft tissue tumors or medullary resorption from intraosseous lesions. In the mandible, lesions most commonly arise from the mandibular nerve and may result in pain or paresthesia. In such cases of mandibular involvement, an accompanying radiographic sign may be the formation of a flaring of the inferior alveolar foramen, the so-called blunderbuss foramen. Involvement of the spine is frequently seen and may result in kyphoscoliosis, which may eventually cause spinal cord compression and paralysis. Some intrabone lesions are believed to be the result of mesodermal dysplasia.

Neurologic abnormalities in neurofibromatosis may result from cranial nerve involvement. Acoustic neuromas, often bilateral, are not uncommon lesions, and they may lead to deafness, dizziness, and headache. Trigeminal nerve involvement may cause facial pain or paresthesia. Other neurologic abnormalities include gliomas, meningiomas, mental retardation, and seizures.

Histopathology. Solitary and multiple neurofibromas have the same microscopic features. They contain spindle-shaped cells, with fusiform or wavy nuclei found in a delicate connective tissue matrix; this matrix may be very myxoid in character (Fig. 7–35). These lesions may be well circumscribed or may blend into surrounding connective tissue. Mast cells are characteristically scattered throughout the lesion. A histologic subtype known as *plexiform neurofibroma* is regarded as being highly characteristic of neurofibromatosis. In this variety, extensive interlacing masses of nerve tissue are supported by a collagen matrix. Small axons may be seen among the proliferating Schwann cells and perineural cells.

Differential Diagnosis. A solitary nodular neurofibroma should be considered in a clinical differential diagnosis with other submucosal lumps of connective tissue origin such as traumatic fibroma, granular cell tumor, and lipoma. Biopsy is the only way to definitively separate these lesions. A diffuse neurofibroma resulting in macroglossia may require differentiation from lymphangioma and possibly amyloidosis.

Treatment. Solitary neurofibromas are treated by surgical excision and have little chance of recurrence. Multiple lesions of neurofibromatosis may be treated in the same way but may be so numerous that this becomes impractical. In this case the importance of lesions is the high risk of malignant transformation. Cosmetic factors are also significant. The prognosis for a patient who has had neurosarcomatous change of a pre-existing lesion is poor.

Mucosal Neuromas of Multiple Endocrine Neoplasia Syndrome, Type III

Etiology. Multiple endocrine neoplasia syndrome, type III (MEN III), of which mucosal neuromas are a prominent part, is inherited as an autosomal dominant trait. The clinical stigmata of this syndrome are related to a defect in neuroectodermal tissue.

Clinical Features. MEN III consists of medullary carcinoma of the thyroid, pheochromocytoma of the adrenal, and mucosal neuromas (Table 7–6). Café-au-lait macules and neurofibromas of the skin may also be seen in this condition. MEN I and II are related to MEN III in that patients with types I and II syndromes have neoplasms of various endocrine organs, but they do not have the oral manifestation of mucosal neuromas.

The mucosal neuromas of MEN III usually appear early in life as small discrete nodules on conjunctiva, labia, larynx, or oral cavity (Fig. 7–36). The oral lesions are seen on tongue, lips, and buccal mucosa.

Histopathology. Mucosal neuromas are composed of serpiginous bands of nerve tissue surrounded by normal connective tissue. Axons have been found in the proliferating nerve tissue. The microscopic appearance has suggested to some that these lesions may be hamartomatous rather than neoplastic.

Differential Diagnosis. The soft tissue masses of mucosal neuromas may share clinical features with neurofibromatosis or multiple papillomas. There may also be some similiarity to the mucosal presentation seen in amyloidosis and hyalinosis cutis et mucosae (lipoid proteinosis). Because the endocrine neoplasia associated with this syndrome is often manifest very early in life, biopsy should be done to establish diagnosis.

Treatment. Mucosal neuromas are surgically excised and are not expected to recur. The neuromas themselves are relatively trivial, but they are of considerable significance because they may be the first sign of this potentially

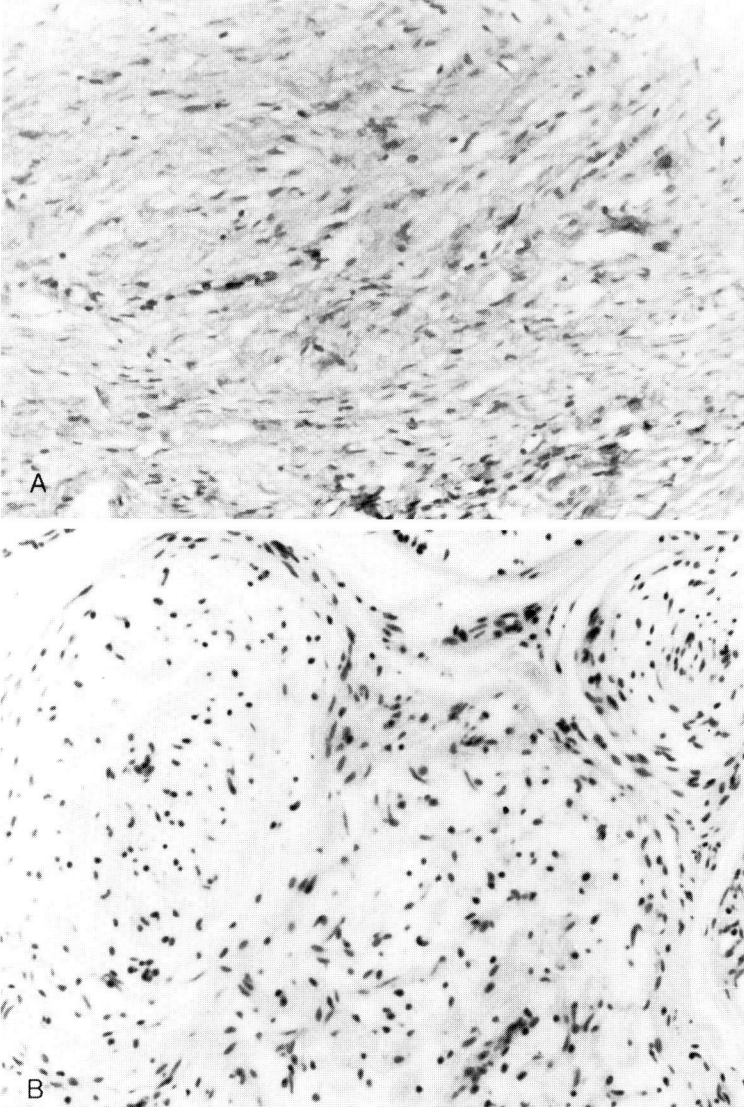

Figure 7–35. *A* and *B*, Two histologic patterns of neurofibroma.

Figure 7–36. Mucosal neuromas of MEN III syndrome. (Courtesy of Dr. R. M. Courtney.)

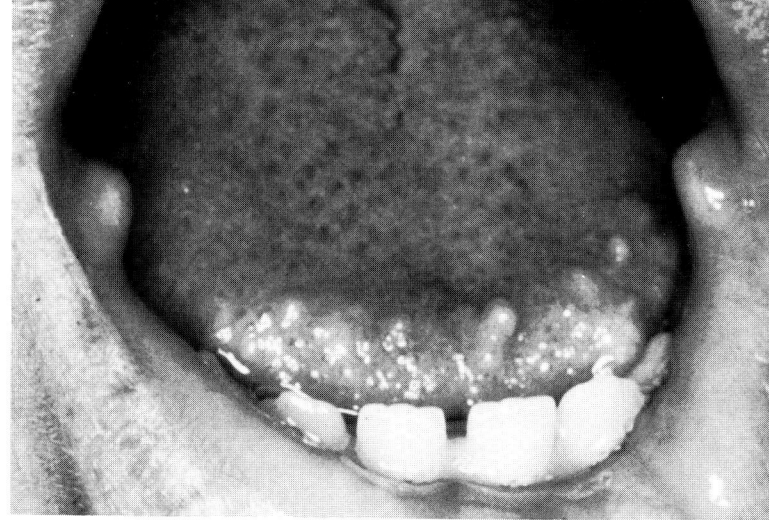

fatal syndrome. The medullary carcinoma of the thyroid is a progressive malignancy that invades locally and has the ability to metastasize to local lymph nodes and distant organs. The 5-year survival rate of this malignancy is about 50%. Pheochromocytoma is a benign neoplasm that produces catecholamines that may cause significant hypertension and other cardiovascular abnormalities. Early detection of the mucosal neuromas is therefore of utmost importance in follow-up screening of these patients.

Neurogenic Sarcoma

Neurogenic sarcoma is a rare malignancy that develops either from a pre-existing lesion of neurofibromatosis or *de novo*. The cell of origin is believed to be the Schwann cell and possibly other nerve sheath cells.

In soft tissues, this neoplasm appears as an expansile mass that is usually asymptomatic. In bone, where it is believed to arise most often from a mandibular nerve, it presents as a dilatation of the mandibular canal or as a diffuse lucency. Pain or paresthesia may accompany the lesion in bone; this is also the case for other malignancies within the mandible or maxilla.

Microscopically, neurogenic sarcoma can be seen arising from a neurofibroma or from a nerve trunk. The lesion is very cellular and is composed of abundant spindle cells with variable numbers of abnormal mitotic figures. Streaming and palisading of nuclei is often seen, and nuclear pleomorphism may also be prominent (Fig. 7–37). Microscopic separation of this lesion from fibrosarcoma and leiomyosarcoma may be difficult, making electron mi-

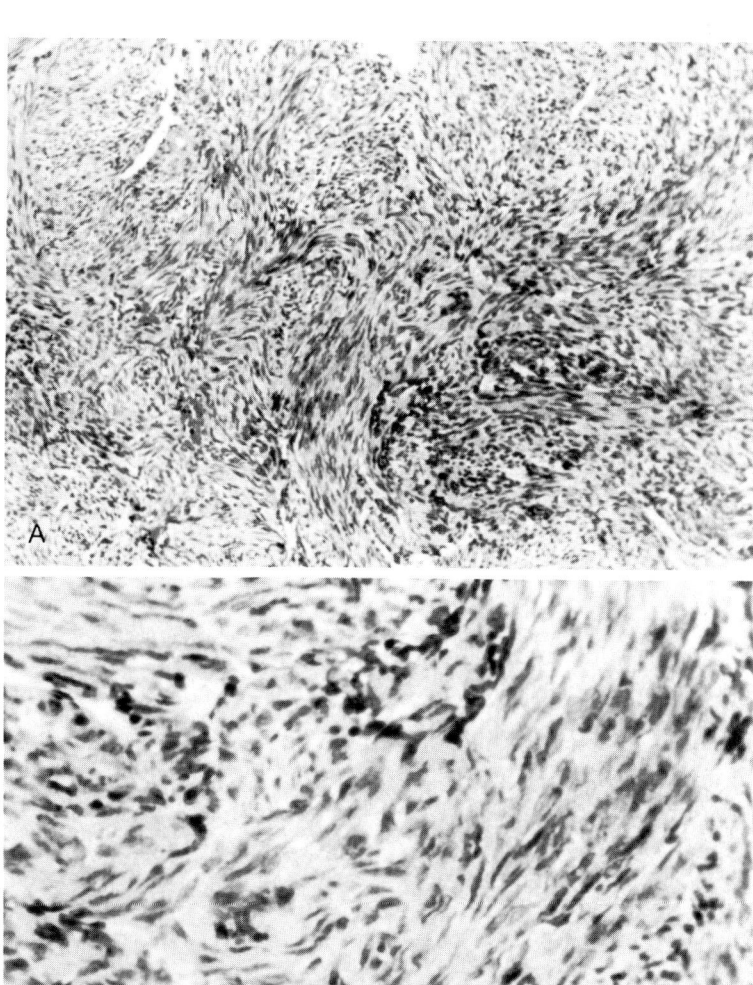

Figure 7–37. *A* and *B*, Neurogenic sarcoma showing high cellularity and slight pleomorphism.

croscopy and immunohistochemistry important diagnostic adjuncts.

The primary method of treatment is wide surgical excision. However, recurrence is common, and metastases are frequently seen. Prognosis varies from fair to good, depending upon clinical circumstances.

Esthesioneuroblastoma

This malignancy, also known as olfactory neuroblastoma, is a rare lesion that arises from olfactory tissue in the superior portion of the nasal cavity. This lesion, typically occurring in young adults, may cause epistaxis, rhinorrhea, or nasal obstruction, or it may present as polyps in the roof of the nasal cavity. It may also result in a nasopharyngeal mass or an invasive maxillary sinus lesion.

Microscopically, this lesion consists of small, undifferentiated, round cells with little visible cytoplasm (Fig. 7–38). Compartmentalization and rosette formation are often seen. Electron microscopy can be used to confirm the light microscopic diagnosis by identifying neurosecretory granules. Microscopic differential diagnosis would include lymphoma and some small round cell sarcomas and carcinomas.

Surgery or radiation is used to treat esthesioneuroblastoma. Recurrences are not uncommon, appearing in about half the patients. Metastases, usually to local nodes or lung, are infrequently encountered.

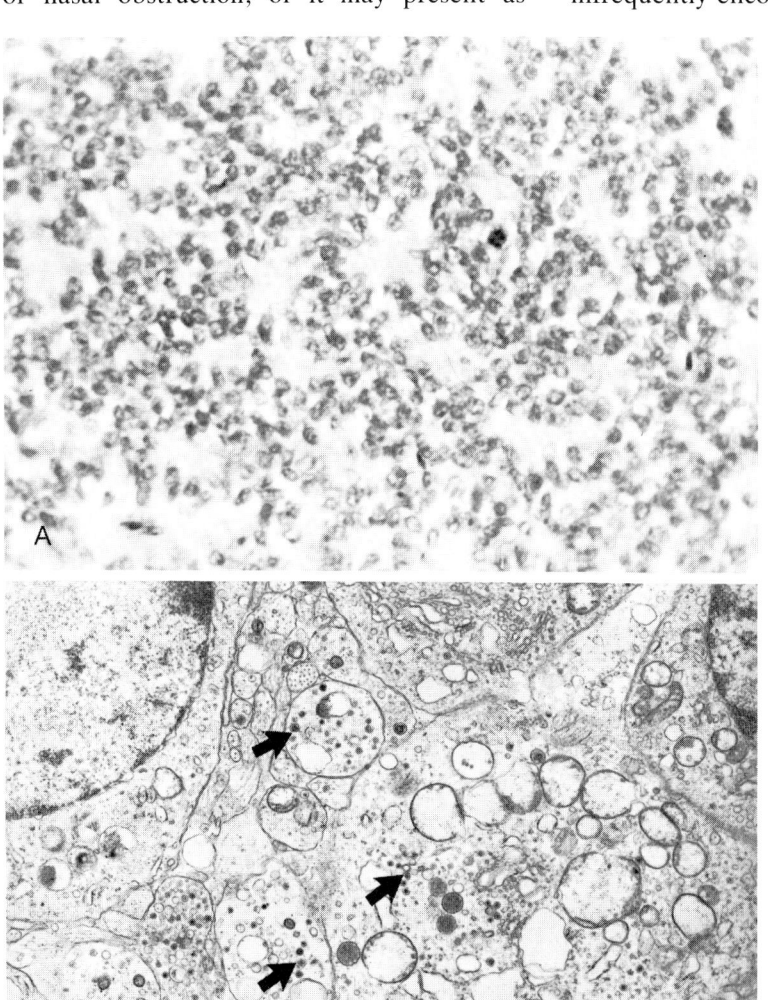

Figure 7–38. *A* and *B*, Esthesioneuroblastoma. Electron micrograph *(B)* show numerous cytoplasmic neurosecretory granules (arrows).

LESIONS OF MUSCLE AND FAT

Reactive Lesions

Myositis Ossificans

This is an uncommon reactive lesion of skeletal muscle. It may appear in the muscles of the head and neck. As the name implies, the condition is an intramuscular inflammatory process in which ossification occurs. The reason for the appearance of bone in the muscle reparative process has not been fully explained.

Muscle ossification may be seen in either of two forms: as a progressive systemic disease (myositis ossificans progressiva) of unknown etiology, or as a focal single-muscle disorder (traumatic myositis ossificans) of traumatic origin. In the latter form, acute or chronic trauma may be responsible for the muscular change. The masseter and the sternocleidomastoid muscles are most commonly affected. As the lesion matures, soft tissue radiographs show a delicate feathery opacification. The actively proliferating osteoblasts have occasionally been confused with osteosarcoma microscopically. Maturation and organization of the osseous tissue peripheral to the central cellular zone is felt to be an important diagnostic feature of myositis ossificans. The lesion is treated with surgical excision.

Neoplasms

Leiomyoma and Leiomyosarcoma

Smooth muscle neoplasms, in general, are relatively common. They may arise anywhere in the body from muscle cells or their precursors in the media of blood vessels, in the muscularis layer of the gut, and in the body of the uterus. In the oral cavity, these neoplasms are rarely encountered.

Oral *leiomyomas* present as slow-growing, asymptomatic submucosal masses, usually in the tongue, hard palate, or buccal mucosa. They may be seen at any age and are usually discovered when they are 1 to 2 cm in diameter.

Microscopic diagnosis may occasionally be difficult because the spindle cell proliferation has many similarities with neurofibroma, schwannoma, and fibromatosis (Fig. 7–39). Special stains that identify collagen may be helpful in distinguishing these lesions. Ultrastructural demonstration of myofilaments and immunohistochemical staining of desmin-type intermediate filaments or actin and myosin antigens may also be useful in establishing a definitive diagnosis. A microscopic subtype known as *vascular leiomyoma* has numerous thick-walled vessels associated with well-differentiated smooth muscle cells. Leiomyomas are surgically excised, and recurrence is unexpected.

Oral *leiomyosarcomas* have been reported in all age groups and most intraoral regions. Microscopic diagnosis is a considerable challenge because of similarities to other spindle cell sarcomas. As with the benign neoplasms, electron microscopy and immunohistochemistry can be valuable diagnostic tools. This malignancy is usually treated with wide surgical excision. Metastasis to lymph nodes or lung is not uncommon.

Rhabdomyoma and Rhabdomyosarcoma

Rhabdomyomas are rare lesions, but they have a predilection for the soft tissues of the head and neck. The oral sites most frequently reported are floor of the mouth, soft palate, tongue, and buccal mucosa. The mean age is about 50 years, and the age range extends from children to older adults. Presentation is as an asymptomatic, well-defined submucosal mass.

Two microscopic variants are recognized. In the adult type, the neoplastic cells closely mimic their normal counterpart (Fig. 7–40); in the fetal type, the neoplastic cells are elongated and less differentiated and exhibit fewer cross striations. The latter type may be confused with rhabdomyosarcoma. Treatment is excision, and recurrence is unlikely.

Rhabdomyosarcomas are subdivided into pleomorphic, embryonal, and alveolar types, depending upon microscopic appearance. The pleomorphic type, the most well differentiated, contains strap or spindle cells that often exhibit cross striations. The embryonal type consists of primitive round cells in which striations are rarely found. The alveolar variant is also composed of round cells but in a compartmentalized pattern.

Rhabdomyosarcoma, when it occurs in the head and neck, is primarily found in children. When occurring outside the head and neck, it is seen typically in adults. Rhabdomyosarcoma presents as a rapidly growing mass, which, if there is jaw involvement, may cause pain or paresthesia. The most commonly affected oral sites are the tongue and soft palate (Fig. 7–41). The embryonal type of rhabdomyosar-

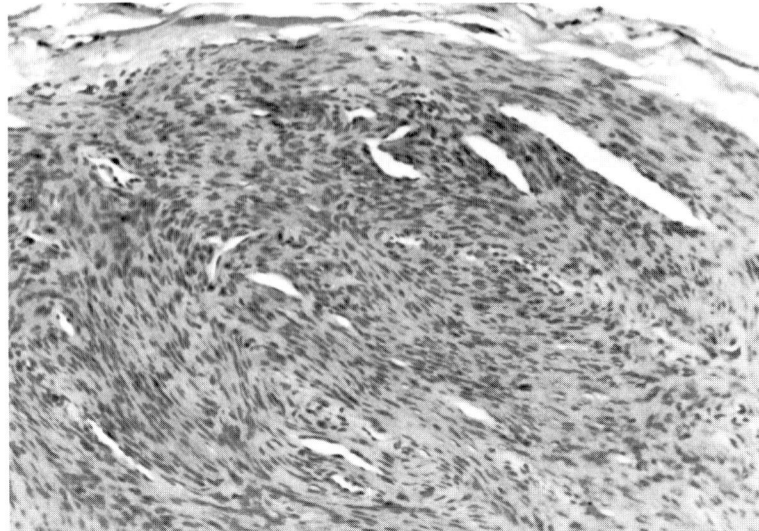

Figure 7-39. Leiomyoma of oral soft tissues. Note capsule (top).

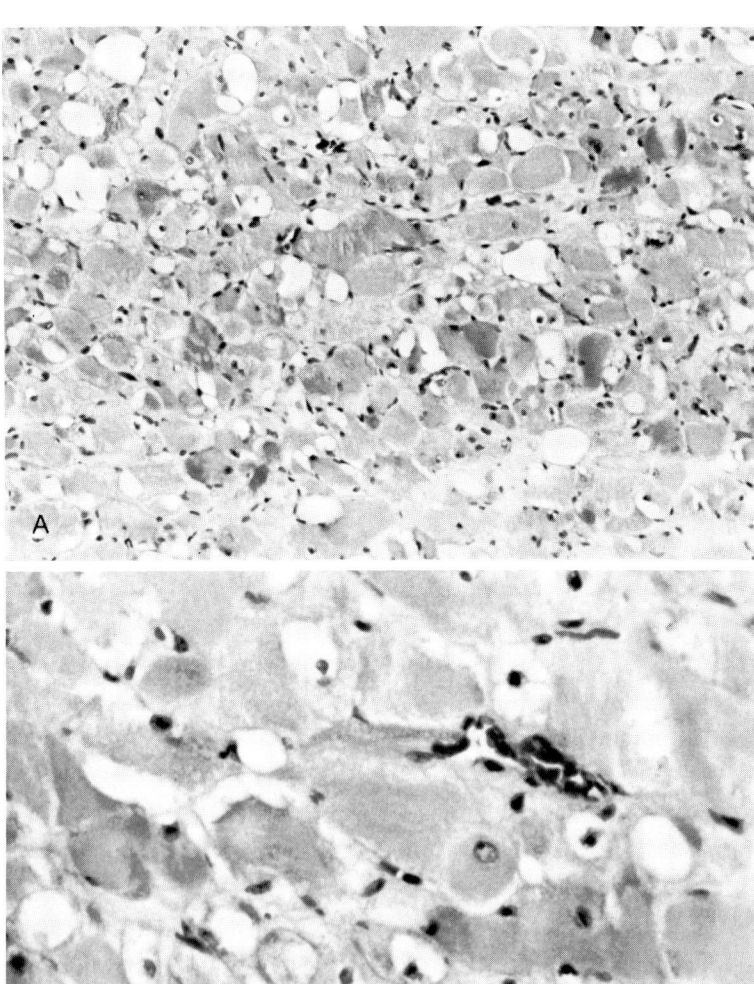

Figure 7-40. Rhabdomyoma, adult type. Note resemblance to normal muscle.

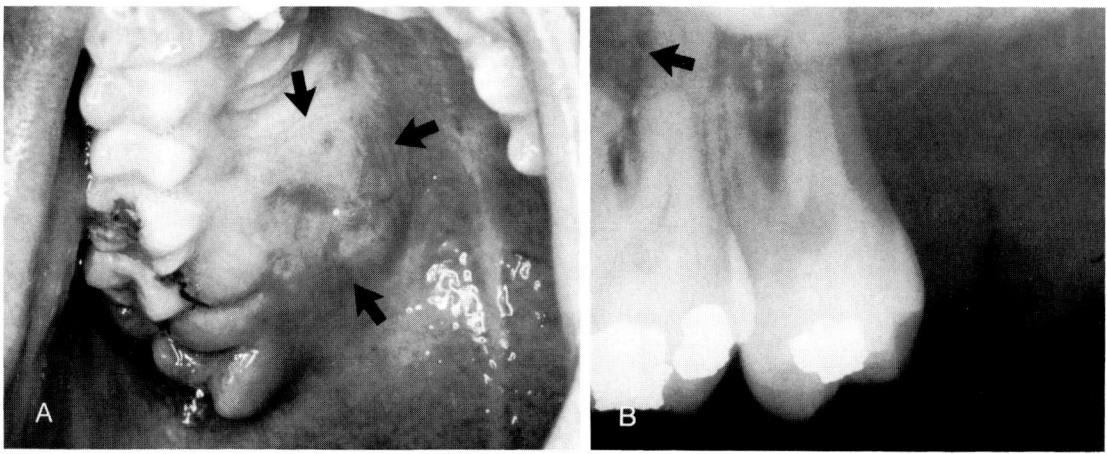

Figure 7–41. *A*, Rhabdomyosarcoma of the maxilla (arrows). *B*, Radiograph showing bone loss and uniformly widened periodontal membrane space (arrow).

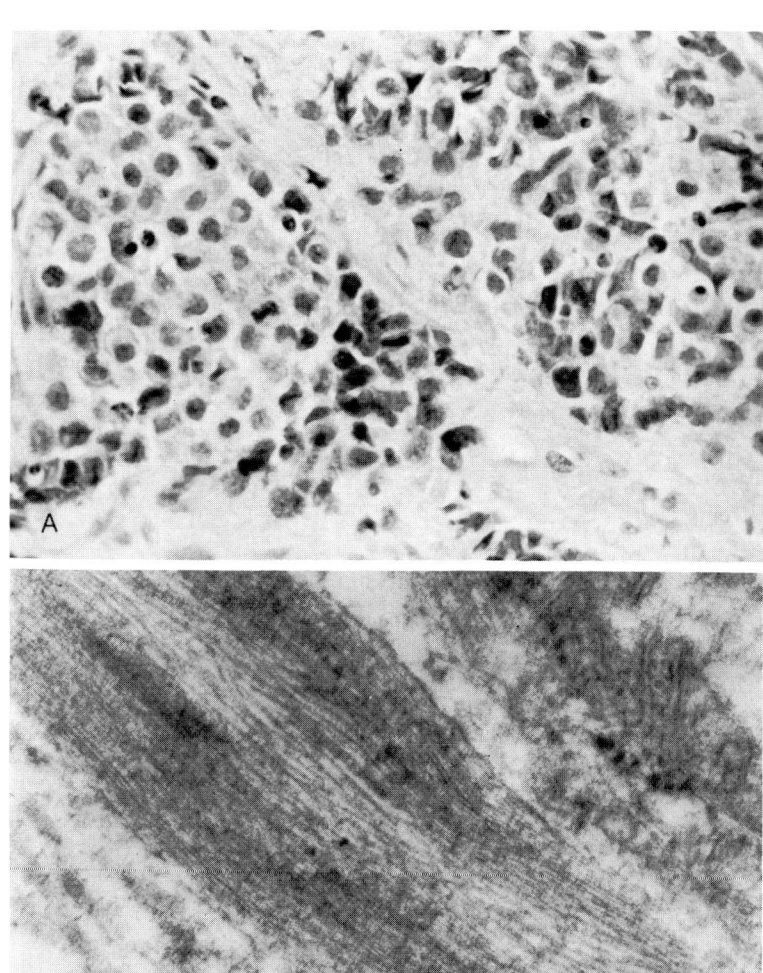

Figure 7–42. *A* and *B*, Rhabdomyosarcoma, embryonal type. Electron micrograph *(B)* showing cytoplasm containing myofilaments with cross-banding.

222 CONNECTIVE TISSUE LESIONS

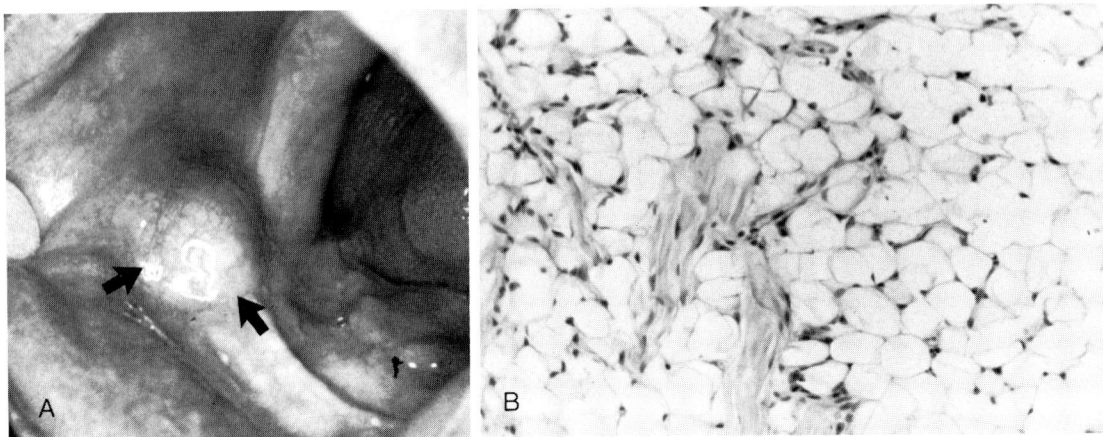

Figure 7–43. *A*, Lipoma of buccal mucosa (arrows). *B*, Micrograph showing close resemblance to normal tissue.

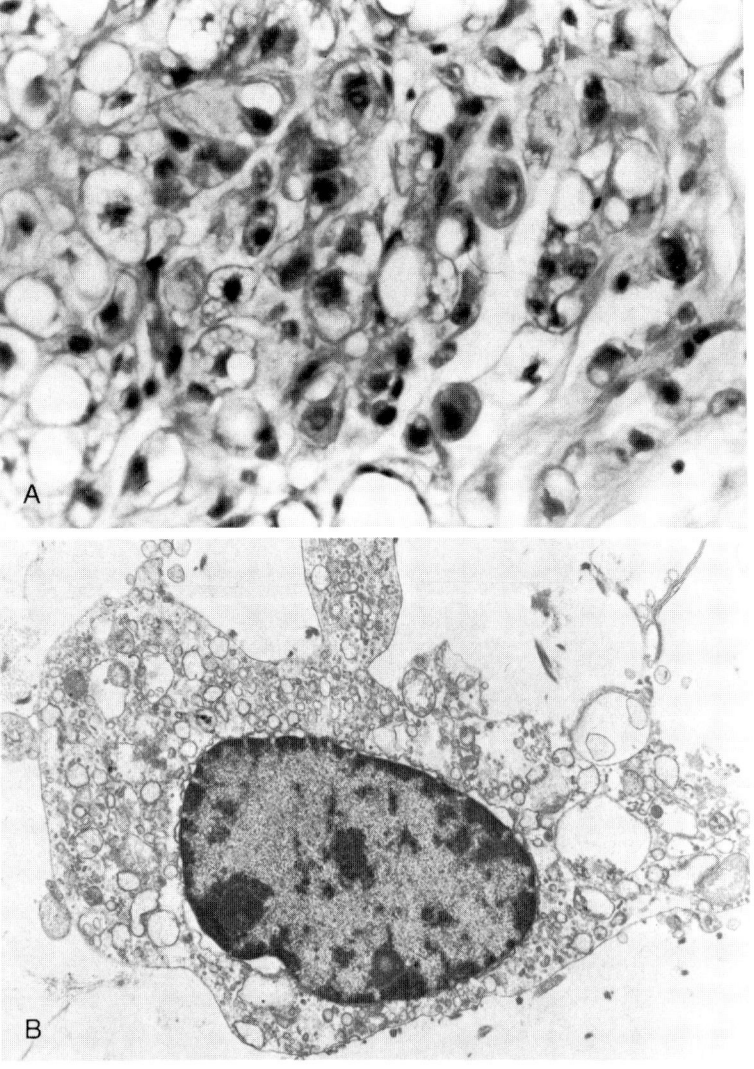

Figure 7–44. *A* and *B*, Liposarcoma of oral soft tissues. Note vacuolation of cytoplasm in both light and electron micrographs.

coma is the variety most commonly seen in the head and neck. Because of the relatively undifferentiated nature of this microscopic subtype, electron microscopy or immunohistochemistry or both are often used to support light microscopic interpretations (Fig. 7–42).

The combination of surgery, radiation, and chemotherapy has been shown to produce far better clinical results than any one of these treatment methods alone. Survival rates have increased from less than 10% to better than 60% with this more aggressive treatment approach.

Lipoma and Liposarcoma

Lipomas are uncommon neoplasms of the oral cavity that may occur in any region. Buccal mucosa, tongue, and floor of the mouth are among the more common locations (Fig. 7–43). Clinical presentation is typically as an asymptomatic, yellowish submucosal mass. The overlying epithelium is intact, and superficial blood vessels are usually evident over the tumor. Other benign connective tissue lesions such as granular cell tumor, neurofibroma, traumatic fibroma, and salivary gland lesions (mucocele and mixed tumor) might be included in a differential diagnosis.

Numerous microscopic subtypes have been described, but they are primarily of academic interest. All types will have adipocytes of varying maturity. The usual simple lipoma consists of a well-circumscribed, lobulated mass of mature fat cells. The lesions are excised and are not expected to recur.

Liposarcoma is rarely encountered in soft tissues of the head and neck. It is a lesion of adulthood and may potentially occur in any site. It is generally slow growing and thus may be mistaken for a benign process. Considerable microscopic variation in these malignancies has led to subclassification into at least four types (well-differentiated, myxoid, round cell, pleomorphic) (Fig. 7–44). The degree of tumor cell differentiation coupled with identification of microscopic subtype is an important factor in predicting clinical behavior. These neoplasms may be treated with surgery or radiation, and prognosis is fair to good.

Bibliography

Fibrous Connective Tissue Lesions

Abdul-Karim F, Ayala A, Chawla S, et al. Malignant fibrous histiocytoma of jaws. A clinicopathologic study of 11 cases. Cancer 56:1590–1596, 1985.

Bernstein K, Lattes R. Nodular (pseudosarcomatous) fasciitis, a nonrecurrent lesion. Cancer 49:1668–1678, 1982.

Bertoni F, Capanna R, Biagini R, et al. Malignant fibrous histiocytoma of soft tissue. Cancer 56:356–367, 1985.

Bras J, Batsakis J, Luna M. Malignant fibrous histiocytoma of the oral soft tissues. Oral Surg Oral Med Oral Pathol 64:57–67, 1987.

Cook C, Lund B, Carney J. Mucocutaneous pigmented spots and oral myxomas: the oral manifestations of the complex of myxomas, spotty pigmentation, and endocrine overactivity. Oral Surg Oral Med Oral Pathol 63:175–183, 1987.

Daley T, Wysocki G, Day C. Clinical and pharmacologic correlations in cyclosporine-induced gingival hyperplasia. Oral Surg Oral Med Oral Pathol 62:417–421, 1986.

Daou R, Attia E, Viloria J. Malignant fibrous histiocytomas of the head and neck. J Otolaryngol 12:383–388, 1983.

Deliliers G, Santoro F, Polli N. Light and electron microscopic study of cyclosporin A–induced gingival hyperplasia. J Periodontol 57:771–775, 1986.

Ellis G, Brannon R. Focal myositis of the perioral musculature. Oral Surg Oral Med Oral Pathol 48:337–341, 1979.

Freedman P, Lumerman H. Intravascular fasciitis: report of two cases and review of the literature. Oral Surg Oral Med Oral Pathol 62:549–554, 1986.

Fujiwara K, Watanabe T, Katsuki T, et al. Proliferative myositis of the buccinator muscle: a case with immunohistochemical and electron microscopic analysis. Oral Surg Oral Med Oral Pathol 63:597–601, 1987.

Gardner D. The peripheral odontogenic fibroma: an attempt at clarification. Oral Surg Oral Med Oral Pathol 54:40–48, 1982.

Gould A, Escobar V. Symmetrical gingival fibromatosis. Oral Surg Oral Med Oral Pathol 51:62–67, 1981.

Handlers J, Abrams A, Melrose R, et al. Fibrosarcoma of the mandible presenting as a periodontal problem. J Oral Pathol 14:351–356, 1985.

Kabot T, Goldman M, Bergman S, et al. Juvenile nasopharyngeal angiofibroma: an unusual presentation in the oral cavity. Oral Surg Oral Med Oral Pathol 59:453–457, 1985.

Keith D. Side-effects of diphenylhydantoin: a review. J Oral Surg 36:206–209, 1978.

McMillan M, Smillie A, Ferguson J. Malignant fibrous histiocytoma of the tongue: report of a case and ultrastructural observations. J Oral Pathol 15:255–260, 1986.

Melrose R, Abrams A. Juvenile fibromatosis affecting the jaws. Oral Surg Oral Med Oral Pathol 49:317–324, 1980.

Orlowski W, Freedman P, Lumerman H. Proliferative myositis of the masseter muscle. Cancer 52:904–908, 1983.

Rapidis A, Triantafyllou A. Myxoma of the oral soft tissues. J Oral Maxillofac Surg 41:188–192, 1983.

Regezi J, Zarbo R, Tomich C, et al. Immunoprofile of benign and malignant fibrohistiocytic tumors. J Oral Pathol 16:260–265, 1987.

Rodu B, Weathers R, Campbell W. Aggressive fibromatosis involving the paramandibular soft tissues. Oral Surg Oral Med Oral Pathol 52:395–403, 1981.

Shimizu S, Hashimoto H, Enjoji M. Nodular fasciitis: an analysis of 250 patients. Pathology 16:161–166, 1984.

Sist T, Greene G. Benign nerve sheath myxoma: light and electron microscopic features of two cases. Oral Surg Oral Med Oral Pathol 47:441–444, 1979.

Suit H, Mankin H, Wood W, et al. Preoperative, intraoperative, and postoperative radiation in the treatment of primary soft tissue sarcoma. Cancer 55:2659–2667, 1985.

Thompson S, Shear M. Fibrous histiocytomas of the oral and maxillofacial regions. J Oral Pathol 13:282–294, 1984.

Tomich C. Oral focal mucinosis. Oral Surg Oral Med Oral Pathol 38:714–724, 1974.

Weiss S, Enzinger F. Malignant fibrous histiocytoma. Cancer 41:2250–2266, 1978.

Werning J. Nodular fasciitis of the orofacial region. Oral Surg Oral Med Oral Pathol 48:441–446, 1979.

Neural Lesions

Chen S, Miller A. Neurofibroma and schwannoma of the oral cavity. Oral Surg Oral Med Oral Pathol 47:522–528, 1979.

Khansur T, Balducci L, Tavassoli M. Granular cell tumor. Cancer 60:220–222, 1987.

Lifshitz M, Flotti T, Greco A. Congenital granular cell epulis. Cancer 53:1845–1848, 1984.

Matthews J, Mason G. Oral granular cell myoblastoma: an immunohistochemical study. J Oral Pathol 11:343–352, 1982.

McCoy J, Mincer H, Turner J. Intra-oral ancient neurilemmoma (ancient schwannoma). Oral Surg Oral Med Oral Pathol 56:174–184, 1983.

Mills S, Frierson H. Olfactory neuroblastoma. A clinicopathologic study of 21 cases. Am J Surg Pathol 9:317–327, 1985.

Monteil R, Loubiere R, Charbit Y, et al. Gingival granular cell tumor of the newborn: immunoperoxidase investigation with anti-S-100 antiserum. Oral Surg Oral Med Oral Pathol 64:78–81, 1987.

Mukai M. Immunohistochemical localization of S-100 protein and peripheral nerve myelin proteins (P2 protein, P0 protein) in granular cell tumors. Am J Pathol 112:139–146, 1983.

Regezi J, Batsakis J, Courtney R. Granular cell tumors of the head and neck. J Oral Surg 37:402–406, 1979.

Regezi J, McClatchey K, Batsakis J. Diagnostic electron microscopy of head and neck tumors. In Trump B, Jones R (eds). Diagnostic Electron Microscopy, Vol 4. John Wiley & Sons, New York, 1983.

Rubenstein A. Neurofibromatosis, a review of the clinical problem. Ann NY Acad Sci 486:1–13, 1986.

Sciubba J, D'Amico E, Attie J. The occurrence of multiple endocrine neoplasia, Type IIB, in two children of an affected mother. J Oral Pathol 16:310–316, 1987.

Seo I, Azzarelli B, Warner T, et al. Multiple visceral and cutaneous granular cell tumors. Cancer 53:2104–2110, 1984.

Shapiro S, Abramovitch K, Van Dis M, et al. Neurofibromatosis: oral and radiographic manifestations. Oral Surg Oral Med Oral Pathol 58:493–498, 1984.

Sist T, Green G. Traumatic neuroma of the oral cavity. Oral Surg Oral Med Oral Pathol 51:394–402, 1981.

Vincent S, Williams T. Mandibular abnormalities in neurofibromatosis. Oral Surg Oral Med Oral Pathol 55:253–258, 1983.

Wright B, Jackson D. Neural tumors of the oral cavity. Oral Surg Oral Med Oral Pathol 49:509–522, 1980.

Zarbo R, Lloyd R, Beals T, et al. Congenital gingival granular cell tumor with smooth muscle cytodifferentiation. Oral Surg Oral Med Oral Pathol 56:512–520, 1983.

Lesions of Muscle and Fat

Brooks J. Immunohistochemistry of soft tissue tumors. Cancer 50:1757–1763, 1982.

Chen S, Fantasia J, Miller A. Myxoid lipoma of oral soft tissue. Oral Surg Oral Med Oral Pathol 57:300–307, 1984.

Corio R, Lewis D. Intra-oral rhabdomyomas. Oral Surg Oral Med Oral Pathol 48:525–531, 1979.

Damm D, Neville B. Oral leiomyomas. Oral Surg Oral Med Oral Pathol 47:343–348, 1979.

Gardner D, Corio R. Fetal rhabdomyomas of the tongue, with a discussion of the two histologic variants of this tumor. Oral Surg Oral Med Oral Pathol 56:293–300, 1983.

Geiger S, Czernobilsky B, Marshak G. Embryonal rhabdomyosarcoma: immunohistochemical characterization. Oral Surg Oral Med Oral Pathol 60:517–523, 1985.

Kratochvil F, MacGregor S, Hewan-Lowe K, et al. Leiomyosarcoma of the maxilla. Oral Surg Oral Med Oral Pathol 54:647–654, 1982.

McMillan M, Ferguson J, Kardos T. Mandibular vascular leiomyoma. Oral Surg Oral Med Oral Pathol 62:427–433, 1985.

Natella J, Neiders M, Greene G. Oral leiomyoma. J Oral Pathol 11:353–365, 1982.

Osborn M, Weber K. Biology of disease—tumor diagnosis by intermediate filament typing. Lab Invest 48:372–394, 1983.

Sadeghi E, Sauk J. Liposarcoma of the oral cavity. Clinical, tissue culture, and ultrastructure study of a case. J Oral Pathol 11:263–275, 1982.

Chapter 8

Salivary Gland Diseases

REACTIVE LESIONS (NON-INFECTIOUS)
Mucus Extravasation Phenomenon
Mucus Retention Cyst
Ranula
Mucocele of the Maxillary Sinus
Maxillary Sinus Retention Cyst and Pseudocyst
Necrotizing Sialometaplasia
Radiation-Induced Salivary Gland Pathology
INFECTIOUS CONDITIONS
Viral Diseases
   Mumps
   Cytomegalic Sialadenitis
Bacterial Sialadenitis
Sarcoidosis
METABOLIC CONDITIONS
CONDITIONS ASSOCIATED WITH IMMUNE DEFECTS
Benign Lymphoepithelial Lesion
Sjögren's Syndrome
BENIGN NEOPLASMS
Benign Mixed Tumor (Pleomorphic Adenoma)
Monomorphic Adenomas
   Basal Cell Adenomas
   Sebaceous Tumors
   Oncocytic Tumors
Sialadenoma Papilliferum and Inverted Ductal Papilloma
Myoepithelioma
MALIGNANT NEOPLASMS
Mucoepidermoid Carcinoma
Adenocystic Carcinoma
Acinic Cell Carcinoma
Carcinoma Ex-mixed Tumor/Malignant Mixed Tumor
Epimyoepithelial Carcinoma of Intercalated Ducts
Terminal Duct Carcinoma
Salivary Duct Carcinoma
Adenocarcinoma
Squamous Cell Carcinoma

Diseases of the salivary glands may be broadly subdivided into neoplastic and non-neoplastic categories. In the latter, several groups test the clinician's diagnostic and therapeutic skills, because reactive, metabolic, immunologic, infectious, and iatrogenic etiologies may all produce similar clinical appearances or symptoms. Physical examination is only one component of the diagnostic process, since by itself it is often insufficient to answer a clinical problem. History and laboratory tests are often equally important in this process. The number and sophistication of tests can vary widely depending on clinical differential diagnosis. For example, assessing the immune system of a patient suspected of having Sjögren's syndrome may require numerous studies, whereas a simple radiograph may suffice to establish the diagnosis in an individual with a sialolith.

Neoplastic diseases, although quite varied in their specific histologic patterns and frequently presenting diagnostic difficulties at the microscopic level, are generally straightforward in their clinical presentation, with much overlap noted from one group of lesions to another. Histologically, various classifications of neoplasms have permitted the identification of a large number of different entities, essentially having little or no clinical distinction. Major and minor salivary gland neoplasms typically present as asymptomatic masses or chronic ulcers. In terms of frequency, rates of malignancy, and management, however, lesions of major and minor salivary glands show distinct differences.

REACTIVE LESIONS (NON-INFECTIOUS)

Mucus Extravasation Phenomenon

Mucus extravasation phenomenon, commonly known by the clinical term, "mucocele," is separated from mucus retention cyst because each has a distinctive pathogenesis and microscopy. Several clinical features also separate these lesions.

Etiology and Pathogenesis. The etiology of mucus extravasation phenomenon is considered to be related to mechanical trauma to the minor salivary gland excretory duct, resulting in its transection or severance (Fig. 8–1). Following this, there is spillage or extravasation of mucus into the surrounding connective tissue stroma. The pool of extravasated mucus induces a secondary inflammatory reaction in the surrounding connective tissue, with neutrophils followed by an influx of macrophages flooding into the area. A granulation tissue response ensues, resulting in the formation of a wall around the mucin pool, giving a pseudocyst-like quality to the lesion. The adjacent salivary gland tissue undergoes a non-specific inflammatory change secondary to mucus retention. With persistent lesions, permanent changes may be noted within the salivary parenchymal tissue, with a corresponding decrease in or absence of secretory activity by the involved gland.

Clinical Features. Although the lower lip is the most frequent site of mucus extravasation phenomenon (Fig. 8–2), the buccal mucosa, ventral surface of the tongue (where the glands of Blandin-Nuhn are located), floor of the mouth, and retromolar region are often affected. Lesions are infrequently found in other intraoral regions where salivary glands are located (Fig. 8–3), probably because of the relative absence of trauma to these areas.

Presentation tends to be away from the midline of the mucosal side of lip, frequently being midway between the midline and the commissural angle. These lesions are painless and smooth surfaced, with an overall bluish hue or translucency associated with a more superficial location. They range from a few millimeters to a few centimeters in diameter. The more deeply placed mucoceles appear as a less discrete, diffuse swelling with no associated translucent or bluish hue. Adolescents and children are most commonly affected, with nearly half of reported cases presenting under 21 years of age and more than one fourth between the ages of 11 and 20 years.

Subsequent to the initiating traumatic event, the clinical swelling may decrease in size, because of resorption of pooled mucin. Further production of mucin often continues in a rather dynamic process that leads to fluctuation in size of the lesion. Maximum size is usually reached within several days after injury, and a viscous material is found if aspiration is attempted.

In another variety of mucus extravasation, focal subepithelial accumulation of mucin is seen (Fig. 8–4). This type of *superficial mucocele* is usually not related to trauma or a process in which actual ductal transection has

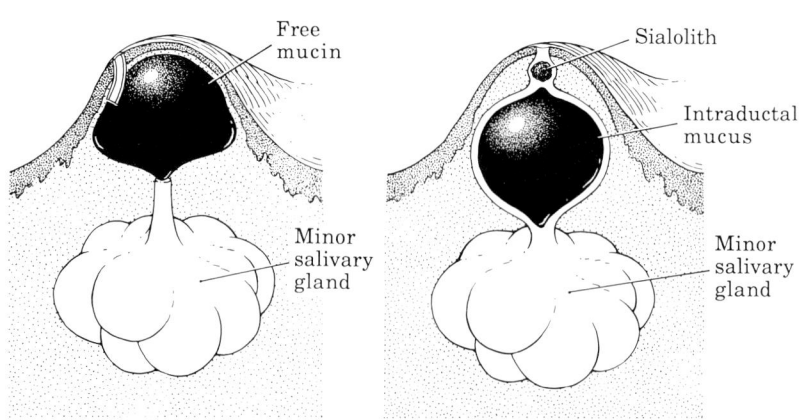

Figure 8–1. *Left*, Mucus extravasation phenomenon—note severed duct at upper left. *Right*, Mucus retention cyst.

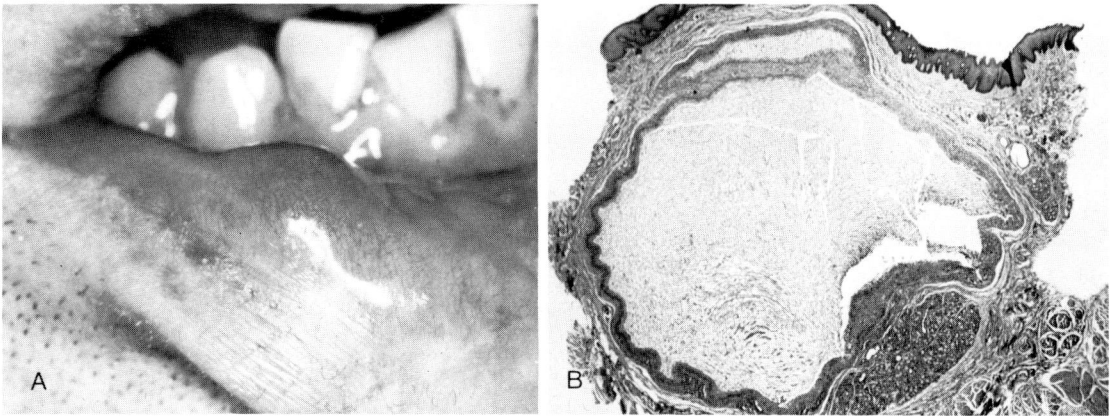

Figure 8–2. *A* and *B*, Mucocele (mucus extravasation phenomenon). Note mucin pool surrounded by granulation tissue in *B*.

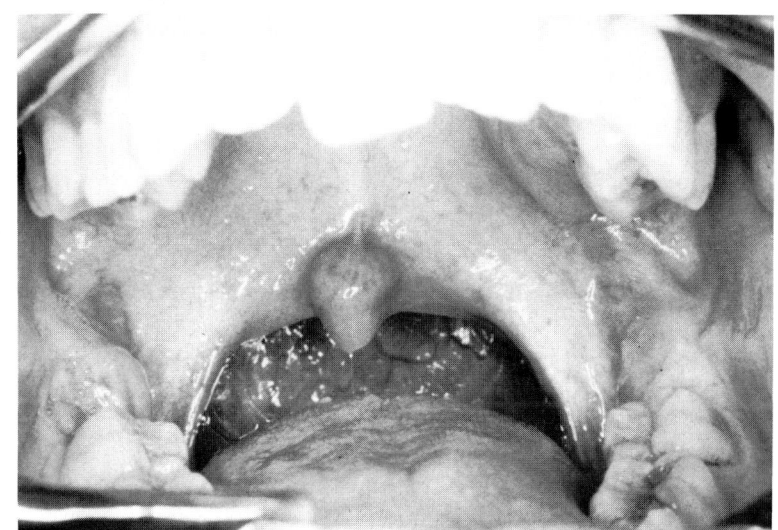

Figure 8–3. Mucocele (mucus extravasation phenomenon) of soft palate.

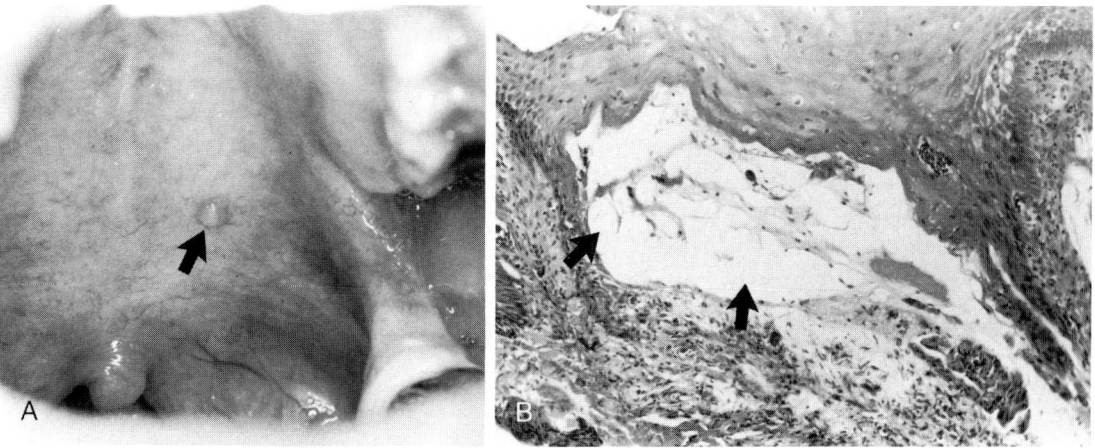

Figure 8–4. *A*, Superficial mucocele (arrow). *B*, Biopsy showing extravasated mucin between epithelium and connective tissue (arrows).

occurred. These lesions are asymptomatic and multiple. Their clinical appearance suggests a vesculo-bullous disease, but the lesions persist for an extended length of time. Other than being a diagnostic challenge, they are apparently of little significance.

Histopathology. The mucus extravasation phenomenon will generally demonstrate a well-circumscribed cavity containing pooled mucin (Fig. 8–5). The overlying epithelium is often thinned and is separated from the mucin pool by a thin wall of compressed granulation tissue. The pool of mucin itself is likewise surrounded by well-formed compressed fibrous and granulation tissue that is infiltrated by large numbers of neutrophils, macrophages, lymphocytes, and occasionally, plasma cells. Extension of the inflammatory process into the surrounding stromal tissue is seen; it decreases in intensity at a distance from the mucin pool.

The adjacent or surrounding salivary parenchymal elements, especially those related to the transected or severed duct, will demonstrate changes consisting of ductal dilatation and acinic degeneration. A combination of interstitial fibrosis and inflammatory infiltrate may also be seen in the recurrent or chronic lesions (Fig. 8–6).

Differential Diagnosis. Although a history of a traumatic event followed by rapid development of a bluish translucency of the lower lip is characteristic of mucus extravasation phenomenon, other lesions might be considered when a typical history is absent. These include salivary gland neoplasms, vascular malformations, venous varices, and soft tissue neoplasms such as neurofibromas and lipomas. If a mucocele appears in the alveolar mucosa, an eruption cyst or gingival cyst should be included in the differential diagnosis.

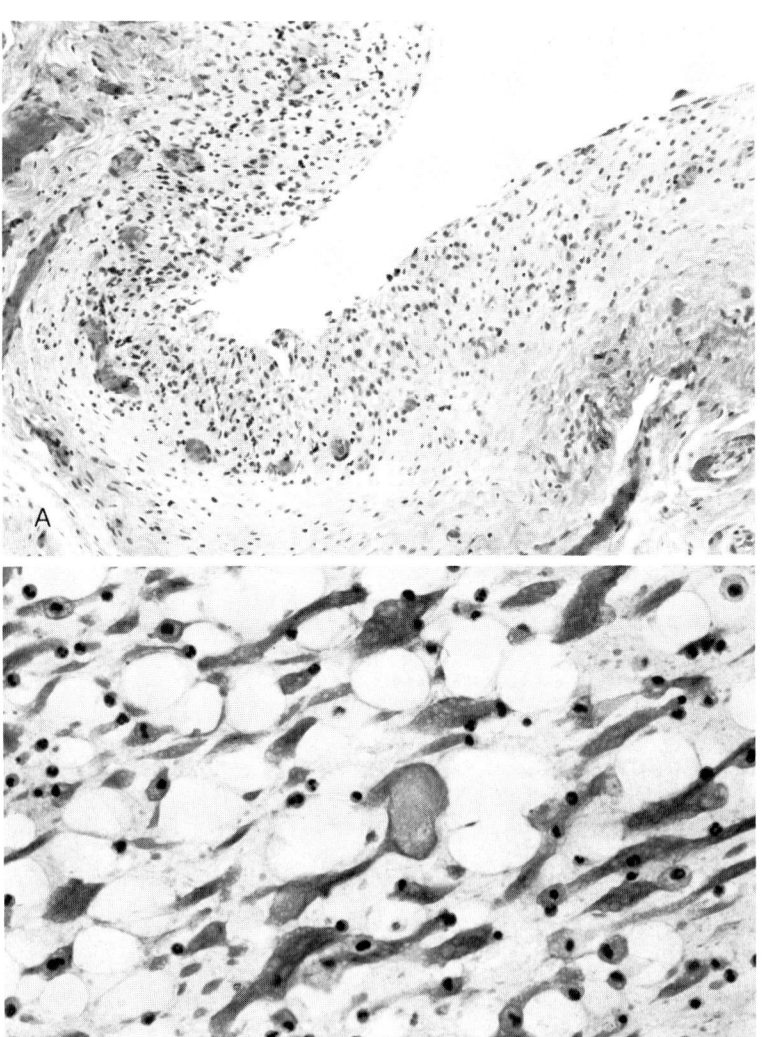

Figure 8–5. Mucus extravasation phenomenon. *A*, Granulation tissue sac surrounding mucin space. *B*, Free mucin containing the usual inflammatory cells, macrophages, and neutrophils.

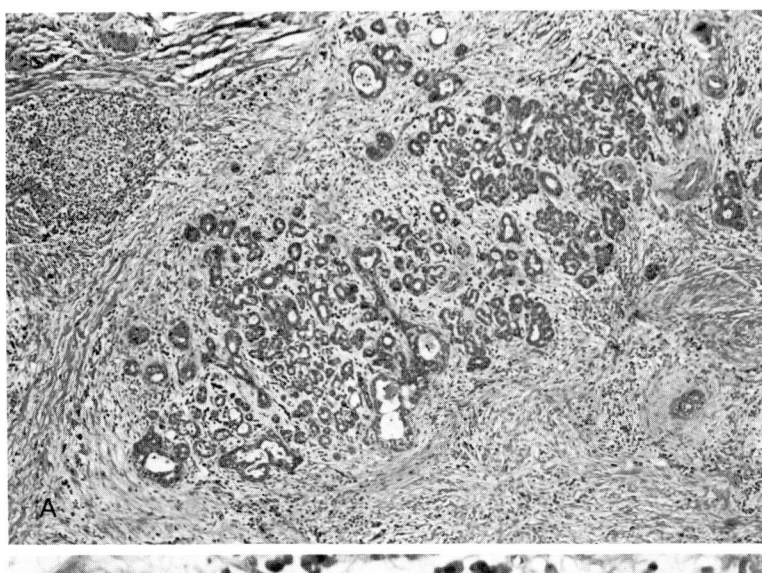
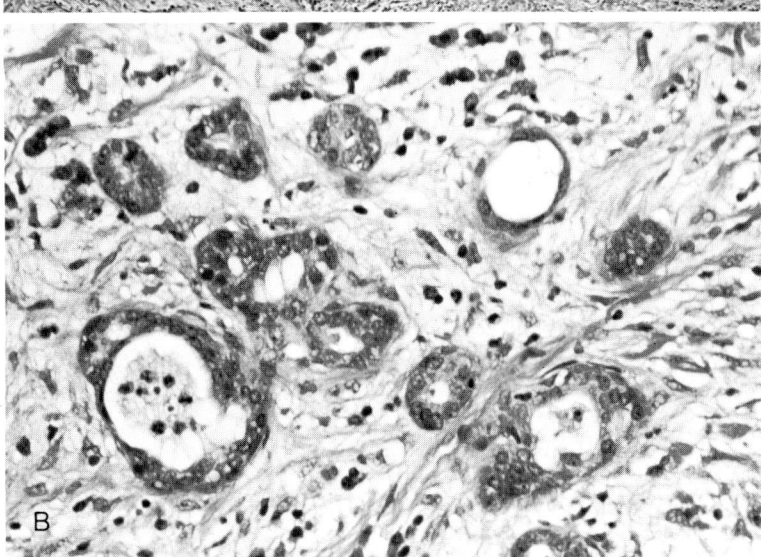

Figure 8–6. *A* and *B*, Non-specific inflammatory changes in minor salivary gland. Note fibrosis, inflammatory cells, and acinic atrophy.

Treatment and Prognosis. The treatment of choice for mucus extravasation phenomenon is surgical excision. Aspiration of the fluid content usually provides no lasting clinical benefit, although this may be used as a diagnostic process. On cytologic preparation of the aspirate, neutrophils and phagocytic cells are dominant, thus helping to characterize the process as inflammatory rather than neoplastic. Removal of the associated minor salivary glands along with the pooled mucus is necessary to prevent recurrence.

Mucus Retention Cyst

Mucus retention cyst is regarded as a cyst because it is lined by an epithelium—unlike mucus extravasation phenomenon, which contains a mucus pool surrounded by granulation tissue. "Mucocele" is used in the clinical setting as a generic term (before microscopic diagnosis) to refer to both the retention cyst and the extravasation phenomenon.

Etiology and Pathogenesis. The mucus retention cyst results from obstruction of salivary flow. Although duct blockage is believed to be the reason for the development of retention mucoceles, there are no specific studies or models to support such a theory.

Clinical Features. The mucus retention type mucocele is less common than the extravasational type. The retention type usually appears after 50 years of age, it rarely presents in the lower lip. Instead, it is found in the palate, cheek, and floor of the mouth, as well as in the maxillary sinus (Fig. 8–7).

Clinical presentation is characterized by an asymptomatic swelling, often without antecedent trauma. The lesions vary in size from 3

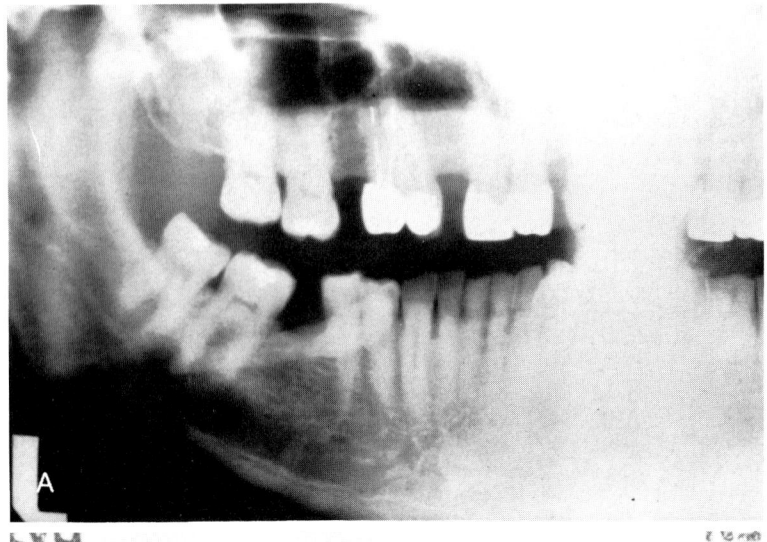

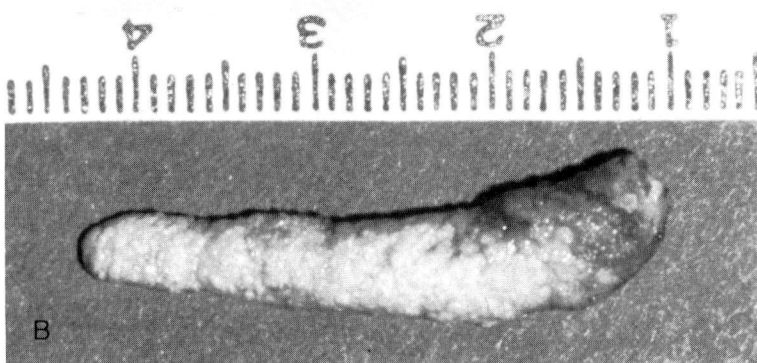

Figure 8–7. *A* and *B*, Sialolithiasis of submandibular gland. Duct stone *(B)* can be seen superimposed on the bicuspid-molar area.

to 10 mm and, on palpation, are mobile, nontender, and generally without peripheral inflammatory change, which is seen in the extravasation type mucocele. The overlying mucosa is intact and of normal color. Lesions situated deeper tend to be firmer and more diffuse in their presentation. When the lining of the maxillary sinus is involved, a dome-shaped, semilunar radiopacity will be noted along the floor of the sinus (see the following discussion).

Histopathology. The cystic cavity of mucus retention cyst is lined by ductal epithelial cells, many of which may be oncocytes. The type of lining formed by the epithelial cells ranges from pseudostratified to a double layer of columnar or cuboidal cells (Fig. 8–8). In some areas, a single row of cuboidal epithelium containing a scant amount of eosinophilic cytoplasm may be noted. Mucous cells may be present among eosinophilic oncocytic elements. The cyst lumen will contain variable amounts of secretion, generally a viscous or inspissated product. Mucus plugs or sialoliths may be found within the ductal system. The supportive connective tissue forming the remainder of the cyst wall characteristically lacks an inflammatory cell infiltrate.

Differential Diagnosis. Salivary gland neoplasms, including mucoepidermoid carcinoma, adenocystic carcinoma, and benign mixed tumor, should be included in a clinical differential diagnosis of this lesion. An extravasation type mucocele could also be considered, as could connective tissue neoplasms.

Treatment and Prognosis. Complete removal of the mucus retention cyst and the associated lobules of minor salivary gland elements is indicated. Removal of any residual acinic elements projecting into the surgical bed is encouraged in order to avoid post-operative mucus extravasation phenomenon occurring at the surgical site.

With adequate treatment, the prognosis is excellent. No recurrence of the cystic element is expected if the associated gland is removed.

Figure 8–8. Mucus retention cyst. A, Lumen space (above) is lined by ductal epithelium. B, Salivary stone (left) fills excretory duct (right).

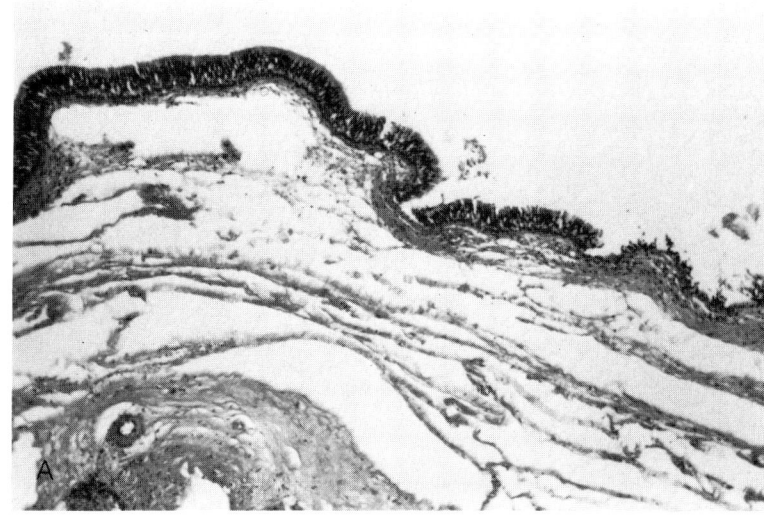
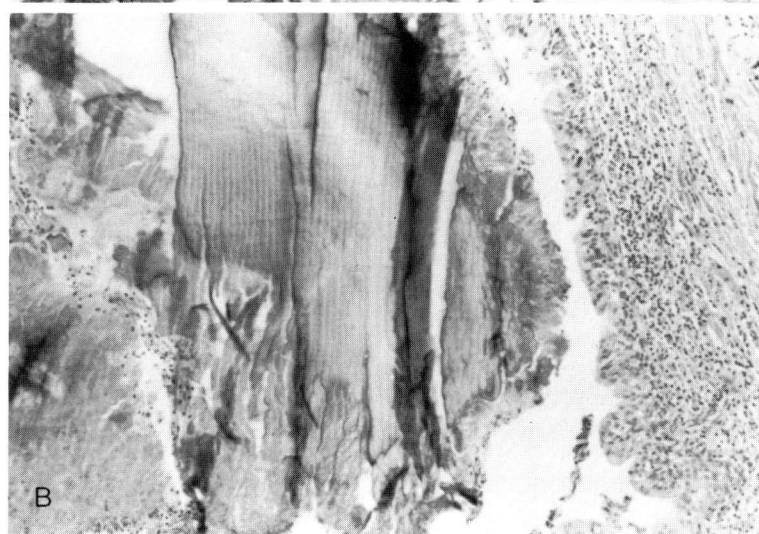

Ranula

"Ranula" is a clinical term that is used to designate a mucocele that occurs specifically in the floor of the mouth. Pathogenetically and microscopically, it may be either mucus extravasation phenomenon or mucus retention cyst. The ranula is associated with the duct system of the sublingual salivary glands and, less commonly, the submandibular glands.

Etiology and Pathogenesis. Although trauma is often the cause for the development of a ranula, ductal obstruction is frequently cited as a significant factor. Obstruction is usually due to a salivary stone or sialolith that may be found anywhere in the ductal system from the gland parenchyma to the excretory duct orifice. Sialoliths represent precipitation of calcium salts (predominantly calcium carbonate and calcium phosphate) around a central nidus of cellular debris or inspissated mucin. Although this phenomenon is most commonly associated with the submandibular glands, it is often seen in the parotid glands and, less frequently, in the sublingual and minor salivary glands.

Clinical Features. The ranula presents as a fluctuant, unilateral, soft tissue mass (Fig. 8–9). It typically has a bluish-white appearance that has been compared to a frog's belly, hence the term "ranula." A wide variation in size has been noted. When it is significantly large, it can produce medial and superior deviation of the tongue. It may also cross the midline if the extravasation process dissects through the underlying soft tissue. When the lesion is deeper in the connective tissue, the typical bluish translucent pattern may not be evident.

In cases due to blockage by a sialolith(s) (Fig. 8–10), radiographs may demonstrate the

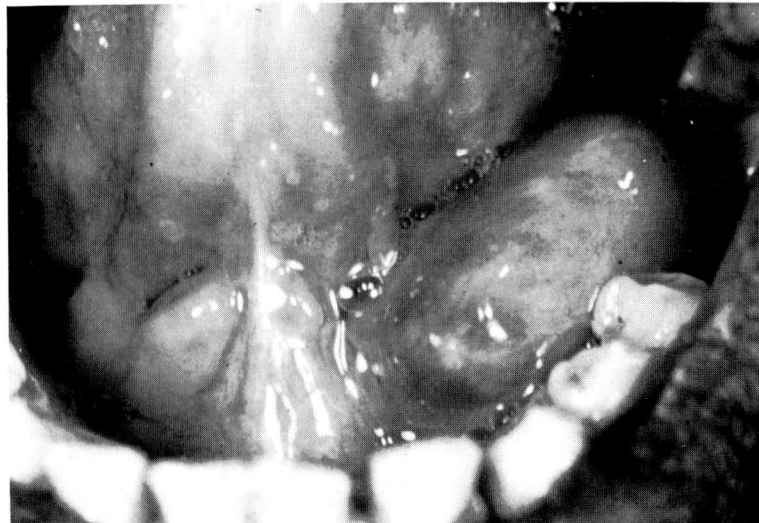

Figure 8-9. Ranula on the floor of mouth.

stone(s). Soft tissue x-rays in an occlusal view may provide diagnostic information. The deep or so-called *plunging ranula* develops as a result of mucus extravasation (herniation) through the mylohyoid muscle and along the fascial planes of the neck (Fig. 8-11). If the process is allowed to continue, the dissection along fascial planes will extend inferiorly. On rare occasions, it may progress into the mediastinum.

Histopathology. Depending on pathogenesis, microscopy of the ranula is the same as for mucus extravasation phenomenon or mucus retention cyst. The majority of the extravasation mucocele specimens are characterized by thick mucoserous fluid surrounded by granulation tissue. The retention mucocele features a lining derived from duct epithelium. A concentrically layered, acellular, calcified salivary stone (sialolith) may also be seen.

Differential Diagnosis. Clinical differential diagnosis of floor of the mouth swellings would include dermoid cyst. However, this lesion is "doughy" in consistency and is more toward the midline in location. Salivary gland tumors and benign mesenchymal neoplasms would be considerations. Deep ranulas must be distinguished from cystic lesions of cervical sinus origin. On rare occasions, thymic cysts may present in a similar fashion in the anterior cervical area.

Treatment. For extravasation type mucoceles, surgery is the preferred therapy. Marsupialization may be performed prior to a definitive excision in an attempt to reduce the overall size of the lesion through natural de-

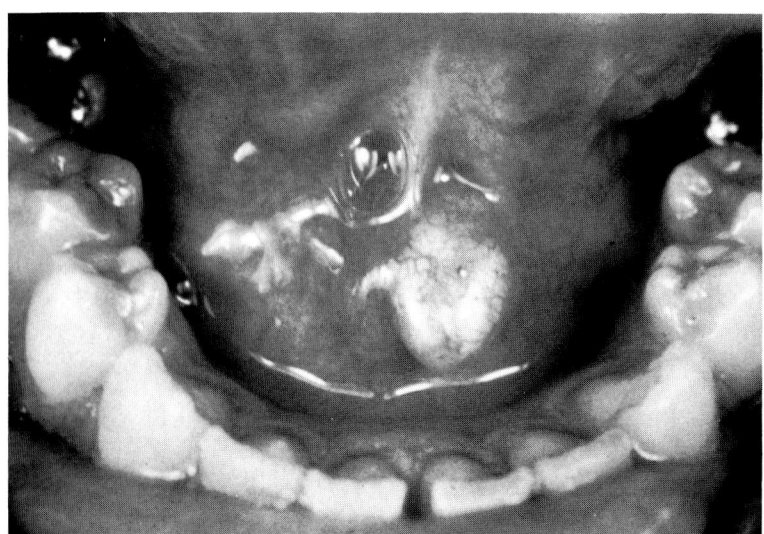

Figure 8-10. Sialolith near orifice of submandibular duct.

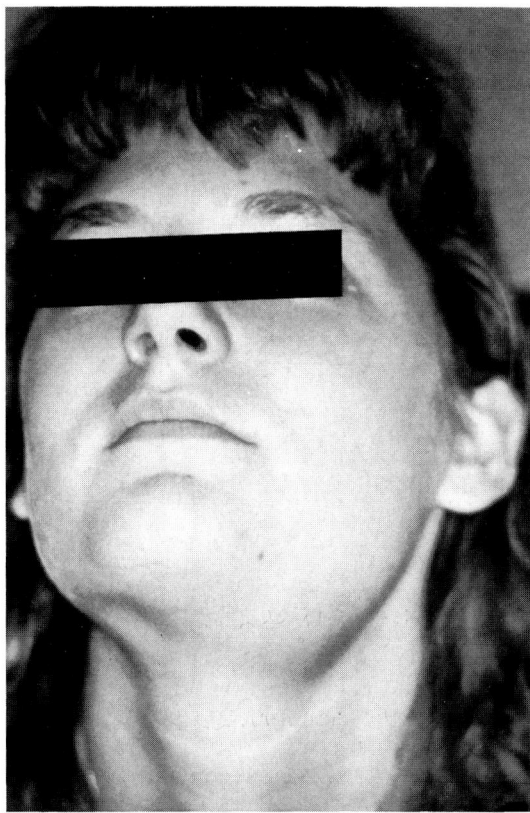

Figure 8–11. Plunging ranula.

compression. Excision of the involved gland (usually the sublingual gland) is generally performed as well.

In the case of sialolithiasis, the stone is either surgically removed or "milked" through the duct orifice. If a duct is surgically entered, special precautions are used to aid the healing process so that duct scarring is minimized. Constriction of the duct through excessive scar formation could result in recurrence.

Mucocele of the Maxillary Sinus

Mucocele of the maxillary sinus is generally regarded as the most common solitary benign lesion of this structure. It is separated from pseudocyst and retention cyst of the maxillary sinus because of differences in etiology and biologic behavior.

Etiology and Pathogenesis. The exact etiology and pathogenesis of mucoceles arising within the paranasal sinuses are uncertain. However, the most acceptable theory relates to blockage or obstruction at a sinus outlet that results in retention of mucus within the sinus cavity. Other factors that may be involved include chronic inflammatory disease producing mucosal thickening, osseous trauma, and tumors located near the ostium. Also, cystic fibrosis may be an important factor in the development of sinus mucoceles in children.

Clinical Features. Paranasal sinus mucoceles are rare in children, since they usually occur between 13 and 80 years. Approximately 65% of mucoceles are found within the frontal sinus; the maxillary sinus is involved in 10% or less of cases.

In the maxillary sinus, slow expansion may lead to obstruction of the ostium and, in time, erosion of the normal anatomic boundaries of the sinus. If infection supervenes, an acute inflammatory mass containing abscesses may form, thus the term "pyocele."

Mucoceles of the maxillary sinus have been reported in approximately 10% of routine sinus radiographs. The radiographic findings show clouding of the sinus because of a soft tissue mass. The involved sinus becomes opacified by entrapped secretions that replace the entire air space if they are not treated. Gradually, decalcification of the mucoperiosteal margin produces loss of the normal osseous borders; the end result is a destructive, smooth, expanded mass surrounded by a zone of sclerosing osteitis. A small percentage of sinus mucoceles contain visible dystrophic calcifications within their walls. Computerized tomography (CT) is helpful in evaluating the character and extent of these lesions.

Histopathology. The lining of the sinus mucocele is variable. Some linings demonstrate goblet and mucous cell hyperplasia, whereas others show a cuboidal type epithelium that forms secondary to pressure atrophy. Mucus may escape or herniate into the underlying lamina propria, producing a concomitant inflammatory reaction. The contents of the mucocele itself may vary from thick and mucoid to firm and gelatinous. This material may also solidify within the connective tissue supportive elements and produce, in a small minority of cases, a so-called mucus impaction tumor. In cases of significant intracavitary or submucosal hemorrhage, cholesterol clefts, hemosiderin deposits, and lipid accumulation may be noted.

Differential Diagnosis. Inflammatory processes of odontogenic origin must be distinguished from the antral or sinus mucocele. Large odontogenic cysts that become infected are capable of producing a similar clinical and radiographic presentation. Primary neoplasia of the maxillary sinus must likewise be considered, especially in view of the occasional destructive nature of the mucocele.

Treatment and Prognosis. Management of the maxillary sinus mucocele is surgical. In contrast to retention cysts of the maxillary sinus, the mucocele must be managed by thorough curettage and débridement of the sinus cavity. Surgical approaches vary from nasal antrostomy to a more definitive Caldwell-Luc procedure, which allows for removal of the antral contents. With adequate surgical management, the overall prognosis is excellent.

Maxillary Sinus Retention Cyst and Pseudocyst

Benign mucosal cysts of the retention type as well as pseudocysts involving the maxillary antrum are common and well-documented findings in periapical and panoramic radiographs. They generally are discovered incidentally, often being of greater curiosity than of clinical significance. Confusion has resulted since many terms have been applied to this particular entity. It is important to separate retention cysts and pseudocysts of the maxillary sinus from the sinus mucocele, since the latter may be destructive and require extensive surgical intervention.

Etiology and Pathogenesis. Retention cysts, sometimes called secretory cysts, may arise from partial blockage of an antral seromucous gland, producing dilatation of the duct and thus forming an epithelium-lined cystic structure. An alternative explanation for retention cyst formation involves a possible invagination of respiratory epithelium into the underlying supportive tissue, which subsequently separates from the antral air space. This theory would account for cyst formation in the absence of seromucous glands. Pseudocysts, also known as non-secreting cysts, are probably inflammatory in origin, possibly resulting from infection or allergy. Damage to the capillary investment by bacterial toxins, anoxia, or other factors may allow loss of protein into surrounding soft tissue, thus raising the osmotic pressure. Subsequent secondary fluid accumulation with coalescence could then account for the clinical growth of these cysts.

Clinical Features. With the exception of a possible relationship to an allergy, retention cysts and pseudocysts are usually unrelated to signs or symptoms of local, antral, or oral disease. The great majority of these lesions are asymptomatic, although the minority may demonstrate slight tenderness or buccal expansion in the region of the mucobuccal fold.

In panoramic and periapical radiographs, retention cysts and pseudocysts of the maxillary sinus are hemispheric, homogeneous, and well delineated (Fig. 8–12). Unlike the antral mucocele, they spare bony structures and landmarks. Mucosal cysts usually demonstrate an attachment to the floor of the antrum, with size being a function of the anatomic space rather than of duration. In unusual circumstances, these lesions may appear bilaterally.

Histopathology. The pathogenesis of the two forms of antral cysts is reflected in the histologic presentaton. The retention cyst is lined by pseudostratified columnar ductal epithelium with occasional mucous cells interspersed. The supportive elements are minimally inflamed, and a collagenous background is evident. In the pseudocyst, there is no evidence of an epithelial lining but rather pools of mucin surrounded by a slightly compressed connective tissue element, which is very similar, if not identical, to the extravasation type mucocele of the oral mucosa.

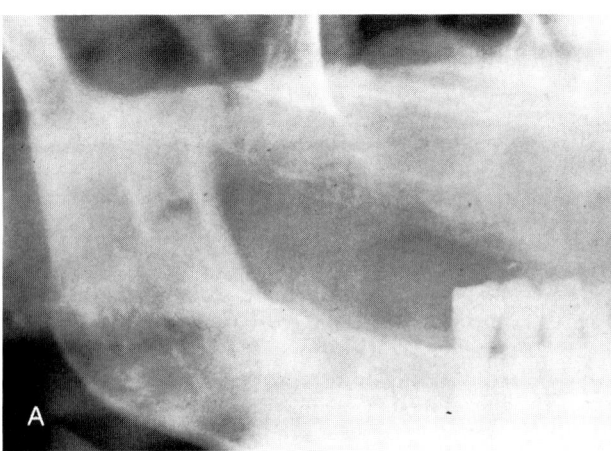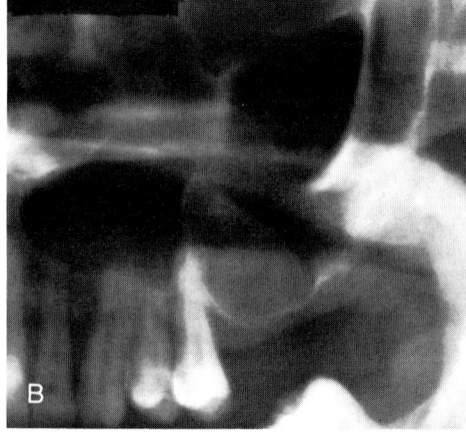

Figure 8–12. *A* and *B*, Maxillary sinus retention cysts.

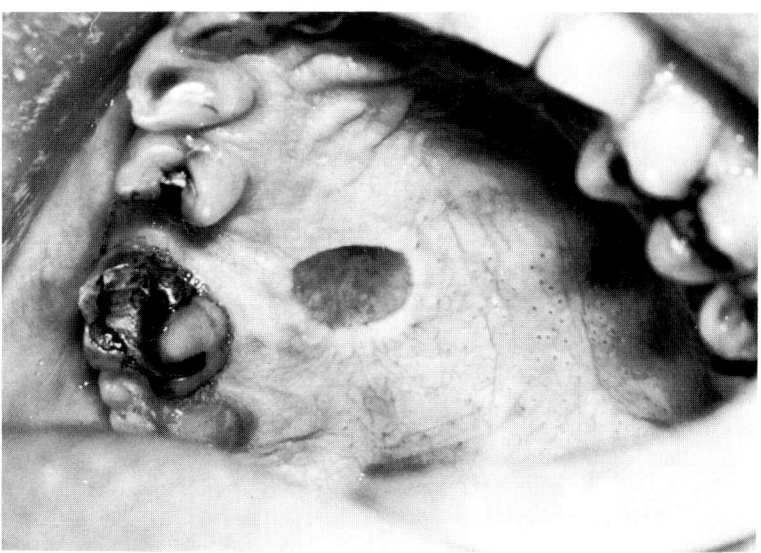

Figure 8–13. Necrotizing sialometaplasia.

Differential Diagnosis. Clinical differential diagnosis of cysts and pseudocysts arising within the mucosa of the maxillary sinus should include inflammatory polypoid disease, hyperplasia of the sinus lining secondary to odontogenic infection, maxillary sinusitis, and neoplasms arising within the soft tissues of the antral lining.

In contrast to the maxillary sinus cyst, sinus or antral polyps are more commonly noted in areas other than the floor of the sinus. The smooth and even elevation of the sinus floor likewise favors antral cysts rather than polyps. Along with an uneven thickening of the sinus lining, sinus polyps will often erode bone in contrast to antral cysts, which do not.

Treatment. Antral cysts and pseudocysts are generally left untreated, because they are limited in growth and not destructive. Periodic observation is all that is required, after informing the patient of the presence of the lesion.

Necrotizing Sialometaplasia

Necrotizing sialometaplasia is a benign condition that may be found in any site containing salivary gland elements, including salivary glands within the oral cavity, major salivary glands, sinonasal tract, and respiratory tract. The condition was first described in 1973, and numerous cases have been reported subsequently. The importance of recognizing this entity relates to the fact that it mimics a malignancy both clinically and microscopically. Failure to recognize necrotizing sialometaplasia has resulted in numerous cases of unnecessary radical surgery because of erroneous preoperative diagnoses of squamous cell carcinoma or mucoepidermoid carcinoma.

Etiology and Pathogenesis. The initiating event in the production of necrotizing sialometaplasia is believed to be related to ischemia, secondary to blockage of local blood supply. After the production of a localized infarct of salivary gland lobules, presumably secondary to vascular compromise and almost always in the absence of arteriosclerotic vascular changes, the acinic elements quickly undergo ischemic necrosis. Ductal preservation is usually noted within the infarcted lobules. Squamous metaplasia of ductal remnants eventually appears, presumably representing an early phase of the healing process.

This condition may be due to local trauma, including surgical manipulation in the area. In cases in which prior surgery has been noted, approximately 3 weeks or longer is required for the lesion to become clinically evident. Intraorally, necrotizing sialometaplasia usually appears spontaneously, often with no history of a prior traumatic precipitating event. No particular oral condition or habit may be associated with this entity.

Clinical Features. Intraorally, this condition is characterized by its spontaneous appearance at its most common site of involvement, the junction of the hard and soft palates (Fig. 8–13). Early in its evolution, the lesion may be noted as a tender swelling, often with a dusky erythema of the overlying mucosa. Subsequently, the mucosa breaks down with the formation of a sharply demarcated deep ulcer with a yellowish-gray lobular base. In the palate, the lesion may be unilateral or bilateral, with individual lesions ranging from 1 to 3 cm in diameter. Symptoms are generally in disproportion to the size of the lesion, with most patients indicating surprisingly mild complaints of tenderness or dull pain. Healing is generally slow, with a protracted clinical course being the rule. Such healing is by secondary intention, ranging from 6 to 10 weeks in duration.

Histopathology. The microscopic features of necrotizing sialometaplasia are consistent and unique. The overlying mucosa is ulcerated in the early phases. Lobular necrosis of the salivary glands, pseudoepitheliomatous hyperplasia of adjacent epithelium, and prominent squamous metaplasia of salivary duct epithelium are typically seen (Figs. 8–14 and 8–15). The recognition of lobular necrosis and the preservation of lobular architecture serve to distinguish this process from neoplasia. The characteristic squamous metaplasia of ductal elements may be misinterpreted as squamous cell carcinoma. When it is seen in the presence of residual viable salivary gland, it may be mistaken for mucoepidermoid carcinoma. In these entities, there is no preservation of lobular architecture but rather extension or infiltration across lobular boundaries.

Differential Diagnosis. Clinically, squamous cell carcinoma or other malignant conditions of minor salivary gland origin must be ruled out. Syphilitic gummas and deep fungal infections may likewise present as punched-out lesions of the palate with sharp margination. In medically compromised patients, such as those with poorly controlled diabetes, opportunistic fungal infections may cause a similar clinical picture.

Treatment and Prognosis. This condition is a benign, self-limiting process that does not require specific treatment. However, incisional biopsy should be done to establish a definitive diagnosis. Healing will take place over several weeks by secondary intention. Patient reassurance and wound irrigation are the only management steps necessary. Recurrence is not expected, and no functional impairment is anticipated subsequent to healing.

Radiation-Induced Salivary Gland Pathology

Head and neck cancer patients who have received tumoricidal levels of radiation often develop a wide range of immediate, interme-

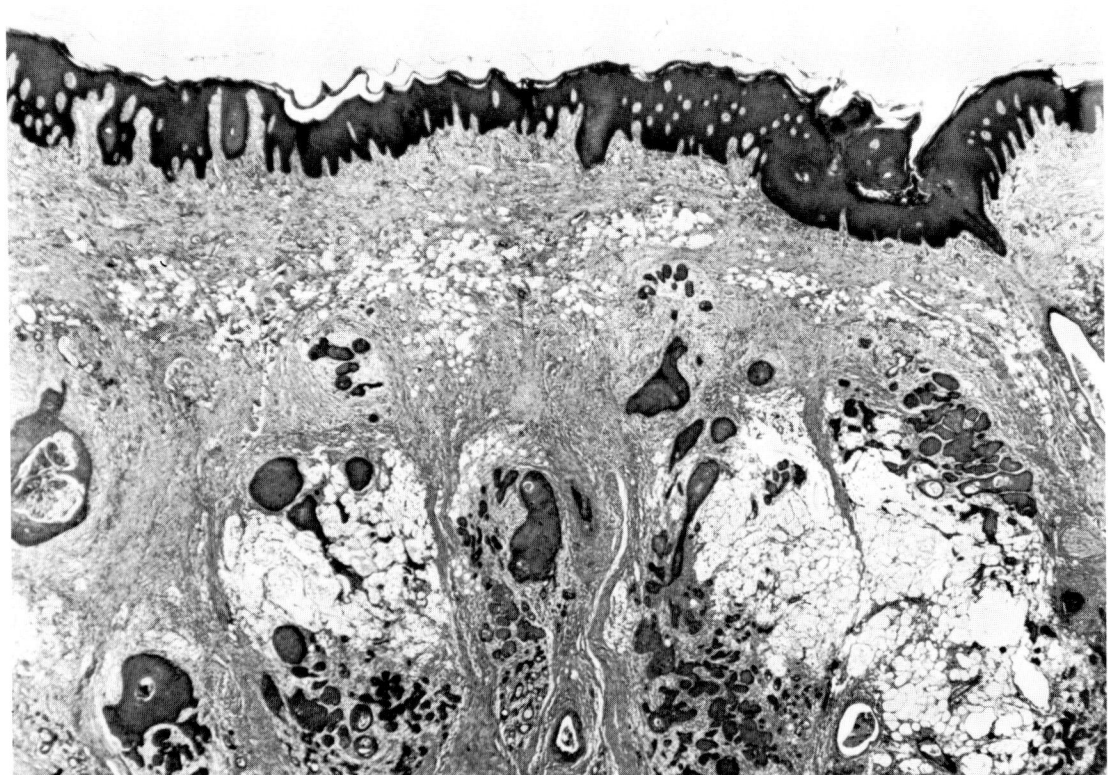

Figure 8–14. Necrotizing sialometaplasia. Note acinic necrosis and squamous metaplasia of ducts.

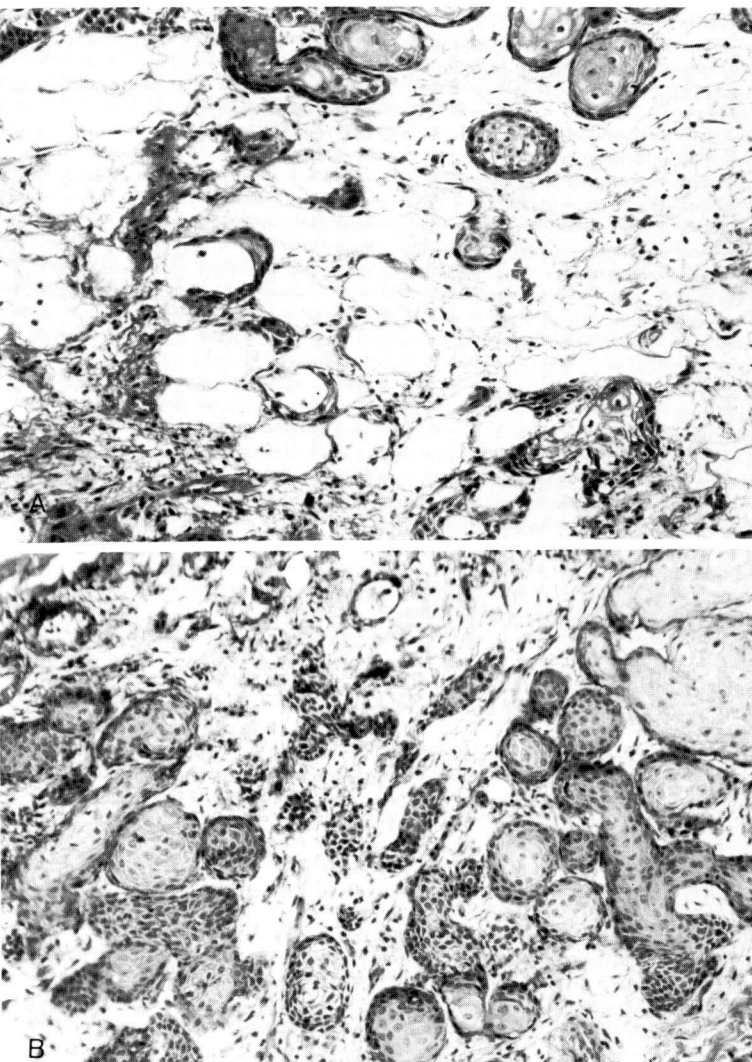

Figure 8-15. Necrotizing sialometaplasia showing necrotic gland *(A)* and squamous metaplasia of ducts *(B)*.

diate, and long-term changes of many tissues and structures in the region of irradiation. When salivary glands are in the radiation path, changes in saliva volume, viscosity, and pH as well as alterations of inorganic and organic components become evident. Such changes predispose individuals to increased caries rates and periodontal disease. There is general agreement that the effect of irradiation on teeth is indirect and results primarily from significant depression of salivary gland function.

Etiology and Pathogenesis. The major biologic effect of irradiation on salivary gland tissues, as well as tissues in general, is produced by ionization. The energy source, be it from cobalt 60, linear accelerator, or other high-energy form, causes release of photons that ultimately strike biologically important molecules within the tissues being irradiated, producing ionization effects. Basically, ionization energy causes expulsion of an electron from an atom, producing a positive ion; the expelled electron (beta particle) attaches to another atom nearby, creating a negative ion. The net result is an ion pair. With gamma rays as the energy source, the resultant beta particle has enough energy to produce more than one ion pair before being absorbed. The unstable molecules generated can also produce secondary biochemical reactions that alter enzyme functions within tissues. Radiosensitivity will vary from tissue to tissue, but the effect on cells is generally greater when mitotic activity of a cell group is high, when the mitotic process is prolonged, and when differentiation or function is not highly established.

One important cell type that is susceptible to therapeutic irradiation is the endothelial cell. Long-term effects on the organ system in which it resides can be profound. Endothelial cell changes include swelling, degeneration, and necrosis. This results in bulging of endothelial cells, producing lumen narrowing and, ultimately, circulatory impedance and obstruction. Consequently, there is parenchymal damage, resulting in decreased function.

With irradiation of salivary glands, the time-dose relationship relative to salivary function is well known. As levels of radiation increase, there is a corresponding decrease of salivary gland flow. Elements of the serous portion of the glands are most severely affected and are lost initially. Mucous cells, more resistant than serous cells, are affected after serous cells but earlier and more acutely than ductal elements, which tend to persist longer than all other glandular epithelial elements. Minor salivary glands suffer similar changes as do the major glands, although apparently less so. During radiotherapy and for a few months post treatment, some recovery of glandular function may be evident; however, the process of degeneration proceeds slowly, secondary to alteration of fine vasculature and fibrosis of interstitial tissues. The fibrosis eventually leads to marked degeneration of the acinic secretory elements, with severe xerostomia being the clinical result.

Clinical Features. Of patients exposed to 6000 rad (6000 cGy) or more, an extremely large percentage develop severe xerostomia (Table 8–1). Not only does the volume of saliva fall drastically but also there are qualitative changes in viscosity, pH, immunoglobulin concentration, and electrolytes. From this comes a significant shift in the oral microflora, with an increase in the proportion of cariogenic bacteria at the expense of non-cariogenic bacteria. The result is the potential for rapidly progressive dental caries in addition to an increased incidence and severity of periodontal disease. The alteration in the physical nature of salivary fluid, including greater viscosity and reduced flow rate, may produce difficulties in deglutition. Restitution of salivary gland function is usually not possible, although the drugs antholetrithione and pilocarpine may be of some benefit to some patients.

Histopathology. Early changes may be noted in the serous acinic tissue after delivery of approximately 1000 to 2500 rad. Such changes include neutrophil and eosinophil cellular infiltrates within the glandular interstitium. Degenerative changes appear within the serous acini, consisting of nuclear pyknosis, cytoplasmic vacuolization, and loss of zymogen granules. At this early stage, mucous glands show little alteration. A dearth of surgical pathology material of irradiated glands has prevented detailed sequential studies of salivary alterations through the course of the treatment phase of head and neck malignancies. It has been shown, however, at 26 days after the final dose of radiation and 75 days after the initial dose of a course of 7000 rad (7000 cGy), there is severe focal loss of serous glands and distortion of remaining elements. Loss of cells, residual nuclear fragments, atrophy and degranulation of cells, pyknosis, prominent basement membranes, and other features may be noted. Of significance is the finding of nearly normal intercalated duct elements with minimal loss of nuclear polarity. Excretory ducts may be dilated and often contain necrotic cell debris. Arterial changes include some contraction and thickening of walls.

During therapy and for short periods thereafter, some signs of recovery may be noted within the acinic component of the glands. However, as time progresses there is continued degeneration of the secretory capacity subsequent to degeneration of fine vasculature and progressive fibrosis. Ultimately, the parenchyma decreases in bulk, with the glands becoming smaller and adhering to surrounding soft tissues. Fibrosis within the interstitial and interlobular elements progresses, with continued and concomitant degeneration of acinic tissue. Variable levels of regeneration may take place, depending upon the design of the fields of therapy, ultimate dosage, and age of the patient.

Treatment and Prognosis. In many patients, return of salivary function is not significant. Consequently, the risk of periodontal disease and rampant caries is high and will persist indefinitely. The prudent course is to begin a program of prevention prior to the initiation of radiotherapy and to carry this through for the lifetime of the patient. Use of a fluoride-

---

Table 8–1. DIFFERENTIAL DIAGNOSIS OF XEROSTOMIA

Sjögren's syndrome
Emotional and anxiety states
Anemia
Negative fluid balance
Polyuria states
Selected nutritional or hormonal deficiencies
Drugs or medications with anticholinergic effect
Acquired immunodeficiency syndrome (AIDS)
Therapeutic radiation through salivary glands

containing preparation is the mainstay of ongoing caries management. Additionally, patients should receive frequent dental prophylaxis and maintain high levels of oral hygiene. Use of remineralizing solutions has a role in the continued management of individuals showing the earliest signs of this process. Saliva substitutes have been recommended for symptomatic relief of xerostomia, although their approximation to normal saliva is less than ideal at this time. Special considerations must relate to management of soft tissues as well as teeth and bone within the irradiated field. The possibility of osteoradionecrosis developing in such circumstances must be kept in mind throughout the lifetime of the patient.

INFECTIOUS CONDITIONS

Viral Diseases

Mumps

Mumps is an infectious, acute viral sialadenitis primarily affecting the parotid glands. Considered the most common of all salivary gland diseases, it has a year-round endemic pattern, although seasonal peaks are noted in the late winter and spring months.

Etiology and Pathogenesis. The causative agent in mumps is a paramyxovirus. A 2- to 3-week incubation period precedes clinical symptoms. Transmission is by direct contact with salivary droplets.

Clinical Features. Patients will develop fever, malaise, headache, and chills in addition to preauricular pain. Salivary glands, usually the parotid, demonstrate a 70% incidence of bilateral infection. The parotid swelling tends to be asymmetric at the outset, reaching maximum proportion within 2 to 3 days. Perceptible diminution of swelling is noted approximately 10 days after the onset of symptoms. The disease affects males and females equally, especially young adults and children.

Potentially serious complications can occur in adults who may develop orchitis or oophoritis, which can occasionally result in sterility. Mumps is a systemic infection, as evidenced by the widespread involvement of glandular and other tissues in the body, including liver, pancreas, kidney, and nervous system.

Severe local pain is often noted, especially on movement of jaws in talking and chewing. Stensen's duct may become partially occluded as the gland swells, with sharp pain noted secondary to the stimulation of the secretory mechanism by food or drink. This is a variable sign, since not all cases will be associated with partial duct obstruction. Papillae at the orifice of Stensen's duct or Wharton's duct may be reddened and enlarged, but this also is not a common or consistent finding.

Differential Diagnosis. Bacterial infections may be considerations in a clinical differential diagnosis. Acute bacterial infection in the form of suppurative parotitis will present with marked tenderness, redness of the skin overlying the glands, and suppuration from the ductal opening. Salivary calculi with obstructive features can also produce similar symptoms. The salivary glands may be enlarged in conditions such as sarcoidosis, lymphoma, benign lymphoepithelial lesion, and certain metabolic diseases, but in these conditions the acute signs and symptoms of mumps will not be seen. Neoplastic states will usually present in a unilateral fashion, with few, if any, symptoms.

Treatment and Prognosis. Management relates to symptomatic therapy as well as bed rest. Analgesics often form the mainstay of treatment. In severe cases, corticosteroids have been prescribed, with variable success.

Complete recovery is generally the rule, although fatalities have been associated with viral encephalitis, myocarditis, and nephritis. Nerve deafness and bilateral testicular atrophy have been noted, but they are uncommon.

Prevention of the disease is now possible using a live attenuated vaccine that induces a non-communicable, subclinical infection. Antibody conversion occurs in approximately 90% of susceptible individuals, and immunity is lifelong.

Although mumps is the most common form of viral sialadenitis, it is important to note that parotitis may also be caused by other viral agents, including Coxsackie A virus, echovirus, choriomeningitis virus, cytomegalovirus, and parainfluenza virus types I and II.

Cytomegalic Sialadenitis

Until recently, cytomegalovirus infection of salivary glands, or so-called cytomegalic inclusion disease, was a rare condition that usually affected neonates because of a transplacental infection. It is also now seen in adults who are in an immunosuppressed state.

Fetal infections may cause fetal debilitation, developmental retardation, and premature birth. Clinically, this disease is characterized by fever, salivary gland enlargement, hepatosplenomegaly, and lymphocytosis. Immunologic abnormalities may also be induced during the infectious period.

Cases of cytomegalovirus infection have been noted in adults who are functionally myelosuppressed owing to leukemia or immunosuppressive medication. Cytomegalovirus has also been cultured from parotid secretion as well as from whole saliva in individuals with human immunodeficiency virus (HIV) infection.

Bacterial Sialadenitis

Etiology and Pathogenesis. Bacterial infections of salivary glands may be subdivided into acute and chronic forms. Regardless of etiology, the involved gland becomes enlarged and painful; disruption of salivary flow is a frequent phenomenon. Concomitant with flow interruptions are changes in the quality and character of salivary secretion.

Acute bacterial infections of the major salivary glands are not uncommon in clinical practice. A reduction in salivary flow is the primary predisposing factor. Such reduction in flow may be noted subsequent to dehydration and debilitation. Numerous drugs associated with decreased salivary flow rate likewise contribute to infections of the major salivary glands, especially the parotid. Other possible causes include trauma to the duct system and hematogenous spread of infection from other areas.

Clinical Features. Clinical features are chiefly characterized by the presence of a painful swelling, low-grade fever, malaise, and headache. Laboratory studies will disclose an elevated erythrocyte sedimentation rate and leukocytosis, often with a characteristic shift to the left. The involved gland is extremely tender, with the patient often demonstrating guarding during examination. Trismus is often noted, and purulence at the duct orifice may be produced by gentle pressure on the involved gland or duct.

The most commonly isolated organism in acute septic parotitis is penicillin-resistant *Staphylococcus aureus*. It is of interest to note that there was a marked reduction in the overall incidence of acute parotitis after the introduction of antibiotics and sulfonamide preparations. As resistant strains have appeared, the prevalence of acute parotitis has increased.

If the infection is not eliminated early, suppuration may extend beyond the limiting capsule of the parotid gland. Extension into surrounding tissues along fascial planes in the neck or extension posteriorly into the external auditory canal may follow. Cases have been reported in which there was extension of the process toward the face with the establishment of a draining cutaneous fistula. Similar considerations also apply to acute sialadenitis of the submandibular salivary glands.

Treatment and Prognosis. The primary role of the clinician is to eliminate the causative organism, coupled with rehydration of the patient and drainage of purulence, if present. Culture and sensitivity testing of the exudate at the orifice of the duct is the first step in antibiotic management. Subsequent to obtaining a culture, all patients should be empirically placed on a penicillinase-resistant antibiotic such as semi-synthetic penicillin. Along with rehydration and attempts at establishing and encouraging salivary flow, moist compresses, analgesics, and rest are in order. Medications containing parasympathomimetic agents should be reduced or eliminated.

Biopsy and retrograde sialography should be avoided when attempting to achieve a diagnosis. The former may cause sinus tract formation, and the latter may allow infection to proceed beyond the boundaries of the gland into surrounding soft tissues. With prompt and effective treatment, recurrence is generally avoided. In cases of recurrent parotitis, considerable destructive glandular changes can be seen.

In the so-called juvenile variant of parotitis, intermittent unilateral or bilateral painful swelling is accompanied by fever and malaise. The initial attack usually occurs in individuals between the second and sixth years, with numerous recurrences thereafter. Gross destruction of the parenchymal and ductal elements may be noted on sialographic examination. Absence of secretory acinic components and a damaged ductal system with numerous punctate globular spaces may be seen. Spontaneous regeneration of parotid salivary tissue has been reported in this condition.

Sarcoidosis

Etiology. Sarcoidosis represents a granulomatous disease of obscure etiology. Although cutaneous manifestations of this disease were recognized as early as 1875, it was later demonstrated that sarcoidosis was a systemic disorder involving visceral tissues as well.

Although no specific cause has been identified, there are certain geographic and immunologic considerations that suggest potential causes. At one point, pine pollen and beryllium were considered as non-infectious agents, but this theory is no longer supported. It is possible that this disease evolved as a hypersensitivity response to atypical mycobacteria—up to 90% of patients in some studies showed significant titers of serum antibodies in these organisms. Studies of a similar nature dispute such findings, however. In some patients with sarcoidosis, a transmissible agent from human sarcoid tissue has been identified as well as a protoplast or L-form tubercle bacillus. To date, however, a definitive etiologic agent remains elusive.

Susceptibility related to human leukocyte antigens (HLA) has been studied. Patients with some histocompatibility antigens (HLA-B7, HLA-B5, HLA-A9) may have a greater frequency of sarcoidosis than do others. It has also been found that most sarcoidosis patients are anergic, demonstrating decreased levels of cutaneous sensitization to dinitrochlorobenzene (DNCB), as well as to tuberculin, mumps virus, Candida antigen, and pertussis antigen. Of interest is the fact that the humoral response is intact, with IgE levels generally higher than in controls.

Decreased numbers of circulating T lymphocytes have been noted during the active phase of sarcoidosis, with some cells demonstrating atypical morphology that suggests an acute viral process. Decreased lymphocyte transformation with phytohemagglutinin (PHA), purified protein derivative (PPD), and concanavalin A (ConA) has also been demonstrated. This has been attributed, to some extent, to a monocyte suppressor effect, possibly related to prostaglandin synthesis.

Clinical Features. The protean manifestations of this disease are well known; a variable clinical course ranges from spontaneous resolution to chronic progression. The disease may affect individuals at any age, although a peak in the second and fourth decades is the rule. Females show a higher incidence than do males, and blacks are more frequently affected than are whites.

Sarcoidosis is usually a self-limiting, benign disease with an insidious onset and protracted course. Patients may complain of lethargy, chronic fatigue, and anorexia, with specific signs and symptoms related to the organ involved.

Pulmonary manifestations are generally considered to be the most characteristic of this disease. They are typified by thoracic alterations that are radiographically seen as bilateral, hilar, and less commonly, paratracheal lymphadenopathy. The disease may stabilize at this point, or it may advance to pulmonary fibrosis and a more ominous prognosis. The most serious complications of sarcoidosis are related to the pulmonary alterations, including pulmonary hypertension, respiratory failure, and cor pulmonale.

The skin may be involved in approximately 25% of cases; most commonly, an erythema nodosum of acute onset and short duration is seen. Skin plaques characterized by non-tender, dark purple, elevated areas on limbs, abdomen, and buttocks may appear. Another form of cutaneous pathology includes lesions known as lupus pernio, a term used to describe symmetric, infiltrative, violaceous plaques on the nose, cheeks, ears, forehead, and hands.

Ocular involvement may be seen but is variable in extent. Inflammation of the anterior uveal tract is the most common occurrence. This may be associated with parotid gland swelling and fever, so-called uveoparotid fever or Heerfordt's syndrome.

Hepatic involvement is quite common, with approximately 60% of patients showing granulomatous lesions on liver biopsy. However, clinical evidence of hepatic involvement appears in less than 50% of patients as demonstrated in abnormal liver function tests.

Osseous lesions are uncommonly noted, with a 5% occurrence rate in most studies. When present, punched-out lesions involving the distal phalanges with erosions of cancellous bone and an intact cortex are characteristic. Destruction of alveolar bone with tooth mobility may be seen within the maxilla and mandible.

Oral soft tissue lesions of sarcoidosis are nodular and generally indistinguishable from those seen in Crohn's disease. Parotid swelling may occur either unilaterally or bilaterally with about equal frequency (Fig. 8–16 and Table 8–2). This is often associated with lassitude, fever, gastrointestinal upset, joint pains, and night sweats, which may precede glandular involvement by several days to weeks. Other salivary glands may also be involved by the granulomatous inflammatory process, leading to xerostomia and its attendant problems.

The upper aerodigestive tract may be involved, with lesions developing in the nasal mucosa, especially in the inferior turbinate and septal regions. Granulomas may also occur in the nasal sinuses, pharynx, epiglottis, and larynx.

Serum chemistry, radiographic studies, and biopsy are useful laboratory tests. Serum

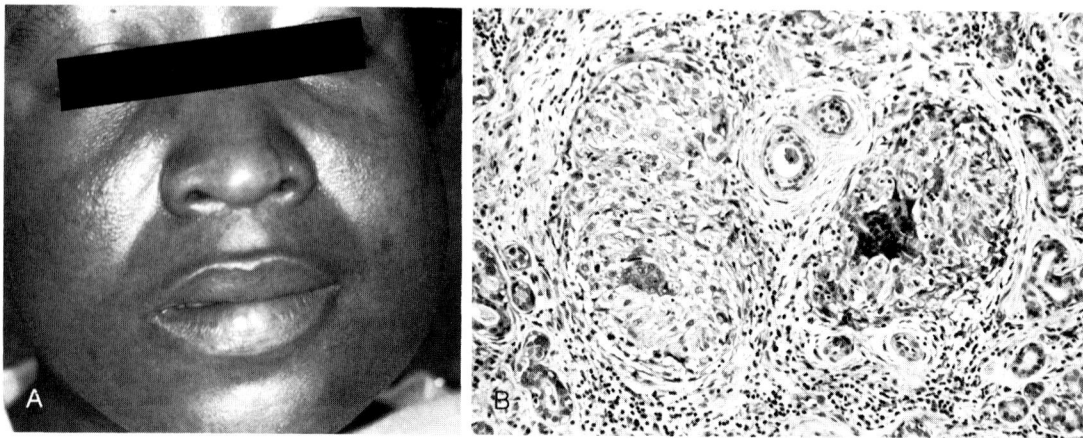

Figure 8–16. *A*, Sarcoidosis of parotid. *B*, Microscopy showing non-caseating granulomas, epithelioid histiocytes, and giant cells.

chemistry studies should include calcium (for evidence of hypercalcemia) and angiotensin-I converting enzyme, lysozyme, and adenosine deaminase levels (for evidence of macrophage activity within granulomas). Gallium scintiscanning and routine chest radiographs and intraoral films may be used to demonstrate bone involvement.

Recently, activity of sarcoidosis has been assessed and gauged by measuring serum angiotensin-I converting enzyme levels in association with gallium lung scan and bronchoalveolar lavage. Although much has yet to be learned regarding the ultimate usefulness of these tests, they remain valid indicators of progression or remission.

Histopathology. The consistent microscopic finding of sarcoidosis is the non-caseating granuloma (Fig. 8–16). The granulomas may be well demarcated and discrete or coalescent. Within the granulomas are macrophage-histiocytes with variable numbers of multinucleated giant cells, usually of the Langhans type. A diffuse lymphocytic infiltrate may be seen around the periphery of the granulomas. Absent is the caseation type necrosis that is typical of tuberculosis (TB).

On occasion, when clinical and radiographic findings suggest sarcoidosis and when there are no readily accessible lesions, a lip biopsy may be done. This random approach may provide a relatively high yield of sarcoid involvement of minor salivary glands and may support initial clinical impressions.

Diagnosis. The Kveim test has traditionally been used to establish the diagnosis of sarcoidosis. An antigenic extract of spleen tissue is prepared from a patient with confirmed sarcoidosis and injected intradermally into the forearm of an undiagnosed patient. In positive circumstances, a nodule develops at the injection site in 4 to 6 weeks. When this nodule is excised, it may show the typical non-caseating granulomas. An 80 to 85% level of positivity is noted in patients with pulmonary involvement; a 2% chance of false positive results exists in individuals with other granulomatous diseases.

The histologic differential diagnosis of the sarcoid granuloma is a significant one in that the granulomatous element of sarcoidosis is similar to that found in many other conditions including TB; leprosy; cat-scratch disease; fungal infections such as blastomycosis, coccidioidomycosis, and histoplasmosis; and parasitic diseases such as toxoplasmosis. Granulomas seen in association with beryllium and talc exposure must also be considered. Localized granulomatous reactions simulating sarcoidal

Table 8–2. CONDITIONS ASSOCIATED WITH CHRONIC SALIVARY GLAND ENLARGEMENT

Sjögren's syndrome
    Benign lymphoepithelial lesion
Neoplasms
    Epithelial: adenomas, carcinoma
    Lymphoma
Sarcoidosis
Infections
    Bacterial
    Actinomycosis
    Tuberculosis (TB)
Metabolic conditions
    Malnutrition, including anorexia and bulimia
    Diabetes mellitus
    Chronic alcoholism

granulomas may be present in lymph nodes draining an area of carcinoma, lymphoma, and Crohn's disease. These patients, however, do not display any clinical evidence of multisystem sarcoidosis or altered serum chemistries typical of sarcoidosis.

Treatment and Prognosis. Spontaneous resolution occurs in a significant number of patients. Corticosteroids are generally considered beneficial and remain the drugs of choice in treating symptomatic pulmonary sarcoidosis. Other agents may be used in addition to or instead of corticosteroids. Chloroquine has been found useful in the management of this disease, either alone or in combination with corticosteroids. Immunosuppressive drugs have been used with good results in individuals not responding to corticosteroid management. Immunomodulators such as levamisole may be useful in the management of arthritic symptoms caused by sarcoidosis.

In general, the prognosis for sarcoidosis is good, but the patient must be monitored periodically with chest radiographs and serum angiotensin-I converting enzyme levels. Clinical relapses are not usually seen in cases in which spontaneous resolution has occurred.

METABOLIC CONDITIONS

There is a group of disorders characterized by salivary gland enlargement, usually the parotid, in the absence of inflammatory symptoms that are of systemic or metabolic origin. Conditions such as chronic alcoholism, dietary deficiency, obesity, diabetes mellitus, hypertension, and hyperlipidemia have been linked to this clinical salivary gland abnormality. It should be noted, however, that conditions are often intermixed, and identification of any one process is often difficult.

The relationship between alcoholic cirrhosis or chronic alcoholism and asymptomatic enlargement of the parotid glands is accepted and documented—incidence levels vary between 30 and 80%. Salivary enlargement has been attributed to chronic protein deficiency rather than to any other metabolic disturbance associated with excessive alcohol consumption. Comparable parotid gland enlargement in individuals with cirrhosis due to other causes does not apparently occur, however. This enlargement may also be related to similar enlargement associated with severe anorexia or bulimia, reflecting nutritional or protein deprivation.

In diabetes mellitus, reduced flow rates have been reported in addition to bilateral parotid gland enlargement. The mechanism of acinic hypertrophy in this condition is unknown. Reduced flow rates from the parotid and other major salivary glands may lead to an increased risk of bacterial sialadenitis.

In cases of type I hyperlipoproteinemia, a sicca-like syndrome has been described. This is characterized primarily by parotid enlargement with mild oral or ocular sicca symptoms; it is generally attributed to the presence of fatty infiltration or replacement of functional salivary gland parenchyma.

Another endocrine-related salivary enlargement may be seen in acromegaly. This may merely be a reflection of a generalized organomegaly seen in this endocrine-mediated disturbance. Apparent parotid enlargement and increased levels of parotid flow have also been noted in patients having chronic relapsing pancreatitis with histologic evidence of acinic hypertrophy.

CONDITIONS ASSOCIATED WITH IMMUNE DEFECTS

Benign Lymphoepithelial Lesion

The term "benign lymphoepithelial lesion" (Mikulicz's disease), was coined in 1952 to characterize a unilateral or bilateral swelling of the parotid glands, resulting from a benign infiltration of lymphoid cells. Originally, the lesion was believed to be inflammatory in origin. Later, neoplastic or pseudoneoplastic processes were believed to be responsible for this condition. The most recent evidence points to an immunologic abnormality. Benign lymphoepithelial lesion may be seen as only a salivary gland abnormality, or it may be one of the manifestations of Sjögren's syndrome. Although the vast majority of lymphoepithelial lesions remain benign, malignant transformation of the lymphoid or the epithelial component has been described.

Etiology. The etiology of the benign lymphoepithelial lesion is obscure. The most likely possibility involves genetic abnormalities or susceptibilities within the cell-mediated arm of the immune system. Postulated is either excessive T helper-cell function or a depression of suppressor-cell function, permitting T cell activation. An alternative theory relates to an antigenic challenge caused by viral alteration of glandular cell surface antigens. This in turn may result in stimulation of B cell antibody production that is directed to glandular tissue. This disorder may result from activation of both these events. The result is an immune-mediated process and a loss of salivary parenchymal tissue with subsequent alteration in function.

Clinical Features. Although the overall incidence of the benign lymphoepithelial lesion is low, it is most frequently noted in middle-aged females as a progressive, asymptomatic enlargement of the affected salivary glands. The process may initially be a unilateral one, but over time, it becomes bilateral. A frequent clinical marker is the appearance of superimposed bacterial infections secondary to reduction in flow rate. In this event, the gland involved becomes enlarged and firm. With repeated bouts of superimposed bacterial infections, it tends to become nodular.

Histopathology. Microscopically, this process occurs within and around intralobular ducts, producing a lymphocytic sialadenitis or parotitis. The result is dilatation of ducts and periductal lymphocytic sialadenitis (Fig. 8–17). Acinic atrophy, a consequence of ductal damage, is progressive and proportional to the degree of lymphocytic infiltration. As this takes place, squamous metaplasia occurs within the ductal segment, ultimately causing luminal obliteration and hyperplasia of duct lining cells. As a result of this process, so-called epimyoepithelial islands appear (Fig. 8–18). This is the histologic cornerstone for the diagnosis of benign lymphoepithelial lesion. A bright eosinophilic cuffing at the interface of the epimyoepithelial islands and the surrounding lymphocytic infiltrates may be striking at times. Late in this stage of the disease, increased interstitial fibrosis occurs, producing a

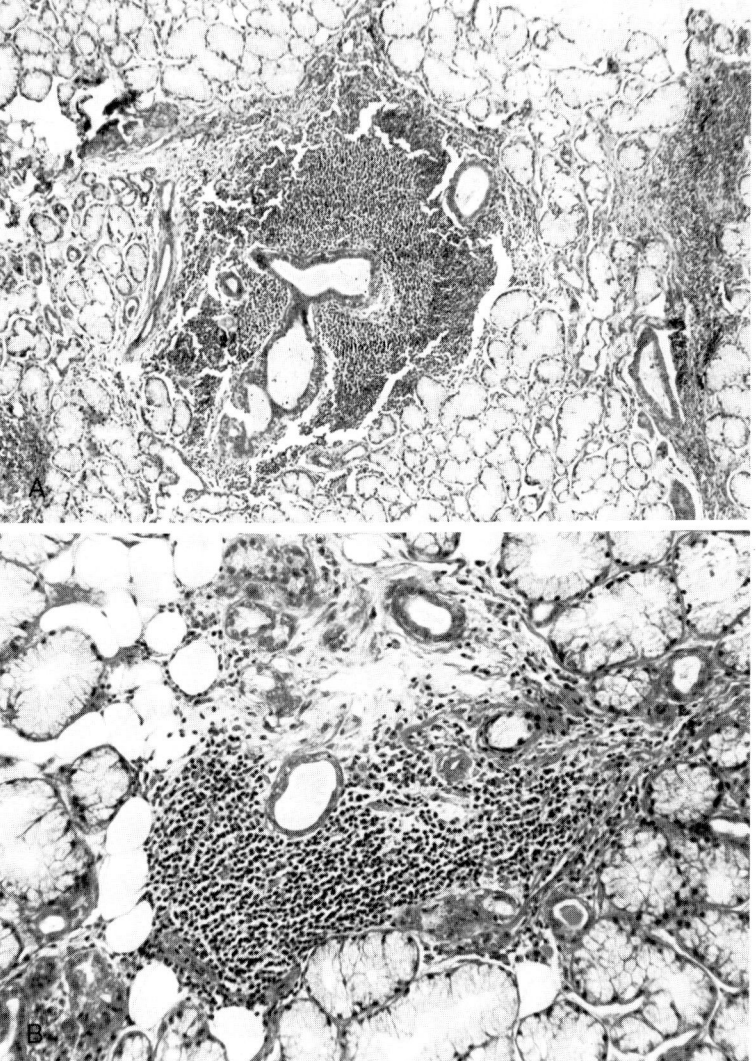

Figure 8–17. *A* and *B*, Early benign lymphoepithelial lesion showing periductal inflammation.

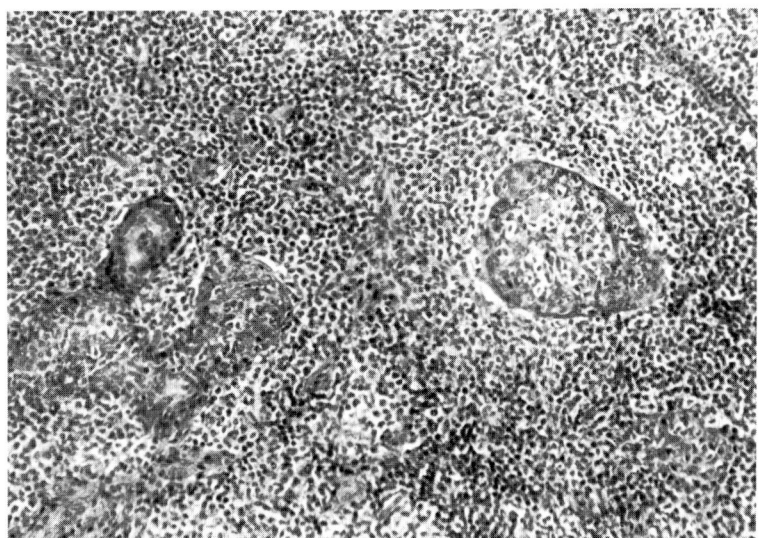

Figure 8–18. Advanced benign lymphoepithelial lesion showing residual epimyoepithelial islands surrounded by lymphocytes.

chronic punctate or cavitary form of sialadenitis on sialographic examination. Rarely, amyloid deposits may be seen. The end result is complete loss of acinic tissues and secretory function.

Differential Diagnosis. Chronic bilateral enlargement of the salivary glands as a result of benign lymphoepithelial lesion must be separated from similar findings seen in sarcoidosis, lymphoma, gout, leukemia, diabetes mellitus, chronic alcohol abuse, and, rarely, hypertension. History and clinical examination are important in identifying the correct process. Serum chemistry studies may help separate sarcoidosis and gout from the other conditions. Peripheral blood counts will help identify leukemia.

Treatment and Prognosis. There is no specific treatment for benign lymphoepithelial lesion. Follow-up observation must be maintained because of a predisposition to neoplastic transformation and a possible relationship to Sjögren's syndrome.

Sjögren's Syndrome

This syndrome is the expression of an autoimmune process that principally causes dry eyes (keratoconjunctivitis sicca) and dry mouth (xerostomia) owing to destruction of lacrimal and salivary glands. Microscopically, the glandular changes are identical to those of benign lymphoepithelial lesion. In some patients, this syndrome may present with vague symptoms related only to xerostomia and xerophthalmia; in others, the autoimmune process may take the form of severe multisystem illness. The lacrimal and salivary gland involvement is often one expression of a generalized exocrinopathy that is lymphocyte or autoimmune mediated.

Etiology. Although the specific cause of this syndrome is unknown, numerous immunologic alterations indicate a disease of great complexity. The generalized alteration relates to a polyclonal B cell hyperactivity that reflects a lack of regulation by T cell subpopulatons. As with the benign lymphoepithelial lesion, the specific causes of this immunologic defect remain speculative.

This syndrome appears to be primarily a chronic inflammatory reaction of autoimmune origin that may be limited to exocrine glands, or it may extend to include systemic connective tissue disorders. In instances of only exocrine involvement, Sjögren's syndrome is considered to be the primary type. If, in addition to the xerostomia and xerophthalmia, there is an associated connective tissue disorder, regardless of the specific type, the appellation of secondary Sjögren's syndrome is used.

Clinical Features. Sjögren's syndrome occurs in all ethnic and racial groups. The peak age of onset is 50 years, and 90% of cases occur in women. Although children are only rarely affected, cases have been reported to arise in late adolescence. Distinguishing between primary and secondary forms of the syndrome, especially those associated with rheumatoid arthritis, is usually not difficult. This may be important because of an increased risk of lymphoreticular malignancy developing in the primary form—the relative risk is estimated to be approximately 44 times that of the general population. An interesting associated sign is a decrease in serum immunoglobulin levels accompanying or preceding the malignant change.

The chief oral complaint in Sjögren's syndrome is xerostomia, which may be the source of eating and speaking difficulties (Table 8–1). These patients are also at greater risk for dental caries, periodontal disease, and oral candidiasis (Fig. 8–19). Parotid gland enlargement, which is often recurrent and symmetric, is seen in approximately 50% of patients (Fig. 8–20 and Table 8–2). A significant percentage of these patients will also present with complaints of arthralgia, myalgia, and fatigue.

The salivary component of Sjögren's syndrome may be assessed by sialochemical studies, nuclear imaging of the glands, contrast sialography, flow rate analysis, and minor salivary gland biopsy. Currently the most commonly used method is labial salivary gland biopsy.

Nuclear medicine techniques utilizing a technetium pertechnetate isotope and subsequent scintiscanning can yield important functional information relative to the uptake of the isotope by salivary gland tissue. Contrast sialography will aid in detecting filling defects within the gland being examined. A punctate sialectasia is characteristic in individuals with Sjögren's syndrome (Fig. 8–21). This latter finding reflects significant ductal and acinic damage, with only the interlobular ducts remaining in cases of moderate to advanced disease. Over time, with further parenchymal and ductal damage, focal areas of narrowing or stenosis of larger ducts takes place and may be seen on the sialogram. Other forms of sialectasia may also be noted, including globular and cavitary types. Least common are atrophic glandular changes in individuals with the sicca syndrome.

Other laboratory findings commonly found in primary and secondary Sjögren's syndrome include mild anemia, leukopenia, eosinophilia, elevated erythrocyte sedimentation rate, and diffuse elevation of serum immunoglobulins. Additionally, numerous autoantibodies may be found, including rheumatoid factor, antinuclear antibodies, and precipitating antinuclear antibodies such as anti–Sjögren's syndrome-A (SS-A) and anti–Sjögren's syndrome-B (SS-B). Antibodies SS-A and SS-B may be seen in association with both primary and secondary Sjögren's syndrome. Patients who have SS-B antibodies are more likely to develop extraglandular disease or the so-called secondary form of the syndrome.

In the secondary form, rheumatoid arthritis is the most common systemic autoimmune disease, although systemic lupus erythematosus is not infrequently seen. Less commonly, diseases such as scleroderma, primary biliary cirrhosis, polymyositis, vasculitis, parotitis, and chronic active hepatitis may be associated with secondary Sjögren's syndrome (Table 8–3).

Immunogenetic typing studies have indicated statistically significant expressions of various histocompatibility antigens in patients with primary and secondary forms of the syndrome. HLA-DR4 antigen is often seen in patients with secondary Sjögren's syndrome; those antigens seen in those with the primary form are frequently HLA-B8, HLA-DR3 types.

Histopathology. In all the major salivary

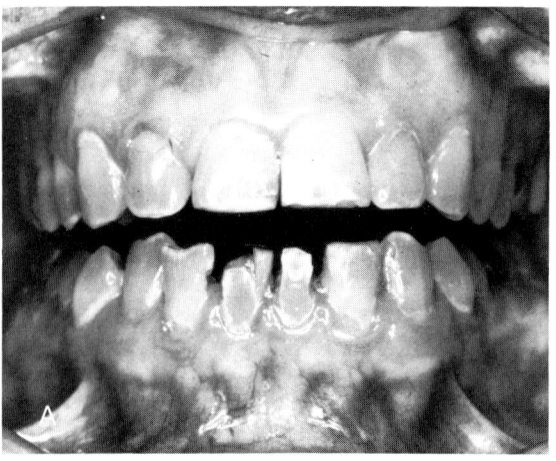 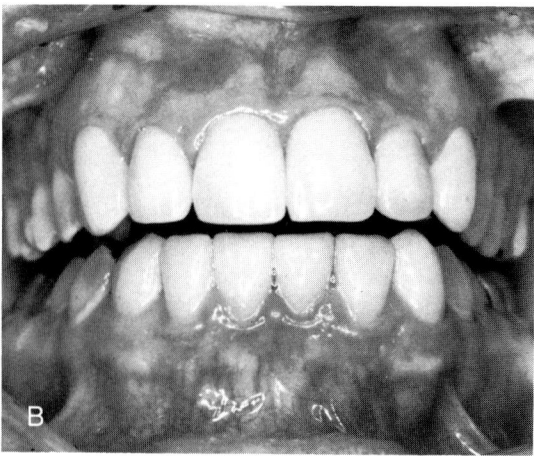

Figure 8–19. *A*, Patient exhibiting extensive cervical caries secondary to xerostomia of Sjögren's syndrome. *B*, Same patient after dental restorations. (Courtesy of Dr. R. M. Courtney.)

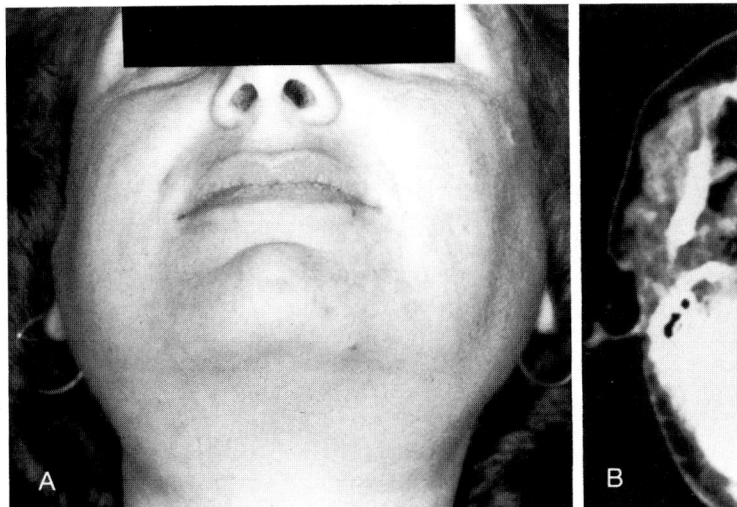

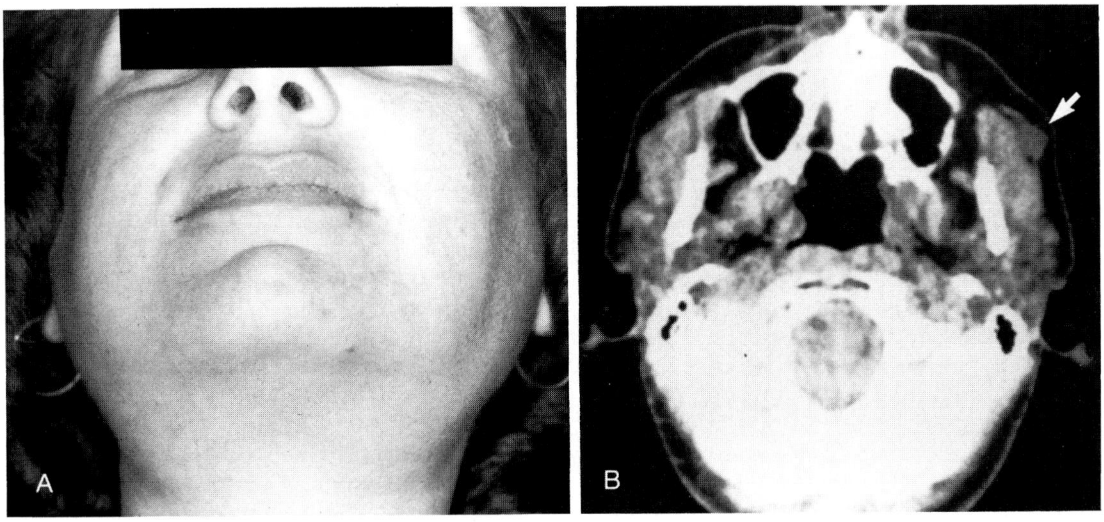

Figure 8–20. *A*, Bilateral parotid swelling associated with Sjögren's syndrome. *B*, Axial tomogram demonstrating symmetric bilateral parotid gland enlargement and unilateral periparotid lymph node enlargement (arrow) in a patient with Sjögren's syndrome.

glands, the microscopic features of Sjögren's syndrome are well known, and these have been described under the rubric of the benign lymphoepithelial lesion. In individuals with Sjögren's syndrome, the benign lymphocytic infiltrate replaces major salivary gland parenchyma. Epimyoepithelial islands are present in approximately 40% of cases. Much less commonly, epimyoepithelial islands are seen in affected minor salivary glands.

The routine preparation of minor salivary gland tissue demonstrates a wide range in the degree of inflammatory cell infiltration and acinic replacement. The initial lesion is represented by a focal periductal aggregate of lymphocytes and fewer plasma cells. As inflammatory foci enlarge, a corresponding level of

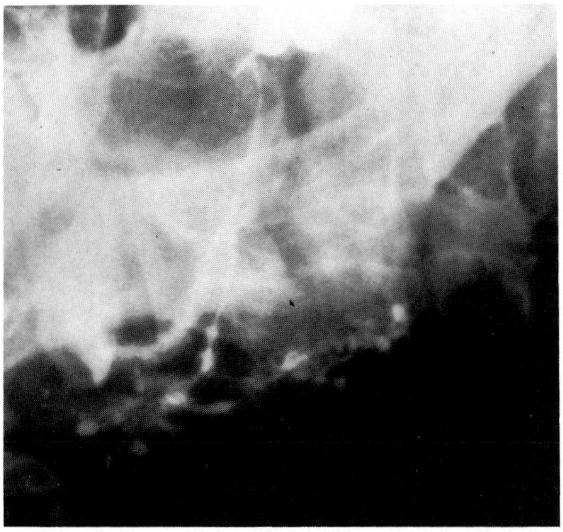

Figure 8–21. A parotid sialogram indicating severe globular and punctate sialectasia. The absence of functional acinic elements in addition to interstitial fibrosis prevents radiographic contrast medium from entering the intralobular portion of the gland. Duct wall damage presents as globular outpouch formation in this patient with Sjögren's syndrome.

Table 8–3. SYSTEMIC FINDINGS IN SJÖGREN'S SYNDROME
Skin
Dryness and reduced sweat production
Scleroderma
Vasculitis
Salivary and lacrimal glands
Enlargement
Xerostomia or xerophthalmia
Atrophy
Gastrointestinal tract
Dental caries
Oral candidiasis
Hypochlorhydria
Hepatosplenomegaly
Biliary cirrhosis
Respiratory
Rhinitis
Pharyngitis
Obstructive pulmonary disease
Cardiovascular or hematopoietic system
Raynaud's disease
Purpura
Anemia (megaloblastic, microcytic-hypochromic)
Thrombocytopenia
Leukopenia
Hypergammaglobulinemia
Hypersedimentation

Modified from Bertram, U. Xerostomia: Clinical aspects, pathology and pathogenesis. Acta Odontol Scand 25:Suppl 49, 1967.

acinic degeneration is seen. With increasing levels of lymphocytic infiltration, confluence of inflammatory foci occurs. Periductal and perivascular hyaline deposition may also be noted. Studies have also shown a positive correlation in pattern and extent of infiltration between labial salivary glands and submandibular and parotid glands in patients with Sjögren's syndrome.

A grading system has been developed to indicate severity of involvement. Grade 0 represents a salivary gland that is free of lymphocytic and plasmacytic infiltration; a grade 4 focus score indicates 50 or more round cells in a 4 mm^2 area of the section. Interpretation of labial gland biopsies should be done with the knowledge that infiltrates may be seen both in normal glands and in glands that are inflamed for other reasons.

Diagnosis. Diagnosis is dependent upon laboratory data, clinical examination, and a detailed history. The classic triad of xerostomia, xerophthalmia, and rheumatoid disease remains valid. Recently it has been proposed that labial salivary gland biopsy should be performed and must demonstrate at least two foci of periductal lymphocytes per 4 mm^2.

Treatment. Sjögren's syndrome and the complication of the sicca component are best managed symptomatically. Artificial saliva and artificial tears are available for this purpose. Preventive oral measures are extremely important relative to xerostomia. Scrupulous oral hygiene, dietary modification, topical fluoride therapy, and remineralizing solutions are important in maintaining oral and dental tissues. Use of sialagogues, such as pilocarpine, remains of limited value and may be contraindicated in some cases.

The prognosis of Sjögren's syndrome is complicated by an association with malignant transformation to lymphoma. This may be a complicating factor in approximately 6 to 7% of cases; it is more common in those with only the sicca components of the syndrome. A predisposing factor in development of lymphoid neoplasia appears to be related to prolonged immunologic and lymphoid hyperreactivity. Less frequently observed is the transformation of the epithelial component to undifferentiated carcinoma.

Generally speaking, the course for Sjögren's syndrome is one of chronicity requiring long-term symptomatic management. Careful follow-up and management by the dentist, ophthalmologist, and rheumatologist, among others, are critical.

BENIGN NEOPLASMS

All salivary glands are felt to develop in essentially the same way, with the anlagen arising initially as ectodermal buds from the lining of the stomodeum or the primitive oral cavity. Solid buds of ectoderm proliferate deep into the subjacent mesenchyme below with a delimiting basal lamina noted at the interface of the ectoderm and mesenchyme. As advancement proceeds, a series of epithelial-mesenchymal or tissue-to-tissue interactions permit the progress of two major developmental steps, cytodifferentiation and morphodifferentiation. Concurrently, the main duct primordium develops between the surface and the budding end of the primordia.

At approximately 5 months of development, the characteristic lobular architecture of the glands becomes established. As branching morphogenesis continues, terminal tubular elements differentiate toward acinic cell formation (Fig. 8–22). Coinciding with acinic granule formation is the early presence of flattened cellular elements, presumptive myoepithelial cells, which form between the acinic cells and surrounding basal lamina. These cells vary in configuration from strap-like to stellate. Early in their development, myoepithelial cells lack their characteristic myofilaments and are often optically clear. The origin of the myoepithelial cell is controversial; most investigators favor origin from terminal tubular cells.

Terminal tubular elements are ultimately responsible for the formation of striated intralobular ducts and intercalated ducts as well as acini and myoepithelial cells. Intralobular and interlobular ducts of the excretory system arise from the remaining progenitor stalk cells.

The microanatomy and the embryogenesis of the salivary glands are related to histogen-

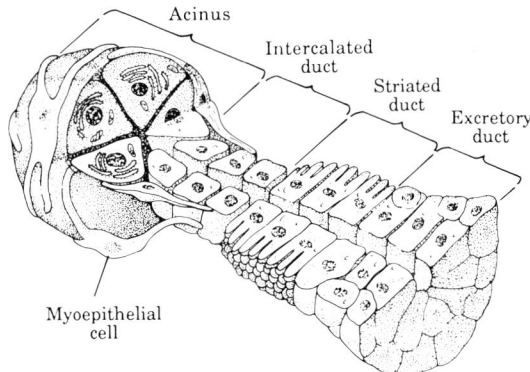

Figure 8–22. The basic mature salivary gland unit.

esis of neoplasia as well as classification schemes of epithelial salivary gland tumors. Numerous classification systems exist based upon morphology, cytologic features, and biologic behavior. No universal opinion exists relative to cell of origin for many tumors. One theory favors the concept of a stem cell or reserve cell within the salivary duct system as being responsible for production of neoplasms. In this scheme, two forms of reserve cells associated with the intercalated and excretory ducts are those that undergo neoplastic transformation following carcinogenic stimulation. The role of the myoepithelial cell in the composition and growth of numerous epithelial salivary tumors is believed to be considerable. Although it is not considered the primary cell of origin of any salivary gland tumor, with the exception of the myoepithelioma, the myoepithelial cell has been shown to be an important participant in mixed tumor, adenocystic carcinoma, salivary duct carcinoma, and epimyoepithelial carcinoma of intercalated duct origin.

Another histogenetic concept relates to the regenerative capacity of acinic cells within the functional gland unit. Animal models suggest that acinic cells are capable of regeneration and therefore might serve as the source of some salivary tumors. An argument against this theory is that the acinic cell is a terminally differentiating cell. It may be incapable of regeneration and therefore not able to serve as the progenitor of neoplasms.

The three major paired salivary glands—parotid, submandibular, and sublingual—plus the hundreds of small minor salivary glands located within the submucosa of the oral cavity and oropharynx are capable of giving rise to a wide range of neoplasms. The majority of salivary neoplasms are epithelial in origin and are considered to be of either ductal or acinic derivation. In addition to epithelial neoplasms, benign lesions may arise from salivary interstitial connective tissue elements, especially within the parotid gland.

The overall incidence of minor salivary gland neoplasia is relatively low. The parotid gland, the most frequent site of salivary gland neoplasia, is more often involved with benign than with malignant neoplasms. On the other hand, submandibular gland and minor salivary gland neoplasms have a greater likelihood of being malignant. The overall figure relative to the incidence of malignancy in the parotid gland is 25%, in the submandibular gland 50%, and in minor salivary glands 60 to 75%. Although tumors of the sublingual glands are extremely uncommon, when they are present, they are almost always malignant.

Benign Mixed Tumor (Pleomorphic Adenoma)

The benign mixed tumor, or pleomorphic adenoma, is the most common tumor of major and minor salivary glands (Table 8–4). Most large series indicate that the parotid gland accounts for approximately 85% of these tumors, whereas the submandibular gland and the intraoral minor salivary glands account for 8% and 7%, respectively. Of those tumors arising within the oral cavity, the majority are noted in the hard and soft palates.

The histogenesis of this lesion relates to a simultaneous proliferation of variable numbers of cells with ductal and myoepithelial features. The myoepithelial cell assumes an important role in determining the overall composition and appearance of mixed tumors. Most studies indicate a range of cell types in mixed tumors—those that are completely epithelial are on one end of a spectrum, and those that are completely myoepithelial are on the other. Between these two extremes, less well developed cells with features of both myoepithelial and

Table 8–4. BENIGN SALIVARY GLAND TUMORS

Type	Parotid	Submandibular	Sublingual	Minor	Total
Benign mixed tumor	3196	266	0	346	3808
Papillary cystadenoma lymphomatosum	431	6	0	0	437
Oncocytoma	45	2	0	0	47
Other monomorphic adenomas	131	5	1	48	185
Total	3803	279	1	394	4477

Compiled from Batsakis JG et al. Head Neck Surg 1:260, 1979; Dardick I et al. Hum Pathol 13:62, 1982; Eneroth CM. Cancer 27:1415, 1971; and Headington JT et al. Cancer 39:2460, 1977.

ductal elements may be seen. It has been theorized that, rather than simultaneous proliferation of neoplastic epithelial and myoepithelial cells, a single cell with the potential to differentiate toward either epithelial or myoepithelial cells may be responsible for these tumors.

Clinical Features. Mixed tumors occur at any age, favor women slightly more than men, and are most prevalent in the second decade of life. They constitute approximately 50% of all intraoral minor salivary gland tumors. Generally, they are mobile except when they occur in the hard palate. They appear as firm, painless swellings and, in the vast majority of cases, do not cause ulceration of the overlying mucosa (Fig. 8–23). The palate is the most common intraoral site, followed by the upper lip and buccal mucosa. Intraoral mixed tumors, especially those noted within the palatal region, lack a well-defined capsule. Within the submandibular gland, mixed tumors present as discrete masses. It is clinically impossible to distinguish these from malignant salivary gland tumors during early stages of growth. They may also be difficult to distinguish from enlarged lymph nodes within the submandibular triangle.

When they arise within the parotid gland, mixed tumors are generally painless, non-tender, and slow growing. They are usually located below the ear and posterior to the mandible. Some tumors may be grooved by the posterior extent of the mandibular ramus, with long-standing lesions capable of producing pressure atrophy on this bone. When they are situated within the inferior pole or tail of the parotid, the tumors may present below the angle of the mandible and anterior to the sternocleidomastoid muscle.

Mixed tumors generally range from a few millimeters to several centimeters in diameter and are capable of reaching giant proportions in the major salivary glands, especially the parotid. The tumor is typically lobulated and enclosed within a connective tissue pseudocapsule that varies in thickness and is often incomplete. In areas where the capsule is deficient, neoplastic tissue lies in direct contact with adjacent salivary tissue.

Histopathology. Microscopically, the mixed tumors demonstrate a wide spectrum of characteristics. The variable patterns within individual tumors are responsible for the synonym "pleomorphic adenoma." Approximately one third of mixed tumors show an almost-equal ratio of epithelial and mesenchymal elements (Fig. 8–24). The epithelial component may be arranged in numerous patterns, including those forming glands, tubules, ribbons, and solid sheets (Fig. 8–25). An occasional finding is the presence of metaplastic epithelial change to squamous, sebaceous, or oncocytic elements. Adding to the histologic complexity are stromal admixtures of myxoid, chondroid, hyaline, and rarely, adipose and osseous tissues (Fig. 8–26).

Myoepithelial cells also add to the complex patterns seen in benign mixed tumors. The myoepithelial component may be of two morphologic types—plasmacytoid cells (Fig. 8–27) and spindle cells. Plasmacytoid cells often tend to aggregate; grouped spindle cells tend to appear in parallel.

Examination of the limiting compressed fibrous connective tissue or pseudocapsule sur-

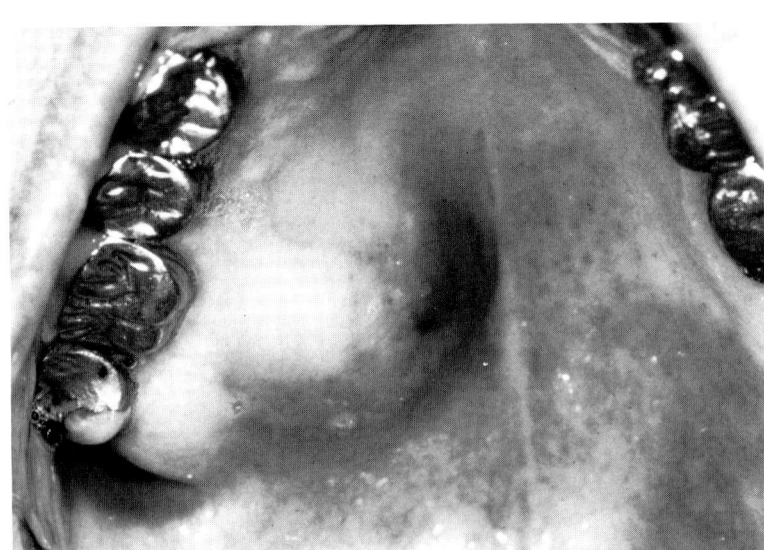

Figure 8–23. Mixed tumor of hard palate.

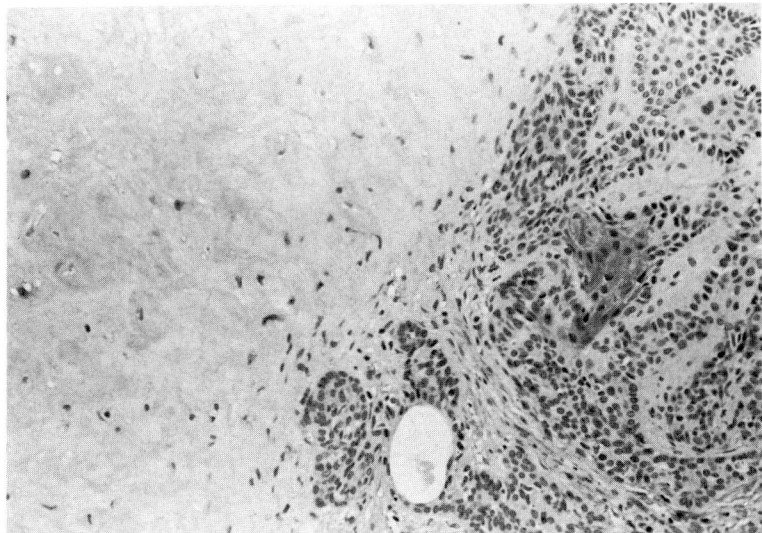

Figure 8–24. Mixed tumor showing mesenchymal component (left) and epithelial component (right).

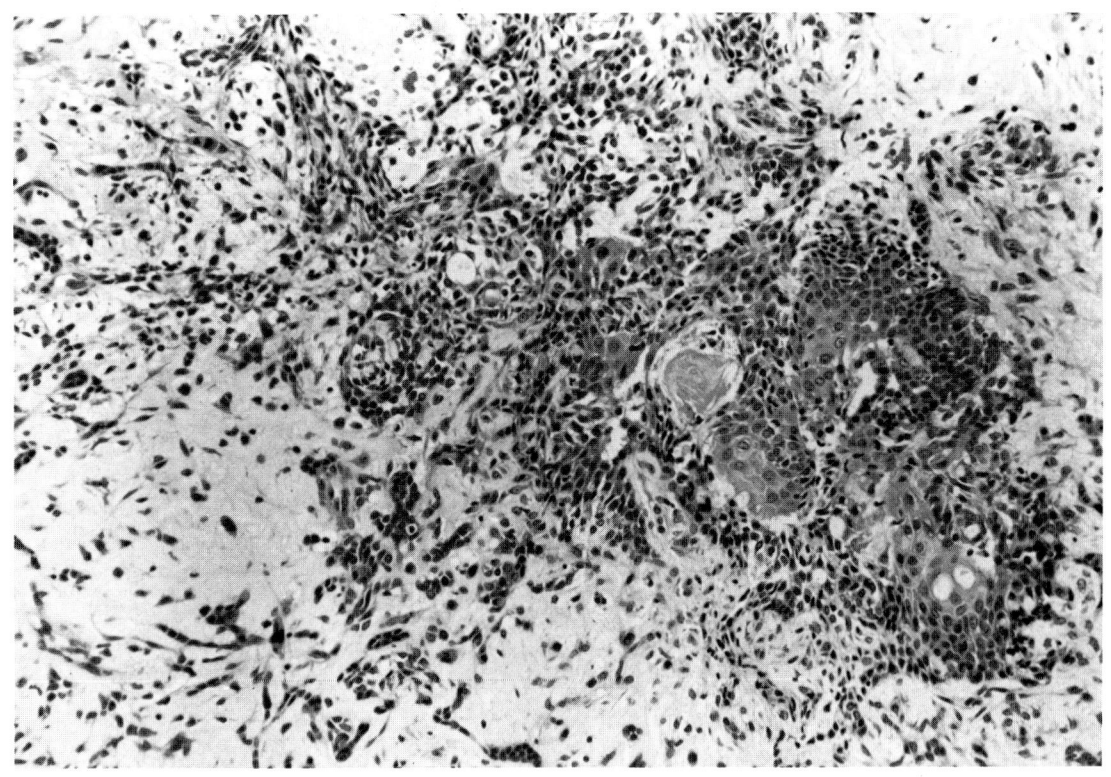

Figure 8–25. Mixed tumor showing both ductal and squamous elements in the epithelial component.

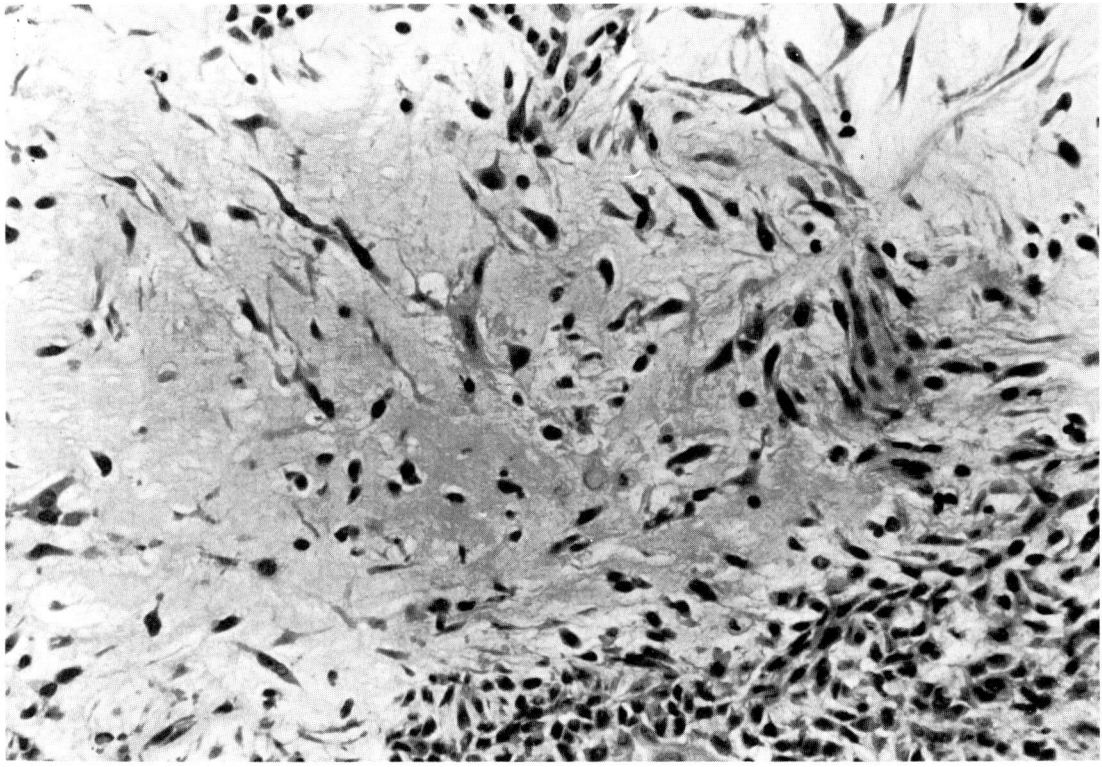

Figure 8–26. Myxoid area in a mixed tumor.

rounding the tumor may demonstrate islands of tissue within it or extending through it. Such islands may appear as satellite nodules at a variable distance from the main tumor mass. Serial sectioning usually demonstrates that such satellites are, in fact, outgrowths or pseudopods continuous with the main tumor mass.

The histologic appearance of the mixed tumor in some cases resembles the monomorphic adenoma; in other cases an adenocystic carcinoma type pattern may be seen. Features that must be kept in mind in assessing the possibility of malignant change include the presence of focal areas of necrosis, invasion, atypical mitoses, and extensive hyalinization.

Treatment and Prognosis. The treatment of choice for benign mixed tumor of minor or major salivary glands is surgical excision. Enu-

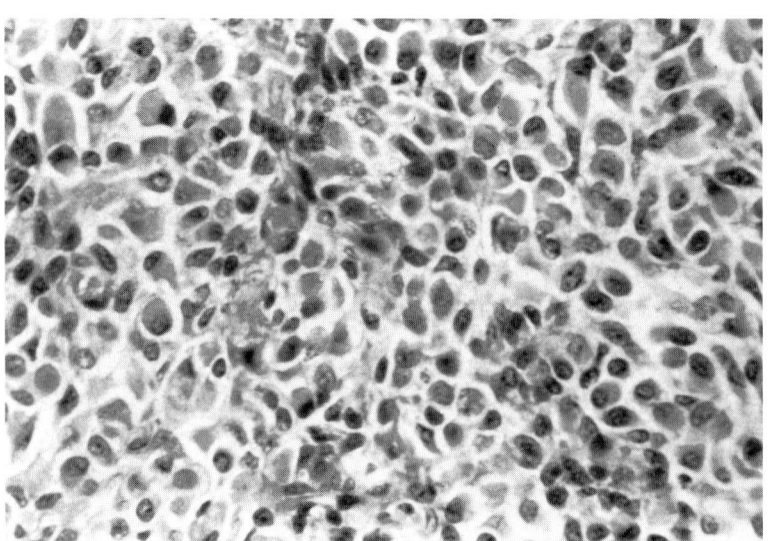

Figure 8–27. Plasmacytoid or oncocytoid cells in mixed tumor.

cleation of parotid mixed tumors is not advisable because of risk of recurrence. Removal of mixed tumors arising within the parotid gland is complicated by the presence of the facial nerve. Any surgical approach, therefore, must include preservation of the uninvolved facial nerve. In most cases, superficial parotidectomy with preservation of the facial nerve is the most appropriate management for mixed tumors arising within the parotid. Resection of the submandibular gland is the preferred treatment for benign mixed tumors in this location. Lesions of the palate or gingiva frequently involve periosteum or bone, making removal difficult. Other oral benign mixed tumors can be more easily removed, but such removal should include tissue beyond the pseudocapsule.

Inadequate initial removal of the mixed tumor in major glands may result in recurrence, often with multiple discrete tumor foci. These recurrent lesions may be widely distributed within the area of previous surgery and may occur in association with the surgical scar. Frequency of recurrence appears to be independent of completeness of a capsule, types of tumor cells involved, and degree of cellularity. The prime determinant of non-recurrence is adequate surgical treatment at the initial phase. In most instances, the recurrent tumor maintains the original pathology; however, with each recurrence there is an increased possibility of malignant transformation. Also, approximately 25% of benign mixed tumors will undergo malignant transformation if lesions are untreated for an extended length of time. The probability of such malignant change also increases if the area has previously been treated with radiotherapy.

Monomorphic Adenomas

The category of benign salivary gland tumors designated as monomorphic adenoma was at one time included under the larger term "mixed tumor." Because it is composed of cells predominantly of one type and because of the absence of connective tissue changes, monomorphic adenoma has been separated from mixed tumors. Some classification schemes have been devised according to overall histologic pattern; others have stressed the histogenetic concept. They all address the variety of cellular and architectural patterns that may be seen under the term "monomorphic adenoma" (Table 8–5).

Table 8–5. HISTOGENETIC CLASSIFICATION OF MONOMORPHIC ADENOMA

Terminal duct origin
  Basal cell adenomas
    Solid
    Trabecular-tubular
    Canalicular
    Membranous (dermal analogue tumor)
Terminal or striated duct origin
  Sebaceous adenoma
  Sebaceous lymphadenoma
Striated duct origin
  Oncocytoma
  Papillary cystadenoma lymphomatosum
Excretory duct origin
  Sialadenoma papilliferum/inverted ductal papilloma

Basal Cell Adenomas

The most common subset within the monomorphic adenoma group is the basal cell or basaloid group of lesions. These tumors are further subdivided into solid, canalicular, trabecular-tubular, and membranous types (dermal analogue tumor). In the basaloid group of lesions, there is little myoepithelial cell participation and little evidence of stromal differentiation or metaplasia.

Clinical Features. Monomorphic adenomas are found predominantly in the parotid gland. Although basal cell adenomas may be found in all salivary tissues, there is a definite preference for the parotid gland and the minor salivary glands of the upper lip. This is in contrast to the mixed tumor, which occurs very infrequently in the upper lip but is found quite commonly in the palate. Basal cell adenomas are generally slow growing and painless. The age range of patients is between 35 and 80 years, with a mean of approximately 60 years. A distinct male predilection is noted.

The *canalicular* and *trabecular-tubular* variants most often present within the upper lip as freely movable masses that are painless and non-tender. These particular variants are rarely located within the parotid gland. Patients in their seventh decade and beyond are most commonly affected.

The *membranous adenoma (dermal analogue tumor)* occurs in the parotid gland in over 90% of cases, with no cases reported in the intraoral minor glands. These lesions vary from 1 to 5 cm in greatest dimension and generally present in the parotid gland as an asymptomatic swelling. Several patients with this particular finding in the parotid gland have presented with synchronous or metachronous adnexal cutaneous tumors, including dermal cylindroma, trichoepithelioma, and eccrine spiradenoma.

Histopathology. Generally, the isomorphic pattern and absence of chondroid metaplasia and mucoid to myxoid stroma help to differentiate this lesion from the benign mixed tumor. In the *solid* variety, islands or sheets of basaloid cells frequently show peripheral palisading, with individual cells at the periphery appearing cuboidal to low columnar in profile (Fig. 8–28). Mitotic activity is inconspicuous. Nuclei are regular in shape and uniformly basophilic, and the amount of cytoplasm is generally minimal.

The *canalicular* and *trabecular-tubular* forms of basal cell adenoma present with a distinctive morphology. In the latter type, trabeculae or solid cords of epithelial cells alternate with ductal or tubular elements composed of two distinctive cell types (Fig. 8–29). The luminal surfaces of the small formed ducts are lined by cuboidal cells with a minimal amount of cytoplasm. A cuboidal basal cell layer separates the epithelial lining elements from the stroma. Often, the trabeculae are outlined by a prominent or thickened basement membrane. In the canalicular type, narrow interconnecting ductal spaces or canals are seen; these occasionally become cystic (Fig. 8–30). The cells lining the ducts range from cuboidal to columnar. An eosinophilic coagulum may be seen, within the cystic spaces. The stroma is loose and pale staining and contains a discrete but delicate endothelium-lined vascular network. This variant of basal cell adenoma is very similar to adenocystic carcinoma. Cribriform patterns within adenocystic carcinoma lack vascularity within microcystic areas; thus this entity can usually be distinguished from canalicular adenoma.

Histologically, the *membranous adenoma* differs from other subtypes in that it is generally multilobular, and it encapsulates in approximately 50% of cases. The tumor grows in a nodular fashion, with individual nodes often separated by normal salivary gland tissue (Fig. 8–31). Variable-sized islands of tumor tissue are embedded in and separated from each other by a thick hyaline and eosinophilic, periodic acid–Schiff (PAS) positive membrane or investment. Similar, if not identical, eosinophilic hyaline material is also noted in droplet form within the intercellular areas of the tumor islands. Individual droplets may coalesce,

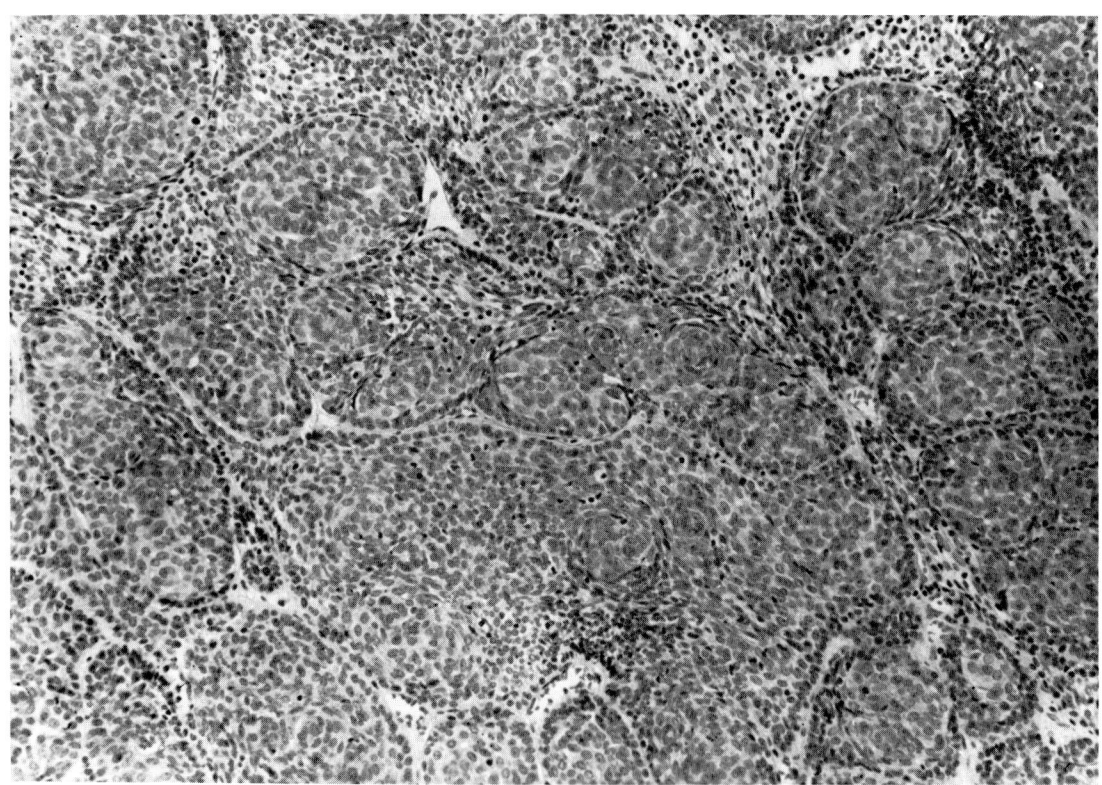

Figure 8–28. Solid variant of basal cell monomorphic adenoma.

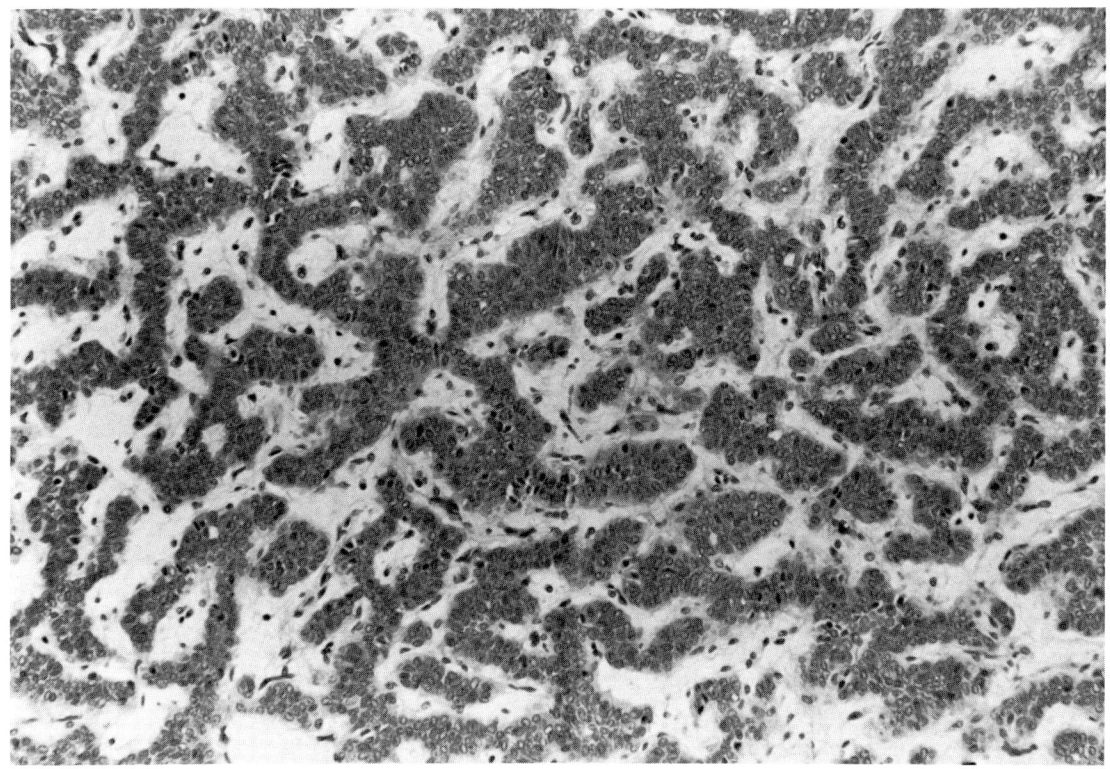

Figure 8–29. Trabecular-tubular variant of basal cell monomorphic adenoma.

Figure 8–30. Canalicular variant of basal cell monomorphic adenoma.

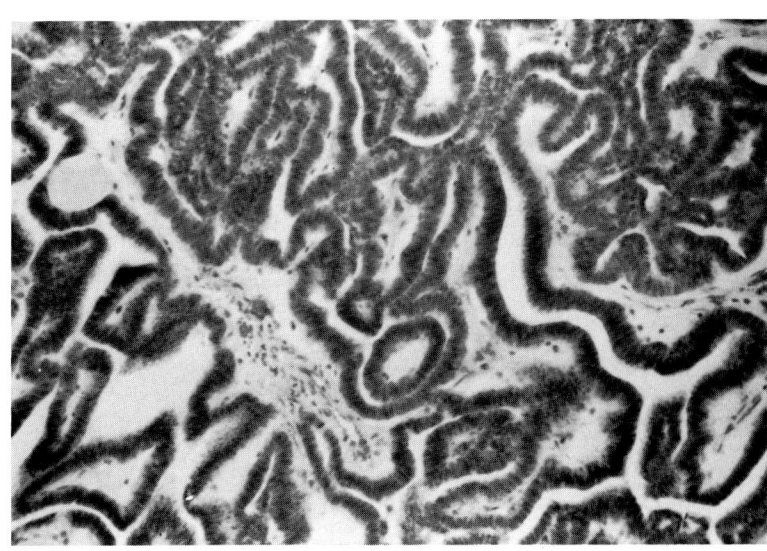

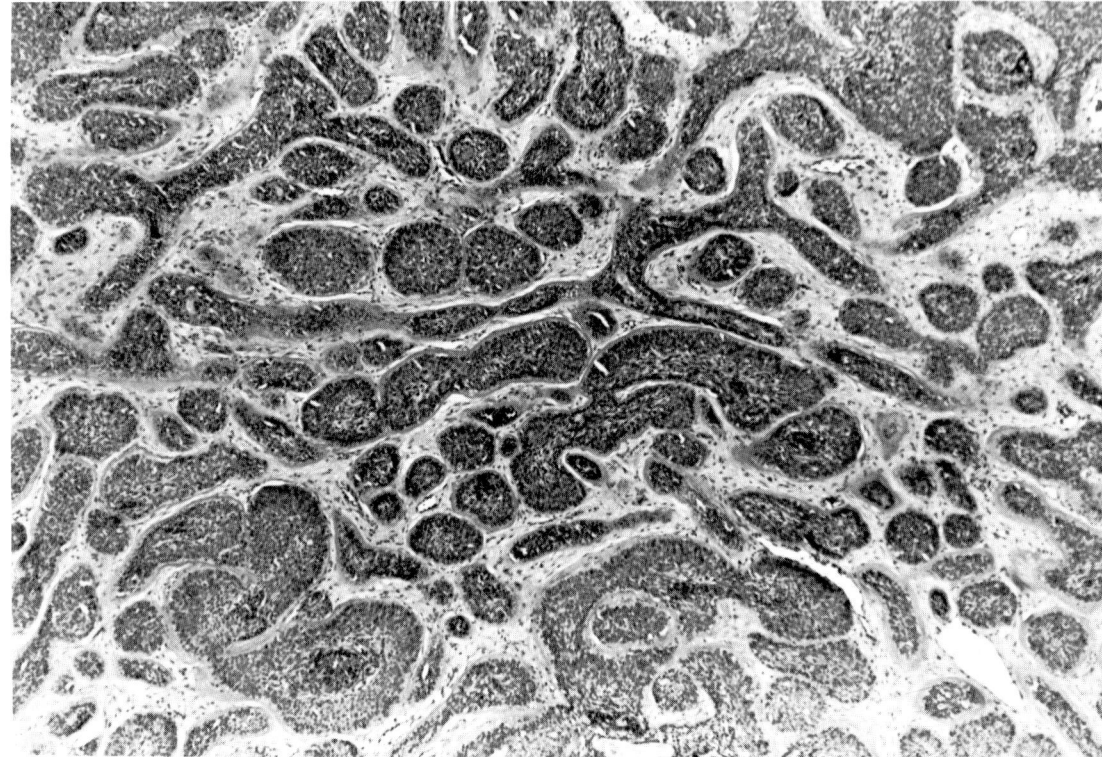

Figure 8–31. Membranous variant of basal cell monomorphic adenoma.

often entrapping densely staining or pyknotic tumor cells.

Treatment and Prognosis. Generally, the lesions qualifying as monomorphic adenoma are benign and rarely recur. The membranous form of the basal cell adenoma, however, demonstrates a significant rate of recurrence because its growth pattern and multifocal nature make complete removal difficult.

Preferred management is conservative surgical excision including a rim or margin of normal uninvolved tissue, paralleling that which would be done in managing a mixed tumor. As with mixed tumors, recurrences may be multinodular and multifocal.

Sebaceous Tumors

The presence of sebaceous glands or evidence of sebaceous differentiation has been noted in submandibular and parotid salivary glands. This particular tissue, thought to originate in intralobular ducts, gives rise to various sebaceous neoplasms designated as sebaceous adenoma, sebaceous lymphadenoma, sebaceous carcinomas, and sebaceous lymphadenocarcinomas. These are rare lesions composed predominantly of sebaceous gland–derived cells; they are well differentiated in the benign forms and moderately to poorly differentiated in the malignant forms. In the lymphadenoma forms, a benign lymphoid component is seen. The parotid gland is the site of chief involvement, although intraoral examples have been reported. These lesions range from a few millimeters to several centimeters in diameter. Parotidectomy is the treatment of choice when lesions arise in this gland. Surgical excision is used in cases of intraoral neoplasms.

Oncocytic Tumors

Oncocytoma

The oncocytoma or oxyphilic adenoma is a rare lesion arising within salivary gland tissue, predominantly in the parotid gland. As the name implies, this lesion is composed of cellular elements termed oncocytes, which are large granular acidophilic cells. Such cells are normally found in salivary glands in the intralobular ducts, and they usually increase in number with age. Oncocytes are found in mucous glands of the aerodigestive tract as well as in minor and major salivary glands of the oral and perioral regions. These cells contain large numbers of mitochondria and are rich in oxidizing enzymes. The histogenetic origin of this lesion is believed to be from the salivary duct epithelium, in particular the striated duct.

Clinically, the oncocytoma tends to be a solid, round to ovoid encapsulated lesion usually less than 5 cm in diameter when it is noted within major salivary glands. These lesions are rarely seen intraorally. In some instances, bilateral occurrence may be noted; within individual glands (most often the parotid) multicentricity or so-called oncocytosis may be seen.

Microscopically, the oncocytic cells are characterized as swollen or enlarged, with granular eosinophilic cytoplasm (Fig. 8–32). The outline of the cells is generally polyhedral, with a pyknotic hyperchromatic nucleus. Ultrastructural studies will often provide an unequivocal diagnosis by finding abundant numbers of mitochondria within the cytoplasm of the tumor cells. Careful examination of the mitochondria shows them to be abnormal with unusual or atypical outlines and large numbers of cristae.

Owing to the near-universal benign course and slow growth rate, treatment is generally conservative, with a superficial parotidectomy the treatment of choice for parotid lesions. In minor salivary glands, removal of the tumor with a margin of normal tissue is deemed to be adequate. Recurrence is rarely noted; if it happens, it will usually be evident within 5 years after the primary surgical procedure.

The malignant oncocytic tumor or so-called malignant oncocytoma is rare, with only a handful of cases reported.

Papillary Cystadenoma Lymphomatosum (Warthin's Tumor)

The papillary cystadenoma lymphomatosum, also known as Warthin's tumor, accounts

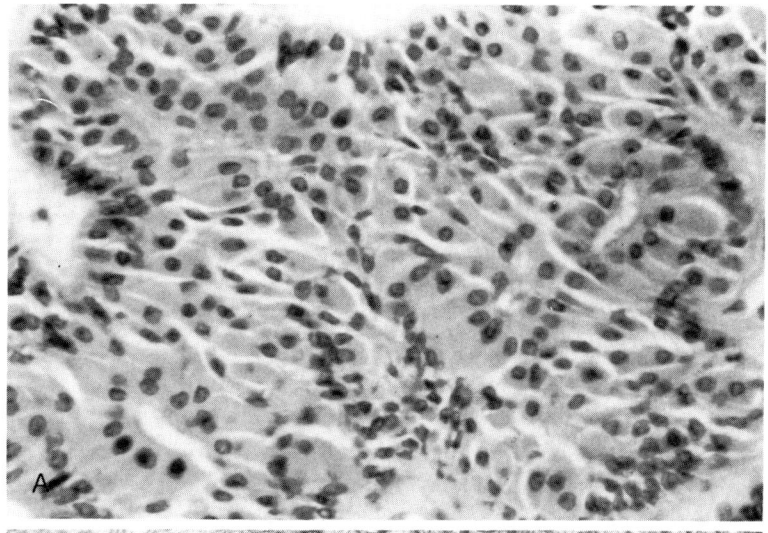
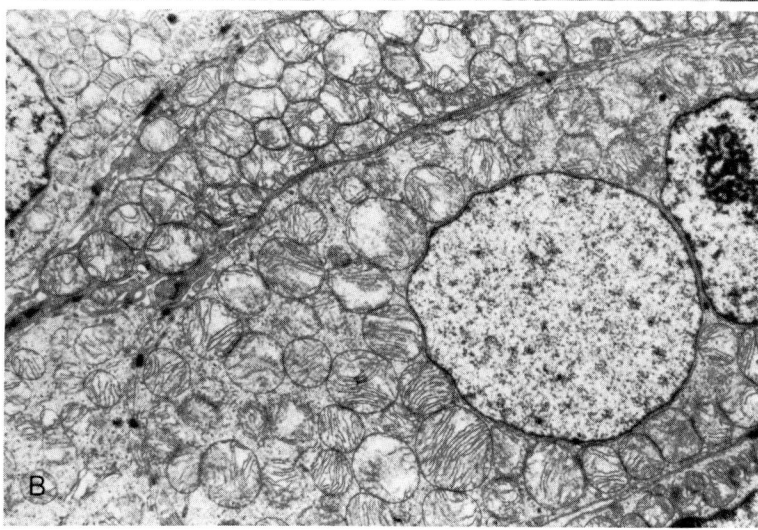

Figure 8–32. *A*, Oncocytoma. *B*, Ultrastructure of the same lesion showing tumor cells with abundant cytoplasmic mitochondria.

for approximately 7% of epithelial neoplasms of salivary glands, with the vast majority occurring within the parotid gland. Intraorally, this lesion is rare. The papillary cystadenoma lymphomatosum is thought to arise within lymph nodes as a result of entrapment of salivary gland elements early in development. This theory is supported by the occasional case of multicentricity as well as normal lymph node architecture surrounding many early or developing tumors. Intraoral lesions may arise in an area of reactive lymphoid hyperplasia secondary to chronic inflammation.

When it occurs in the parotid, this tumor presents typically as a doughy to cystic mass in the inferior pole of the gland, adjacent and posterior to the angle of the mandible (Fig. 8–33). In this situation, the proximity of the submandibular gland may give the impression that the lesion has developed within this gland rather than within the parotid.

There is a distinct male predilection for Warthin's tumor, with an average male to female ratio of 5 to 1 noted in many older series. More recently, however, case studies and larger series have reported more equal gender distribution, with only slight male predominance. The average age of onset is generally between the fifth and eighth decades. When bilaterality is noted (2 to 6% of cases), the growths may be multiple and synchronous or metachronous.

This lesion is also characterized upon nuclear scan as being capable of technetium-99 uptake, and therefore it may appear as a so-called hot nodule.

This tumor is encapsulated and has a smooth to lobulated surface and a round outline. When it opens into the cystic cavity, a brown viscid fluid containing ceroid pigment may be noted.

Microscopically, numerous cystic spaces of irregular outline contain papillary projections lined by columnar eosinophilic cells (oncocytes) (Fig. 8–34). The lining cells are supported by reserve cells that are cuboidal and centrally nucleated. Occasionally, squamous metaplasia of the lining cells may be seen. At the base of the cuboidal cell layer, a basement membrane separates the epithelium from an underlying lymphoid stroma. Germinal centers and sinusoidal spaces are typically seen.

The basis for the cytoplasmic granularity of the epithelial component relates to the presence of a large number of mitochondria within the cytoplasm. The lymphoid element is overwhelmingly composed of B lymphocytes.

Recurrences have been documented but are believed to represent second primary lesions or an expression of multiple lesions. Malignant transformation or carcinoma arising within this lesion is rarely seen, but it may follow radiotherapy of the region. The type of malignancy arising in the majority of cases is squamous cell carcinoma, with fewer cases of adenocarcinoma and mucoepidermoid carcinoma reported.

Sialadenoma Papilliferum and Inverted Ductal Papilloma

Sialadenoma papilliferum is an unusual benign salivary gland neoplasm first reported in 1969 as a distinct entity of minor and major salivary gland origin. The majority of cases reported subsequently have been found intraorally, with the buccal mucosa and palate the most common sites.

Sialadenoma papilliferum usually presents as a painless exophytic papillary lesion; the patient is often unaware of the duration or presence of the lesion. Most cases have been reported in males between the fifth and eighth decades. In most reported cases, the clinical

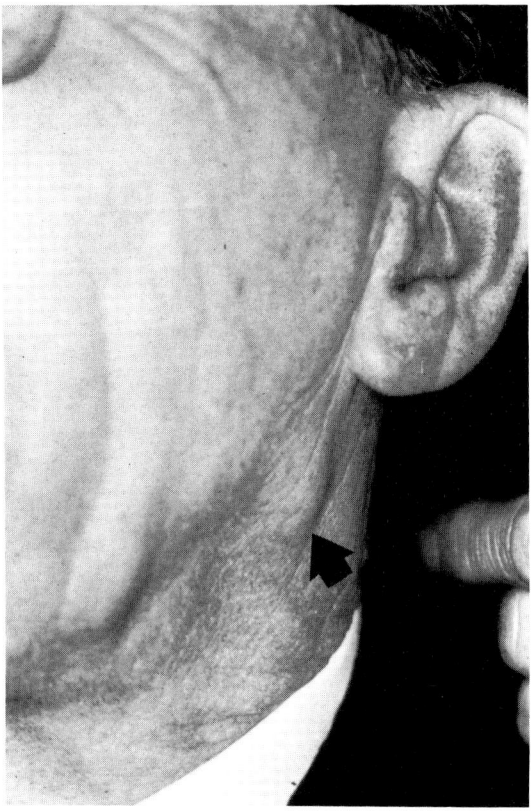

Figure 8–33. Warthin's tumor in tail of parotid gland (arrow).

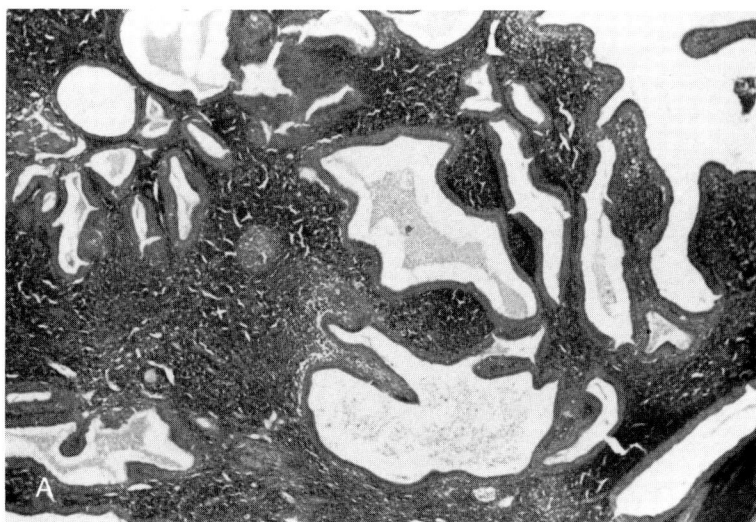
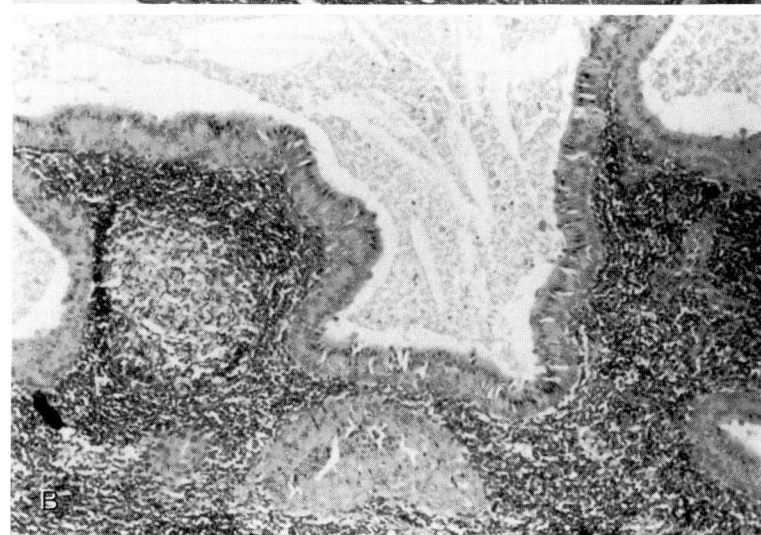

Figure 8-34. *A* and *B*, Warthin's tumor. Note cystic spaces lined by columnar cells supported by lymphoid tissue.

impression prior to removal is that of a simple papilloma, owing to its frequent keratotic appearance and papillary surface configuration.

This tumor appears to originate from the superficial portion of the salivary gland excretory duct. Papillary processes develop, forming convoluted clefts and spaces (Fig. 8–35). Each papillary projection is lined by a layer of epithelium approximately two to three cell layers thick and is supported by a core of fibrovascular connective tissue. The more superficial portions of the lesion demonstrate a squamous epithelial lining; deeper portions show more cuboidal to columnar cells, often oncocytic in appearance. As growth continues, the overlying mucous membrane becomes papillary to verrucous in nature, much like a squamous papilloma. If the origin of the processes is deeper within the duct system, a submucosal nodular swelling may be the presenting sign. This lesion generally resembles the syringadenoma papilliferum of the scalp, a lesion of eccrine sweat gland origin.

The behavior of this lesion is benign, with no reports of malignant transformation or malignant variations. Management is by conservative surgery; there is little chance for recurrence.

A related papillary lesion of salivary duct origin is the *inverted ductal papilloma*. This is a rare entity of minor salivary gland origin that presents as a nodular submucosal mass resembling a fibroma or lipoma. It is seen in adults and has an equal gender distribution.

Microscopically, the inverted ductal papilloma resembles the sialadenoma papilliferum (Fig. 8–36). Below an intact surface, a marked proliferation of ductal epithelium into the surrounding stromal tissue is noted. Crypts and cyst-like spaces lined by columnar cells with

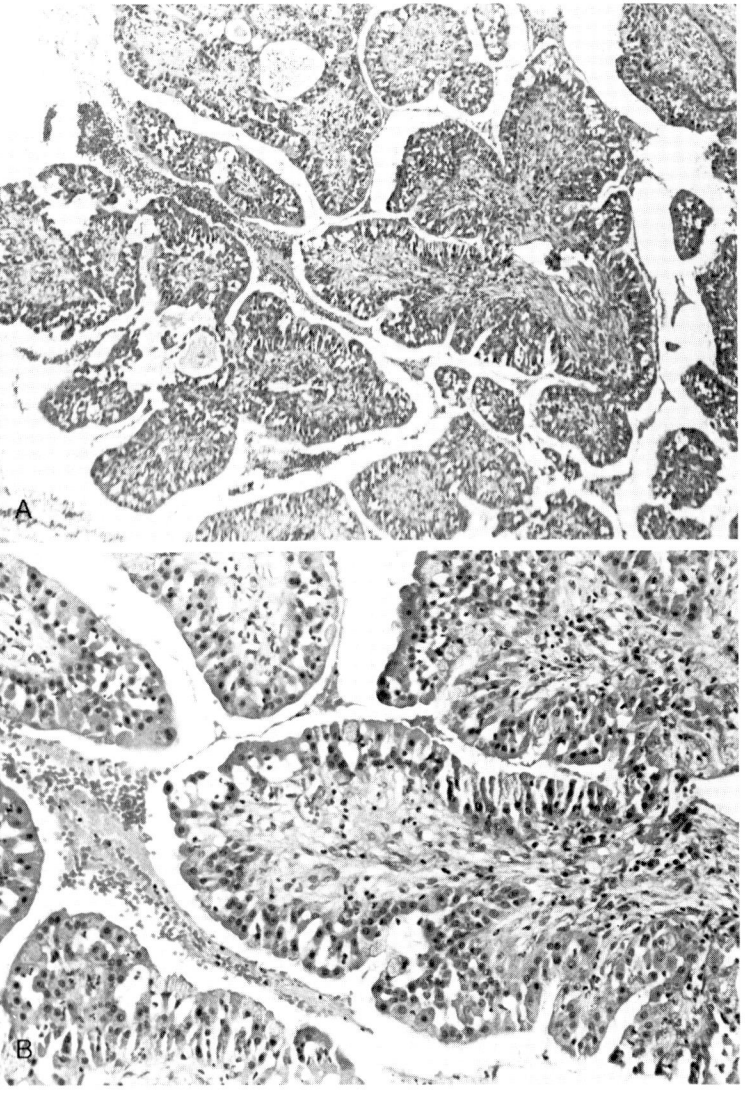

Figure 8–35. *A* and *B*, Sialadenoma papilliferum composed of epithelium-lined papillary projections.

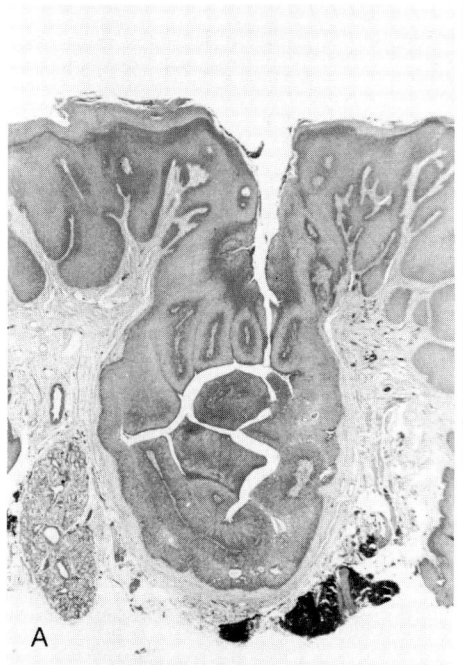

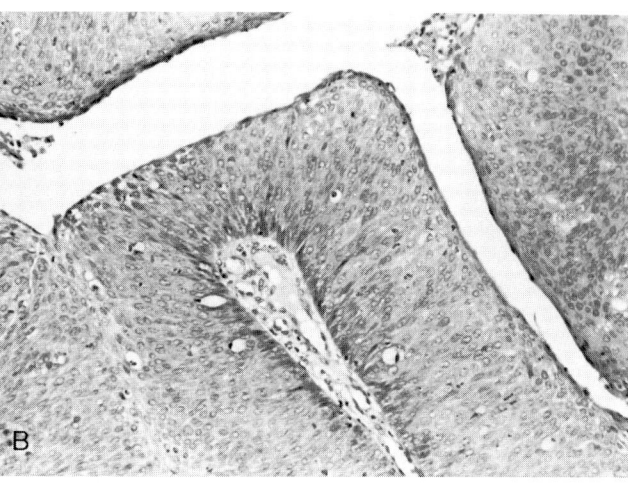

Figure 8–36. *A* and *B*, Inverted ductal papilloma.

polarized nuclei are interspersed with goblet cells and transitional forms of cuboidal to squamous cells.

Histologically, the inverted ductal papilloma resembles the inverted papilloma of the sinonasal tract. There is, however, a more benign course associated with the intraoral lesion; conservative but complete removal is sufficient to prevent recurrence.

Myoepithelioma

Benign salivary gland tumors composed entirely of myoepithelial cells have been described. Although of epithelial origin or derivation, the phenotypic and functional expression of the tumor cells is more closely related to smooth muscle. This is also reflected in the immunoreactivity for myosin and S-100 protein as well as keratins.

Most myoepitheliomas arise within the parotid gland and, less frequently, in the submandibular gland and intraoral minor salivary glands (Fig. 8–37). Clinically, myoepitheliomas present as circumscribed painless masses within the affected gland. An equal gender occurrence has been noted. A range of presentation from the third through ninth dec-

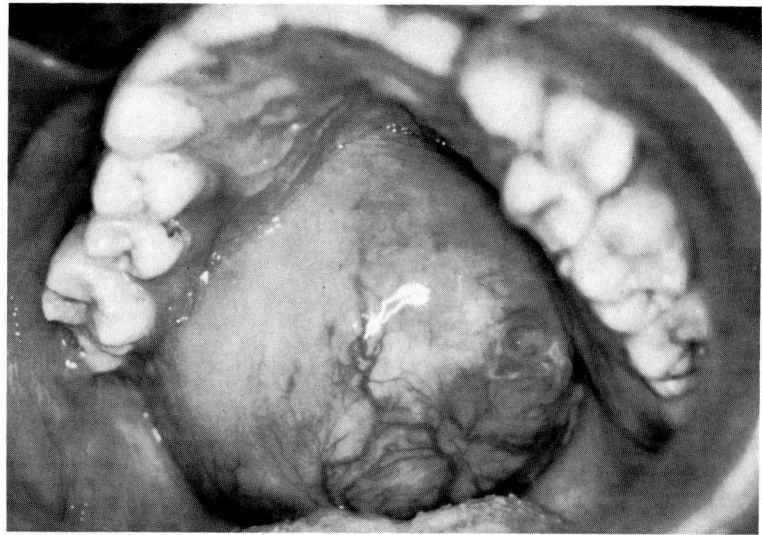

Figure 8–37. Myoepithelioma of the hard palate.

ades, with a median of 53 years, has been reported.

Microscopically, clusters of either plasmacytoid or spindle cells make up these lesions. Approximately 70% of cases contain spindle cell elements, and approximately 20% are composed of plasmacytoid cells (Fig. 8–38). In one study, 13% of myoepitheliomas were seen to contain both cell forms in approximately equal quantity. Growth patterns range from predominantly solid lesions with little background stroma to those with significant levels of mucoid or myxoid elements interspersed between myoepithelial cells.

Ultrastructurally, a thin basal lamina will be found between the tumor cells and the supportive stroma. Occasional hemidesmosomes and pinocytotic vesicles may be noted along the stromal aspect of the plasma membrane of the bordering cell population. Pools or dispersed forms of glycogen may be noted peripherallly. Centrally, filamentous or fibrillar material within the spindle cells is arranged parallel to the long axis of the cells, producing an overall resemblance to smooth muscle cells. Within the plasmacytoid type of myoepithelial cell, filaments tend to be randomly scattered.

Treatment of this benign lesion is identical to that of the benign mixed tumor. Conservative excision of lesions arising in minor salivary glands is advised, including a thin rim of surrounding normal tissue. When lesions are noted within the parotid gland, superficial parotidectomy is indicated. Overall prognosis is excellent, and recurrences are not expected.

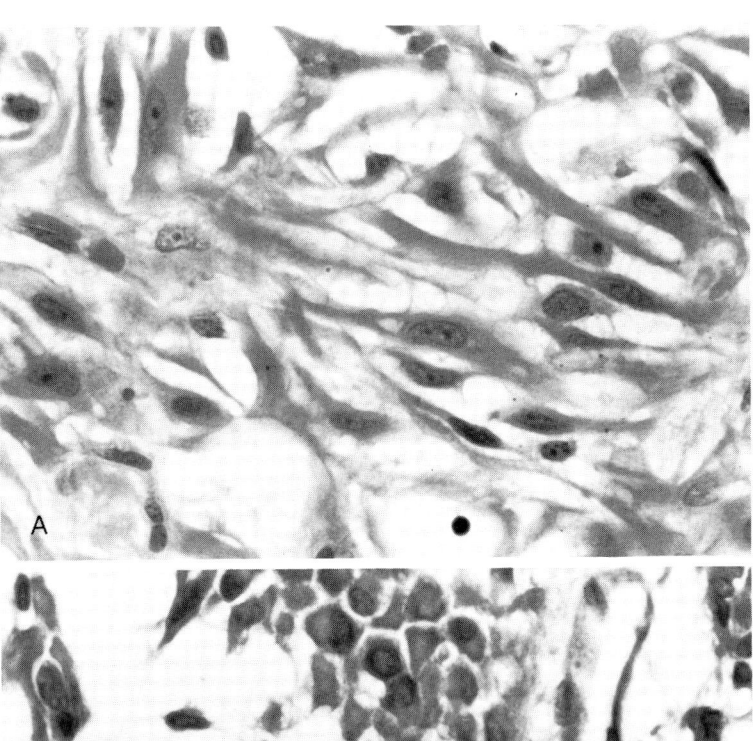

Figure 8–38. *A*, Myoepithelioma composed of spindle cells. *B*, Myoepithelioma composed of plasmacytoid cells.

MALIGNANT NEOPLASMS

Mucoepidermoid Carcinoma

The mucoepidermoid carcinoma has been a somewhat controversial lesion of salivary gland origin with respect to its biologic behavior and natural history. Evidence supports the opinion that all such lesions are carcinomas and have the potential to metastasize. However, the so-called low-grade mucoepidermoid carcinomas often pursue a locally invasive, relatively non-aggressive course. As the name implies, mucoepidermoid carcinomas are epithelial mucin-producing tumors. They are believed to arise from the interlobular and intralobular segments of the salivary duct system. The name of this tumor accurately reflects its biphasic structure, implying a mixed epidermoid and mucus-secreting cell population. The origin of the lesion is likewise reflected in the epidermoid and mucous cell differentiation that is seen in normal duct epithelium. The neoplastic mucous cells contain neutral glycoproteins, acidic mucins, and sulfomucins; the epidermoid cells contain keratin intermediate filaments.

Clinical Features. The most common site of the mucoepidermoid carcinoma is the parotid gland, where 60 to 90% of such lesions are encountered. This lesion represents the most common malignant tumor of salivary gland origin, composing between 6 and 9% of all salivary gland tumors. Based on review of several large series of salivary gland tumors, mucoepidermoid carcinoma accounts for approximately 34% of parotid malignancies, 20% of submandibular gland malignancies, and 29% of salivary tumors within the oral cavity (Table 8–6 and Figs. 8–39 and 8–40). This lesion may also arise centrally within the mandible (Fig. 8–41), presumably from embryonically entrapped salivary elements or from neoplastic transformation of mucous cells in odontogenic cysts. Central intraosseous mucoepidermoid carcinomas may clinically resemble an ameloblastoma, in terms of both radiographic appearance and rate of progression.

The prevalence of mucoepidermoid carcinoma is noted to be highest in the third to fifth decades, and there is an equal gender representation. This neoplasm represents the most common salivary malignancy of childhood. The mean duration between onset and diagnosis varies depending upon the histologic grade of the lesion—one study indicated a 6-year hiatus between onset and treatment. High-grade lesions demonstrate a 1.5-year interval prior to diagnosis.

The clinical manifestations of the mucoepidermoid carcinoma depend greatly upon the grade of malignancy. Tumors of low-grade malignancy will present in a manner similar to the benign mixed tumor, with a prolonged period of painless expansion or enlargement. Within the oral cavity, the mucoepidermoid carcinoma often resembles an extravasation or retention type mucocele that, at times, may be fluctuant as a result of cyst formation. Palatal masses may be diagnosed clinically as a periapical cyst or periodontal abscess. Tumors of high-grade malignancy, on the other hand, grow rapidly and are often accompanied by pain and mucosal ulceration. Within the major salivary glands, high-grade tumors may present with evidence of facial nerve involvement or obstructive signs. In unusual circumstances in which mucoepidermoid carcinomas arise within the mandible or maxilla, they generally

Table 8–6. MALIGNANT SALIVARY GLAND TUMORS

Tumor	Parotid	Submandibular	Sublingual	Minor	Total
Mucoepidermoid carcinoma	593	73	8	253	927
Adenocystic carcinoma	180	148	7	388	723
Acinic cell carcinoma	241	8	8	25	282
Malignant mixed tumor	257	54	–	66	377
Adenocarcinoma	318	53	–	243	614
Squamous cell carcinoma	83	23	1	5	112
Other	60	17	–	38	115
Total	1732	376	24	1018	3150

Compiled from Chaudhry AP, et al. Cancer 58:72, 1986; Chen SY, et al. Cancer 42:678, 1978; Ellis GL, et al. Cancer 52:542, 1983; Evans HL, et al. Cancer 53:935, 1985; Luna MA, et al. Oral Surg Oral Med Oral Pathol 59:482, 1985; Perzin KH, et al. Cancer 42:265, 1978; Ranko RM, et al. Am J Surg 118:790, 1969; Spiro RH, et al. Am J Surg 130:452, 1975; and Spiro RH, et al. Cancer 39:388, 1977.

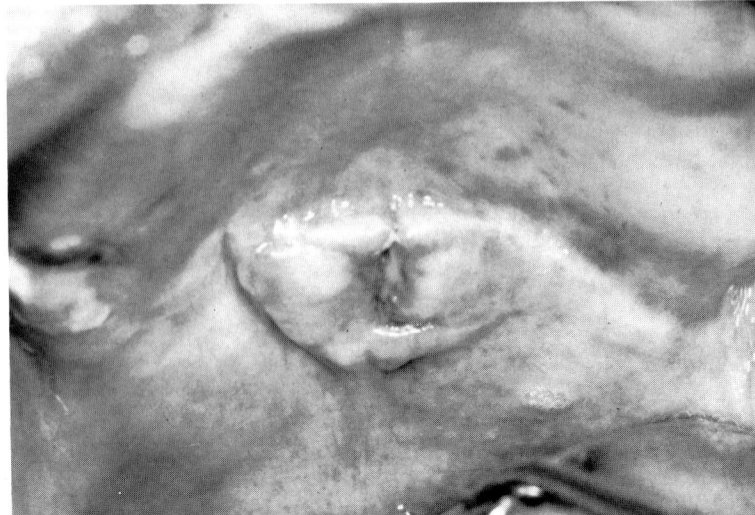

Figure 8–39. Mucoepidermoid carcinoma at the junction of the hard and soft palate.

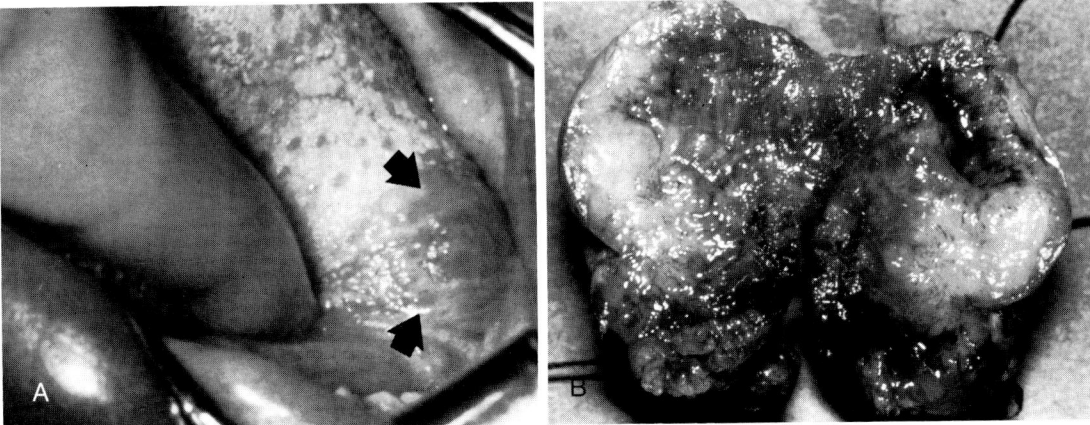

Figure 8–40. *A*, Mucoepidermoid carcinoma in the posterolateral aspect of the tongue (arrows). *B*, Gross specimen showing infiltrative tumor as lighter colored areas.

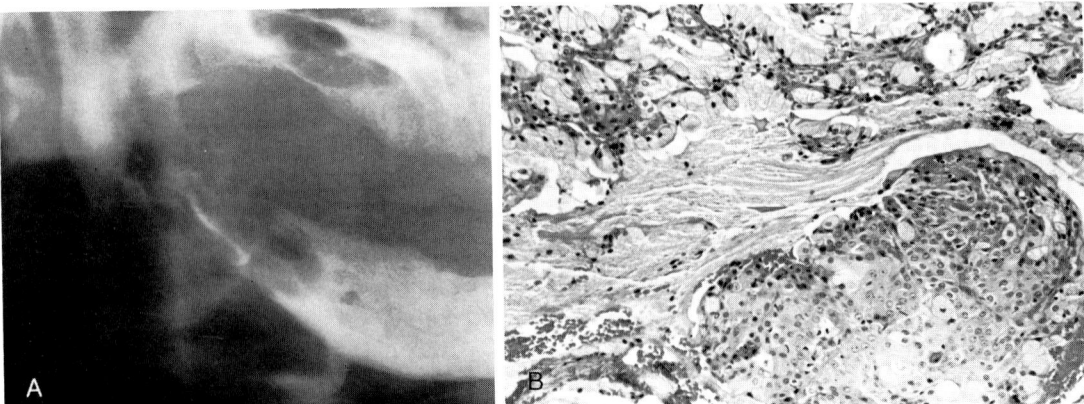

Figure 8–41. *A*, Central mucoepidermoid carcinoma of molar-ramus area of the mandible. *B*, Biopsy showing mucous and epidermoid cells in a low-grade tumor.

are detected as radiolucent lesions that are expansile and situated within the molar and premolar area. Radiographically, they must be separated from giant cell granuloma, odontogenic cysts, ameloblastoma, and other odontogenic tumors.

Histopathology. The mucoepidermoid carcinoma is often well circumscribed and occasionally may be partially encapsulated. The lesion typically demonstrates infiltration of adjacent tissue. A solid growth pattern may be noted in some tumors, although cyst formation is a common finding, especially in low-grade lesions.

Most low-grade mucoepidermoid carcinomas are composed of mucus-secreting cells arranged around microcystic structures, often with an intermingling of intermediate or epidermoid cellular elements (Figs. 8–42 and 8–43). The mucin-containing cells are characterized by intracellular mucin, which may be demonstrated by PAS and mucicarmine positivity (Figs. 8–44 and 8–45). Coalescence of small cysts into large cystic spaces is typical of low-grade malignancy. These cysts may distend the surrounding supportive tissue and rupture, allowing escape of mucus into the surrounding tissues, with a concomitant reactive inflammatory response. At the margin of low-grade tumors, the pattern is often one of broad pushing fronts, a testament to the tumor's low-level invasiveness.

High-grade malignancies, on the other hand, are characterized by variable levels of local infiltration and invasion. Neoplastic cell clusters are more solid with fewer cystic spaces and mucous cells (Fig. 8–46). Larger numbers of epidermoid cells and intermediate elements are seen at the expense of more differentiated mucous cell elements. Cellular pleomorphism, nuclear hyperchromatism, and mitotic figures may be noted within the intermediate and high-grade tumors. In many high-grade mucoepidermoid carcinomas, much of the lesion may resemble squamous cell carcinoma, with small numbers of mucous cells evident. In high-grade lesions, infiltration in the form of cords and strands of cells may be noted well beyond the obvious clinical focus of the tumor.

The pattern and proportion of mucous to epidermoid elements in metastatic foci may not resemble the primary lesion. Extremes of cellular type may be evident, with either mucous or epidermoid cells forming the predominant component.

Some debate exists regarding the number of cell types in the mucoepidermoid carcinoma. Some authorities feel that up to six morpho-

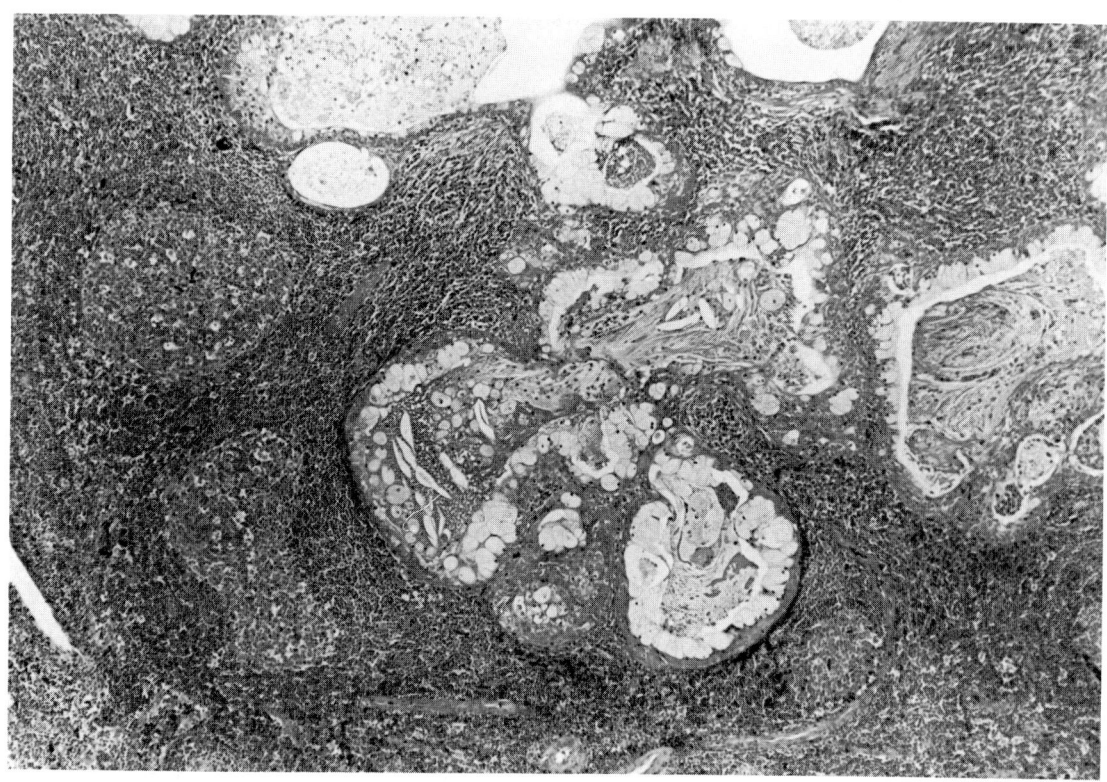

Figure 8–42. Low-grade mucoepidermoid carcinoma metastatic to a cervical lymph node.

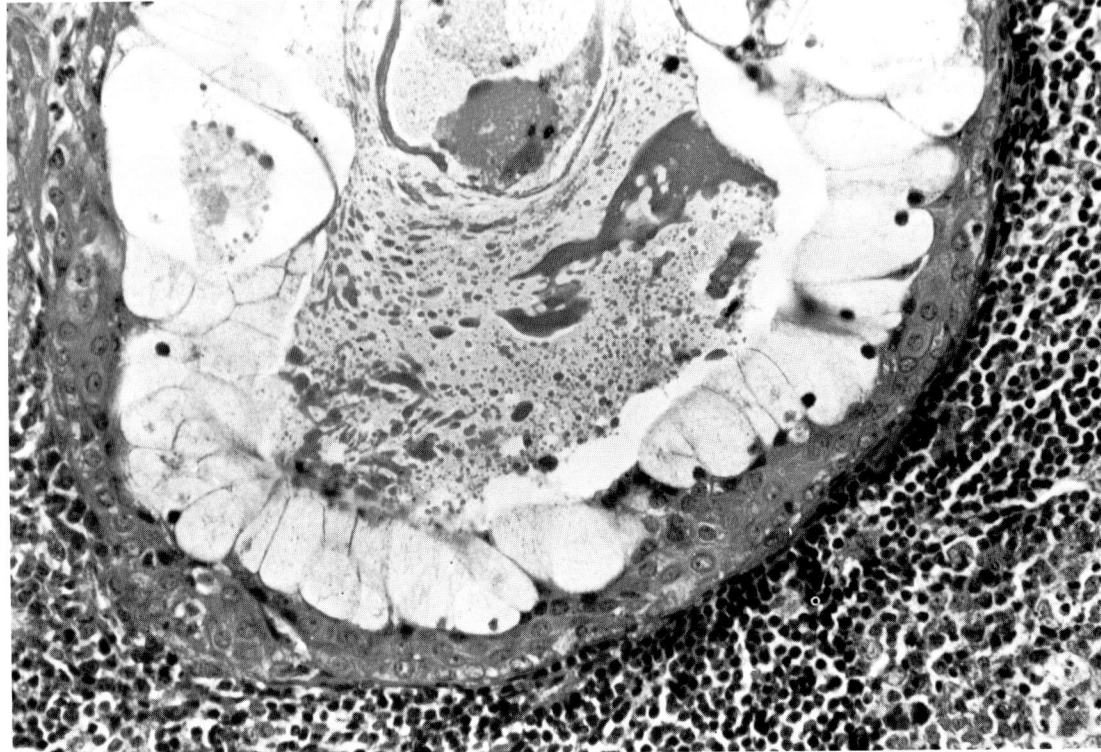

Figure 8-43. High magnification of tumor in Figure 8-42 showing mucin goblet cell differentiation.

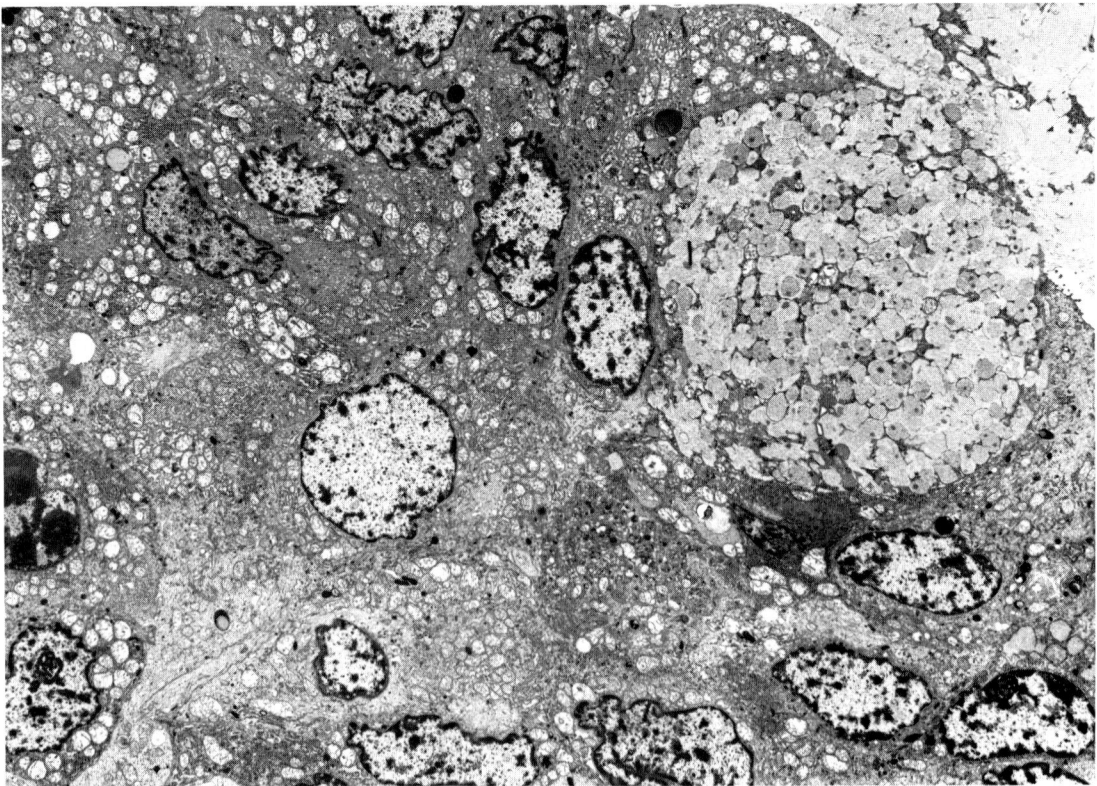

Figure 8-44. Electron micrograph of low-grade mucoepidermoid carcinoma. Note mucous cell in upper right.

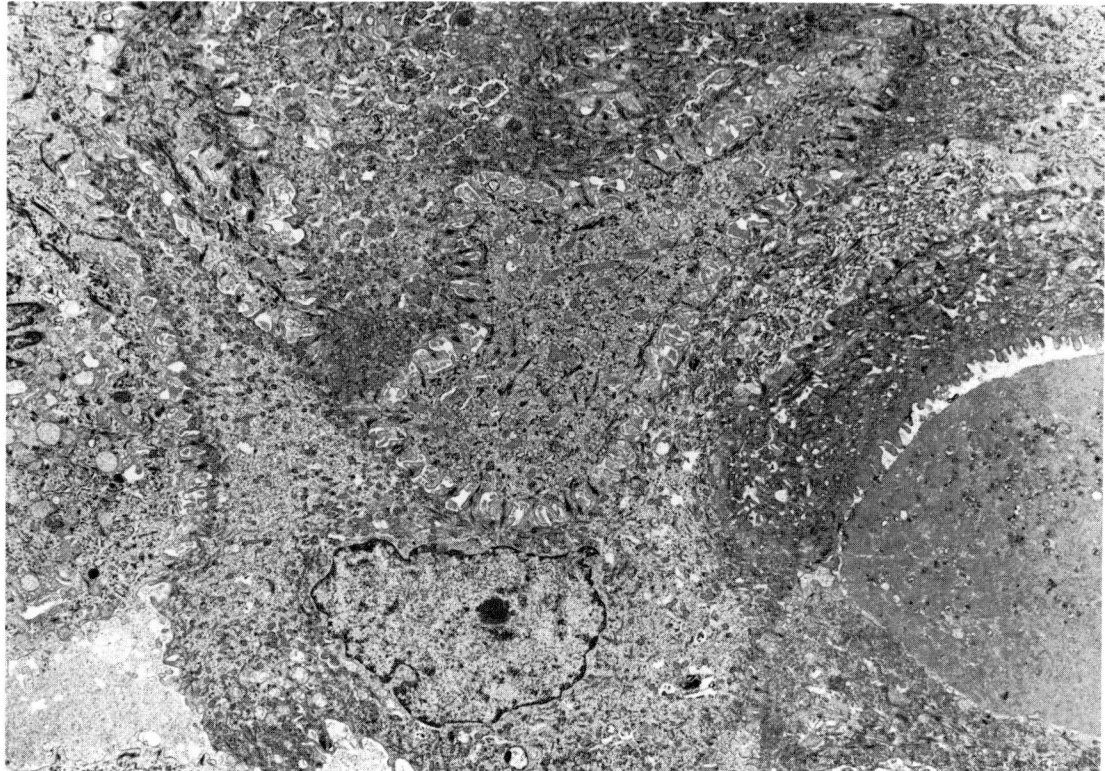

Figure 8-45. Electron micrograph of low-grade mucoepidermoid carcinoma. Tonofilaments can be seen in the cytoplasm of most cells, and desmosomes can be seen between cells.

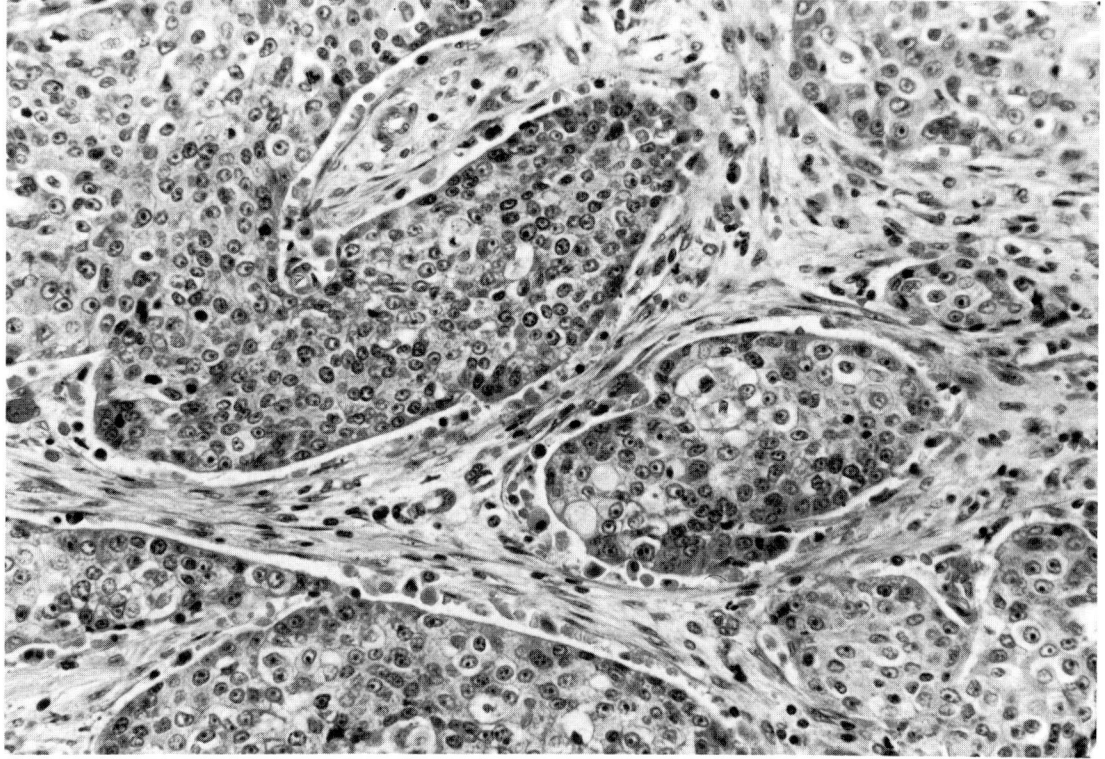

Figure 8-46. High-grade mucoepidermoid carcinoma.

logically distinct types of cells may be present; most others indicate that epidermoid, mucous, and intermediate cells will be found in varying proportion relative to the level or grade of differentiation.

Owing to the variable histologic composition of mucoepidermoid carcinomas, differential diagnosis may range from benign ductal dilatation of developmental or inflammatory origin with metaplastic features to several forms of carcinoma, including squamous cell carcinoma, for lesions of high-grade character.

Prognosis and Treatment. Prognostic significance may be ascribed to histologic grades of malignancy from low to high grade. Characteristically, low-grade mucoepidermoid carcinomas generally follow a benign clinical course similar to that noted for the benign mixed tumor. There have been, however, several instances of low-grade lesions that have metastasized widely and have proved fatal. Clinical confirmation of the aggressiveness of high-grade carcinomas generally is evident within the first 5 years after the initial treatment, with local and distant metastases being evident in up to 60% of cases. Incidences of metastases to cervical lymph nodes from mucoepidermoid carcinomas of the parotid gland (excluding low-grade lesions) have reached 44%. When all patients with mucoepidermoid carcinomas are considered, a 5-year survival of nearly 90% has been recorded. For high-grade lesions, however, survival rates of approximately 40% have been noted in two large series. In follow-up periods extended to 15 years, the cure rate for low-grade carcinomas has been stated to be 98% as compared with 25% or less for higher grade mucoepidermoid carcinomas.

Treatment of the primary malignancy is surgical. Higher grade malignancies are usually managed with surgery plus post-operative radiotherapy to the primary site. Radical neck dissection is rarely performed in small lesions of low-grade malignancy; high-grade tumors usually will require this form of management.

Adenocystic Carcinoma

The adenocystic or adenoid cystic carcinoma has been portrayed as one of the most biologically deceptive and frustrating of all tumors in the head and neck region. This form of adenocarcinoma is distinctive and merits separation from other forms of glandular neoplasia because of its microscopic appearance, behavioral characteristics, high rate of local recurrence, and systemic spread.

The origin of adenocystic carcinoma is thought to be from the intercalated duct reserve cell or terminal tubule complex. Differentiation is believed to be along the intercalated duct cell line.

Clinical Features. This lesion accounts for approximately 23% of all salivary gland carcinomas. It is the most common salivary gland malignancy noted within the minor intraoral glands and submandibular glands. It constitutes almost one third of malignancies occurring within the sublingual glands. The minor salivary glands, including those of the sinonasal tract, account for approximately 50 to 70% of all reported cases of adenocystic carcinoma in the head and neck region. In the major salivary glands, the parotid gland is most often affected.

The bulk of the patients with adenocystic carcinoma are between the fifth and seventh decades. There is no gender predilection, although a slight female predominance is noted for lesions arising in the submandibular gland.

In the major salivary glands, the clinical appearance is usually that of a unilobular mass that is firm on palpation and may be associated with some pain or tenderness. These lesions generally are characterized by a slow growth rate; they have often been present for several years prior to the patient's seeking treatment.

Bone invasion occurs frequently, initially without radiographic changes because of infiltration through marrow spaces. Rarely, this lesion may arise within the mandible. Distant spread to the lungs is more common than is metastasis to regional lymph nodes. Also of interest is the tendency for tumor invasion of perineural spaces, with the neoplasm often presenting well beyond the site of clinical disease. A frequent feature of intraoral lesions, particularly those arising on the palate, is ulceration of the overlying mucosa, a point often used to help clinically distinguish this lesion from the more common benign mixed tumor (Fig. 8–47).

Histopathology. The standard and well-accepted light microscopic features of adenocystic carcinoma are characterized by a cribriform or cylindromatous pattern (Figs. 8–48 and 8–49), a tubular-trabecular pattern, a solid basaloid pattern of growth, or a combination of these. There is some controversy regarding an overall behavioral prediction relative to these histologic variants, but it is felt that the solid basaloid type of growth is associated with a poorer overall prognosis. Areas of central necrosis within solid clusters of cells may indicate a more aggressive form of disease. More im-

Figure 8–47. *A* and *B*, Adenocystic carcinomas of the hard palate (arrows).

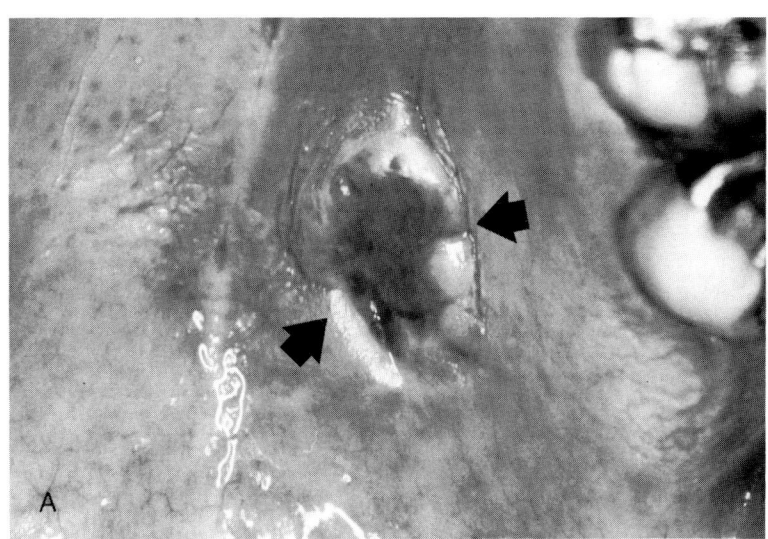
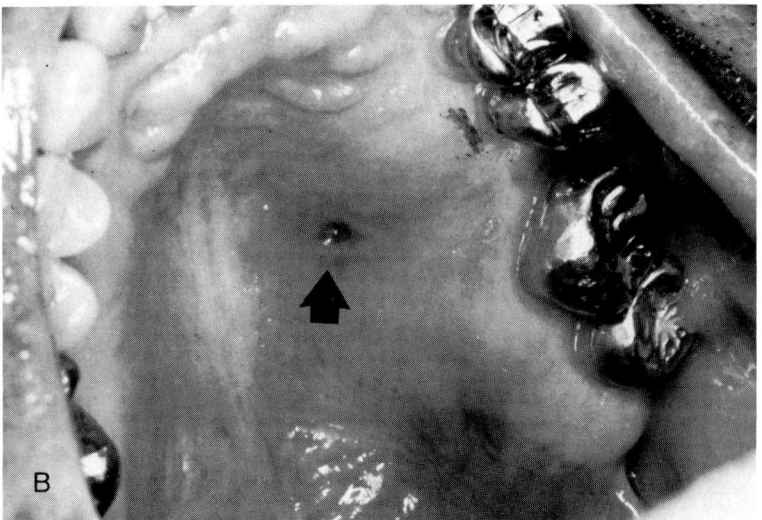

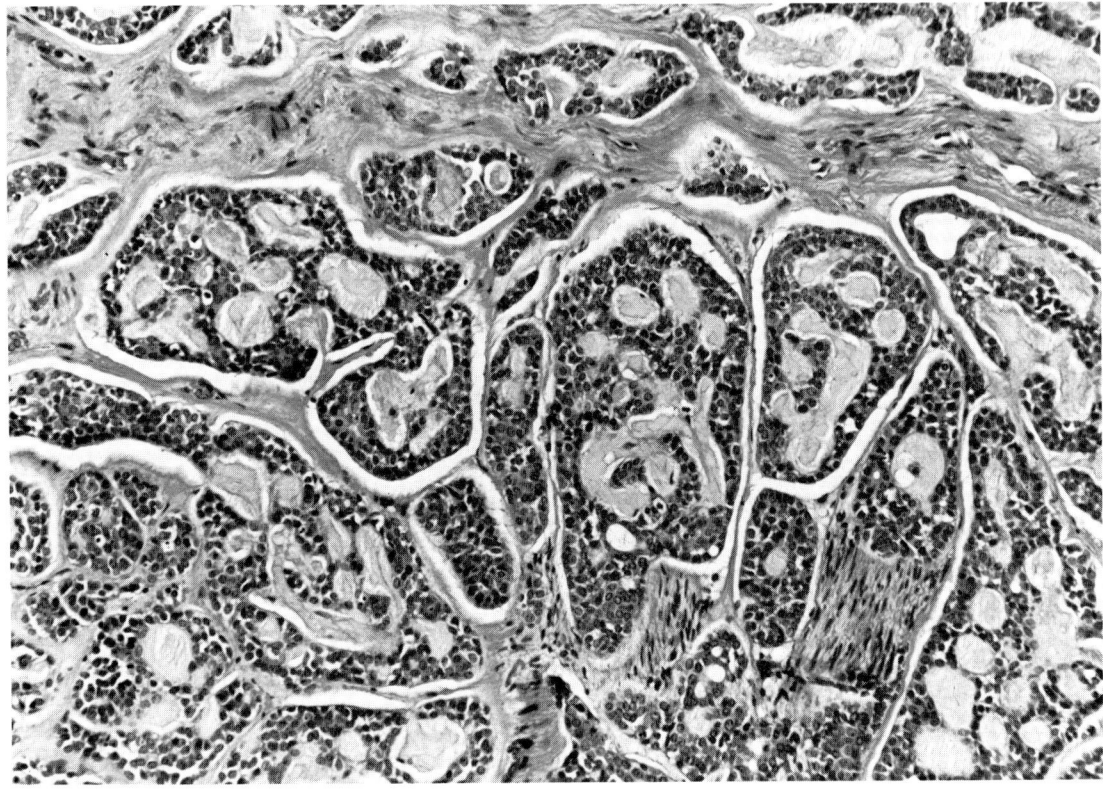

Figure 8-48. Adenocystic carcinoma, cribriform pattern.

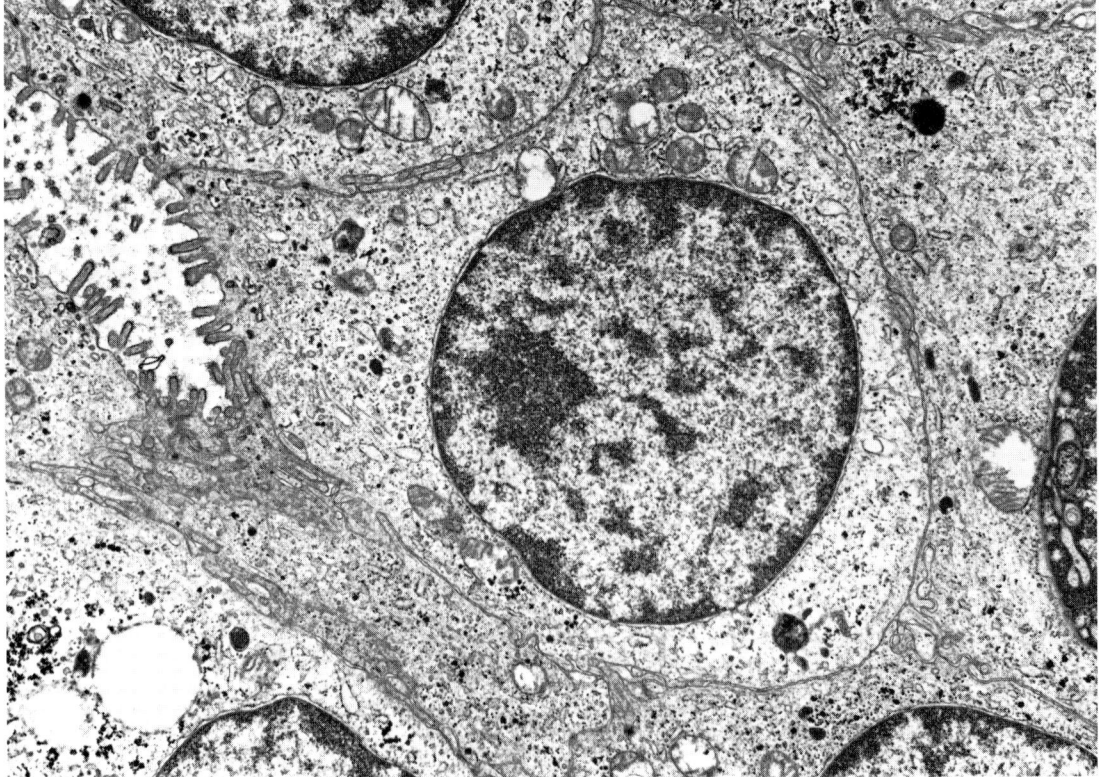

Figure 8-49. Electron micrograph of adenocystic carcinoma composed of small undifferentiated cells.

portant factors regarding prediction of behavior include size of the primary lesion, anatomic location, presence or absence of metastatic disease at diagnosis, and for parotid lesions, facial nerve involvement.

Individual cells composing the tumor are small and cuboidal with disproportionately large isomorphic nuclei. Nuclear atypia is absent or minimal, and mitotic activity is usually not seen. Chromatin aggregation is dense, and nuclear contours are even.

The distinctive morphology of this neoplasm relates to formation of pseudocystic spaces that contain a variety of acellular substances. This material consists chiefly of sulfated mucopolysaccharides that are ultrastructurally characterized by multilayered or replicated basal lamina material. Myoepithelial cells may represent a small fraction of the cellular component of adenocystic carcinomas. Occasionally, both myoepithelial and ductal elements may be arranged similarly to normal ducts in which there is an inner row of small cuboidal cells surrounded by larger myoepithelial cells. A final distinctive microscopic feature is perineural and intraneural invasion (Fig. 8–50).

Treatment and Prognosis. Regardless of the site of the primary lesion, surgery is regarded as the treatment of choice for adenocystic carcinomas. When the parotid glands are involved, wide resection in the form of a superficial parotidectomy or superficial and deep lobectomy is recommended. In the parotid region, debate exists as to whether or not the facial nerve should be spared; most investigators recommend resection only if the tumor surrounds or invades this nerve.

Intraorally, wide excision, often with removal of underlying bone, is the treatment of choice. Radical surgical excision is frequently used to obtain surgical margins that are free of tumor.

Post-surgical radiation therapy has shown promising results and has a role in the management of recurrence. Currently, chemotherapy is regarded as ineffective for long-term management of recurrent or metastatic adenocystic carcinoma. However, multiple agent chemotherapy has shown some promise in management of widely metastatic disease.

The prognosis in adenocystic carcinoma must be judged not in terms of 5-year survival rates but rather in terms of 15- to 20-year survival rates. Survival rates at 5 years approximate 70%; at 15 years the rate is only 10%. An additional factor that negatively influences prognosis is the presence of tumor in the lines of surgical excision.

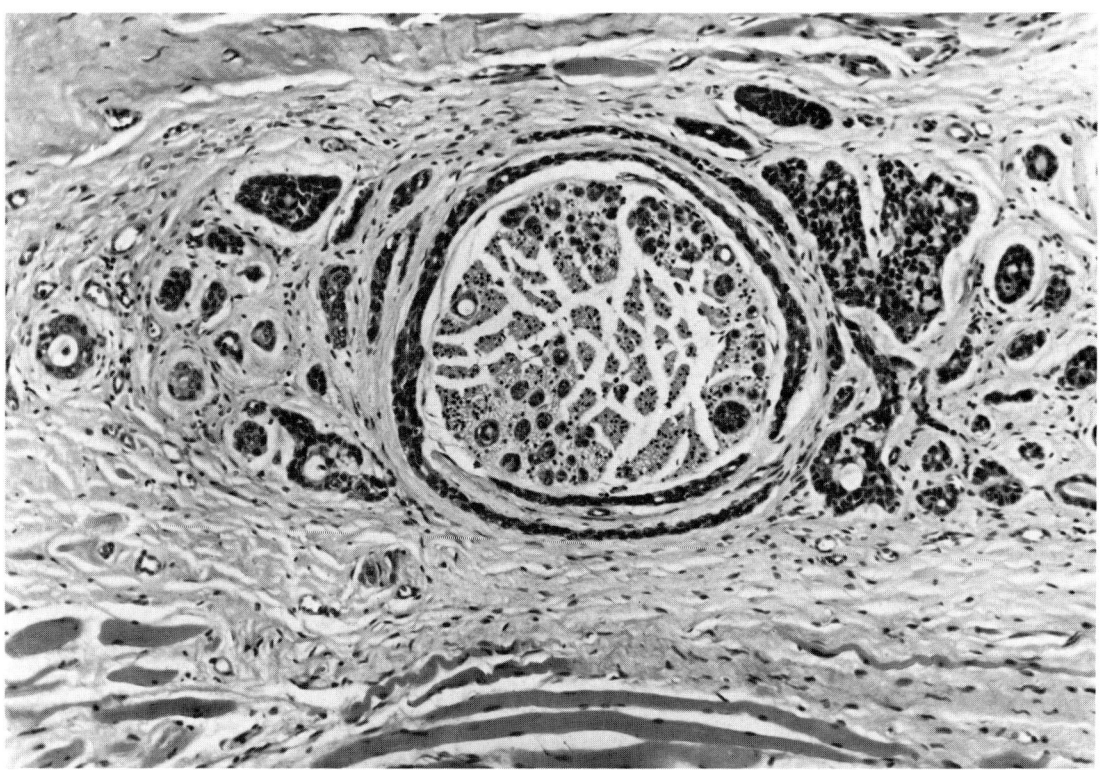

Figure 8–50. Adenocystic carcinoma showing perineural invasion.

Recurrence patterns often relate to local extension of the primary lesion—distant metastasis is seen in about 40% of all cases. Regional lymph node involvement is less common than is distant metastatic disease resulting from vascular or hematogenous spread. Lung metastases are approximately three times as common as regional lymph node metastases.

Acinic Cell Carcinoma

The acinic cell carcinoma is a distinctive neoplasm of salivary gland origin. The preponderance of cases are reported in major salivary glands, especially the parotid. The putative origin of the acinic cell carcinoma is from the intercalated duct reserve cell, although there is reason to believe that the acinic cell itself retains the potential for neoplastic transformation in adults. It has been suggested that the acinic cell carcinoma may represent an integrated proliferation of intercalated and acinic precursors and, less commonly, myoepithelial cells. The neoplastic elements may be organized in a fashion simulating the acinic intercalated duct unit.

Clinical Features. The acinic cell carcinoma may be found in all age groups, including children, with the peak incidence noted within the fifth and sixth decades. There appears to be no gender predilection.

This lesion accounts for 14% of all parotid gland tumors and 9% of the total of salivary gland carcinomas of all sites. An unusual feature is its frequency of bilateral parotid gland involvement in approximately 3% of cases. Most cases develop within the superficial lobe and inferior pole of the parotid gland. Far fewer cases have been reported within the submandibular and minor salivary glands. Within the oral cavity, most cases occur in the palate and buccal mucosa.

Acinic cell carcinomas usually present as slow-growing lesions less than 3 cm in diameter. Although it is not indicative of prognosis, pain is a frequent presenting symptom. The interval between the initial appearance of the mass and treatment varies from 6 months to 5 years. In nearly half of all cases, the clinical impression is that of a benign lesion.

Histopathology. In at least one third of acinic cell carcinomas, a marked cystic growth pattern can be noted. Large lobules or nests of tumor cells with little intervening stroma are characteristic. The arrangement of neoplastic cells is quite variable, with several growth patterns evident. Generally, cells are arranged in solid masses with blunted or pushing margins. The solid pattern of growth is the most common (Fig. 8–51), followed closely by a trabecular pattern. Other variations include microcystic, papillary cystic, and follicular forms.

The most predominant cell type is the well-differentiated acinic cell containing cytoplasmic granules varying from finely diffuse to large and coarse. Granules are PAS-positive and identical to those found in normal acinic cells. Intercalated duct type cells are seen in approximately one third of cases, and nonspecific and vacuolated cells are seen in nearly one fourth of cases. Many acinic cell carcinomas demonstrate occasional clear cell elements, and rare examples are found that are composed entirely of clear cells.

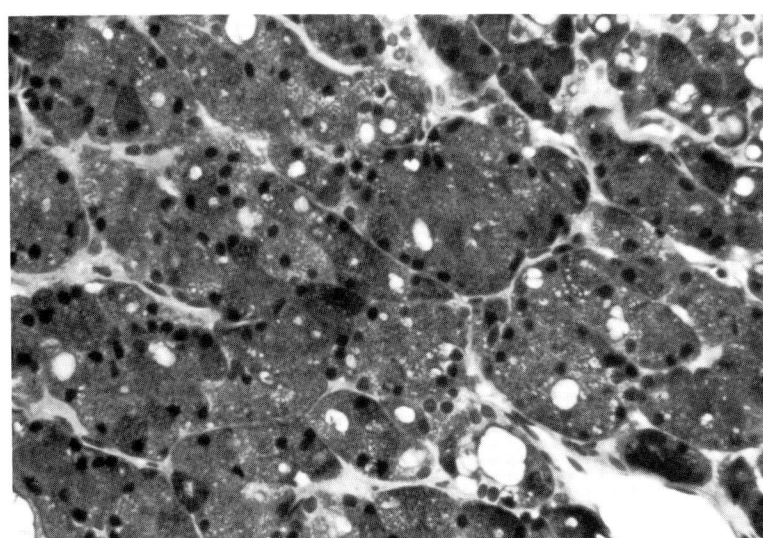

Figure 8–51. Acinic cell carcinoma. Tumor cell cytoplasm is granular and basophilic.

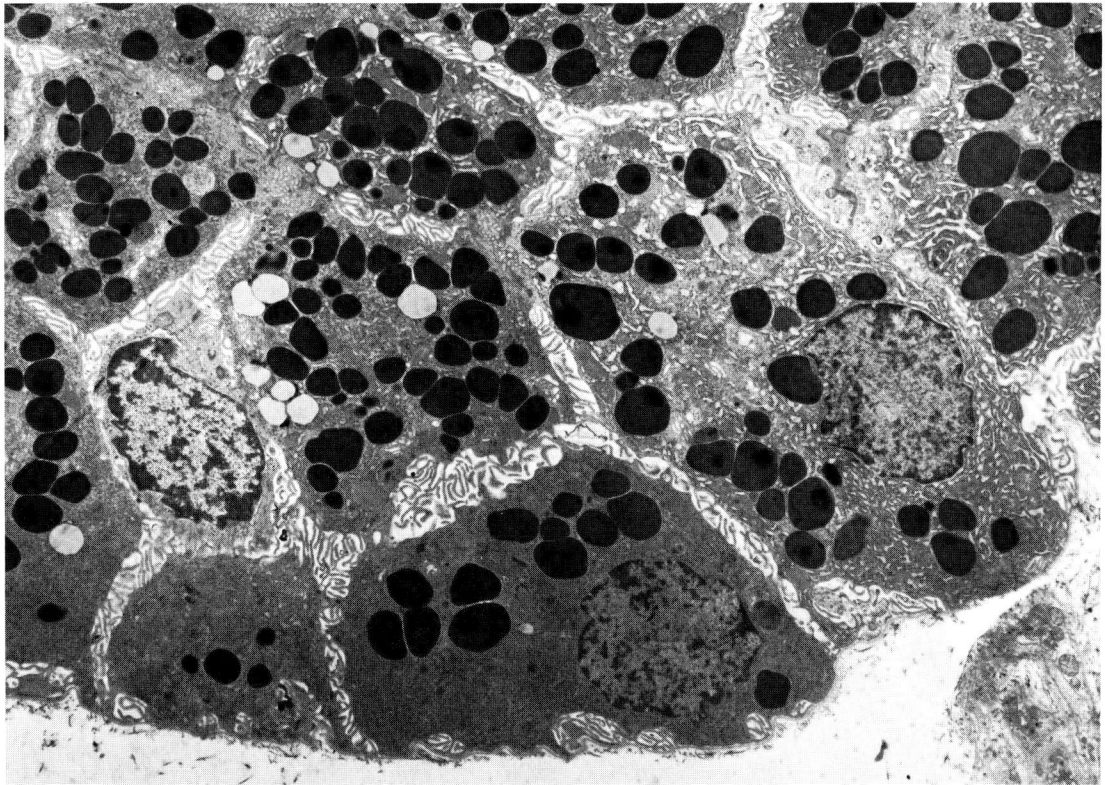

Figure 8–52. Electron micrograph of acinic cell carcinoma. Tumor cells contain dark secretory granules.

Ultrastructurally, acinic tumor cells reflect normal acinic elements with large accumulations of rough endoplasmic reticulum, well-developed Golgi complexes, and secretory granule formation (Fig. 8–52). The granules demonstrate maturation as they approach the apical portion of the cytoplasm, where ultimately they fuse with the plasma membrane and lose contents through exocytosis.

Treatment and Prognosis. Surgery is the preferred management. In general, acinic cell carcinomas seldom metastasize, yet they have a strong tendency to recur. Determinant survival rates of 89% at 5 years and 56% at 20 years indicate its overall malignant nature. Metastases to regional lymph nodes occur in approximately 10% of cases, whereas distant metastases occur in approximately 15% of cases.

Carcinoma Ex-mixed Tumor/ Malignant Mixed Tumor

The term "carcinoma ex-mixed tumor" has been used interchangeably with "malignant mixed tumor." This reflects the literature, although each designation represents a different histopathologic entity. For purposes of this discussion, *carcinoma ex-mixed tumor* is used to represent an epithelial malignancy arising in a pre-existing mixed tumor where such remnants may be identified. When metastatic disease supervenes, only the malignant component metastasizes. This is more common than the so-called malignant mixed tumor.

Two types of *malignant mixed tumor* have been recognized. One type is a malignancy in which both the epithelial and the mesenchymal components are malignant; hence a carcinosarcoma designation could be used. In metastatic instances, both elements are present. The second type of malignant mixed tumor is characterized by a histologically benign mixed tumor that for some reason metastasizes while still retaining its bland or benign histologic character.

Clinical Features. The carcinoma ex-mixed tumor usually arises from a benign mixed tumor known to be present for several years (Fig. 8–53) or from a benign mixed tumor that has had multiple recurrences over many years. Malignancy occurring within a previously benign tumor is heralded by rapid growth after an extremely long period of minimally perceptible increase.

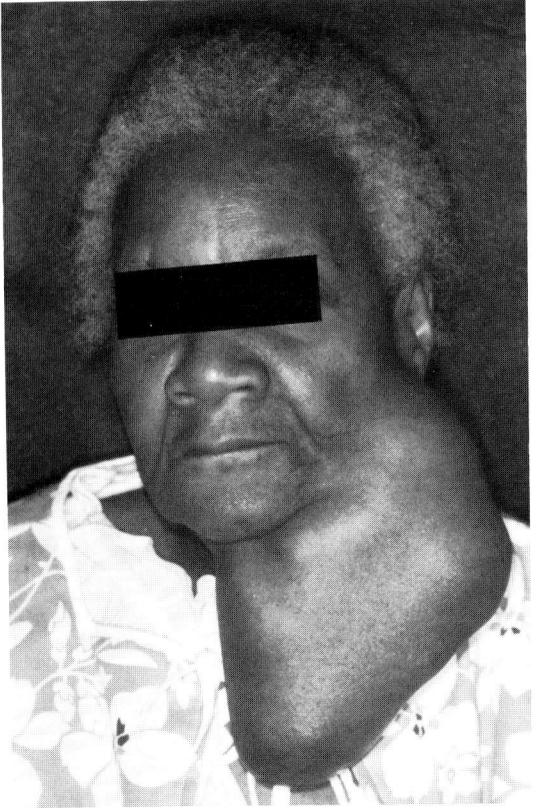

Figure 8–53. Carcinoma ex-mixed tumor occurring in a long-standing mixed tumor.

Approximately 68% of carcinoma ex-mixed tumors and malignant mixed tumors are found in the parotid gland, and 18% are found in the minor intraoral salivary glands. The average age when malignancy becomes evident is 60 years, approximately 20 years beyond the age noted for benign mixed tumor. Suspicious signs of malignancy include fixation of the mass to surrounding tissues or overlying mucosa, cutaneous ulceration, and regional lymphadenopathy.

Histopathology. The margins of carcinoma ex-mixed tumors and malignant mixed tumors are generally well defined, although infiltrative areas are likely to be present. Necrosis and hemorrhage with areas of dystrophic mineralization are frequently noted. Most areas of malignancy appear as adenocarcinoma or undifferentiated carcinoma, or a combination of both (Fig. 8–54). Uncommonly the histologic picture of the benign mixed tumor may be noted with minimal areas of carcinomatous change. Non-invasive carcinoma or carcinoma *in situ* may also be infrequently found within the benign mixed tumor.

When they are present, metastatic deposits mimic the primary lesion. Chondroid patterns may be evident in metastatic deposits, also mimicking the primary tumor.

Treatment and Prognosis. Treatment is almost exclusively surgical, with radical neck dissection part of the initial treatment in patients with evidence of cervical lymph node involvement.

Local recurrence remains a problem in nearly half of patients with primary parotid neoplasms and nearly three fourths of patients with submandibular and minor salivary gland tumors. Approximately 10% of cases present with uncontrollable lymphatic disease, with nearly one third showing metastasis to distant sites, usually to lung and bone.

Determinant cure rates at 5, 10, and 15 years post treatment in one study were 40%, 24%, and 19%, respectively; in another study, 30% of those followed for 10 years were free of disease.

Epimyoepithelial Carcinoma of Intercalated Ducts

Salivary gland tumors composed of optically clear cells may be derived from intercalated duct cells, reserve cells, myoepithelial cells, mucous cells, sebaceous cells, and acinic cells. Cytoplasmic optical clarity is thought to result from minimal cellular differentiation and lack of organelles; from storage or accumulation of cytoplasmic elements such as glycogen, mucin, or lipid or clear secretory granules; or from fixation artifact. Clear cells may therefore be encountered in numerous salivary gland tumors, including mucoepidermoid carcinomas and sebaceous neoplasms, and in organelle-poor cells within benign mixed tumors, acinic cell carcinomas, and monomorphic adenomas. When these tumors are eliminated in a differential diagnosis of a clear cell tumor, most of the remainder probably belong in the epimyoepithelial carcinoma category. The epimyoepithelial or intercalated duct carcinoma is one of several lesions that have recently been separated from the larger, less well defined adenocarcinoma group. Until 1972, the epimyoepithelial carcinoma had also been classified as a member of clear cell salivary gland neoplasms. Origin of this lesion is believed to be from the intercalated ducts of the salivary gland unit, with the reserve cells of this duct—modified by epigenetic events—serving as progenitors. Differentiation toward both epithelial

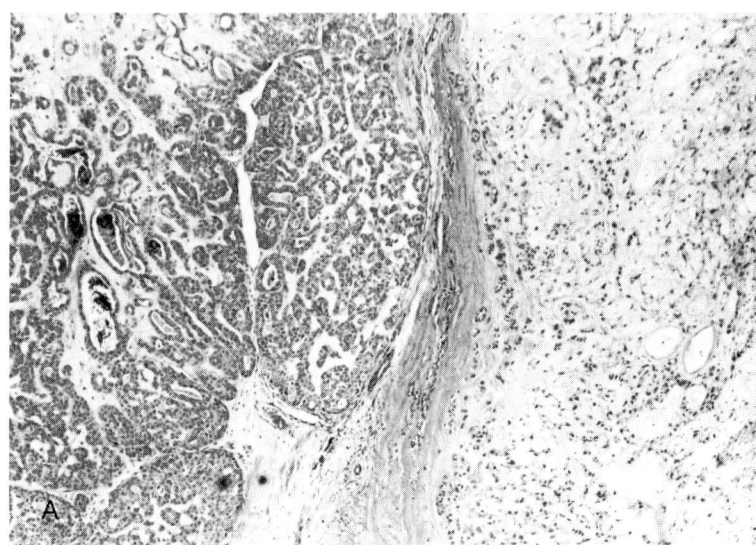
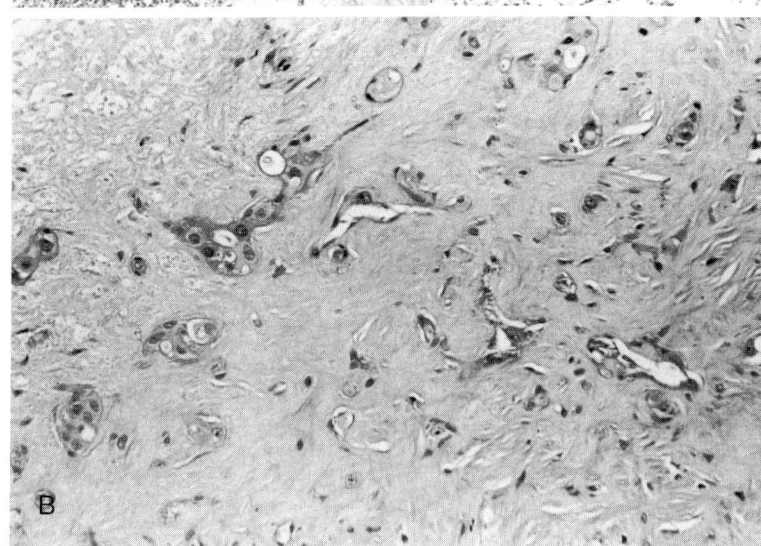

Figure 8–54. *A* and *B*, Carcinoma ex-mixed tumor. Neoplastic cells are hyperchromatic and pleomorphic.

and myoepithelial cells in this tumor is evident from morphologic and immunologic studies.

Microscopically, a multinodular growth pattern is characteristic. Nodules of tumor are composed of two cell types, generally in a duct-like arrangement (Fig. 8–55). A row of cuboidal, darkly staining cells form a lumen, often containing PAS-positive material. These ductal cells are surrounded by one or several layers of myoepithelial cells that are characterized by a columnar to ovoid outline with pale or clear cytoplasm. Large concentrations of cytoplasmic glycogen may be present in these cells. Immunohistochemical studies have shown the presence of contractile proteins and S-100 protein in the clear cell component, supporting their myoepithelial origin. Clusters or lobules of tumor epithelium are surrounded by a hyalinized, poorly cellular matrix. Extensions of tumor are frequently noted, with areas of necrosis also evident on occasion.

Ultrastructurally, both ductal and myoepithelial elements have been confirmed and substantiate the earlier conclusions regarding histogenesis and cellular origins of this lesion. Microscopic differential diagnosis of salivary gland clear cell tumors would include the so-called clear cell myoepithelioma, the glycogen-rich clear cell adenoma, and the glycogen-rich carcinoma. Although such lesions usually appear in the parotid, they make up less than 1% of parotid gland neoplasms.

Treatment of this lesion is essentially surgical. When it occurs in the parotid gland, superficial parotidectomy is the treatment of choice; neck dissection is reserved for patients

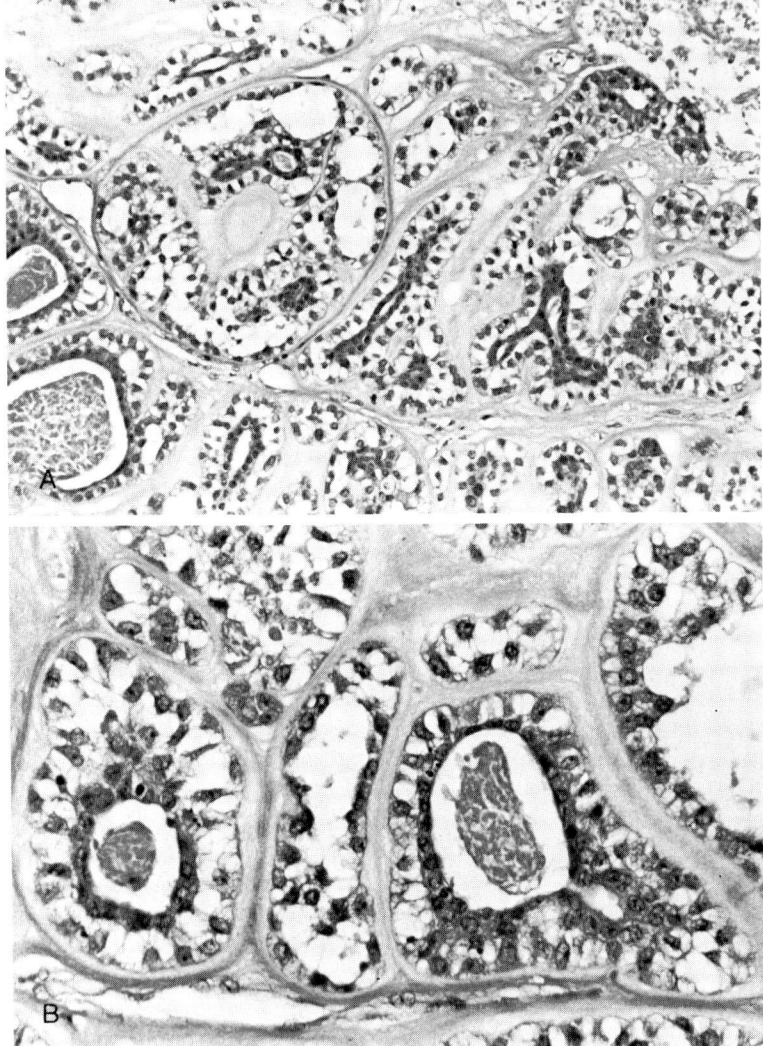

Figure 8–55. *A* and *B*, Epimyoepithelial carcinoma of intercalated ducts.

demonstrating lymphadenopathy. Recurrences are common, but death as a direct result of widespread tumor is uncommon.

Terminal Duct Carcinoma

Until recently, a heterogeneous group of salivary gland neoplasms were classified simply as salivary gland adenocarcinomas for lack of a better designation. A lesion called terminal duct carcinoma (lobular carcinoma, polymorphous low-grade adenocarcinoma) has been segregated from the others in this group because of its distinctive clinical, histomorphologic, and behavioral aspects. The terminal duct carcinoma is generally considered to be a low-grade malignancy with a relatively indolent course and low risk of metastasis.

The origin of the terminal duct adenocarcinoma is believed to be the most proximal portion of the salivary duct. Both myoepithelial and ductal elements appear to participate in the growth of this tumor. In some areas, these lesions resemble other forms of salivary neoplasia that histogenetically arise from the intercalated duct reserve cell system.

Clinical Features. This neoplasm arises from the fifth through eighth decades, with a mean age of 59 years. Gender predilection is not evident. The lesion tends to occur in minor salivary glands, with the palate being the most frequently reported site (Table 8–7). Terminal duct carcinomas typically present as firm, elevated, non-ulcerated, nodular swellings that are usually non-tender. A wide range of size has been noted, but most are between 1 and 4 cm in diameter. The slow growth rate is evi-

Table 8–7. TERMINAL DUCT CARCINOMA (1987)

Location	Number	Per cent
Palate	39	62
Buccal mucosa	8	13
Upper lip	6	10
Retromolar	4	6
Base of tongue	2	3
Pterygomandibular raphe	2	3
Mandibular mucosa	1	1.5
Maxillary tuberosity	1	1.5

Compiled from Batsakis JG. Ann Oto Rhinol Laryngol 89:196, 1980; Eneroth CM. Cancer 27:1415, 1971; Eveson JW, et al. J Pathol 146:51, 1985; Freedman P, et al. Oral Surg Oral Med Oral Pathol 56:157, 1983; and Spiro RH. Head Neck Surg 8:177, 1986.

denced by the long duration—many months to years—prior to diagnosis and treatment. Neurologic symptoms have not been reported in association with clinical presentation.

Histopathology. Absence of encapsulation and a generalized lobular morphology characterize this group of low-grade adenocarcinomas. Infiltration into the surrounding salivary gland and connective tissue is evident at low-power examination (Fig. 8–56). In most areas, the tumor is composed of a homogeneous population of cells with prominent, bland nuclei and minimal cytoplasm. These cells are arranged in lobules as well as in solid nests (Fig. 8–57). At the periphery, tubules form; they are lined by a single layer of cells that often produce cribriform type structures bearing a close resemblance to adenocystic carcinoma. Tumor cells, often spindled, are also arranged in trabeculae and narrow cords in the so-called Indian-file arrangement. The spindle cell element is representative of myoepithelial cell participation and helps confirm the terminal duct origin of these lesions. Striking patterns may be noted in which concentric arrangements of individual cells appear around blood vessels and nerves. The perineural pattern of growth is similar to that seen in the adenocystic carcinoma. In the latter, larger nerve trunks are generally involved; terminal duct adenocarcinoma seems to chiefly affect small nerve twigs. The epithelial and myoepithelial components of the lesion are scattered in a stroma that may be hyalinized or mucohyalinized with an overall basophilic hue to the background. Striking is the absence both of necrosis and of significant numbers of mitoses.

Treatment and Prognosis. The indolent nature of this disease as well as its low level of mitotic activity mandates conservative surgical excision. To date, radiotherapy has not been utilized frequently enough to define its role in the treatment of terminal duct carcinoma. Perineural invasion in the pattern associated with this malignancy does not appear to affect prognosis. In the rare cases in which cervical lymph node involvement is noted, appropriate surgical dissection is indicated.

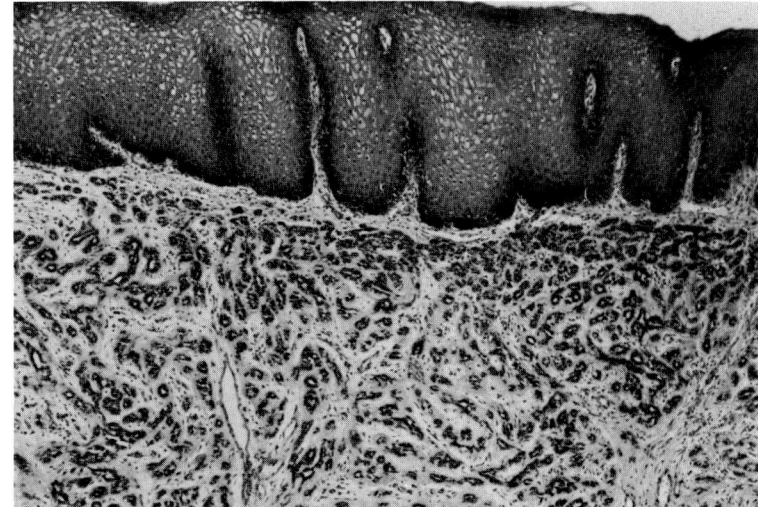

Figure 8–56. Terminal duct carcinoma in oral mucous membrane.

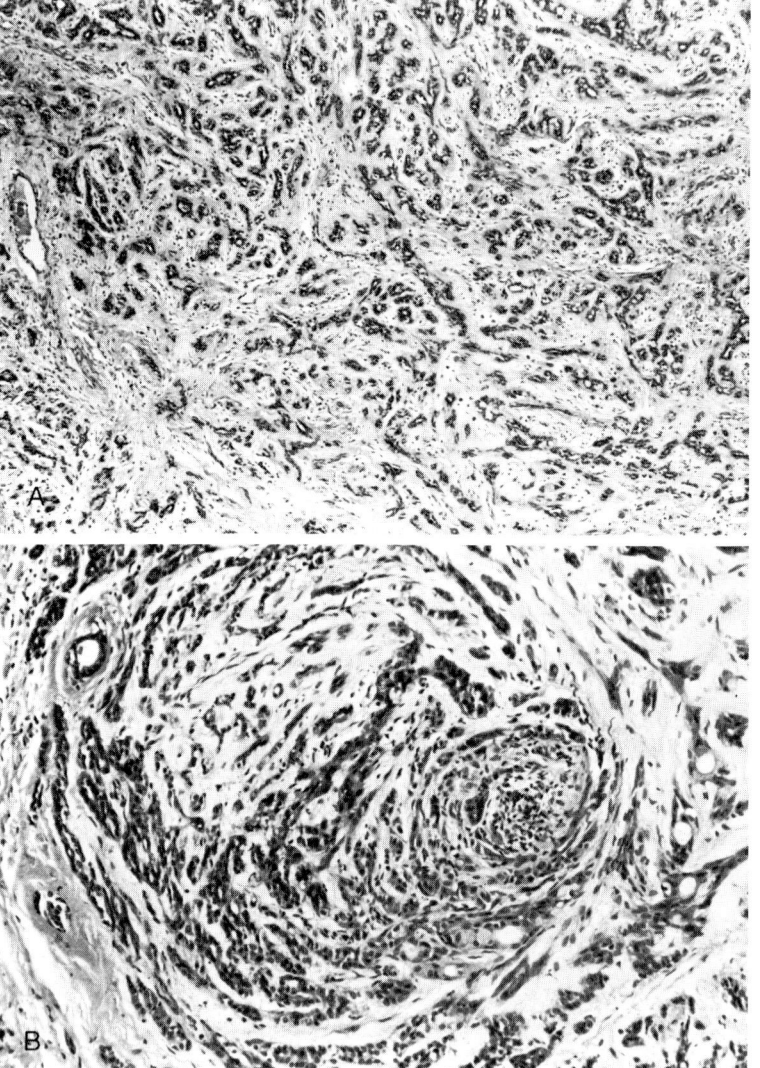

Figure 8–57. *A* and *B*, Terminal duct carcinoma.

The prognosis of this low-grade malignancy is generally good, although long-term follow-up should be part of patient management.

Salivary Duct Carcinoma

Salivary duct carcinoma is another recently recognized lesion that was previously included under the general heading of "adenocarcinoma."

The salivary duct carcinoma is characterized clinically by a distinctive predominance in the parotid gland (over 80% of cases); the submandibular gland accounts for the balance. Nearly 80% of cases have been recorded in males, and the overall peak incidence is in the seventh decade. The lesions arise as firm, painless masses. They are generally brought to the clinician's attention within 1 year of onset.

A striking microscopic resemblance to ductal carcinomas originating in the breast is noted, with architectural features that include papillary cribriform and solid growth patterns along with a desmoplastic stroma and comedo necrosis (Fig. 8–58). Cellular features include an apocrine type appearance with eosinophilic cytoplasm and occasional accumulations of intracytoplasmic mucin. A variable level of nuclear atypia is noted. In general, few mitoses are seen. Most tumors contain infiltrative margins, with neural invasion present in approximately 50% of cases (Fig. 8–59).

Surgical excision is indicated for this lesion, with concomitant neck dissection or post-operative irradiation, or both. The role of chemotherapy is yet to be determined. In cases of advanced disease, combination therapy has not altered prognosis. Large series indicate that over 50% of patients die from their disease within 5 months to 6 years after treatment. Pulmonary and osseous metastases are frequently noted.

Adenocarcinoma

By definition, any malignancy arising from salivary duct epithelium or within salivary glands of epithelial origin is an adenocarcinoma. This term, however, is less commonly used as a specific diagnostic entity, since most classification systems have broken down this complex group of neoplasms into discrete entities. The entities may be defined primarily by structure but also by behavior. Following recognition of terminal duct carcinoma, salivary duct carcinoma, and epimyoepithelial carcinoma, the small remaining group of salivary carcinomas with no specific designation may be categorized as adenocarcinomas. Included in this group are rare examples of undifferentiated carcinoma, neuroendocrine carcinoma, small cell carcinoma, and mucus-producing adenopapillary carcinoma.

The utility of the "not otherwise specified" adenocarcinoma heading relates to the undifferentiated carcinoma. Owing to a near-total lack of differentiation, placement in existing categories becomes impossible. High-grade malignancies, such as salivary duct carcinomas and mucoepidermoid carcinomas, may have similar features but also may have other microscopic elements that permit their diagnosis.

Microscopically, undifferentiated carcinomas vary from solid to trabecular with cell types ranging from spindle to round and small. The small cell carcinoma, although suggesting a neuroectodermal origin, has yet to be shown to possess the appropriate neurosecretory granular component necessary for that diagnosis. Most authorities feel that the small cell carcinoma of salivary gland origin merely represents a variant of anaplastic carcinoma. Since undifferentiated adenocarcinomas are of a high-grade type, a correspondingly poor prognosis is seen, even with radical or combination therapy.

Squamous Cell Carcinoma

Squamous cell carcinoma arising within the salivary glands is a rare event. The submandibular gland is most commonly involved, followed by the parotid. Obstructive sialadenitis (more common in the submandibular gland) has been thought to be a predisposing condition. Most patients tend to be in the seventh decade of life or beyond.

Squamous cell carcinomas of the parotid gland and submandibular glands are generally well to moderately well differentiated with no evidence of mucin production. Metastatic squamous cell carcinoma and high-grade mucoepidermoid carcinoma are usually alternative diagnoses.

Local recurrence and regional lymph node metastasis are common events, and distant metastasis is unusual. Surgery is the treatment of choice. As with most other salivary gland malignancies, ultimate survival relates more to the clinical stage than to histologic differentiation.

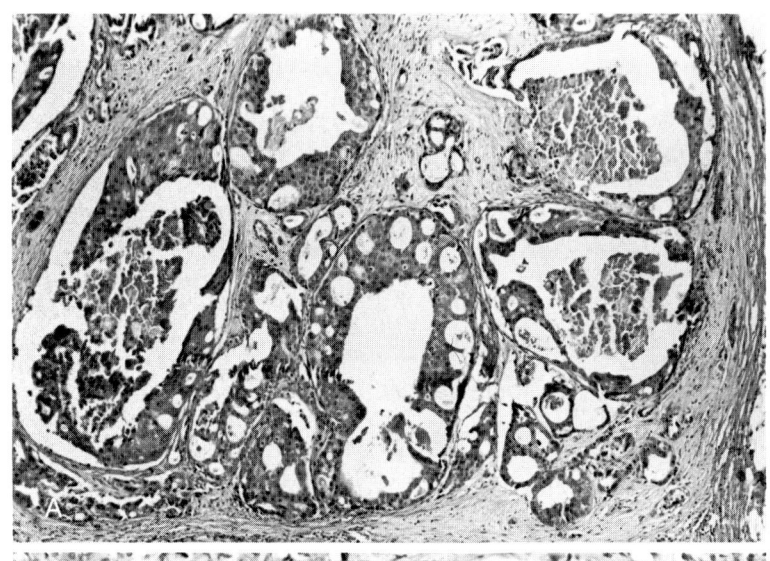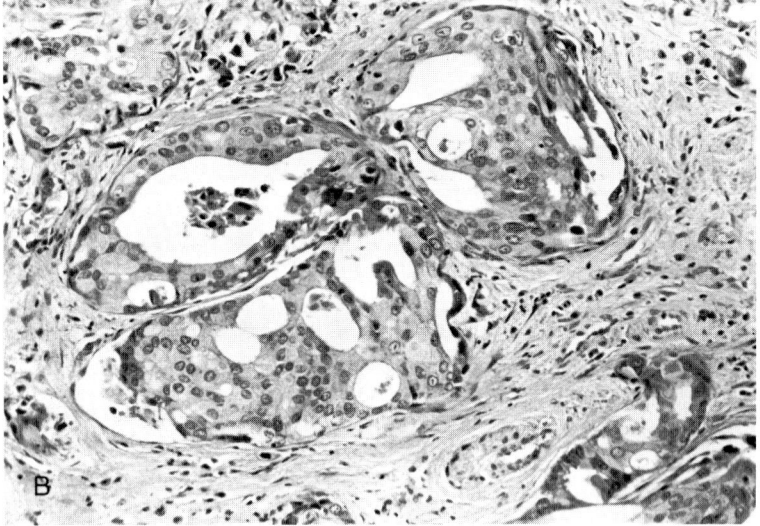

Figure 8–58. *A* and *B*, Salivary duct carcinoma.

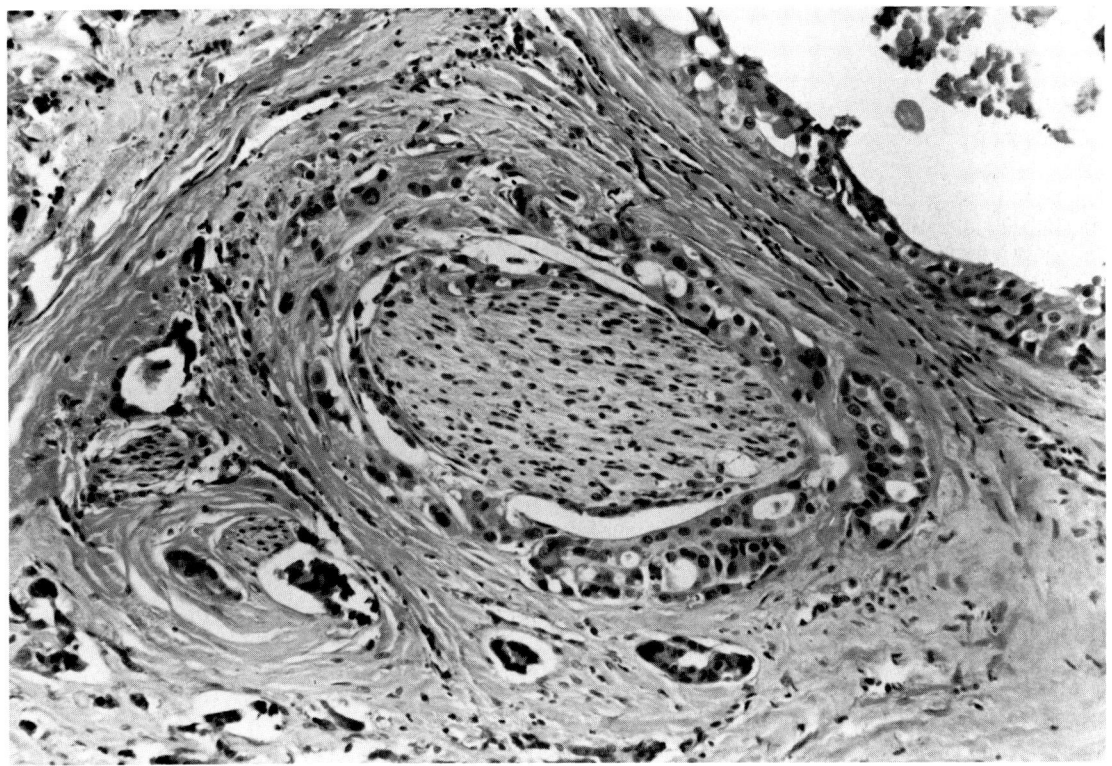
Figure 8–59. Salivary duct carcinoma showing perineural invasion.

Bibliography

Reactive Lesions (Non-infectious)

Abrams AM, Melrose RJ, Howell FV. Necrotizing sialometaplasia—a disease simulating malignancy. Cancer 32:130–135, 1973.

Akker HP, van der Bags RA, Becker AE. Plunging or cervical ranula: review of the literature and report of four cases. J Maxillofac Surg 6:286–293, 1978.

Allard RHB, van der Kwast WAM, van der Waal I. Mucosal antral cysts: review of the literature and report of a radiographic survey. Oral Surg Oral Med Oral Pathol 51:2–9, 1981.

Beumer J, Curtis T, Harrison RE. Radiation therapy of the oral cavity: sequelae and management, part 1. Head Neck Surg 1:301–312, 1979.

Dreizen S, Brown LR, Daley TR, et al. Prevention of xerostomia-related dental caries in irradiated cancer patients. J Dent Res 56:99–104, 1977.

Epstein J, Schubert M. Synergistic effect of sialogogues in management of xerostomia after radiation therapy. Oral Surg Oral Med Oral Pathol 64:179–182, 1987.

Fajardo LF, Berthrong M. Radiation injury in surgical pathology—part III. Salivary glands, pancreas, and skin. Am J Surg Pathol 5:153–178, 1981.

Fechner RE. Necrotizing sialometaplasia. A source of confusion with carcinoma of the palate. Am J Clin Pathol 67:315–317, 1977.

Gardner DG. Pseudocysts and retention cysts of the maxillary sinus. Oral Surg Oral Med Oral Pathol 58:561–567, 1984.

McClatchey KD, Appelblatt NH, Zarbo RJ. Plunging ranula. Oral Surg Oral Med Oral Pathol 57:408–412, 1984.

Natvig K, Larsen TE. Mucocele of the paranasal sinuses. A retrospective clinical and histological study. J Laryngol Otol 92:1075–1082, 1978.

Quick CA, Lowell SH. Ranula and the sublingual salivary glands. Arch Otolaryngol 103:397–400, 1977.

Rothwell BR. Prevention and treatment of the orofacial complications of radiotherapy. J Am Dent Assoc 114:316–322, 1987.

Infectious Conditions

Cohen C, Krutchkoff DJ, Eisenberg E. Systemic sarcoidosis: report of two cases with oral lesions. J Oral Surg 39:613–618, 1981.

DeLuke DM, Sciubba JJ. Oral manifestations of sarcoidosis: report of a case masquerading as a neoplasm. Oral Surg Oral Med Oral Pathol 59:184–188, 1985.

Galili D, Marmary Y. Spontaneous regeneration of parotid gland following juvenile recurrent parotitis. Oral Surg Oral Med Oral Pathol 60:605–607, 1985.

Gronhagen-Riska C, Fyhrquist F, von Willebrand E. Angiotensin I–converting enzyme: a marker of highly differentiated monocytic cells. Ann NY Acad Sci 465:242–249, 1986.

James DG, Williams-Jones W. Immunology of sarcoidosis. Am J Med 72:5–8, 1982.

Lazarus AA. Sarcoidosis. Otolaryngol Clin North Am 15:621–633, 1982.

Marder M, Barr C, Mandel I. Cytomegalovirus presence and salivary composition in acquired immunodeficiency syndrome. Oral Surg Oral Med Oral Pathol 60:372–376, 1985.

Nessan VJ, Jacoway JR. Biopsy of minor salivary glands in the diagnosis of sarcoidosis. N Engl J Med 301:922–928, 1979.

Sharma OP. Diagnosis of sarcoidosis. Arch Intern Med 143:1418–1419, 1983.

Metabolic Conditions

Batsakis JG, McWhirter JD. Non-neoplastic diseases of the salivary glands. Am J Gastroenterol 57:226–247, 1972.

Peinertsen JL, Schaefer EJ, Brewer HB, et al. Sicca-like syndrome in type V hyperlipoproteinemia. Arthritis Rheum 23:114–118, 1980.

Conditions Associated with Immune Defects

Alexander EL, Hirsch TJ, Arnett FC, et al. Ro (SSA) and La (SSB) antibodies in the clinical spectrum of Sjögren's syndrome. J Rheumatol 9:239–246, 1982.

Batsakis JG. The pathology of head and neck tumors: the lymphoepithelial lesion and Sjögren's syndrome. Head Neck Surg 5:150–163, 1982.

Caselitz J, Osborn M, Wustrow J, et al. Immunohistochemical investigations on the epimyoepithelial islands in lymphoepithelial lesions. Lab Invest 55:427–432, 1986.

Daniels TE. Labial salivary gland biopsy in Sjögren's syndrome. Arthritis Rheum 27:147–156, 1984.

Ferlito A, Cattai N. The so-called "benign lymphoepithelial lesions"—part II. Clinical and pathological considerations with regard to evolution. J Laryngol Otol 94:1283–1301, 1980.

Fox PC, van der Ven PF, Sonies BC, et al. Xerostomia evaluation of a symptom with increasing significance. J Am Dent Assoc 110:519–525, 1985.

Fox RI, Howell FV, Bone RC, et al. Primary Sjögren's syndrome: clinical and immunopathologic features. Semin Arthritis Rheum 14:77–105, 1984.

Fox RI, Robinson CA, Curd JG, et al. Sjögren's syndrome: proposed criteria for classification. Arthritis Rheum 29:577–585, 1986.

Reichlin M. Significance of the Ro antigen system. J Clin Immunol 6:339–348, 1986.

Rooney E, Lindsley HB. Sjögren's syndrome—an update. J Kans Med Soc 84:482–485, 1983.

Benign Neoplasms

Batsakis JG, Brannon RB, Sciubba JJ. Monomorphic adenomas of salivary glands: a histologic study of 96 tumors. Clin Otolaryngol 6:129–143, 1981.

Batsakis JG, Regezi JA, Block D. The pathology of salivary gland tumors, part 3. Head Neck Surg 1:260–273, 1979.

Chau MNY, Radden BG. Intraoral salivary gland neoplasms: a retrospective study of 98 cases. J Oral Pathol 15:339–342, 1986.

Dardick I, van Nostrand PAW, Philips MJ. Histogenesis of salivary gland pleomorphic adenoma (mixed tumor) with an evaluation of the role of the myoepithelial cell. Hum Pathol 13:62–75 1982.

Eneroth CM. Salivary gland tumors in the parotid gland, submandibular gland, and the palate region. Cancer 27:1415–1418, 1971.

Eveson JW, Cawson RA. Salivary gland tumors. A review of 2,410 cases with particular reference to histologic types, site, age, and sex distribution. J Pathol 146:51–58, 1985.

Headington JT, Batsakis JG, Beals TF, et al. Membranous basal cell adenoma of parotid gland, dermal cylindromas and trichoepitheliomas. Cancer 39:2460–2469, 1977.

Main JHP, Orr JA, McGurk FM, et al. Salivary gland tumors: review of 643 cases. J Oral Pathol 5:88–102, 1976.

Spiro RH. Salivary neoplasms: overview of a 35-year experience with 2,807 patients. Head Neck Surg 8:177–184, 1986.

Malignant Neoplasms

Aberle AM, Abrams AM, Bowe R, et al. Lobular (polymorphous low-grade) carcinoma of minor salivary glands. Oral Surg Oral Med Oral Pathol 60:387–395, 1985.

Abrams AM, Melrose RJ. Acinic cell tumors of minor salivary gland origin. Oral Surg Oral Med Oral Pathol 46:220–233, 1978.

Batsakis JG. Clear cell tumors of salivary glands. Ann Otol Rhinol Laryngol 89:196–197, 1980.

Batsakis JG, Pinkston GR, Luna MA, et al. Adenocarcinomas of the oral cavity: a clinicopathologic study of terminal duct carcinomas. J Laryngol Otol 97:825–835, 1983.

Batsakis JG, Regezi JA, Repola DA. The pathology of head and neck tumors. Salivary glands, part 2. Head Neck Surg 1:167–180, 1978.

Budd GT, Groppe CW. Adenoid cystic carcinoma of the salivary gland. Sustained complete response to chemotherapy. Cancer 51:589–590, 1983.

Chau MNY, Radden BG. Intraoral salivary gland neoplasms: a retrospective study of 98 cases. J Oral Pathol 15:399–342, 1986.

Chaudhry AP, Leifer C, Cutler LS, et al. Histogenesis of adenoid cystic carcinoma of the salivary glands. Light and electron microscopic study. Cancer 58:72–82, 1986.

Chen SY, Brannon RB, Miller AS, et al. Acinic cell adenocarcinoma of minor salivary glands. Cancer 42:678–681, 1978.

Conley J, Meyers E, Cole R. Analysis of 115 patients with tumors of the submandibular gland. Ann Otol Rhinol Laryngol 81:323–330, 1972.

Corio RL, Sciubba JJ, Brannon RB, et al. Epithelial-myoepithelial carcinoma of intercalated duct origin. Oral Surg Oral Med Oral Pathol 53:280–287, 1982.

Dardick I, George D, Jeans MTD, et al. Ultrastructural morphology and cellular differentiation in acinic cell carcinoma. Oral Surg Oral Med Oral Pathol 63:325–334, 1987.

Ellis GL, Corio RL. Acinic cell adenocarcinoma. A clinicopathologic analysis of 294 cases. Cancer 52:542–549, 1983.

Eneroth CM. Salivary gland tumors in the parotid gland, submandibular gland, and the palate region. Cancer 27:1415–1418, 1971.

Evans HL, Batsakis JG. Polymorphous low-grade adenocarcinomas of minor salivary glands: a study of 14 cases of a distinctive neoplasm. Cancer 53:935–942, 1985.

Eveson JW, Cawson RA. Salivary gland tumors. A review of 2,410 cases with particular reference to histologic types, site, age, and sex discrimination. J Pathol 146:51–58, 1985.

Freedman P, Lumerman H. Lobular carcinoma of intraoral minor salivary gland origin. Report of 12 cases. Oral Surg Oral Med Oral Pathol 56:157–165, 1983.

Frierson HF, Mills SE, Garland TA. Terminal duct carcinoma of minor salivary glands. Am J Clin Pathol 84:8–14, 1985.

Garland TA, Innes DJ, Fechner RE. Salivary duct carcinoma: an analysis of four cases with a review of the literature. Am J Clin Pathol 81:436–441, 1984.

Hickman RE, Cawson RA, Duffy SW. The prognosis of salivary gland tumors. Cancer 54:1620–1624, 1984.

Hui KK, Batsakis JG, Luna MH, et al. Salivary duct adenocarcinoma: a high-grade malignancy. J Laryngol Otol 100:105–114, 1986.

LiVolsi VA, Perzin KH. Malignant mixed tumors arising in salivary glands. I. Carcinomas arising in benign mixed tumors: a clinicopathologic study. Cancer 39:2209–2230 1977.

Luna MA, Batsakis JG, Ordonez NG, et al. Salivary gland adenocarcinomas. A clinicopathologic analysis of three distinctive types. Semin Diagn Pathol 4:117–135, 1987.

Luna MA, Ordonez NG, MacKay B, et al. Salivary epithelial-myoepithelial carcinoma of intercalated ducts: a clinical, electron microscopic, and immunocytochemical study. Oral Surg Oral Med Oral Pathol 59:482–490, 1985.

Main JHP, Orr JA, McGurk FM, et al. Salivary gland tumors: review of 643 cases. J Oral Pathol 5:88–102, 1976.

Nagao K, Matsuzaki O, Saiga H, et al. Histologic studies on carcinoma in pleomorphic adenoma of the parotid gland. Cancer 48:113–121, 1981.

Nascimento AG, Amaral ALP, Prado ALF, et al. Adenoid cystic carcinoma of salivary glands. A study of 61 cases with clinicopathologic correlation. Cancer 57:312–319, 1986.

Perzin KH, Gullane P, Clairmont AC. Adenoid cystic carcinomas arising in salivary glands. A correlation of histologic features and clinical course. Cancer 42:265–282, 1978.

Ranko RM, Mignona F. Cancer of the sublingual gland. Am J Surg 118:790–795, 1969.

Spiro RH. Salivary neoplasms: overview of a 35-year experience with 2,807 patients. Head Neck Surg 8:177–184, 1986.

Spiro RH, Huvos AG, Berk R, Strong EW. Mucoepidermoid carcinoma of salivary gland origin. A clinicopathologic study of 367 cases. Am J Surg 136:461–468, 1978.

Spiro RH, Huvos AG, Strong EW. Cancer of the parotid gland. A clinicopathologic study of 288 primary cases. Am J Surg 130:452–459, 1975.

Spiro RH, Huvos AG, Strong EW. Malignant mixed tumor of salivary origin. A clinicopathologic study of 196 cases. Cancer 39:388–396, 1977.

Spiro RH, Koss LG, Hajdu SI, et al. Tumors of minor salivary gland origin. A clinicopathologic study of 492 cases. Cancer 31:117–129, 1973.

Stephen J, Batsakis JG, Luna MA, et al. True malignant mixed tumors (carcinosarcoma) of salivary glands. Oral Surg Oral Med Oral Pathol 61:597–602, 1986.

Szanto PA, Luna MA, Tortoledo ME, et al. Histologic grading of adenoid cystic carcinoma of the salivary glands. Cancer 54:1062–1069, 1984.

Chapter 9

Lymphoid Lesions

REACTIVE LESIONS
Lymphoid Hyperplasia
Angiolymphoid Hyperplasia with
  Eosinophilia (ALHE)
DEVELOPMENTAL LESIONS
Lymphoepithelial Cyst
NEOPLASMS
Lymphoma
  Hodgkin's Lymphoma
  Non-Hodgkin's Lymphoma
Myeloma/Plasmacytoma

REACTIVE LESIONS

In assessing the overall group of lymphoid lesions of the oral cavity, a wide array of diagnostic entities must be considered. In this section, three primary groupings—reactive, developmental, and neoplastic—will be considered. Use of the term "lymphoid" is less precise than "lymphocytic," but it does permit integration of several new entities into the discussion. Also important in the discussion of any lymphoid lesion involving the oral cavity and its adjacent areas is the fact that many such lesions, especially those arising in lymph nodes, are capable of simulating malignancy, although this will not always be the case.

Lymphoid Hyperplasia

It may be difficult to distinguish reactive from neoplastic lymphoid proliferations, both clinically and microscopically. When these lesions occur in unusual sites such as the peritonsillar area, the palatal region, and lymph node tissue within the cheek, diagnosis is more difficult. Within salivary glands, lymphoproliferation may also occur, usually associated with involvement of ductal structures. Concomitant disturbances of intraductal and interstitial architecture make diagnosis challenging in this tissue as well. Critical to a diagnosis of lymphoid lesions are the pattern of involvement within the affected site and the cytologic detail of the proliferative elements.

Prior to discussion of various entities involving lymph node or lymphoid tissue, the location of lymphoid aggregates normally present within the oral cavity will be considered briefly. Normal sites include the posterolateral portion of the tongue, mesially anterior to the palatoglossus muscle. The aggregations of lymphoid tissue within this area are also known as foliate papillae. Tissues in this area have also been designated as lingual tonsil. They may be distinguished from other lymphoid tissues by deep crypts lined by stratified squamous epithelium. Foliate papillae occasionally become inflamed or irritated, with associated enlargement and tenderness. In such instances, patients often become symptomatic. Upon examination, these areas are enlarged and somewhat lobular in outline with an intact overlying mucosa. Prominent superficial vascular elements may be evident. In the rare instances in which such lesions are removed for diagnostic purposes, the chief finding is reactive hyperplasia with enlargement of germinal centers and hyperplasia of interfollicular and medullary zones. Occasional plasma cells may be noted as well. Within the enlarged germinal centers, mitotic activity and macrophages containing cellular debris may be seen. In addition to the foliate papillae, other zones where lymphoid tissue is found include the anterior floor of the mouth on either side of the lingual frenum, the anterior tonsillar pillar, and the posterior portion of the soft palate. Since lymphoid tissues are not always found in these areas, they are usually regarded as ectopic. The term "oral tonsil" also refers to this tissue, especially when it is hyperplastic. Microscopy of lymphoid tissue for all such areas is similar.

From a clinical perspective, reactive lymphoid hyperplasia (oral tonsil) has been shown to have a distinct male predominance, with a significant incidence noted within the second and third decades. In one study, a mean of 23 years was found. The lesions range from 1 to 15 mm in diameter and may last up to 2 years.

The *buccal* or *facial lymph node* is often the site of a reactive hyperplastic process. This lesion is characterized as a freely movable submucosal nodule often adjacent to the second premolar and first molar teeth. The cause of the process is unknown, but it may be attributed to non-specific irritation or localized trauma. Occasionally, focal areas of gingivitis or periapical pathology may stimulate or initiate enlargement of this particular lymph node.

Management should be directed toward elimination of the cause of the problem if it can be identified and followed by simple observation.

A recently described condition involving the soft tissues covering the hard palate has been designated *follicular lymphoid hyperplasia*, which must be separated from *lymphoproliferative disease of the palate*. The latter condition is associated with malignancy, whereas the former is a process that presents as and remains reactive in nature.

Immunologically, follicular lymphoid hyperplasia has been characterized as a polyclonal proliferation of lymphocytes and therefore not a neoplastic entity. Of importance is the fact that cases of follicular lymphoid hyperplasia in the palate show great histologic similarity to nodular lymphoma. In the latter condition, however, a single cell type and monoclonality occur along with cytologic atypia.

Histologically, follicular lymphoid hyperplasia of the palate is characterized by irregularly sized, well-demarcated germinal centers with a crisply defined rim or mantle of small, mature lymphocytes (Fig. 9–1). Within the germinal centers, cells in various stages of development may be seen that are characterized as follicular center cell transformation. Mitotic figures are often abundant but are normal and remain restricted to the germinal centers. Occasionally, a "starry-sky" type appearance may be noted secondary to the ingestion of nuclear debris by macrophages. Stromal elements between follicles tend to be well vascularized and contain a population of well-differentiated, mature lymphocytes and scattered plasma cells.

Of importance to a differential diagnosis is the similarity between follicular lymphoid hyperplasia and palatal lymphoproliferative disease and lymphoma. These entities can present as unilateral or bilateral enlargements with an intact surface. On palpation, the lesions may be soft to firm and non-tender. Rarely, if ever, is there underlying bone resorption or alteration. Other clinical entities to be distinguished from follicular lymphoid hyperplasia of the palate include benign lymphoepithelial lesion and salivary gland neoplasia. Management of follicular lymphoid hyperplasia consists of careful periodic follow-up and observation.

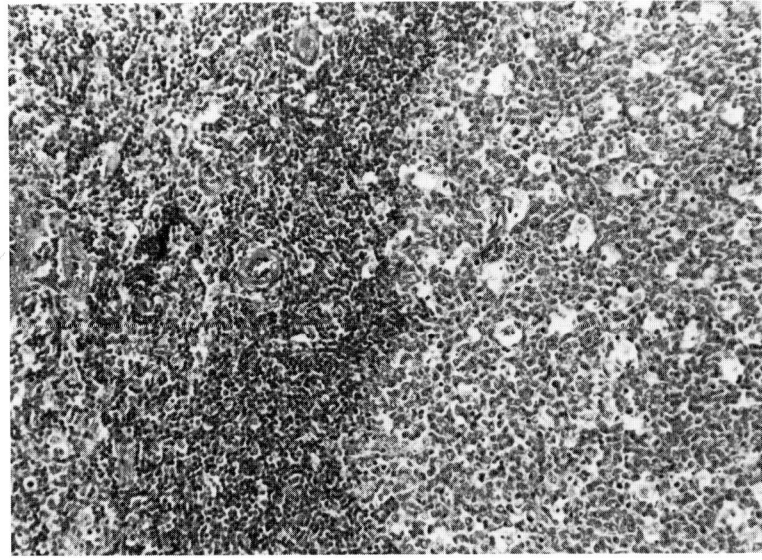

Figure 9–1. Lymphoid hyperplasia. Note germinal center (right) with numerous light-staining macrophages.

Angiolymphoid Hyperplasia with Eosinophilia (ALHE)

This condition was first described in 1948 as a nodular subcutaneous benign disease in young men. Later, however, cases with the same clinical and histologic features were reported to occur in the oral cavity. In addition to nodular aggregates of lymphocytes and eosinophils, regional lymphadenopathy and blood eosinophilia are noted. Soon after the original description, similar findings were noted under the headings of Kimura's disease, eosinophilic granuloma of soft tissue, and eosinophilic lymphofolliculosis. Because Kimura's disease was originally described as having a distinct male predilection and as occurring in older individuals without the associated regional lymphadenopathy, some clinicians believe that the two conditions represent different entities. Some histologic differences have also been described, adding to the confusion over the splitting of ALHE into two separate but related entities.

Etiology. Because a proliferating vascular component along with an intensive inflammatory infiltrate tends to dominate the microscopic picture of ALHE, a reactive etiology has been suggested. Studies demonstrating a marked increase in serum IgE levels as well as deposition of IgE within the lymphoid follicles in typical cases further suggested that the immune system may be primarily involved. Also demonstrated has been the presence of anti–*Candida albicans* antibody within the lesions and improvement after hyposensitization to this allergen.

Other investigators have suggested that ALHE falls along a spectrum of benign vascular lesions and have designated this as *histiocytoid hemangioma*. Support for this concept has been seen in intraoral cases in which there is arterial involvement suggesting aneurysm formation and subsequent capillary proliferation from the involved vessel(s). Inflammatory infiltration over time also dominates the histologic picture.

Clinical Features. When considering all cases of ALHE, oral mucous membrane involvement is rare. When intraoral cases are included, however, this predominance is less clear-cut. Within this context, the labial mucosa is the oral site most commonly involved. In Asians, there is a distinct male predominance. There is a wide age range from 7 to 79 years and a mean age of 35 years. The head and neck area predominates, accounting for 86% of all cases. Lesions generally are solitary, with a mean size of 1.7 cm reported. Eosinophilia greater than 4% has been noted in 60% of the cases in which peripheral blood counts have been included. The clinical course is characterized by the presence of a painless, mobile, submucosal nodule that enlarges gradually. Multiple lesions have been reported in over 40% of cases.

Histopathology. Lesions are circumscribed and usually are grossly separable from surrounding tissue. A nodular mass of hyperplastic lymphoid tissue with well-developed lymphoid follicles containing germinal centers may be seen. Proliferating capillaries with plump endothelial cells are found in a dense, patchy infiltrate of lymphocytes, with eosinophils and fewer numbers of macrophages noted as well. Toward the periphery, this infiltrate may extend into surrounding soft tissue. Small arteries may be involved. Arterial intimal proliferation and disruption of the internal elastic lamina may be seen. Early lesions, or those in an active growth phase, may be dominated by a vascular element; older or quiescent lesions may contain a larger percentage of inflammatory cells.

Differential Diagnosis. When it involves the labial mucosa, ALHE's characteristic nodule may be indistinguishable from a minor salivary gland neoplasm or a mucus retention cyst or mucocele. Other benign soft tissue neoplasms, such as lipoma and schwannoma, might be included in the differential diagnosis.

Because of the presence of eosinophils within tissue, microscopic differential diagnosis should include eosinophilic granuloma and traumatic eosinophilic granuloma with stromal eosinophilia.

Treatment. Excision is the treatment of choice. Intralesional steroid injections have also been used with variable results. Recurrences are occasionally seen. The presence of blood or peripheral eosinophilia has generally been reported with multiple or recurrent lesions.

DEVELOPMENTAL LESIONS

Lymphoepithelial Cyst

The lymphoepithelial cyst arising within the oral cavity is an uncommon lesion; it is found much more frequently in major salivary glands. This entity is thought to arise from an entrapment of oral epithelium within lymph nodes or lymphoid tissue during development. Subsequent epithelial proliferation results in a clinically evident mass.

The oral lymphoepithelial cyst (see also ectopic lymphoid tissue in Chapter 3) presents as an asymptomatic mucosal elevation that is well defined and yellowish-pink in color. The site most commonly affected is the floor of the mouth, where approximately 50% of cases are found. The ventral and posterolateral portions of the tongue constitute an additional 40% of the cases; the balance is shared among the soft palate, mucobuccal fold, and anterior faucial pillars. A wide age range is noted from adolescence to the seventh decade. The gender distribution is essentially equal. Except for the small central cystic space, these lesions are identical to ectopic lymphoid aggregates.

Histopathology. The lymphoepithelial cyst is lined by stratified squamous epithelium that is often parakeratotic. There may be focal areas of pseudostratified columnar cells or mucous cells. The epithelial lining is surrounded by a discrete, well-circumscribed lymphoid component, often with germinal center formation and a sharply defined zone of mantle lymphocytes. Occasionally, continuity of the cyst lining with the surface oral epithelium may be noted.

Differential Diagnosis. In the anterior floor of the mouth, a sialolith may be similar in appearance to a lymphoepithelial cyst. However, a history of pain and swelling would be expected with a salivary duct stone. Developmental anomalies such as teratoma or dermoid cyst, benign mesenchymal neoplasms, and salivary gland tumors might also be considered in a differential diagnosis for submucosal soft tissue mass.

Treatment. Conservative excisional biopsy is generally used for definitive diagnosis as well as for treatment. Recurrence is not expected.

NEOPLASMS

Lymphoma

Lymphomas arising within the oral cavity account for less than 5% of oral malignancies. In the head and neck, lymphomas may be seen within regional lymph nodes and within extranodal lymphoid sites in areas known as the gut-associated lymphoid tissue, which extend from the oral cavity to the anal region. Within the oral cavity, the gut-associated lymphoid tissue is chiefly represented as Waldeyer's ring; elsewhere within the oral cavity it is unencapsulated lymphoid tissue within the base of the tongue and soft palate.

Lymphoid tumors often present difficulty in microscopic interpretation, resulting in the proliferation of many histologic classifications. Lymphomas basically are derived from lymphocytes of bursal or thymic lineage; they may rarely be of macrophage origin. Some schemes of categorization of cells composing the various lymphomas have taken into account immunologic characteristics of neoplastic cells. As a consequence, several such classifications have been suggested that include new terminology to reflect biologic as well as morphologic features. Regardless of which classification scheme is employed, reproducibility, accuracy, and clinical significance are of greatest importance. A fundamental aim is also to separate lymphomas into two groups: those of Hodgkin's type and those considered non-Hodgkin's lymphomas.

Hodgkin's Lymphoma

Although Hodgkin's disease involving the oral cavity is considered a rarity, there are numerous cases in which this disease has appeared in the soft tissues as well as in the mandible and maxilla. On occasion, the oral manifestations may represent the initial and only site of involvement; in other cases, associated cervical lymphadenopathy or more widespread Hodgkin's disease may be noted concurrently.

Clinical Features. Generally, Hodgkin's disease is found across a wide age spectrum, with clustering of patients within the 15- to 35-year-old group and a second cluster beyond 55 years. There is a slight male predilection. Clinically, Hodgkin's disease is characterized by painless enlargement of lymph nodes or extranodal lymphoid tissue. Within the oral cavity, concomitant tonsillar enlargement, usually unilateral, may be seen in the early phases. When extranodal sites are involved, submucosal swellings may be seen, sometimes with mucosal ulceration or erosion of underlying bone. Subsequent to microscopic diagnosis, clinical staging must be undertaken. This consists of physical examination, laboratory studies, radiographic studies, and laparotomy. Following the staging procedure, a definitive treatment plan is established. Table 9–1 provides details of the Ann Arbor system of clinical staging.

Histopathology. Common to all forms of Hodgkin's disease is the presence of malignant lymphoid cells and non-neoplastic inflammatory cells, including lymphocytes, macrophages, eosinophils, and plasma cells. Of greatest significance is the identification of the

Table 9–1. ANN ARBOR STAGING CLASSIFICATION OF HODGKIN'S DISEASE (MODIFIED)	
Stage I:	Involvement of a single lymph node region. I_e—Involvement of single extralymphatic site.
Stage II:	Involvement of two or more lymph node regions on the same side of the diaphragm. II_e—Involvement of an extralymphatic site or organ and one or more lymph node regions on the same side of the diaphragm.
Stage III:	Regional involvement of lymph nodes on both sides of the diaphragm. III_e—Involvement of localized extralymphatic organ.
Stage IV:	Disseminated involvement of one or more extralymphatic organs or tissues with or without associated lymph node enlargement.

Reed-Sternberg cell, which must be present for the diagnosis of Hodgkin's disease to be established. This cell is characterized by its large size and bilobed nucleus; each lobe contains a large amphophilic or eosinophilic nucleolus (Fig. 9–2). The nuclear chromatin pattern is vesicular and condensed at the periphery. Other Reed-Sternberg cells may be characterized by two nuclei with a prominent nucleolus or by multiple nuclei. Cells similar to Reed-Sternberg cells may be seen in certain viral diseases such as infectious mononucleosis and Burkitt's lymphoma, and in patients with treated lymphocytic lymphoma, chronic lymphocytic leukemia, and some benign immunoblastic proliferations.

The Lukes-Butler histologic classification of Hodgkin's disease that was modified by Rye recognizes four subtypes (Table 9–2): (1) lymphocyte predominance, (2) nodular sclerosis, (3) mixed cellularity, and (4) lymphocyte depletion. The lymphocyte-predominant type has the most favorable prognosis, and the lymphocyte-depletion form carries with it the least favorable prognosis. In the lymphocyte-predominant form, a small mature lymphocyte is the most prevalent cell, but it is mixed with scattered macrophages (Fig. 9–3). The key diagnostic element, the Reed-Sternberg cell, is rare in this form of the disease. Eosinophils and plasma cells are also rare.

The most frequent form of Hodgkin's disease is the nodular-sclerosing type. It is characterized by bands of collagen that originate from the periphery and penetrate into the lymph node, subdividing it into islands of tumor that contain Reed-Sternberg cells (Fig. 9–4).

The mixed-cellularity type of Hodgkin's disease contains a combination of lymphocytes, eosinophils, neutrophils, plasma cells, and macrophages without bands of collagen typical of the nodular-sclerosing form. The mixed-cellularity type of Hodgkin's disease carries the third best prognosis, intermediate between the nodular-sclerosing type and the lymphocyte-depletion form.

In the lymphocyte-depletion form of Hodgkin's disease, the chief microscopic characteristic is that of highly pleomorphic malignant

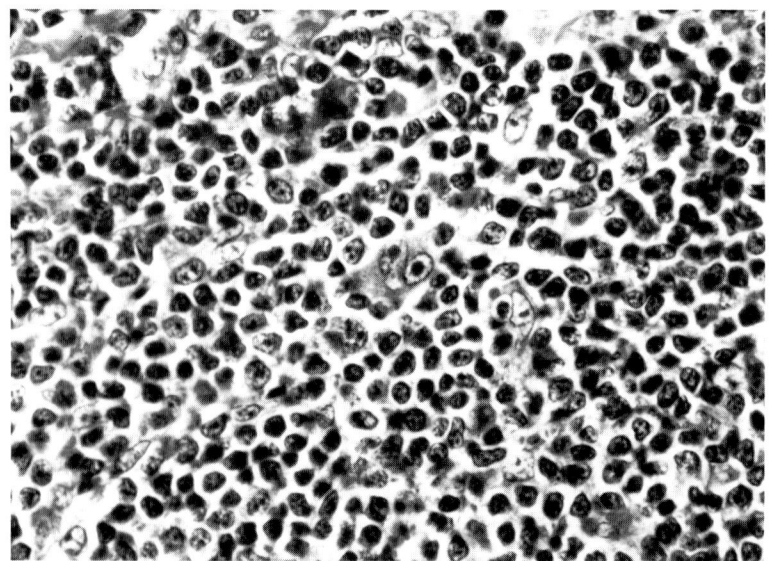

Figure 9–2. Reed-Sternberg cell (center) in Hodgkin's disease.

Table 9-2. HODGKIN'S DISEASE (LUKES-BUTLER HISTOLOGIC CLASSIFICATION [RYE MODIFICATION])

Lymphocyte predominance
Nodular sclerosis
Mixed cellularity
Lymphocyte depletion
Unclassified

reticulum cells. The microscopic depletion of lymphocytes signifies a poor prognosis.

Differential Diagnosis. Presentation as cervical lymphadenopathy should suggest a large array of conditions ranging from inflammatory to neoplastic. Specified entities that can produce lymph node enlargement include tuberculosis, other granulomatous diseases such as sarcoidosis and chlamydial infections, fungal infections, and parasitic diseases such as toxoplasmosis. In the young patient, infectious mononucleosis should be separated from Hodgkin's disease. The young patient on anticonvulsive medication (phenyltoin) may demonstrate lymphadenopathy, which may or may not regress when the drug is discontinued. Finally, a benign cervical lymph node disease of unknown etiology that commonly affects children, termed sinus histiocytosis with massive lymphadenopathy, may require separation from lymphoma.

Treatment and Prognosis. The clinical staging and histologic classification of Hodgkin's disease (and non-Hodgkin's lymphoma) are critical in determining prognosis. Stage and

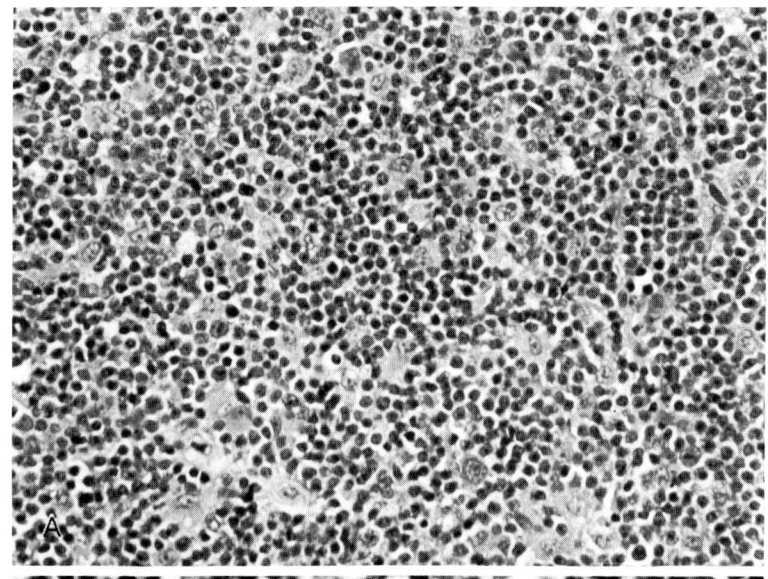
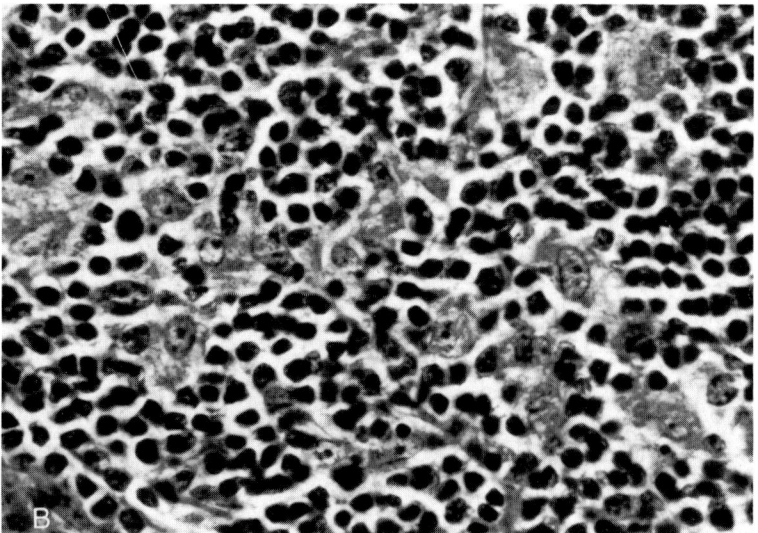

Figure 9-3. *A* and *B*, Hodgkin's disease, lymphocyte predominance.

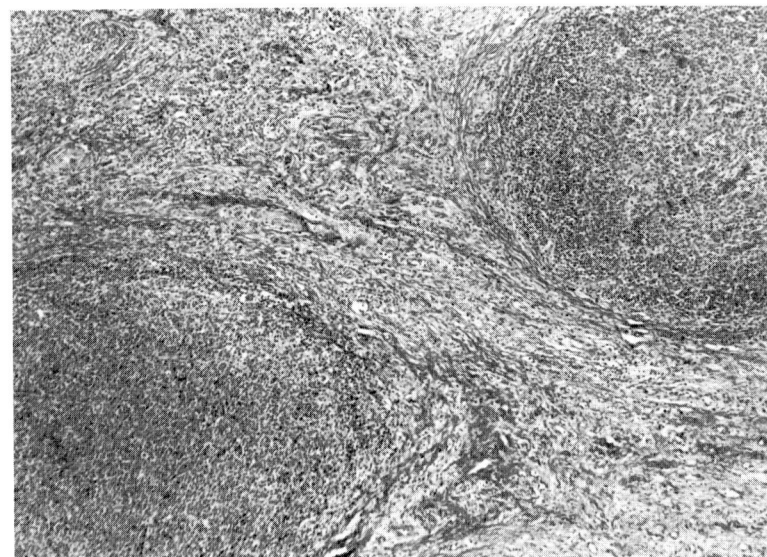

Figure 9–4. Hodgkin's disease, nodular sclerosing type.

classification also dictate appropriate therapy. As already stated, the lymphocyte-predominant form of the disease carries with it the most favorable prognosis, and the lymphocyte-depletion form the worst prognosis. Stage I of the disease has the best prognosis; the disseminated disease in stage IV has the worst. Generally, clinical stage has a greater influence on overall prognosis than does histologic subtype.

Management of patients with Hodgkin's disease consists of external radiation therapy and multiple-agent chemotherapy. What was once a fatal illness with poor survival statistics has become a curable disease. At least half of all patients with Hodgkin's disease are cured, regardless of stage, because of treatment with intensive radiotherapy or chemotherapy, or both.

Non-Hodgkin's Lymphoma

Non-Hodgkin's lymphoma is representative of a group of lymphoid neoplasms that are diverse in history, manner of presentation, response to therapy, and ultimate prognosis. In the head and neck, extranodal presentation is relatively common compared with nodal disease in other areas of the body. Although primary presentation of intraoral non-Hodgkin's lymphoma is uncommon, it is important to be aware of this possibility, since primary intraoral manifestations may represent the start of a progression of involvement of other lymph nodes and reticuloendothelial organs. In general, the oral manifestations of non-Hodgkin's lymphoma occur secondary to a more widespread distribution throughout the body. As with Hodgkin's disease, extranodal presentation occurs at a higher incidence in this region owing to the presence of rich lymphoid deposits such as Waldeyer's ring and other submucosal sites.

Clinical Features. The middle-aged and elderly are most commonly affected by non-Hodgkin's lymphoma. Studies show that males have a slight preponderance over females. In extraoral sites, nodal disease is characterized by gradual focal enlargement which is asymptomatic and which may remain static for a considerable period prior to diagnosis (Fig. 9–5). Without intervention, additional lymph nodes will become involved. The rate of enlargement will depend upon the type of lymphoma and the level of overall differentiation. When primary oral lesions are present, they are characterized by an absence of symptoms and by a relatively soft character, often with overlying ulceration (Figs. 9–6 and 9–7 and Table 9–3).

Table 9–3. ORAL SOFT TISSUE SITES AFFECTED BY NON-HODGKIN'S LYMPHOMA	
Tonsil	55%
Palate	30%
Buccal mucosa	10%
Tongue	2%
Floor of mouth	2%
Retromolar region	2%

Compiled from Eisenbud L et al. Oral Surg 56:151, 1983; and Fierstein JT et al. Laryngoscope 88:582, 1978.

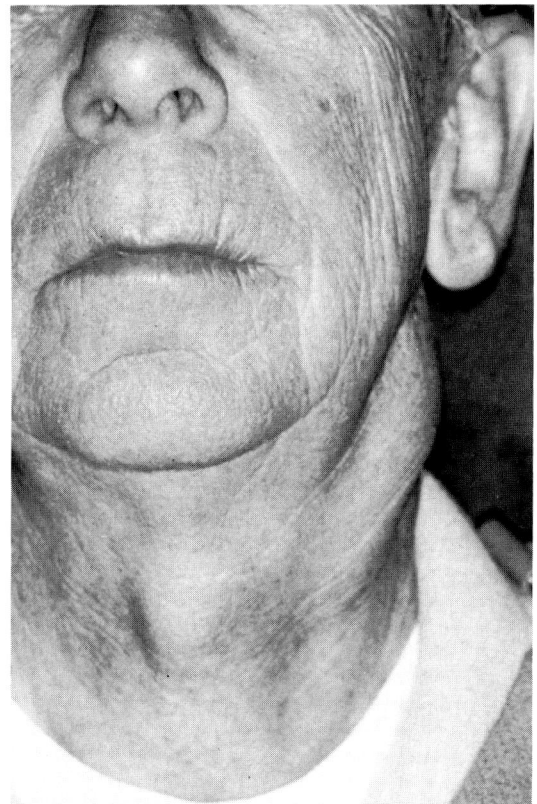

Figure 9–5. Lymphoma (non-Hodgkin's) of cervical lymph nodes.

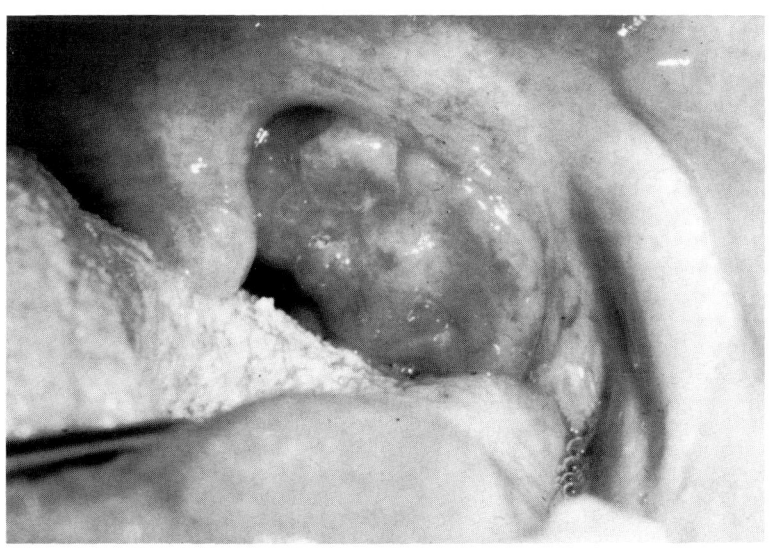

Figure 9–6. Lymphoma (non-Hodgkin's) of left tonsil.

292 LYMPHOID LESIONS

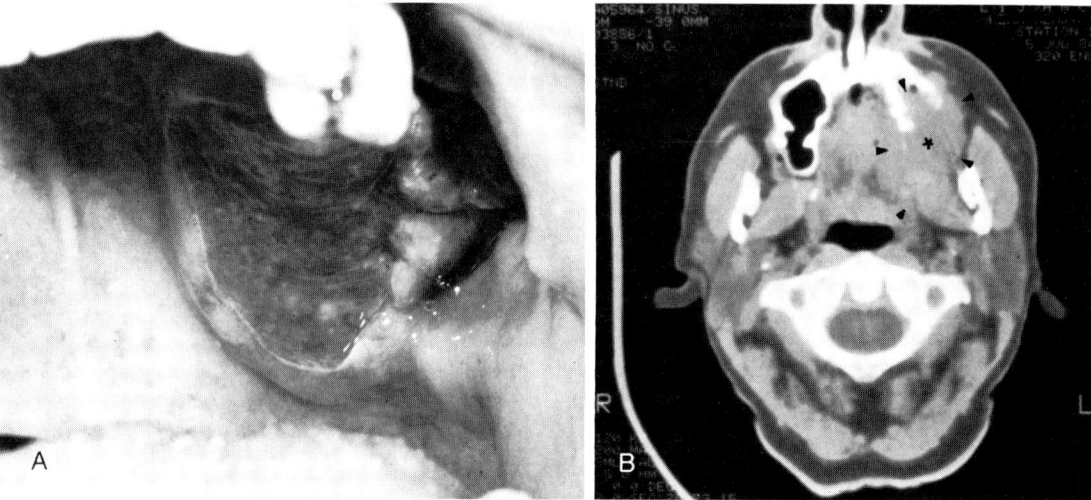

Figure 9–7. *A*, Lymphoma (non-Hodgkin's) of sinus with oral presentation. *B*, Computerized axial tomographic scan showing large destructive mass (*). Lateral, medial, and posterior walls of the maxillary sinus have been destroyed by the tumor.

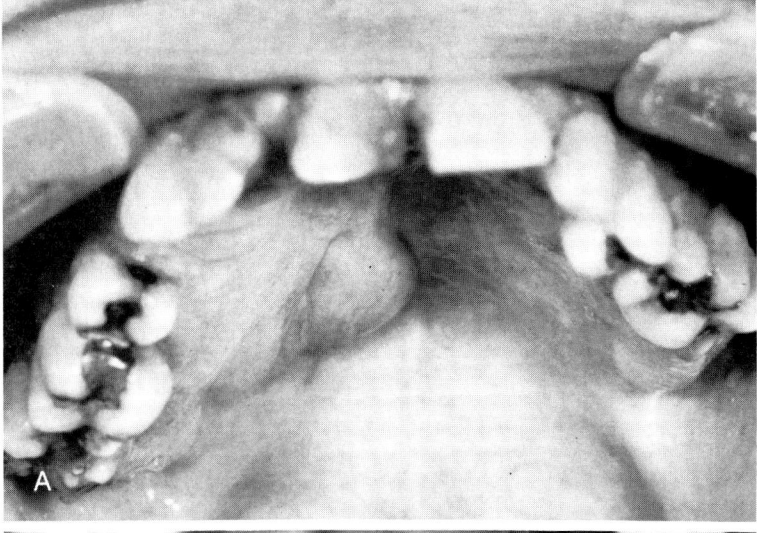

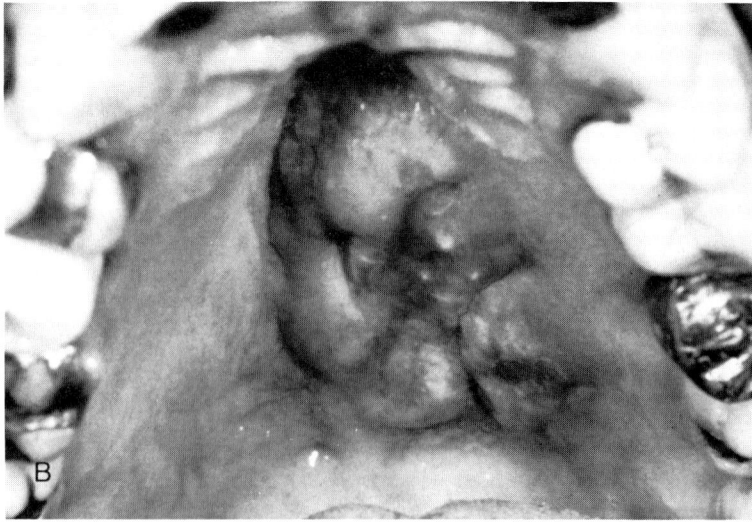

Figure 9–8. *A* and *B*, Lymphomas (non-Hodgkin's) of the hard palate.

If bone is the primary site, alveolar bone loss and tooth mobility are often presenting signs. Swelling, pain, numbness of the lip, and pathologic fracture may also be associated with bone lesions. The entity originally reported as *lymphoproliferative disease of the hard palate* is now considered to represent a bona fide lymphoma (Fig. 9–8). Microscopically, this condition may be difficult to separate from lymphoid hyperplasia (Fig. 9–9).

Subsequent to establishing the diagnosis of lymphoma, a staging procedure similar to that used in Hodgkin's lymphoma is performed. Most treatment centers utilize the so-called Ann Arbor classification, with stage I disease representing involvement of a single lymph node region or a single extralymphatic site. Stage II disease involves two or more lymph node chains; stage III involvement demonstrates positive disease on both sides of the diaphragm. Stage IV correlates with diffuse or disseminated involvement of one or more extralymphatic organs, other than spleen, spine, Waldeyer's ring, or appendix. The involvement of bone marrow or liver likewise indicates a stage IV disease.

Histopathology. For non-Hodgkin's lymphoma, numerous classification schemes have evolved. Those most commonly used include classifications of Lukes and Collins, the World Health Organization, and Rappaport (Table 9–4). Most schemes concern themselves with architectural arrangement of neoplastic cells and cytologic variations from normal.

In general, two basic groups of lymphoma are accepted, nodular (follicular) and diffuse

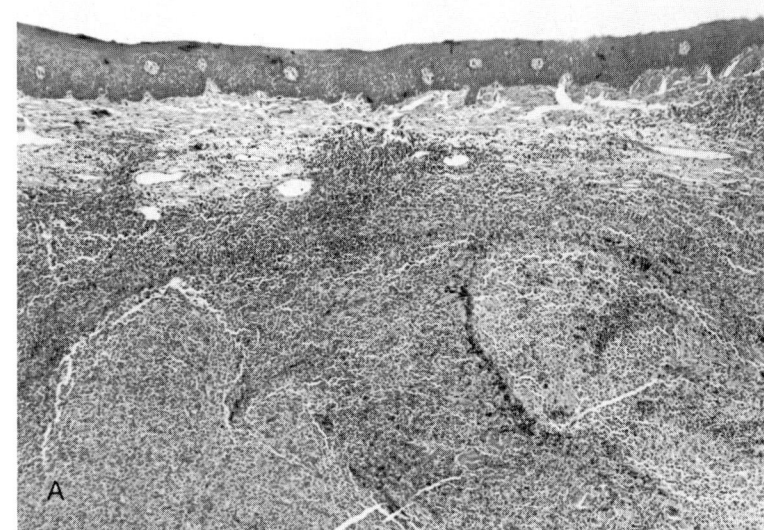
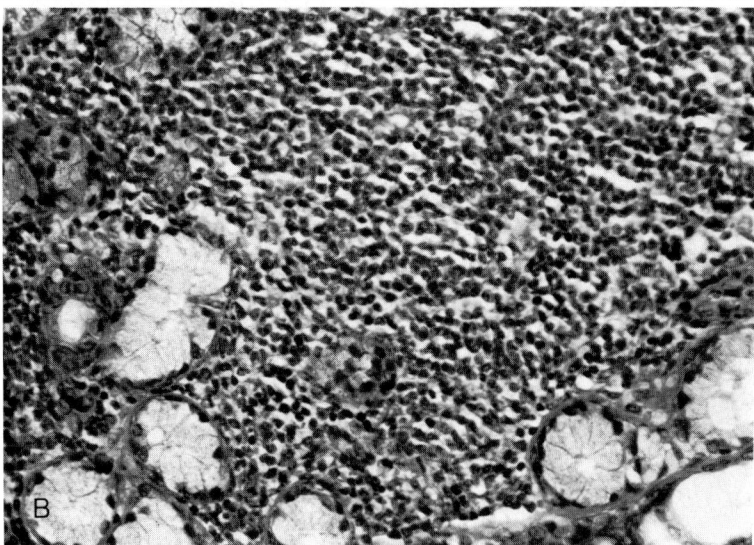

Figure 9–9. *A* and *B*, Lymphoproliferative disease (lymphoma) of the hard palate.

Table 9–4. MICROSCOPIC CLASSIFICATION OF NON-HODGKIN'S LYMPHOMA

Nodular
  Poorly differentiated lymphocytic
  Mixed lymphocytic-"histiocytic"*
  "Histiocytic"
Diffuse
  Well-differentiated lymphocytic
  Poorly differentiated lymphocytic
  "Histiocytic"
  Mixed lymphocytic-"histiocytic"
  Lymphoblastic
  Undifferentiated (includes Burkitt's lymphoma)

*Histiocytes are large (transformed) lymphocytes, as determined from immunologic markers.

Nodular Lymphomas. Nodular lymphomas may be divided into three subtypes based upon cytologic characteristics within the nodules: poorly differentiated lymphocytic, mixed lymphocytic-"histiocytic," and "histiocytic." Common to all subtypes are varying numbers of atypical small lymphoid cells and large lymphoid cells ("histiocytes"). The small cells show scanty cytoplasm and an irregular cleaved or indented nucleus along with coarse condensed chromatin. The large cells are frequently two or three times the diameter of normal lymphocytes, with vesicular nuclei containing one to three nucleoli. Because of the size and nuclear characteristics of the larger cells, they were originally considered histiocytes but more recently have been shown to represent transformed B lymphocytes.

It is important to subdivide nodular lymphomas because of clinical and prognostic considerations. It has been shown that patients with nodular lymphoma, poorly differentiated lymphocytic type, usually present with generalized disease; yet, despite extensive disease, these patients have a relatively favorable prognosis. The least favorable prognosis is associated with the so-called histiocytic or large cell subtype. Despite the fact that these tumors are more often localized at the time of diagnosis, they are most prone to progress from a nodular to a diffuse pattern, which has a significantly poorer prognosis. Immunologic studies have shown through antigenic markers that nodular lymphomas are neoplasms of follicular B lymphocytes, with the majority composed of follicular center cells.

Diffuse Lymphomas. Diffuse lymphomas are a heterogeneous group of tumors, both

forms; the former shows a more favorable prognosis (Figs. 9–10 and 9–11). Nodular lymphomas show malignant cells arranged in a pattern characterized by regular nodules distributed throughout a lymph node or extranodal site. In lymphomas showing a diffuse pattern, abnormal cells are not clustered or aggregated but rather are distributed uniformly throughout the involved lymph node or extranodal site. In either case, the normal architecture of the lymphoid tissue is destroyed. In addition to nodular and diffuse patterns, cytology or predominant cell type within the lesion is of great significance. Several parameters of cell morphology, including nuclear size and configuration and the general heterogeneity of the cellular population, must be evaluated.

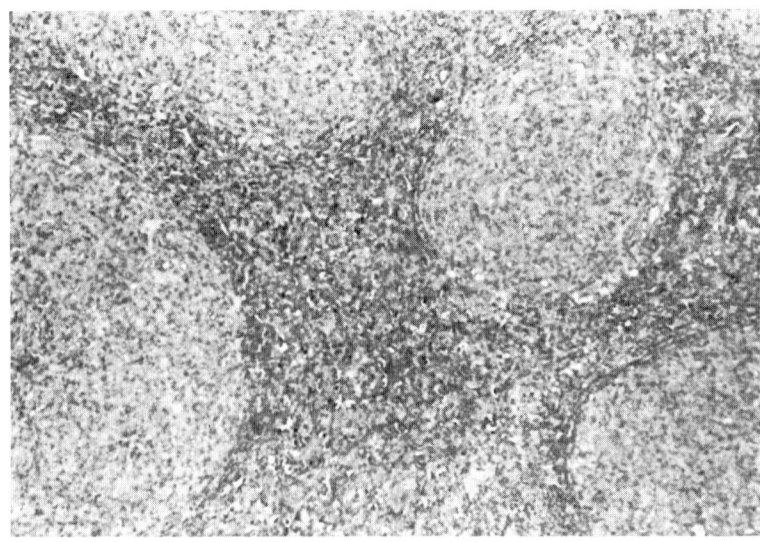

Figure 9–10. Nodular lymphoma.

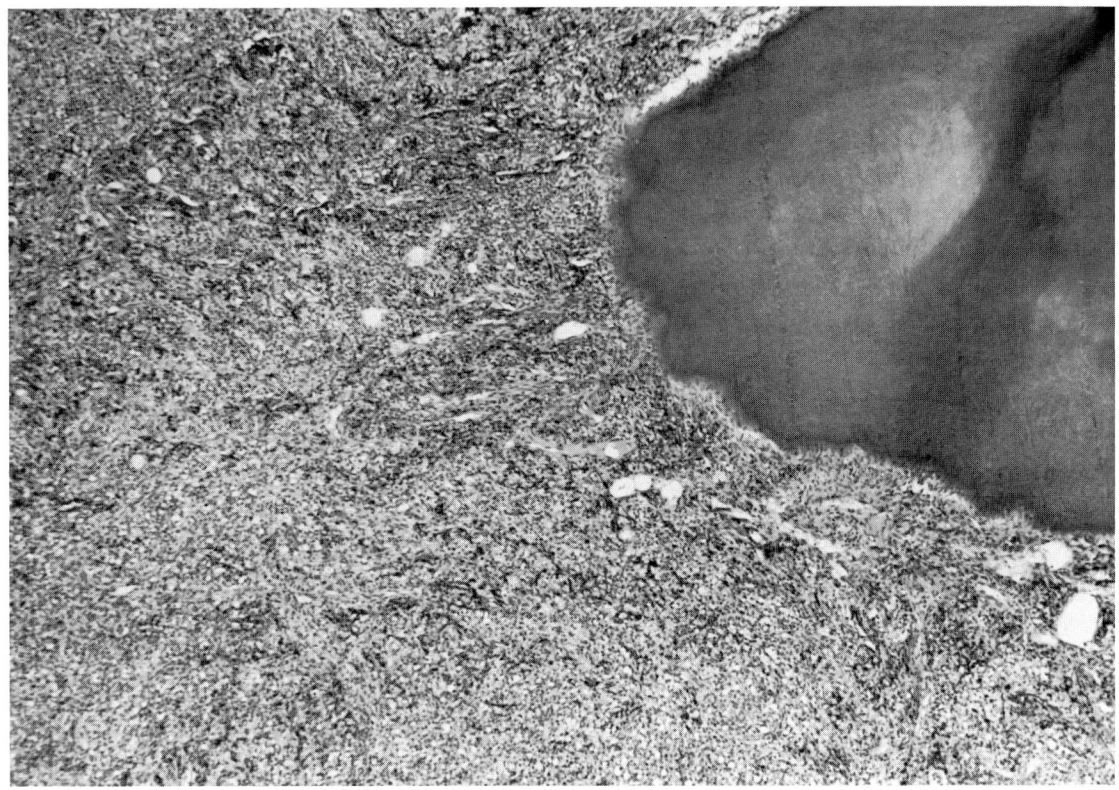

Figure 9–11. Diffuse lymphoma.

morphologically and clinically. Various cell types participate in these neoplasms, which allows subclassification into several groups: lymphocytic (well and poorly differentiated types) (Fig. 9–12), "histiocytic" (large cell) (Fig. 9–13), mixed lymphocytic-"histiocytic," lymphoblastic, and undifferentiated (includes Burkitt's lymphoma).

The "histiocytic" or diffuse large cell lymphoma is the most common type in the head and neck region. As a general rule, the incidence of large cell lymphomas increases with age. The clinical course is usually aggressive, and there is a poor prognosis, although this type frequently presents with disease limited to one side of the diaphragm. Histologically, the neoplastic cell is a large lymphocyte that exhibits considerable variation in nuclear shape and cellular size. Frequently, cells contain two or more nuclei, often with a single large eosinophilic nucleolus. The nuclear chromatin tends to be vesicular, and mitotic figures are often numerous with a high proliferation rate. The presence of macrophages containing cytoplasmic inclusions known as tingible bodies is characteristic.

The frequency with which diffuse large cell lymphomas present in extranodal sites is much greater than that of the nodular counterpart. The latter rarely presents in non-nodal locations outside the gastrointestinal tract. This explains, in part, the predominance of the diffuse large cell type lymphoma in the oral and head and neck regions.

Treatment and Prognosis. The treatment of non-Hodgkin's lymphoma depends upon the outcome of the clinical staging procedure. Although general agreement exists for local radiation therapy in stage I disease, there is wide variation of opinion for the treatment of other stages of lymphoma. Some centers have demonstrated excellent results with radiation only; other institutions have done very well with radiation therapy and multiple-agent chemotherapy. Cumulative relapse-free 5-year survival rates in stage I non-Hodgkin's lymphoma treated with primary radiation have ranged from 50 to 90%. Patients with more advanced disease (stages II, III, and IV) are generally treated initially with multiple-agent chemotherapy; long-term survival has been noted in 37 to 65% of cases in which histologically aggressive or so-called unfavorable lymphomas were diagnosed. In histologically indolent or so-called favorable lymphomas, long-term cures may be difficult to achieve if treatment

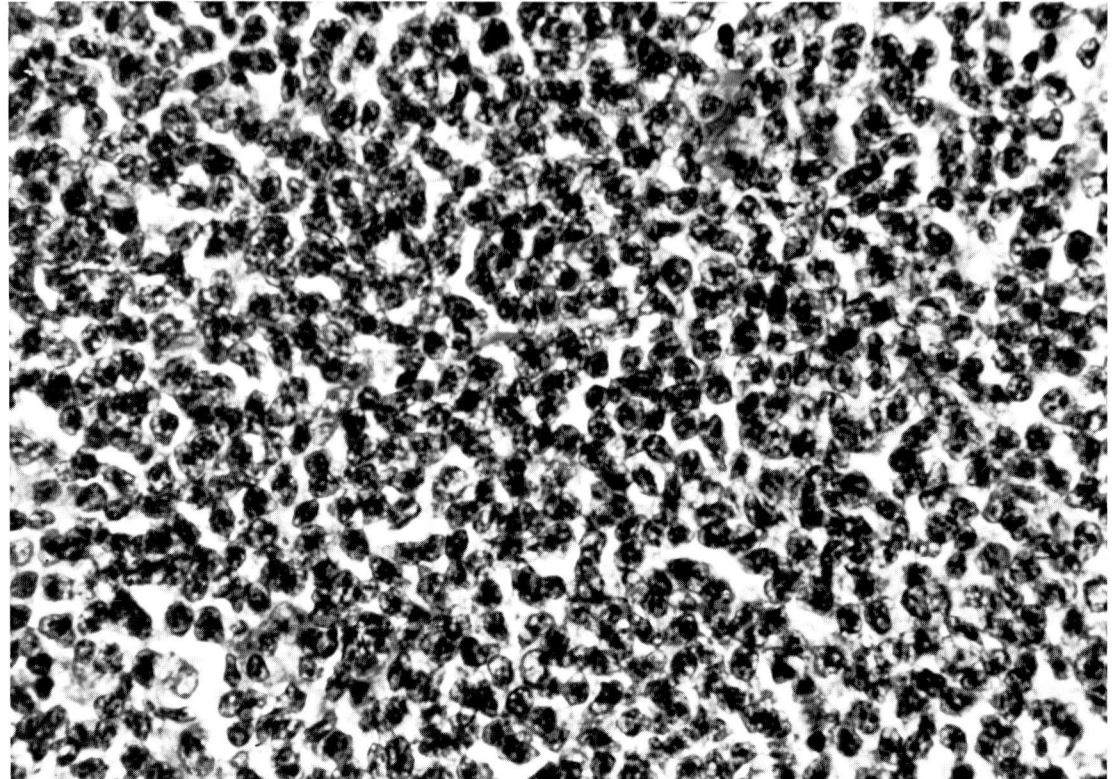

Figure 9–12. Lymphocytic lymphoma.

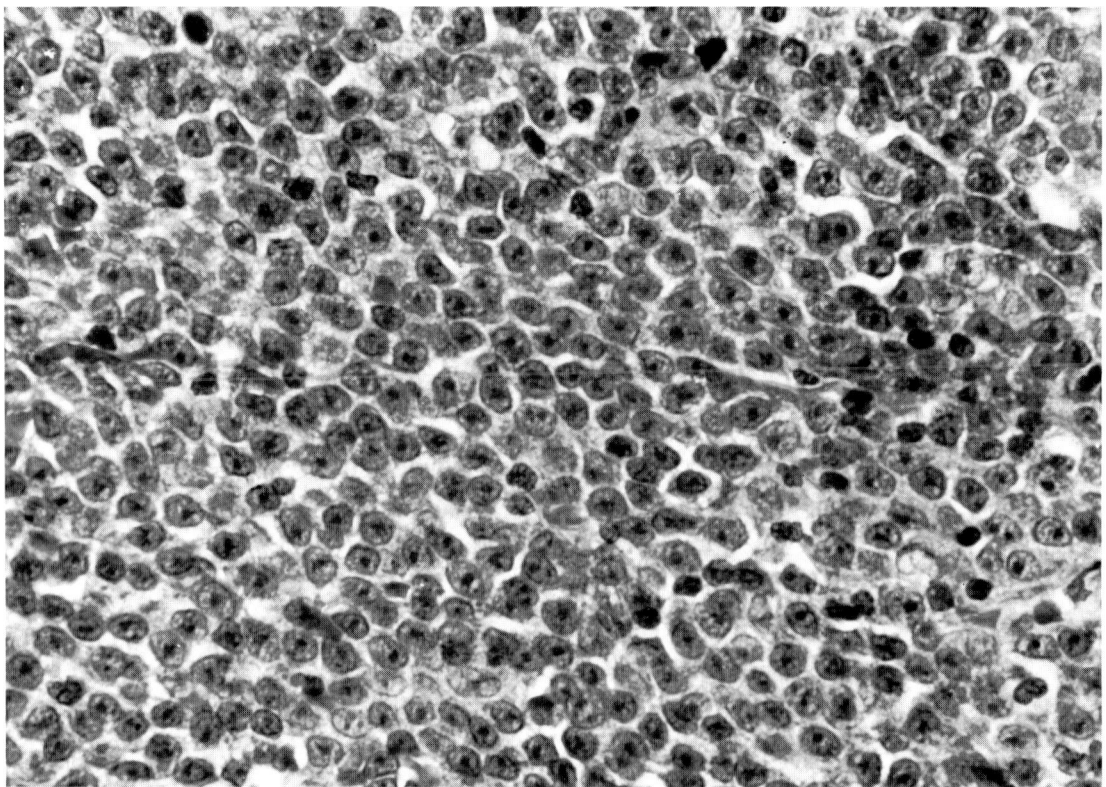

Figure 9–13. "Histiocytic" (large cell) lymphoma.

is initiated when the disease becomes progressive or when systemic symptoms develop.

The use of monoclonal antibodies directed against antigens or within malignant lymphocytes is a newer approach to therapy that shows some promise. The injection of interferons has also shown encouraging results.

Burkitt's Lymphoma

This form of non-Hodgkin's lymphoma is separated from the other forms because it occurs as a distinctive clinical-pathologic entity in children (Figs. 9–14 and 9–15). It was originally described in tropical Africa but is now known to occur elsewhere in the world. In the head and neck, this condition occurs in the mandible and maxilla and is therefore described in Chapter 14.

Myeloma/Plasmacytoma

Myeloma represents a tumor group composed of terminally differentiated B lymphocytes or plasma cells that generally present as multiple bone lesions (multiple myeloma, myelomatosis) (Fig. 9–16). The neoplastic population of plasma cells is termed monoclonal because the cells produce an identical or homogeneous immunoglobulin composed of a single class of heavy and light chains (Fig. 9–17). Plasma cell tumors are subclassified into three types: solitary plasmacytoma of bone (Fig. 9–18), multiple myeloma, and extramedullary (soft tissue) plasmacytoma. The bone lesions are discussed in detail in Chapter 14.

Extramedullary plasmacytomas typically occur in the soft tissue of the upper respiratory tract and, rarely, the oral cavity. They present as lobulated masses in a broad age range that includes children and young adults. Generally, laboratory studies are negative for extramedullary plasmacytoma.

In multiple myeloma, chemotherapy, including use of alkylating agents and prednisone, is a mainstay of treatment, either alone or in combination with local radiation. For solitary plasmacytoma and extramedullary plasmacytoma, radiation or surgery is the standard mode of therapy. Progression of the solitary bone lesions to multiple myeloma is the rule,

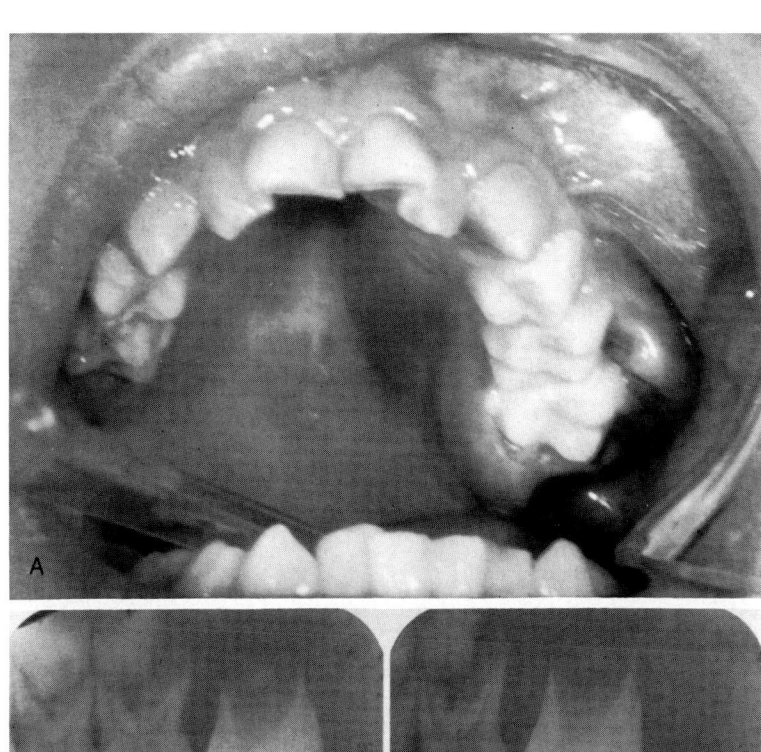

Figure 9–14. *A* and *B*, Burkitt's lymphoma.

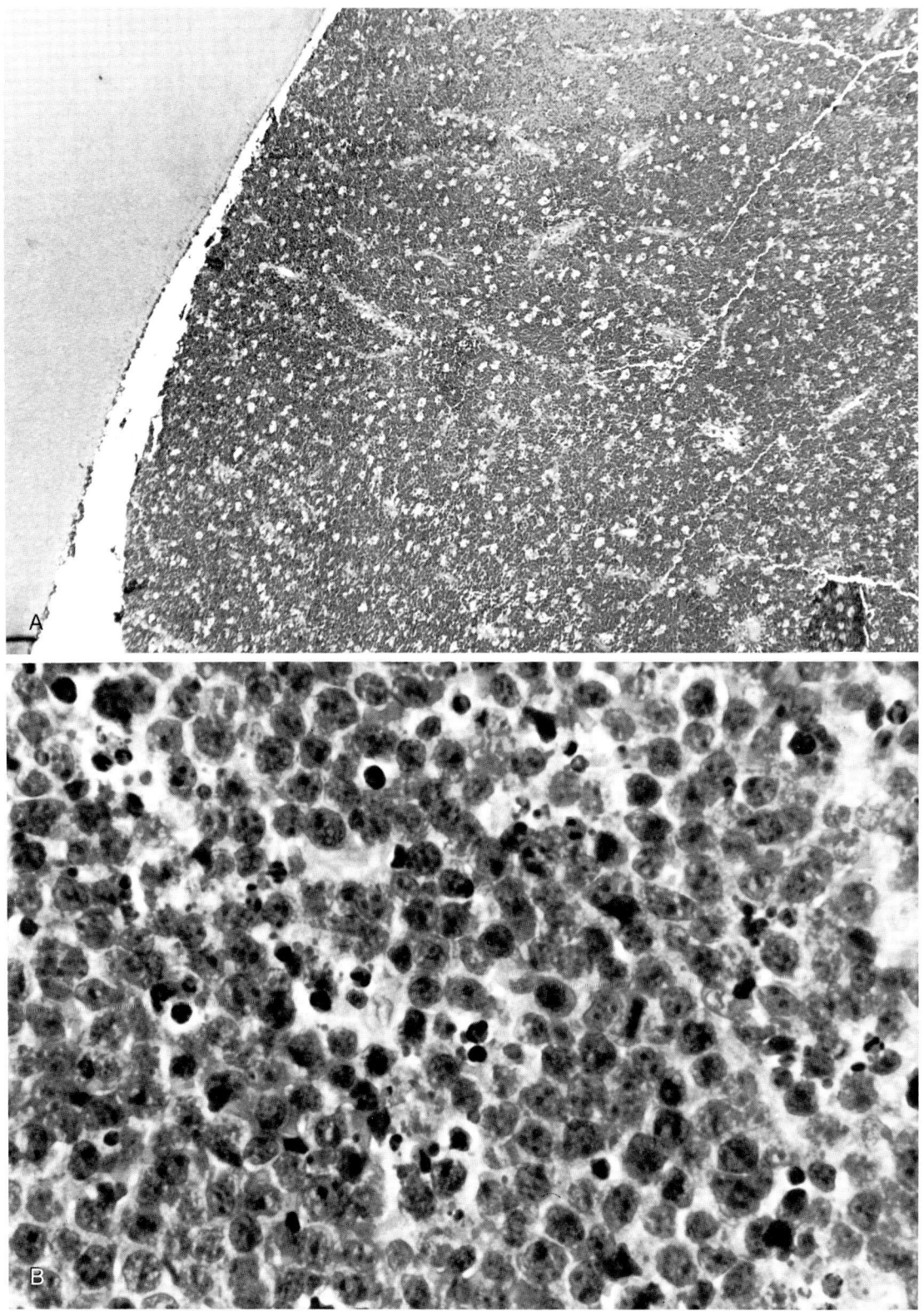

Figure 9–15. *A* and *B*, Burkitt's lymphoma.

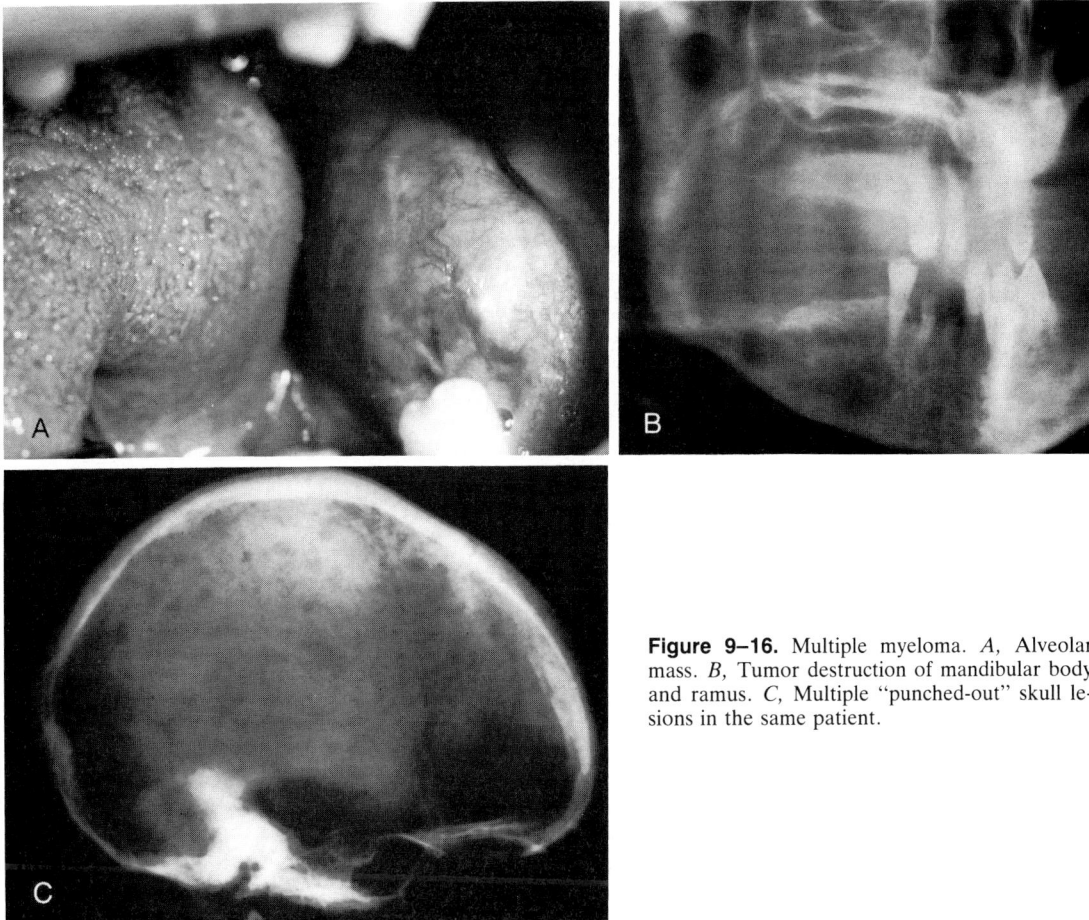

Figure 9–16. Multiple myeloma. *A*, Alveolar mass. *B*, Tumor destruction of mandibular body and ramus. *C*, Multiple "punched-out" skull lesions in the same patient.

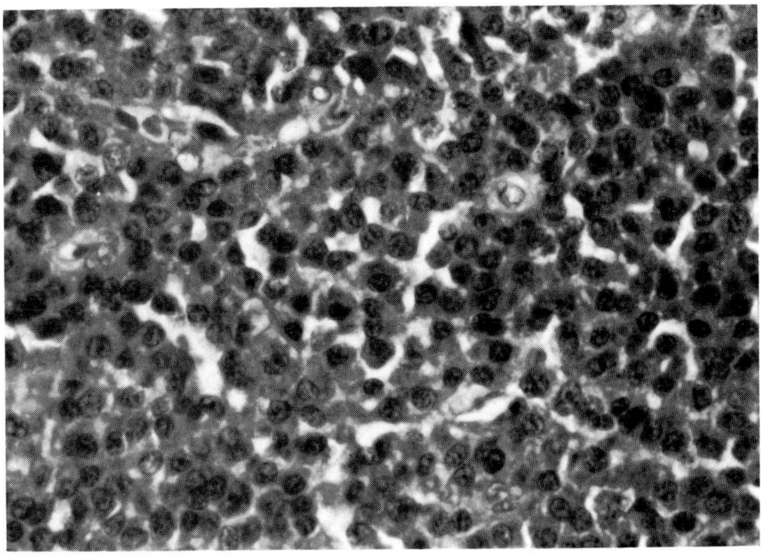

Figure 9–17. Multiple myeloma showing neoplastic plasma cells.

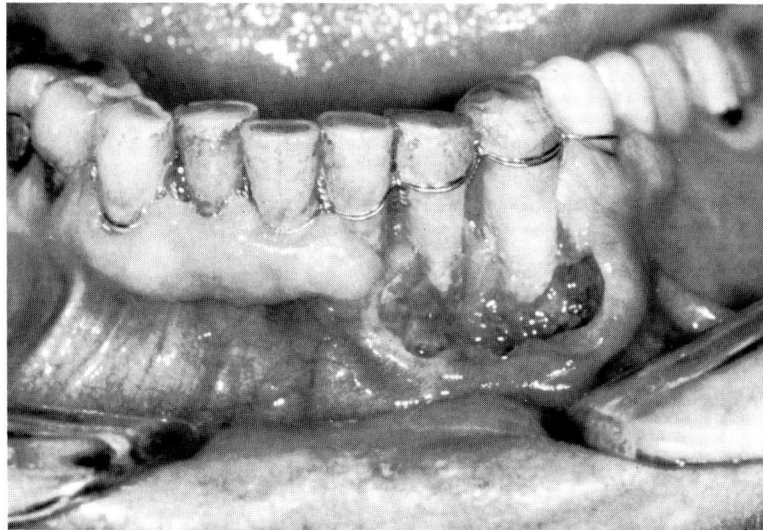

Figure 9–18. Plasmacytoma of mandibular alveolar bone.

and progression of extramedullary lesions to multiple myeloma is the exception.

Bibliography

Reactive Lesions

Bradley G, Main JHP, Birt BD, et al. Benign lymphoid hyperplasia of the palate. J Oral Pathol 16:18–26, 1987.

Buchner A, Silverman S, Wara WM, et al. Angiolymphoid hyperplasia with eosinophilia (Kimura's disease). Oral Surg Oral Med Oral Pathol 49:309–313, 1980.

Elzay RP. Traumatic ulcerative granuloma with stromal eosinophilia (Riga-Fede's disease and traumatic eosinophilic granuloma). Oral Surg Oral Med Oral Pathol 55:497–509, 1983.

Googe P, Harris N, Mihm M. Kimura's disease and angiolymphoid hyperplasia with eosinophilia: two distinct histopathological entities. J Cutan Pathol 14:263–271, 1987.

Harsanyi BL, Ross J, Fee WE Jr. Follicular lymphoid hyperplasia of the hard palate simulating lymphoma. Otolaryngol Head Neck Surg 88:349–356, 1980.

Peters E, Altini M, Kola AH. Oral angiolymphoid hyperplasia with eosinophilia. Oral Surg Oral Med Oral Pathol 61:73–79, 1986.

Rosai J. Angiolymphoid hyperplasia with eosinophilia of the skin. Am J Dermatopathol 4:175–184, 1982.

Tomich CE, Shafer WG. Lymphoproliferative disease of the hard palate: a clinicopathologic entity. Oral Surg 39:754–768, 1975.

Wright JM, Dunsworth AR. Follicular lymphoid hyperplasia of the hard palate: a benign lymphoproliferative process. Oral Surg 55:162–168, 1983.

Developmental Lesions

Knapp MJ. Oral tonsils: location, distribution, and histology. Oral Surg 29:155–161, 1970.

Neoplasms

Batsakis JG. Plasma cell tumors of the head and neck. Ann Otol Rhinol Laryngol 92:311–313, 1983.

Bonadonna G, Lattuada A, Monfardini S, et al. The role of combined radiotherapy in the primary management of non-Hodgkin's lymphomas. In Rosenberg SA, Kaplan HS (eds). *Malignant Lymphomas*. Academic Press, New York, 1982, pp 537–551.

Byrne GE Jr. Rappaport classification of non-Hodgkin's lymphoma: histologic features and clinical significance. Cancer Treat Rep 61:934–935, 1977.

Carbone PR, Rappaport H, Rosenberg SA, et al. Symposium (Ann Arbor): staging in Hodgkin's disease. Cancer Res 31:1707, 1971.

Chabner BA, Johnson RE, Young RC, et al. Sequential surgical and non-surgical staging of non-Hodgkin's lymphoma. Ann Intern Med 85:149–154, 1976.

Eisenbud L, Sciubba JJ, Mir R, et al. Oral presentations in non-Hodgkin's lymphoma: a review of 31 cases. Part I. Data analysis. Oral Surg 56:151–156, 1983.

Fierstein JT, Thawley SE. Lymphoma of the head and neck. Laryngoscope 88:582–593, 1978.

Handlers JP, Howell RE, Abrams AM, et al. Extranodal oral lymphoma. Part I. A morphologic and immunoperoxidase study of 34 cases. Oral Surg Oral Med Oral Pathol 61:362–367, 1986.

Jaffe ES, Shevach EM, Frank MM, et al. Nodular lymphoma: evidence for origin from follicular B lymphocytes. N Engl J Med 290:813–819, 1974.

Kaplan HS. Hodgkin's Disease. 2nd ed. Harvard University Press, Cambridge, Mass, 1980.

Mann RB, Jaffe ES, Berard CW. Malignant lymphomas—a conceptual understanding of morphologic diversity. Am J Pathol 94:105–192, 1979.

Portlock CS. Deferral of initial therapy for advanced indolent lymphomas. Cancer Treat Rep 66:417–419, 1982.

Streuli RA, Ultmann JE. Non-Hodgkin's lymphomas: historical perspective and future prospects. Semin Oncol 7:223–233, 1980.

Chapter 10

Cysts of the Oral Region

ODONTOGENIC CYSTS
Radicular (Periapical) Cyst
Dentigerous Cyst
 Eruption Cyst
Lateral Periodontal Cyst
Gingival Cyst of the Newborn
Odontogenic Keratocyst
Calcifying Odontogenic Cyst (COC)
NON-ODONTOGENIC CYSTS
"Globulomaxillary" Cyst
Nasolabial Cyst
Median Mandibular Cyst
Nasopalatine Canal Cyst
PSEUDOCYSTS
Aneurysmal Bone Cyst
Traumatic (Simple) Bone Cyst
Static Bone Cyst
Focal Osteoporotic Bone Marrow Defect
SOFT TISSUE CYSTS OF THE NECK
Branchial Cyst
Dermoid Cyst
Thyroglossal Tract Cyst

Cysts of the maxilla, mandible, and perioral regions comprise several entities from the standpoint of histogenesis, relative rates of frequency, behavior, and treatment. The overriding majority of cysts in this anatomic region are found within the maxilla and mandible, and they are generally inflammatory in origin. A cyst may be defined as an epithelium-lined pathologic cavity that may contain fluid or cellular debris. Although most cysts in this region are true cysts (they have an epithelial lining), some entities designated as such may not be epithelium-lined and therefore do not satisfy the criterion for a true cyst. The classification system used here accounts for true cysts, with an additional category of non-epithelial cysts designated as pseudocysts because of the absence of the requisite lining.

ODONTOGENIC CYSTS

Radicular (Periapical) Cyst

Radicular (referring to root) cysts are by far the most common of the oral and perioral regions. This cyst has been designated also as the apical periodontal cyst or the periapical cyst. This inflammatory cyst derives its epithelial lining from proliferation of small odontogenic epithelial residues (rests of Malassez) within the periodontal ligament.

Etiology and Pathogenesis. The radicular or periapical cyst develops within a pre-existing *periapical granuloma* (Fig. 10–1). A periapical granuloma represents a discrete focus of chronically inflamed granulation tissue in bone at the apex of a tooth. It develops in response to pulpal death and subsequent tissue necrosis. Stimulation of the epithelial rests relates to the inflammatory process within the periapical granuloma. Cystification occurs as epithelial elements proliferate, ultimately forming a lining.

Remnants of cellular debris are found within the cyst lumen, producing an increase in oncotic or osmotic pressure. The result is fluid transport across the epithelial lining and connective tissue that act as a semipermeable membrane. The direction and rate of transfer is determined by the difference between osmotic and hydrostatic pressures in the cyst fluid and plasma. Fluid ingress into the lumen ultimately results in outward growth of the

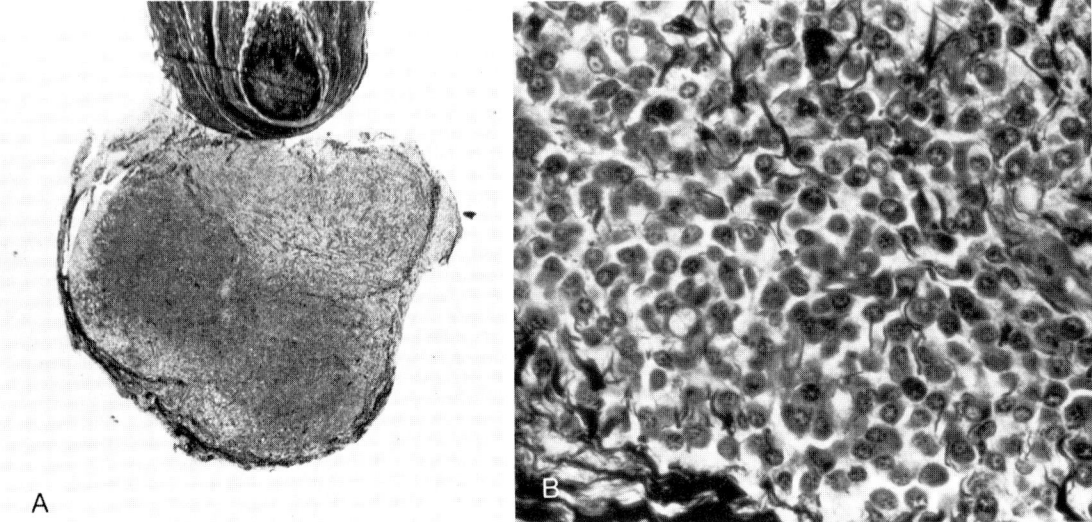

Figure 10–1. *A*, Low-magnification photomicrograph of periapical granuloma. Note root tip at top of photo. *B*, High magnification shows inflammatory cells, mostly plasma cells.

cyst. The outward or centrifugal growth is enhanced by osteoclastic bone resorption. There is also a direct effect on bone by prostaglandins and other bone-resorbing factors from inflammatory cells and cellular elements within the peripheral portion of the lesion.

The fluid present within the cyst lumen contains proteins primarily derived from plasma. A relatively low concentration of non-immunoglobulin proteins indicates an absence of free passage of plasma proteins into cyst fluid. Some immunoglobulins present in cyst fluid are produced locally; others are derived from plasma. The free passage of large plasma proteins is probably related to restricted vascular permeability and a molecular sieve effect produced by soluble collagenous proteins within the cyst capsule. Further accumulation of fluid is encouraged by inadequate lymphatic and venous drainage of the cyst cavity contents.

Clinical Features. Radicular cysts and the related residual cysts (to be described later) form the largest group within the jaw cyst category. They constitute approximately half to three fourths of all cysts in most large series. The age distribution peaks in the third through sixth decades. Of interest is the relative rarity of radicular cysts in the first decade even though caries and non-vital teeth are rather frequent in this age group. A majority of cases have been noted in males. Most cysts are located in the maxilla, especially the anterior region.

Most radicular cysts are asymptomatic and are often discovered incidentally during routine dental radiographic examination (Fig. 10–2). Most cysts do not produce bone expansion. When they are present, they tend to favor labial or buccal locations. By definition, the presence of a non-vital pulp is necessary for the clinical diagnosis of a radicular cyst to be made.

Radiographically, there are no distinctive differences between a radicular cyst and a periapical granuloma. In the past, undue emphasis was placed on the presence of a thin radiopacity at the circumference of the radiolucent lesion. This, once thought to indicate a cyst, has proved not to be the case, since periapical granulomas can present with a similar if not identical radiographic appearance. Size also is not an accurate indicator of the cyst versus granuloma diagnosis.

The radiolucency associated with a radicular cyst is generally round to ovoid, with a narrow, opaque margin that is contiguous with the lamina dura of the involved tooth. This radiopaque component may not be apparent if the cyst is actively enlarging. The cyst ranges from 5 mm or less to several centimeters in diameter, although the majority tend to be less than 1.5 cm. In long-standing cysts, root resorption of the offending tooth and occasionally adjacent teeth may be noted (Fig. 10–3).

Histopathology. The radicular cyst is lined by stratified squamous epithelium (Fig. 10–4). It is usually hyperplastic, exhibiting proliferating rings and arcades over well-vascularized connective tissue (Fig. 10–5). The actual thickness of the lining varies—in some areas, it may be attenuated or absent; in other areas, it may be 20 or more cell layers deep. Variable

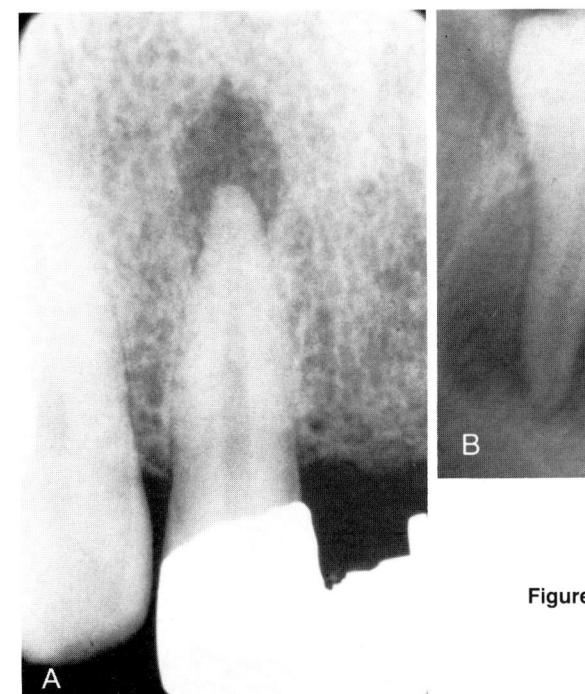
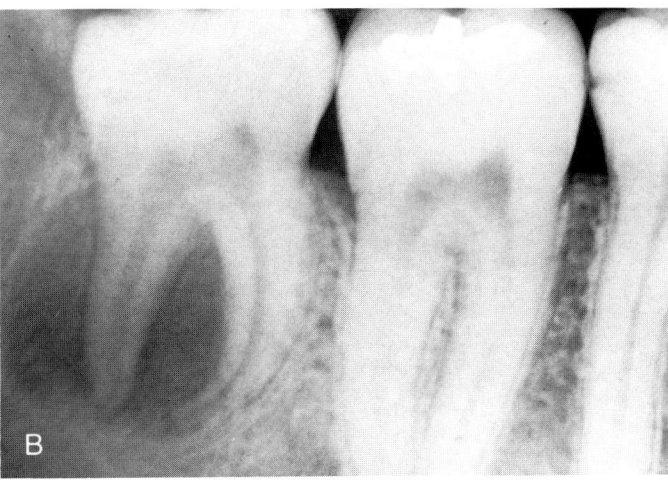

Figure 10–2. *A* and *B*, Radicular (periapical) cysts.

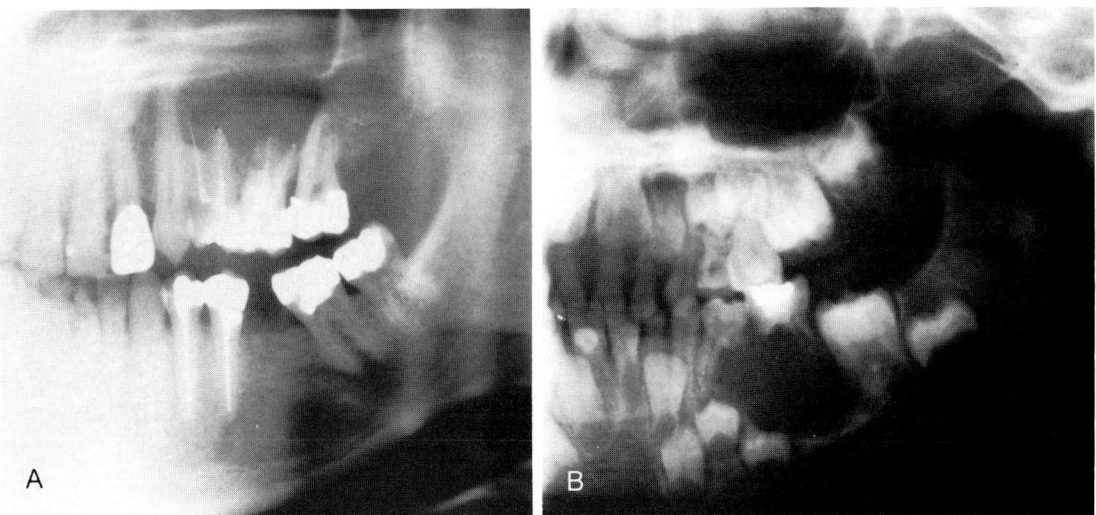

Figure 10–3. *A*, Radicular cyst of the maxilla. (Lesion did not resolve after endodontic therapy.) *B*, Radicular cyst associated with a primary molar.

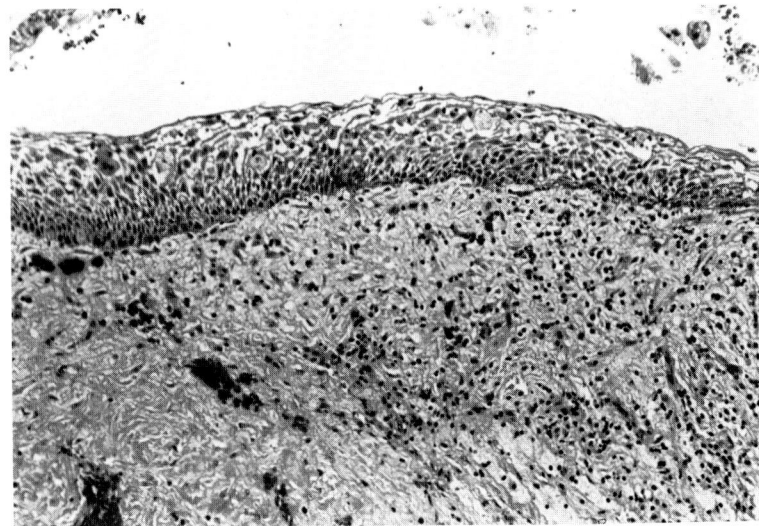

Figure 10–4. Radicular cyst lined by non-keratinized stratified epithelium.

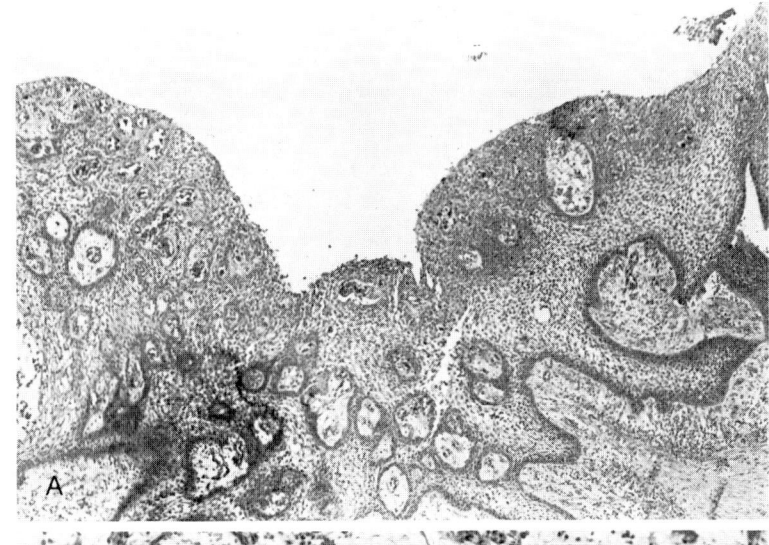

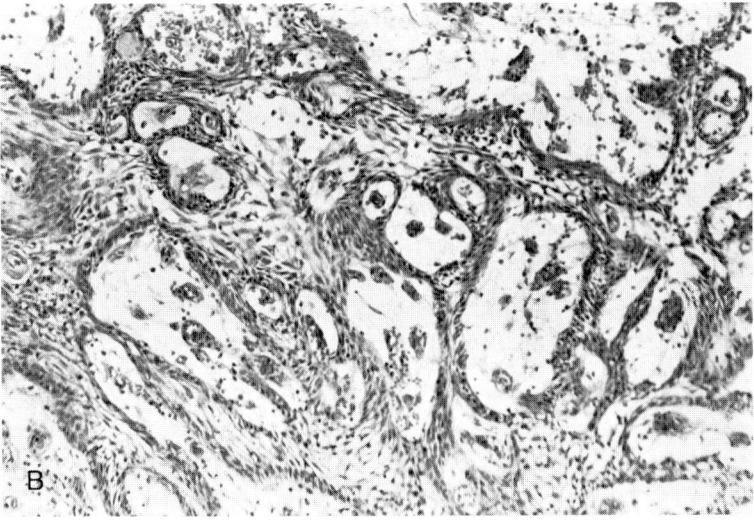

Figure 10–5. *A* and *B*, Hyperplastic epithelium lining a radicular cyst.

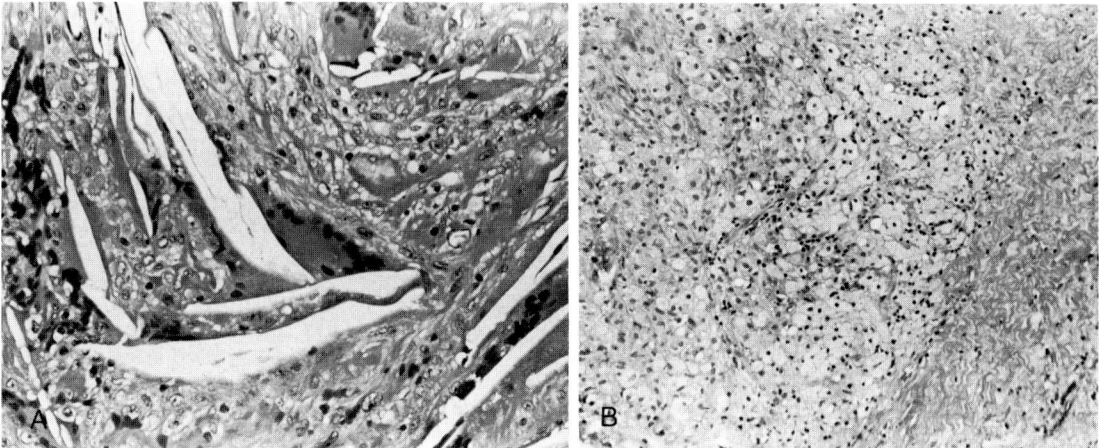

Figure 10–6. Cholesterol clefts and giant cells *(A)*, and lipid-filled macrophages *(B)* in the wall of a radicular cyst.

degrees of spongiosis (intercellular edema) may be seen. Transmigration of inflammatory cells through the epithelium is a common finding, with large numbers of polymorphonuclear leukocytes and fewer numbers of lymphocytes involved in this process. The underlying supportive connective tissue may be focally or diffusely infiltrated with a mixed inflammatory cell population. Toward the epithelium, polymorphonuclear leukocytes dominate; deeper within the connective tissue, lymphocytes are more common. Plasma cells and associated Russell bodies are found frequently, as are foci of dystrophic calcification, cholesterol clefts, and engorged blood vessels. Multinucleated foreign body type giant cells may frequently be seen in close approximation to cholesterol clefts and hemosiderin within the connective tissue wall (Fig. 10–6). Both the cholesterol and the hemosiderin deposits are felt to be related to hemolysis of red blood cells and necrosis of other cells participating in the inflammatory and healing processes.

Microscopic variations of the radicular cyst epithelium include the presence of ciliated or mucous cells. The presence of a keratinized lining of either the orthokeratotic or the parakeratotic type is very uncommon. In a small percentage of radicular cysts (and dentigerous cysts), hyaline bodies, so-called Rushton bodies, may be found (Fig. 10–7). Such bodies within the epithelial lining are characterized by a hairpin or slightly curved shape, concentric lamination, and occasional basophilic mineralization. They tend to be predominantly eosinophilic. However, with mineralization, basophilic changes may extend from the central portion to the periphery. The origin of

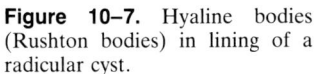

Figure 10–7. Hyaline bodies (Rushton bodies) in lining of a radicular cyst.

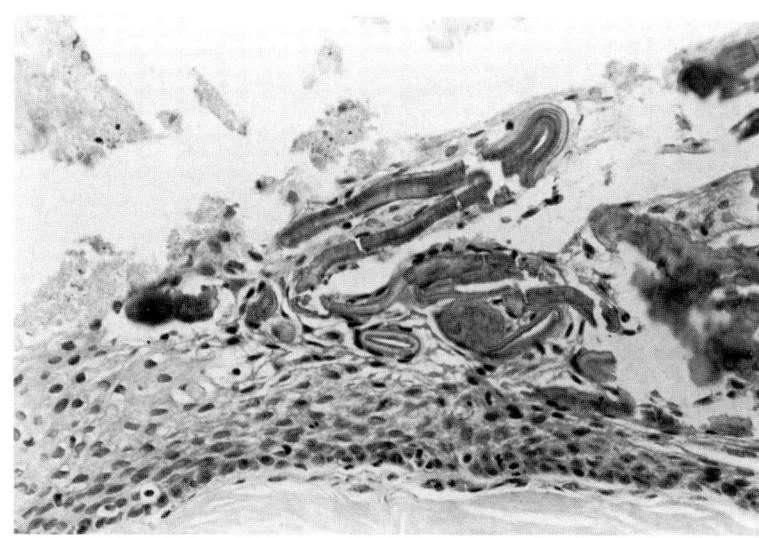

such bodies is controversial. Some believe that they have a hematogenous origin; others believe that they have an odontogenic origin, representing a type of keratin or enamel cuticle. These structures are also interesting in that they appear to be almost unique to odontogenic cysts.

Differential Diagnosis. Radiographically, the differential diagnosis of the radicular cyst must include the periapical granuloma. In areas of previously treated apical pathology, a surgical defect or periapical scar must also be considered. In the anterior mandibular areas, a periapical radiolucency should be distinguished from the early phase of periapical cemental dysplasia. In the posterior quadrants, apically placed radiolucencies must be distinguished from the traumatic bone cyst. In the posterior cases, adjacent teeth test vital with pulp testing. Occasionally, giant cell lesions, metastatic disease, and primary osseous tumors may mimic a radicular cyst.

Treatment and Prognosis. The radicular cyst may be successfully managed by extraction of the associated non-vital tooth and curettage of the epithelium in the zone of apical pathology. Alternatively, endodontic therapy may be performed in association with an apicoectomy to permit direct curettage of the cystic lesion. In cases of extremely large radicular cysts, exteriorization or marsupialization has proved beneficial. This decompression procedure will usually allow for shrinkage of the cystic cavity; this may then be followed by more sparing enucleation of the cyst and extraction of the non-vital tooth.

With adequate removal of this cyst, recurrence is unexpected. With incomplete removal, however, a *residual cyst* may develop from months to years after the initial treatment (Fig. 10–8). If either a residual cyst or the original radicular cyst remains untreated, continued growth can cause significant destruction and weakening of the mandible or maxilla. Complete bone repair is usually seen in adequately treated radicular and residual cysts.

Dentigerous Cyst

The dentigerous or follicular cyst is the second most common type of odontogenic cyst. By definition, a dentigerous cyst must be associated with the crown of an unerupted or developing tooth (the term "dentigerous" means "containing teeth"). The cyst enclosing the crown of the unerupted tooth is also attached to the tooth along the cervical region, which helps differentiate this cyst from the primordial cyst.

Etiology and Pathogenesis. The dentigerous cyst develops following an accumulation of fluid between the remnants of the enamel organ and the subjacent tooth crown. The enamel organ remnant or reduced enamel epithelium forms one of the delimiting surfaces of the cyst, and the mature tooth crown forms the other. Fluid accumulates between the reduced enamel epithelium and the crown and, occasionally, within the enamel organ itself.

An alternative pathogenetic mechanism suggests that there is initially partial enamel organ degeneration. If this occurs, it may be possible for cysts to develop by separation of the elements of enamel epithelium. Degeneration within the enamel organ, in particular the stellate reticulum, at an early stage of odontogenesis would probably be associated with enamel hypoplasia. Alternatively, crown completion may occur, followed by fluid accumulation between the component structures of the reduced enamel epithelium. The latter theory would not account for any concomitant enamel hypoplasia in the associated unerupted tooth.

Expansion of the dentigerous cyst is related to a secondary increase in cyst fluid osmolality as a result of passage of inflammatory cells and desquamated epithelial cells into the cyst lumen. As with the radicular cyst, the increased intracystic osmotic pressure results in a net ingress of fluid and secondary centrifugal growth of the cyst. Concomitant compensatory epithelial proliferation also occurs. This is felt to be a slow process, since the mitotic index for dentigerous cysts is rather low in comparison with primordial or odontogenic keratocysts.

Clinical Features. The most common sites for dentigerous cysts are the third molar regions of the mandible and maxilla and the maxillary canine regions (Fig. 10–9). Correspondingly, these teeth are the most frequently impacted. The highest incidence of dentigerous cysts occurs during the second and third decades. There is a greater frequency in males, with a ratio of 1.6 to 1 reported.

Symptoms are generally absent, with late eruption the usual indication of possible dentigerous cyst formation. This particular cyst, however, is capable of achieving significant size, occasionally with associated bone expansion. Lesions may rarely achieve such a size as to predispose to a pathologic fracture through erosion of cortical bone. As the cortex thins, a crackling or crepitus-type sensation may be

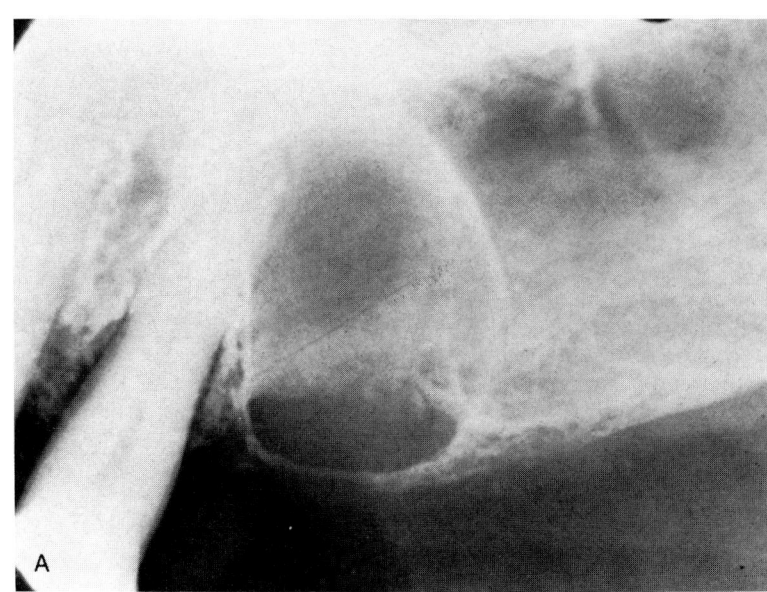

Figure 10–8. *A* and *B,* Residual cysts.

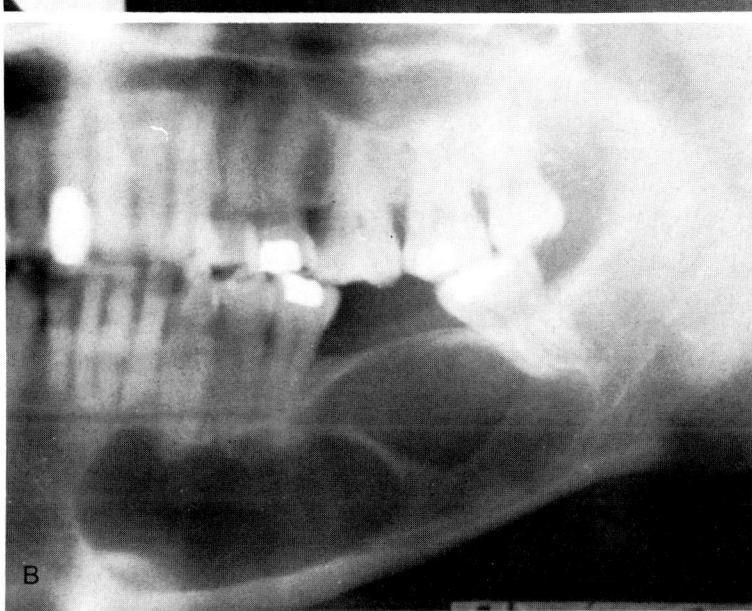

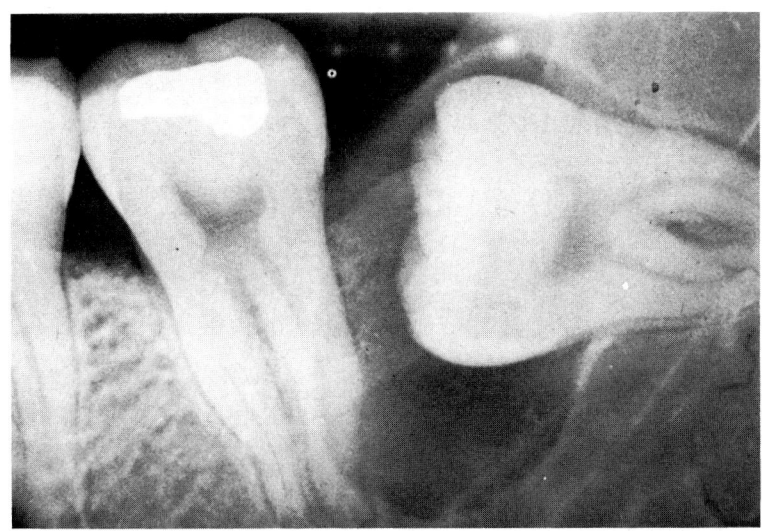

Figure 10–9. Dentigerous cyst.

elicited upon digital compression; in the complete absence of limiting cortical bone, a soft doughy to spongy sensation may be noted.

Radiographically, the dentigerous cyst presents as a well-defined, usually unilocular radiolucency in association with the crown of an unerupted tooth (Fig. 10–10). The envelopment of the crown is generally symmetric, although less frequently, lateral radiolucencies may be noted. Concomitant displacement of the unerupted tooth is frequent and may be noted in any plane or position. In the mandible, the associated radiolucency may extend superiorly from the third molar site into the ramus or anteriorly and inferiorly along the body of the mandible. In maxillary dentigerous cysts involving the canine region, extension into the maxillary sinus or to the orbital floor may be noted as well as extension toward the nasal fossa. Maxillary third molar dentigerous cysts may expand distally and superiorly, often compromising the maxillary sinus space.

Other radiographic features include the presence of a demarcation between the lucency of the cyst and the surrounding uninvolved bone. Unless they are involved by infection, the radiographic margins are discrete and further characterized by a thin radiopaque outline. In long-standing dentigerous cysts extending toward the roots of adjacent erupted teeth, root resorption may occur (approximately 50% of cases).

Histopathology. The supporting fibrous connective tissue wall of the cyst is lined by stratified squamous epithelium (Fig. 10–11). The stroma is collagenous, and its intervening ground substance is rich in acidic glycoproteins and mucopolysaccharides. In an uninflamed dentigerous cyst, the epithelial lining tends to be approximately two to four cell layers thick. The epithelium–connective tissue junction is generally flat, although in cases in which there is chronic inflammation or secondary infection, epithelial hyperplasia may be noted. Of importance is the fact that the epithelial lining is non-keratinized (Fig. 10–12). In at least 25% of mandibular dentigerous cysts and approximately 50% of maxillary dentigerous cysts, focal areas of mucous cells may be noted. Uncommonly, ciliated cells or hyaline bodies may be seen. Rarely, sebaceous cell elements may be detected within the lining structure. In some cases, a keratinizing element, representative of a metaplastic process, must be differentiated from an odontogenic keratocyst lining. Such nuances of histologic presentation reflect the multipotentiality of the odontogenic epithelial lining of the dentigerous cyst.

Differential Diagnosis. Differential diagnosis of pericoronal radiolucency must include, in addition to the dentigerous cyst, the ameloblastoma. The unicystic ameloblastoma represents the most important lesion to be distinguished from an uncomplicated dentigerous cyst radiographically. Ameloblastic transformation of a dentigerous cyst lining should also be part of the differential diagnosis. An odontogenic keratocyst presenting in a dentigerous relationship is another important possibility. With anterior maxillary pericoronal radiolucencies, the adenomatoid odontogenic tumor (AOT) is a consideration. Finally, the ameloblastic fibroma should be included with a dentigerous cyst when it occurs in the posterior region of the mandible or maxilla in young patients.

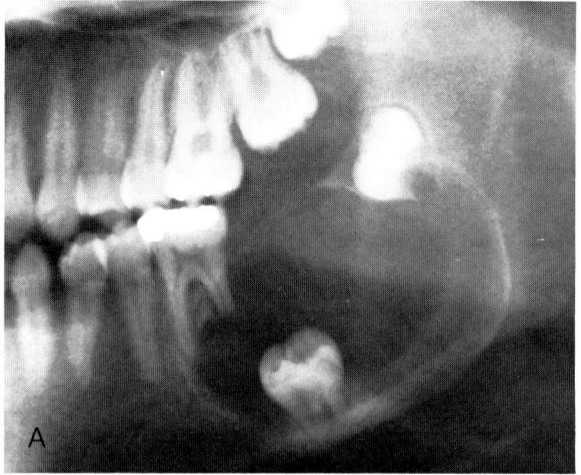
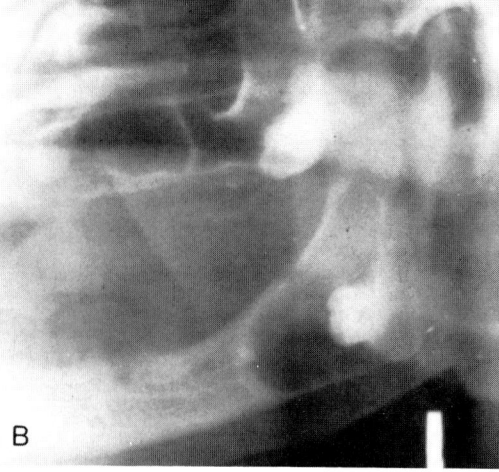

Figure 10–10. *A* and *B*, Dentigerous cysts.

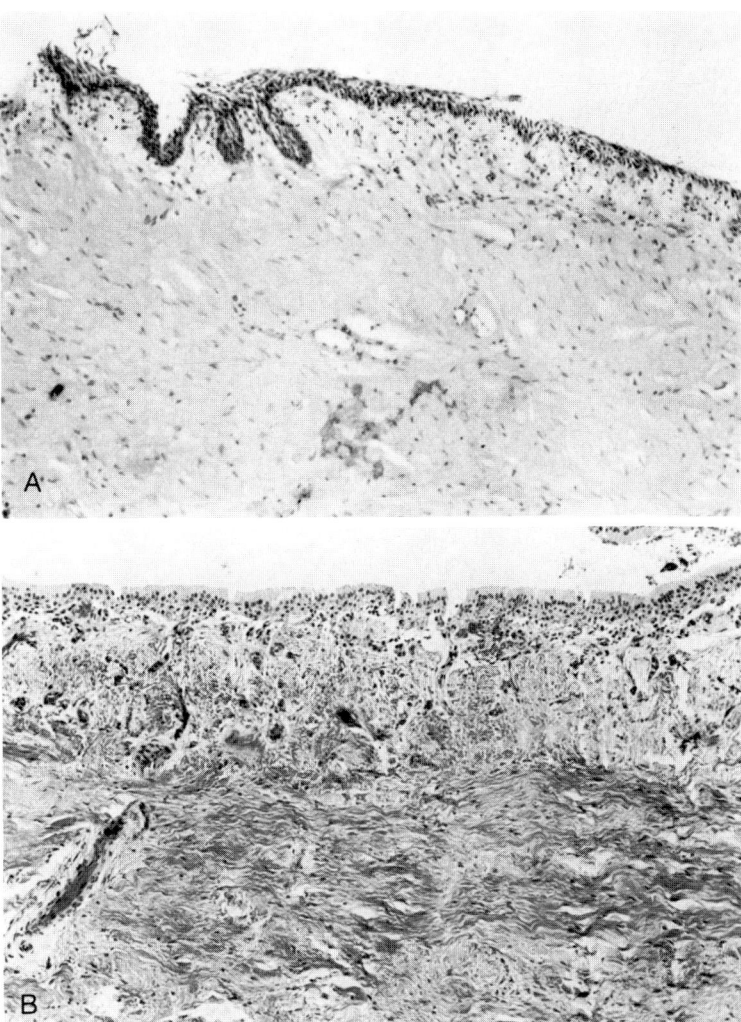

Figure 10–11. *A,* Stratified squamous epithelial lining of a dentigerous cyst. *B,* Reduced enamel epithelial lining of a follicular sac over the crown of an unerupted tooth.

Treatment. Removal of the associated tooth and careful enucleation of the soft tissue component is definitive therapy in most instances. In cases in which cysts affect significant portions of the mandible, an acceptable early treatment approach involves exteriorization or marsupialization of the cyst lumen to allow for decompression and subsequent shrinkage of the bone defect, thereby reducing the extent of surgery to be done at a later date.

Potential complications of the untreated dentigerous cyst are of considerable significance. Transformation of the epithelial lining of the dentigerous cyst into an ameloblastoma is a familiar occurrence. Rarely, dysplastic or carcinomatous transformation of the lining epithelium may be noted. Finally, in cases in which mucous cells are present, potential is believed to exist for development of the rarely seen intraosseous mucoepidermoid carcinoma. The dentigerous cyst has a much higher rate of these complications than do other odontogenic cysts (with the exception of the odontogenic keratocyst).

The specific complication of ameloblastoma arising in a dentigerous cyst is frequently a difficult histopathologic problem. Identification of early ameloblastomatous transformation has, however, been associated with the following microscopic findings:

1. Nuclear hyperchromatism of the basal cell nuclei.
2. Palisading of the basal cells with nuclear polarization away from the basement membrane.
3. Cytoplasmic vacuole formation within the basal cells, generally between the nuclei and basement membrane.
4. Increased width of intercellular space within the epithelial layers.

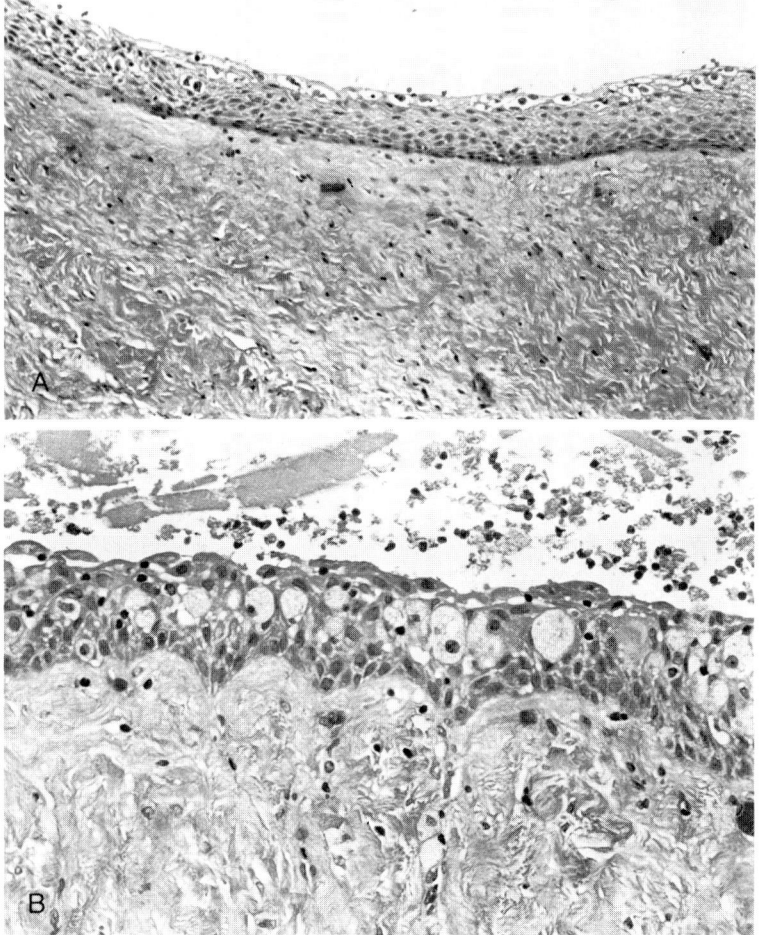

Figure 10–12. *A* and *B*, Epithelial linings of dentigerous cysts. Note mucous cells in *B*.

Eruption Cyst

The eruption cyst is a separate form of dentigerous cyst, found in children and, rarely, in adolescents. This soft tissue cyst results from fluid accumulation within the follicular space of an erupting tooth (Fig. 10–13). The clinical manifestation is a soft tissue swelling on the alveolar ridge immediately superior to the erupting tooth. If the cyst is aspirated, a clear fluid may be found. At times, such fluid may be blood tinged owing to secondary trauma. In other circumstances, if trauma is intense, blood may appear within the tissue space, forming a so-called eruption hematoma. No treatment is needed because the tooth erupts through the lesion. Subsequent to eruption, the cyst will disappear spontaneously without complication.

Lateral Periodontal Cyst

The lateral periodontal cyst may be defined as a non-keratinized, non-inflammatory developmental cyst occurring adjacent or lateral to the root of a tooth. Discussion of the *gingival cyst of adulthood* appears with the discussion of lateral periodontal cyst because of the close relationship between these lesions.

Etiology and Pathogenesis. It was once thought that the lateral periodontal cyst arose from the reduced enamel epithelium or the epithelial rests of Malassez within the periodontal ligament. Histologic observations, however, have militated against this concept, suggesting instead that the origin is related to proliferation of rests of dental lamina. This would pathogenetically link the lateral periodontal cyst and the gingival cyst, since the

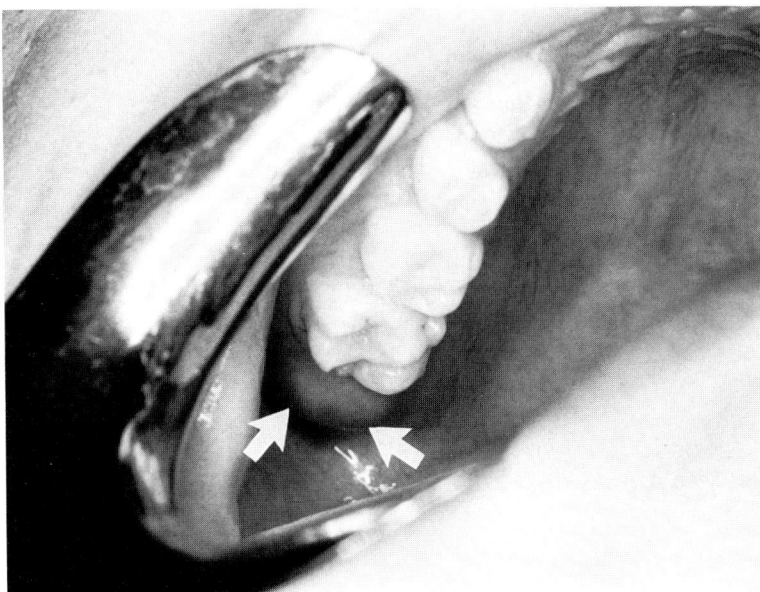

Figure 10–13. Eruption cyst over molar (arrows).

latter arises from dental lamina remnants in soft tissue between the oral epithelium and the periosteum. Dental lamina remnants within bone and separate from the periodontal ligament would give rise to the lateral periodontal cyst. The relationship between the gingival and lateral periodontal cysts is further supported by their similar distribution patterns along the facial portion of the alveolus. This corresponds to the higher concentration of dental lamina remnants in this region rather than of rests of Malassez, which are more plentiful around the apices of teeth.

Clinical Features. The majority of lateral periodontal cysts and gingival cysts of the adult occur in the mandibular premolar and cuspid region with fewer in the incisor area (Fig. 10–14). In the maxilla, similar lesions are noted primarily in the lateral incisor region. A distinct male predilection is noted for the lateral periodontal cyst, with a greater than 2 to 1 distribution the adult gingival cyst shows a nearly equal gender predilection. The median age for both the lateral periodontal and the gingival cysts occurs between the fifth and sixth decades, with a range of 20 to 85 years for the

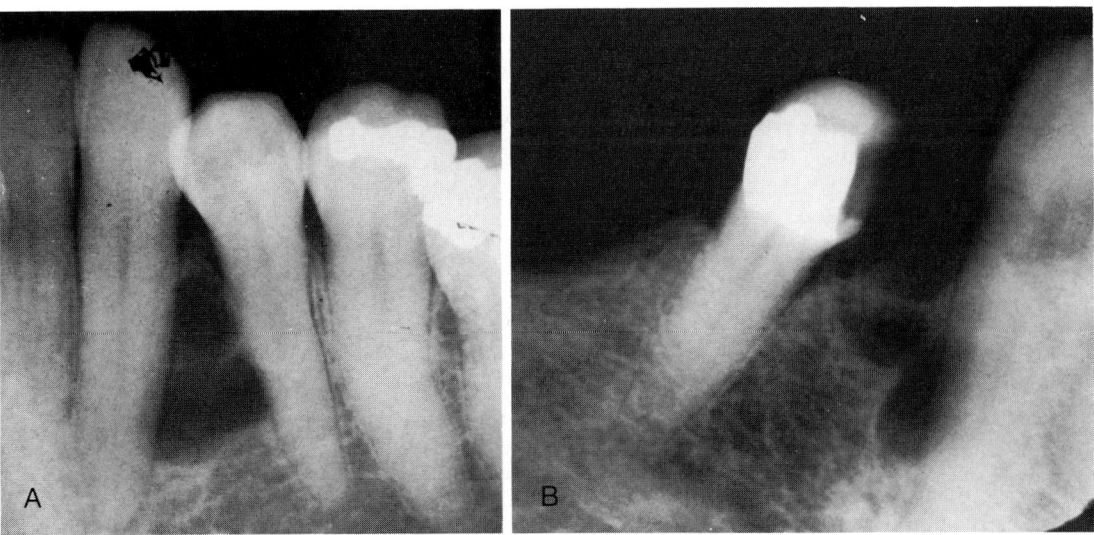

Figure 10–14. *A* and *B*, Lateral periodontal cysts. Note multilocularity.

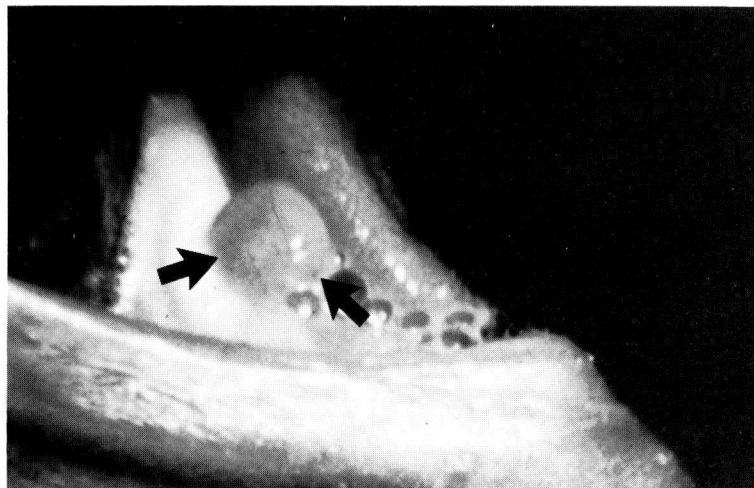

Figure 10–15. Gingival cyst of an edentulous adult (arrows).

lateral periodontal cyst and 40 to 75 years for the gingival cyst of the adult.

Clinically, the gingival cyst will appear as a small soft tissue swelling within or slightly inferior to the interdental papilla. It may assume a slightly bluish discoloration when it is relatively large. Most cysts are less than 1 cm in diameter (Fig. 10–15).

The lateral periodontal cyst will present radiographically as a well-delineated radiolucency with an opaque margin along the lateral surface of the tooth root with no associated clinical symptoms. The area of involvement is generally between adjacent roots with rare root divergence.

Histopathology. Both the lateral periodontal cyst and the gingival cyst of the adult are lined by a thin non-keratinized epithelium (Fig. 10–16). Clusters of clear cells may be noted as nodular thickenings within the cyst lining and also within the connective tissue wall. These cells have been shown to contain aggregates of glycogen, which can be demonstrated with appropriate stains. Less commonly, the gingival cyst may assume a polycystic or so-called botryoid type of morphology. When a similar sort of polycystic morphology is noted in an intrabony location, as with the lateral periodontal cyst, the term "botryoid odontogenic cyst" has been used. A possible explanation of multilocularity is that several clusters of dental lamina remnants undergo cystic degeneration and subsequent fusion. Of interest is the fact that the botryoid odontogenic cyst has a histologic appearance and location similar to the lateral periodontal cyst. This supports the concept that it merely represents a multilocular variant.

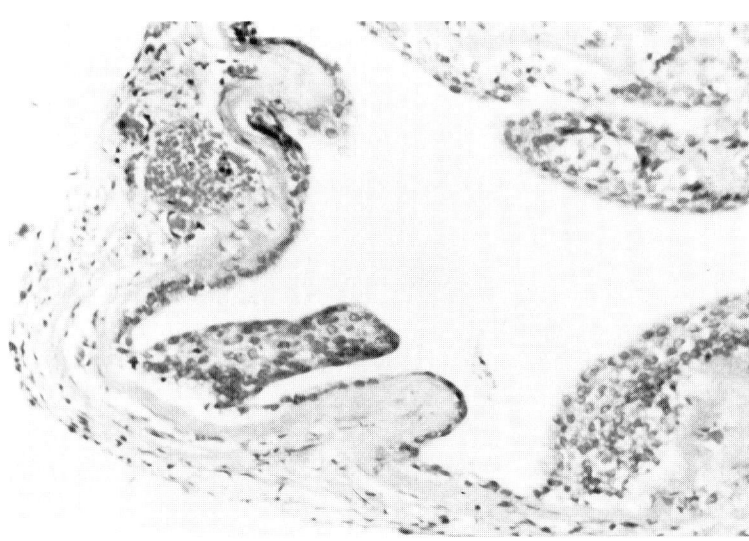

Figure 10–16. Epithelial lining of a lateral periodontal cyst. Note occasional epithelial tufts in an otherwise thin lining.

Differential Diagnosis. The lateral periodontal cyst must be distinguished from a cyst forming secondary to severe periodontitis, a lateral radicular cyst, a primordial cyst along the lateral root surface, and any radiolucent odontogenic tumor. The differential diagnosis for the gingival cyst would include gingival mucocele, Fordyce's granules, and possibly a peripheral odontogenic tumor.

Treatment and Prognosis. Local excision of both the gingival and the lateral periodontal cysts is curative, with little or no tendency for recurrence. Caution must be exercised, however, in management of the lateral periodontal cyst to avoid damaging the adjacent root structure.

Gingival Cyst of the Newborn

The gingival cyst of the newborn has also been designated as the dental lamina cyst of the newborn or Bohn's nodules. Such cysts appear typically as multiple nodules along the alveolar ridge in neonates. As the alternative terminology indicates, there is consensus that fragments of the dental lamina that remain within the alveolar ridge mucosa after tooth formation proliferate to form small keratinized cysts. It is important to note that such proliferation is limited in its overall extent and potential. In the vast majority of cases, these cysts degenerate and involute.

Upon histologic examination, an intact cyst will contain keratin debris and a thin epithelial lining, usually two to three cell layers thick (Fig. 10–17). On occasion, epithelium-lined tracts may be seen between the cyst and the surface mucosa. Treatment is not necessary, since nearly all involute spontaneously before 3 months of age.

Similar epithelial inclusional cysts may occur along the midline of the palate *(palatine cysts of the newborn* or *Epstein's pearls)*. These are of developmental origin but are not derived from odontogenic epithelium. This epithelium originates in inclusions in the fusion line between the palatal shelves and the nasal processes. These cysts also contain keratin and show a thin attenuated epithelial lining. No treatment is indicated, since such cysts will usually fuse with the overlying oral epithelium and discharge their contents into the oral cavity during the neonatal period.

Odontogenic Keratocyst

The odontogenic keratocyst has engendered a great deal of discussion in terms of classification and its relationship to the *primordial cyst* that occurs in place of a tooth owing to cystic degeneration of an enamel organ. In 1956, the term "odontogenic keratocyst" was introduced to apply to any jaw cyst containing keratin. Subsequently, it was shown that primordial cysts were, microscopically, odontogenic keratocysts. Confusion arose because other odontogenic cysts, including dentigerous, radicular, and residual cysts, occasionally contain keratinized cells. The odontogenic keratocyst, however, has been shown to be a distinctive entity that is worthy of separation because of its specific histology and behavior. Therefore, although keratinization may be present in many other types of cysts, the spe-

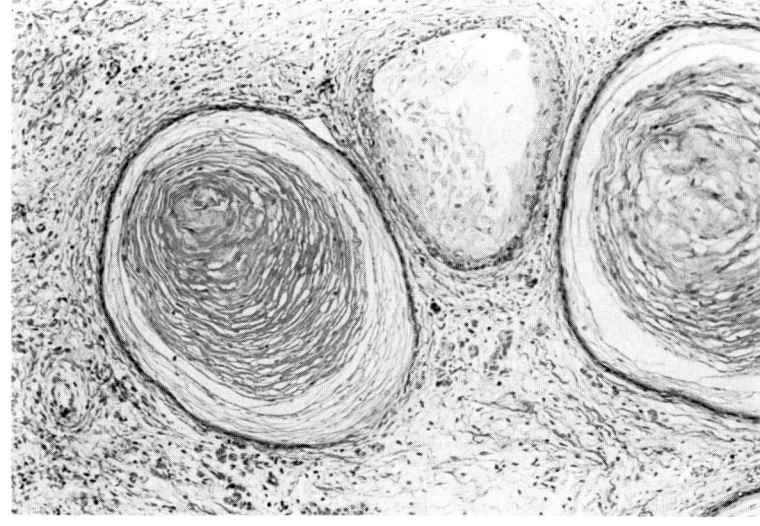

Figure 10–17. Gingival cysts of the newborn.

cific histologic pattern of the odontogenic keratocyst separates it from all others.

Etiology and Pathogenesis. There is general agreement that the origin of the odontogenic keratocyst resides with dental lamina remnants in the mandible and maxilla. However, convincing arguments may also be made for origin of this cyst from extension of basal cell components of the overlying oral epithelium.

Clinical Features. There is a wide age range within which the odontogenic keratocyst occurs. The peak incidence is within the second and third decades. Lesions found in children are often reflective of multiple odontogenic keratocysts as a component of the *nevoid basal cell carcinoma syndrome*. In the context of multiple odontogenic keratocysts, this particular syndrome must be ruled out. This will be discussed in further detail.

The chief site of involvement is the mandible, in approximately a 2 to 1 ratio. In the mandible, most odontogenic keratocysts occur within the posterior portion of the body and ramus region. Maxillary odontogenic keratocysts are noted chiefly in the third molar area; the canine region is the next most frequent site.

Radiographically, the odontogenic keratocyst characteristically presents as a well-circumscribed radiolucency with smooth margins and thin radiopaque borders (Fig. 10–18). Multilocularity may be present and tends to be seen more frequently in larger lesions. Most lesions, however, are unilocular, with up to 40% noted adjacent to the crown of an unerupted tooth. A significant percentage of odontogenic keratocysts will produce bone expansion. Approximately 30% of maxillary lesions produce buccal rather than palatal expansion. As many as one half of mandibular lesions show buccal expansion, and one third show lingual enlargement.

Histopathology. The fibrous connective tissue component of the cyst wall is often free of an inflammatory cell infiltrate and is relatively thin (Fig. 10–19). The epithelium–connective tissue interface is characteristically flattened, with no epithelial ridge formation. The epithelial lining generally ranges from eight to ten cell layers in thickness. The basal layer is quite characteristic—it is palisaded with prominent, polarized, and intensely staining nuclei of uniform diameter. The surface is characteristically uneven or corrugated, with a parakeratotic surface layer that can often be seen shedding individual or clusters of squames into the cyst lumen. The lumen may contain large amounts of keratin debris or clear fluid similar to serum transudate. Elevated levels of osmolarity of cyst contents and increased epithelial cell turnover are believed to contribute to enlargement of the cyst.

The parakeratotic type forms 85 to 95% of all odontogenic keratocysts; the balance is made up of the *orthokeratinized variant* (Fig. 10–20). Histologic distinction between the para- and orthokeratinized variants is made because there is a difference in behavior; the latter is less aggressive, with a much lower rate of recurrence. In the orthokeratotic odontogenic keratocyst, a prominent granular layer is found immediately below a flat non-corrugated surface. The basal cell layer is less prominent, with a more flattened or squamous appearance in comparison with the parakeratotic type.

Histologic variations of the parakeratinized odontogenic keratocyst include budding of the basal layer of the epithelium into the support-

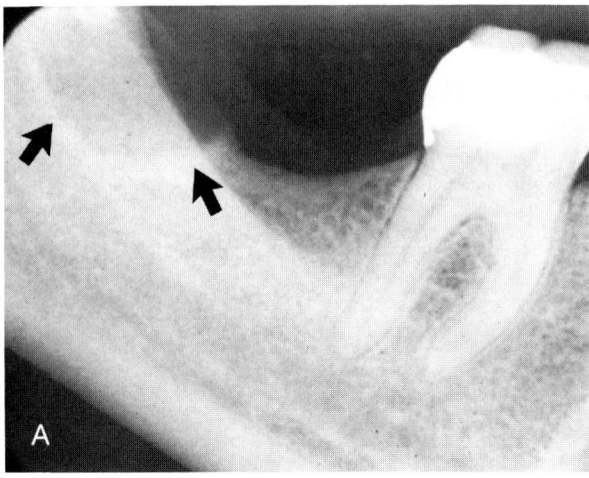
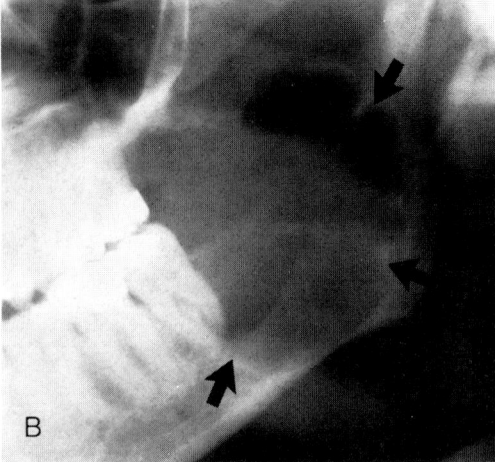

Figure 10–18. *A* and *B*, Odontogenic keratocysts (arrows).

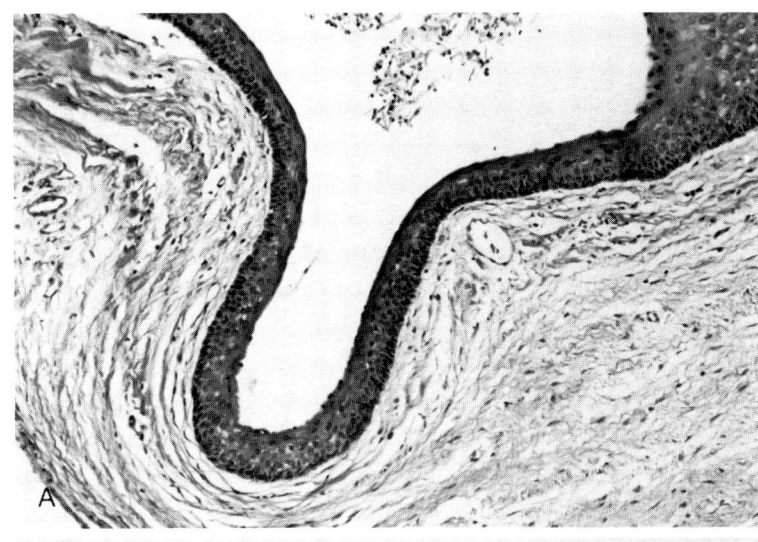
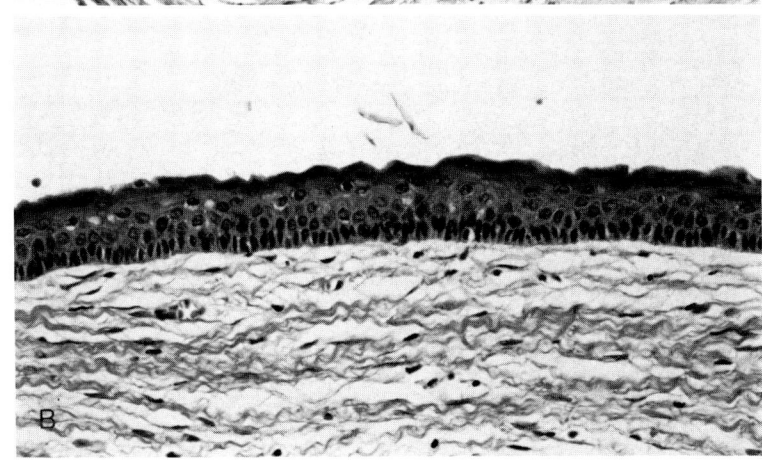

Figure 10–19. A and B, Parakeratotic epithelium typical of odontogenic keratocysts.

ing connective tissue (Fig. 10–21). On occasion, these proliferative buds may appear slightly dysplastic and dyskeratotic. Within the walls of some cysts, there may be islands of epithelial cells exhibiting central keratinization or microcyst formation. Such microcysts or so-called satellite cysts have been noted in 7 to 26% of cases.

Differential Diagnosis. As with any well-circumscribed radiolucency of the mandible or maxilla in a pericoronal relationship, several entities must be considered, including the dentigerous cyst, ameloblastoma, minimally calcified calcifying odontogenic cyst, AOT, and ameloblastic fibroma. The possible clinical considerations of pericoronal radiolucencies become significant in terms of overall numbers if all potential rarities are considered as well.

Of importance, however, is the solitary radiolucency separate from impacted or erupted teeth. The odontogenic keratocyst may well present in such a manner and must therefore be separated from the traumatic bone cyst, central giant cell granuloma, lateral periodontal cyst, and various forms of fissural cysts. Non-odontogenic tumors, such as vascular abnormalities, benign bone tumors, plasmacytoma/myeloma, and metastatic low-grade carcinoma, may also present in a similar fashion.

Treatment and Prognosis. Surgical excision with peripheral osseous curettage or ostectomy is the preferred method of management. This more aggressive approach for a cystic lesion is based upon the fact that a high recurrence rate is associated with this form of odontogenic cyst. The reason for such high recurrence rates, ranging from 5 to 62%, remains unclear. Several possibilities have been suggested, however. The friable thin connective tissue wall of the cyst may lead to the leaving behind of small epithelial fragments or satellites after removal. It is possible that small dental lamina remnants reside in the bone adjacent to the

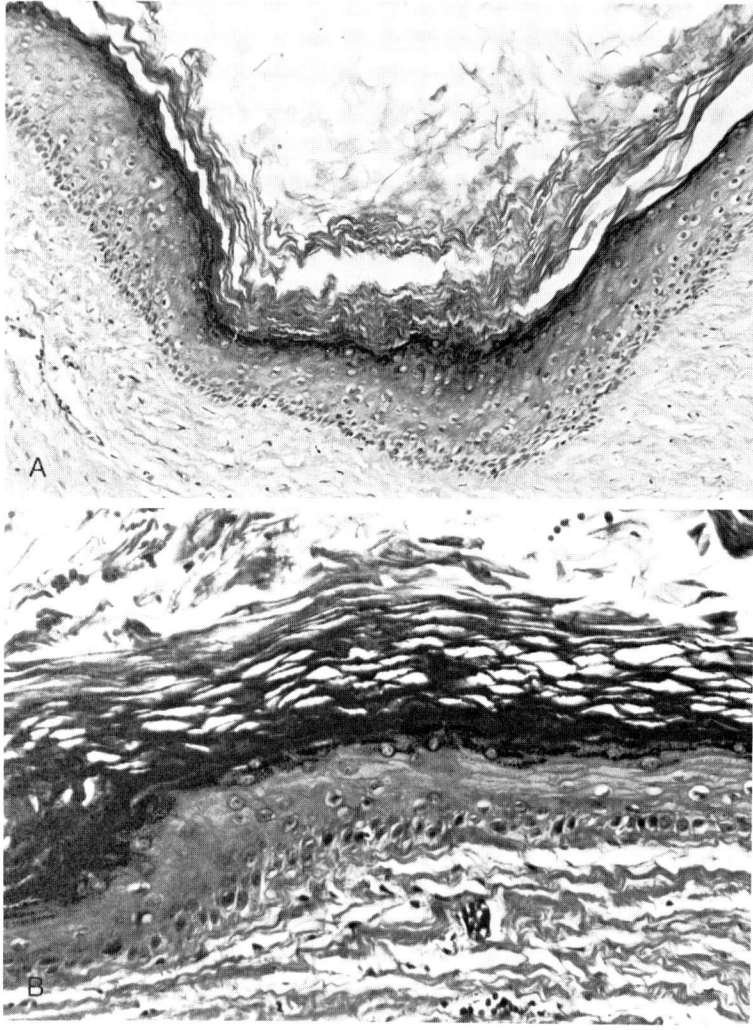

Figure 10–20. A and B, Orthokeratinized variant of the odontogenic keratocyst.

primary lesion. Recurrences have also been proposed to be related to cystic proliferation of the overlying oral epithelial basal cell layer. The actual biologic qualities of the cyst epithelium have also been mentioned. The mitotic index of keratocyst lining epithelial cells has been shown to be greater than that in other forms of odontogenic cysts, with values approximating those seen within the epithelial component of the ameloblastoma or actively growing dental lamina.

Follow-up, therefore, is an important component of overall management of this lesion so that any recurrent cysts can be detected early. Most recurrences become clinically evident within 5 years of treatment, although in one large series, recurrences at 8 or more years after original treatment were identified. Aside from recurrence potential, neoplastic changes are possible within the epithelial lining of this cyst as with other types of jaw cysts.

Studies indicate that in patients with multiple keratocysts, there is a significantly higher rate of recurrence than in those with single keratocysts: 35 and 10%, respectively. In such circumstances, it is necessary to rule out the presence of the nevoid basal cell carcinoma syndrome. Approximately 7% of patients with multiple odontogenic keratocysts are afflicted with this syndrome.

Briefly stated, the nevoid basal cell carcinoma syndrome is characterized by cutaneous abnormalities including palmar and plantar keratotic pitting, multiple basal cell carcinomas, multiple milia, and dermal calcinosis. In addition to the keratocyst component, bifid ribs are frequently seen as well as vertebral and metacarpal abnormalities. Mild mandibular prognathism has been recorded in a small percentage of cases. Facial dysmorphogenesis may be seen. Features include a broad nasal bridge with corresponding ocular hypertelor-

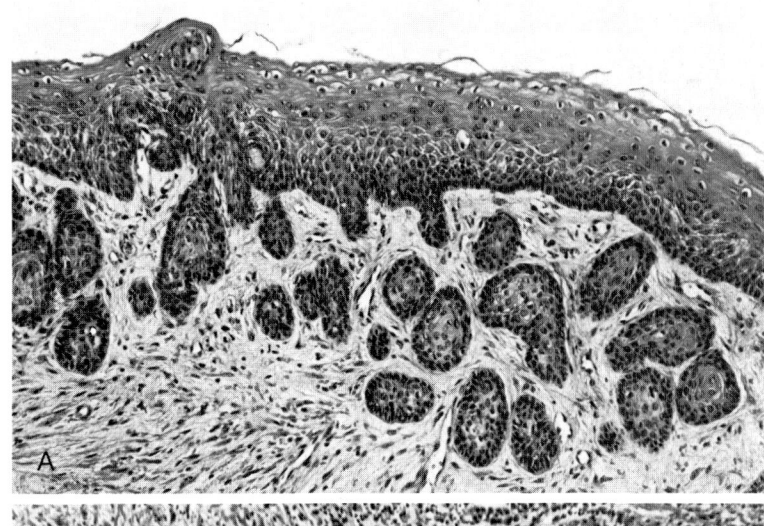
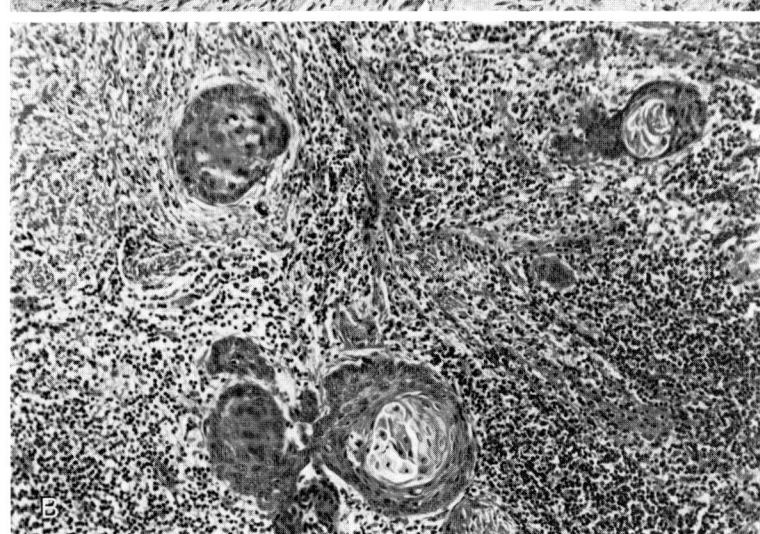

Figure 10–21. Odontogenic keratocyst histologic variations. *A* shows budding, and *B* shows satellite cysts in the cyst wall.

ism and laterally displaced inner ocular canthi (dystopia canthorum). Neurologic abnormalities including medulloblastoma, dysgenesis or agenesis of the corpus callosum, calcification of the falx cerebri and, less frequently, of the falx cerebelli have also been documented.

Calcifying Odontogenic Cyst (COC)

It is generally agreed that the COC is a developmental odontogenic lesion. However, because occasional aggressive behavior has been documented, some have proposed that it is instead a neoplasm, prompting the term "odontogenic ghost cell tumor."

Etiology and Pathogenesis. The COC is believed to be derived from odontogenic epithelial remnants within the gingiva or within the mandible or maxilla. Ghost cell keratinization, the characteristic microscopic feature of the COC, is also often associated with the epithelial element of odontomas, ameloblastomas, AOTs, ameloblastic fibro-odontomas, and ameloblastic fibromas. Whether these represent two unrelated lesions developing simultaneously or a single lesion with ghost cell change is open to question and awaits further study.

Clinical Features. There is a wide age range for this cyst with a peak incidence in the second decade. It usually appears in individuals less than 40 years of age and has a decided predilection for females. Over 70% of COCs are associated with the maxilla. Approximately one fourth of these lesions present extraosseously as localized masses involving the gingiva. A proportion of these may secondarily involve alveolar bone by pressure resorption.

Radiographically, the central or intraosseous

COC may present as a unilocular or multilocular radiolucency with discrete, well-demarcated margins. Within the radiolucency may be scattered irregularly sized calcifications producing variable degrees of opacity (Fig. 10–22). Such opacities may be seen as a "salt and pepper" type of pattern, with an equal and diffuse distribution. In some cases, mineralization may develop to such an extent that the radiographic margins of the lesion are difficult to determine. When the cyst is seen in conjunction with an odontoma of the complex type, an overlapping or blending of the opaque components of the cyst and odontoma may be seen.

Associated expansion of the alveolar bone, or soft tissues in the case of an extraosseous lesion, may be the presenting complaint in approximately 50% of cases. A wide range in size has been reported, from 1 to 8 cm with a 3 cm diameter mean in one study. Absence of tenderness and pain are characteristic, with the majority of patients noting duration for 6 months or less.

Histopathology. Most lesions present as multicystic well-delineated processes with a fibrous connective tissue wall surrounding a lumen lined by odontogenic epithelium. In the more solid lesions, significant intraluminal epithelial proliferation will obscure or compromise the cyst lumen, thereby producing the impression of a solid tumor (Fig. 10–23). The epithelial layer is irregular and of variable thickness. The lining is very similar to an ameloblastic type of epithelium. The basal epithelium may focally be quite prominent, with hyperchromatic nuclei and cuboidal to columnar morphology. Above the basal layer are more loosely arranged epithelial cells bearing similarity to the stellate reticulum of the enamel organ.

The most prominent and unique microscopic feature of the epithelial element within this lesion is the presence of so-called ghost cells, which are often intermingled within the stellate reticulum–like areas. A gradation of changes may be noted, from the basal cells to cells bearing an initially hyaline homogeneous cytoplasm that eventually becomes deeply eosinophilic. The nucleus undergoes karyolysis as keratinization progresses. Careful examination of the ghost cell element will show individual cells or clusters of cells with dystrophic mineralization characterized by extremely fine basophilic granularity. This granularity may increase in size and intensity, eventually forming, in some cases, large sheets of calcified material. In other areas within the cyst lining and in the fibrous connective tissue wall, there may be irregular eosinophilic masses considered by some as dentinoid. On occasion, ghost cells may have broken through the cystic lining, coming into contact with the connective tissue component of the cyst and eliciting a foreign body giant cell response. The ghost cell keratinization, dystrophic calcification, and foreign body reaction are also typical of a cutaneous lesion known as calcifying epithelioma of Malherbe or pilomatricoma.

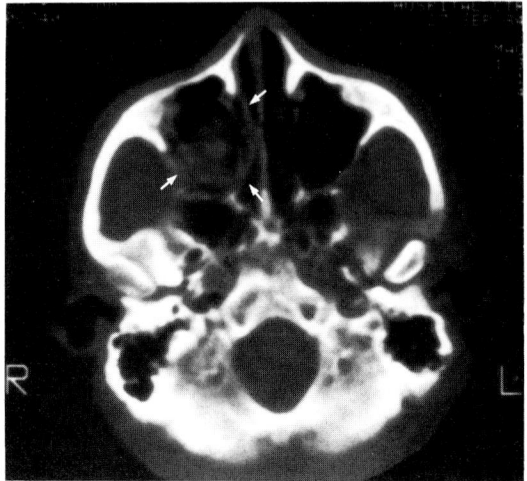

Figure 10–22. Axial computer-assisted tomogram of a maxillary (right) calcifying odontogenic cyst (arrows).

Differential Diagnosis. In the early stages of formation, the COC may have little or no mineralization, and it therefore may present as a radiolucency with cyst-like features. It must then be distinguished from a dentigerous cyst, odontogenic keratocyst, or unicystic ameloblastoma. In later phases of growth, when a mixed radiolucent-radiopaque appearance is present, this lesion must be separated from the AOT, a partially mineralized odontoma, and a calcifying epithelial odontogenic tumor. An ameloblastic fibro-odontoma may also be included within this differential diagnosis.

Treatment and Prognosis. When the COC is associated with no other lesion, simple enucleation is sufficient treatment, and there is little risk of recurrence. This likewise applies in cases of a COC in association with an odontoma of either the complex or the compound type. If it is seen, however, in combination with an ameloblastoma, the lesion must be treated as if it were an ameloblastoma, with appropriate considerations for that particular entity.

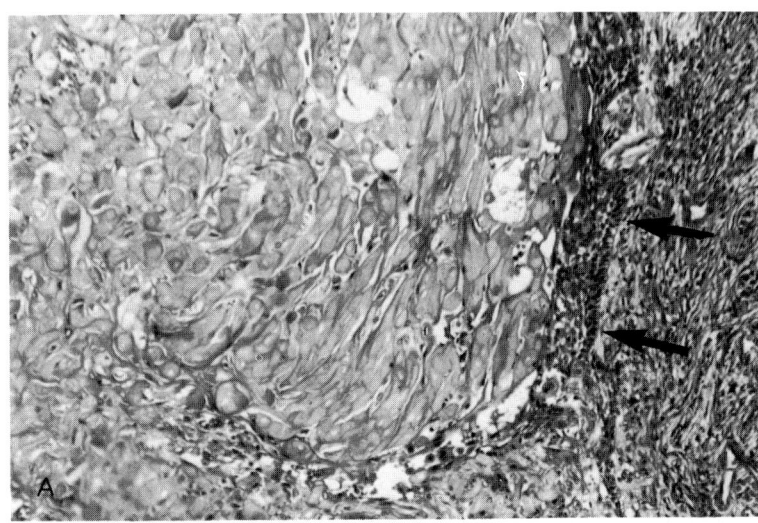
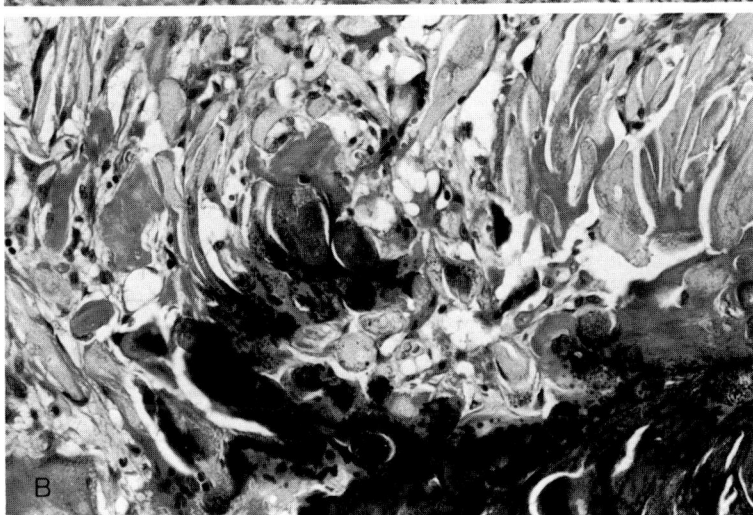

Figure 10–23. Calcifying odontogenic cyst. *A,* Epithelium (arrows) is thin, and lumen (left) is filled with ghost cells. *B,* Ghost cell keratinization showing a focus of dystrophic calcification (bottom).

NON-ODONTOGENIC CYSTS

"Globulomaxillary" Cyst

The globulomaxillary cyst was once considered a fissural cyst, with the theory of origin relating to epithelial entrapment within a line of embryologic closure and subsequent cystic degeneration. More recent evidence, however, shows that the derivation of this type of cyst is probably from odontogenic epithelium located between the maxillary lateral incisor and canine teeth. Current embryologic principles emphasize that fusion of the secondary palatal processes is the only circumstance permitting sequestration of surface epithelium that would not relate anatomically to this particular cyst.

In a large case series in which 37 globulomaxillary cysts were re-examined, revised diagnoses included radicular cysts, periapical granulomas, lateral periodontal cysts, odontogenic keratocysts, central giant cell granuloma, a COC, and an odontogenic myxoma. Because of this and related studies, it has been suggested that the term "globulomaxillary" be abandoned or used only as a clinical term.

Clinical Features. Radiologically, the so-called globulomaxillary cyst presents as a well-defined radiolucency, often producing divergence of the roots of the maxillary lateral incisor and canine teeth. Assuming the adjacent teeth to be vital, a radicular cyst or an abnormally placed periapical granuloma could be ruled out. Symptoms may vary from those associated with periapical pathology to no symptoms at all.

Histopathology. As judged by the array of potential diagnoses discussed, the histology may vary considerably from case to case. Specific histologic features of the differential diagnoses offered previously are to be found in the more definitive discussions of these entities.

Treatment and Prognosis. Treatment is enucleation of the cyst and curettage of the surrounding bone. If the surrounding teeth are non-vital, appropriate endodontic therapy is necessary. Surgical excision of the cyst in instances in which vital teeth are present in the surgical field may necessitate endodontic therapy preoperatively in order to avoid postoperative complications.

Recurrence rates of this lesion vary relative to the specific entity that is diagnosed histologically. For example, an odontogenic keratocyst will have a considerably higher recurrence potential than will a radicular cyst. If an odontogenic tumor, such as an AOT or an odontogenic myxoma, is present, the prognosis is quite variable. The reader is referred to each specific section for details.

Nasolabial Cyst

The nasolabial cyst has been called, inaccurately, nasoalveolar cyst. This latter designation is inappropriate because the entity is not a true cyst of the maxilla. Rather, it represents a soft tissue cyst without involvement of the alveolus, hence the preference for the designation "nasolabial cyst."

Etiology and Pathogenesis. The pathogenesis of the nasolabial cyst is unclear, although in the past it was considered to arise from epithelial enclavement at the site of fusion between the globular portions of the lateral nasal and maxillary processes. It was thought to represent the non-osseous equivalent of the globulomaxillary cyst. This is no longer tenable, since the embryologic basis, as previously stated, has been refuted. The currently accepted pathogenesis relates to development from the inferior and anterior portion of the nasolacrimal duct. It is felt that remnants of the solid cord of cells that ultimately form the caudal end of the nasolacrimal duct give rise to the nasolabial cyst. Alternatively, the lower anterior portion of the mature duct may produce this soft tissue cyst. The occurrence of bilateral nasolabial cysts also helps support this particular theory of developmental origin.

Clinical Features. The nasolabial cyst is a rare lesion with a peak incidence noted in the fourth and fifth decades. There is a distinct female predilection of nearly 4 to 1. The chief clinical sign is a soft tissue swelling that may present in the canine region. Occasionally, the patient may complain of discomfort or some minor degree of nasal obstruction. The mass may present intraorally in the mucobuccal fold with a soft to doughy consistency. If it is untreated, the cyst will continue to grow at a slow rate and ultimately distort the ala of the nose laterally and superiorly.

Radiographically, bone alteration may result from pressure resorption along the labial aspect of the anterior maxilla.

Histopathology. Mature fibrous connective tissue forms the wall of the cyst, with variable amounts of collagen deposited. The epithelial lining is characteristically pseudostratified columnar type with numerous goblet cells (Fig. 10–24). Stratified squamous epithelium may be present in addition to cuboidal epithelium in a minority of cases.

Differential Diagnosis. A radicular cyst may present on occasion as a swelling within the mucobuccal fold in this region; vitality tests of the adjacent teeth are helpful in this case. Odontogenic cysts of the non-inflammatory type may also rarely present in this fashion. Alternatively, salivary gland neoplasms, cutaneous or adnexal inclusion cysts, and sebaceous cysts must be ruled out.

Treatment and Prognosis. Management is surgical excision. In uncomplicated cases, this procedure has little morbidity associated with it. Recurrence is unexpected.

Median Mandibular Cyst

The median mandibular cyst, like the globulomaxillary cyst, was once considered a fissural cyst. Justification for a fissural origin would have to be based on epithelial entrapment within the midline of the mandible during the fusion process of each side of the mandibular arch. Embryologic evidence refutes this. Instead of a midline gap or space between lateral mesenchymal masses, there is an isthmus of mesenchyme that is gradually eliminated as growth continues. There is no fusion, therefore, of epithelium-covered embryologic processes and therefore no possibility of epithelial enclavement.

Cases diagnosed as median mandibular cysts were re-evaluated by Buchner and Ramon and were reported to demonstrate a diagnostic pattern similar to that seen with globulomaxillary cysts. Radicular cysts, lateral periodontal cysts, odontogenic keratocysts, and residual cysts were noted in this area. Detection of mucous cells and ciliated epithelium in cysts found in the midline of the mandible does not

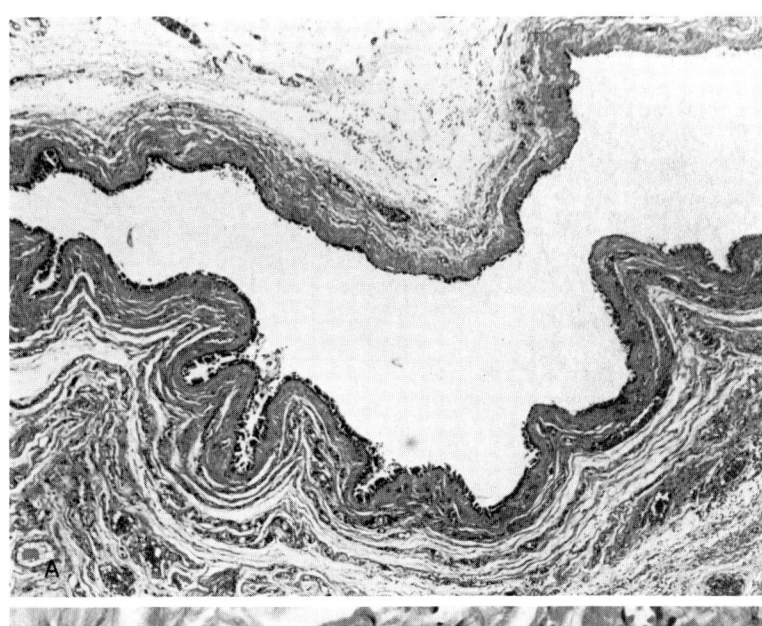
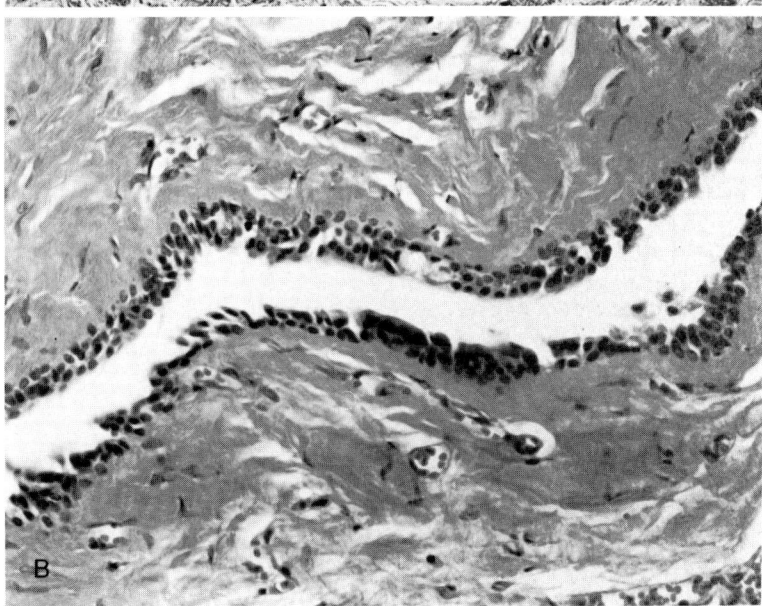

Figure 10–24. *A* and *B*, Nasolabial cysts.

preclude an odontogenic origin, since both mucous cell elements and ciliated epithelial cells may be found in odontogenic cysts in both the mandible and maxilla.

Nasopalatine Canal Cyst

The nasopalatine canal cyst, also known as incisive canal cyst, may be located within the nasoplatine canal or within the palatal soft tissues at the point of the opening of the canal (in this location, it is called a *cyst of the palatine papilla*). A growing trend is to report all maxillary midline developmental cysts as nasopalatine duct cysts, thereby encompassing the so-called *median palatine cyst*. Many now believe that this latter entity represents a more posterior presentation of a nasopalatine canal cyst rather than cystic degeneration of epithelial rests at the line of fusion of the palatine shelves. To be separated, however, from the nasopalatine canal cyst is the rare *median alveolar cyst*, which has been reported in the alveolar process anterior to the incisive canal. This cyst in all probability represents an odontogenic cyst, possibly a primordial cyst of supernumerary (mesiodens) tooth bud origin.

Etiology and Pathogenesis. The development of the nasopalatine canal cyst relates to the presence of epithelial remnants of paired embryonic nasopalatine ducts within the incisive canal. The canal itself forms secondary to the fusion of the premaxilla with the right and left palatal processes. The anatomic exit of the canal is slightly posterior to the incisive papilla.

The exact etiology of cyst formation from the epithelial remnants of the nasopalatine canals is uncertain. Most theories of pathogenesis are, however, related to bacterial infections or trauma that stimulate epithelial remnants to proliferate. Alternatively, it has been suggested that the presence of mucous glands within the lining may relate to secondary cyst formation as a result of mucin secretion within this enclosed structure.

The soft tissue, and far less common, variant of the nasopalatine canal cyst is the *cyst of the palatine papilla*. The anatomic precursor is identical to that of its intrabony counterpart. The mechanism for cyst development within this area is similar in nature, although traumatic stimulation of epithelial remnants has a more probable etiologic role in this situation.

Clinical Features. A symmetric swelling in the anterior region of the palatal midline is characteristic of this lesion. In cases of more substantial cyst formation, a midline swelling of the labial aspect of the maxillary alveolar ridge may be noted.

The overall frequency of nasopalatine canal cysts in the general population ranges from 0.08% to 1.3% as determined from analysis of specimen skulls. The majority of cases occur between the fourth and sixth decades. Several large series of cases indicate that males are more frequently affected than females—differences ranged as high as 3 to 1.

Most cases are asymptomatic, with the clinical sign of swelling usually calling attention to the lesion. Symptoms may follow infection, resulting in a noticeable swelling within a short time. Sinus formation is not uncommon and usually occurs at the most prominent portion of the palatine papilla.

Radiographically, the nasopalatine canal cyst is purely radiolucent with sharply defined margins (Fig. 10–25). It may produce divergence of the roots of the maxillary incisor teeth and less commonly induce external root resorption. The anterior nasal spine is often centrally superimposed on the lucent defect, producing a rather characteristic heart shape, but this is by no means always evident. Occasionally, the radiolucency may be unilateral, with the midline forming the most medial aspect of the radiolucency. Infrequently, separate but adjacent radiolucent cystic defects may be noted on a radiograph in either a periapical or an occlusal projection.

Histopathology. A wide variation in the epithelial lining features of the nasopalatine canal cyst is often noted. Epithelium ranging from stratified squamous to cuboidal to pseudostratified columnar may be noted (Fig. 10–26). In many instances, a mixture of two or more types of epithelial lining is seen. Goblet cells are not infrequently noted in relation to the pseudostratified columnar type lining (which may also be ciliated). The variation in epithelial lining is felt to reflect both the inferior-superior relationships of the canal itself and

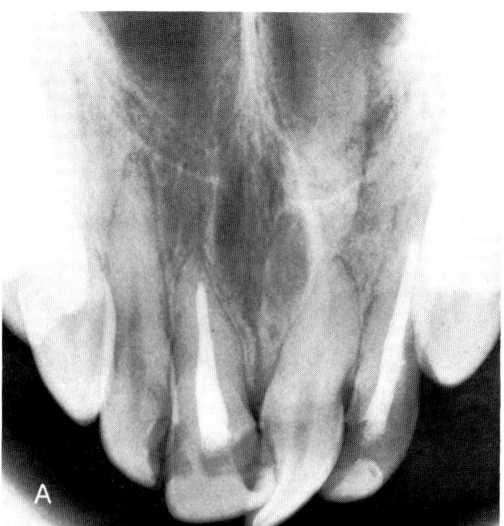 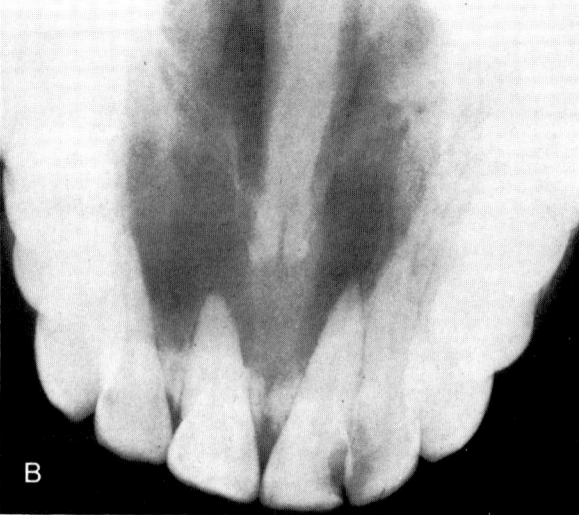

Figure 10–25. *A* and *B,* Nasopalatine canal cysts. Large lesion in *B* extends to the mid-palate.

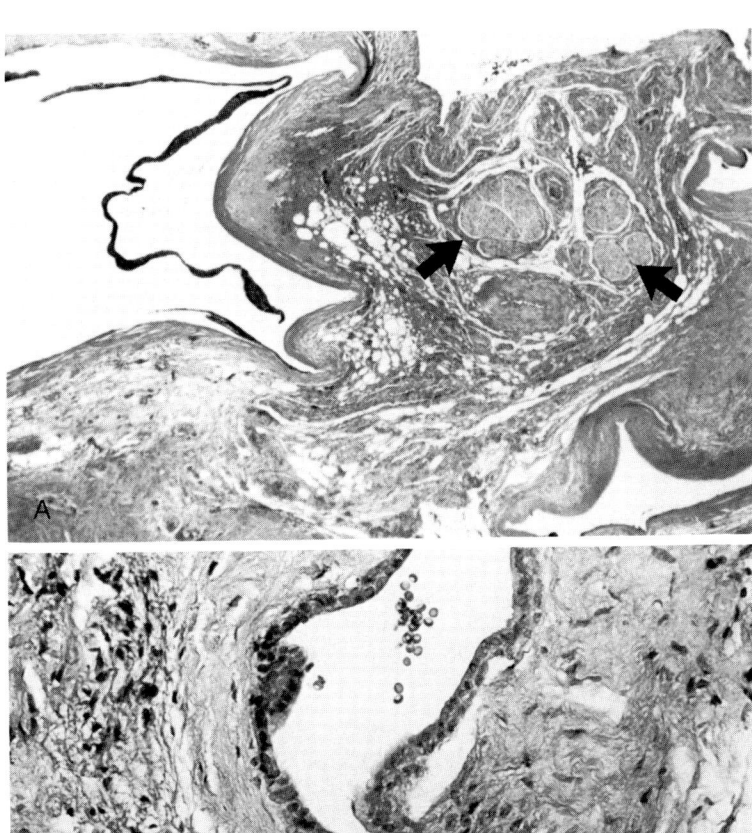

Figure 10–26. *A* and *B*, Nasopalatine canal cysts. Note nerve bundles (arrows) and vascular channels in cyst wall *(A)*.

the proximity of the nasal cavity on the one hand and the oral cavity on the other. An alternative to an anatomic explanation of the variation concerns a multipotential epithelium giving rise to several subtypes including stratified squamous epithelium.

The connective tissue portion of the fibrous capsule often contains small arterioles and nerve structures. In some instances, prominent neurovascular bundles may be noted, reflecting the presence of the sphenopalatine nerve and associated vessels that normally course through the incisive canal.

Differential Diagnosis. Periapical granuloma and odontogenic cysts of the radicular type must be separated from the nasopalatine canal cyst. This can be done simply by determining tooth vitality. That the canal is normal must also be established. Additionally, primordial cysts resulting from degradation of a mesiod-

ens or supernumerary tooth may potentially present in a similar fashion.

Treatment and Prognosis. The treatment of choice is surgical enucleation. In cases of large cysts, marsupialization may be considered prior to definitive enucleation.

PSEUDOCYSTS

Aneurysmal Bone Cyst

The aneurysmal bone cyst is classified as a pseudocyst because it appears radiographically as a cyst-like lesion but microscopically exhibits no epithelial lining. It represents a benign lesion of bone that may arise in the mandible, maxilla, or other bones. The incidence in the cranial and maxillofacial area is approximately

5% of bone lesions; in all other sites this cyst represents 3% of all bone lesions.

Etiology and Pathogenesis. Although the pathogenesis of the aneurysmal bone cyst is obscure, it is generally regarded as representative of a reactive rather than a neoplastic or cystic process. Frequently, an unrelated antecedent primary lesion of bone exists that is believed to initiate a vascular, presumably arteriovenous malformation, causing significant alteration of hemodynamic forces and resulting in a secondary lesion or aneurysmal bone cyst. The observation is strengthened by reports documenting pre-existing fibrous dysplasia in some cases and central giant cell granuloma in others. Less commonly, the aneurysmal bone cyst may arise in association with a non-ossifying fibroma, chondroblastoma, or central hemangioma.

Clinical Features. The age group in which the aneurysmal bone cyst is typically seen is under 30 years. The peak incidence occurs within the second decade. There is a slight female predilection.

When the mandible and maxilla are involved, the more posterior regions are affected, chiefly the molar areas. Pain is described in approximately half the cases, and a firm non-pulsatile swelling is a frequent clinical sign. On auscultation, a bruit is not heard, and on firm palpation, crepitus may be noted.

Radiographic features include the presence of a destructive or osteolytic process within the mandible and maxilla (Fig. 10–27). A multilocular pattern is noted in some instances, although usually a unilocular radiolucency is found. Slightly irregular margins may be noted in comparison with the smooth margins of a benign cystic process of odontogenic origin. When the alveolar segment of the mandible and maxilla is involved, teeth may be displaced with or without concomitant external root resorption.

Histopathology. A fibrous connective tissue

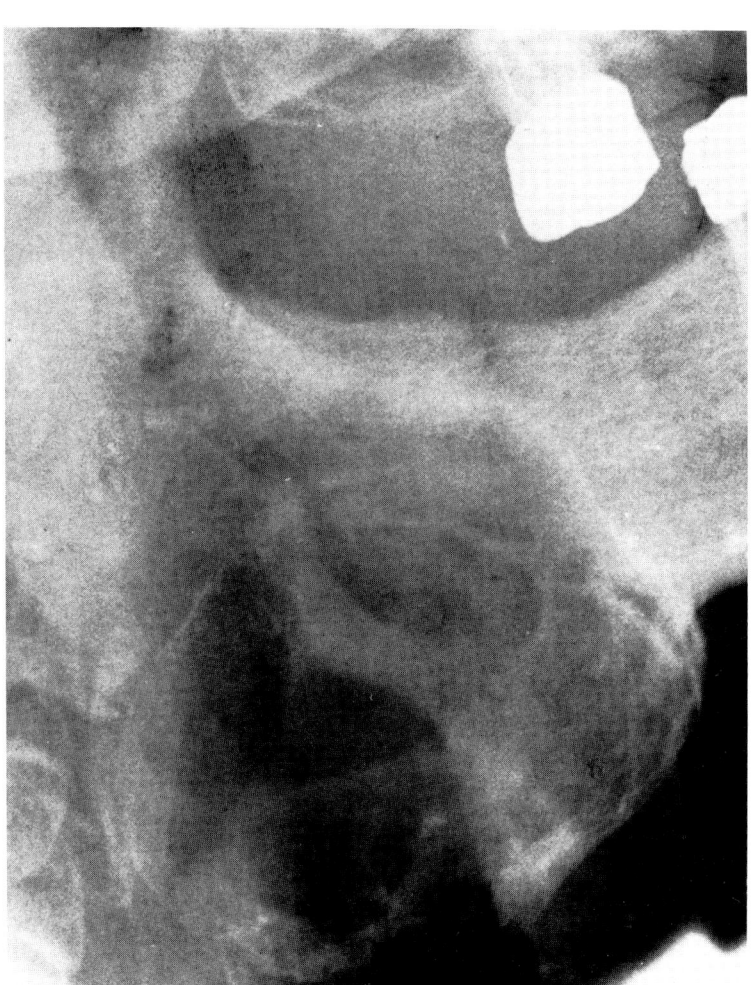

Figure 10–27. Aneurysmal bone cyst located in the angle of the mandible.

stroma containing variable numbers of multinucleated giant cells in relation to sinusoidal blood spaces is noted (Fig. 10–28). That the sinusoidal spaces are not lined by endothelial cells has been confirmed by ultrastructural and immunohistochemical studies. Instead, fibroblasts and macrophages (histiocytes) line the sinusoids. The tissue between the vascular or sinusoidal elements often contains large numbers of multinucleated giant cells, fibroblastic elements, extravasated erythrocytes, and hemosiderin in a pattern reminiscent of central giant cell granuloma. New bone formation akin to that seen in ossifying fibroma or fibrous dysplasia is frequently noted. In some instances, bony arcades are disposed around larger sinusoidal spaces with large amounts of osteoid present. This appears to be a reaction to the vascular proliferation with the bone elements acting apparently in a supportive fashion.

Differential Diagnosis. When the aneurysmal bone cyst is present in the posterior mandible, ameloblastoma is a logical diagnosis to include in a clinical differential, especially in cases with a multilocular appearance. Similarly, the central giant cell granuloma may be impossible to distinguish radiographically. A central vascular lesion must also be excluded, although this may be ruled out upon auscultation since a bruit is often heard. Upon aspiration, brisk bleeding is likely to be encountered in a hemangioma as well.

Treatment and Prognosis. In relatively small lesions, curettage may be attempted, although a high recurrence rate of aneurysmal bone cyst has been associated with this form of management. Adequate curettage of mandibular lesions may necessitate an extraoral approach or supplementation with cryotherapy. Although some cases have been treated by radiotherapy, this is not felt to be appropriate owing to the benign nature of the lesion. Because of the potential for recurrence, follow-up examinations are important.

Traumatic (Simple) Bone Cyst

The traumatic bone cyst lacks an epithelial lining and cannot be classified as a true cyst. The designation of this as a pseudocyst relates to its cystic radiographic appearance and its gross surgical presentation. This lesion is quite uncommon in the mandible and maxilla, but it is relatively frequent in the humerus and other long bones.

Pathogenesis. The pathogenesis of this lesion is not known, although most believe that it is associated with an antecedent traumatic event. Assuming this to be the case, it has been hypothesized that a traumatically induced hematoma forms within the intramedullary portion of bone. Rather than the clot's being organized, it breaks down, leaving an empty cavity within the bone. Secondary to altered or obstructed lymphatic or venous drainage, it has been hypothesized that a steady expansion of the lesion occurs until cortical bone is reached; then expansion stops.

Alternative pathways of development that have been suggested include cystic degeneration of primary tumors of bone, such as central giant cell granuloma, disorders of calcium metabolism, and ischemic necrosis of bone marrow. Of significance is the fact that in one large series, 80% of affected patients provided evidence of prior trauma to the area of involvement.

Clinical Features. A wide age range of from 2.5 to 75 years has been noted, with the peak frequency within the second decade. Most series show a strong predilection for individuals under 40 years of age. An equal gender distribution has been noted.

The most frequent site of occurrence is the mandible, with an equal distribution of cases noted in the body and the ramus region. Rare bilateral cases have been described.

The clinical presentation in approximately one fourth of cases includes swelling. Pain is a presenting symptom in less than 10% of cases.

Radiographically, a well-delineated area of radiolucency with an irregular but defined edge will be noted, usually in the posterior portion of the mandible (Fig. 10–29). Minimal to prominent inter-radicular scalloping may be noted with or without the presence of lamina dura. Of interest is the occasional finding of minimal external root resorption.

In cases of florid osseous dysplasia, there is a disproportionate number of associated traumatic bone cysts. The association between these two entities is not understood. It is interesting to note that there is increased incidence of both entities in black females over 30 years of age.

Histopathology. Often, a gross specimen will be minimal in extent, although at surgery a relatively large cavity is found (Fig. 10–30). Occasionally, the lesion may contain blood or serosanguineous fluid; the lining itself is usually composed of a thin and attenuated fibrous membrane or granulation tissue.

When the soft tissue component is examined, delicate, well-vascularized, fibrous con-

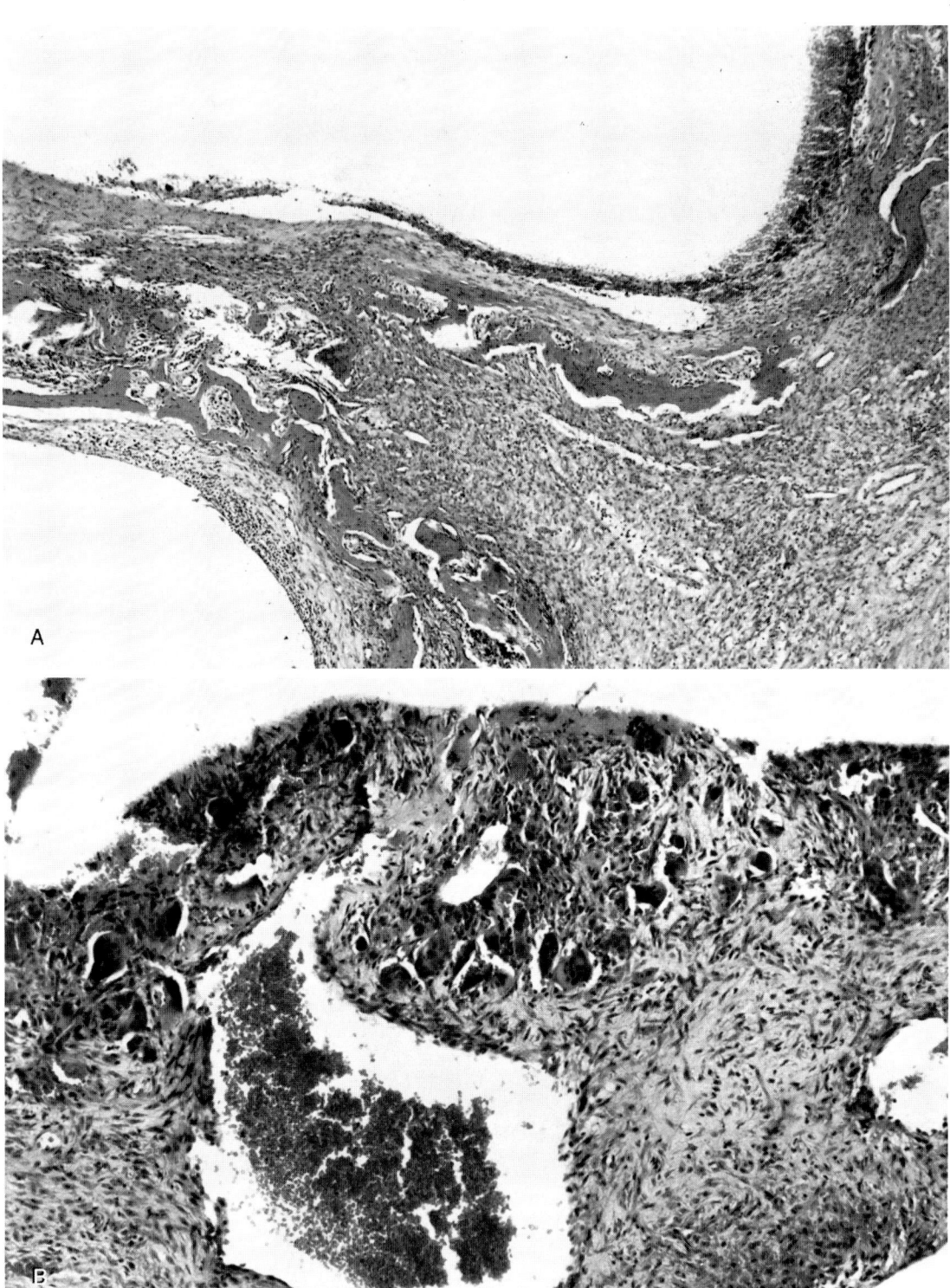

Figure 10–28. *A* and *B*, Aneurysmal bone cysts. Note large sinusoidal blood spaces. Multinucleated giant cells are found in the supporting connective tissue *(B)*.

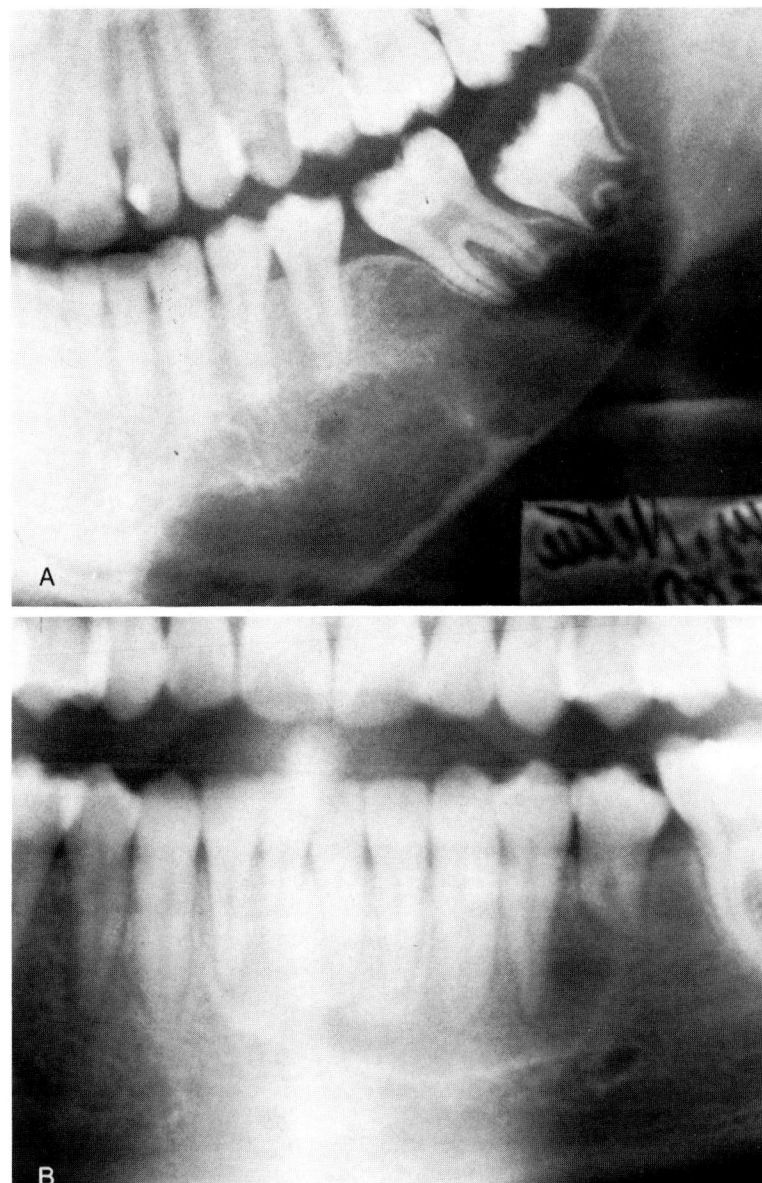

Figure 10–29. *A* and *B*, Traumatic bone cysts.

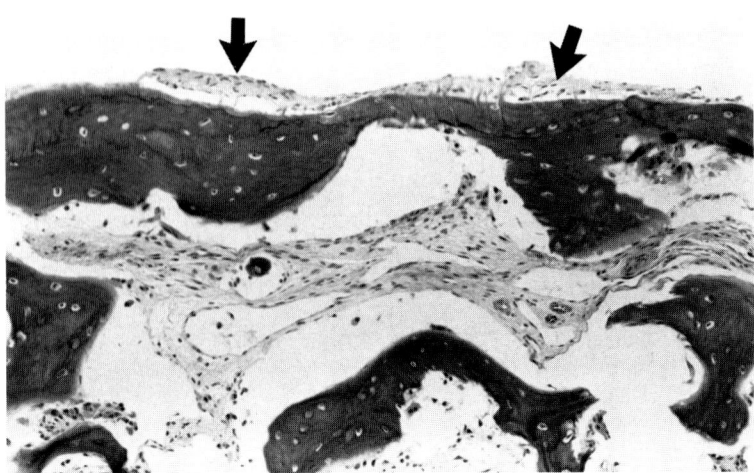

Figure 10–30. Wall of a traumatic bone cyst. Note connective tissue lining the lesion (arrows).

nective tissue without evidence of an epithelial component is identified. Extravasated erythrocytes and hemosiderin may be seen as well as small osteoclast type multinucleated cells.

Treatment and Prognosis. Once entry into the cavity is accomplished, the clinician need merely establish bleeding into the lesion prior to closure. Subsequent to organization of the clot, it is anticipated that bone repair will occur, with little chance of recurrence.

The potential for recurrence in individuals with multiple lesions and in patients with multiple lesions who demonstrated a bluish discoloration of overlying bone at surgery must be emphasized. This discoloration is produced by secondary cortical erosion and therefore indicates an increased level of clinical aggressiveness, conceivably predisposing to higher recurrence rates.

Static Bone Cyst

The static bone cyst represents an entity that appears cystic on radiographic examination but in fact contains no epithelial lining. The actual origin and definition of the process is one of a developmental depression of the mandible secondary to (1) entrapment of salivary gland parenchyma during the development of the mandible, (2) accentuation of a cavity, or (3) indentation along the lingual aspect of the mandible within which there is extension of the submandibular gland. Occasionally, these defects may be noted bilaterally, and rarely, anterior to the first molar region of the mandible.

This lesion is entirely asymptomatic and is often observed incidentally upon extraoral roentgenographic examination. The location and character of the static bone cyst are distinctive and essentially are pathognomonic. When it is observed over time, there is rarely a change in size, hence the term "static." With the use of extraoral panoramic radiographic techniques, the reported frequency of such an entity has increased.

The radiographic presentation is one of a sharply circumscribed radiolucency beneath the level of the inferior alveolar canal, with encroachment on the inferior border of the mandible immediately anterior to the mandibular angle (Fig. 10–31). The lesion is round to oval and sharply circumscribed with a radiopaque margin. Other depressions of the cortical surface of the mandible have been reported, albeit rarely, in association within the parotid gland along the lateral or facial aspect of the mandibular ramus.

Salivary gland inclusion presenting as a static bone cyst has not been reported in the maxilla. Cystic lesions, however, may occur in the anterior portion of the maxilla, which contains salivary gland tissue. This is probably representative of a nasopalatine duct cyst, which contains salivary gland tissue within the cystic wall.

The microscopic examination of material from these defects typically reveals normal submandibular salivary gland tissue. Because the static bone cyst is diagnostic radiographically, biopsy is not necessary. Similarly, no treatment is required.

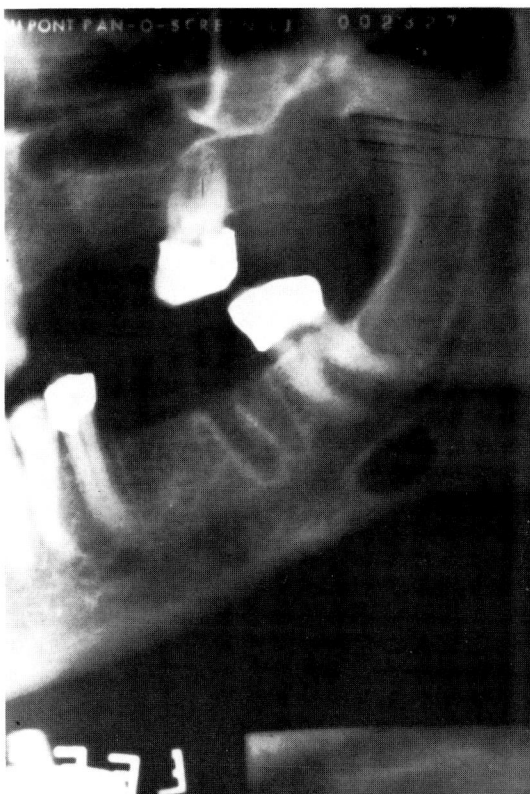

Figure 10–31. Static bone cyst in characteristic location inferior to the mandibular canal.

Focal Osteoporotic Bone Marrow Defect

The focal osteoporotic defect is an uncommon lesion that typically presents as a focal radiolucency in areas away from normal hematopoietic marrow (angle of the mandible and maxillary tuberosity). Approximately 70% occur in the posterior mandible; 70% occur in females.

The pathogenesis of the osteoporotic marrow defect is unknown, although three theories have been proposed. One theory states that tooth extraction in the area and abnormal healing may be responsible. The fact that most lesions are noted within areas of previous extractions supports this theory of aberrant bone regeneration (Fig. 10–32). Another theory states that residual remnants of fetal marrow may persist into adulthood, thus presenting as a focal lucency. The third theory suggests that these defects are actually foci of marrow hyperplasia that are responsive in nature.

Microscopic findings in most cases are those of a cellular hematopoietic marrow with cell to fat ratios greater than 1 to 1. Within the cellular marrow, small lymphoid aggregates may be found as well as megakaryocytes. Bony trabeculae found in biopsy specimens usually show an absence of osteoblastic rimming and osteoclastic activity.

The differential diagnosis should include osteomyelitis, traumatic bone cyst, and ameloblastoma. Owing to the radiographically non-specific findings, most clinicians opt for establishment of a diagnosis by incisional biopsy. Subsequent to this diagnosis, no further management is necessary.

SOFT TISSUE CYSTS OF THE NECK

Branchial Cyst

The branchial (cleft) cyst or cervical lymphoepithelial cyst is located in the lateral portion of the neck, usually anterior to the sternomastoid muscle (Fig. 10–33).

The most widely accepted theory regarding the genesis of the branchial cyst relates to incomplete obliteration of the branchial clefts, arches, and pouches, with remnants of buried epithelial rests ultimately undergoing cystic degeneration. The majority of such cysts arise from either the cervical sinus or the second branchial cleft or pouch. Branchial cysts arising within this area are found deep to the sternomastoid muscle or along its anterior border, usually at the level of or immediately below the angle of the mandible.

An alternative theory of origin has been suggested. This proposes entrapment of epithelium within cervical lymph nodes, with subsequent cystic change. The epithelium is thought to be of salivary origin.

The branchial cyst has an intraoral counterpart known as the *lymphoepithelial cyst*. The floor of the mouth is the most common site for these lesions, followed by the tongue (Fig. 10–34). Rarely, lymphoepithelial cysts have also been reported in the parotid gland. The lesions are generally asymptomatic, and they are discovered incidentally.

Clinical Features. Cysts usually become clinically apparent in late childhood or adulthood with enlargement because of infection or for unknown reasons. In cases of infection, abscesses and draining sinuses may form. Presentation is usually as a small opening with drainage along the anterior margin of the ster-

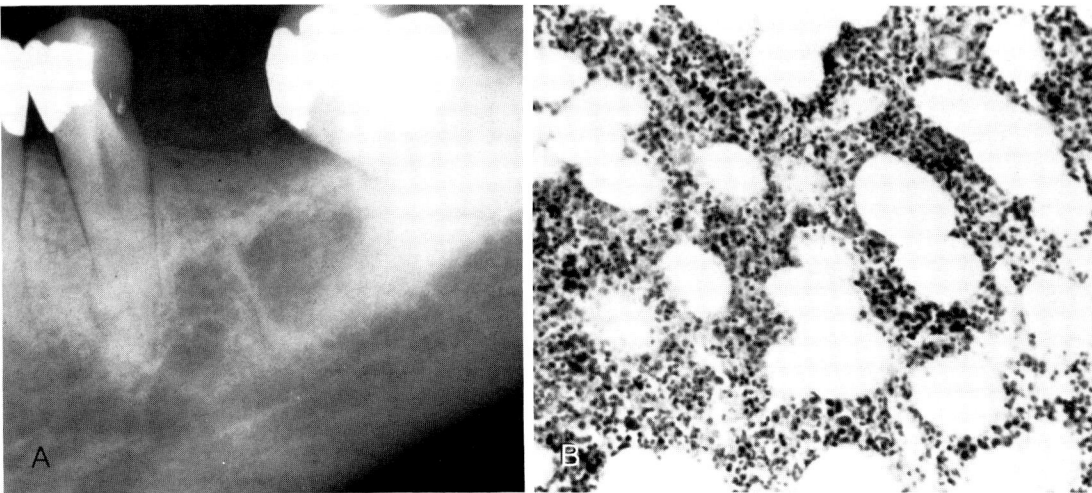

Figure 10–32. *A,* Focal osteoporotic bone marrow defect in edentulous area of the mandible. *B,* Hematopoietic marrow from the defect.

nomastoid muscle. The branchial cyst is one particular manifestation of branchial cleft anomalies. Other branchial arch anomalies may extend into the ear as well as along the anterior and lateral neck regions. Such anomalies may take the form of cysts, sinuses, and fistulas; the second branchial arch is the most commonly involved structure.

The branchial cyst is lined with stratified squamous epithelium or pseudostratified columnar epithelium, or both (Fig. 10–35). The epithelial component is supported by lymphoid aggregates usually demonstrating well-formed germinal centers. The cyst wall is composed of mature fibrous connective tissue, and the contents of the cyst space will vary from serous to gelatinous.

Treatment is surgical excision.

Dermoid Cyst

"Dermoid cyst" is a rather imprecise term that, in effect, refers to cystic lesions that are disorders of development. They may occur in many areas of the body, and when they are found in the oral cavity, are usually in the anterior portion of the floor of the mouth at

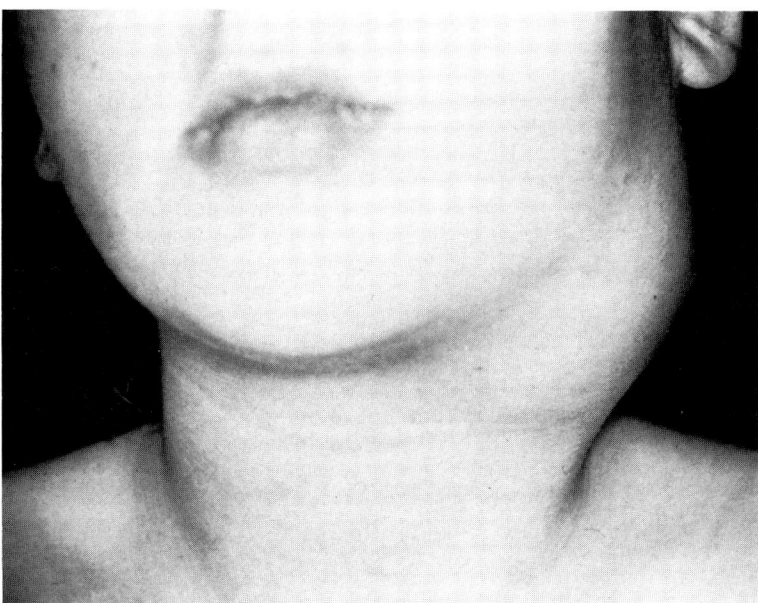

Figure 10–33. Branchial (lymphoepithelial) cyst.

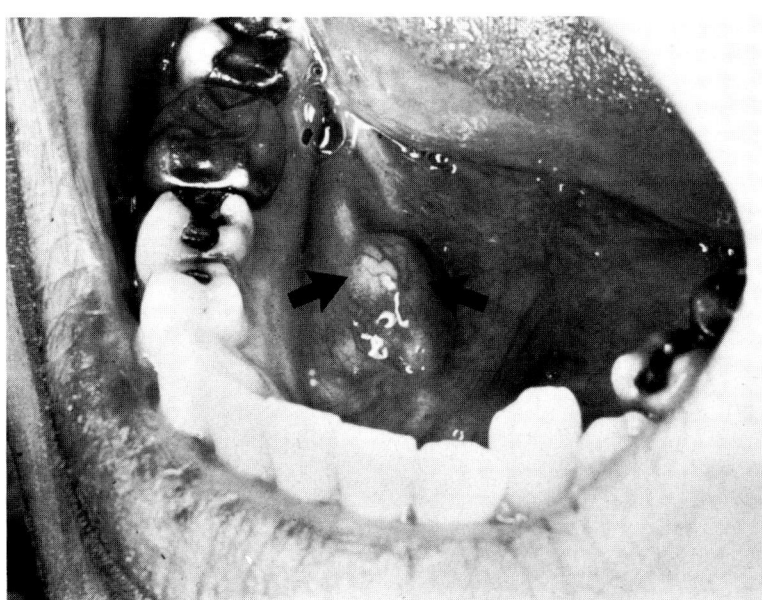

Figure 10–34. Oral lymphoepithelial cyst (arrows).

or on either side of the midline. The overall incidence of this type of cyst in the head and neck is rather low, accounting for less than 2% of all dermoid cysts. The etiology of the dermoid cyst in this area is related either to implantation of epithelium with subsequent cystic breakdown or to developmental entrapment of multipotential cells.

Clinically, these cysts, when located above the mylohyoid muscle, displace the tongue superiorly and posteriorly, with resultant difficulties in function. When they are located below the mylohyoid muscle, a midline swelling of the neck occurs (Fig. 10–36). These cysts are painless and slow growing; there is no gender predilection. Lesions are generally less than 2 cm in diameter; however, extreme examples may range up to 8 cm to 12 cm. On palpation, the cysts are soft to fluctuant, with a pale yellowish-pink color noted beneath the thinned but intact epithelium; when keratin debris and sebum fill the lumen, they may have a doughy consistency on palpation.

Microscopically, this developmental cyst is lined by stratified squamous epithelium supported by a fibrous connective tissue wall. Numerous ectodermal derivatives may be seen including dermal adnexa, such as hair follicles, sebaceous glands, and sweat glands, and occasionally teeth (Fig. 10–37).

Treatment is surgical, and complete excision is required. Most lesions can be removed through the mouth with little risk of recurrence.

Thyroglossal Tract Cyst

The thyroglossal tract cyst is the most common developmental cyst of the neck, accounting for nearly three fourths of such lesions. The basis of this cystic pathology relates to thyroid gland development. The thyroid origin occurs in the fourth week of gestation where derivatives of first and second branchial arches form the posterior portion of the tongue in the region of the foramen caecum. The thyroid anlage grows downward to its permanent location in the neck from what will become the foramen caecum. Between the foramen caecum and the cervical location of the thyroid gland is the embryonic tract of the thyroid tissue. The developing gland passes through the base of the tongue and the hyoid bone to the midneck. By the tenth week of gestation, the tract or duct breaks up or involutes. Residual epithelial elements that do not completely atrophy may give rise to cysts in childhood or adult life that may present in the posterior portion of the tongue (*lingual thyroid*) or in the neck itself.

Approximately 30% of cases are found in patients older than 30 years, with a similar percentage in patients under 10 years. Most cysts occur in the midline, with 60% over the thyrohyoid membrane and only 2% within the tongue itself (Fig. 10–38). The overriding majority (70 to 80%) occur below the level of the hyoid bone. These cysts are generally asymptomatic; when they are attached to the hyoid

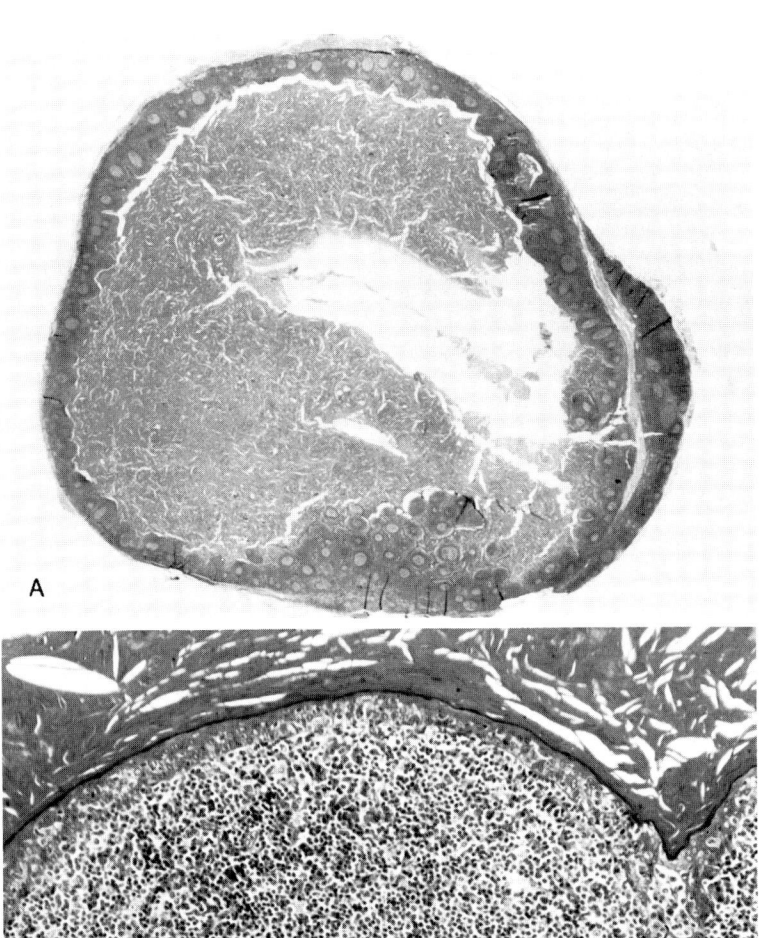

Figure 10–35. *A* and *B*, Branchial cysts. Note lymphoid tissue subjacent to thin epithelial lining.

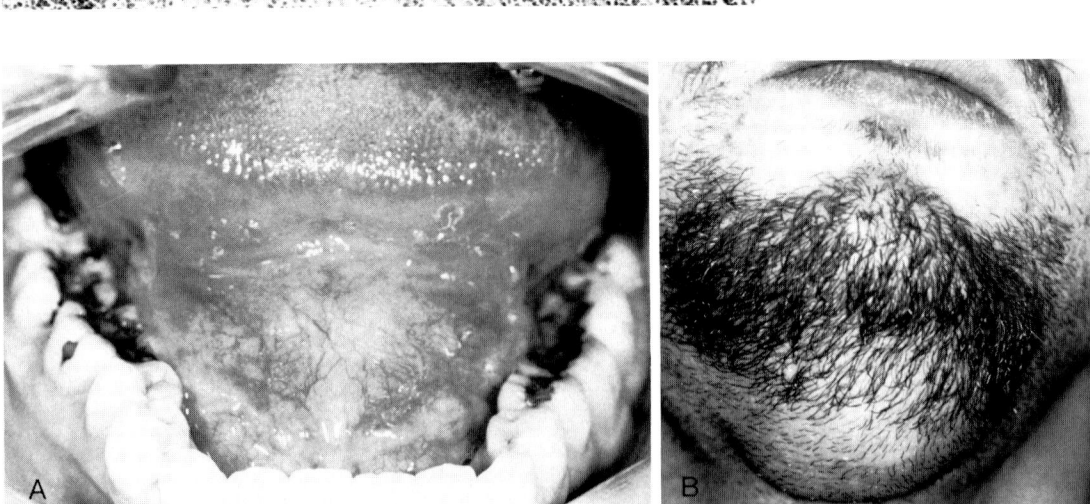

Figure 10–36. *A*, Dermoid cyst presenting in the midline of the floor of the mouth. *B*, Dermoid cysts presenting in the midline of the neck.

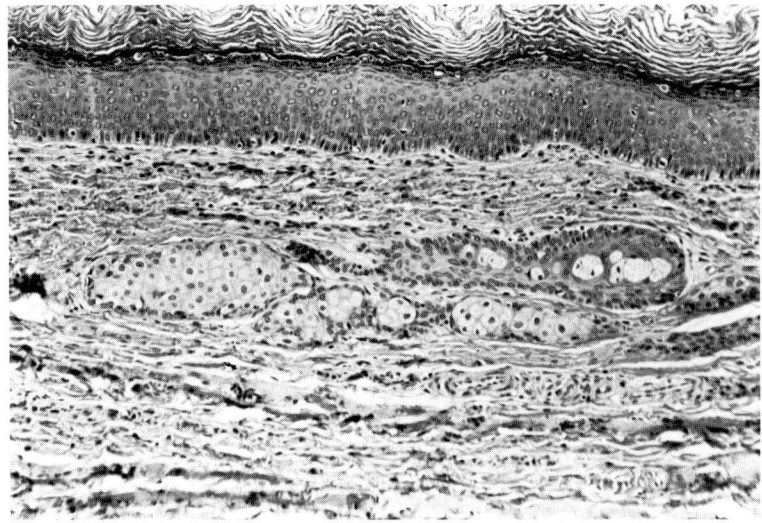

Figure 10–37. Dermoid cyst. Note keratinized epithelium and sebaceous elements in supporting connective tissue.

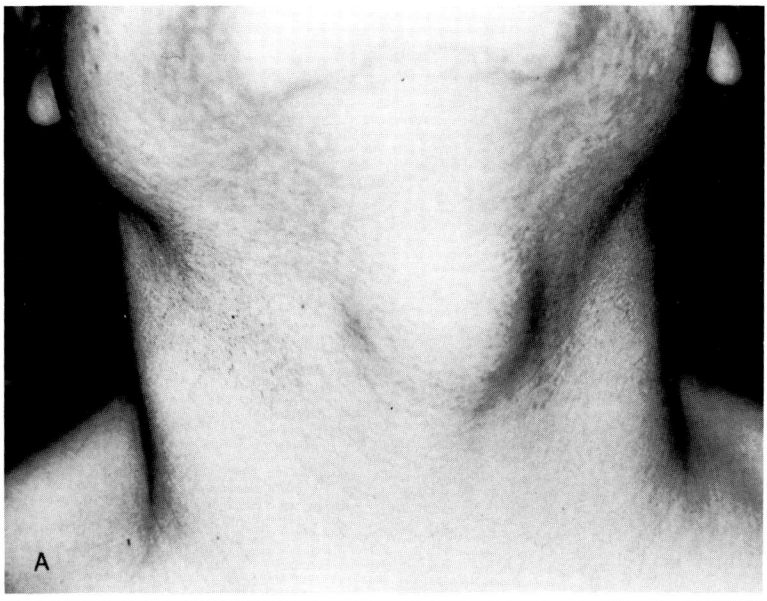

Figure 10–38. *A* and *B*, Thyroglossal tract cysts in the midline of the neck. Cyst in *B* is secondarily infected.

bone and tongue, they may retract on swallowing or extension of the tongue. If they are infected, drainage through a sinus tract may occur.

Microscopic findings vary depending upon the location of the cyst. Lesions occurring above the level of the hyoid bone will demonstrate a lining chiefly of stratified squamous epithelium. A ciliated or columnar type epithelium usually is found in cysts occurring below the hyoid bone (Fig. 10–39). However, wide variation may be seen within a single cyst. Occasionally, thyroid tissue may be seen within the connective tissue wall. Malignancy arising within the thyroglossal tract cyst may occur, usually in the form of papillary adenocarcinoma.

The differential diagnosis of the thyroglossal tract cyst should include a branchial cyst as well as a sebaceous cyst. When a draining lesion is encountered, however, a wider range of entities must be considered, including osteomyelitis or a draining abscess of cutaneous origin.

Treatment is complete surgical excision. It is often recommended that the central portion

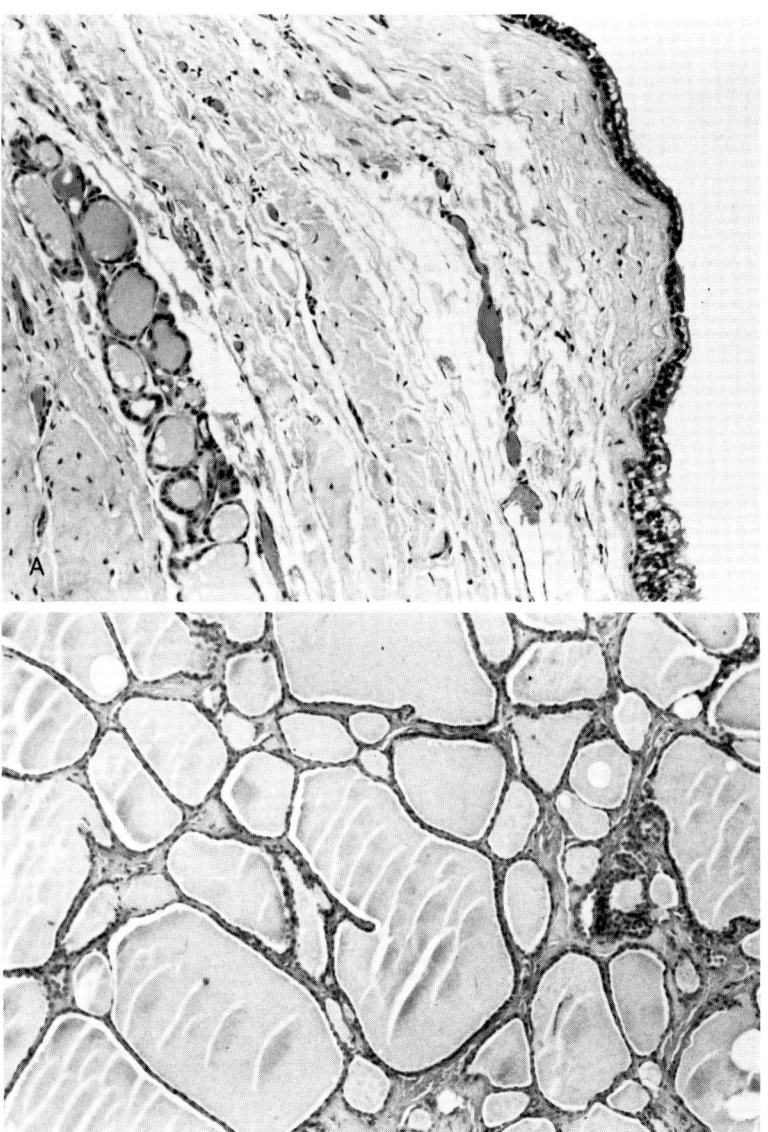

Figure 10–39. *A*, Thyroglossal tract cyst. Note lumen (right) and thyroid acini (left). *B*, Thyroid tissue in a lingual thyroid.

of the hyoid bone be removed in an effort to eliminate any residual thyroglossal tract epithelium and avoid recurrence.

Bibliography

Odontogenic Cysts

Alfors E, Larson A, Sjögren S. The odontogenic keratocyst—a benign cystic tumor? J Oral Maxillofac Surg 42:10–19, 1984.

Al-Talabani NG, and Smith CJ. Experimental dentigerous cysts and enamel hypoplasia: their possible significance in explaining the pathogenesis of dentigerous cysts. J Oral Pathol 9:82–91, 1980.

Barsky SH, and Hanna JB. Extracellular hyaline bodies are basement membrane accumulations. Am J Clin Pathol 87:45–46, 1987.

Brannon RB. The odontogenic keratocyst—a clinicopathologic study of 312 cases. Part I. Clinical features. Oral Surg 42:54–72, 1976.

Brannon RB. The odontogenic keratocyst—a clinicopathologic study of 312 cases. Part II. Histologic features. Oral Surg 43:233–255, 1977.

Buchner A, and Hansen LS. The histomorphologic spectrum of the gingival cyst in the adult. Oral Surg 48:532–539, 1979.

Fantasia JE. Lateral periodontal cyst. An analysis of 46 cases. Oral Surg 48:237–243, 1979.

Fejerskov O, Krogh J. The calcifying ghost cell odontogenic tumor—or the calcifying odontogenic cyst. J Oral Pathol 1:273–287, 1972.

Freedman PD, Lumerman H, Gee JK. Calcifying odontogenic cyst. Oral Surg 40:93–106, 1975.

Gardner DG, Sapp JP, Wysocki GP. Odontogenic and fissural cysts of the jaws. Pathol Annu 13:177–200, 1978.

Gold L. The keratinizing and calcifying odontogenic cyst. Oral Surg 16:1414–1424, 1963.

Gorlin RJ, Pindborg JJ, Redman RS, et al. The calcifying odontogenic cyst. A new entity and possible analogue of the cutaneous calcifying epithelioma of Malherbe. Cancer 17:723–729, 1964.

Killey HC, Kay LW, Seward GR. Benign Cystic Lesions of the Jaws, Their Diagnosis and Treatment. 3rd ed. Churchill-Livingstone, Edinburgh, 1977.

Main DMG. Epithelial jaw cysts: a clinicopathologic reappraisal. Br J Oral Surg 8:114–125, 1970.

Main DMG. Epithelial jaw cysts: ten years of the WHO classification. J Oral Pathol 14:1–7, 1985.

Partridge M, and Towers JF. The primordial cyst (odontogenic keratocyst): its tumor-like characteristics and behavior. Br J Oral Maxillofac Surg 25:271–279, 1987.

Praetorius F, Hjørting-Hansen E, Gorlin RJ, et al. Calcifying odontogenic cyst. Range, variations, and neoplastic potential. Acta Odontol Scand 39:227–240, 1981.

Shear M. Cysts of the Oral Regions. 2nd ed. John Wright & Sons, Bristol, Eng, 1983, pp 114–141.

Shear M. Cysts of the jaws: recent advances. J Pathol 14:43–59, 1985.

Skaug N. Intracystic fluid pressure in non-keratinizing jaw cysts. Int J Oral Surg 5:59–65, 1976.

Skaug N. Soluble proteins in fluid from non-keratinizing jaw cysts in man. Int J Oral Surg 6:107–121, 1977.

Stoelinga PJW. Studies on the dental lamina as related to its role in the etiology of cysts and tumors. J Oral Pathol 5:65–73, 1976.

Stoelinga PJW, Cohen MM, Morgan AF. The origin of keratocysts in the basal cell nevus syndrome. Int J Oral Surg 33:659–663, 1973.

Struthers PJ, and Shear M. Root resorption produced by enlargement of ameloblastomas and cysts of the jaws. Int J Oral Surg 5:128–132, 1976.

Torabinejad M, Bakland LK. Immunopathogenesis of chronic periapical lesions. Oral Surg Oral Med Oral Pathol 46:685–699, 1978.

Torabinejad M, Kettering J D: Detection of immune complexes in human dental periapical lesions by anticomplement immunofluorescence technique. Oral Surg 48:256–261, 1979.

Weathers DR, Waldron CA. Unusual multilocular cysts of the jaws (botryoid odontogenic cysts). Oral Surg 36:235–241, 1973.

Wright JM. The odontogenic keratocyst: orthokeratinized variant. Oral Surg 51:609–618, 1981.

Wysocki GP, Brannon RB, Gardner DG, et al. Histogenesis of the lateral periodontal cyst and the gingival cyst of the adult. Oral Surg 50:327–334, 1980.

Non-odontogenic Cysts

Browne RU. Metaplasia and degeneration in odontogenic cysts in man. J Oral Pathol 1:145–148, 1972.

Buchner A, and Ramon Y. Median mandibular cyst—a rare lesion of debatable origin. Oral Surg 37:431–437, 1974.

Chamda RA, Shear M. Dimensions of incisive fossae on dry skulls and radiographs. J Oral Pathol 9:452–457, 1980.

Christ TF. The globulomaxillary cyst—an embryologic misconception. Oral Surg 30:515–526, 1970.

DiFiore PM, Hartwell GR. Median mandibular lateral periodontal cysts. Oral Surg Oral Med Oral Pathol 63:545–550, 1987.

Gardner DG. An evaluation of reported cases of median mandibular cysts. Oral Surg Oral Med Oral Pathol 65:208–213, 1988.

Killey AC, Kay LW, Seward GR. Benign Cystic Lesions of the Jaws, their Diagnosis and Treatment. 3rd ed. Churchill-Livingstone, Edinburgh, 1977.

Main DMG. The enlargement of epithelial jaw cysts. Odont Rev 21:29–49, 1970.

Tenca JI, Guinta JL, Norris LH. The median mandibular cyst and its endodontic significance. Oral Surg Oral Med Oral Pathol 60:316–321, 1985.

Ten Cate AR. Oral Histology: Development, Structure, and Function. CV Mosby Co, St. Louis, 1980, pp 22–25.

Wysocki GP. The differential diagnosis of globulomaxillary radiolucencies. Oral Surg 51:281–286, 1981.

Zegarelli DJ, Zegarelli EV. Radiolucent lesions in the globulomaxillary region. J Oral Surg 31:767–771, 1973.

Pseudocysts

Alles JU, Schulz A. Immunocytochemical markers (endothelial and histiocystic) and ultrastructure of primary aneurysmal bone cysts. Hum Pathol 17:39–45, 1986.

Barker GR. A radiolucency of the ascending ramus of the mandible associated with invested parotid salivary gland material and analogous with a Stafne bone cavity. Br J Oral Maxillofac Surg 26:81–84, 1988.

Biesecker JL, Marcove RC, Huvos AG, Mike V. Aneurysmal bone cysts. A clinicopathological study of 66 cases. Cancer 26:615–625, 1970.

Correll RW, Jensen JL, Rhyne RR. Lingual cortical mandibular defects: a radiographic incidence study. Oral Surg Oral Med Oral Pathol 50:287–291, 1980.

Eisenbud LE, Attie JN, Gaslick J, et al. Aneurysmal bone cyst of the mandible. Oral Surg Oral Med Oral Pathol 64:202–206, 1987.

Feinberg SE, Finkelstein MW, Page HL, et al. Recurrent "traumatic" bone cysts of the mandible. Oral Surg Oral Med Oral Pathol 57:418–422, 1984.

Gorab GN, Brahney C, Aria AA. Unusual presentation of a Stafne bone cyst. Oral Surg Oral Med Oral Pathol 61:213–220, 1986.

Hanson LS, Sapone J, Sproat RC. Traumatic bone cysts of jaws. Oral Surg 37:899–910, 1974.

Kaugars GE, Cale AE. Traumatic bone cyst. Oral Surg Oral Med Oral Pathol 63:318–324, 1987.

Moule I. Unilateral multiple solitary bone cysts. J Oral Maxillofac Surg 46:320–323, 1988.

Ruiter DJ, van Rijssel TG, van der Velde EA. Aneurysmal bone cysts. A clinicopathological study of 105 cases. Cancer 39:2231–2239, 1977.

Struthers PJ, Shear M. Aneurysmal bone cyst of the jaws. I. Clinicopathologic features. Int J Oral Surg 13:85–91, 1984.

Struthers PJ, Shear M. Aneurysmal bone cyst of the jaws. II. Pathogenesis. Int J Oral Surg 13:92–100, 1984.

Soft Tissue Cysts of the Neck

Bhaskar SN, Bernier JL. Histogenesis of branchial cysts. Am J Pathol 35:407–423, 1959.

Buchner A, Hansen LS. Lymphoepithelial cysts of the oral cavity. A clinicopathologic study of 38 cases. Oral Surg 50:441–449, 1980.

Himalstein MR. Correlation of surgical anatomy and embryology in lateral cervical anomalies. Trans Am Acad Ophthalol Otolaryngol 75:974–982, 1971.

Work WP. New concepts of first branchial cleft defects. Laryngoscope 82:1581–1593, 1972.

Chapter 11

Odontogenic Tumors

EPITHELIAL TUMORS
Ameloblastoma
Squamous Odontogenic Tumor
Calcifying Epithelial Odontogenic Tumor (CEOT)
Clear Cell Odontogenic Tumor
Adenomatoid Odontogenic Tumor (AOT)
MESENCHYMAL TUMORS
Odontogenic Myxoma
Central Odontogenic Fibroma
Cementifying Fibroma
Cementoblastoma
Periapical Cemental Dysplasia
MIXED (EPITHELIAL AND MESENCHYMAL) TUMORS
Odontoma
Ameloblastic Fibroma and Ameloblastic Fibro-odontoma

Odontogenic tumors are lesions derived from epithelial or mesenchymal elements, or both, that are part of the tooth-forming apparatus. They are therefore found exclusively in the mandible and maxilla (and gingiva on rare occasions) and must be considered in differential diagnoses of lesions involving these sites.

For the group, etiology and pathogenesis are totally obscure—no cause or stimulus has been elucidated. Clinically, odontogenic tumors are typically asymptomatic, but they may cause jaw expansion, movement of teeth, and bone loss. Knowledge of typical basic features such as age, location, and radiographic appearance of the various odontogenic tumors can be extremely valuable in developing a differential diagnosis (Table 11–1).

Like neoplasms elsewhere in the body, odontogenic tumors tend to mimic microscopically the cell or tissue of origin. Histologically, they may resemble soft tissues of the enamel organ or dental pulp, or they may contain hard tissue elements of enamel, dentin, or cementum, or a mixture or composite of these.

Lesions in this group range from hamartomatous proliferations to malignant neoplasms with metastatic capabilities. An understanding of the biologic behavior of the various odontogenic tumors is of fundamental importance to the overall treatment of patients.

Several histologic classifications have been devised to help comprehend this complex group of lesions. Common to all schemes is the division of tumors into those that are composed of odontogenic epithelial elements, those that are composed of odontogenic mesenchyme, and those that are proliferations of both epithelial and mesenchymal tissues. A vast array of microscopic types of odontogenic lesions have been reported. However, many represent histologic variants of one of the major tumor groups. Since these variants are not biologically different, recognition as separate entities is cumbersome and unimportant. In the classification used in this chapter, histologic variants are discussed briefly under major entities.

EPITHELIAL TUMORS

Ameloblastoma

Historically, this lesion has been known for many years, with reports dating back to the early nineteenth century. Its persistent local growth in the maxillofacial area and its ability to produce marked deformity before leading to serious debilitation probably account for its early recognition and numerous subsequent reports. Recurrence, especially after conservative treatment, has also contributed to the awareness of this lesion. Ever since the ame-

Table 11-1. TYPICAL CLINICAL FEATURES OF MAJOR ODONTOGENIC TUMORS

Tumor	Mean Age	Usual Location	Radiograph
Ameloblastoma	40 years	Molar-ramus, mandible	Lucent, frequently multilocular
Calcifying Epithelial Odontogenic Tumor	40 years	Molar-ramus, mandible	Lucent or with opaque foci
Adenomatoid Odontogenic Tumor	18 years	Anterior jaws	Lucent or with opaque foci
Myxoma	30 years	Any region	Lucent, often multilocular
Cementifying fibroma	40 years	Mandible	Lucent or with opaque foci
Cementoblastoma	25 years	Posterior mandible	Opaque
Periapical cemental dysplasia	40 years	Anterior mandible	Lucent to mixed to opaque
Odontoma	18 years	Any region	Opaque
Ameloblastic fibroma and fibro-odontoma	12 years	Molar-ramus, mandible	Lucent or with opaque focus

loblastoma was appreciated for its locally aggressive behavior, recurrence rate, and slight metastatic potential, controversy has centered around the most appropriate form of treatment. As clinical pathologic subtypes have been better defined, a rational basis for treatment has developed that provides an optimal cure rate with minimal patient morbidity.

This neoplasm originates within the mandible or maxilla from epithelium that is involved in the formation of teeth. Potential epithelial sources include enamel organ, odontogenic rests (rests of Malassez, rests of Serres), reduced enamel epithelium, and the epithelial lining of odontogenic cysts, especially the dentigerous cyst. The trigger or stimulus for neoplastic transformation of these otherwise trivial epithelial structures is totally unknown.

Clinical Features. This is a lesion of adults that occurs predominantly in the fourth and fifth decades (Figs. 11-1 to 11-3). The age range is very broad, extending from childhood to late adulthood. Mean ages have been most commonly between 35 and 45 years. The rare lesions occurring in children are typically unicystic and appear clinically as odontogenic cysts. There appears to be no gender predilection for this tumor.

Ameloblastomas may occur anywhere in the mandible or maxilla, although the mandibular molar-ramus area is the most favored site (Fig. 11-4). In the maxilla, the molar area is more

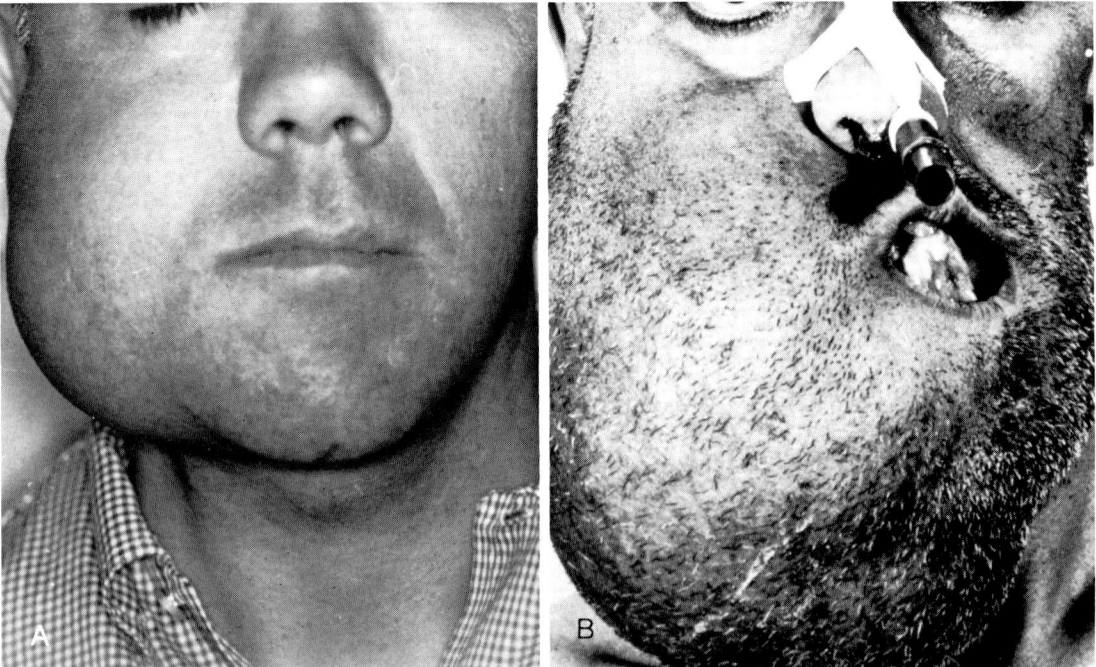

Figure 11-1. *A*, Ameloblastoma of the mandible (patient refused treatment). *B*, Same patient 7 years later.

Figure 11-2. *A*, Intraoral view of patient in Figure 11-1 showing movement of teeth and filling of vestibule. *B*, Lateral jaw radiogram showing multilocular radiolucency *(arrows)*.

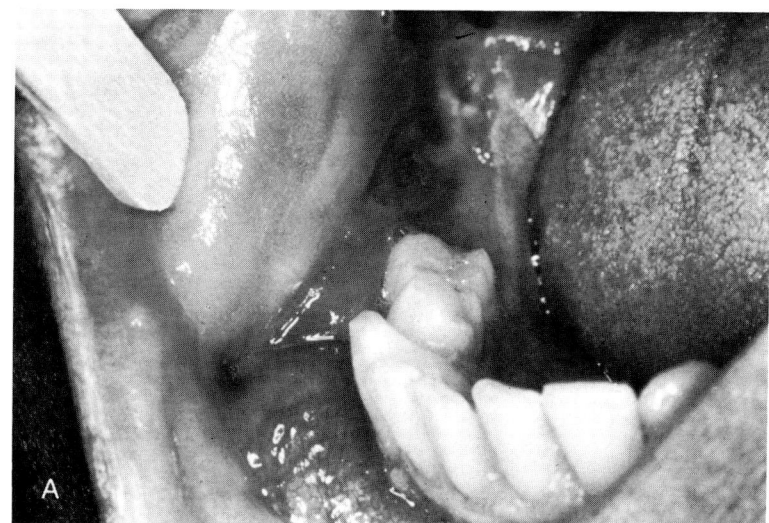
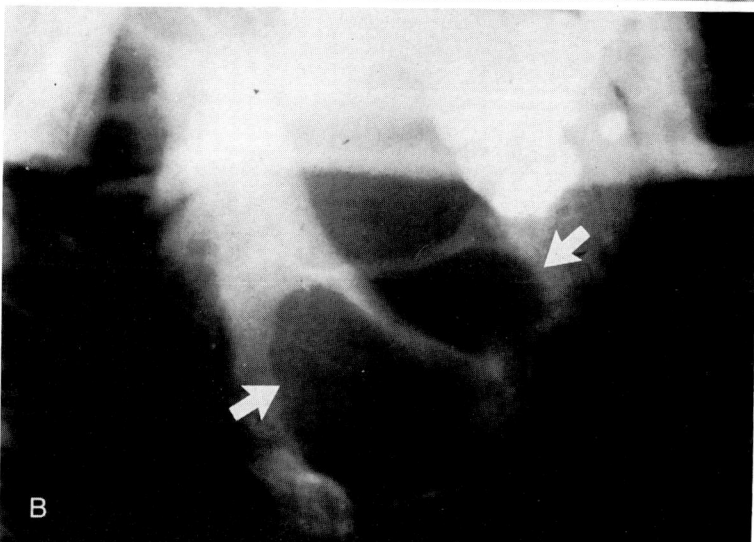

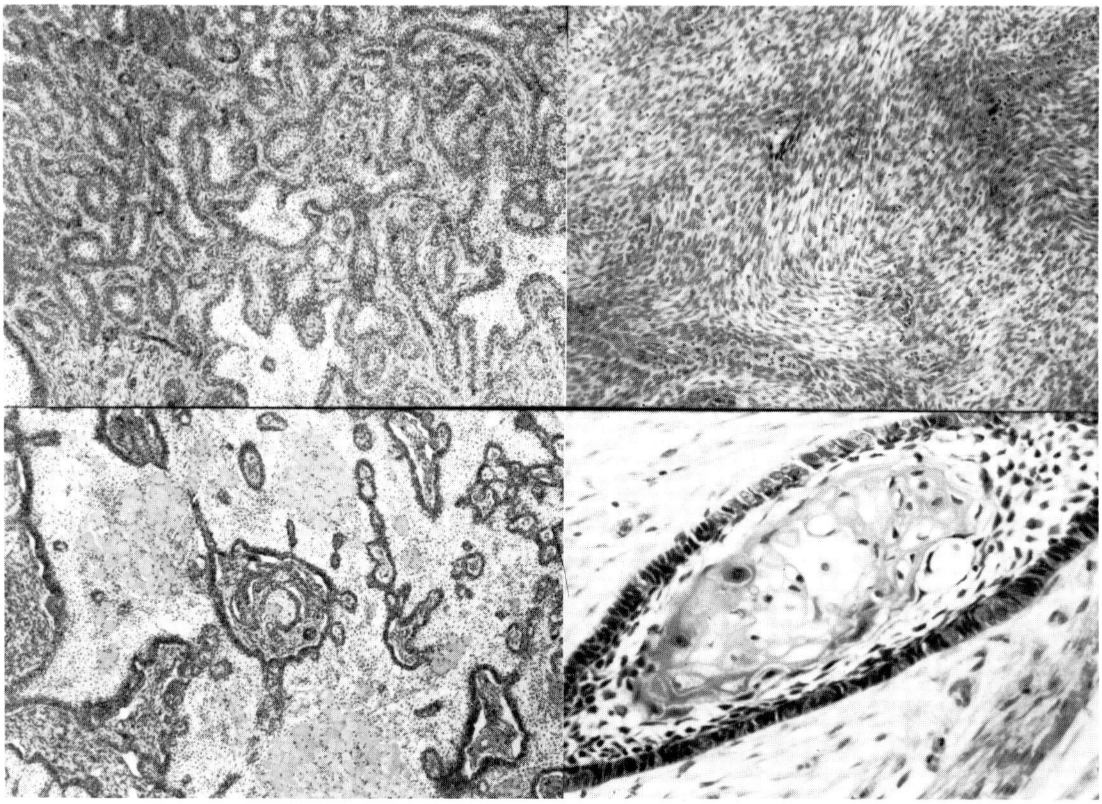

Figure 11-3. Microscopy of ameloblastoma from patient in Figure 11-1B. *Upper left,* Follicular pattern. *Upper right,* Spindle pattern. *Lower left,* Granular cell change. *Lower right,* Keratinization of tumor island.

commonly affected than are the premolar or anterior regions. Rarely, *extraosseous peripheral ameloblastomas* are found in the gingiva. These are seen in older adults, usually between 40 and 60 years of age. They arise from overlying epithelium and exhibit a benign nonaggressive course. Peripheral lesions generally do not invade underlying bone, and they recur infrequently. Ameloblastomas are usually asymptomatic and are discovered either during routine radiographic examination or because of asymptomatic jaw expansion. Occasional tooth movement or malocclusion may be the initial presenting sign.

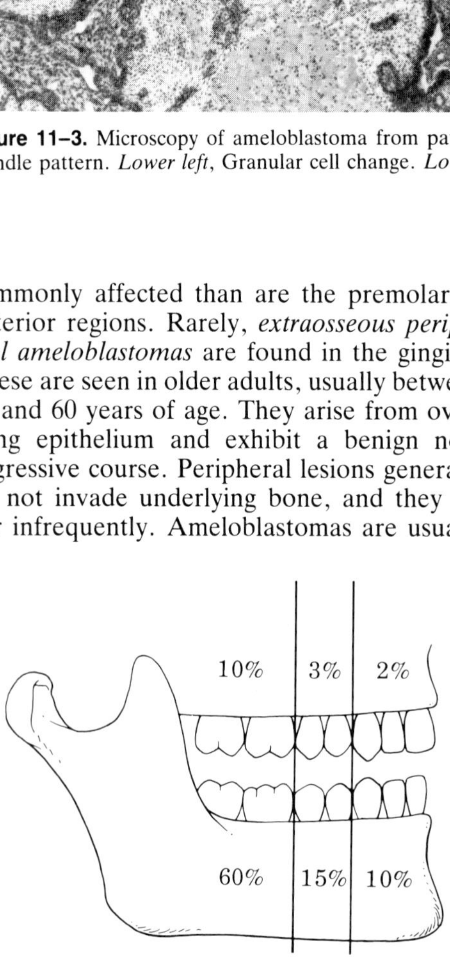

Radiographically, ameloblastomas appear as osteolytic processes (Fig. 11-5). These tumors, typically found in the tooth-bearing areas of the jaws, may exhibit a unilocular or multilocular appearance (Fig. 11-6). Because ameloblastomas are slow growing, the radiographic margins are usually well defined and sclerotic. In cases in which connective tissue desmoplasia occurs in conjunction with tumor proliferation, ill-defined radiographic margins are typically seen (this variety also has a predilection for the anterior jaws). The generally slow tumor growth rate is also responsible for the movement of tooth roots. Root resorption may appear in association with ameloblastoma growth, but this is an uncommon phenomenon.

Histopathology. Numerous histologic patterns have been described in ameloblastomas. Some may exhibit a single histologic subtype; others may display several histologic patterns

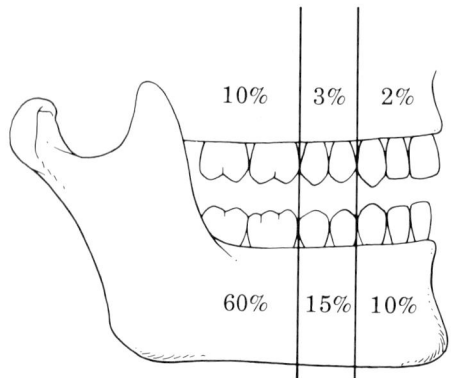

Figure 11-4. Approximate regional distribution of ameloblastomas.

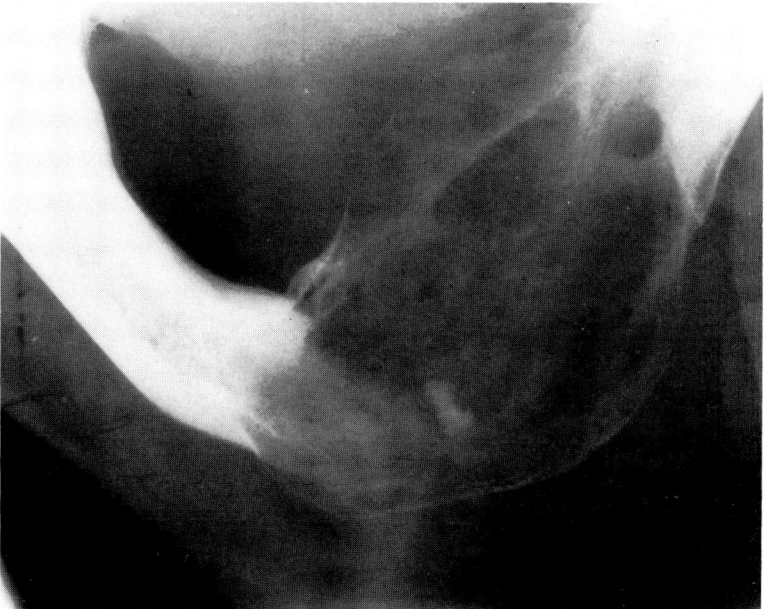

Figure 11–5. Ameloblastoma of the anterior mandible.

within the same lesion. Common to all subtypes is the polarization of cells around the proliferating nests in a pattern similar to ameloblasts of the enamel organ. Central to these cells are loosely arranged cells that mimic the stellate reticulum of the enamel organ. Another typical feature is the budding of tumor cells from neoplastic foci in a pattern reminiscent of tooth development.

The microscopic subtype most commonly seen is the follicular type (Fig. 11–7). It is composed of islands of tumor cells that mimic the normal dental follicle. Central cystic degeneration of the follicular islands leads to a pattern with the name *cystic ameloblastoma* (Fig. 11–8). Occasionally, the neoplastic cells develop into a network of epithelium, prompting the term *plexiform ameloblastoma*. When the central portions of the tumor islands become squamoid or elongated, the adjectives *acanthomatous* and *spindle* are sometimes used to modify the term ameloblastoma. Some tumors exhibit a pattern that is microscopically similar to basal cell carcinoma of the skin; these are *basal cell ameloblastomas*.

A subtype in which the central neoplastic cells exhibit prominent cytoplasmic granularity has been designated *granular cell ameloblastoma* (Fig. 11–9). Although one report suggested that this subtype of ameloblastoma may be more aggressive and may have a higher recurrence rate, this has not been substanti-

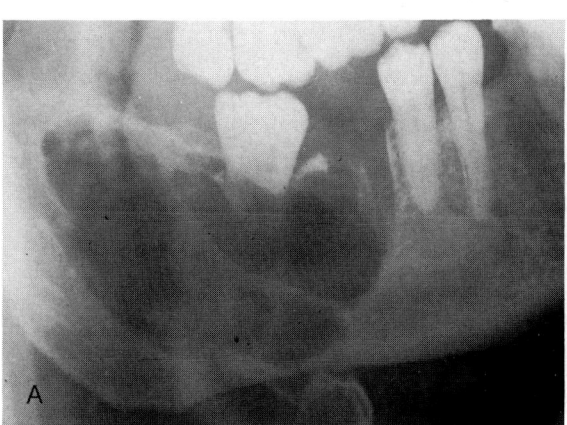 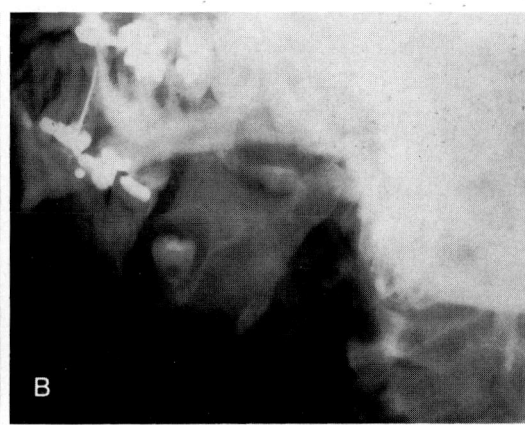

Figure 11–6. *A*, Ameloblastoma of molar-ramus area. *B*, Ameloblastoma in wall of a dentigerous cyst.

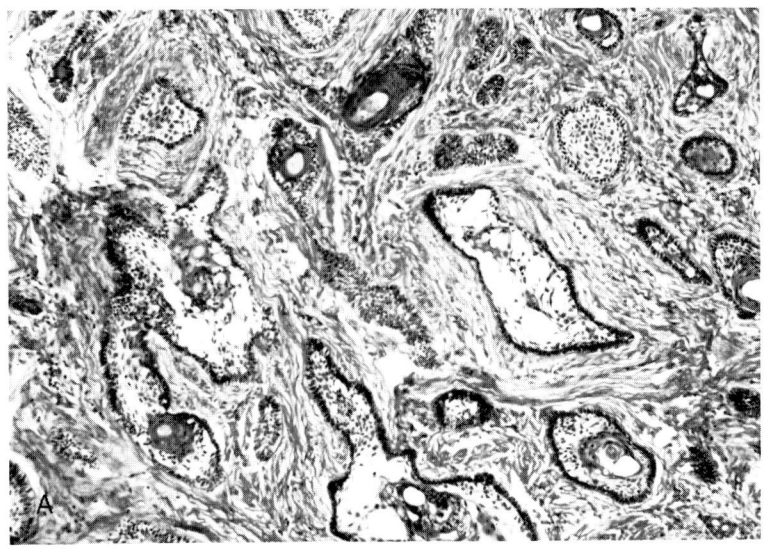
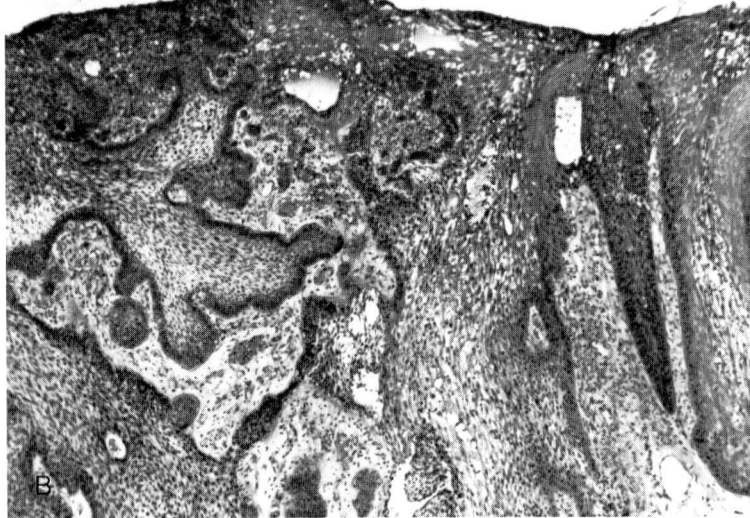

Figure 11–7. *A*, Ameloblastoma, follicular type. *B*, Peripheral (gingival) ameloblastoma.

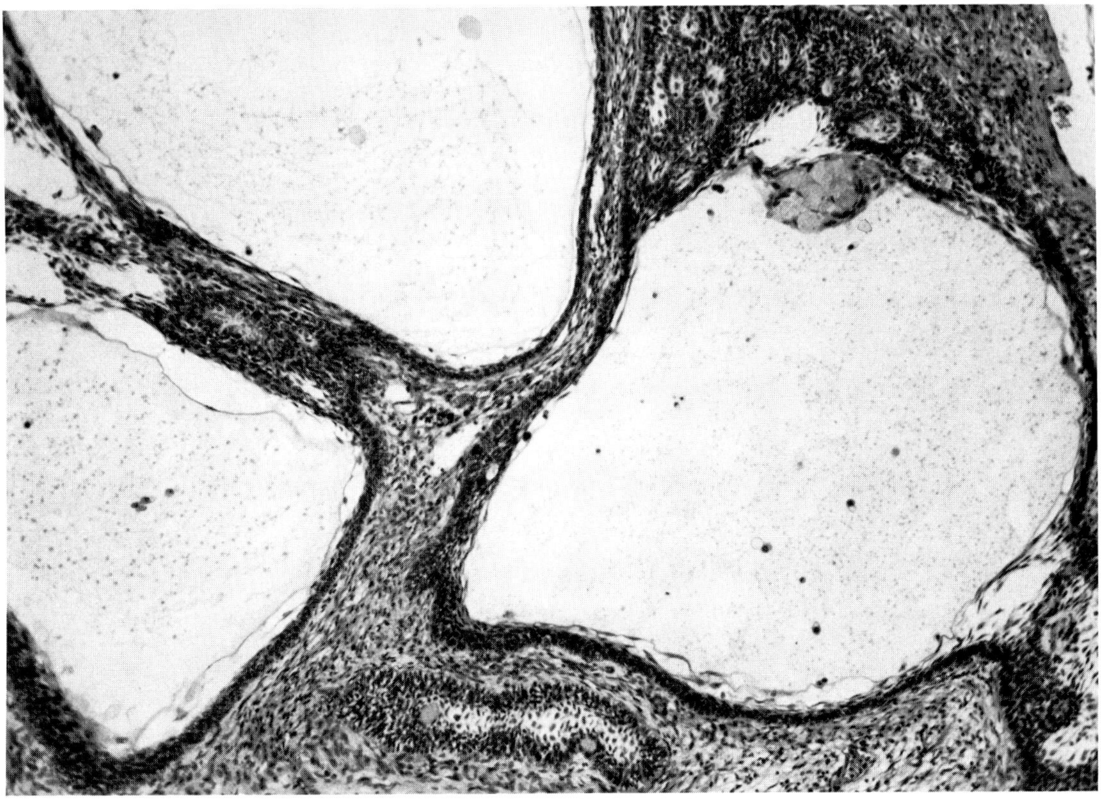

Figure 11-8. Ameloblastoma with cystic change.

Figure 11-9. Ameloblastoma with granular cells.

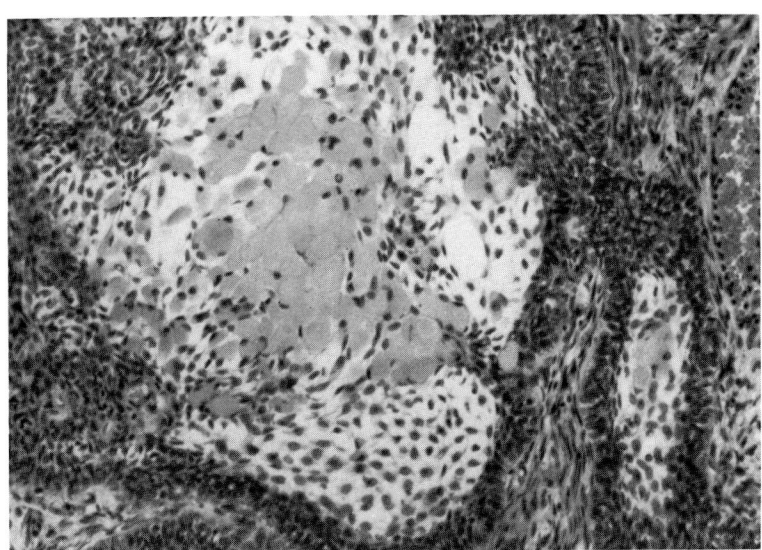

ated. Optically clear tumor cells and cells expressing "ghost cell" type keratinization have also been seen in ameloblastomas (Fig. 11–10); the significance of this remains to be determined. Separation of ameloblastomas into the various microscopic groups described is essentially an academic exercise, since there appears to be no correlation between clinical behavior and these microscopic patterns.

Ameloblastomas have been subdivided into two biologic-microscopic subtypes—*solid* or *multicystic* and *unicystic*. There is significant justification for such subdivision, because treatment and prognosis differ markedly. The solid or multicystic ameloblastoma, which may exhibit any or all of the microscopic patterns discussed, is more aggressive and requires more extensive treatment than its unicystic counterpart. It also has a relatively high recurrence rate (50 to 90%) if treated with curettage.

The unicystic lesion, in contrast, is an ameloblastoma that has a single cystic space in which there is intraluminal or mural growth. It may represent an ameloblastoma that is unilocular, or it may represent an odontogenic cyst in which there has been ameloblastic transformation of the epithelial lining. A histologic variant of this type is the *plexiform unicystic ameloblastoma* in which the cyst wall exhibits an epithelial network of ameloblastic proliferation (Fig. 11–11). Uncystic ameloblastoma is seen in a younger age group (second to third decades) and typically in the mandibular molar area. It has a recurrence rate of less than 10% when curettage is the primary form of treatment. Diagnosis is usually retrospective after enucleation for what appeared clinically as an

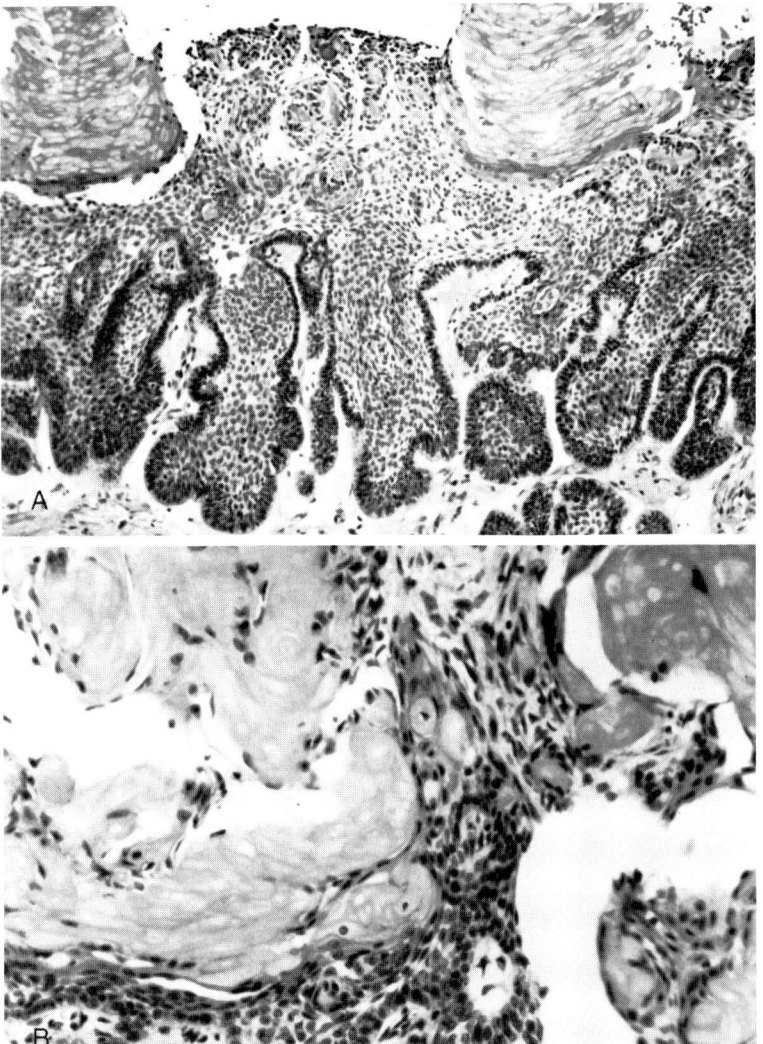

Figure 11–10. *A* and *B*, Ameloblastoma with "ghost cell" type of keratinization.

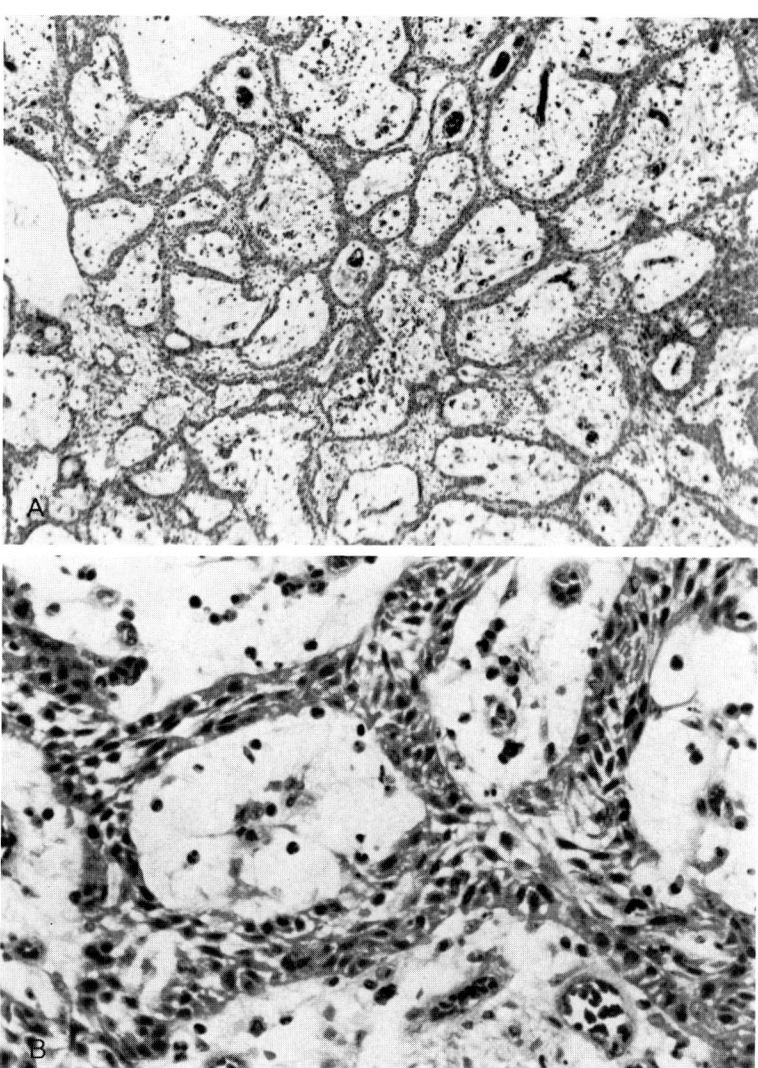

Figure 11–11. *A* and *B*, Plexiform unicystic ameloblastoma.

odontogenic cyst. No additional treatment is required after enucleation or curettage, although follow-up is indicated.

Differential Diagnosis. When considering age, location, and radiographic features together, the clinical differential diagnosis can generally be limited to several entities in the three categories of jaw disease—odontogenic tumors, cysts, and benign non-odontogenic lesions. Among the odontogenic tumors, the calcifying epithelial odontogenic tumor (CEOT) (radiolucent variety) and odontogenic myxomas are prime considerations. The dentigerous cyst and the odontogenic keratocyst can also be included. In relatively young individuals, lesions that are radiographically similar to ameloblastoma include non-odontogenic lesions such as central giant cell granuloma, ossifying fibroma, central hemangioma, and possibly idiopathic histiocytosis.

Microscopically, some ameloblastomas, especially the plexiform unicystic and multicystic lesions, may be confused with odontogenic cysts in which there is hyperplasia of the lining. In the ameloblastoma, basal cell palisading is evident, and inflammatory cells are usually scant. Maxillary ameloblastomas occasionally appear less differentiated, requiring separation from adenocarcinomas and squamous cell carcinomas of maxillary sinus origin (Fig. 11–12).

Treatment and Prognosis. No single standard type of therapy should be advocated for patients with ameloblastoma. Rather, each case should be judged on its own merits. Of prime consideration is whether the lesion is a solid-multicystic, unicystic, or extraosseous le-

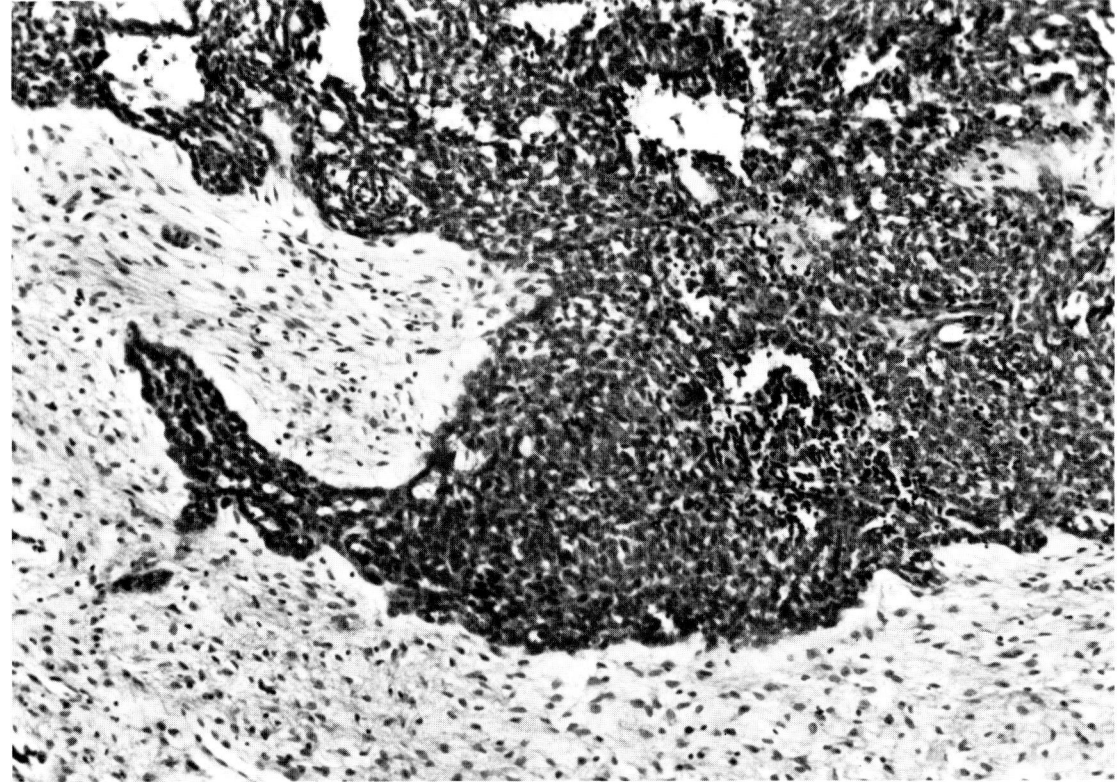

Figure 11-12. Maxillary ameloblastoma.

sion. The solid-multicystic lesions require at least surgical excision, since recurrence follows curettage in 50 to 90% of cases. Block excision or resection should generally be reserved for larger lesions. Unicystic lesions, especially the smaller ones, require only enucleation and should not be overtreated. Peripheral amelo-blas-tomas should also be treated in a similar conservative fashion.

Radiotherapy has been used to a very limited extent in the treatment of ameloblastomas, because it is generally felt that these tumors are radioresistant. There has been some evidence, however, that radiation levels of 4500 rad may produce significant therapeutic results. Until more is known about tumor responsiveness, radiation should be used in the exceptional case in which surgery may be unacceptably destructive, primarily maxillary lesions.

Malignant behavior by ameloblastomas is rarely encountered. By definition, these are lesions that metastasize to local lymph nodes or distant organs (Fig. 11-13). Direct extension into contiguous areas does not qualify for a malignant classification. Malignant lesions have been divided into two subtypes: the *malignant ameloblastoma*, in which the primary and metastatic lesions are microscopically well differentiated; and *ameloblastic carcinoma*, in which the metastatic deposits exhibit poor microscopic differentiation. It has also been proposed that ameloblastic carcinoma include all ameloblastomas, either primary or recurrent, that have histologic signs of malignancy (Fig. 11-14). Metastasis from malignant varieties of ameloblastoma appear usually in the lung, presumably owing to aspiration of tumor cells. Regional lymph nodes are the second most common metastatic site, followed by skull, liver, spleen, kidney, and skin.

Another epithelial odontogenic malignancy of the mandible and maxilla that is believed to arise from odontogenic rests has been designated as *primary intraosseous carcinoma*. This rare adult lesion affects men more than women, and it is seen in the mandible more than the maxilla. Microscopically, about half these lesions exhibit keratin formation and about half show peripheral palisading of epithelial cell nests. Prognosis is poor, with a 2-year survival rate reported at 40%.

A lesion known as *craniopharyngioma* is related to the ameloblastoma through similar

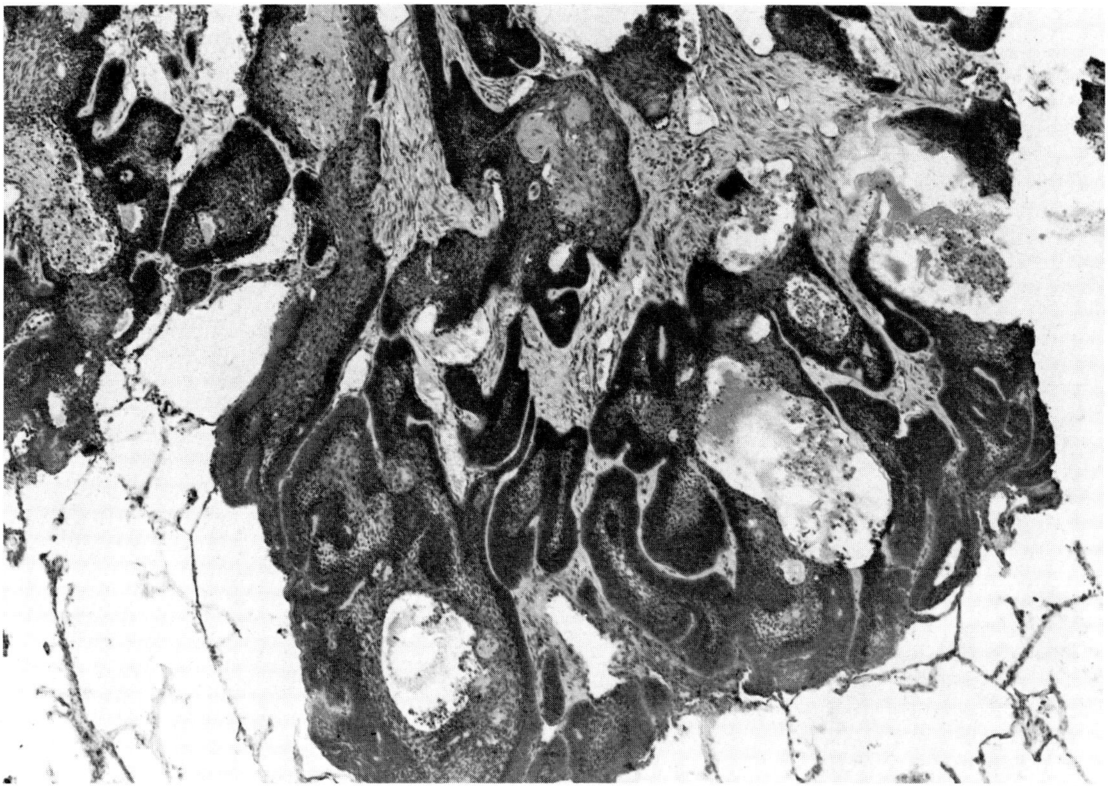

Figure 11–13. Metastatic ameloblastoma. Note lung alveoli at lower right and left.

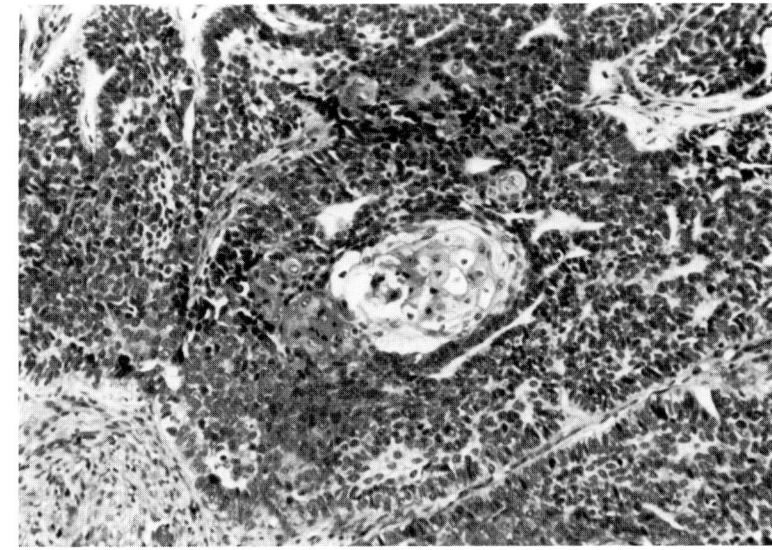

Figure 11–14. Ameloblastic carcinoma. Note hypercellularity and nuclear hyperchromatism.

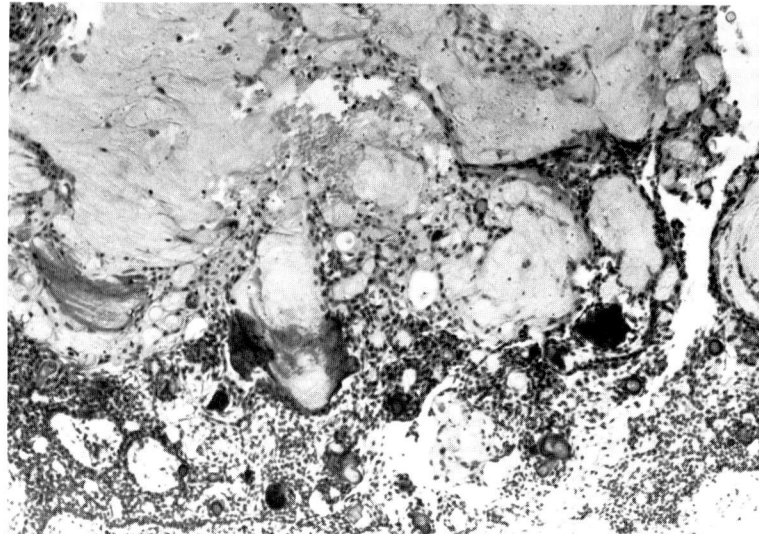

Figure 11–15. Craniopharyngioma. "Ghost cell" keratinization above and dark calcific deposits below.

origins. Both are ultimately derived from oral ectoderm—the ameloblastoma by way of dental lamina, and the craniopharyngioma by way of Rathke's pouch. The invagination of oral ectoderm (Rathke's pouch) is the initial embryonic expression of the development of part of the hypophysis. As the epithelium migrates to its final position in the base of the skull, epithelial rests may be left behind along the tract known as the craniopharyngeal duct. The rests, through some unknown mechanism, may proliferate to produce the rare neoplasm called craniopharyngioma. Biologically, this is a benign, slow-growing, infiltrative tumor similar to the ameloblastoma. Obviously, the location in the base of the skull makes this of greater significance relative to treatment and prognosis. Microscopically, the craniopharyngioma exhibits features of the ameloblastoma (Fig. 11–15). It also bears a striking resemblance to the calcifying odontogenic cyst through ghost cell keratinization and calcific deposits.

Another lesion known as *adamantinoma of tibia* was thought to be related to the ameloblastoma because of some histologic similarities. The adamantinoma (also an obsolete synonym for ameloblastoma) was also at one time thought to be endothelial, synovial, or mesenchymal in origin. However, based on the ultrastructural demonstration of desmosomes and tonofilaments, and on the immunohistochemical demonstration of keratin (and negativity for factor VIII), an epithelial origin, most likely in basal epithelial cells or eccrine cells, appears most probable.

Squamous Odontogenic Tumor

Because this tumor involves the alveolar process, it is believed to be derived from neoplastic transformation of the rests of Malassez (Fig. 11–16). It occurs in the mandible and maxilla with equal frequency, favoring the anterior region of the maxilla and the posterior region of the mandible. Multiple lesions are occasionally seen.

The age range in which squamous odontogenic tumor has been described extends from the second through the seventh decades, with a mean of 40 years. There is no gender predilection. Patients usually experience no symptoms, although tenderness and tooth mobility have been reported. Radiographically, this lesion is typically a well-circumscribed, often semilunar lesion associated with the roots of teeth. Microscopically, there is some similarity to ameloblastoma, although the squamous odontogenic tumor lacks the columnar peripherally palisaded layer of epithelial cells.

This lesion has some invasive capacity and, infrequently, recurs following conservative therapy. Curettage or excision is the treatment of choice.

Calcifying Epithelial Odontogenic Tumor (CEOT)

This neoplasm, also known as Pindborg tumor after the oral pathologist who first described the entity, shares many features with

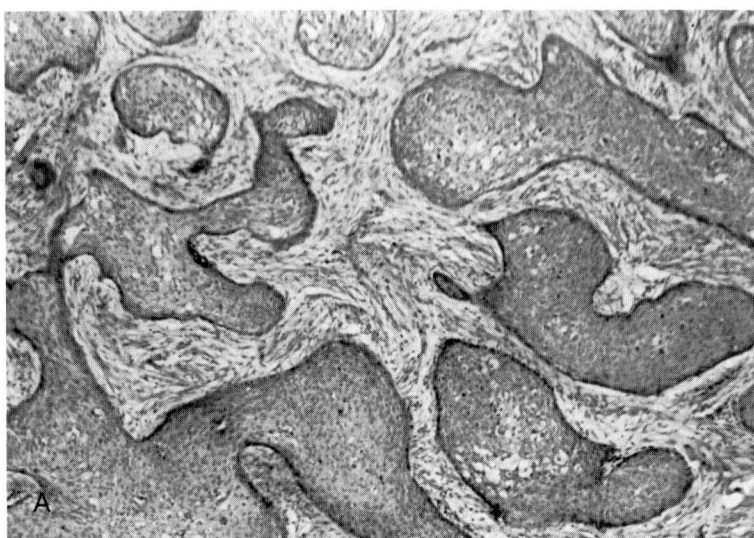
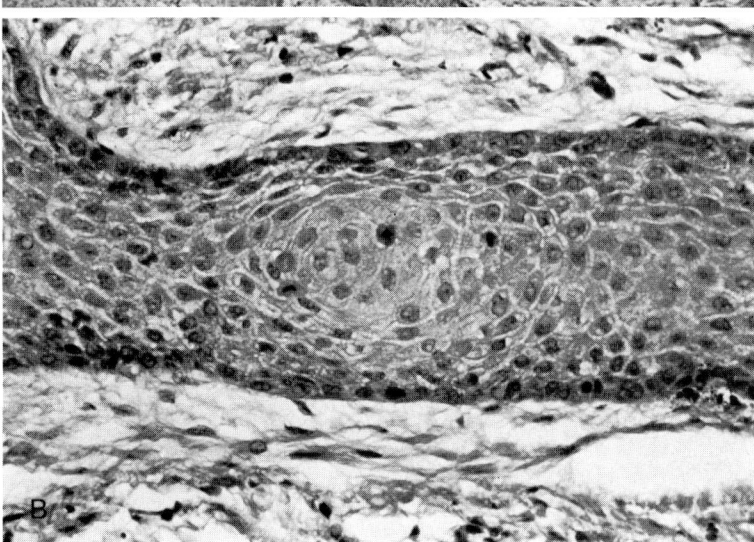

Figure 11–16. *A* and *B*, Squamous odontogenic tumor.

the ameloblastoma. Microscopically, however, there is no resemblance to the ameloblastoma, and occasionally radiographically distinct differences may be noted. The CEOT is of odontogenic origin. The specific cell from which it is derived and the stimulus for growth are unknown, although the stratum intermedium of the enamel organ has been mentioned.

Clinical Features. The CEOT is seen in patients ranging in age from the second to the tenth decade, with a mean around 40 years. There is no gender predilection.

The mandible is affected twice as often as is the maxilla. There is a predilection for the molar-ramus region, although any site may be affected. Peripheral lesions, usually in the anterior gingiva, have occasionally been identified.

Jaw expansion or incidental observation on routine radiographic survey is the usual way in which these lesions are discovered (Fig. 11–17). Radiographically, lesions are frequently associated with impacted teeth. The lesions may be unilocular or multilocular. Small loculations in some lesions have prompted the use of the term "honeycombed" to describe this lucent pattern. The CEOT may be completely radiolucent, or it may contain opaque foci—a reflection of the calcified islands seen microscopically. The lesions are usually well circumscribed radiographically, although sclerotic margins may not be evident.

Histopathology. A unique microscopic pattern typifies the CEOT. Sheets of large polygonal epithelial cells are usually seen (Fig. 11–18). Nuclei show considerable variation in size,

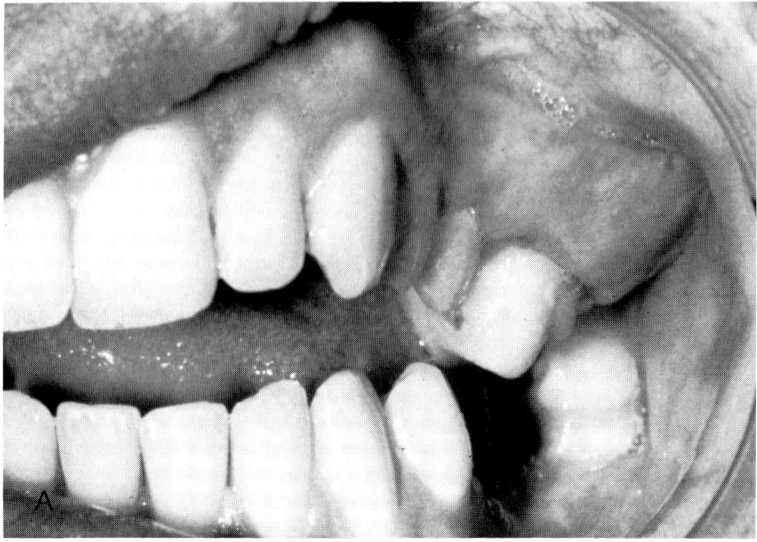
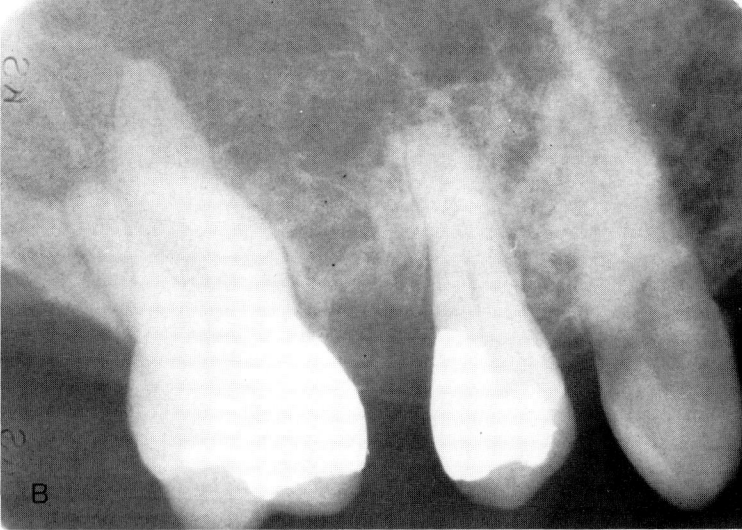

Figure 11–17. *A*, Calcifying epithelial odontogenic tumor of maxilla. *B*, Radiogram showing poorly defined lucency. (Courtesy of Dr. T. Pickens.)

shape, and number. Mitotic figures are rare. The cytoplasm is abundant and eosinophilic. Occasionally, focal zones of optically clear cells can be seen in the microscopic clear cell variant.

Varying amounts of an extracellular product that most investigators believe is amyloid is also typical of these tumors (Fig. 11–19). This homogeneous, pale-staining eosinophilic material stains positive for amyloid with Congo red stain in polarized light and with thioflavine T in ultraviolet light. Concentric calcific deposits (Liesegang rings) may be seen in the amyloid material. These rings, if sufficiently dense and large, are responsible for radiopacities.

Differential Diagnosis. When this lesion is radiolucent, it must be separated clinically from the dentigerous cyst, odontogenic keratocyst, ameloblastoma, and odontogenic myxoma. Some benign non-odontogenic jaw tumors might also be considered, but these would be less likely, based on age and location.

When a mixed radiolucent-radiopaque pattern is encountered, the calcified odontogenic cyst should be considered in a clinical differential diagnosis. Other less likely possibilities include adenomatoid odontogenic tumor (AOT), ameloblastic fibro-odontoma, ossifying fibroma, and osteoblastoma.

Treatment. This tumor has invasive potential but apparently not to the extent of the ameloblastoma. It is a slow-growing tumor and compromises the patient through direct extension. Metastases have not been reported. Various forms of surgery, ranging from enuclea-

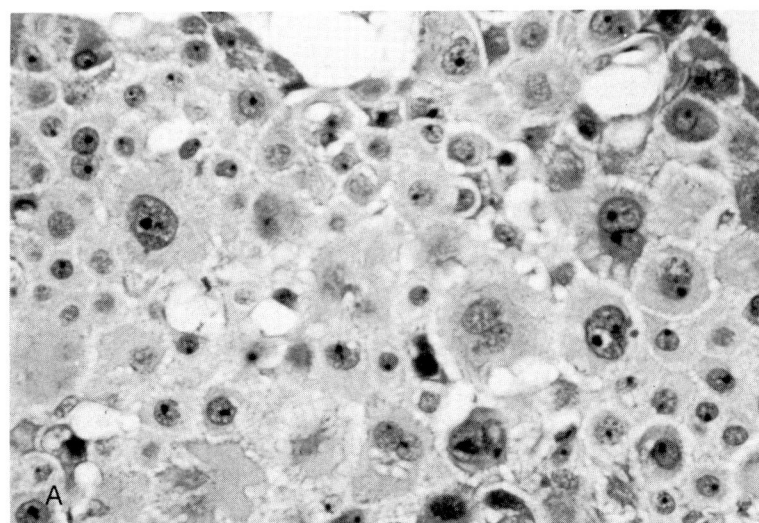
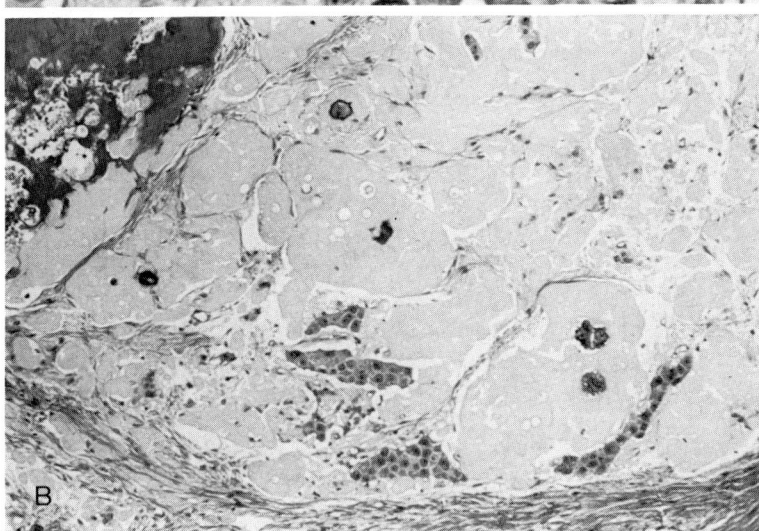

Figure 11–18. Calcifying epithelial odontogenic tumor. *A*, Bizarre epithelial cells. *B*, Amyloid component showing calcification (upper left).

tion to resection, have been used to treat CEOTs. The overall recurrence rate has been under 20%, indicating that aggressive surgery is not indicated for the management of most patients with this benign neoplasm.

Clear Cell Odontogenic Tumor

This is a rare neoplasm of the mandible and maxilla. It has been found in women over 60 years of age. It is a locally aggressive, poorly circumscribed neoplasm composed of sheets of optically clear cells. Microscopic differential diagnosis includes other jaw tumors that may have a clear cell component, such as CEOT, central mucoepidermoid carcinoma, metastatic acinic cell carcinoma, metastatic renal cell carcinoma, and ameloblastoma. Whether this neoplasm should be regarded as a clear cell variant of the ameloblastoma or should be recognized as a distinct and separate entity will depend upon further documentation and follow-up of a larger number of cases.

Adenomatoid Odontogenic Tumor (AOT)

Although the AOT is of odontogenic origin, the presence of unusual duct-like or gland-like structures has given rise to numerous names that have been modified by "adeno." Until its distinctive characteristics were fully appreciated, the AOT was thought to be a subtype of ameloblastoma and was known by the name

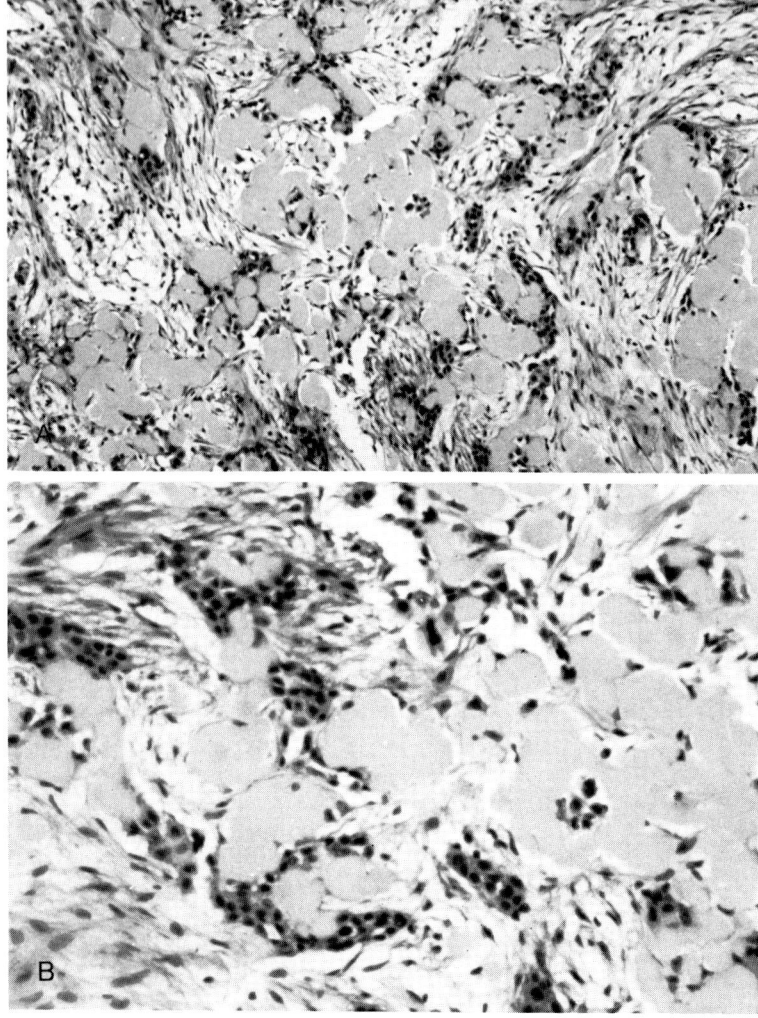

Figure 11–19. A and B, Calcifying epithelial odontogenic tumor showing strands of epithelium and globules of amyloid.

"adenoameloblastoma." Clinically, microscopically, and behaviorally, it is clearly different from ameloblastoma. Some would classify this lesion as a hamartoma rather than a neoplasm.

Clinical Features. The AOT is seen in a rather narrow age range between 5 and 30 years, with most cases appearing in the second decade. Females tend to be more commonly affected than males. Most lesions appear in the anterior portion of the jaws and more frequently in the anterior maxilla, generally in association with the crowns of impacted teeth (Fig. 11–20). From this position, the tumor tissue typically proliferates into the lumen of a well-encapsulated cyst-like space.

Radiographically, the AOT is a well-circumscribed unilocular lesion usually around the crown of an impacted tooth (Fig. 11–21). The lesions are typically radiolucent but may have small opaque foci distributed throughout, reflecting the presence of enameloid islands in the tumor tissue. When they are located between anterior teeth, divergence of roots may be seen (Fig. 11–22).

Histopathology. An epithelial proliferation is composed of polyhedral to spindle cells. The pattern is often lobular but may appear as a reticulum (Fig. 11–23). Rosettes or duct-like structures of columnar epithelial cells give the lesion its characteristic microscopic feature (Fig. 11–24). Foci of enameloid material are scattered throughout the lesion. The number, size, and degree of calcification of these foci determines how the lesion presents radiographically.

Differential Diagnosis. Other lesions that

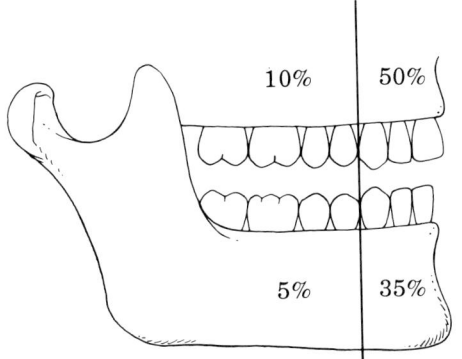

Figure 11–20. Approximate regional distribution of adenomatoid odontogenic tumor.

might be included in a differential diagnosis of AOT are dentigerous cyst, because of frequent association with impacted teeth, and lateral root cyst, because of occasional location adjacent to roots of anterior teeth. If opacities are evident, the calcifying odontogenic cyst and the CEOT should receive consideration.

Treatment. Conservative treatment (enucleation) is all that is required for this lesion. The AOT is a totally benign encapsulated lesion that does not recur.

MESENCHYMAL TUMORS

Odontogenic Myxoma

This odontogenic tumor is mesenchymal in nature and origin, mimicking microscopically the dental pulp or follicular connective tissue. When relatively large amounts of collagen are evident, the term "myxofibroma" may be used to designate this entity. This is a benign neoplasm that may be infiltrative and aggressive and may recur.

Clinical Features. The age range in which this lesion appears extends from 10 to 50 years, with a mean of about 30. There is no gender predilection, and the lesions are seen anywhere in the mandible and maxilla, with about equal frequency (Fig. 11–25).

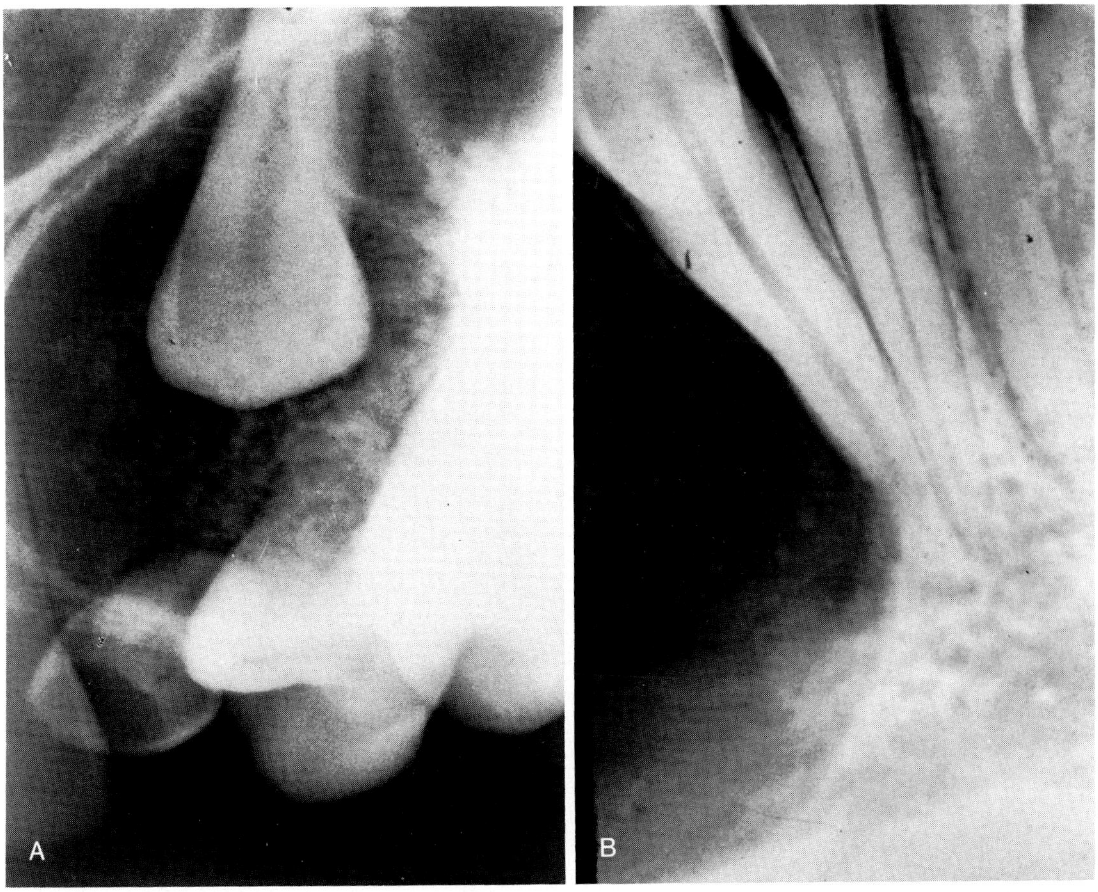

Figure 11–21. *A* and *B*, Adenomatoid odontogenic tumors. Note opaque foci within the radiolucent lesions.

354 ODONTOGENIC TUMORS

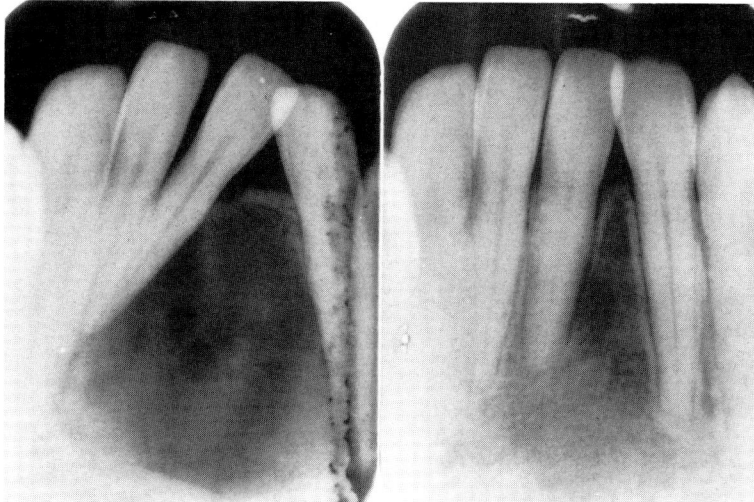

Figure 11–22. Adenomatoid odontogenic tumor (left). One year after enucleation (right).

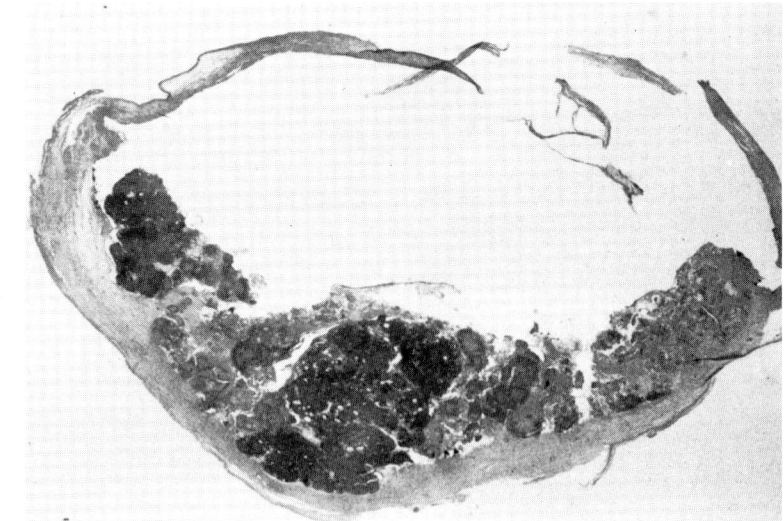

Figure 11–23. Adenomatoid odontogenic tumor proliferating into the lumen of cystic space.

Figure 11–24. *A* and *B*, Two microscopic patterns of adenomatoid odontogenic tumor.

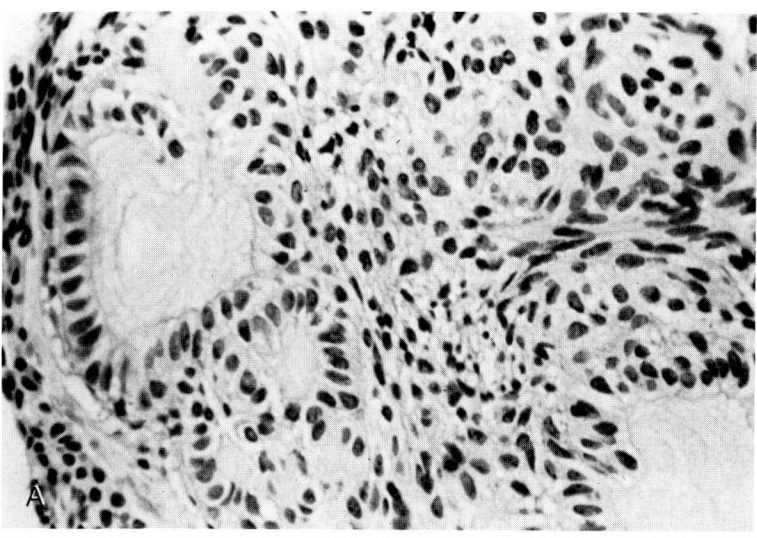
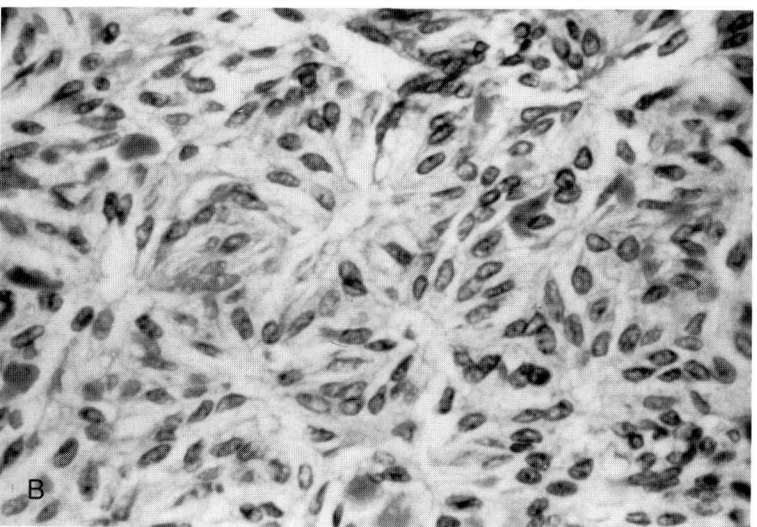

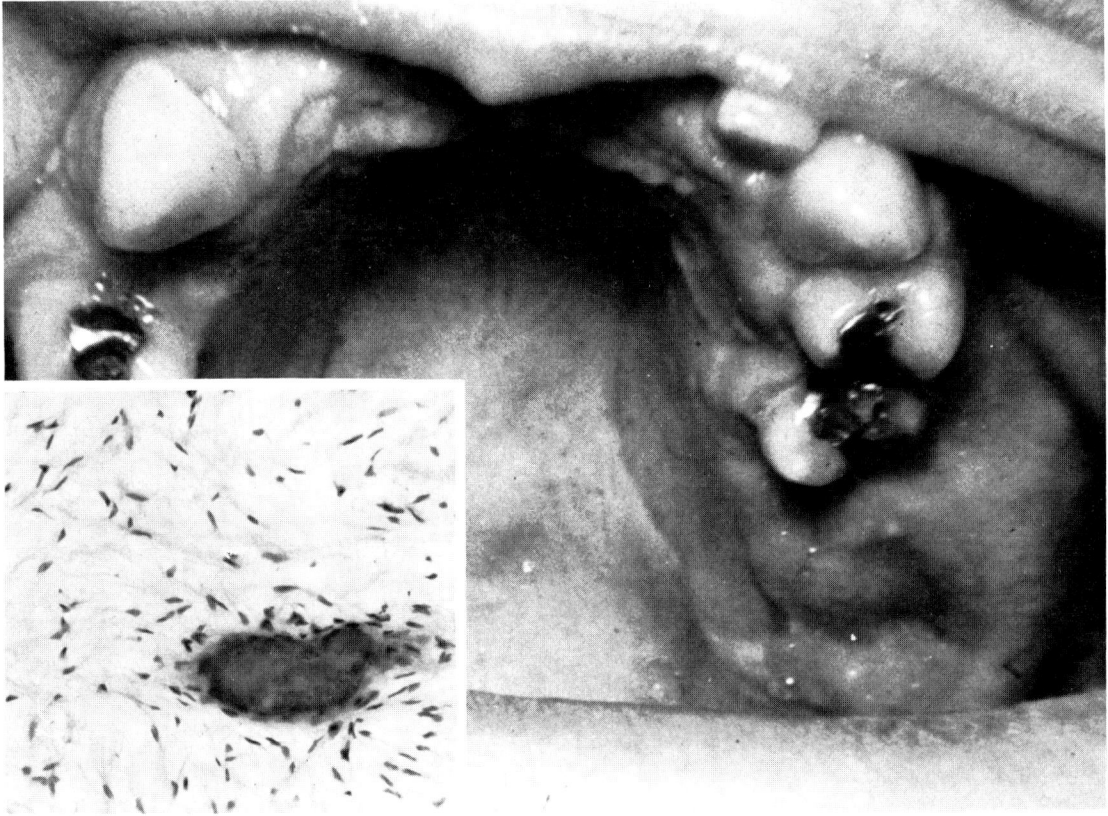

Figure 11–25. Myxoma of the left maxilla. Inset shows myxomatous tissue with bony island.

Radiographically, this lesion is always lucent, although the pattern may be quite variable. It may appear as a well-circumscribed lesion or as a diffuse lesion. It is often multilocular, frequently with a "honeycombed" pattern (Fig. 11–26). Cortical expansion (rather than perforation) and root displacement (rather than resorption) are the rule.

Histopathology. This tumor is composed of bland, relatively acellular myxomatous connective tissue (Fig. 11–27). Benign fibroblasts and myofibroblasts with variable amounts of collagen are found in a mucopolysaccharide matrix. Bony islands, representing residual trabeculae, and capillaries are found scattered throughout the lesion. Odontogenic rests are very uncommmon in these tumors. Their absence should not preclude the diagnosis.

Differential Diagnosis. Clinical differential diagnosis is essentially the same as that described for the ameloblastoma. Additionally, the central hemangioma is a serious consideration in lesions that are "honeycombed." Important to consider microscopically when confronted with a myxomatous lesion from the central jaws are normal dental pulp and follicular connective tissue surrounding an impacted developing or mature tooth. This connective tissue may be a hyperplastic follicle and myxoid in character, closely mimicking the neoplasm (Fig. 11–28). History and radiographs are important aids in the definitive diagnosis of odontogenic myxomas.

Treatment. Surgical excision is the treatment of choice. Because of an often loose, gelatinous consistency, curettage may result in incomplete removal of viable neoplasm. The absence of encapsulation may also contribute to recurrence if the lesion is treated too conservatively. Although these lesions exhibit some aggressiveness and have a moderate recurrence rate, the prognosis is very good. Repeated surgical procedures do not appear to stimulate growth or cause metastasis.

Central Odontogenic Fibroma

This rare lesion is regarded as the central counterpart to the peripheral odontogenic fi-

ODONTOGENIC TUMORS 357

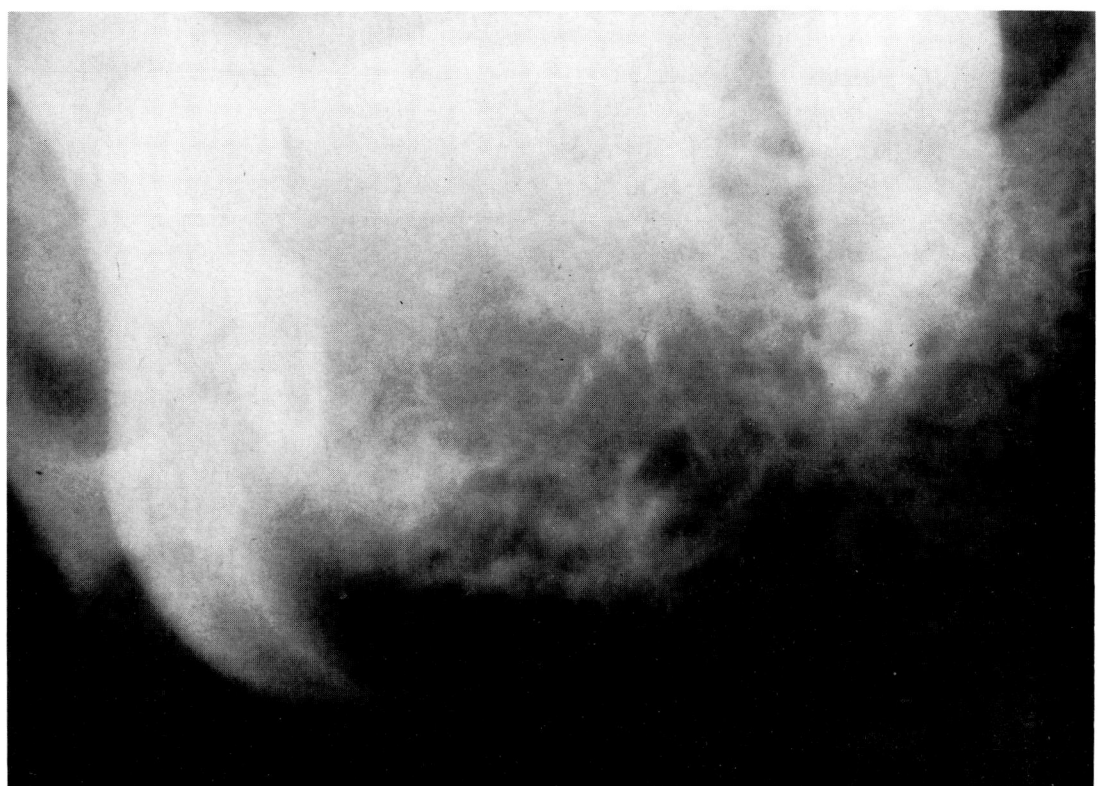

Figure 11-26. Lateral jaw radiogram showing an odontogenic myxoma of the body of the mandible. Symphysis to the left and molar to the right.

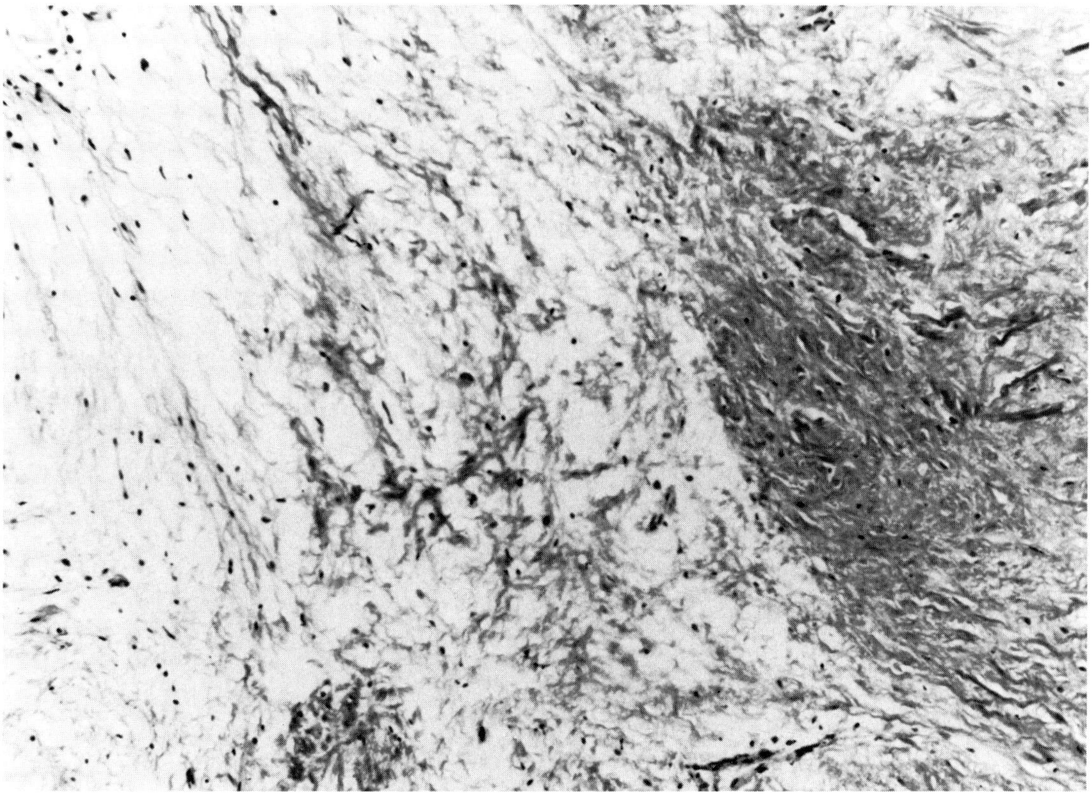

Figure 11-27. Odontogenic myxoma showing variable amount of collagen.

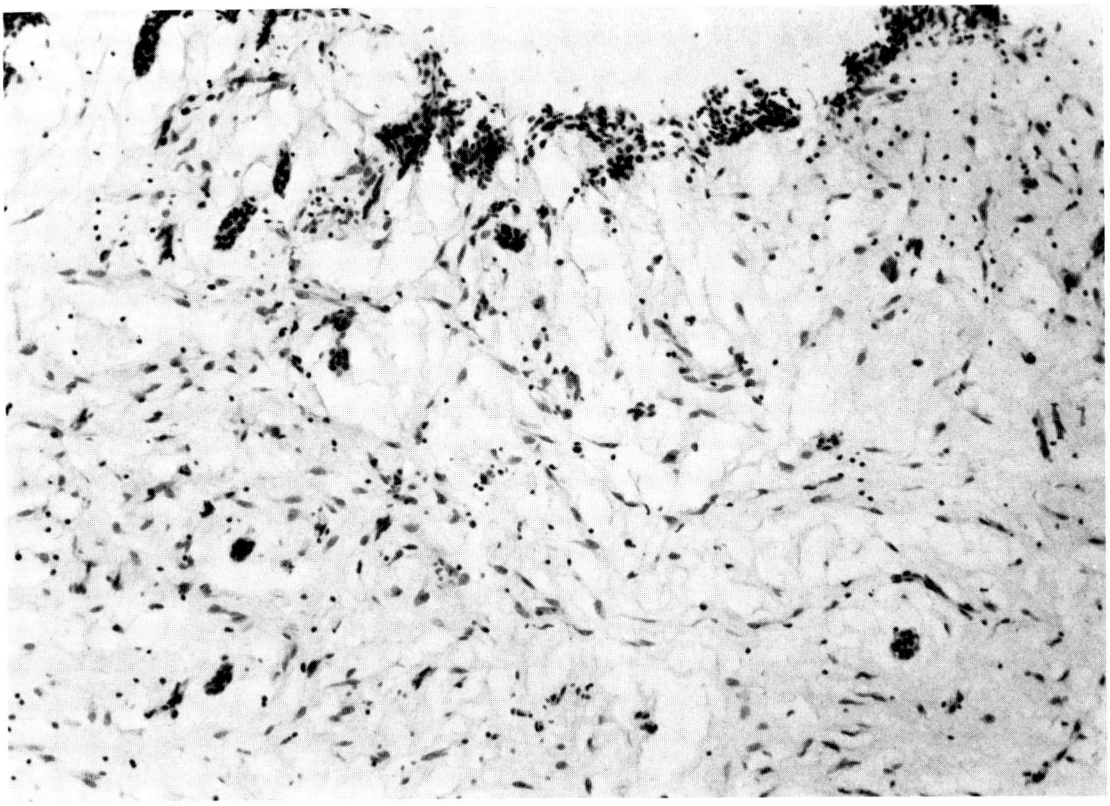

Figure 11-28. Myxomatous dental follicle. Note remnants of reduced enamel epithelium (top).

broma. It has been seen in all age groups, and it is found in both the mandible and the maxilla. It results in a radiolucent lesion that is usually multilocular, often causing cortical expansion. Clinical differential diagnosis is similar to that described for ameloblastoma.

Microscopically, two patterns are generally ascribed to central odontogenic fibroma. In the simple type, the lesion is composed of a mass of mature fibrous tissue containing few epithelial rests. In the WHO (World Health Organization) type, mature connective tissue contains abundant rests and calcific deposits of what is regarded as dentin or cementum (Fig. 11-29). This microscopic differentiation may be academic, as there appears to be no differ-

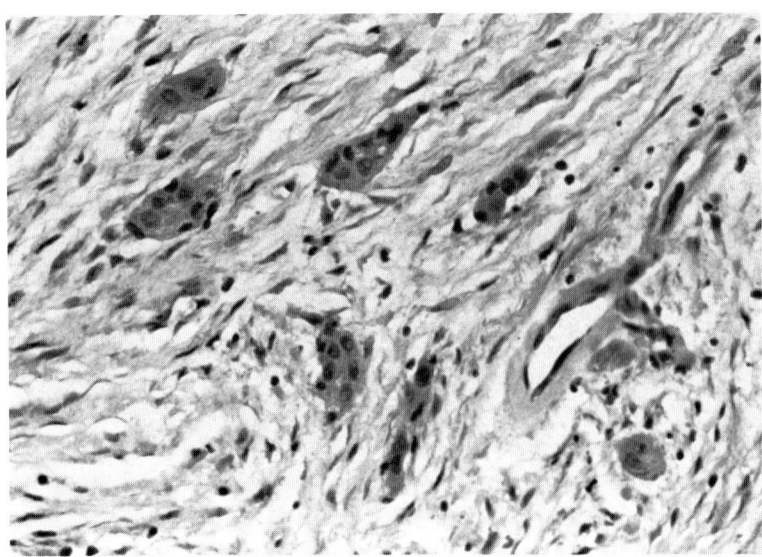

Figure 11-29. Central odontogenic fibroma. Note fibrous stroma containing several odontogenic rests.

ence in clinical behavior between the two subtypes. Treatment is excision, and recurrence is unexpected.

Cementifying Fibroma

This lesion may be impossible to separate from ossifying fibroma and may in fact be just part of a spectrum of central fibrous lesions that contain calcified material. The only feature that has served to separate the two is the microscopic identification of cementum or bone in the lesion, a distinction that is unfortunately strictly subjective using current diagnostic tools. In any event, the separation appears to be essentially an academic exercise.

Clinical Features. The cementifying fibroma occurs chiefly in adults around the age of 40 years, but it has a fairly wide age range. There are predilections for the mandible and for females. The lesion may cause tooth movement or cortical expansion. Radiographically, it may appear relatively radiolucent (Fig. 11–30), lucent with opaque foci, or diffusely opaque. The radiographic appearance is dependent upon the size of the islands of cementum and the extent of calcification. The lesions are usually well circumscribed and are surrounded by a sclerotic margin.

Histopathology. A benign fibroblastic stroma typifies these lesions (Fig. 11–31). Cellularity may be high, but mitoses are rare. Cementum is usually identified as globules or oval islands of calcified material that are frequently surrounded by eosinophilic cementoid and cementoblasts. The cemental islands are evenly distributed throughout the lesion, but they may on occasion converge to form lobulated masses. Inflammatory cells are rarely seen.

Differential Diagnosis. Clinical differential diagnosis of cementifying fibroma should include cementoblastoma, ossifying fibroma, chronic osteomyelitis, and fibrous dysplasia. Fibrous dysplasia and, occasionally, chronic osteomyelitis are less likely possibilities, because of their lack of radiographic circumscription. If the cementifying fibroma is relatively lucent, central giant cell granuloma and odontogenic tumors such as ameloblastoma and odontogenic myxoma are viable diagnostic considerations.

Treatment. Because of the well-circumscribed nature of this lesion, conservative treatment is all that is required. Enucleation or excision should be curative. Recurrence is unexpected.

Cementoblastoma

Clinical Features. The cementoblastoma, also known as true cementoma, is a rare benign neoplasm of cementoblast origin. It occurs predominantly in the second and third decades, typically before 25 years of age. There is no gender predilection. It is more often seen in the mandible than in the maxilla and more often in posterior than in anterior regions. It is intimately associated with the root of a tooth, and the tooth remains vital. The cementoblastoma may cause cortical expansion and, occasionally, low-grade intermittent pain.

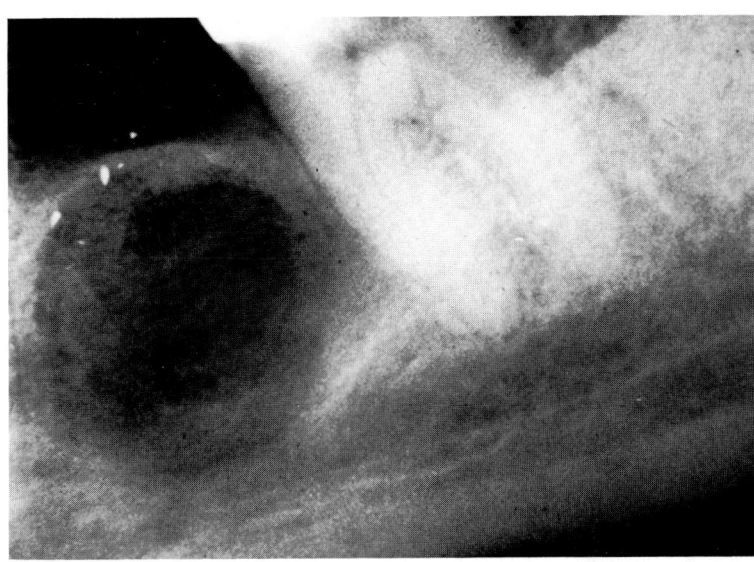

Figure 11–30. Cementifying fibroma in body of the mandible.

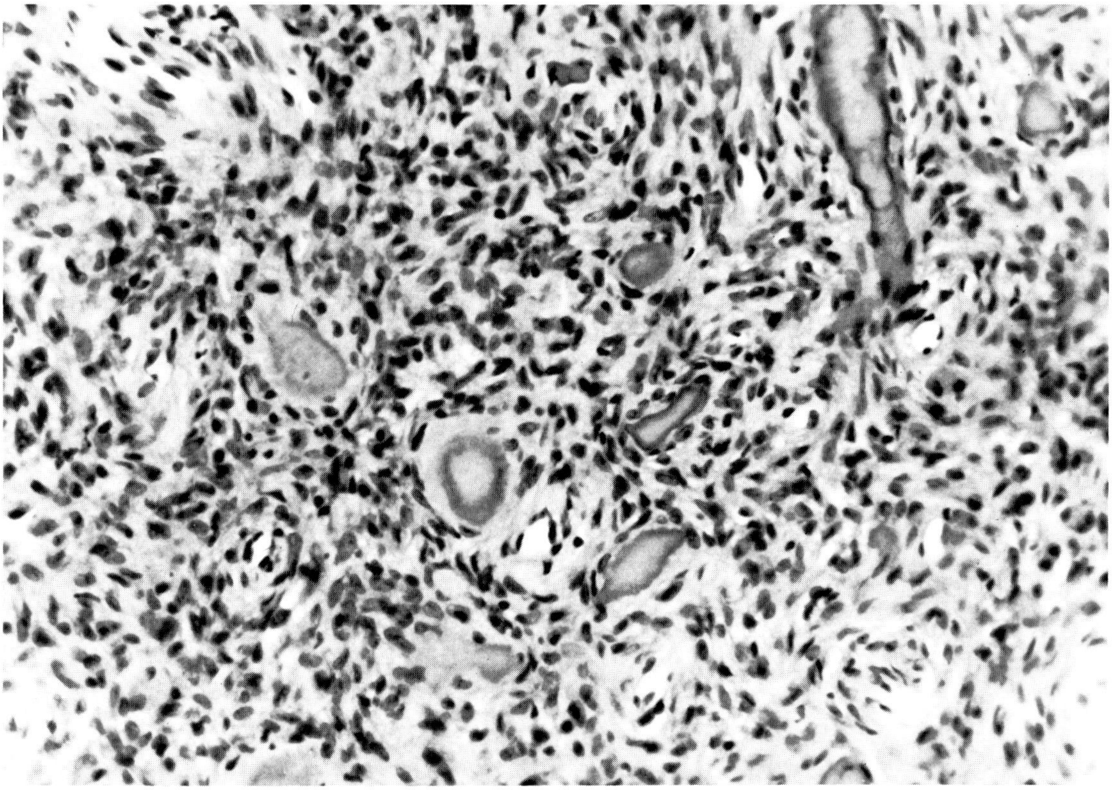

Figure 11-31. Cementifying fibroma composed of benign fibroblasts and islands of cementum.

Radiographically, this is an opaque lesion that replaces the root of the tooth (Fig. 11-32). It is usually surrounded by a radiolucent ring.

Histopathology. This lesion appears microscopically as a conglomeration of cementum-like material with numerous reversal lines. Intervening well-vascularized soft tissue contains cementoblasts, often numerous, large, and hyperchromatic. Cementoclasts are also evident.

Differential Diagnosis. The characteristic radiographic appearance of this lesion is usually diagnostic. Other opaque lesions that share some features include odontoma, osteoblastoma, focal sclerosing osteomyelitis, and hypercementosis.

Treatment. Because of the intimate associ-

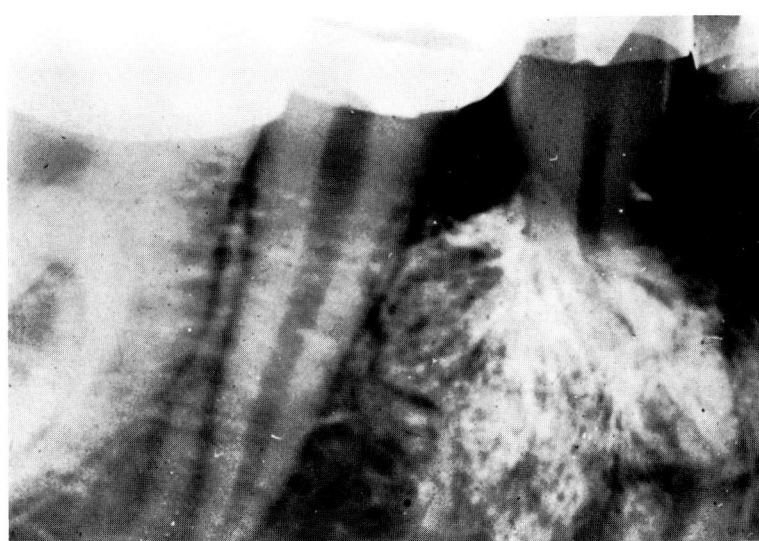

Figure 11-32. Cementoblastoma.

ation of neoplasm with tooth root, this lesion cannot be removed without sacrificing the tooth. Bone relief is typically required to remove this well-circumscribed mass. Recurrence is not seen.

Periapical Cemental Dysplasia

As the name implies, this lesion (formerly known as cementoma) represents a reactive rather than a neoplastic process. This lesion appears to be an unusual response of periapical bone and cementum to some local factor. Although the precise cause of this condition is unknown, trauma and infection are suspected.

Clinical Features. This is a relatively common phenomenon that occurs at the apex of vital teeth. Biopsy is unnecessary because the condition is usually diagnostic by clinical and radiographic features. Women, especially black women, are affected more than are men. Periapical cemental dysplasia appears in middle age (around 40 years) and rarely under the age of 20. The mandible, especially the anterior periapical region, is far more commonly affected than is the maxilla. More often, the apices of two or more teeth are affected.

This condition is typically discovered on routine radiographic examination, since patients are asymptomatic. This condition appears first as a periapical lucency that is continuous with the periodontal ligament space (Fig. 11–33). Although this initial pattern simulates radiographically a periapical granuloma or cyst, the teeth are always vital. As the condition progresses or matures, the lucent lesion develops into a mixed or mottled pattern owing to bone repair. The final stage appears as a solid opaque mass often surrounded by a thin lucent ring. This process takes months to years to reach final stages of development and, obviously, may be discovered at any stage.

A rare condition described as *florid osseous dysplasia* (FOD) appears to be an exuberant form of periapical cemental dysplasia. FOD would represent the severe end of the spectrum of this unusual process. There is no apparent cause, and patients are asymptomatic except when the complication of osteomyelitis occurs. Females, especially black females, are predominantly affected, usually between 25 and 60 years of age. The condition is typically bilateral and may affect all four quadrants. A curious finding has been the concomitant appearance of traumatic (simple) bone cysts in affected tissue. Radiographically, FOD appears as diffuse radiopaque masses throughout the jaw (Fig. 11–34). A "ground-glass" or cyst-like appearance may also be seen (Fig. 11–35).

Clinical differential diagnosis includes diffuse sclerosing osteomyelitis and Paget's disease. Paget's disease can be ruled out with biopsy and determination of serum alkaline

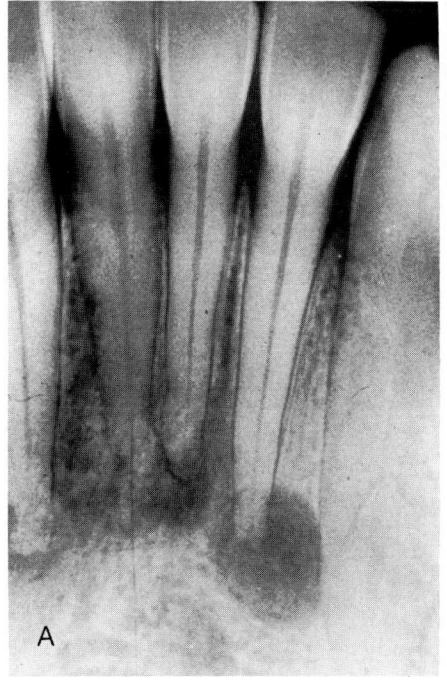

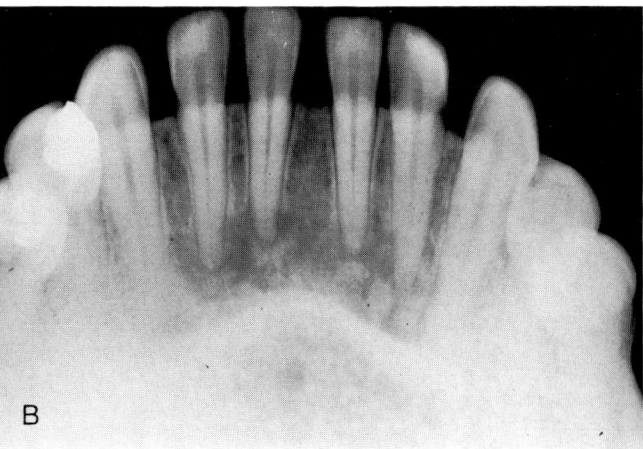

Figure 11–33. Periapical cemental dysplasia. *A*, Early lesions. *B*, More mature lesions.

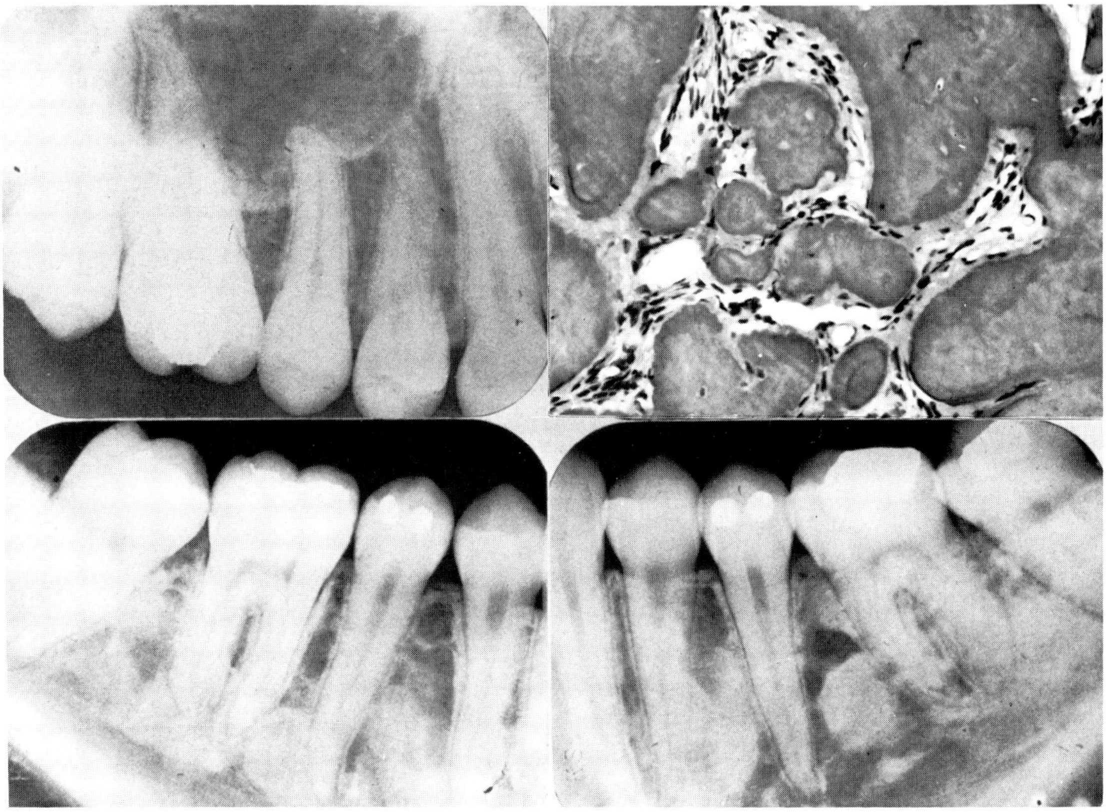

Figure 11-34. Florid osseous dysplasia. Maxilla is unaffected. Low-power photomicrograph shows irregular bony trabeculae in benign fibrous matrix.

phosphatase (normal in FOD). Chronic diffuse sclerosing osteomyelitis would be symptomatic. It may have a different radiographic appearance, and inflammatory cells would appear in biopsy tissue.

Microscopically, FOD consists of a benign fibrous stroma containing irregular trabeculae of mature bone and cementum-like material. Inflammatory cells are not a feature of this condition. Because FOD is an asymptomatic self-limited process, no treatment is required. In cases in which secondary infection occurs,

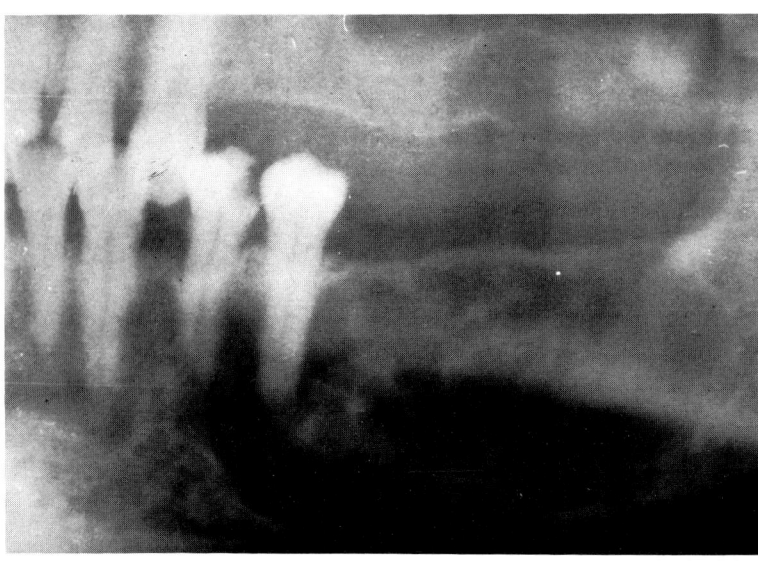

Figure 11-35. Florid osseous dysplasia. Note lesions at apex of anterior teeth.

antibiotics and sequestrectomy may be necessary.

Histopathology. Periapical cemental dysplasia is a mixture of benign fibrous tissue, bone, and cementum. The calcified tissue is arranged in trabeculae, spicules, or larger irregular masses. Reversal lines are eventually seen, and osteoblasts or cementoblasts, or both, line the islands of hard tissue. Chronic inflammatory cells may also be seen. Microscopically, periapical cemental dysplasia may appear very similar to chronic osteomyelitis and ossifying fibroma.

Differential Diagnosis. Age, gender, location, radiographic appearance, and tooth vitality considered together are diagnostic of this condition. When one or more of these factors are atypical, other diagnostic considerations include chronic osteomyelitis, ossifying fibroma, and periapical granuloma or cyst. In the opaque stage, odontoma, osteoblastoma, and focal sclerosing osteomyelitis are diagnostic possibilities.

Treatment. No treatment is required for this condition. Once the opaque stage is reached, the lesion stabilizes and causes no complications. Because teeth remain vital throughout the entire process, they should not be extracted, and endodontic procedures should not be done. Once clinical diagnosis is established, only observation is necessary.

MIXED (EPITHELIAL AND MESENCHYMAL) TUMORS

Odontoma

Odontomas are known as mixed odontogenic tumors because they are composed of tissue that is of both epithelial and mesenchymal origin. These tissues become fully differentiated, resulting in deposition of enamel by ameloblasts and dentin by odontoblasts. Although these cells and tissues appear normal, the architecture is defective. This abnormal organization of otherwise normal mature tissues has led to the opinion that odontomas should be regarded as hamartomas rather than as neoplasms.

These calcified lesions take one of two general configurations. They may appear as multiple miniature or rudimentary teeth, in which case they are known as compound odontomas, or they may appear as amorphous conglomerations of hard tissue, in which case they are known as complex odontomas. As a group, they are the most common odontogenic tumors.

Clinical Features. Odontomas are lesions of children and young adults; most are discovered in the second decade of life. The range does, however, extend into later adulthood. The maxilla is affected slightly more often than the mandible. There is also a tendency for compound odontomas to occur in the anterior jaws and for complex odontomas to occur in the posterior jaws. There does not appear to be a significant gender predilection. Clinical signs that reflect the presence of an odontoma are a retained deciduous tooth (Fig. 11–36), an impacted tooth, and alveolar swelling. These lesions generally produce no symptoms.

Radiographically, the compound odontoma appears as several, and occasionally tens of, mature teeth in a single focus. This focus is typically in a tooth-bearing area, between roots or over the crown of an impacted tooth. Complex odontomas appear in the same regions but as amorphous opaque masses (Fig. 11–37). Lesions discovered during early stages of tumor development are primarily radiolucent, with focal areas of opacity representing early calcification of dentin and enamel.

Histopathology. Normal-appearing enamel, dentin, cementum, and pulp may be seen in these lesions (Fig. 11–38). Prominent enamel matrix and associated enamel organ are often seen before final maturation of hard tissues. So-called ghost cell keratinization is seen in epithelial cells of the enamel of some odontomas. This microscopic feature appears to have no significance other than to indicate the potential of these epithelial cells to keratinize.

Differential Diagnosis. Compound odontomas are diagnostic on radiographic examination. Complex odontomas usually present a typical radiographic appearance because of their solid opacification in relationship to teeth. However, differential diagnosis might include other opaque jaw lesions such as focal sclerosing osteomyelitis, osteoma, periapical cemental dysplasia, ossifying fibroma, and cementoblastoma.

Treatment. Odontomas have very limited growth potential, although an occasional complex lesion may cause considerable bone expansion. Enucleation is curative, and recurrence is not a problem.

A rare variant known as *ameloblastic odontoma* has been described. This is essentially an ameloblastoma in which there is focal differentiation into an odontoma. Until more is known of the behavior of this uncommon lesion, it should be treated as an ameloblastoma.

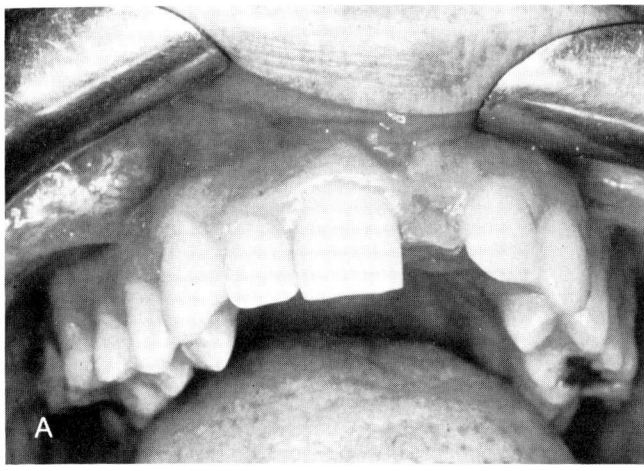
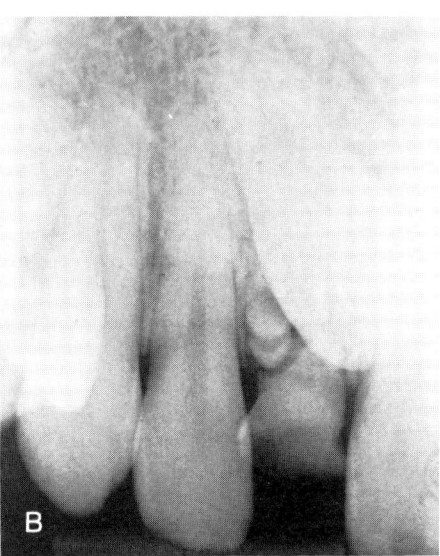

Figure 11-36. *A*, Retained deciduous tooth. *B*, Radiogram showing retained tooth and compound odontoma blocking impacted central incisor.

Ameloblastic Fibroma and Ameloblastic Fibro-odontoma

These two lesions are considered together because they appear to be variations of the same process. The occurrence of an odontoma(s) is characteristic of the ameloblastic fibro-odontoma; otherwise, the two lesions share similar features of age, gender, and location. Their biologic behaviors are also similar. Both are mixed odontogenic tumors composed of neoplastic epithelium and mesenchyme with microscopically identical soft tissue components. Both are regarded as benign neoplastic processes of odontogenic origin.

Clinical Features. These neoplasms occur predominantly in children and young adults. The mean age is about 12 years, and the upper age limit may extend as high as 40 years. The mandibular molar-ramus area is the favored location for these lesions, although any region may be affected. There is no gender predilection.

Radiographically, these lesions are well circumscribed and are usually surrounded by a sclerotic margin. They may be either unilocular or multilocular and may be associated with the crown of an impacted tooth. An opaque focus appears within the ameloblastic fibro-odontoma owing to the presence of an odontoma (Fig. 11–39). This lesion therefore presents as a combined lucent-opaque lesion; the ameloblastic fibroma is completely lucent radiographically.

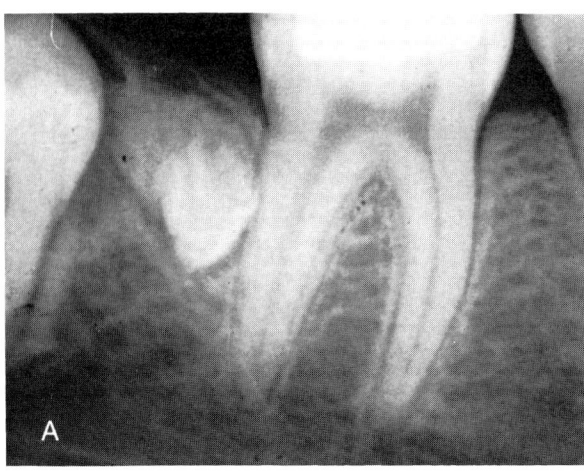
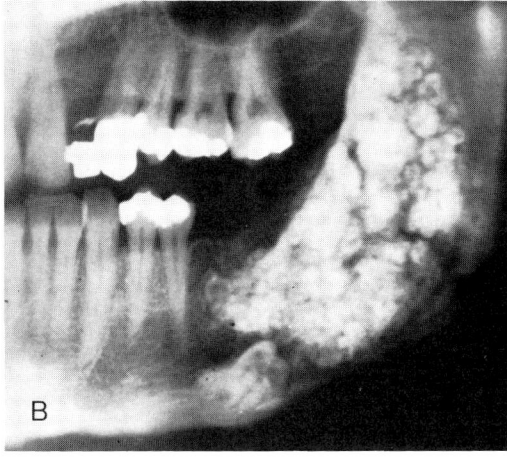

Figure 11-37. *A* and *B*, Complex odontomas. Note impacted molar in *B* (bottom).

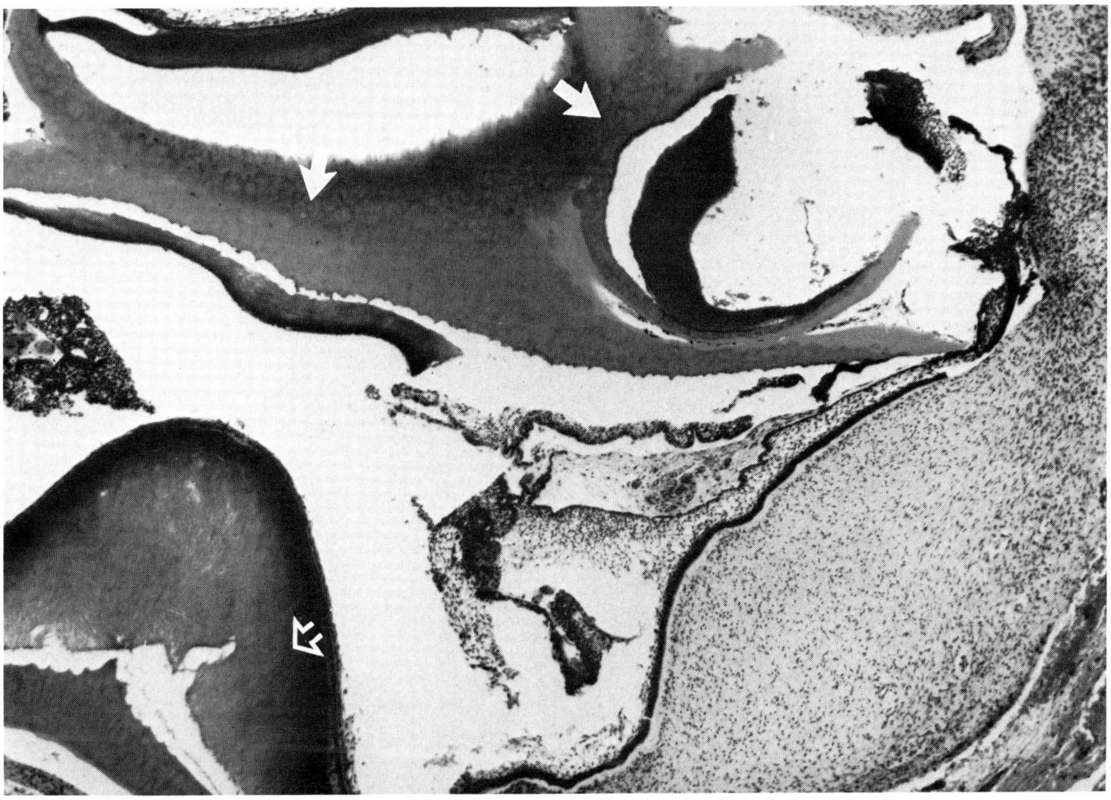

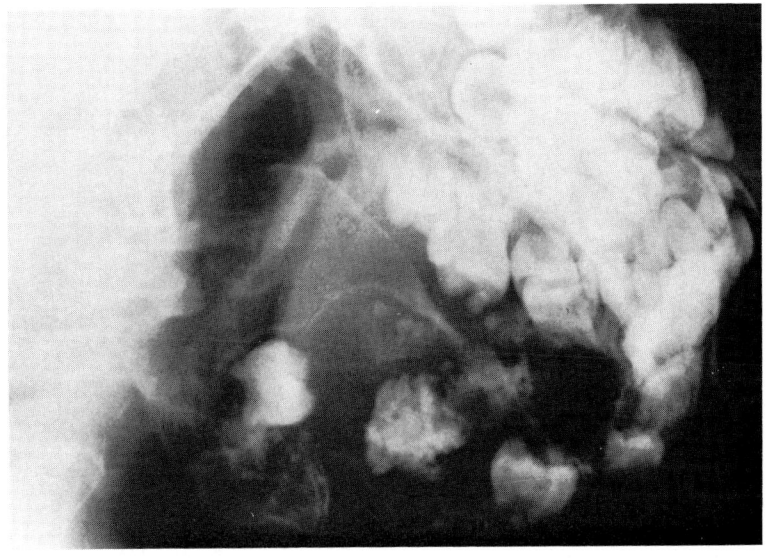

Figure 11–38. Complex odontoma composed of enamel matrix *(open arrow)* against dentin *(closed arrows)* and pulp tissue (lower right).

Figure 11–39. Lateral jaw radiogram from an 11-year-old male showing ameloblastic fibro-odontoma of body and ramus of the mandible. (Courtesy of Dr. R. Hannah.)

Histopathology. These lesions are lobulated in general configuration and usually surrounded by a fibrous capsule. The tumor mass is composed predominantly of a primitive-appearing myxoid connective tissue (Fig. 11–40). The general absence of collagen gives this component a resemblance to dental pulp. Evenly distributed throughout the tumor mesenchyme are ribbons or strands of odontogenic epithelium that are typically two cells wide. The epithelial component has been compared microscopically with the dental lamina that proliferates from oral epithelium in the early stages of tooth development.

In the ameloblastic fibro-odontoma, cells in one or more foci continue the differentiation process and produce enamel and dentin. This may be in the form of a compound or complex odontoma, the presence of which does not alter the treatment or prognosis.

Differential Diagnosis. When ameloblastic fibroma (fibro-odontoma) presents with the age, location, and radiographic pattern typical for these lesions, diagnosis is usually apparent. When clinical features are outside the usual boundaries, a differential diagnosis for ameloblastic fibroma should include ameloblastoma, odontogenic myxoma, dentigerous cyst, odontogenic keratocyst, central giant cell granuloma, and histiocytosis. The differential diagnosis for ameloblastic fibro-odontoma includes lesions with mixed radiographic patterns

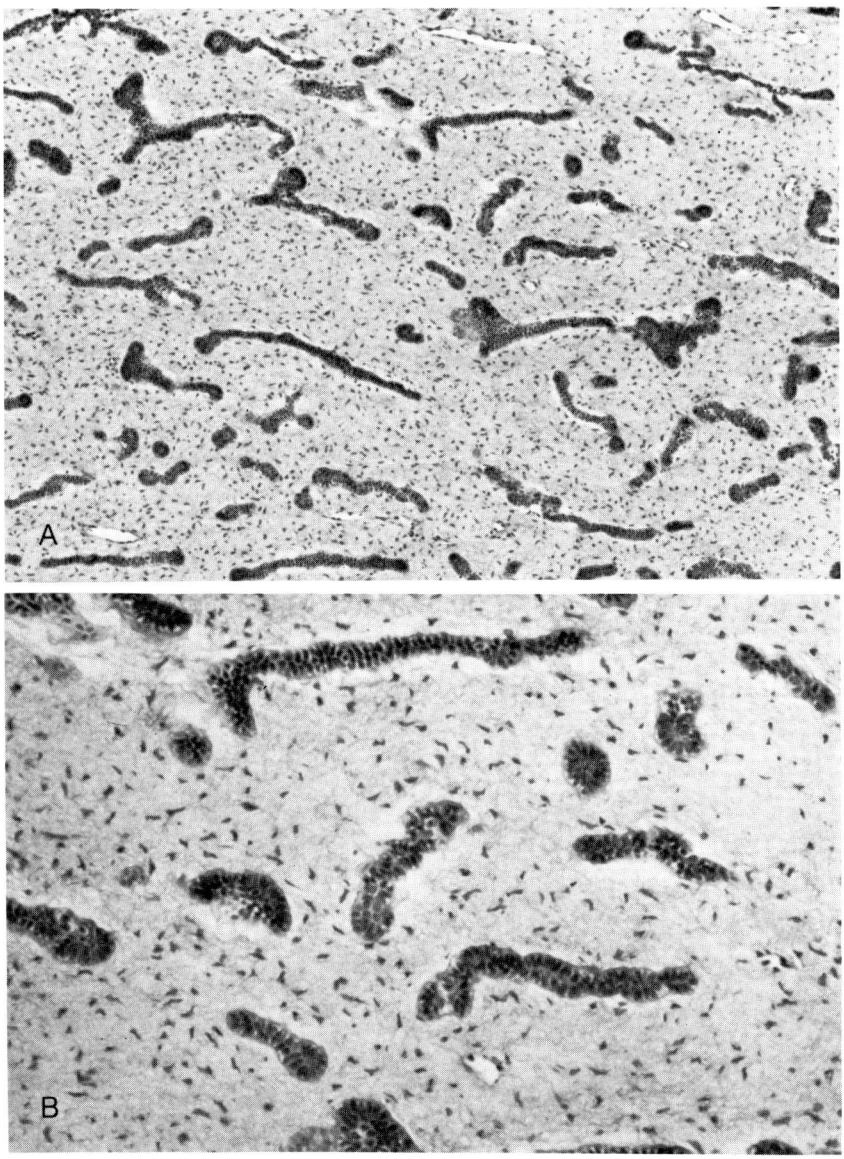

Figure 11–40. *A* and *B*, Myxomatous stroma of ameloblastic fibroma containing strands of odontogenic epithelium.

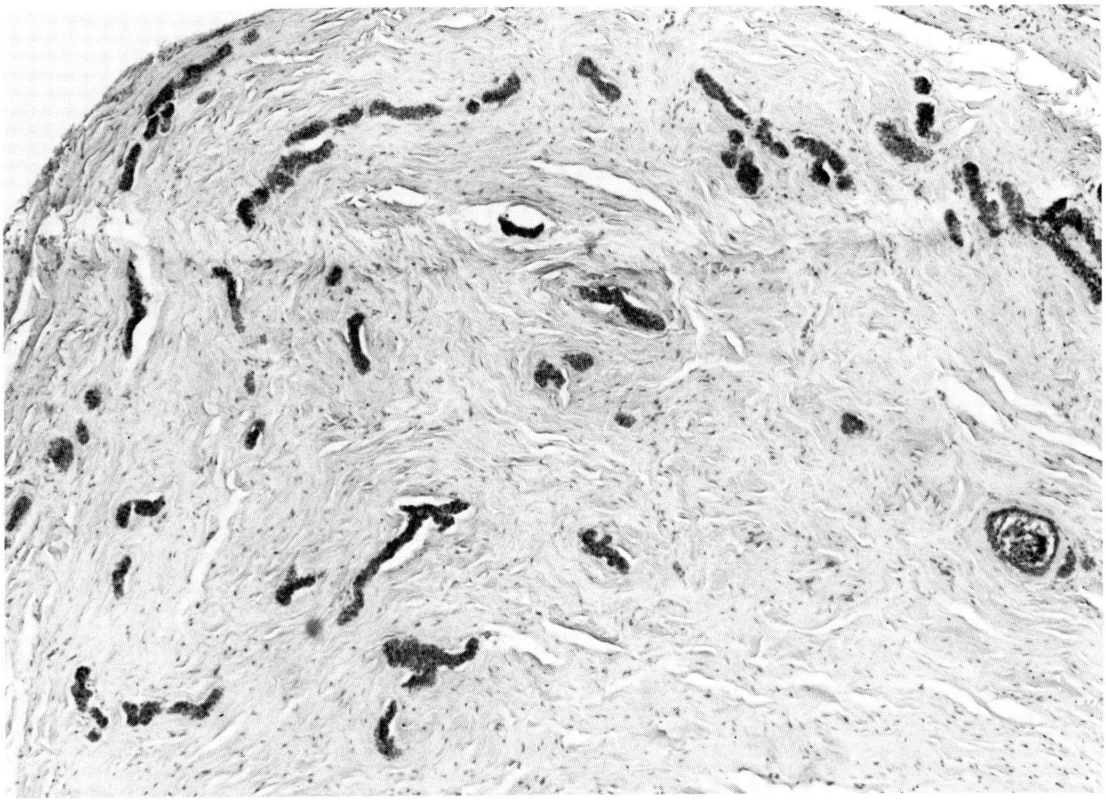

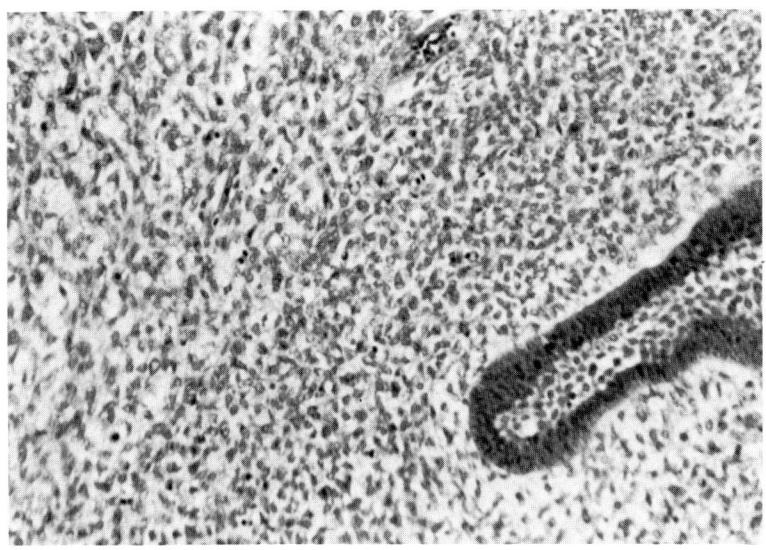

Figure 11-41. Fibrous sac (dental follicle) containing proliferative odontogenic rests.

such as CEOT, calcifying odontogenic cyst, developing odontoma, and possibly AOT. Microscopically, this lesion must be differentiated from the more fibrous hyperplastic follicular sac, in which there is proliferation of odontogenic rests (Fig. 11–41).

Treatment. Because of tumor encapsulation and the general lack of invasive capacity, this lesion is treated with a conservative surgical procedure such as curettage or excision. Recurrences have been documented, but they are uncommon.

A rare malignant counterpart to these odontogenic tumors known as *ameloblastic fibrosarcoma* has been documented as arising in the jaws either de novo or from pre-existing or

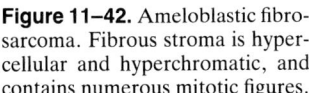

Figure 11-42. Ameloblastic fibrosarcoma. Fibrous stroma is hypercellular and hyperchromatic, and contains numerous mitotic figures.

recurrent ameloblastic fibroma. In this lesion, the mesenchymal component has the appearance of a fibrosarcoma, and the epithelial component appears as it does in the benign lesion (Fig. 11–42). Clinically, the ameloblastic fibrosarcoma occurs at an older age, around 30 years, and it appears more often in the mandible than in the maxilla. Symptoms of pain and paresthesia may be present. This is a locally aggressive lesion that has metastatic potential. Resection is therefore the treatment of choice.

Bibliography

Ameloblastoma

Adekeye E, McCallum K. Recurrent ameloblastoma of the maxillofacial region. J Maxillofac Surg 14:153–157, 1986.

Atkinson C, Harwood A, Cummings B. Ameloblastoma of the jaw: a reappraisal of the role of megavoltage irradiation. Cancer 53:869–873, 1984.

Corio R, Goldblatt L, Edwards P, et al. Ameloblastic carcinoma: a clinicopathologic study and assessment of eight cases. Oral Surg Oral Med Oral Pathol 64:570–576, 1987.

Eversole R, Leider A, Hansen L. Ameloblastomas with pronounced desmoplasia. J Oral Maxillofac Surg 43:735–740, 1984.

Gardner D. A pathologist's approach to the treatment of ameloblastoma. J Oral Maxillofac Surg 42:161–166, 1984.

Gardner D, Corio R. Plexiform unicystic ameloblastoma: a variant of ameloblastoma with a low recurrence rate after enucleation. Cancer 53:1730–1735, 1984.

Keszler A, Dominguez F. Ameloblastoma in childhood. J Oral Maxillofac Surg 44:609–613, 1986.

Leider A, Eversole L, Barkin M. Cystic ameloblastoma. Oral Surg Oral Med Oral Pathol 60:624–630, 1985.

Muller H, Slootweg P. The ameloblastoma, the controversial approach to therapy. J Maxillofac Surg 13:79–84, 1985.

Muller H, Slootweg P. Clear cell differentiation in an ameloblastoma. J Maxillofac Surg 14:158–160, 1986.

Slootweg P, Muller H. Malignant ameloblastoma or ameloblastic carcinoma. Oral Surg 57:168–176, 1984.

White R, Patterson J. Distant skin metastases in a long-term survivor of malignant ameloblastoma. J Cutan Pathol 13:383–389, 1986.

Tsaknis P, Nelson J. The maxillary ameloblastoma: an analysis of 24 cases. J Oral Surg 38:336–342, 1980.

Ueno S, Nakamura S, Mushimoto K, et al. A clinicopathologic study of ameloblastoma. J Oral Maxillofac Surg 44:361–365, 1986.

Waldron C, El-Mofty S. A histopathologic study of 116 ameloblastomas with special reference to the desmoplastic variant. Oral Surg Oral Med Oral Pathol 63:441–451, 1987.

Waldron C, Small I, Silverman H. Clear cell ameloblastoma—an odontogenic carcinoma. J Oral Maxillofac Surg 43:707–717, 1985.

Woo S, Smith-Williams J, Sciubba J, et al. Peripheral ameloblastoma of the buccal mucosa: case report and review of the English literature. Oral Surg Oral Med Oral Pathol 63:78–84, 1987.

Other Epithelial Odontogenic Tumors

Ai-Ru L, Zhen L, Jian S. Calcifying epithelial odontogenic tumors. J Oral Pathol 11:399–406, 1982.

Bernstein M, Buchino J. The histologic similarity between craniopharyngioma and odontogenic lesions: a reappraisal. Oral Surg Oral Med Oral Pathol 56:501–510, 1983.

Buchner A, Sciubba J. Peripheral epithelial odontogenic tumors: a review. Oral Surg Oral Med Oral Pathol 63:688–697, 1987.

Eisenstein W, Pitcock J. Adamantinoma of the tibia. Arch Pathol Lab Med 108:246–250, 1984.

Ellis G, Shmookler B. Aggressive (malignant?) epithelial odontogenic ghost cell tumor. Oral Surg Oral Med Oral Pathol 61:471–478, 1986.

Elzay R. Primary intraosseous carcinoma of the jaws. Oral Surg Oral Med Oral Pathol 54:299–303, 1982.

Eversole L, Belton C, Hansen L. Clear cell odontogenic tumor: histochemical and ultrastructural features. J Oral Pathol 14:603–614, 1985.

Goldblatt L, Brannon R, Ellis G. Squamous odontogenic tumor. Oral Surg Oral Med Oral Pathol 54:187–196, 1982.

Grodjesk J, Dolinsky H, Schneider L, et al. Odontogenic ghost cell carcinoma. Oral Surg Oral Med Oral Pathol 63:576–581, 1987.

Hansen L, Eversole L, Green T, et al. Clear cell odontogenic tumor—a new histologic variant with aggressive potential. Head Neck Surg 8:115–123, 1985.

Kristensen S, Andersen J, Jacobsen P. Squamous odontogenic tumor. J Laryngol Otol 99:919–924, 1985.

Mills W, Davila M, Beuttenmuller E, et al. Squamous odontogenic tumor. Oral Surg Oral Med Oral Pathol 61:557–563, 1986.

Mori H, Yamamoto S, Hiramatsu K, et al. Adamantinoma of the tibia. Clin Orthop 190:299–310, 1984.

Norris L, Baghaei-Rad M, Maloney P. Bilateral maxillary squamous odontogenic tumors and the malignant transformation of a mandibular radiolucent lesion. J Oral Maxillofac Surg 42:827–834, 1984.

Perez-Atayde A, Kozakewich H, Vawter G. Adamantinoma of the tibia. Cancer 55:1015–1023, 1985.

Mesenchymal and Mixed Odontogenic Tumors

Altini M, Thompson S, Lownie J, et al. Ameloblastic sarcoma of the mandible. J Oral Maxillofac Surg 43:789–794, 1985.

Dahl E, Wolfson S, Haugen J. Central odontogenic fibroma. J Oral Surg 39:120–124, 1981.

Dunlap C, Barker B. Central odontogenic fibroma of the WHO type. Oral Surg Oral Med Oral Pathol 57:390–394, 1984.

Melrose R, Abrams A, Mills B. Florid osseous dysplasia. Oral Surg Oral Med Oral Pathol 41:62–82, 1976.

Regezi J, Kerr D, Courtney R. Odontogenic tumors: analysis of 706 cases. J Oral Surg 36:771–778, 1978.

Vincent S, Hammond H, Ellis G, et al. Central granular cell odontogenic fibroma. Oral Surg Oral Med Oral Pathol 63:715–721, 1987.

Zachariades N, Skordalaki A, Papanicolaou S, et al. Cementoblastoma: review of the literature and report of a case in a seven-year-old girl. Br J Oral Maxillofac Surg 23:456–461, 1985.

Chapter 12

Benign Non-odontogenic Tumors

Jeffery C. B. Stewart

OSSIFYING FIBROMA
FIBROUS DYSPLASIA
OSTEOBLASTOMA
OSTEOID OSTEOMA
CHONDROMA
OSTEOMA
CENTRAL GIANT CELL GRANULOMA
GIANT CELL TUMOR
HEMANGIOMA OF BONE
IDIOPATHIC HISTIOCYTOSIS (LANGERHANS CELL DISEASE)
TORI AND EXOSTOSES
CORONOID HYPERPLASIA

OSSIFYING FIBROMA

Ossifying fibroma is a benign, slow-growing lesion of the jaws that is often clinically and microscopically similar, if not identical, to cementifying fibroma. This tumor is classified as one of the benign fibro-osseous lesions of the jaws and historically has been referred to as fibro-osteoma, osteofibroma, and benign fibro-osseous lesion of periodontal ligament origin.

Etiology and Pathogenesis. The ossifying fibroma is considered by many investigators to be a benign neoplasm that develops from undifferentiated cells of periodontal ligament origin. Others regard this lesion as an example of a localized dysplastic process in which bone metabolism is altered. The similarities between this lesion and the cementifying fibroma are numerous. Both tumors occur in similar age groups and locations and manifest comparable clinical characteristics. The microscopic features are also indistinguishable in many instances. The distinction between these processes, most often based on the nature of the calcified product in the tumor, may in fact be academic, since their biologic behavior is identical.

Clinical Features. The ossifying fibroma is a slow-growing, expansile lesion that is usually asymptomatic when discovered. The lesions, with rare exceptions, arise in the tooth-bearing regions of the jaws, most often in the mandibular premolar-molar area. Some cases of ossifying fibroma have been reported in craniofacial bones other than the jaws. The slow growth of the tumor may ultimately produce expansion and thinning of the buccal and lingual cortical plates, although perforation and mucosal ulceration are rare. Ossifying fibromas are uncommon lesions that tend to occur during the third and fourth decades of life. A definite female predominance has been evident in several studies. These lesions occur most commonly in a solitary fashion, although rare instances of multiple synchronous lesions have been reported.

The most important radiographic feature of this lesion is the well-circumscribed, sharply defined border (Fig. 12–1). Ossifying fibromas otherwise present a variable appearance depending on the maturation or the amount of calcification present (Fig. 12–2). Early lesions may appear as unilocular or multilocular radiolucencies that bear considerable resemblance to odontogenic cysts. The initial radiolucent stage gradually progresses to a mixed radiolucent-radiopaque lesion as calcified ma-

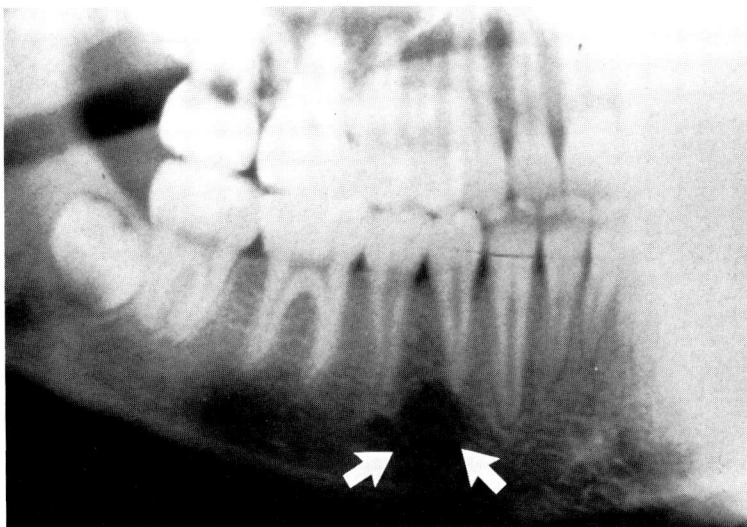

Figure 12–1. Ossifying fibroma in the premolar region of the mandible (arrows).

terial is deposited in the tumor. Mature lesions may consist of a dense, radiopaque mass surrounded by a well-defined, radiolucent rim. Displacement of the roots of teeth may be present, and less commonly, the lesion may resorb tooth roots.

The well-circumscribed appearance of the ossifying fibroma is most evident at the time of surgery, when the lesion may be curetted or enucleated from the normal bone with ease.

Histopathology. The tumor consists of a collagenous stroma that contains varying numbers of uniform spindled or stellate cells (Fig. 12–3). Collagen fibers are often arranged haphazardly although a whorled, storiform pattern may be evident. The stroma is well vascularized in many instances, although in some cases it is relatively fibrotic and avascular.

Calcific deposits are noted throughout the fibrous stroma (Fig. 12–4). The nature of the hard tissue is generally quite variable within a given tumor as well as between lesions. Irregular trabeculae of woven immature bone are most consistently noted in these tumors, although lamellar bone is also present in a large percentage of cases. Osteoblasts may or may not be evident at the periphery of the bone deposits.

Additional patterns of calcified material include small, ovoid to globular, basophilic deposits and anastomosing trabeculae of cementum-like material. The observation of these

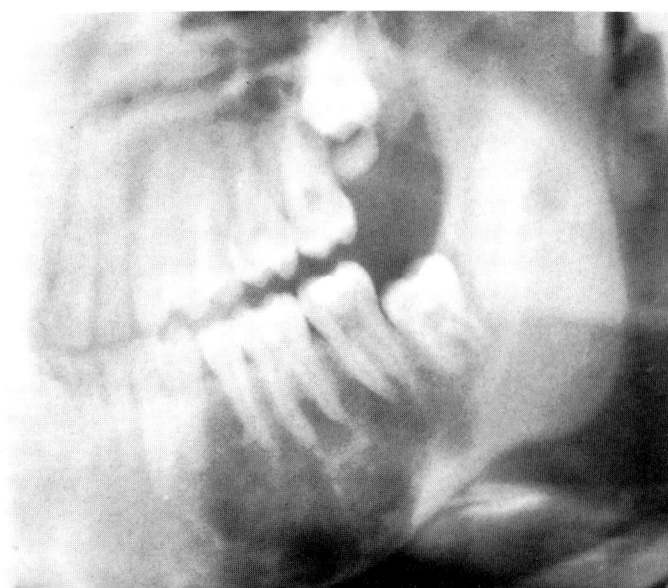

Figure 12–2. Ossifying fibroma of the mandible.

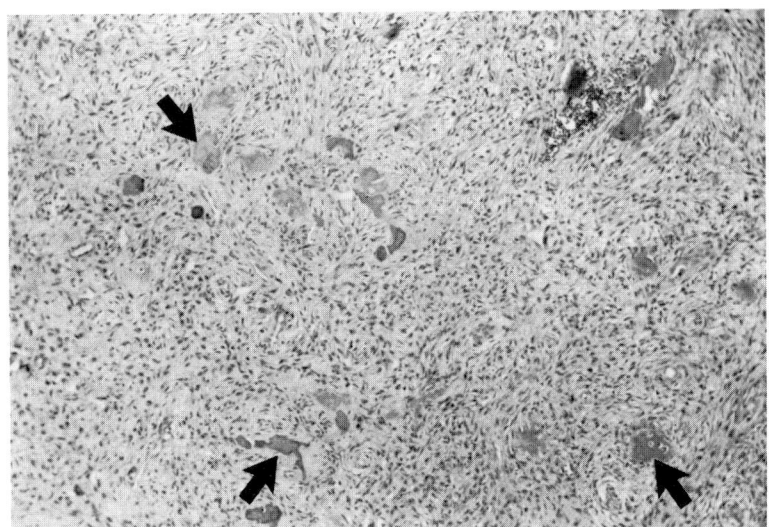

Figure 12–3. Ossifying fibroma composed of evenly distributed fibroblasts and several calcified foci of bone (arrows).

deposits in many of these lesions has led some investigators to conclude that the ossifying fibroma and cementifying fibroma are similar, if not identical, lesions.

Most ossifying fibromas exhibit a mixture of the different types of calcified products, although a single morphologic type is evident in others.

Differential Diagnosis. Distinguishing between ossifying fibroma and fibrous dysplasia is the primary differential diagnostic challenge. Both processes may exhibit similar clinical, radiographic, and microscopic features. The most helpful feature distinguishing the two is the radiographic and clinically well-circumscribed appearance of ossifying fibroma and the ease with which it can be separated from normal bone. In most cases, the well-defined appearance of ossifying fibroma is evident radiographically. Historically, attempts at differentiating the two lesions were based only on histologic criteria. Fibrous dysplasia was reported to contain only woven bone, without evidence of osteoblastic rimming of bone. The presence of mature lamellar bone was felt to be characteristic of ossifying fibroma. Most authorities now acknowledge that these criteria are unreliable, because both types of bone may be found in either lesion.

Osteoblastoma and osteoid osteoma are evident in a slightly younger age group and are often characterized by pain. Additionally, osseous trabeculae in these lesions are rimmed by abundant plump osteoblasts. A central nidus is also evident in these lesions. Cementoblastoma may arise with a similar clinical and radiographic presentation; however, this lesion is fused to the root of the involved tooth.

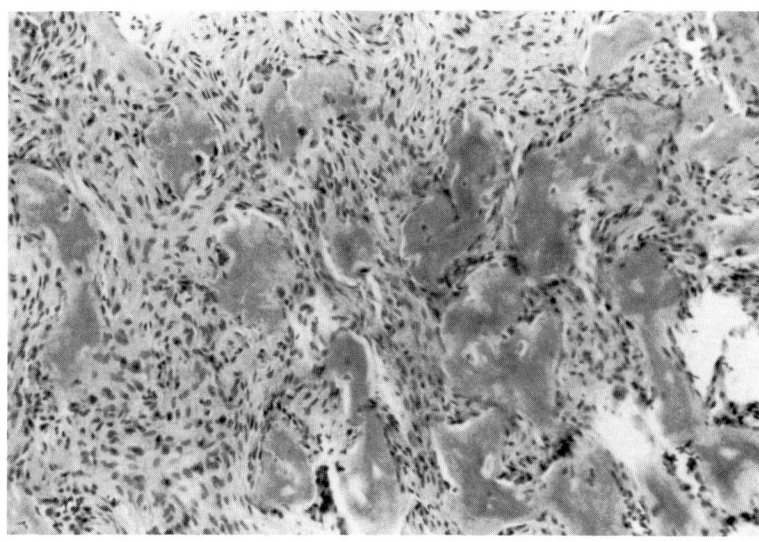

Figure 12–4. Ossifying fibroma composed of benign fibroblasts and irregular islands of new bone.

Occasionally, it may be necessary to distinguish ossifying fibroma from focal sclerosing osteomyelitis. In general, a source of inflammation will be evident, possibly accompanied by pain, tenderness, swelling, or lymphadenopathy.

Treatment and Prognosis. Treatment of ossifying fibroma is most often accomplished by surgical removal utilizing curettage or enucleation. As stated, the lesion can be separated easily from the surrounding normal bone. Recurrence is not expected following removal. A variant of ossifying fibroma, the *juvenile active ossifying fibroma*, has been described in children. This rare lesion behaves in a more aggressive fashion than does the ossifying fibroma, and it may require more extensive therapy when encountered. The true relationship between these lesions awaits elucidation.

FIBROUS DYSPLASIA

Fibrous dysplasia is an idiopathic condition in which normal medullary bone is gradually replaced by an abnormal fibrous connective tissue proliferation. The mesenchymal tissue contains varying amounts of osteoid and osseous material that presumably arises through metaplasia. The resultant fibro-osseous tissue is poorly formed and structurally inadequate.

Subsequent to the original description of this process, confusion developed regarding the criteria necessary for the diagnosis of fibrous dysplasia. As a result, many entities that appear to be distinct from fibrous dysplasia were included under this designation. Attempts to more precisely describe and define fibrous dysplasia continue.

Etiology and Pathogenesis. The etiology of this condition remains unknown, although various theories have been proposed. Many authorities accept the premise that fibrous dysplasia represents a non-neoplastic, hamartomatous growth resulting from deranged mesenchymal cell activity. It has also been proposed that this lesion results from an arrest in the maturation of mesenchymal tissue at the woven bone stage. Another hypothesis suggests that fibrous dysplasia is an abnormal reaction of bone to a localized traumatic episode. Alternatively, focal bone expression of a complicated endocrine disturbance has been suggested as a possible etiology. A hereditary basis for development of fibrous dysplasia has not been found.

Clinical Features. This disease most commonly presents as an asymptomatic, slow enlargement of the involved bone. Fibrous dysplasia may involve one bone or several bones concomitantly. *Monostotic fibrous dysplasia* is the designation used to describe the process as it occurs in one bone; *polyostotic fibrous dysplasia* applies to cases in which more than one bone exhibits evidence of the disorder. Polyostotic fibrous dysplasia is relatively uncommon; however, many patients have lesions of the skull, facial bones, or jaws as a component of the condition. *Albright's syndrome* is a designation that has been applied to patients with polyostotic fibrous dysplasia, cutaneous melanotic pigmentations (café-au-lait macules), and endocrine abnormalities. The most commonly reported endocrine disorder consists of precocious sexual development in females. *Jaffe-Lichtenstein syndrome* has been used to describe patients with multiple bone lesions of fibrous dysplasia and skin pigmentations.

Monostotic fibrous dysplasia is much more common than the polyostotic form, accounting for up to 80% of the cases. Jaw involvement is common in this form of the disease. Other bones frequently affected are the ribs and femur. Fibrous dysplasia occurs within the maxilla more often than the mandible. Maxillary lesions may extend to involve the maxillary sinus, zygoma, sphenoid bone, and floor of the orbit. This form of the disease, with involvement of several adjacent bones, has been referred to as *craniofacial fibrous dysplasia*. The most common site of occurrence with mandibular involvement is in the body portion.

The slowly progressive enlargement of the affected jaw is usually painless and typically presents as a unilateral swelling (Fig. 12–5). As the lesion grows, facial asymmetry becomes evident and may be the initial presenting complaint. The fusiform swelling of the affected jaw most commonly results from buccal cortical plate expansion, and it rarely affects the lingual or palatal aspect. Displacement of teeth with resultant malocclusion and interference with normal eruption patterns may occur, although mobility of erupted teeth is not a feature of fibrous dysplasia.

This condition characteristically has its onset during the first or second decade of life. Rarely, the lesion is not evident until later in life, although this finding may only reflect the insidious, asymptomatic nature of fibrous dysplasia.

Monostotic fibrous dysplasia generally exhibits an equal gender distribution, and the

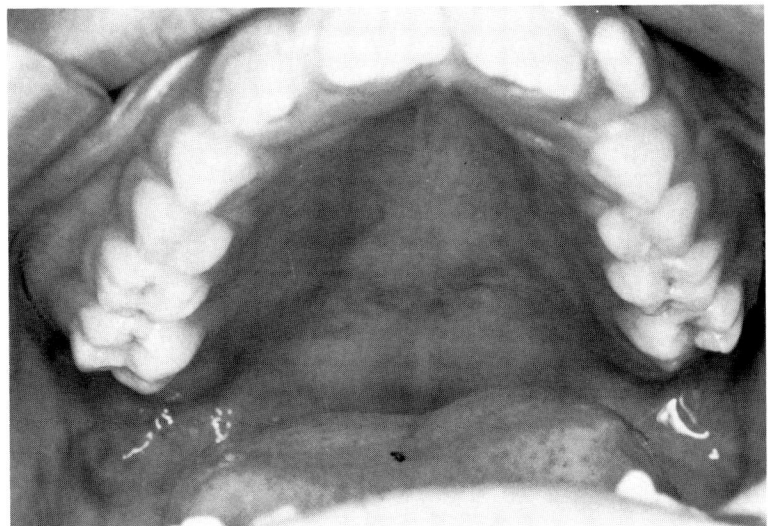

Figure 12–5. Monostotic fibrous dysplasia causing expansion of the right maxilla.

polyostotic form tends to occur more commonly in females.

Fibrous dysplasia has a variable radiographic appearance that ranges from a radiolucent lesion to a densely radiopaque mass (Fig. 12–6). The classic presentation has been described as radiopaque with numerous bony trabeculae imparting a "ground-glass" appearance. This characteristic feature, which becomes most identifiable on intraoral radiographs, is, however, not pathognomonic. Lesions of fibrous dysplasia may also present as unilocular or multilocular radiolucencies. A third pattern is one in which a mottled radiolucent and radiopaque appearance, similar to that noted in Paget's disease, predominates.

An important distinguishing feature of fibrous dysplasia is the poorly defined radiographic and clinical margins of the lesion. The process appears to blend into the surrounding normal bone without evidence of a circumscribed border. Additionally, these lesions are frequently elliptical as opposed to spherical. Laboratory values, specifically serum calcium, phosphorus, and alkaline phosphatase, are within normal ranges for the patient's age group.

Histopathology. The histologic findings in fibrous dysplasia consist of a cellular, fibrous connective tissue proliferation that contains foci of irregularly shaped trabeculae of immature bone. The collagen fibers may completely lack orientation or, alternatively, may be arranged in a storiform pattern of interlacing collagen bundles. The fibroblasts exhibit uniform, spindle- to stellate-shaped nuclei. The bony trabeculae assume bizarre, irregular shapes, likened to Chinese characters (Fig. 12–7). These trabeculae do not display any apparent functional orientation. The bone is predominantly woven bone that appears to arise directly from the collagenous stroma without prominent osteoblastic activity (Fig. 12–8). In a mature fibrous dysplasia lesion, lamellar bone may be found. It should be noted that the microscopic features of fibrous dysplasia share many characteristics with those of ossifying fibroma.

Differential Diagnosis. The primary differential diagnosis for fibrous dysplasia of the jaws is ossifying fibroma. As previously noted, clinical, radiographic, and microscopic features must be considered together in order to most accurately distinguish these processes. The well-circumscribed appearance of ossifying fi-

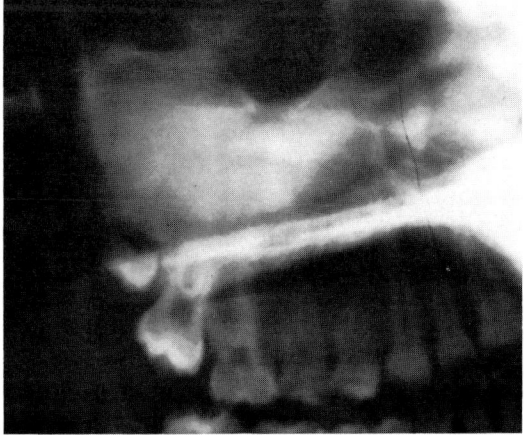

Figure 12–6. Diffuse maxillary opaque mass of fibrous dysplasia.

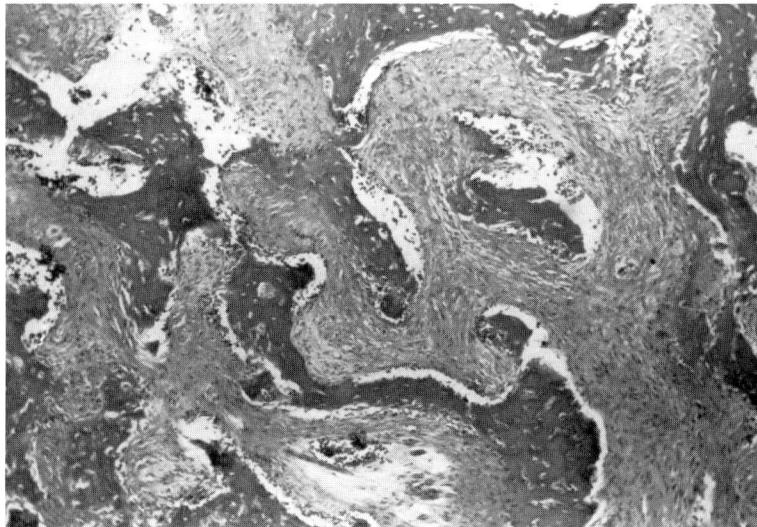

Figure 12–7. Irregular trabeculae of fibrous dysplasia.

broma in comparison with the ill-defined borders of fibrous dysplasia often serves as the differentiating factor. Additional features that aid in distinguishing these processes are listed in Table 12–1.

Paget's disease shares some features with fibrous dysplasia, but it occurs in a much older age group and typically exhibits a bilateral distribution. Alkaline phosphatase levels are characteristically increased in Paget's disease. Chronic osteomyelitis may mimic the mottled radiographic appearance of fibrous dysplasia. Inflammation is generally present and is accompanied by variable symptoms, including tenderness, pain, or purulent drainage. The slowly progressive, asymptomatic nature of fibrous dysplasia usually allows differentiation from malignant tumors of bone.

Treatment and Prognosis. Following a variable period of growth, fibrous dysplasia frequently stabilizes or slows considerably after the onset of puberty. Small lesions may therefore require no treatment other than biopsy confirmation and periodic follow-up. Large lesions that have caused cosmetic or functional deformity may be treated through a process of osseous recontouring. This procedure is generally reserved for the period of time following stabilization of the disease process. *En bloc* resections for complete removal are impractical and unnecessary because the lesions are relatively large and are generally regarded as non-neoplastic.

Malignant transformation is a rare complication of fibrous dysplasia (less than 1% of cases) that has been described usually in pa-

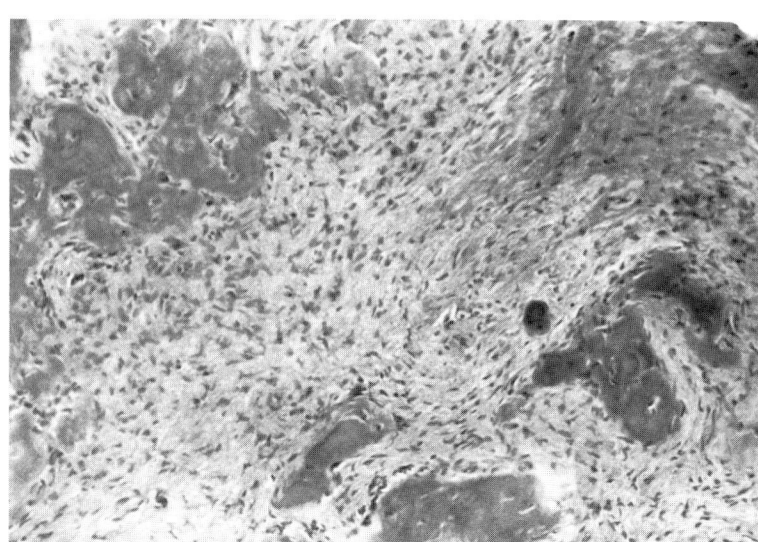

Figure 12–8. Fibrous dysplasia consisting of benign fibrous matrix and "metaplastic" bone.

Table 12–1. DIFFERENTIATING FEATURES OF OSSIFYING FIBROMA AND FIBROUS DYSPLASIA		
Feature	**Ossifying Fibroma**	**Fibrous Dysplasia**
Age	Third and fourth decades	First and second decades
Gender predilection	Females	Equal (monostotic)
Location	Body of mandible favored	Maxilla favored slightly
Radiography	Well-defined margins	Poorly defined margins
Lesion shape	Roughly nodular or spherical jaw expansion	Fusiform or elliptical jaw expansion

tients with the polyostotic type. Many of these patients were treated with radiation therapy, suggesting a role for radiation in the transformation process.

OSTEOBLASTOMA

Osteoblastoma is an uncommon primary lesion of bone that occasionally arises in the maxilla or the mandible. The term "giant osteoid osteoma" has been employed at times to describe this lesion, because it is believed to represent a larger version of the osteoid osteoma. Osteoblastoma is a benign process that may exhibit a seemingly rapid onset and cause pain. These clinical features, as well as histologic findings, may on occasion cause confusion between this lesion and malignant tumors of bone.

Etiology and Pathogenesis. Although the etiology of the osteoblastoma is unknown, most authorities consider this to be a true neoplasm of bone. Reports of regression of lesions following incomplete treatment have led some investigators to postulate that osteoblastoma represents an unusual reactive process within bone.

Clinical Features. Osteoblastoma arises most frequently in the vertebrae and the long bones of the body. These lesions involve the jaws and other craniofacial bones less commonly, but the mandible is the most frequent head and neck site. The posterior tooth-bearing regions of the maxilla or mandible are the usual sites of involvement. The midline areas of the jaws and the coronoid processes are rarely affected.

Most cases occur during the second decade of life, with 90% of osteoblastomas presenting before age 30. Males seem to be affected more commonly than females, by a ratio of approximately 2 to 1.

Osteoblastomas present with a variety of signs and symptoms. Pain, often quite severe, is the most consistent symptom. Localized swelling may occur alone or along with the pain. The bony cortices may be expanded and tender to palpation, although mucosal ulceration is absent. Mobility of adjacent teeth has been noted. Unlike the pain occurring with those lesions that have been reported as osteoid osteoma, the pain associated with osteoblastoma is not often relieved by aspirin. The classic nocturnal pain of osteoid osteoma is also uncommon with these lesions. Duration of signs or symptoms of osteoblastoma ranges from weeks to years.

The radiographic features are variable, consisting of combinations of radiolucent and radiopaque patterns (Fig. 12–9). The designation of osteoblastoma may be used for lesions greater than 2 cm in diameter, in contrast to smaller lesions that are often referred to as osteoid osteomas. The well-circumscribed nature of the process is evident radiographically. A thin radiolucency may be noted, surrounding a variably calcified, central tumor mass. Sclerosis of perilesional bone, a constant feature of the smaller osteoid osteoma, is usually absent in osteoblastoma. A "sun-ray" pattern of new bone production, similar to that described in various malignant bone tumors, may be evident in these lesions.

Histopathology. The histologic appearance of osteoblastoma, like its radiographic appearance, is quite variable. Irregular trabeculae of osteoid and immature bone are present within a stroma containing a prominent vascular network (Fig. 12–10). The bony trabeculae exhibit varying degrees of calcification. Remodeling of the osseous tissue may be evident in the form of basophilic reversal lines. Several layers of plump, hyperchromatic osteoblasts typically line the bony trabeculae. Pleomorphism and abnormal mitotic activity are not fea-

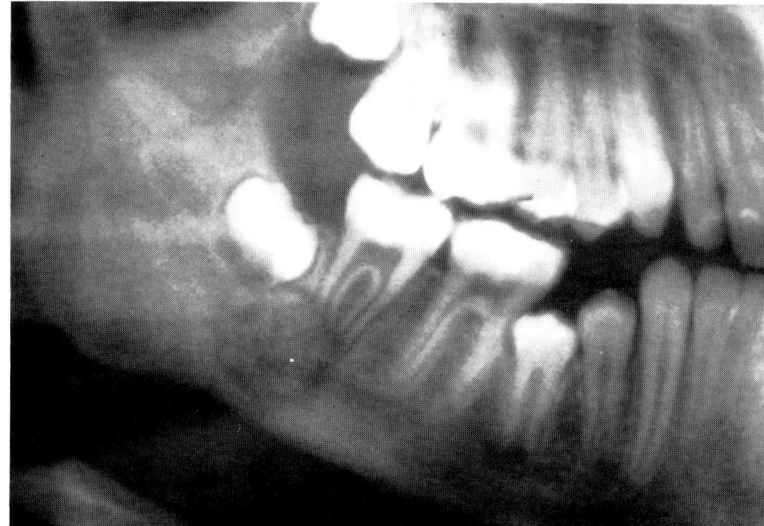

Figure 12–9. Osteoblastoma of the mandible.

tures of these active osteoblasts, however. Stromal cells are generally small and slender, although osteoblast-like cells may be noted in these areas. An additional characteristic of osteoblastoma is the presence of numerous multinucleated giant cells scattered throughout the stroma.

Differential Diagnosis. Osteoblastoma must be differentiated from a number of bone-producing lesions, including osteoid osteoma, cementoblastoma, ossifying fibroma, fibrous dysplasia, and osteosarcoma.

Osteoid osteoma bears considerable clinical, radiographic, and histologic similarity to osteoblastoma. Many experts, in fact, regard the two lesions as identical. Classically, the distinction rests primarily in the size of the lesion: osteoid osteoma, under 2 cm, and osteoblastoma, larger than 2 cm. Nocturnal pain, frequently relieved by aspirin, is more commonly noted in osteoid osteoma. A sclerotic peripheral bone reaction is a significant feature of osteoid osteoma. Cementoblastoma can be differentiated from osteoblastoma since the former lesion arises from the surface of a tooth root and is fused to it. This intimate connection between lesion and tooth is unexpected in osteoblastoma.

Multilayered, plump osteoblasts lining bony trabeculae serve to distinguish osteoblastoma from ossifying fibroma. The clinical and radiographic features of these lesions may be similar, although pain is not a usual symptom of ossifying fibroma. Fibrous dysplasia has a poorly defined margin in contrast to the well-circumscribed appearance of osteoblastoma.

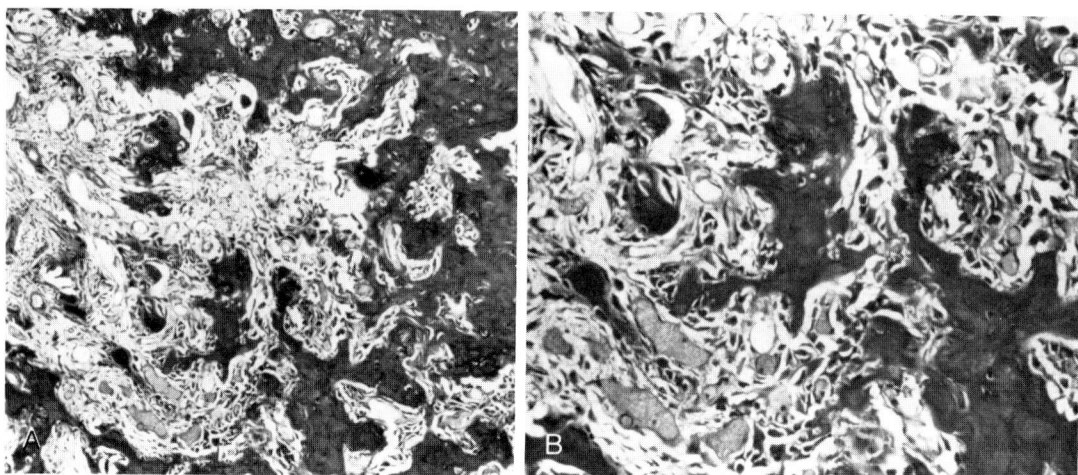

Figure 12–10. *A* and *B,* Osteoblastoma composed of irregular bony trabeculae surrounded by abundant hyperchromatic osteoblasts.

Prominent osteoblastic activity is not a significant microscopic feature of fibrous dysplasia.

The relatively rapid onset and pain associated with some osteoblastomas necessitate differentiation from osteosarcoma. Radiographic and histologic similarities may also exist between given lesions. The hyperchromatic, large osteoblasts noted in osteoblastoma must be distinguished from the malignant tumor cells of osteosarcoma. Cytologic atypia, abnormal mitotic figures, and delicate osteoid adjacent to tumor cells are features of osteosarcoma.

Chondroid differentiation, often noted in osteosarcomas of the jaws, is typically absent in osteoblastoma, unless a previous fracture has occurred through the involved area.

Treatment and Prognosis. Surgical excision of osteoblastoma is the preferred method of treatment. A conservative approach, curettage or local excision, is curative in virtually all cases. Recurrence following surgical intervention is rare.

OSTEOID OSTEOMA

This benign lesion of bone shares many features with osteoblastoma, as previously discussed. Distinction between these lesions has been described on the basis of size, site of occurrence, and radiographic appearance. These lesions, as they present in the jaws, are best regarded as closely related variants of the same process.

Etiology and Pathogenesis. Osteoid osteoma is idiopathic. This lesion is generally regarded as a true neoplasm although the limited growth potential suggests an unusual reactive disorder.

Clinical Features. Osteoid osteoma is an uncommon bone lesion that, like osteoblastoma, occurs predominantly in individuals in the second and third decades of life. A definite male preponderance is also apparent. The tumor arises most commonly in the femur and tibia, with jaw lesions being rare. Any area of the mandible or maxilla may be involved, however.

Pain is the major symptom associated with osteoid osteoma. The pain may be described initially as intermittent, dull, and vague. It is frequently worse during the night and is often relieved with aspirin. Increasing severity of pain with time has been noted. Lesions located near the cortex may produce a localized, tender swelling.

The classic radiographic appearance is that of a small, ovoid radiolucency surrounded by a rim of sclerotic bone. The nidus of the tumor may exhibit varying degrees of calcification, often presenting with a densely opaque center. Osteoid osteoma has a limited growth potential, not exceeding 2 cm in diameter.

Histopathology. Distinction between the histologic features of osteoid osteoma and osteoblastoma is essentially impossible. A richly vascular stroma invests trabeculae of osteoid and immature bone. The bone is rimmed by layers of active, plump osteoblasts. Some studies have suggested that osteoid osteoma contains fewer osteoblasts, reduced vascularity, and broader osseous trabeculae than does osteoblastoma. These differences have been difficult to appreciate in the experience of most pathologists. Electron microscopic studies have shown identical morphologic features in proliferating osteoblastic cells in both lesions.

Differential Diagnosis. The differential diagnosis for osteoid osteoma is similar to that for osteoblastoma. Lesions may occasionally resemble focal osteomyelitis on a radiographic basis. The absence of both inflammatory cells and fibrosis in the biopsy specimen of osteoid osteoma serves to distinguish the two processes.

Treatment and Prognosis. This benign process is treated by conservative surgical excision. Cure is expected following removal, since recurrence is rare. Spontaneous regression following no treatment or incomplete treatment has been reported. Surgical intervention, nonetheless, is the treatment of choice.

CHONDROMA

Chondromas are benign tumors composed of mature cartilage. The etiology of these lesions is unknown. Chondromas are known to occur in the jaws; however, these lesions are rare in this location in comparison with their occurrence in other skeletal sites.

Clinical Features. The chondroma commonly presents as a painless, slow, progressive swelling. The gradual expansion of the lesion rarely results in mucosal ulceration. Most lesions of the craniofacial complex arise in the nasal septum and ethmoid sinuses. Chondromas of the maxilla are most frequently found in the anterior region, where cartilaginous remnants of development are located. Mandibular chondromas have been noted in the body and symphysis areas as well as the coronoid process and the condyle. Chondromas occur with equal incidence in both genders, with the majority of tumors appearing before 50 years of age.

The radiographic appearance of the chondroma is variable, the lesion most often presenting as an irregular radiolucent area. Foci of calcification may be evident within the radiolucent lesion. Resorption of the roots of adjacent teeth has been noted.

Histopathology. The lesion consists of well-defined lobules of mature hyaline cartilage. The cartilage may exhibit areas in which calcification has occurred. The chondrocytes are small cells that contain single, regular nuclei. Degeneration and necrosis may be present focally. The degree of cellularity varies considerably from one area to another within the chondroma.

Differential Diagnosis. The principal diagnostic dilemma rests in distinguishing the chondroma from a well-differentiated chondrosarcoma. Clinical and radiographic features often provide little useful information to distinguish these lesions. Considerable overlap may occur between these lesions histologically as well. Well-differentiated chondrosarcomas may be underdiagnosed as chondromas if the lesions are examined insufficiently.

Treatment and Prognosis. Surgical excision is the appropriate therapy for the chondroma. The difficulty in distinguishing histologically between this lesion and a well-differentiated chondrosarcoma suggests that wide, although not radical, surgical excision may be justified in some instances.

Prognosis for the chondroma is good following therapy, and recurrence is unusual. Recurrence should be cause for reconsidering the original diagnosis for the possibility of low-grade malignancy.

OSTEOMA

Osteomas are benign tumors that consist primarily of mature, compact, or cancellous bone. Because these lesions are often small and asymptomatic, the true incidence involving the jaws is difficult to determine. Osteomas are generally thought to be relatively uncommon in this region, however.

Etiology and Pathogenesis. The etiology of these lesions is unknown. Various causative factors that have been proposed include trauma, response to infection, and developmental abnormalities. None of these has been definitively shown to be the cause of osteomas.

Clinical Features. Osteomas are most commonly identified during the second to fifth decades of life, although they may be found at any age. These tumors are reported to occur in males twice as frequently as in females, although a marked female predominance has been noted in one study of osteomas of the jaws. These lesions most often occur in solitary fashion, except when associated with Gardner's syndrome.

Gardner's syndrome is inherited as an autosomal dominant disorder, characterized by intestinal polyposis, multiple osteomas, fibromas of the skin, epidermal and trichilemmal cysts, and impacted permanent and supernumerary teeth. The majority of patients with Gardner's syndrome will not exhibit the complete spectrum of clinical disease expression. The presence of multiple osteomas of the jaws and facial bones should lead one to investigate the possibility of this syndrome (Fig. 12–11). Osteomas may be found in the jaws, especially the mandibular angle, as well as in facial and long bones. The intestinal polyps associated with Gardner's syndrome are commonly located in the colon and rectum. Significantly, the polyps, found microscopically to be adenomas, exhibit a very high rate of malignant transformation to invasive colorectal carcinoma.

Osteomas present clinically as asymptomatic, slow-growing, bony, hard masses.

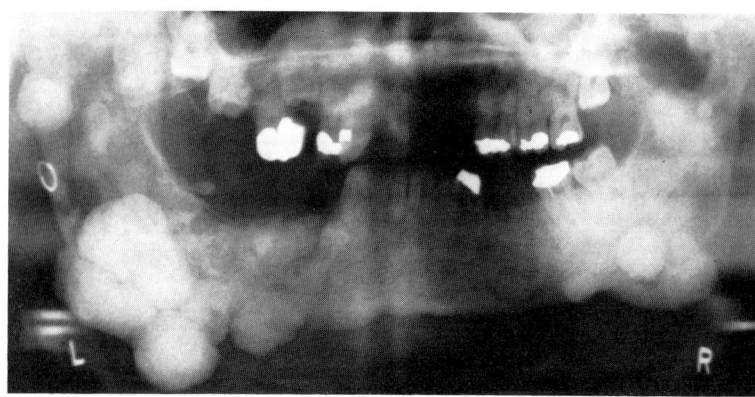

Figure 12–11. Multiple osteomas in Gardner's syndrome. Note impacted teeth.

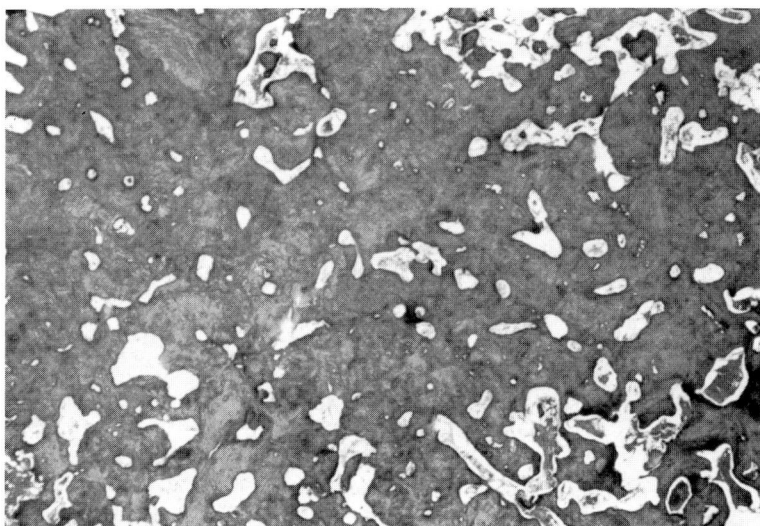

Figure 12–12. Dense, mature bone in an osteoma from a patient with Gardner's syndrome.

Asymmetry may be noted when lesions enlarge to sufficient proportion. Osteomas occurring within medullary bone may be discovered during routine radiographic examination as dense, well-circumscribed radiopacities, since extensive growth must take place before cortical expansion is evident. Osteomas may arise in the maxilla or mandible, as well as in facial and skull bones and within paranasal sinuses. Symptoms occasionally accompany these tumors. Headaches, recurrent sinusitis, and ophthalmologic complaints have been noted, dependent upon lesion location.

Radiographically, both periosteal and endosteal osteomas appear as well-circumscribed, sclerotic, radiopaque masses.

Histopathology. Two distinct histologic variants of osteoma have been described. One form is composed of relatively dense, compact bone with sparse marrow tissue (Fig. 12–12). The other form consists of lamellar trabeculae of cancellous bone with abundant fibrofatty marrow spaces. Osteoblastic activity is usually prominent.

Differential Diagnosis. Osteomas should be distinguished from exostoses of the jaws. Exostoses are bony excrescences that occur on the buccal aspect of alveolar bone. These lesions are of reactive or developmental origin and are not thought to be true neoplasms. Osteoblastomas and osteoid osteomas, which might also be considered in a differential diagnosis, are more frequently painful and may exhibit a more rapid rate of growth than osteomas. Osteomas may also be confused radiographically with odontomas or focal sclerosing osteomyelitis.

Treatment and Prognosis. The treatment of osteomas is surgical excision. Lesions should also be excised for the purpose of establishing the diagnosis. Osteomas do not recur following surgical removal.

CENTRAL GIANT CELL GRANULOMA

The central giant cell granuloma is a benign process that occurs almost exclusively within the jawbones. The tumor typically presents as a solitary, radiolucent lesion of the mandible or maxilla.

Etiology and Pathogenesis. The true nature of the central giant cell granuloma remains unknown, despite considerable discussion and controversy in the literature. It has been proposed that the process represents a reparative response to intrabone hemorrhage and inflammation. Although the clinical progression of these lesions is inconsistent with repair, many investigators regard these lesions as reactive. A previous traumatic or inflammatory episode is not elicited in most cases, however. Other authorities view the central giant cell granuloma as a lesion related to the giant cell tumor of long bones, a lesion considered to be a true neoplasm. A third theory is that this lesion may represent a developmental anomaly closely related to the aneurysmal bone cyst.

Clinical Features. Central giant cell granuloma is an uncommon lesion and occurs less frequently than does peripheral giant cell granuloma. This process is found predominantly in children and young adults, with approximately

75% of cases presenting prior to 30 years of age. Females are affected more frequently than males, with a ratio of 2 to 1.

The central giant cell granuloma is present almost exclusively in the maxilla and mandible, with isolated cases in facial bones having been reported. Lesions occur more frequently in the mandible than in the maxilla. These lesions tend to involve the jaws anterior to the molar teeth, with occasional extension across the midline. Rarely, lesions involve the posterior jaws, including the mandibular ramus and condyle.

The central giant cell granuloma typically produces a painless expansion or swelling of the affected jaw. Cortical plates are thinned; however, perforation with extension into soft tissues is uncommon. The radiographic features of the central giant cell granuloma consist of a multilocular or, less frequently, unilocular radiolucency of bone (Fig. 12–13). The margins of the lesion are relatively well demarcated, often presenting a scalloped border. In some instances, the margins appear less clearly defined. Roots of teeth may be displaced and, less commonly, resorbed.

Histopathology. The lesion is composed of a proliferation of spindled fibroblasts in a stroma containing variable amounts of collagen (Fig. 12–14). Numerous small, vascular channels are evident throughout the lesion. Hemosiderin-laden macrophages are frequently noted as well as extravasated erythrocytes. Multinucleated giant cells are present throughout the connective tissue stroma. The giant cells may be evenly dispersed; however, they are frequently aggregated around vascular channels. Inflammatory cells are not prominent, and when they are seen, most likely they are secondary in nature. Foci of osteoid may be present, scattered throughout the stroma.

Differential Diagnosis. The typical radiographic features of a solitary, multilocular radiolucency indicate that ameloblastoma, odontogenic myxoma, odontogenic keratocyst, and aneurysmal bone cyst must be differentiated from this lesion. Cystic processes of the jaws should also be considered in a differential diagnosis, since some central giant cell granulomas may be unilocular.

The microscopic appearance of central giant cell granuloma is virtually identical to the giant cell lesion associated with hyperparathyroidism. These processes must be differentiated on the basis of biochemical tests. Increased serum calcium and alkaline phosphatase and decreased serum phosphorus values are indicative of hyperparathyroidism; normal serum chemistries are expected with central giant cell granuloma.

The giant cell tumor of bone may present with similar clinical and microscopic features, although many investigators believe careful examination will allow differentiation. The giant cell tumor of bone is regarded as rare in the jaws in comparison with the central giant cell granuloma.

Treatment and Prognosis. Surgical management of these lesions with aggressive curettage is generally regarded as the treatment of choice. Curettage of the tumor mass followed by removal of the peripheral bony margins results in a good prognosis and a low recurrence rate. In some instances, presurgical endodontic therapy of involved teeth or their extraction may be necessary.

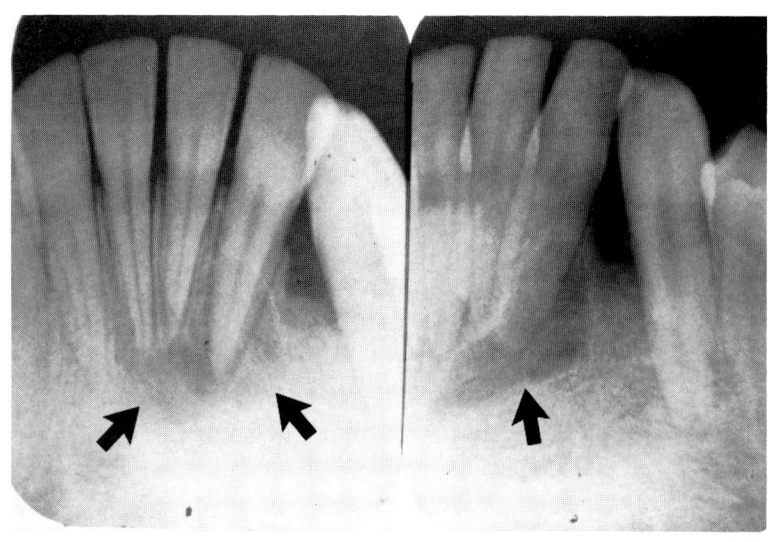

Figure 12–13. Central giant cell granuloma of the anterior mandible (arrows).

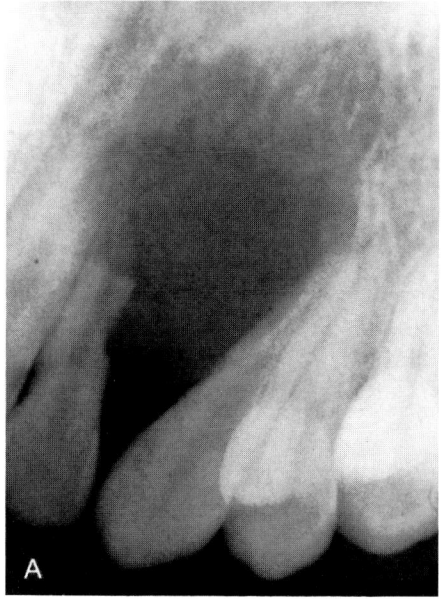
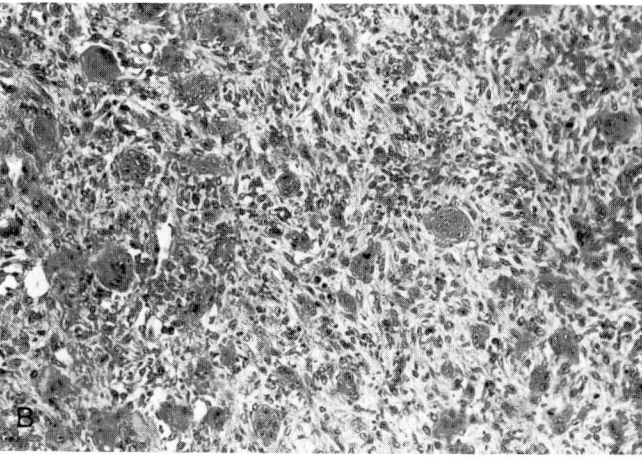

Figure 12–14. *A,* Central giant cell granuloma of the maxilla. *B,* Microscopy shows a benign fibroblastic matrix and numerous multinucleated giant cells.

GIANT CELL TUMOR

Giant cell tumors are true neoplasms that arise most frequently in the long bones, especially in the area of the knee joint. These tumors exhibit a wide spectrum of biologic behavior from benign to malignant. Controversy exists as to the relationship between this lesion and the central giant cell granuloma. Most investigators regard the giant cell tumor as a distinct entity from the central giant cell granuloma, acknowledging the very rare occurrence of the giant cell tumor within jaws.

Etiology and Pathogenesis. These neoplasms are thought to arise from undifferentiated supporting cells of the bone marrow. These neoplastic proliferations are generally regarded as distinct from the central giant cell granuloma, which appears to be reactive. Some authors, however, have considered the giant cell tumor of bone to be representative of a biologically more aggressive variant of the central giant cell granuloma.

Clinical Features. Giant cell tumors, although rare, have been reported to involve the jaws. Other sites of involvement in the head and neck include the sphenoid, ethmoid, and temporal bones. The giant cell tumor has been reported most frequently in the third and fourth decades of life.

These lesions may exhibit a wide range of biologic behavior and, thus, may present a variety of clinical features. Benign variants may exhibit slow growth and bone expansion virtually identical to those of a giant cell granuloma. Aggressive or malignant variants may produce rapid growth, pain, or paresthesia. Radiographically, the giant cell tumor produces a radiolucent lesion similar in appearance to the central giant cell granuloma. Giant cell tumors have been noted in association with pre-existing Paget's disease in both the jaws and the long bones.

Histopathology. The tumor is characterized by the presence of numerous multinucleated giant cells. The giant cells are dispersed evenly among mononuclear stromal cells. Nuclear morphology of both types of cells is virtually identical. Collagen production is generally minimal in these lesions. Several studies have suggested that the giant cells in giant cell tumors are larger and contain more nuclei compared with the corresponding cells of central giant cell granuloma. There is, however, significant variation in these findings, such that any given lesion may present diagnostic difficulty. Giant cell tumors may exhibit a relative absence of hemorrhage and hemosiderin deposition. Osteoid formation is also noted less frequently than in giant cell granulomas.

Differential Diagnosis. Microscopically, the giant cell tumor must be differentiated from other conditions that contain multinucleated giant cells, including central giant cell granuloma, hyperparathyroidism, aneurysmal bone cyst, and cherubism.

Treatment and Prognosis. Surgical excision is the treatment of choice for the giant cell tumor. These lesions exhibit a greater tendency to recur following treatment than that noted for the giant cell granuloma. Although too few cases have been reported in the jaws to predict recurrence rates, it is noteworthy that 30% of lesions in long bones recur following curettage. Finally, the existence of a true malignant giant cell tumor has recently been reported in the jaws.

HEMANGIOMA OF BONE

Hemangiomas of bone are uncommon intraosseous lesions consisting of a proliferation of blood vessels. The central hemangioma occurs most frequently in vertebrae and the skull. The mandible and the maxilla are the next most common sites of occurrence.

Etiology and Pathogenesis. The etiology of central hemangiomas is unknown. Some lesions may represent true neoplasms; others are more probably developmental or traumatic in origin.

Clinical Features. More than half the central hemangiomas of the jaws occur in the mandible, with its posterior region being the most frequent site. The lesion occurs approximately twice as frequently in females as in males. The peak age of incidence is the second decade of life.

A slow-growing, asymmetric expansion of the mandible or maxilla is the most common patient complaint. Spontaneous gingival bleeding around teeth in the area of the hemangioma may also be noted. Paresthesia or pain is occasionally evident as well as mobility of involved teeth. Teeth may exhibit a pumping action such that, when depressed in an apical direction, the teeth rapidly resume their original position. Bruits or pulsation of large hemangiomas may be detected with careful auscultation or palpation of the thinned cortical plates. Significantly, hemangiomas may be present without any signs or symptoms.

Hemangiomas of the mandible and maxilla present a wide variety of radiographic appearances (Fig. 12–15). More than half occur as multilocular radiolucencies that have a characteristic "soap-bubble" appearance. A second form of these lesions consists of a rounded, radiolucent lesion in which bony trabeculae radiate from the center of the lesion, producing angular loculations. Less commonly, hemangiomas appear as cyst-like radiolucencies.

Histopathology. Hemangiomas of bone are composed of a proliferation of blood vessels. Most intrabone hemangiomas are of the cavernous type (Fig. 12–16). Dilated, thin-walled, vascular spaces are lined by benign endothelial cells. Fibrous connective tissue stroma supports the blood-filled vascular spaces. Numerous, small, capillary-sized vascular channels may be the prominent histologic feature. These lesions have been referred to as capillary hemangiomas. Frequently, a mixture of both histologic subtypes is evident. The microscopic appearance of hemangiomas is academic since biologic behavior of the lesions is independent of this factor.

Differential Diagnosis. The differential diagnosis of the multilocular hemangioma of bone includes ameloblastoma, odontogenic myxoma, odontogenic keratocyst, central giant cell granuloma, and aneurysmal bone cyst. A unilocular lesion may be easily confused with other cystic processes that occur within jaws.

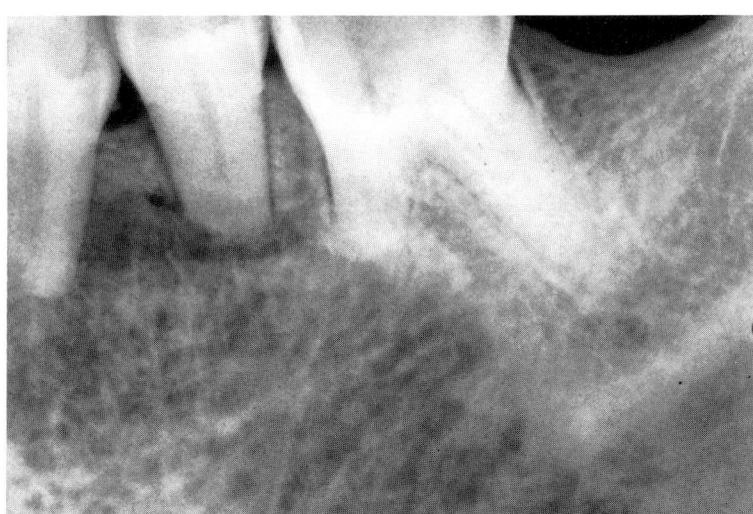

Figure 12–15. Hemangioma of the mandible, causing tooth resorption. (Courtesy of Dr. E. Ellis.)

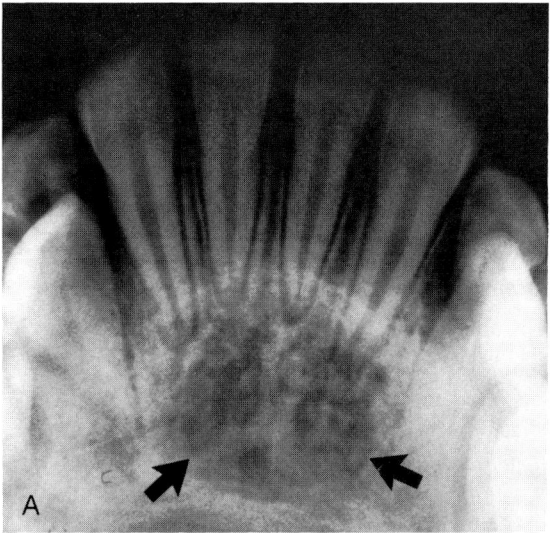 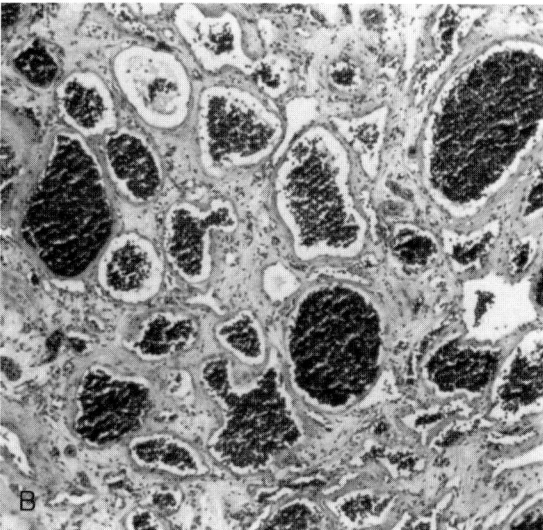

Figure 12–16. *A*, Hemangioma of the anterior mandible (arrows). *B*, Microscopy shows numerous vascular channels.

Treatment and Prognosis. The most significant feature of hemangiomas of bone is that these lesions may prove life threatening if improperly managed. It is imperative to perform needle aspiration of any central lesion that potentially may be of vascular origin prior to performing a biopsy.

Methods utilized in the treatment of hemangioma of bone include surgery, radiation therapy, sclerosing agents, cryotherapy, and presurgical embolization techniques. The vascular supply of a given lesion as well as its size and location must be evaluated prior to the selection of a given treatment method.

IDIOPATHIC HISTIOCYTOSIS (LANGERHANS CELL DISEASE)

Idiopathic histiocytosis or Langerhans cell disease, also formerly known as histiocytosis X, is a disorder characterized by a proliferation of cells exhibiting phenotypic characteristics of Langerhans cells. The clinical manifestations of this process range from solitary or multiple bone lesions to disseminated visceral, skin, and bone lesions.

Traditionally, idiopathic histiocytosis has been used to encompass three disorders: eosinophilic granuloma, Hand-Schüller-Christian syndrome, and Letterer-Siwe syndrome. These entities were grouped together owing to their similar microscopic appearance, in spite of the diverse manner of clinical disease expression. *Eosinophilic granuloma* has referred to patients with solitary or multiple bone lesions only. *Hand-Schüller-Christian syndrome* has represented a specific clinical triad of lytic bone lesions, exophthalmos, and diabetes insipidus. Many of these patients also exhibited lymphadenopathy, dermatitis, splenomegaly, or hepatomegaly. *Letterer-Siwe syndrome* has been characterized by a rapidly progressive, usually fatal, clinical course. Widespread organ, bone, and skin involvement by the proliferative process in infants has been the common presentation.

Most authorities do not currently consider this histiocytosis classification scheme as truly representative of this disease process. Letterer-Siwe syndrome, more recently referred to as the *acute disseminated form* of idiopathic histiocytosis, most likely represents a malignant neoplastic process. A minority of patients actually present with the classic triad of Hand-Schüller-Christian syndrome. This *chronic disseminated form* of the disorder is only one of a variety of presentations in which lymph node, visceral, and bone involvement may occur. Less severe *chronic localized forms* of idiopathic histiocytosis appear to be represented by cases in which only multifocal or unifocal bone lesions are noted.

Etiology and Pathogenesis. The etiology and pathogenesis of idiopathic histiocytosis remain obscure. Recent investigations, however, have elucidated the cell of origin of this process. Ultrastructural and immunohistochemical similarities exist between the proliferative cell of this disorder and the Langerhans cell that normally resides in epidermis and mucosa. The dendritic (Langerhans) cells function in the

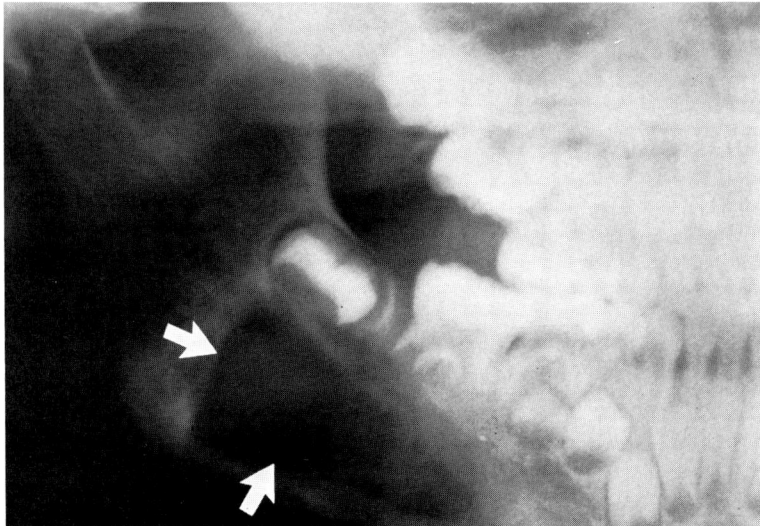

Figure 12–17. Idiopathic histiocytosis of the mandible (arrows). (Courtesy of Dr. J. Hayward.)

processing and presentation of antigens to effector immune cells (T lymphocytes).

The acute form of this disease and some cases of the chronic forms are thought to represent a neoplastic transformation. It has also been suggested that some may result from exuberant reaction to an unknown antigenic challenge. Evidence is emerging that some patients with idiopathic histiocytosis may exhibit defects in certain aspects of the cell-mediated arm of the immune system. These immunologic defects may affect normal regulatory mechanisms with resultant Langerhans cell proliferation.

Clinical Features. Idiopathic histiocytosis is generally regarded as a condition of children and young adults. An increased male predominance has been noted by some investigators. The monostotic and polyostotic forms of the disorder may affect virtually any bone of the body. The skull, mandible, ribs, vertebrae, and long bones are frequently involved. Oral changes may be the initial presentation in all forms of this disorder. Tenderness, pain, and swelling are frequent patient complaints. Loosening of teeth in the area of the affected alveolar bone is a common occurrence. The gingival tissues are frequently inflamed, hyperplastic, and ulcerated.

The jaws may exhibit solitary or multiple radiolucent lesions (Fig. 12–17). The lesions frequently affect the alveolar bone, resulting in the appearance of teeth that are "floating in space" (Fig. 12–18). Bone lesions with a sharply circumscribed, punched-out appearance may also occur in the central aspects of the mandible or maxilla. Occasionally, these lesions are located exclusively in a periapical site. Jaw lesions may be accompanied by bone involvement elsewhere in the skeleton. Radiographic skeletal surveys are useful for detecting widespread involvement. Cervical lymphadenopathy, mastoiditis, and otitis media are head and neck manifestations frequently present with multifocal involvement.

Histopathology. The disorder is character-

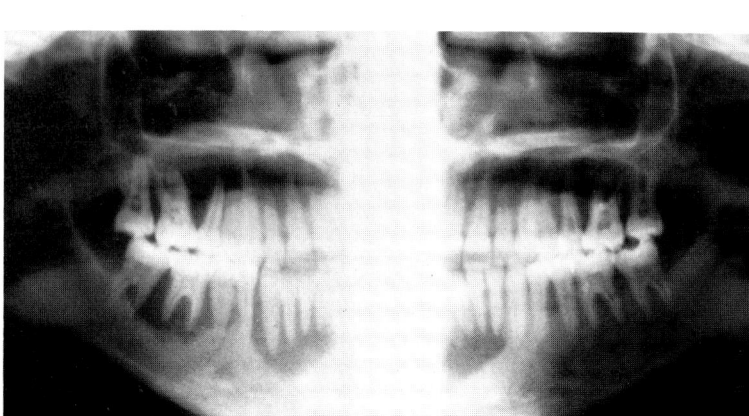

Figure 12–18. Idiopathic histiocytosis of the mandible causing "floating-teeth" appearance.

ized by the proliferation of large cells with abundant cytoplasm, indistinct cell borders, and oval to reniform nuclei. These cells are most often arranged in sheets and may be admixed with varying numbers of eosinophils and other inflammatory cells (Fig. 12–19). A second population of mononuclear phagocytes is frequently evident. These cells exhibit foamy, vacuolated cytoplasm in some cases. Multinucleated giant cells and foci of necrosis may be noted.

Electron microscopic study of the proliferative cells is significant because of the presence of rod-shaped cytoplasmic structures (Figs. 12–20 and 12–21). These Birbeck granules, normally present in Langerhans cells, are lamellated and exhibit central, periodic striations.

Immunohistochemical studies of tumor cells also support an origin from Langerhans cells. Phenotypic expression of T-6 antigens, S-100 protein, and HLA-DR antigens is shared by both normal cells and tumor cells. Identification of these antigenic markers and ultrastructural granules can provide useful diagnostic information.

Differential Diagnosis. Classic presentation of idiopathic histiocytosis in the jaws often results in loosening or premature exfoliation of teeth. Under these conditions, differential diagnosis must include juvenile or diabetic periodontitis, hypophosphatasia, leukemia, cyclic neutropenia, agranulocytosis, and primary or metastatic malignant neoplasms. Lesions located in a periapical site may be confused with inflammatory periapical lesions of pulpal origin. The presence of vital pulp in the involved tooth excludes the possibility of periapical granuloma or cyst.

Solitary radiolucent lesions in the central aspects of the jaws should be differentiated from odontogenic tumors and cysts. Multiple, well-circumscribed radiolucencies may suggest multiple myeloma, although this occurs in a much older age group. Histologic examination of tissue removed for biopsy generally serves to distinguish this disorder from the other entities listed. Disseminated disease will also produce the signs and symptoms mentioned previously.

Treatment and Prognosis. The acute disseminated form commonly occurs during the first years of life and pursues a rapidly progressive course. The primary method of treatment involves use of multiple chemotherapeutic agents. The disease is often fatal in spite of intensive treatment.

Disseminated visceral and bone involvement in somewhat older children often behave in a more chronic fashion. Individual lesions may be effectively managed with surgical curettage or low-dose radiation therapy. Cytotoxic agents such as vincristine sulfate, cyclophosphamide, and methotrexate may be employed for widespread or visceral involvement. The

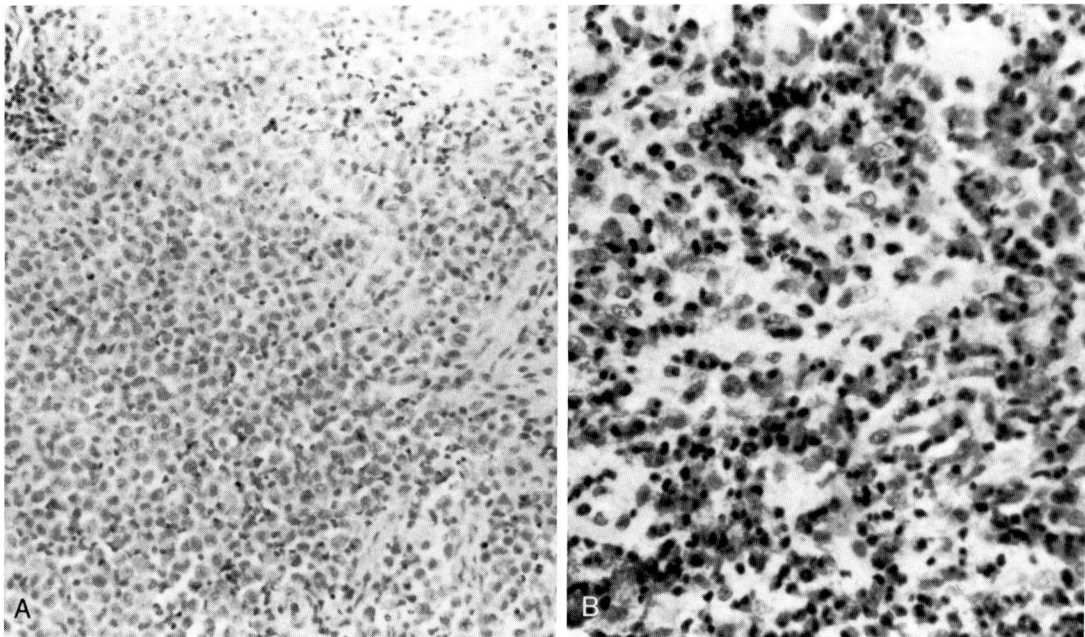

Figure 12–19. Idiopathic histiocytosis, with an infiltrate of pale-staining Langerhans cells *(A)* in one zone and an infiltrate of Langerhans cells and eosinophils in another *(B)*.

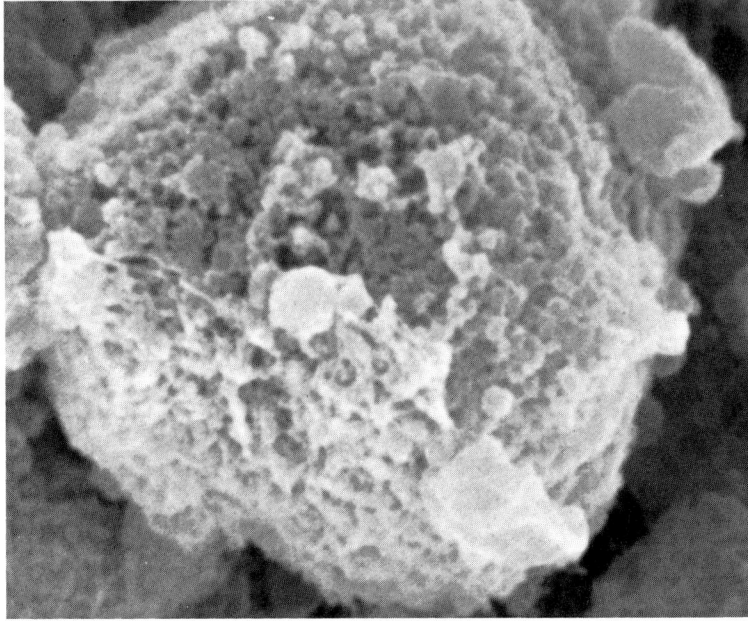

Figure 12–20. Scanning electron micrograph of Langerhans cell of idiopathic histiocytosis. Note the highly irregular cell surface.

prognosis in this form is more optimistic, with half the patients surviving for 10 to 15 years.

The localized form of Langerhans cell disease occurs in older children, teen-agers, and young adults. These lesions may be treated successfully with vigorous surgical curettage. Low-dose radiotherapy is employed for lesions that are inaccessible to surgical treatment. Spontaneous regression of lesions has been reported, although this is rare and unpredictable. Involved teeth are generally sacrificed at the time of surgical therapy owing to the absence of bony support. The prognosis for this form of the disorder is good. These patients must be evaluated for additional bone or visceral involvement, which is usually manifested within the first 6 months following detection of the original lesion. Long-term follow-up is necessary in order to rule out the possibility of recurrent disease.

TORI AND EXOSTOSES

Tori and exostoses are nodular protuberances of mature bone whose precise designation depends on anatomic location. These lesions are of little clinical significance; they are non-neoplastic and rarely are a source of discomfort. Occasionally, the mucosa surfacing

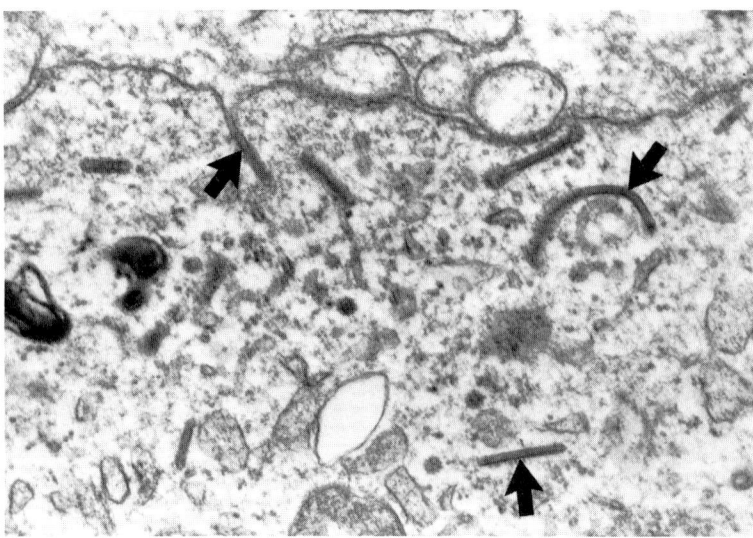

Figure 12–21. Transmission electron micrograph of Langerhans cell of idiopathic histiocytosis. Note intracytoplasmic Langerhans cell granules (arrows). Surface membrane (top) shows infoldings where granules presumably originate.

these lesions may be traumatically ulcerated, producing a slow-healing, painful wound. Surgical removal for the purpose of prosthetic rehabilitation may be necessary.

Etiology and Pathogenesis. The precise etiology of this lesion remains obscure, although evidence has been presented to suggest that the torus may be an inherited condition. The palatal torus is relatively prevalent in certain populations such as Asians, Native Americans, and Eskimos. The incidence in the general population of the United States is between 20 and 25%.

Mandibular tori are seen more commonly in certain groups such as blacks and some Asian populations. The overall incidence in the United States is estimated to be between 6 and 12%.

The etiology of exostoses is unknown. It has been suggested that the bony growths represent a reaction to increased or abnormal occlusal stresses of the teeth in the involved areas.

Clinical Features

Torus Palatinus. The palatal torus is a sessile, nodular mass of bone that presents along the midline of the hard palate (Fig. 12–22). This lesion occurs in females twice as often as it does in males. The palatal torus usually appears during the second or third decade of life, although it may be noted at any age. The bony mass exhibits slow growth and is generally asymptomatic. These lesions are frequently present in a symmetric fashion along the midline of the hard palate. Tori have been noted to form various configurations referred to as nodular, spindled, lobular, or flat. Large tori may be evident on radiographs as diffuse, radiopaque lesions.

Torus Mandibularis. Mandibular tori are bony, exophytic growths that present along the lingual aspect of the mandible superior to the mylohyoid ridge (Fig. 12–23). These tori are almost always bilateral, occurring in the premolar region. Infrequently, a torus may be noted on one side only. These lesions are asymptomatic, exhibiting slow growth during the second and third decades of life.

Mandibular tori may arise as solitary nodules or as multiple nodular masses that appear to coalesce. A significant gender predilection is not evident.

Exostoses. Exostoses are multiple bony excrescences that occur less commonly than do tori (Fig. 12–24). They are multiple, asymptomatic, bony nodules that are present along the buccal aspect of alveolar bone. Lesions are noted most frequently in the posterior portions of both the maxilla and the mandible.

Histopathology. These lesions are composed of hyperplastic bone consisting of mature cortical and trabecular bone. The outer surface exhibits a smooth, rounded contour.

Treatment and Prognosis. Treatment of tori and exostoses is unnecessary, unless required for prosthetic considerations or in cases of frequent trauma to the overlying mucosa. Recurrence following surgical excision is not seen.

CORONOID HYPERPLASIA

Hyperplasia of the coronoid processes of the mandible is an uncommon condition that is frequently associated with limitation of mandibular motion.

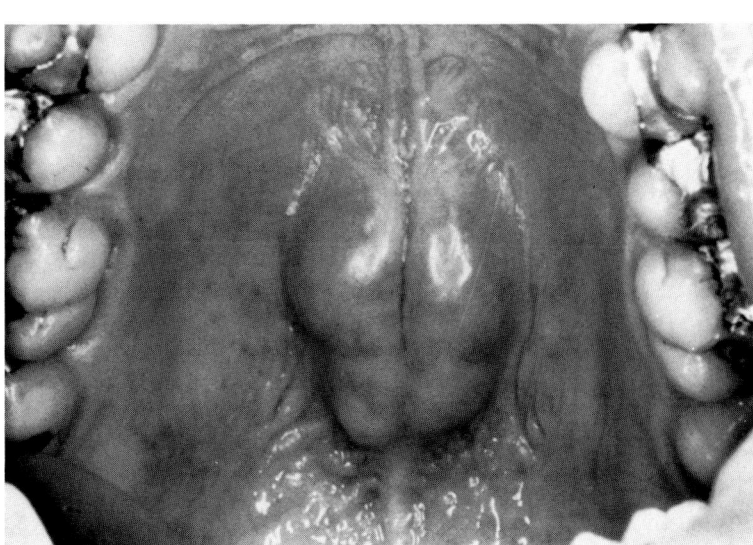

Figure 12–22. Torus palatinus.

BENIGN NON-ODONTOGENIC TUMORS

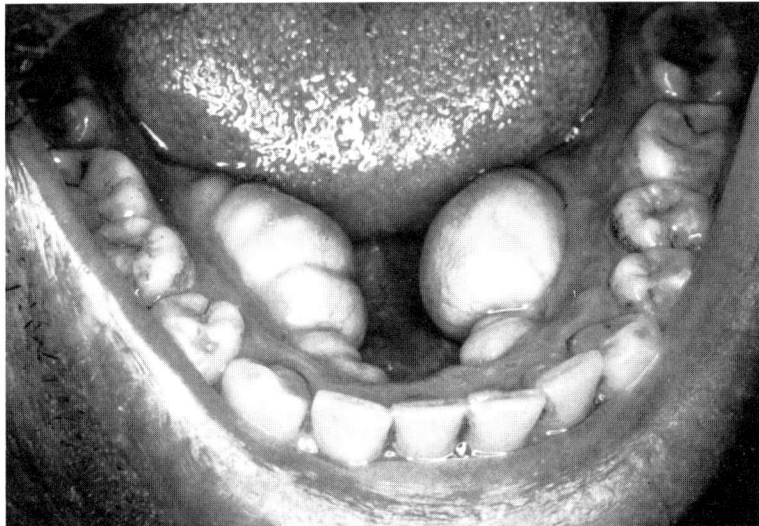

Figure 12–23. Torus mandibularis.

Etiology and Pathogenesis. The etiology of this process remains unknown. A history of trauma is present in many instances; however, the precise relationship between the traumatic episode and the onset of coronoid enlargement has been difficult to establish. The coronoid enlargement appears to represent a hyperplastic process, although it has been suggested that the lesion may be neoplastic. Unilateral coronoid hyperplasia may be the result of a solitary osteochondroma; bilateral coronoid hyperplasia is apparently the result of a different process. The majority of cases have been reported in males, leading some investigators to suggest an X-linked inherited etiology. Subsequent cases have been reported in females, which seems to preclude this possibility. Increased activity of the temporalis muscle with unbalanced condylar support has also been postulated as an etiologic factor.

Clinical Features. Hyperplasia of the coronoid processes is frequently bilateral, although unilateral enlargement has been noted. Bilateral coronoid hyperplasia typically results in limitation of mandibular movement, which is progressive over time.

The disorder is painless and, with a few exceptions, is not associated with facial swelling or asymmetry. Coronoid hyperplasia has been reported most frequently in young male patients. The age of onset is typically around puberty. However, cases have been noted, especially in females, before puberty and during adult life.

Enlarged and elongated coronoid processes are evident radiographically, although the gen-

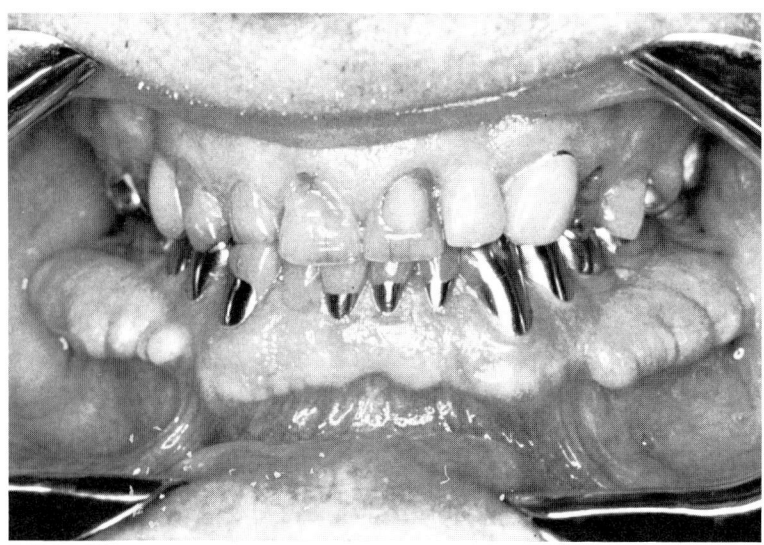

Figure 12–24. Mandibular exostoses.

eral shape of the processes is usually normal. Unilateral coronoid hyperplasia often results in misshapen or mushroom-shaped coronoid processes on radiographs. Temporomandibular joint radiographs are unremarkable.

Histopathology. The enlarged coronoid processes consist of mature, hyperplastic bone. The bone may be partially covered by cartilaginous and fibrous connective tissue.

Differential Diagnosis. Bilateral coronoid hyperplasia rarely presents diagnostic difficulties. However, cases of unilateral coronoid hyperplasia must be differentiated from osseous and chondroid neoplasms.

Treatment and Prognosis. Treatment consists of surgical excision of the hyperplastic coronoid processes. Postoperative physiotherapy is also advocated. Functional improvement is marked following surgical intervention. Recurrence has not been reported.

Bibliography

Barnes L. Surgical Pathology of the Head and Neck. Marcel Dekker, New York, 1985, Chap 17.

Carl W, Herrera L. Dental and bone abnormalities in patients with familial polyposis coli. Semin Surg Oncol 3:77–83, 1987.

Chuong R, Kaban LB, Kozakewich H, Perez-Atayde A. Central giant cell lesions of the jaws: a clinicopathologic study. J Oral Maxillofac Surg 44:708–713, 1986.

Eisenbud L, Stern M, Rothberg M, Sachs SA. Central giant cell granuloma of the jaws: experiences in the management of 37 cases. J Oral Maxillofac Surg 46:376–384, 1988.

Eversole LR, Leider AS, Nelson K. Ossifying fibroma: a clinicopathologic study of 64 cases. Oral Surg Oral Med Oral Pathol 60:505–511, 1985.

Eversole LR, Sabes WR, Rovin S. Fibrous dysplasia: a nosologic problem in the diagnosis of fibro-osseous lesions of the jaws. J Oral Pathol 1:189–220, 1972.

Greer RO, Berman DN. Osteoblastoma of the jaws. Current concepts and differential diagnosis. J Oral Maxillofac Surg 36:304, 1978.

Huvos AG. Bone Tumors. Diagnosis, Treatment, and Prognosis. WB Saunders Co, Philadelphia, 1979.

King DR, Moore GE. An analysis of torus palatinus in a transatlantic study. J Oral Med 31:44–46, 1976.

Kreutz RW, Sanders B. Bilateral coronoid hyperplasia resulting in severe limitation of mandibular movement. Report of a case. Oral Surg Oral Med Oral Pathol 60:482–484, 1985.

Krutchkoff DJ, Jones CR. Multifocal eosinophilic granuloma: a clinical pathologic conference. J Oral Pathol 13:472–488, 1984.

Marra LM. Bilateral coronoid hyperplasia, a developmental defect. Oral Surg Oral Med Oral Pathol 55:10–13, 1983.

Nesbit ME, O'Leary M, Dehner LP, Ramsay NKC. The immune system and the histiocytosis syndromes. Am J Pediatr Hematol Oncol 3:141–149, 1981.

Shatz A, Calderon S, Mintz S. Benign osteoblastoma of the mandible. Oral Surg Oral Med Oral Pathol 61:189–191, 1986.

Smith RA, Hansen LS, Resnick D, Chan W. Comparison of osteoblastoma in gnathic and extragnathic sites. Oral Surg Oral Med Oral Pathol 54:285–298, 1982.

Stewart JCB, Regezi JA, Lloyd RV, McClatchey KD. Immunohistochemical study of idiopathic histiocytosis of the mandible and maxilla. Oral Surg Oral Med Oral Pathol 61:48–53, 1986.

Suzuki M, Sakai T. A familial study of torus palatinus and torus mandibularis. Am J Phys Anthropol 18:263–272, 1960.

Waldron CA. Fibro-osseous lesions of the jaws. J Oral Maxillofac Surg 43:249–262, 1985.

Worth HM, Stoneman DW. Radiology of vascular abnormalities in and about the jaws. Dent Radiogr Photogr 52:1–23, 1979.

Chapter 13

Inflammatory Jaw Lesions

PULPITIS
PERIAPICAL ABSCESS
ACUTE OSTEOMYELITIS
CHRONIC OSTEOMYELITIS
  Garré's Osteomyelitis
  Diffuse Sclerosing Osteomyelitis
  Focal Sclerosing Osteomyelitis

Osteomyelitis, by definition, is inflammation of bone and bone marrow. In the mandible and maxilla, most cases are related to a microbiologic (usually bacterial) infection reaching the bone through non-vital teeth, periodontal lesions, or traumatic injuries. This, coupled with the patient's resistance factors, determines the clinical presentation, extent of the inflammatory process, and speed with which the infection develops. The recognized subtypes of osteomyelitis are closely related and essentially represent differences in etiologic agent and host response. The primary justification for separation of osteomyelitis into the various subtypes lies in the differences in treatment and prognosis for each. It is also important to be aware of clinical and radiographic presentations in making differential diagnoses of bone lesions.

PULPITIS

All the principles of inflammation that apply to any other body organ apply to lesions of the dental pulp. In addition, dental pulp has some unique features that make it unusually fragile and sensitive. First, it is encased by hard tissue (dentin/enamel) that will not allow for the usual swelling associated with the exudate of the inflammatory process. Second, there is no collateral circulation to maintain vitality when the primary blood supply is compromised. Third, biopsy and direct application of medications are impossible without causing necrosis of the entire organ. Fourth, pain is the only sign that can be used to determine the severity of pulpal inflammation.

Because of referred pain, localizing the problem to the correct tooth can often be a considerable diagnostic challenge. Also of significance is the difficulty in relating clinical status of a tooth to histopathology. There are, unfortunately, no reliable symptoms or tests that consistently correlate the two. The level of pulpal inflammation is determined through a combination of clinical criteria. Results of electric, heat, cold, and percussion tests must be added to patient history, clinical examination, and operator experience to arrive at the most appropriate diagnosis for the correct tooth. Generally, the more intense the pain and the longer the duration of symptoms, the greater the damage to the pulp. Severe symptoms usually indicate irreversible damage.

Etiology. In the dental pulp, inflammation is the response to injury, just as it is in any other organ. Additionally, the pulp response includes stimulation of odontoblasts to deposit reparative dentin at the site to help protect the pulp. If the injury is severe, the result is, instead, necrosis of these cells.

Caries is the most frequent form of injury that causes pulpitis. The degree of damage depends upon the rapidity and extent of hard tissue destruction. Entry of bacteria into the pulpal tissue through a carious lesion is not necessary for pulpitis to occur, but this appears to be an important factor in the intensification of the inflammatory response. Operative dental procedures in cavity and crown preparation may also trigger an inflammatory response in the dental pulp. The heat, friction, chemicals, and filling materials associated with restoration of teeth are all potential irritants. It is well known that less damage is done when a water spray is used during tooth preparation than when no water is used. It is also well established that an insulating base can provide significant protection of the pulp from irritating chemicals used with non-metallic restorative materials and from heat transferred through large metallic fillings.

Other types of injury that may trigger pulpitis are trauma, especially when it is severe enough to cause root or crown fracture, and periodontal disease that has extended to an apical or lateral root foramen.

Clinical and Histopathologic Features. Several detailed classifications of pulpitis have been proposed that are based on histopathologic changes. Because of the difficulty in correlating clinical features with microscopy, these schemes have proved to be of little practical value. Instead, most practitioners prefer a simple classification that is helpful in the clinical setting relative to treatment and prognosis (Fig. 13–1).

Focal Reversible Pulpitis. This acute mild inflammatory pulpal reaction typically follows carious destruction of a tooth or placement of a large metallic filling. It causes teeth to be hypersensitive to thermal and electric stimuli. The pain is mild to moderate and is typically intermittent. As the name implies, the changes are focal (subjacent to the injurious agent) and reversible if the cause is removed. Microscopically, the predominant feature is dilatation and engorgement of blood vessels (hyperemia). Exudation of plasma proteins also occurs, but this is difficult to appreciate in microscopic sections.

Acute Pulpitis. This inflammatory response may occur as a progression of focal reversible pulpitis, or it may represent an acute exacerbation of an already established chronic pulpitis. Pulpal damage may range in severity from simple acute inflammation marked by vessel dilatation, exudation, and neutrophil chemotaxis to focal liquefaction necrosis (pulp abscess) (Fig. 13–2) to total pulpal suppurative necrosis. Constant severe tooth-associated pain is the usual presenting complaint. Pain is intensified with the application of heat or cold, although in cases in which liquefaction of the pulp has occurred, cold may, in fact, alleviate the symptoms. If there is an opening from the pulp to the oral environment, symptoms may be lessened because of the escape of the exudate that causes pressure on and chemical irritation of the pulpal and periapical nerve tissues.

In the early phases of acute pulpitis, the tooth may be hyperreactive to electric stimulation, but as pulp damage increases, sensitivity is reduced until there is no response. Because the exudate is confined primarily to the pulp rather than the periapical tissues, percussion tests generally elicit a response little different from normal.

Chronic Pulpitis. Chronic pulpitis is an inflammatory reaction that results from long-term, low-grade injury or occasionally from quiescence of an acute process. Symptoms,

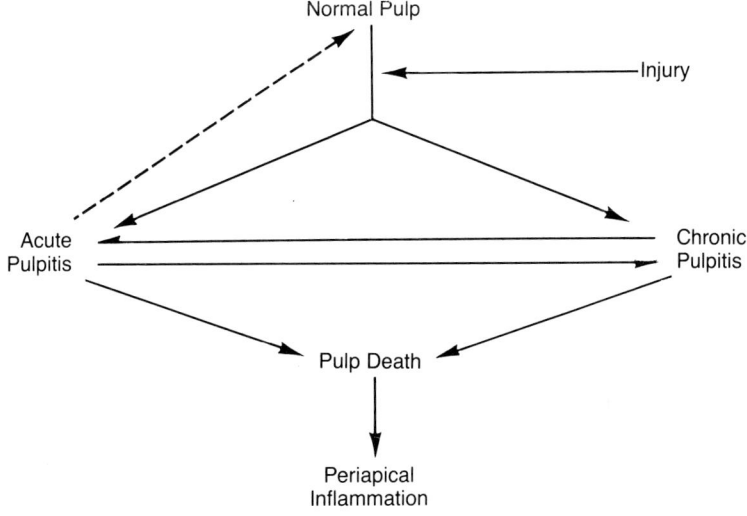

Figure 13–1. Pulpitis pathways.

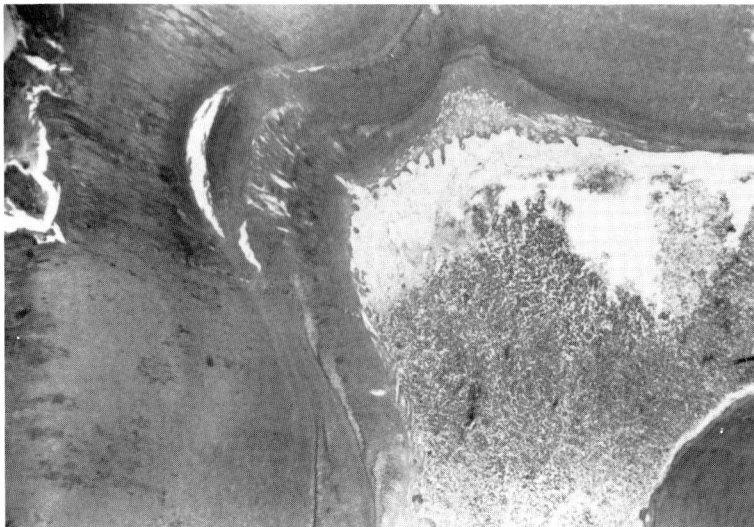

Figure 13–2. Abscess of coronal pulp showing liquefaction and acute inflammatory cell infiltrate. Note carious lesion and reparative dentin (left).

characteristically mild and often intermittent, appear over an extended period of time. A dull ache may be the presenting complaint, or the patient may have no symptoms at all. As the pulp deteriorates, responses to thermal and electric stimulation are reduced. Microscopically, lymphocytes, plasma cells, and fibrosis appear in the chronically inflamed pulp. Unless there is an acute exacerbation of the chronic process, neutrophils are not evident.

Chronic Hyperplastic Pulpitis. This special form of chronic pulpitis occurs in molar teeth (both primary and secondary) of children and young adults (Fig. 13–3). The involved teeth exhibit large carious lesions that open into the coronal pulp chamber. Rather than necrosing, the pulp tissue reacts to the injury by undergoing hyperplasia, producing a red mass of reparative granulation tissue that extrudes through the pulp exposure. This type of reaction is believed to be related to the open root foramen through which a relatively rich blood supply flows.

Symptoms seldom occur because there is no exudate under pressure and generally no nerve tissue proliferating with the granulation tissue. Although the pulp tissue is viable, the process is not reversible and necessitates endodontic therapy or extraction. The well-vascularized granulation tissue mass frequently becomes epithelialized, presumably by autotransplantation of epithelial cells from nearby mucosal surfaces.

Treatment and Prognosis. If the cause is identified and eliminated, focal reversible pulpitis should recede, returning the pulp to a

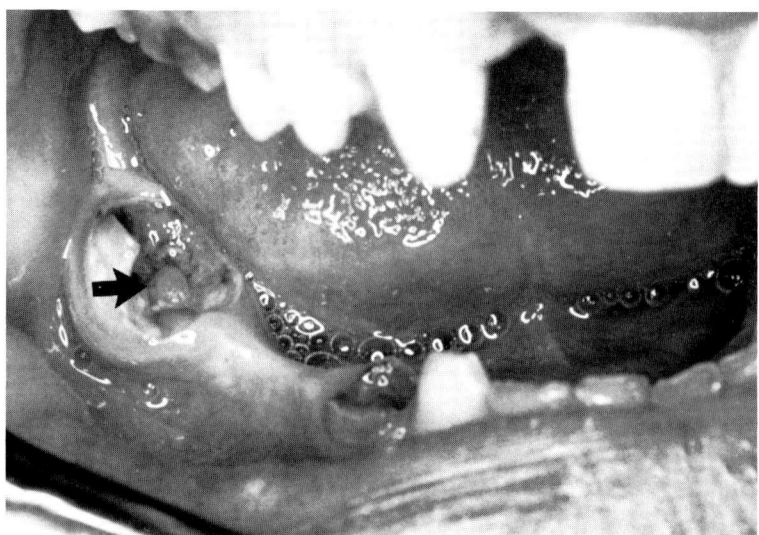

Figure 13–3. Hyperplastic pulpitis of first permanent molar (arrow).

normal state. If the inflammation progresses into an acute pulpitis with neutrophil infiltrates and tissue necrosis, recovery is unlikely regardless of attempts to remove the cause. Endodontic therapy or extraction is the only treatment available at this stage.

With chronic pulpitis, pulpal death is the characteristic end result. Removal of the cause may slow the process or occasionally save the vitality of the pulp. Endodontic therapy or extraction is typically required. Chronic hyperplastic pulpitis is essentially an irreversible end stage that is treated with pulp extirpation and an endodontic filling or extraction.

PERIAPICAL ABSCESS

Etiology. Numerous sequelae may follow untreated pulp necrosis, all of which are dependent upon virulence of microorganisms involved and integrity of the patient's overall defense mechanisms (Fig. 13–4). From its origin in the pulp, the inflammatory process extends into the periapical tissues, where it may present as a granuloma or cyst, if chronic, or an abscess, if acute. Acute exacerbation of a chronic lesion may also be seen. The necrotic pulpal tissue debris, inflammatory cells, and bacteria all serve to stimulate and sustain the periapical inflammatory process.

Clinical Features. Patients with periapical abscesses typically have severe pain in the area of the non-vital tooth because of pressure and the effects of chemical mediators on nerve tissue. The exudate and neutrophilic infiltrate of an abscess cause pressure on the surrounding tissue, frequently resulting in slight extrusion of the tooth from its socket. Pus associated with a lesion, if not focally constrained, will seek the path of least resistance and spread into contiguous structures. The affected area of the jaw may be tender to palpation, and the patient may be hypersensitive to tooth percussion. The involved tooth will be unresponsive to electric and thermal tests owing to pulp necrosis.

Because of the rapidity with which this lesion develops, there is generally insufficient time for significant amounts of bone resorption to occur. Therefore, radiographic changes are slight, usually limited to mild radiographic thickening of apical periodontal membrane space. However, if the lesion develops as an acute exacerbation of a chronic periapical granuloma, a radiolucent lesion will be evident.

Histopathology. Microscopically, this lesion appears as a zone of liquefaction composed of proteinaceous exudate, necrotic tissue, and viable and dead neutrophils (pus). Adjacent tissue containing dilated vessels and a neutrophilic infiltrate surrounds the area of liquefaction necrosis.

The *periapical granuloma* represents the result of chronic inflammation at the apex of a non-vital tooth. It is composed of granulation tissue and scar infiltrated by variable numbers of chronic inflammatory cells (lymphocytes, plasma cells, macrophages). This lesion is to be distinguished from granulomatous inflammation, which is a distinctive type of chronic inflammation that is characteristic of certain diseases (e.g., tuberculosis, sarcoid, histoplas-

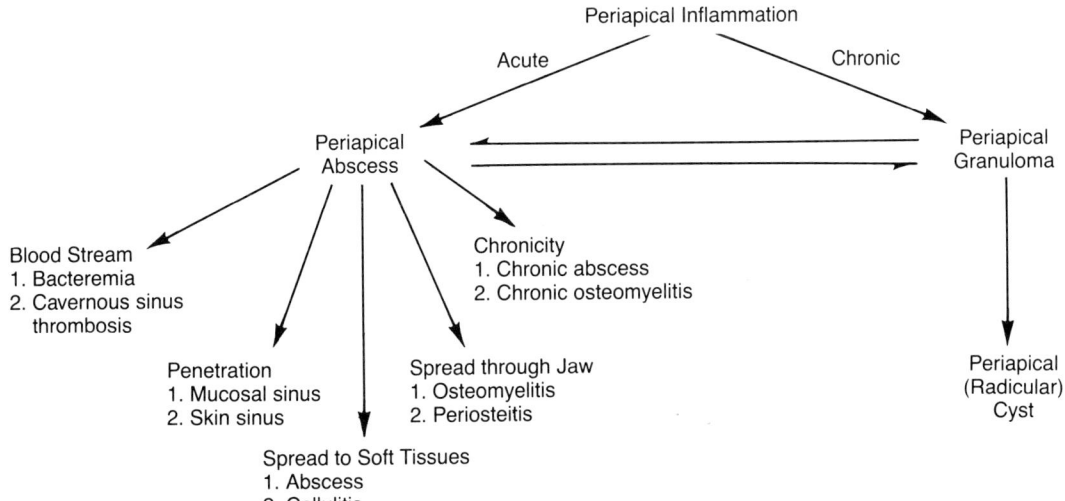

Figure 13–4. Sequelae of periapical inflammation.

mosis) and features a predominance of macrophages (histiocytes) and often multinucleated giant cells. An acute flare of a periapical granuloma would show an abundant neutrophilic infiltrate in addition to granulation tissue and chronic inflammatory cells.

Treatment and Prognosis. Treatment of an acute periapical abscess requires observance of the standard principles of management of acute inflammation. Drainage should be established, either through an opening in the tooth itself or through the soft tissue surrounding the jaw if cellulitis has developed. Antibiotics directed against the offending organism will also be required. Management must be thoughtful and skilled, because the consequences of delayed or inappropriate treatment can be significant and occasionally life threatening.

Spread of an abscess may be through one of several avenues. It may progress through the buccal cortical bone and gingival soft tissue, establishing a natural drain or sinus tract (Fig. 13–5). The same type of situation may occur in the palate or skin; this depends upon the original location of the abscess and the path of least resistance (Fig. 13–6). If a drain is not established, the purulent exudate can cause an abscess (Fig. 13–7) or *cellulitis* (Fig. 13–8) in the soft tissues of the face, oral cavity, or neck. Cellulitis is an acute inflammatory process that is diffusely spread throughout the tissue rather than localized as with an abscess. This variant is the result of infection by virulent organisms that produce enzymes that allow rapid spread through tissue. Cellulitis of the submandibular space has been given the name "Ludwig's angina."

A dangerous situation occurs when the acute infection involves major blood vessels. This may allow bacteria to enter the blood stream, resulting in bacteremia. Also, retrograde spread of the infection through facial veins to the cavernous sinus may set up the necessary conditions for thrombus formation. *Cavernous sinus thrombosis* is an emergency situation that is often fatal.

ACUTE OSTEOMYELITIS

Etiology. Acute inflammation of the bone and bone marrow of the mandible and maxilla results most frequently from extension of a periapical abscess. The second most common cause of acute osteomyelitis is physical injury as seen with fracture or surgery. Osteomyelitis may also result from bacteremia.

Most cases of acute osteomyelitis are infectious. Almost any organism may be part of the etiologic picture, although staphylococci and streptococci have been the most frequently cited.

Clinical Features. Pain is the primary feature of this inflammatory process. Pyrexia, painful lymphadenopathy, leukocytosis, and other signs and symptoms of acute infection are also frequently present. Paresthesia of the lower lip is occasionally seen with mandibular involvement. In the development of a clinical differential diagnosis, the presence of this symptom should also suggest malignant mandibular neoplasms.

Unless the inflammatory process has been present for more than 1 week, radiographic evidence of acute osteomyelitis is usually not

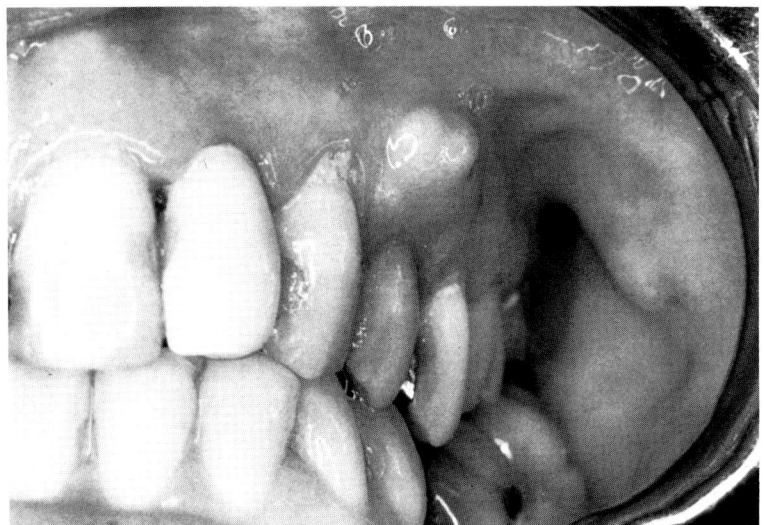

Figure 13–5. Parulis representing pus from apex of non-vital bicuspid.

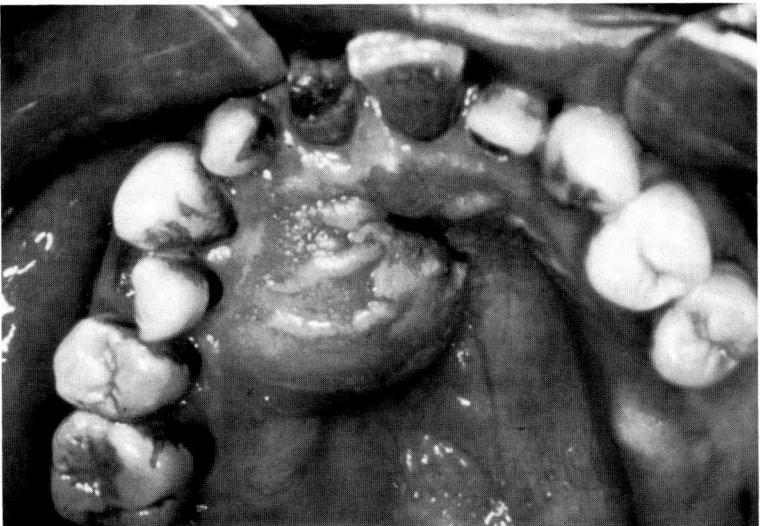

Figure 13–6. Palatal abscess originating from apex of non-vital bicuspid.

present. With time, diffuse radiolucent changes begin to appear.

Histopathology. A purulent exudate occupies the marrow spaces in acute osteomyelitis. Bony trabeculae show reduced osteoblastic activity and increased osteoclastic resorption. If an area of bone necrosis occurs (sequestrum), osteocytes are lost and the marrow undergoes liquefaction.

Treatment. Acute osteomyelitis is usually treated with antibiotics and drainage. Ideally, the causative agent is identified, and an appropriate antibiotic is selected through sensitivity testing in the laboratory. Surgery may also be part of the treatment, and it ranges from simple sequestrectomy to excision with autologous bone replacement. Each case should be judged individually because of variations in disease severity, organisms involved, and patient's overall health.

CHRONIC OSTEOMYELITIS

Etiology. Chronic osteomyelitis may be one of the sequelae of acute osteomyelitis (either untreated or inadequately treated), or it may represent a long-term, low-grade inflammatory

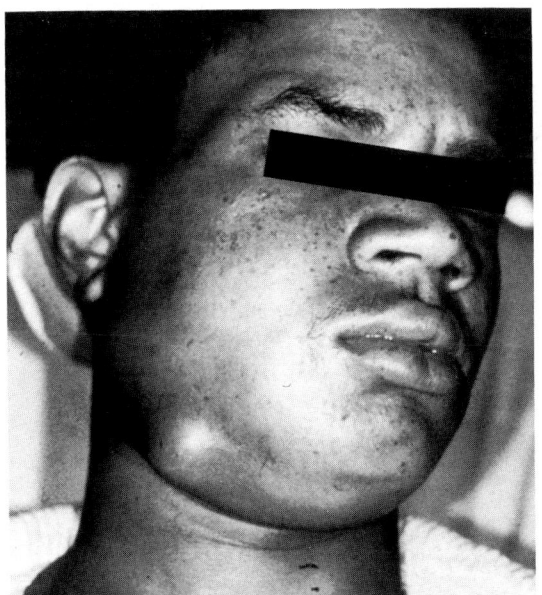

Figure 13–7. Skin abscess of odontogenic origin.

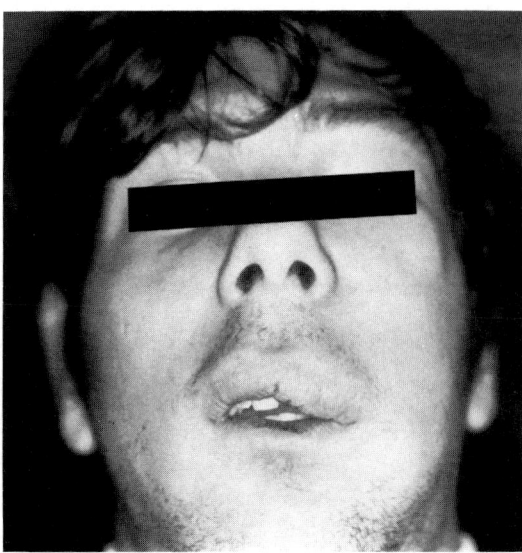

Figure 13–8. Cellulitis of odontogenic origin.

reaction that never went through a significant or clinically noticeable acute phase. In either event, there are many similar etiologic factors in acute and chronic osteomyelitis. Most cases are infectious, and like most infections, the clinical presentation and course are directly dependent upon the virulence of the microorganism involved and the patient's resistance. Anatomic location, immunologic status, nutritional status, patient age, and the presence of pre-existing systemic factors such as Paget's disease, osteopetrosis, and sickle cell disease are other factors affecting presentation and course. Bone irradiated as part of head and neck cancer treatment is particularly susceptible to infection. Because of reduced vascularity and osteocyte destruction, osteoradionecrosis occurs in approximately 20% of patients who have undergone local irradiation (Fig. 13–9). Secondary infection generally follows. Typical precipitating or triggering events include periapical inflammation resulting from non-vital teeth, extractions (Fig. 13–10), periodontal disease, and fractures communicating with skin or mucosa.

Identification of a specific infectious agent involved in chronic osteomyelitis is usually difficult both microscopically and microbiologically. Sample error is significant either because of small, difficult-to-reach bacterial foci or because of contamination of the lesion by resident flora. Previously taken antibiotics will also reduce the chances of culturing the causative organism. Although an etiologic agent is often not confirmed, most investigators believe that bacteria (e.g., staphylococci, streptococci, bacteroides, actinomyces) are responsible for the vast majority of chronic osteomyelitis cases.

Clinical Features. The mandible, especially the molar area, is much more frequently affected than is the maxilla. Pain is usually present but varies in intensity, and it is not necessarily related to the extent of the disease. Duration of symptoms is generally proportional to disease extension. Swelling of the jaw is a commonly encountered sign; loose teeth and sinus tracts are less frequently seen. Anesthesia is very uncommon.

Radiographically, chronic osteomyelitis appears primarily as a radiolucent lesion that may show focal zones of opacification. The lucent pattern is often described as "motheaten" because of its mottled radiographic appearance (Fig. 13–11). Lesions may be very extensive, and margins are often indistinct.

Histopathology. The inflammatory reaction in chronic osteomyelitis can vary from very mild to intense. In mild cases, microscopic diagnosis can be difficult because of similarities to fibro-osseous lesions such as ossifying fibroma and fibrous dysplasia (Fig. 13–12). Few chronic inflammatory cells (lymphocytes and plasma cells) are seen in a fibrous marrow (Fig. 13–13). Both osteoblastic and osteoclastic activity may be seen, along with irregular bony trabeculae—unlikely features of fibro-osseous lesions. In advanced chronic osteomyelitis, necrotic bone (sequestrum) may be present, as evidenced by both necrotic marrow

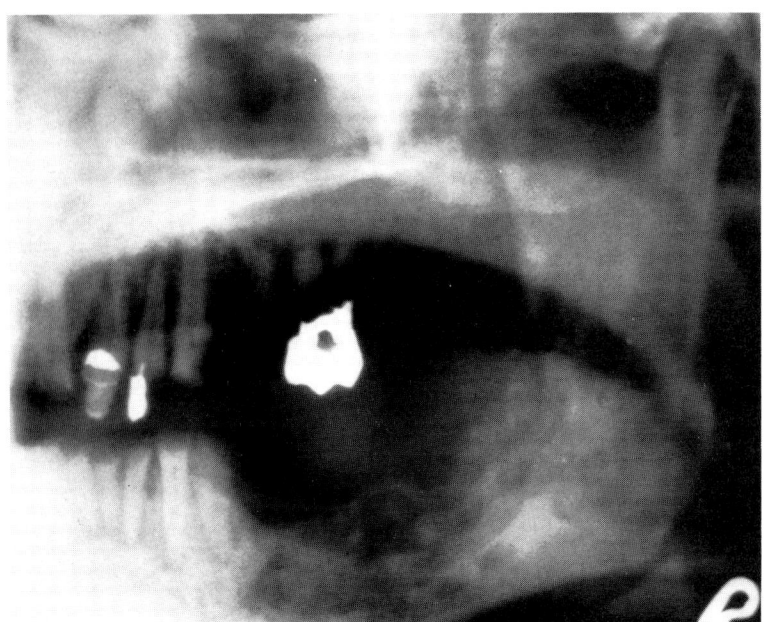

Figure 13–9. Chronic osteomyelitis in mandible of a patient irradiated for oral cancer.

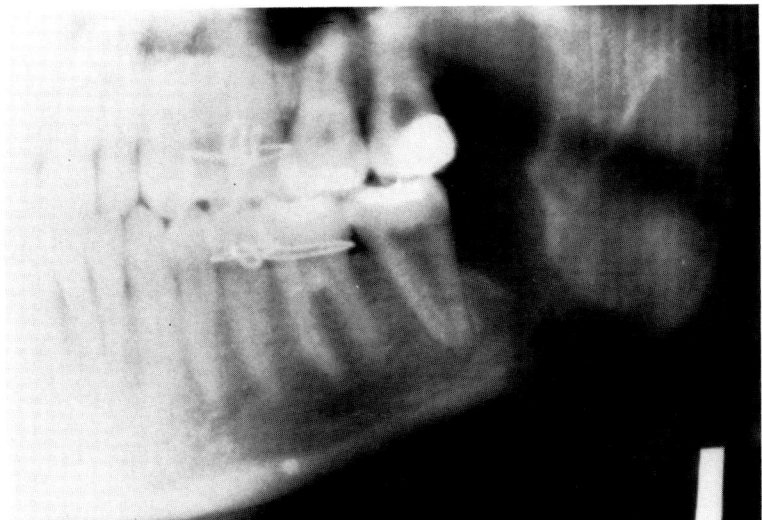

Figure 13–10. Chronic osteomyelitis at the site of a third molar extraction.

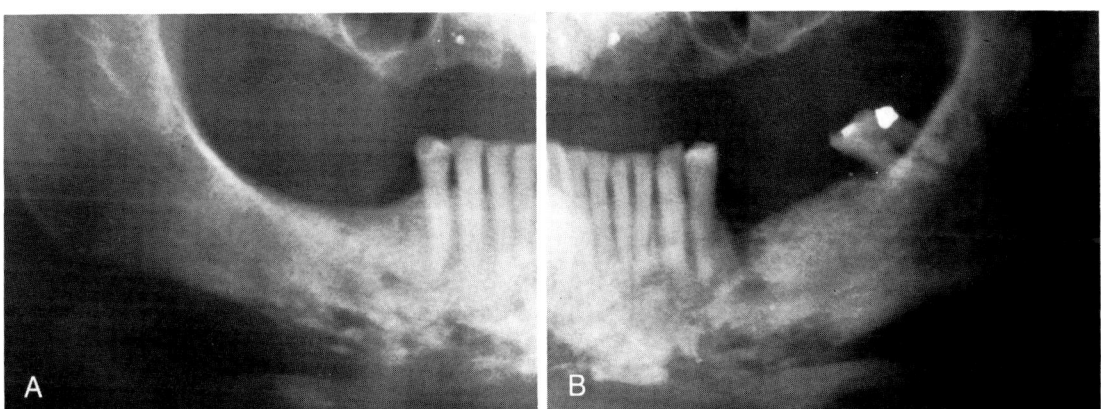

Figure 13–11. *A* and *B*, Chronic osteomyelitis.

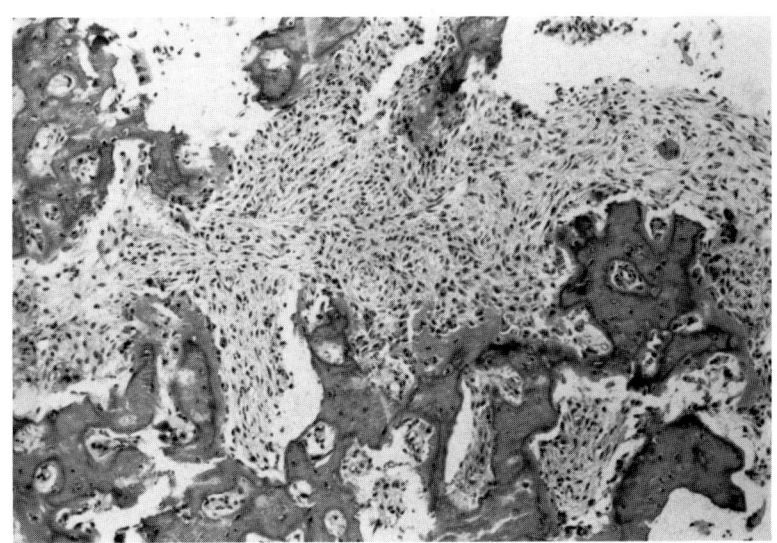

Figure 13–12. Chronic osteomyelitis showing irregular trabeculae and fibrous marrow.

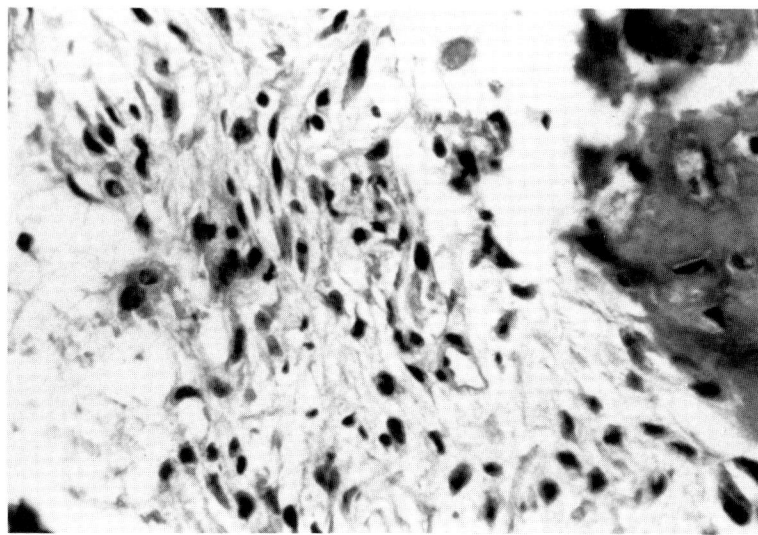

Figure 13–13. Chronic osteomyelitis showing typical scant chronic inflammatory cell infiltrate.

and osteocytes (Fig. 13–14). Reversal lines reflect the waves of deposition and resorption of bone. Inflammatory cells are more numerous and osteoclastic activity more prominent than in mild cases.

Treatment. The basic treatment of chronic osteomyelitis centers around the selection of appropriate antibiotics and the proper timing of surgical intervention. Culture and sensitivity testing should be done. Combinations of antibiotics may, on occasion, be more successful than single agents. Duration of antibiotic administration may also be relatively extended.

Surgery when a sequestrum appears will hasten the healing process. Excision of other non-vital bone, sinus tracts, and scar has also been advocated. In cases in which pathologic fracture is a significant potential, immobilization is required.

In recalcitrant cases of chronic osteomyelitis and osteoradionecrosis, the use of *hyperbaric oxygen* has provided significant patient benefit. In difficult cases, hyperbaric oxygen used in conjunction with antibiotics or surgery appears to be generally better than any of these methods used alone. The rationale for using hyperbaric oxygen is related to its stimulation of vascular proliferation, collagen synthesis, and osteogenesis. Contraindications include presence of viral infections, optic neuritis, known residual or recurrent malignancies, and some lung diseases. The regimen typically used for this treatment adjunct involves placing a patient in a closed chamber with 100% oxygen at 2 atmospheres of pressure for 2 hours per

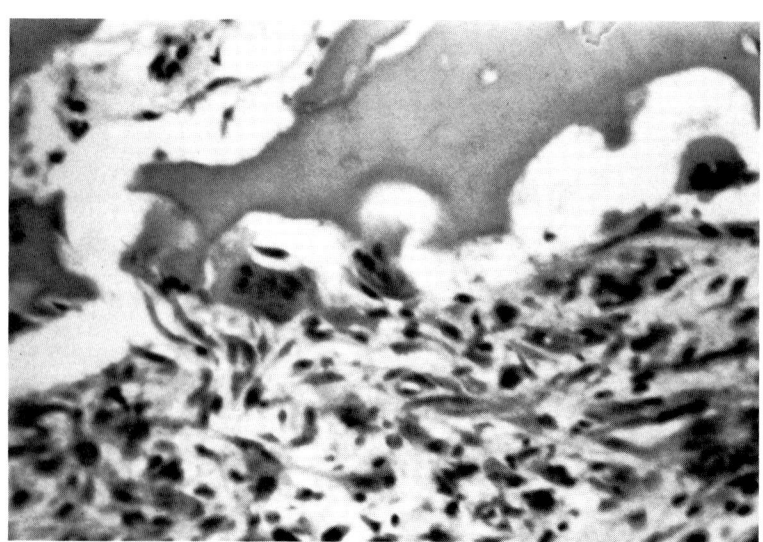

Figure 13–14. Sequestrum showing osteoclastic resorption.

day for several weeks. The elevated tissue oxygen levels achieved with this technique reach a limited maximum level by the end of therapy, but the effects appear to be long lasting.

Garré's Osteomyelitis

Etiology. Garré's osteomyelitis, or chronic osteomyelitis with proliferative periostitis, is essentially a subtype of chronic osteomyelitis in which there is, additionally, a prominent periosteal inflammatory reaction. It most often results from a periapical abscess of a mandibular molar. It has also followed infection associated with tooth extraction or partially erupted molars.

Clinical Features. This variety of osteomyelitis is uncommonly encountered. It has been described in the tibia, and in the head and neck, it is seen in the mandible. It typically involves the posterior mandible and is usually unilateral. Patients characteristically present with an asymptomatic bony hard swelling with normal-appearing overlying skin and mucosa (Fig. 13–15). On occasion, slight tenderness may be noted. This presentation necessitates the differentiation of this process from benign mandibular neoplasms. Radiographs and biopsy will provide a definitive diagnosis.

Radiographically, the lesion appears centrally as a mottled, predominantly lucent lesion in a pattern consistent with chronic osteomyelitis (Fig. 13–16). The feature that provides the distinctive difference is the periosteal reaction. This, best viewed on an occlusal radiograph, appears as an expanded cortex, often with concentric or parallel opaque layers (Fig. 13–17). Trabeculae perpendicular to the "onion skin" layers may also be apparent.

Histopathology. Reactive new bone typifies the subperiosteal cortical response. Perpendicular orientation of new trabeculae to redundant cortical bone is best seen under low magnification (Fig. 13–18). Osteoblastic activity dominates in this area, and both osteoblastic and osteoclastic activity are seen centrally. Marrow spaces contain fibrous tissue with scattered lymphocytes and plasma cells. Inflammatory cells are often surprisingly scant, making microscopic differentiation from fibro-osseous lesions a diagnostic challenge.

Treatment. Identification and removal of the offending agent is of primary importance in Garré's osteomyelitis. This usually requires removal of the involved tooth. Antibiotics are generally included early in this treatment also. The mandible then undergoes gradual remodeling without additional surgical intervention.

Diffuse Sclerosing Osteomyelitis

Etiology. Diffuse sclerosing osteomyelitis represents an inflammatory reaction in the mandible or maxilla, believed to be in response to a microorganism of low virulence. Bacteria are generally suspected as causative agents, although they are seldom specifically identified. Based on histologic changes, it has been suggested that hypersensitivity may be a plausible explanation of the cause. Important in the etiology and progression of diffuse sclerosing osteomyelitis is chronic periodontal disease, which appears to provide a portal of entry for bacteria. Carious non-vital teeth are less frequently implicated.

Clinical Features. This condition may be seen in any age, sex, or race, but it tends to occur most frequently in middle-aged black females. The disease is typified by a protracted

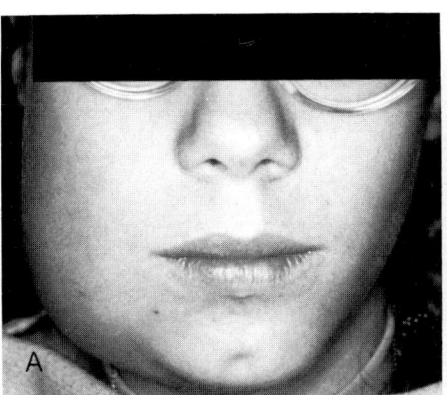
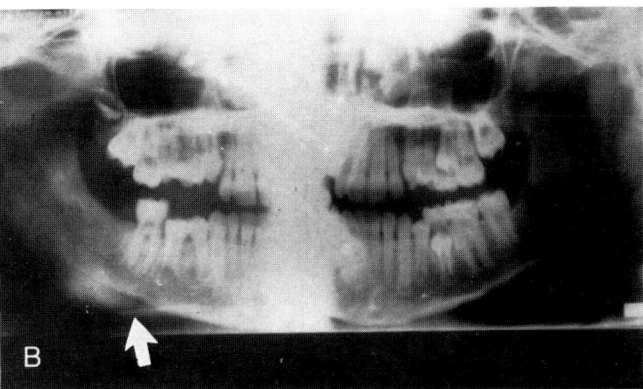

Figure 13–15. *A* and *B*, Garré's osteomyelitis. Note periosteal reaction in radiogram (arrow).

400 INFLAMMATORY JAW LESIONS

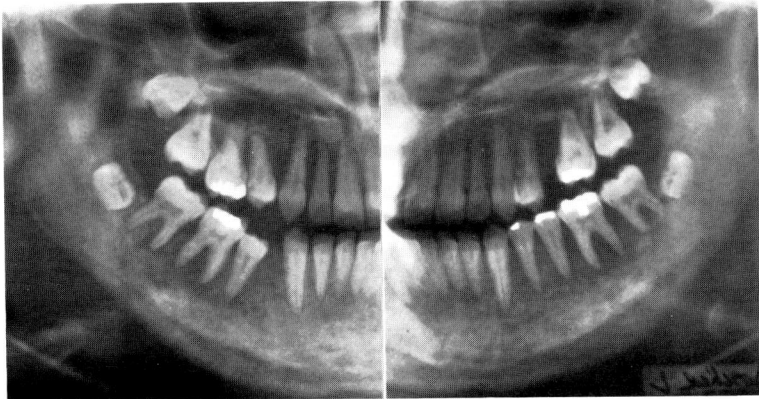

Figure 13–16. Garré's osteomyelitis. Note mottled mandibular bone and expansion of periosteum along the inferior border.

Figure 13–17. Garré's osteomyelitis showing typical periosteal reaction.

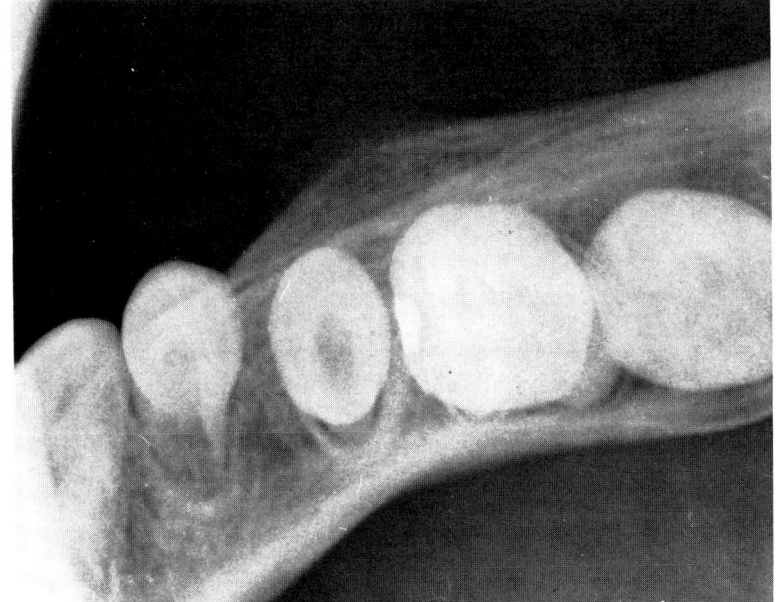

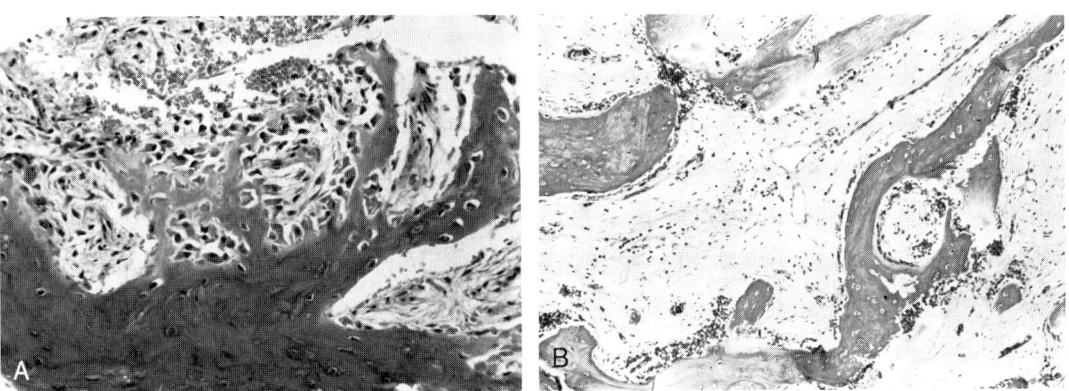

Figure 13–18. Garré's osteomyelitis showing periosteal reaction *(A)* and fibrotic mildly inflamed marrow *(B)*.

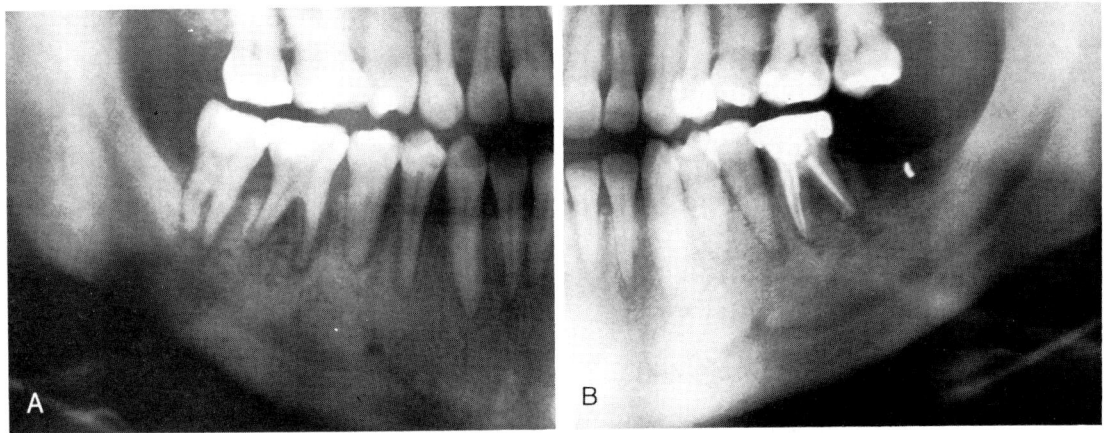

Figure 13–19. *A* and *B*, Diffuse sclerosing osteomyelitis.

chronic course with acute exacerbations of pain, swelling, and occasional drainage.

Radiographically, this process is diffuse, typically affecting a large part of the jaw (Fig. 13–19). The lesion is ill defined. Early lucent zones may appear in association with sclerotic masses. In advanced stages, sclerosis dominates the radiographic picture. Periosteal thickening may also be seen.

Histopathology. The microscopic changes of this condition are inflammatory. There is fibrous replacement of marrow. A chronic inflammatory cell infiltrate and occasionally a neutrophilic infiltrate are also seen. Bony trabeculae exhibit irregular size and shape and may be lined by numerous osteoblasts. Focal osteoclastic activity is also present. The characteristic sclerotic masses are composed of dense bone (Fig. 13–20), often exhibiting numerous reversal lines.

Differential Diagnosis. Chronic sclerosing osteomyelitis shares many clinical, radiographic, and histologic features with florid osseous dysplasia. The two should be separated, since the former is an infectious process and the latter a bony dysplastic process. Treatment and prognosis will therefore be dissimilar. Florid osseous dysplasia appears to be an extensive form of periapical cemental dysplasia and, unlike diffuse sclerosing osteomyelitis, may exhibit anterior periapical lesions and traumatic bone cysts. Further, florid osseous dysplasia is usually asymptomatic and lacks an inflammatory cell infiltrate.

Treatment. The management of diffuse sclerosing osteomyelitis is problematic because of the relative avascular nature of the affected tissue and because of the large size of the lesion. Even with treatment, the course is protracted.

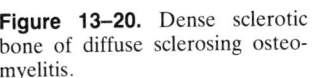

Figure 13–20. Dense sclerotic bone of diffuse sclerosing osteomyelitis.

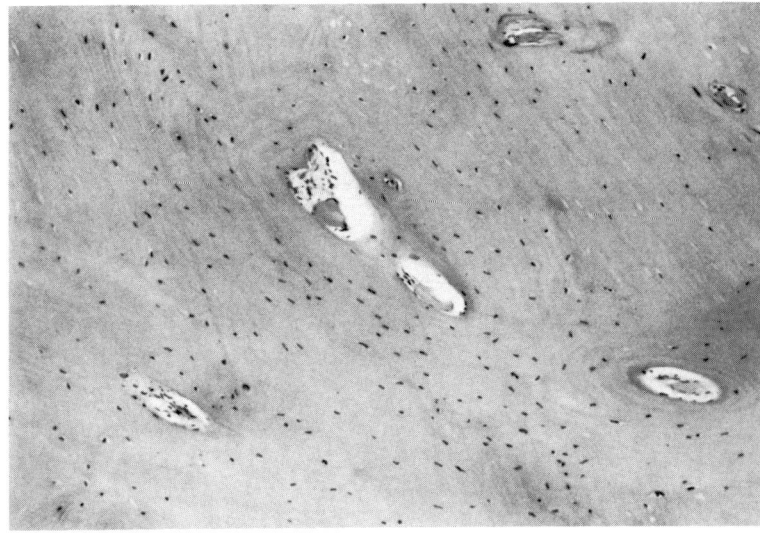

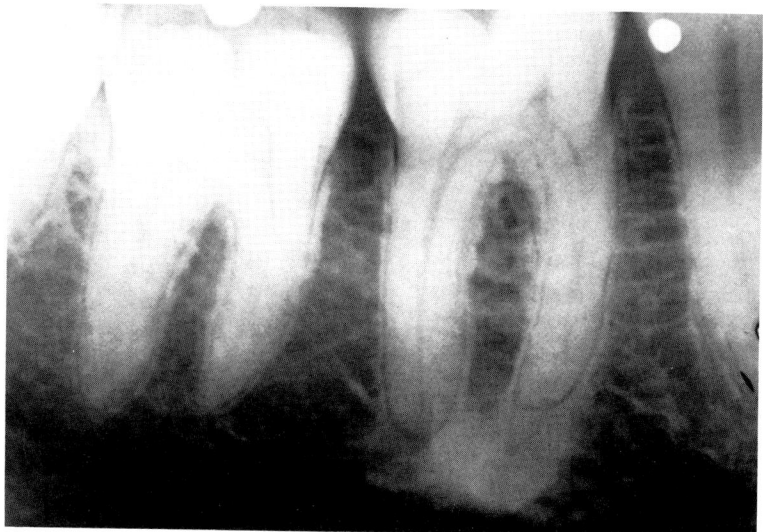

Figure 13–21. Focal sclerosing osteomyelitis, sometimes called focal periapical osteopetrosis when associated with normal teeth.

If an etiologic factor such as periodontal disease or a carious tooth can be identified, it should be eliminated. Antibiotics are the mainstay of treatment and are especially helpful during painful exacerbations. Surgical removal of the diseased area is usually an inappropriate procedure because of the extent of the disease. Decortication of the affected area has resulted in improvement in some cases. Low-dose corticosteroids have also been used with some success. Hyperbaric oxygen therapy may prove to be a valuable adjunct.

Focal Sclerosing Osteomyelitis

Etiology. This is a relatively common phenomenon that is believed to represent a focal bony reaction to a low-grade inflammatory stimulus. It is usually seen at the apex of a tooth in which there has been a long-standing pulpitis. Occasionally, this lesion may be adjacent to a sound unrestored tooth, suggesting that other etiologic factors such as malocclusion may be operative.

Synonyms for focal sclerosing osteomyelitis include bony scar, condensing osteitis, and sclerotic bone. The term *focal periapical osteopetrosis* has also been used to describe the lesions associated with normal caries-free teeth (Fig. 13–21).

Clinical Features. Focal sclerosing osteomyelitis may be found at any age but is typically discovered in young adults. Patients are usually asymptomatic, and most lesions are discovered on routine radiographic examina-

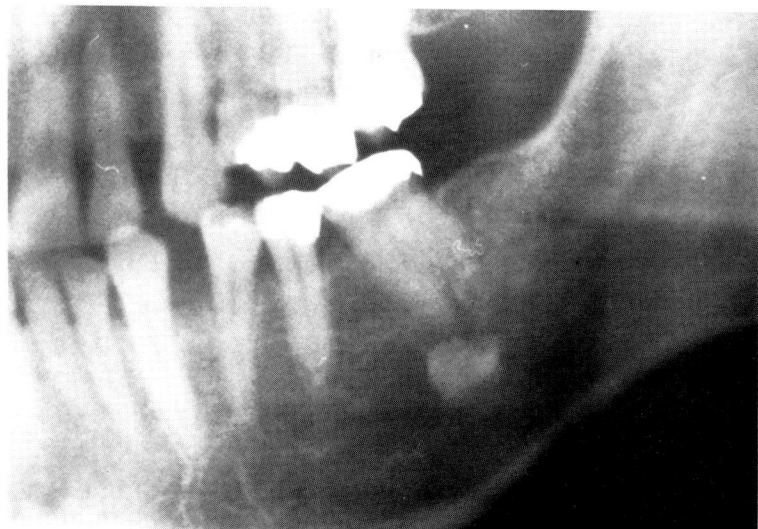

Figure 13–22. Focal sclerosing osteomyelitis.

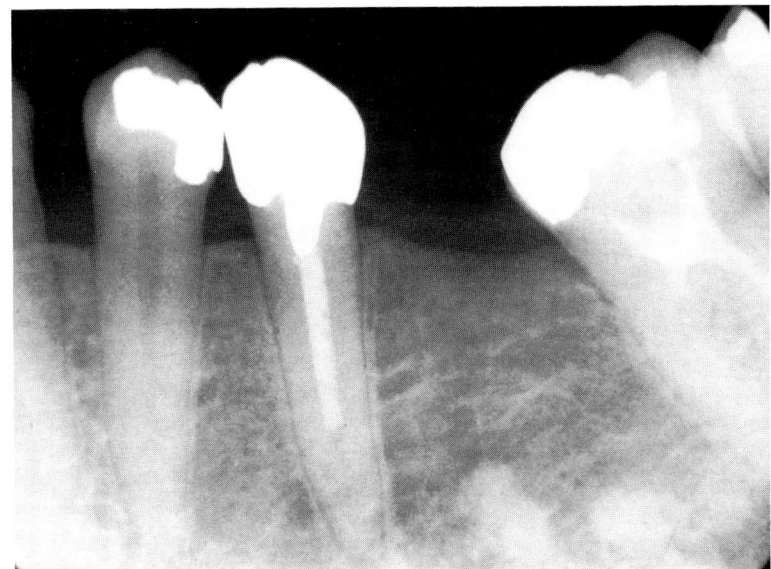

Figure 13–23. Focal sclerosing osteomyelitis.

tion. A majority are found at the apices of mandibular first molars, with a minority associated with mandibular second molars and premolars (Fig. 13–22). When teeth are extracted, these lesions remain behind indefinitely (Fig. 13–23).

Radiographically, one of several patterns may be seen. The lesion may be uniformly opaque; it may have a peripheral lucency with an opaque center; it may have an opaque periphery with a lucent center; or it may be composed of confluent or lobulated opaque masses.

Histopathology. Microscopically, these lesions are masses of dense sclerotic bone (Fig. 13–24). Connective tissue is scant, as are inflammatory cells.

Differential Diagnosis. Differential diagnosis should include periapical cemental dysplasia, osteoma, complex odontoma, cementoblastoma, osteoblastoma, and hypercementosis. In most cases, however, diagnosis can be made with confidence on historical and radiographic features.

Treatment. Because it is believed to represent a physiologic bone reaction to a known stimulus, the lesion need not be removed. Biopsy might be contemplated to rule out more significant lesions that received serious consideration in the differential diagnosis. The in-

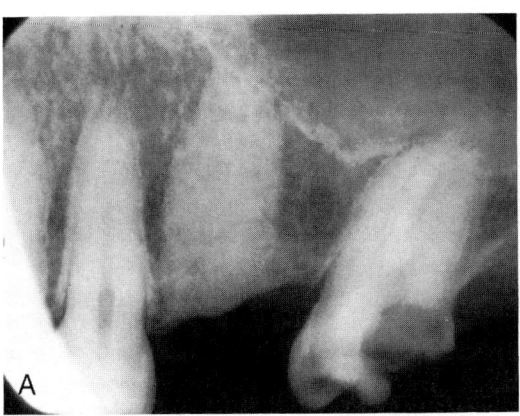
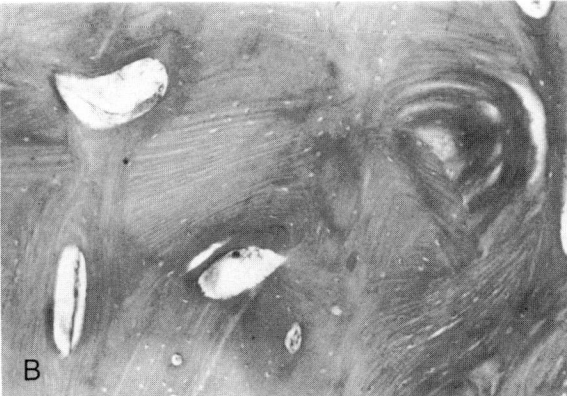

Figure 13–24. *A* and *B*, Focal sclerosing osteomyelitis.

flamed pulp that stimulated the focal sclerosing osteomyelitis should be treated. The decision as to whether the tooth should be restored, treated endodontically, or extracted should be based on findings in a case-by-case basis.

Bibliography

Cecic P, Hartwell G, Bellizzi R. Cold as a diagnostic aid in cases of irreversible pulpitis. Oral Surg Oral Med Oral Pathol 56:647–650, 1983.

Daramola J. Massive osteomyelitis of the mandible complicating sickle cell disease: report of a case. J Oral Surg 39:144–146, 1981.

Daramola J, Ajagbe H. Chronic osteomyelitis of the mandible in adults: a clinical study of 34 cases. Br J Oral Surg 20:58–62, 1982.

Eisenbud L, Miller J, Roberts I. Garré's proliferative periostitis occurring simultaneously in four quadrants of the jaws. Oral Surg 51:172–178, 1981.

Eversole L, Stone C, Strub D. Focal sclerosing osteomyelitis/focal periapical osteopetrosis: radiographic patterns. Oral Surg 58:456–460, 1984.

Fattore L, Strauss R. Hyperbaric oxygen in the treatment of osteoradionecrosis: a review of its use and efficacy. Oral Surg Oral Med Oral Pathol 63:280–286, 1987.

Guernsey L, Clark J. Hyperbaric oxygen therapy with subtotal extirpation surgery in the management of osteonecrosis of the mandible. Int J Oral Surg 10 (Suppl 1):168–177, 1981.

Hyman J, Cohen M. The predictive value of endodontic diagnostic tests. Oral Surg 58:343–346, 1984.

Jacobsson S, Dahlen G, Moller A. Bacteriologic and serologic investigation in diffuse sclerosing osteomyelitis (DSO) of the mandible. Oral Surg 54:506–512, 1982.

Jacobsson S, Heyden G. Chronic sclerosing osteomyelitis of the mandible. Oral Surg 43:357–364, 1977.

Jacobsson S, Hollender L. Treatment and prognosis of diffuse sclerosing osteomyelitis (DSO) of the mandible. Oral Surg 49:7–14, 1980.

Jacobsson S, Hollender L, Lindberg S, et al. Chronic sclerosing osteomyelitis of the mandible. Oral Surg 45:167–174, 1978.

Kerley T, Mader J, Hulet W, et al. The effect of adjunctive hyperbaric oxygen on bone regeneration in mandibular osteomyelitis: report of a case. J Oral Surg 39:619–623, 1981.

Khosla V. Current concepts in the treatment of acute and chronic osteomyelitis: review and report of four cases. J Oral Surg 28:209–214, 1970.

Khosla V, Rosenfield H, Berk L. Chronic osteomyelitis of the mandible. J Oral Surg 29:649–658, 1971.

Lichty G, Langlais R, Aufdemorte T. Garré's osteomyelitis: literature review and case report. Oral Surg 50:310–313, 1980.

Marx R, Johnson R. Studies in the radiobiology of osteoradionecrosis and their clinical significance. Oral Surg Oral Med Oral Pathol 64:379–390, 1987.

Marx R, Johnson R, Kline S. Prevention of osteoradionecrosis: a randomized prospective clinical trial of hyperbaric oxygen versus penicillin. J Am Dent Assoc 111:49–54, 1985.

Morton M. Osteoradionecrosis: a study of the incidence in the northwest of England. Br J Oral Maxillofac Surg 24:323–331, 1986.

Morton M, Simpson W. The management of osteoradionecrosis of the jaws. Br J Oral Maxillofac Surg 24:332–341, 1986.

Smith B, Eveson J. Paget's disease of bone with particular reference to dentistry. J Oral Pathol 10:233–247, 1981.

Steiner M, Gould A, Means W. Osteomyelitis of the mandible associated with osteopetrosis. J Oral Maxillofac Surg 41:395–405, 1983.

Triplett R, Branham G. Treatment of experimental mandibular osteomyelitis with hyperbaric oxygen and antibiotics. Int J Oral Surg 10 (Suppl 1):178–182, 1981.

Wannfors K, Hammarstrom L. Infectious foci in chronic osteomyelitis of the jaws. Int J Oral Surg 14:493–503, 1985.

Chapter 14

Malignant Non-odontogenic Neoplasms of the Jaws

Richard J. Zarbo

OSTEOSARCOMA
Juxtacortical Osteosarcomas
   Parosteal Osteosarcoma
   Periosteal Osteosarcoma
CHONDROSARCOMA
Mesenchymal Chondrosarcoma
EWING'S SARCOMA
BURKITT'S LYMPHOMA
PLASMA CELL NEOPLASMS
Multiple Myeloma
Solitary Plasmacytoma of Bone
METASTATIC CARCINOMA

Malignant non-odontogenic neoplasms of the jaws, both primary and metastatic, are rare compared with tumors arising in the surrounding soft tissues. Despite the infrequent occurrence of these entities, a diagnosis of malignant jaw tumor has serious prognostic implications, often signaling a treatment plan requiring major therapeutic intervention. Tumors to be considered in this chapter are those arising from the hard tissues (osteosarcoma and chondrosarcoma) and those involving the marrow cavity of the mandible and maxilla (Ewing's sarcoma, Burkitt's lymphoma, plasma cell myeloma, and metastatic carcinoma).

OSTEOSARCOMA

Osteosarcomas account for approximately 20% of all sarcomas and, after plasma cell myeloma, are the most common primary bone tumors. Approximately 5% of osteosarcomas occur in the jaws, with an incidence of approximately 1 case in 1.5 million persons per year. Osteosarcomas arise in several clinical settings, including pre-existing bone abnormalities such as Paget's disease, fibrous dysplasia, giant cell tumor, multiple osteochondromas, bone infarct, chronic osteomyelitis, and osteogenesis imperfecta. Some osteosarcomas have also been preceded by radiation therapy to the affected bone for unrelated or antecedent disease. The vast majority of osteosarcomas involve the tubular long bones, especially those adjacent to the knee. Osteosarcomas can also be classified by site of origin into (1) the conventional type, arising within the medullary cavity; (2) the juxtacortical tumors, arising from the periosteal surface; and (3) the extraskeletal osteosarcomas, arising in soft tissue.

Clinical Features. Conventional osteosarcomas involving the mandible and maxilla display a predilection for males (62%). Although the peak incidence of osteosarcomas of the skeleton occurs in the second decade, those arising in the jaws present 1 to 2 decades later, with a mean age of 34 years. There is a nearly equal

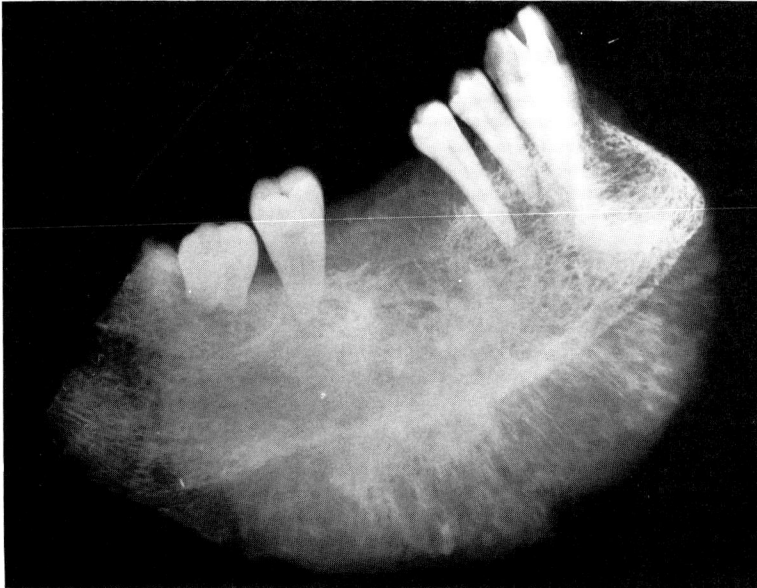

Figure 14–1. Osteosarcoma of the mandible showing radiating spicules of tumor bone in a sunburst pattern.

involvement of the maxilla (51%) and the mandible (49%). The majority (60%) of mandibular osteosarcomas arise in the body of the mandible; the remaining sites of predilection include the symphysis, angle of mandible, ascending ramus, and temporomandibular joint. In the maxilla, there is a nearly equal incidence of tumors involving the alveolar ridge and maxillary antrum, with few affecting the palate.

Osteosarcomas involving the jaws present most commonly with swelling and localized pain. In some cases, there may be loosening and displacement of teeth as well as paresthesia due to involvement of the inferior alveolar nerve. Maxillary tumors display similar clinical symptoms but may cause paresthesia of the infraorbital nerve, epistaxis, nasal obstruction, or eye problems. Skin and mucosal ulceration is usually not a feature of osteosarcoma of the jaws. The average duration of symptoms is 3 to 4 months before diagnosis.

The radiographic appearance of conventional intramedullary osteosarcoma can be quite variable, reflecting the degree of calcification (Fig. 14–1). There appears to be little relationship between the radiographic pattern and the histologic subtype of osteosarcoma. Early osteosarcomas are characterized by localized widening of the periodontal ligament space of one or two teeth (Fig. 14–2). The widened space results from tumor invasion of the periodontal ligament and resorption of the surrounding alveolar bone. Advanced tumors

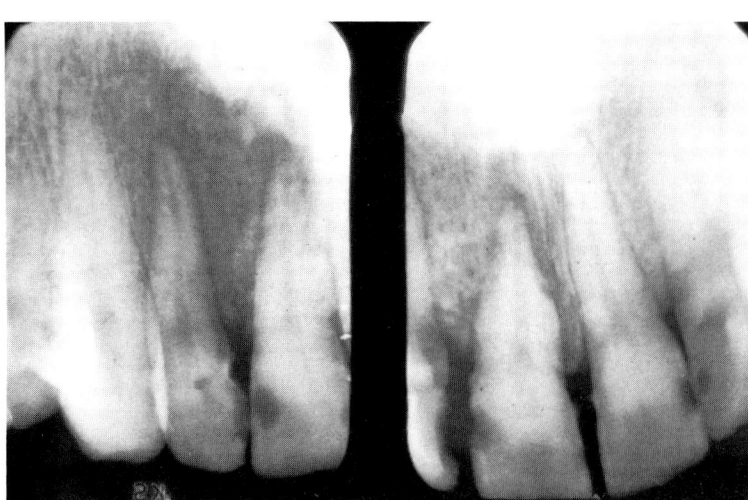

Figure 14–2. Osteosarcoma of the maxilla involving the alveolus of the central and lateral incisors.

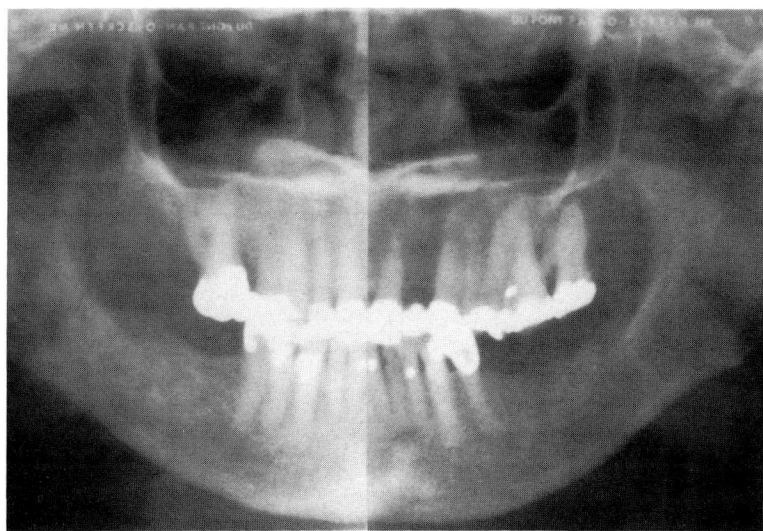

Figure 14–3. Osteosarcoma of the body and ramus of the mandible (left) exhibiting a mottled radiographic pattern.

can be visualized as moth-eaten radiolucencies (Fig. 14–3) or irregular, poorly marginated radiopacities (Fig. 14–4). The majority of these neoplasms have mixed radiographic features. The typical sun ray or sunburst radiopaque appearance due to periosteal reaction may be seen in jaw lesions but is not diagnostic of osteosarcoma.

Histopathology. Histologically, all osteosarcomas have in common a sarcomatous stroma directly producing tumor osteoid. Variable histologic patterns dominate and have been designated osteoblastic (Fig. 14–5), chondroblastic (Fig. 14–6), and fibroblastic (Fig. 14–7). An additional variant has been designated telangiectatic—it displays multiple aneurysmal blood-filled spaces lined by malignant cells. This variant rarely occurs in the head and neck region. All these histologic variants reflect the multipotentiality of the neoplastic mesenchymal cell in producing osteoid, cartilage, and fibrous tissue. Such histologic subclassification, however, bears no prognostic significance. Although osteoblastic histologic variants predominate in the skeleton, chondroblastic osteosarcomas are the most frequent histologic type (48%) occurring in the jaws. Most osteosarcomas of the mandible tend to be lytic (43%); those in the maxilla are osteoblastic (50%).

Overall, jaw osteosarcomas tend to be better

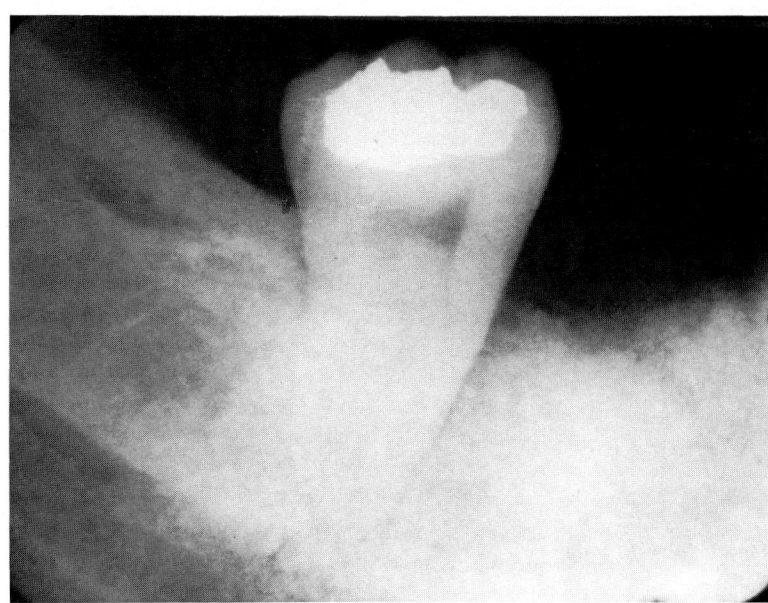

Figure 14–4. Osteosarcoma in edentulous molar area showing extensive calcified tumor bone.

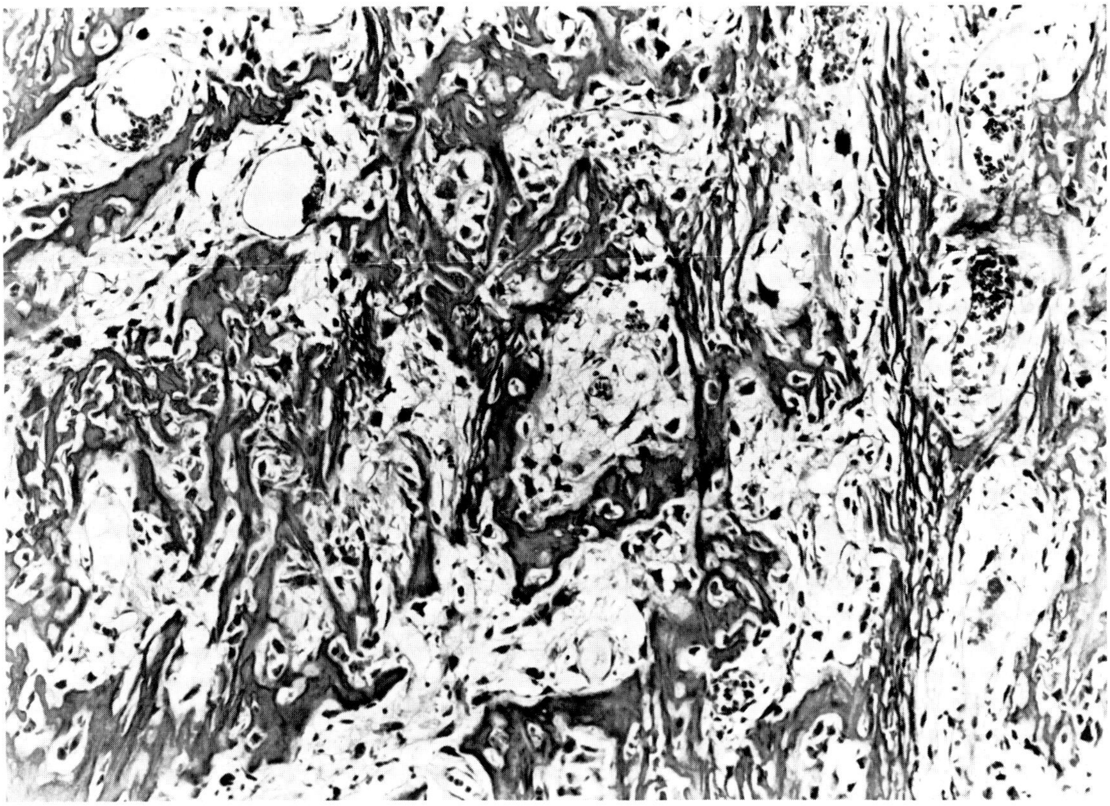

Figure 14–5. Osteoblastic variant of osteosarcoma characterized by irregular network of calcifying osteoid trabeculae.

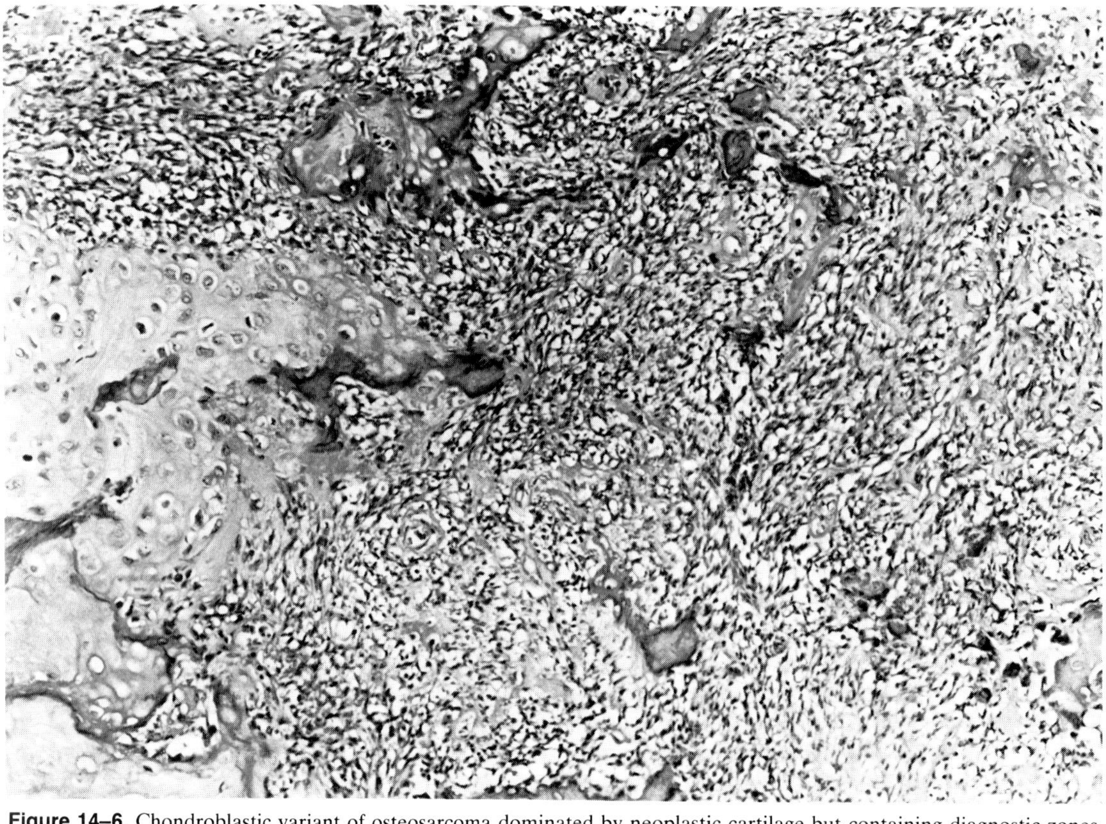

Figure 14–6. Chondroblastic variant of osteosarcoma dominated by neoplastic cartilage but containing diagnostic zones of malignant osteoid production by spindle cell stroma.

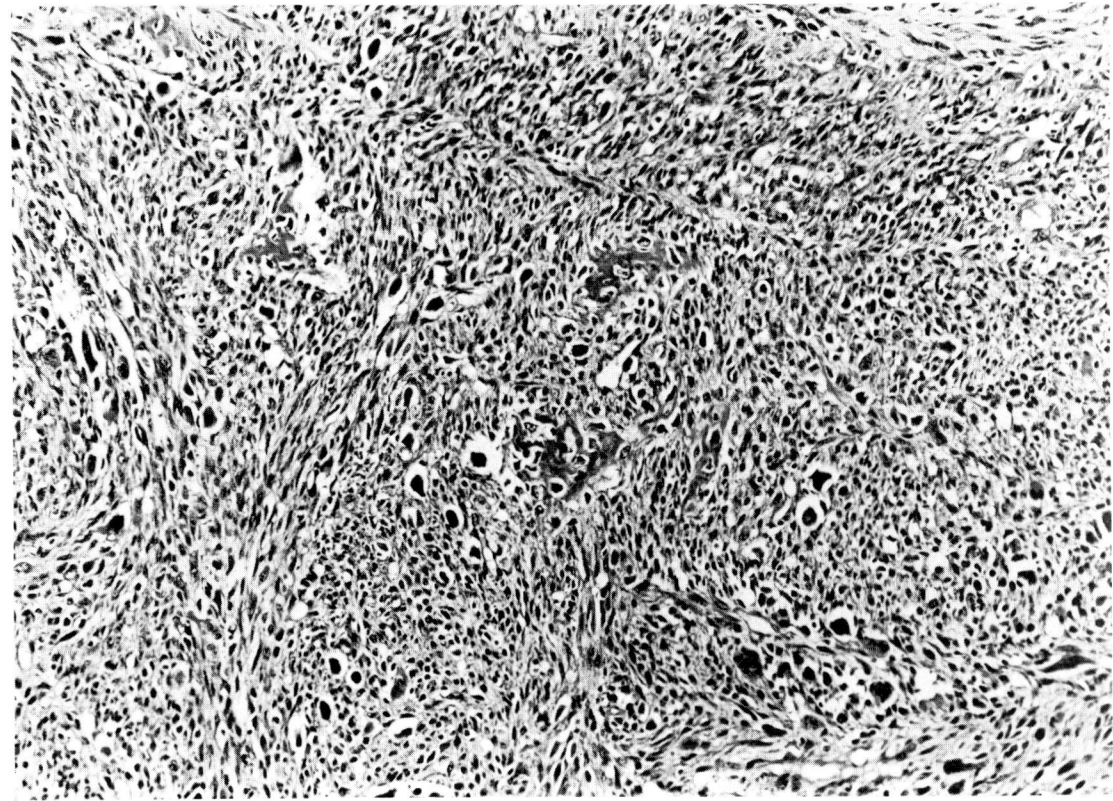

Figure 14–7. Fibroblastic variant of osteosarcoma with a malignant dense spindle cell stroma producing islands of osteoid.

differentiated than those of the skeleton. This difference appears to correspond to the poorer prognosis associated with osteosarcomas arising outside the jaws.

Differential Diagnosis. The uniform widening of the periodontal ligament space of involved teeth appears to be characteristic for early osteosarcoma. However, this focal radiographic defect may also have been seen with other malignancies surrounding teeth. Uniform widening of periodontal ligament spaces surrounding all teeth is seen in scleroderma. Moth-eaten radiolucencies are common to other malignancies, chronic osteomyelitis, and several benign neoplasms. A sclerotic radiographic appearance may be seen with some metastatic carcinomas and in Pindborg tumor, which is also often associated with an impacted tooth.

The histologic diagnosis hinges upon finding the malignant osteoid production. Many jaw osteosarcomas are predominantly chondroblastic, however, and may be misdiagnosed as chondrosarcoma. Osteosarcomas with a predominant fibroblastic component may be misdiagnosed as fibrosarcoma or malignant fibrous histiocytoma of bone. Failure to recognize pathologic features of malignancy in the telangiectatic osteosarcoma has resulted in a misdiagnosis of aneurysmal bone cyst or giant cell tumor.

Treatment and Prognosis. Overall, 5-year survival rates of 25 to 40% are reported for jaw osteosarcomas in various series. Patients with mandibular tumors generally fare better than patients with maxillary tumors. Osteosarcomas are best treated by radical mandibulectomy or maxillectomy, with radiotherapy and chemotherapy for recurrences, soft tissue extension, or metastatic disease. As with most malignant jaw tumors, initial radical surgery results in a superior survival rate of 80% compared with 27% survival for local surgery. Treatment of mandibular osteosarcomas by presurgical insertion of radium needles has resulted in a 76% 5-year survival. Osteosarcomas of the jaws frequently recur (40 to 70%), with a metastatic rate of 25 to 50%. Osteosarcomas rarely metastasize to regional lymph nodes. The most common sites of metastases are lung and brain. Once the disease has become metastatic, the mean survival is 6 months. Nearly 80% of patients dying of the disease do so within the first 2 years. Local recurrences and isolated metastatic deposits are treated by surgical excision and chemotherapy.

Juxtacortical Osteosarcomas

In contrast to the central intramedullary osteosarcomas, juxtacortical osteosarcomas arise at the periphery of bone at the periosteal surface, and they display distinct clinical, histologic, and radiographic features as well as a different biologic behavior. Juxtacortical osteosarcomas are uncommon neoplasms that compose approximately 5% of all osteosarcomas of the skeleton; they are rarely seen in the jaws. Most juxtacortical osteosarcomas arising in the jaws are of the parosteal subtype and rarely of the periosteal subtype.

Parosteal Osteosarcoma

Parosteal osteosarcoma occurs over a wide age range, with a peak incidence at 39 years. When the long bones are affected, there is a female predominance (3:2), but when the jaws are affected, males predominate. This variant of juxtacortical osteosarcoma most commonly involves the distal femoral metaphysis. The tumor presents as a slow-growing swelling or palpable mass, often accompanied by a dull aching sensation. Radiographically, the tumor is frequently radiodense and attached to the external surface of bone by a broad sessile base (Fig. 14-8). It is often more radiodense at the base than at the periphery. The broad pedicle is not continuous radiographically with the underlying marrow cavity. A radiolucent clear space, corresponding to the periosteum, can often be identified between the tumor and the normal bone cortex.

Histologically, parosteal osteosarcomas are well differentiated and characterized by a spindle cell stroma with minimal atypia; rare mitotic figures separate irregular trabeculae of woven bone having foci of osteoid and cartilage (Fig. 14-9). The periphery is less ossified than the base; it may have a lobulated cartilaginous cap or may be irregular because of linear extensions into soft tissue. Medullary involvement is unusual at initial presentation, but approximately 20% of tumors, especially recurrent ones, exhibit invasion of the underlying bone. This does not seem to adversely affect prognosis. The bland histologic appearance of parosteal osteosarcoma raises the possibility of osteoma, osteochondroma, heterotopic ossification, and myositis ossificans.

Periosteal Osteosarcoma

Periosteal osteosarcoma occurs much less often than does parosteal osteosarcoma. There is a 2 to 1 male predominance and a peak age of occurrence of 20 years. These tumors commonly involve the upper tibial metaphysis. They are rarely seen in the jaws.

The radiographic appearance of periosteal osteosarcoma is distinct from that of parosteal osteosarcoma. The cortex of involved bone is

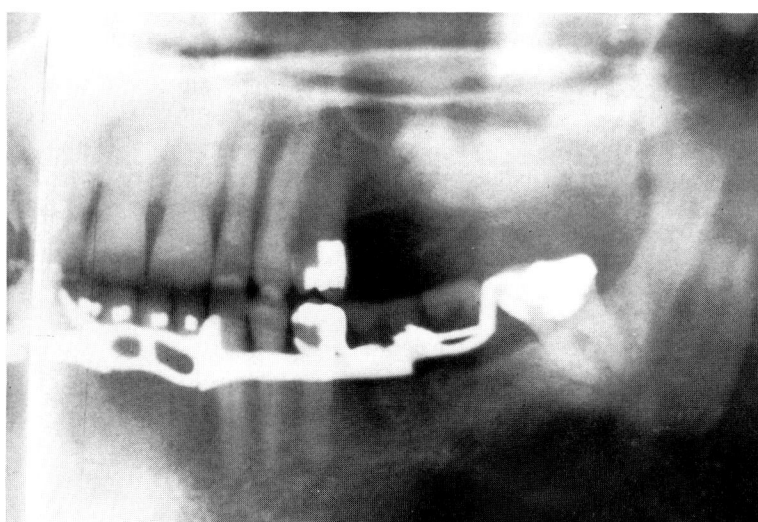

Figure 14-8. Parosteal osteosarcoma of the posterior maxillary alveolus. (Courtesy of Dr. K. Volz.)

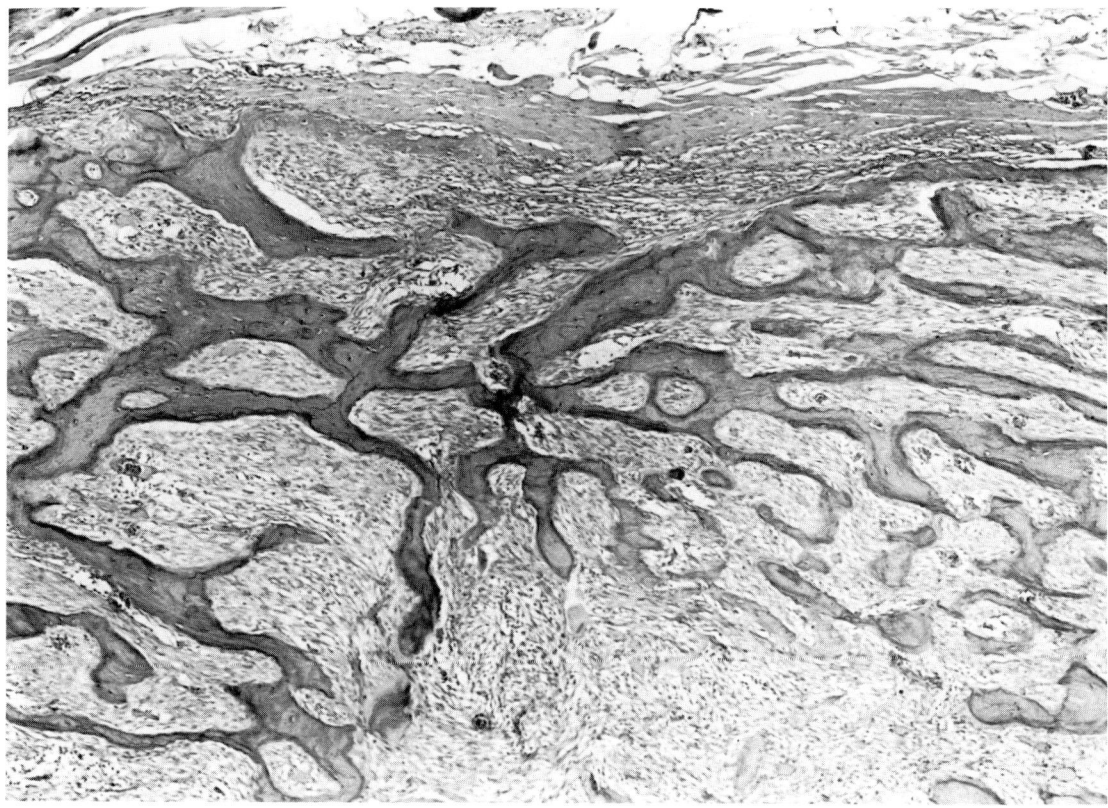

Figure 14–9. Parosteal osteosarcoma has radiating spicules of woven bone in a fibrocellular stroma that displays minimal cytologic atypia.

radiographically intact and sometimes thickened, with no tumor involvement of the underlying marrow cavity (Fig. 14–10). The tumor is most often radiolucent, corresponding to its predominantly cartilaginous component, and has a more poorly defined periphery. On occasion, there is a periosteal reaction in the form of a Codman triangle, and there may be variably sized perpendicular calcified spicules of bone radiating from the cortex. Overall, the periosteal osteosarcoma tumor matrix is not as radiographically dense or homogeneous as that of the parosteal osteosarcoma.

Histologically, periosteal osteosarcoma is composed of lobules of poorly differentiated malignant cartilage; it often shows central ossification. The malignant cartilage and osteoid appear to radiate from an intact cortex (Fig. 14–11). The osteoid present in this variant is fine and lace-like, and it is found in the chondroid islands among intervening malignant spindle cells (Fig. 14–12). These histologic features can be identical to those of intramedullary osteosarcomas; therefore, radiographic correlation is necessary in order to make this diagnosis. The malignant cytologic features also distinguish this variant of juxtacortical osteosarcoma from the parosteal type. In periosteal osteosarcoma, there is typically minimal tumor infiltration into cortical bone without medullary involvement. This feature helps differentiate this lesion from a chondroblastic intramedullary osteosarcoma that has permeated the cortex and formed a soft tissue mass.

The juxtacortical osteosarcoma must be completely removed by either *en bloc* resection or radical excision. A significant local recurrence rate can be expected if the underlying cortical bone is not removed with these lesions. The overall 5-year survival rate for juxtacortical osteosarcomas of the skeleton is 80%. In one series of juxtacortical osteosarcomas, pulmonary metastases developed in 13% of patients with parosteal osteosarcomas and in 22% of patients with periosteal osteosarcomas. Overall, the survival rate for juxtacortical osteosarcomas is superior to that of conventional intramedullary osteosarcomas. However, it is not known if juxtacortical osteosarcomas of

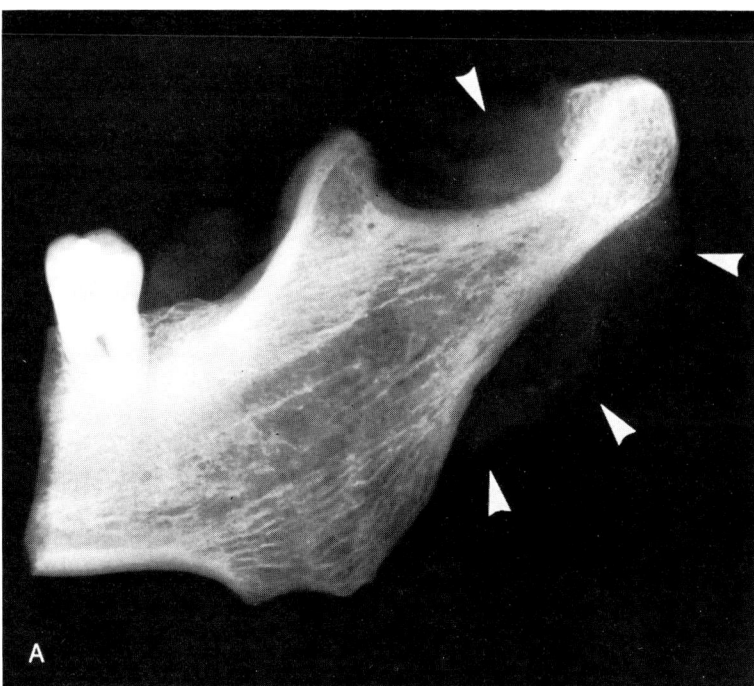
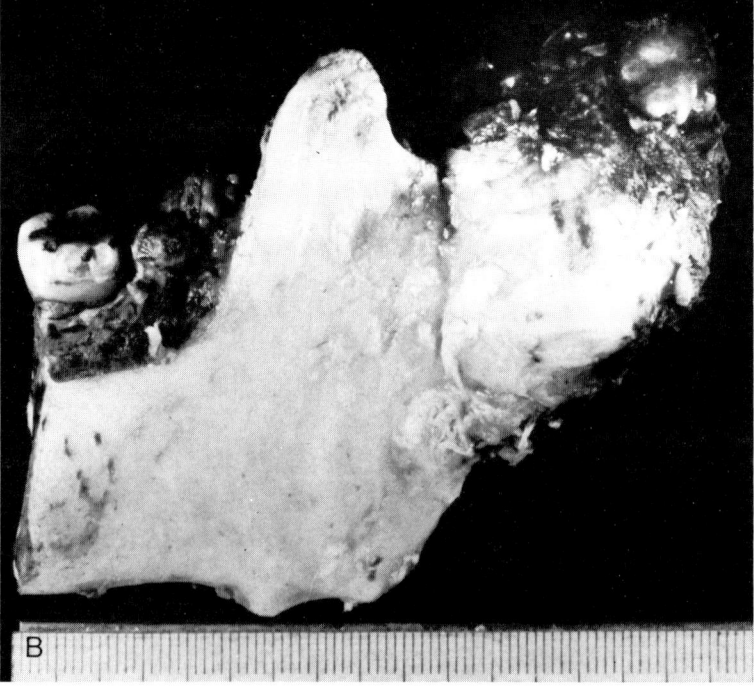

Figure 14–10. *A*, Radiograph of mandibulectomy specimen of periosteal osteosarcoma showing a lucent tumor mass overlying an intact cortex and medulla. *B*, Resected mandibular periosteal osteosarcoma showing white tumor involving ramus but sparing coronoid and condylar processes.

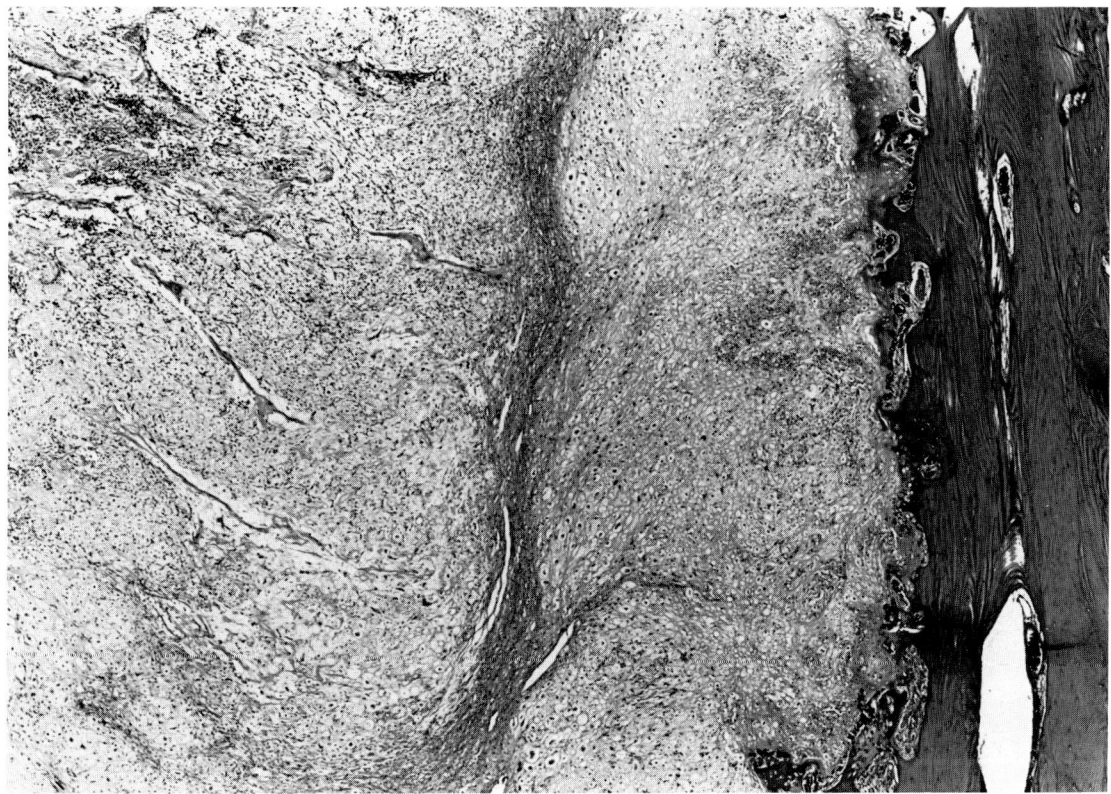

Figure 14–11. Periosteal osteosarcoma is a predominantly cartilaginous neoplasm overlying cortical bone without involvement of marrow cavity. A poorly differentiated spindle cell component (upper left) is farthest from the cortex (right).

the jaws are substantially different in biologic behavior from those occurring in long bones. Meaningful conclusions comparing the treatment and prognosis of parosteal and periosteal osteosarcomas in the jaws cannot be made, because of the few cases reported and the various methods of treatment employed (curettage, local excision, and radical resection).

CHONDROSARCOMA

Chondrosarcomas arising in the mandible and maxilla are extremely rare and have accounted for approximately 1% of chondrosarcomas of the entire body. The existence of benign chondrogenic tumors in the jaws is doubtful. Even in one large series of 162 chondromas of the body, none was reported in the jaws. The histologic distinction between a benign chondroma and a low-grade chondrosarcoma is ill defined, and clinical experience dictates that chondrogenic neoplasms in the jaws be considered potentially malignant and be handled accordingly.

Clinical Features. Chondrosarcomas more frequently involve the maxillofacial area (60%) than the mandible (40%). Lesions arising in the maxilla usually involve the anterior region (lateral incisor–canine region) and the palate. Mandibular chondrosarcomas occur most frequently in the premolar and molar regions, symphysis, coronoid process, and occasionally, condylar process (Fig. 14–13). There is no distinct gender predilection. Chondrosarcomas predominate in adulthood and old age. Although the mean age of occurrence of jaw chondrosarcomas is 60 years, almost half the cases have arisen in the third and fourth decades of life.

The most common signs are a painless swelling and expansion of the affected bones, resulting in loosening of teeth or ill-fitting dentures. Pain, visual disturbances, nasal signs, and headache may result from extension of chondrosarcomas from the jaw bones to contiguous structures.

The radiographic appearance of chondrosarcoma varies from moth-eaten radiolucencies that are solitary or multilocular to diffusely

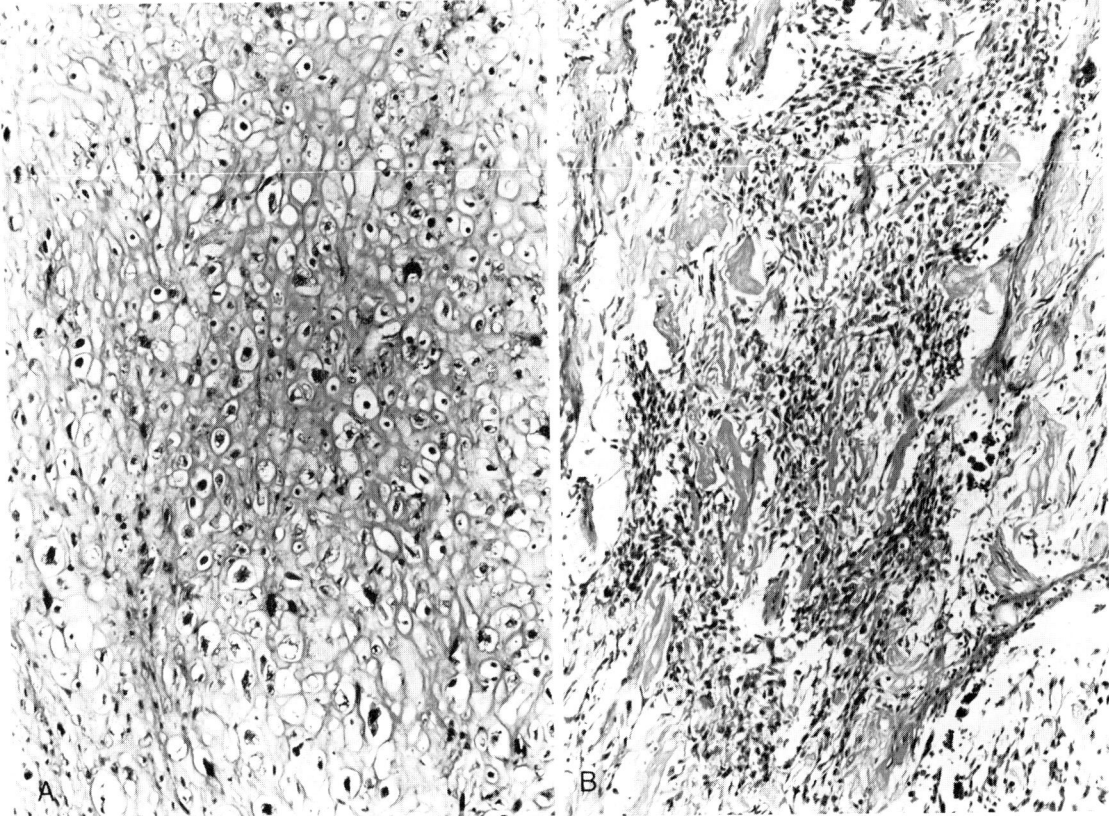

Figure 14–12. Cartilage component *(A)* and fine osteoid component *(B)* produced by spindle cell stroma in periosteal osteosarcoma.

opaque lesions. Many chondrosarcomas contain mottled densities corresponding to areas of calcification and ossification. Localized widening of the periodontal ligament space may also be seen in chondrosarcoma. Computed tomographic visualization of cartilaginous neoplasms appears to be superior in defining the peripheral extent of the tumor compared with panoramic or flat-plate radiographs. A multilocular radiographic appearance may suggest a differential diagnosis of ameloblastoma, central giant cell granuloma, odontogenic myxoma, aneurysmal bone cyst, and keratocyst, whereas other patterns may suggest metastatic carcinoma, osteogenic sarcoma, and calcifying epithelial odontogenic tumor.

Histopathology. The histologic appearance of chondrosarcomas is variable. Most of these tumors arising in the jaws are well differentiated. The prognostic significance of the pathologic grading of chondrosarcomas is well established. The incidence of metastatic disease has been shown to be 0%, 10%, and 71% for chondrosarcomas of grade I, grade II, and grade III, respectively. Grade I chondrosarcomas often have a lobular architecture; they range from proliferations resembling benign cartilage to those with increased numbers of chondrocytes in a chondroid to myxomatous stroma (Fig. 14–14). Grade II tumors often have a myxoid stroma with enlarged chondrocyte nuclei displaying occasional mitotic figures (Fig. 14–15). Frequently, there is increased cellularity at the periphery of the cartilaginous lobules. Grade III chondrosarcomas are markedly cellular, often with a spindle cell proliferation. Mitotic figures may be numerous.

Differential Diagnosis. Histologic differential diagnosis of chondrosarcoma arising in the jaws most commonly includes the chondroblastic variant of osteosarcoma. The latter is recognized when adequate tissue sampling reveals foci of malignant osteoid formation. In addition, chondroid areas of pleomorphic adenoma arising in overlying soft tissues may mimic cartilaginous tumors of bone. Synovial chondromatosis involving the temporomandibular joint may also simulate chondrosarcoma.

Treatment and Prognosis. Because chondrosarcomas are considered to be radioresistant

MALIGNANT NON-ODONTOGENIC NEOPLASMS OF THE JAWS 415

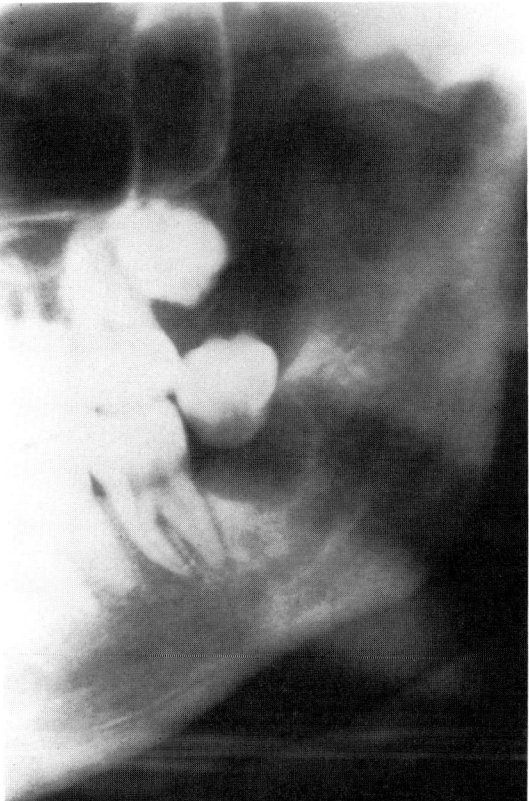

Figure 14–13. Chondrosarcoma of the molar-ramus of the mandible. Note extrusion of third molar by tumor and uniformly widened periodontal membrane space around roots of second molar.

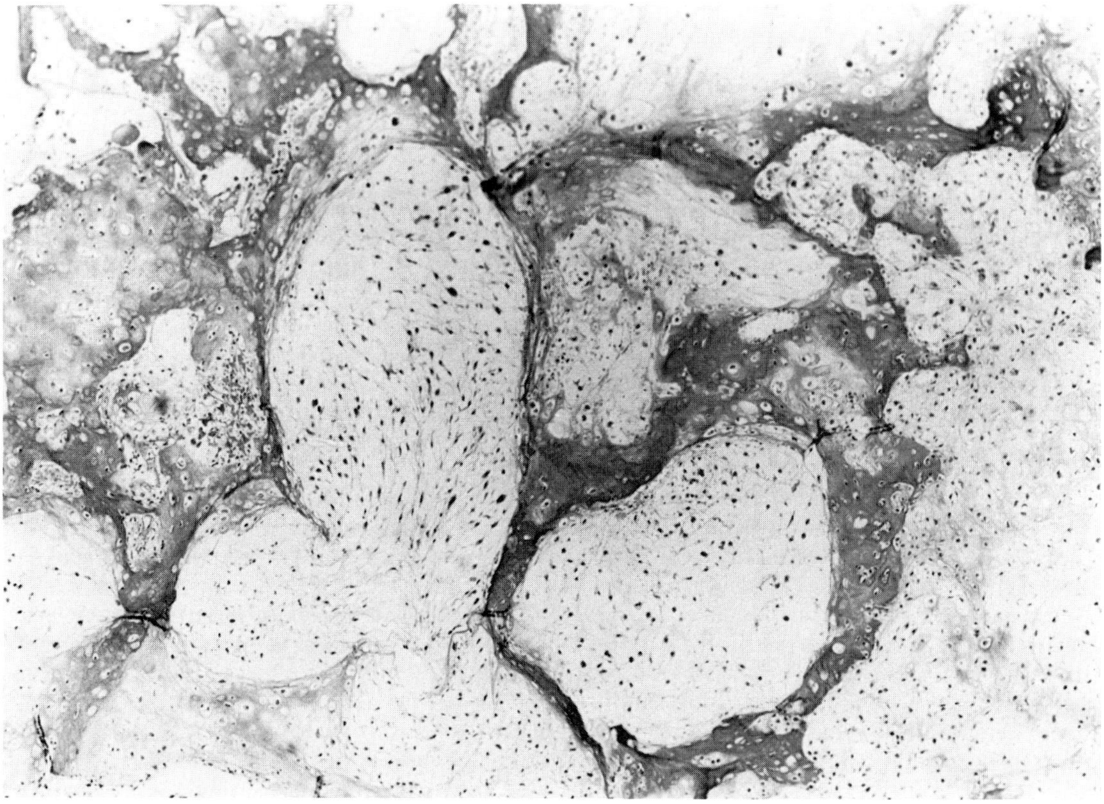

Figure 14–14. Low-grade chondrosarcoma showing lobulated proliferation of neoplastic cartilage.

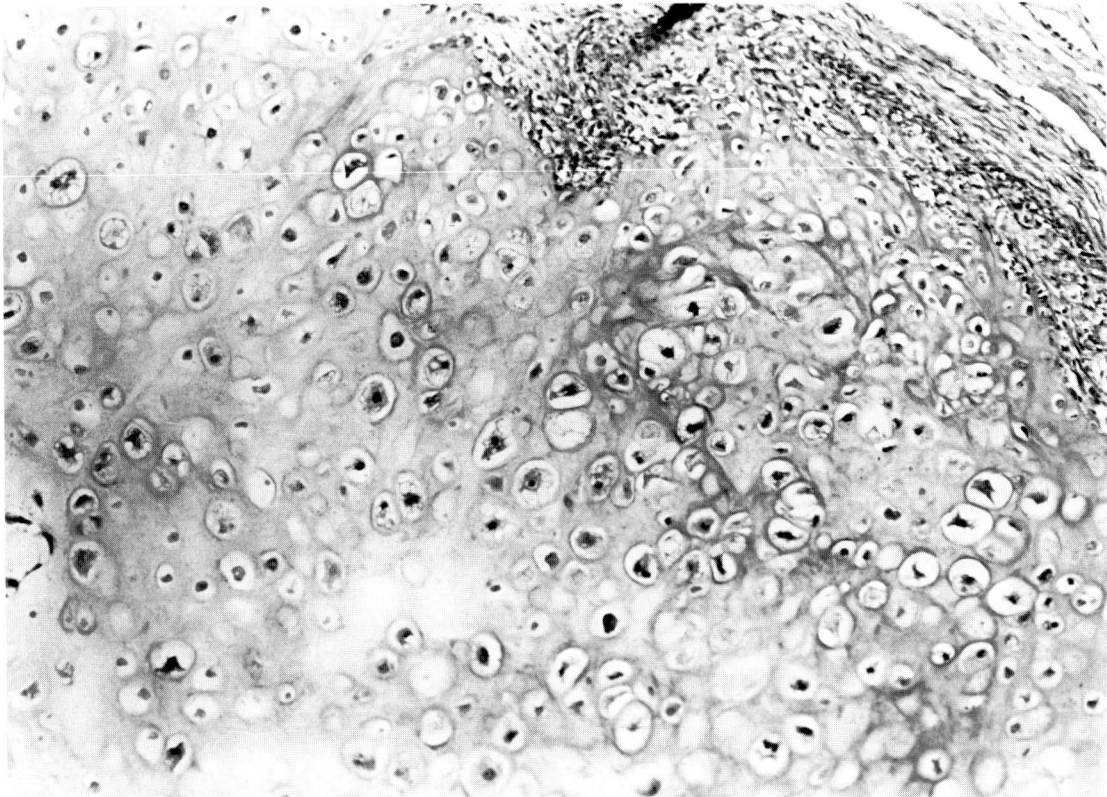

Figure 14–15. High-power micrograph of grade II chondrosarcoma displaying enlarged atypical condrocyte nuclei and occasional binucleate forms.

neoplasms, wide local or radical surgical excision is the treatment of choice. Therefore, location of primary lesion and adequacy of surgical resection (tumor-free margins) are of prime prognostic significance for chondrosarcomas of the jaws. In addition, the pathologic grade of chondrosarcoma is indicative of its innate biologic behavior and propensity for metastasis. The most common cause of death from chondrosarcomas of the jaws is uncontrolled local recurrence and extension into adjacent vital structures. Metastasis, more common with high-grade chondrosarcomas, is generally to lungs or bone. The usual clinical course of chondrosarcomas is long, with recurrences not uncommonly occurring after 5 years and even 10 to 20 years after therapy. The 5-year survival for chondrosarcomas of the jaws and craniofacial bones appears to be poorer than that for chondrosarcomas in other body sites. In addition, the 17% five-year survival for patients with chondrosarcomas of the mandible is extremely poor—even worse than that of osteosarcomas involving the jaws.

Mesenchymal Chondrosarcoma

Mesenchymal chondrosarcoma is a very rare form of chondrosarcoma that is both histologically distinct and clinically unique compared with the chondrosarcomas arising in bone.

Up to one third of the mesenchymal chondrosarcomas arise in soft tissue. Those that arise in bone show a predilection for the maxilla, mandible, and ribs. In one series of 15 mesenchymal chondrosarcomas of bone, one third occurred in the jaws. Most tumors arise between the ages of 10 and 30 years, with a nearly equal gender distribution. This presentation is distinctly different from other forms of chondrosarcoma that occur with a mean age of 60 years.

Similar to the other malignant neoplasms discussed, pain and, at times, swelling are the usual presenting symptoms. The radiologic appearance is of a lytic lesion that may be ill defined or sharply defined. Most contain stippled or large areas of calcification.

The characteristic histologic appearance of

mesenchymal chondrosarcoma is that of anaplastic small cell sarcoma containing zones of readily identifiable and often well-formed malignant cartilage. The undifferentiated small cell proliferation resembles Ewing's sarcoma and often displays a hemangiopericytoma-like growth pattern. It has been suggested that the small cell undifferentiated proliferation represents precartilaginous mesenchyme.

Appropriate sampling of these tumors will demonstrate a bimorphic proliferation of undifferentiated small cells alternating with areas of cartilage. The latter finding distinguishes mesenchymal chondrosarcoma from similar-appearing Ewing's sarcoma, hemangiopericytoma, or even synovial sarcoma.

Mesenchymal chondrosarcoma is a highly malignant neoplasm that requires radical or wide surgical excision. Like other chondrosarcomas, it is relatively radioresistant, but the Ewing's sarcoma–like component may respond to radiation or chemotherapy. This is a highly lethal sarcoma as evidenced by the fact that 80% of the patients in one series died of the disease. In addition to local recurrence, mesenchymal chondrosarcomas show a significant rate of distant metastases, often to lung and bones. Detection of metastatic disease in survivors may be delayed from 12 to 22 years after treatment of the primary tumor.

EWING'S SARCOMA

This is a highly lethal round cell sarcoma that was first described by James Ewing in 1921. The etiology is unknown, the cell of origin uncertain, and even the multipotentiality of antigenic expression controversial. Ewing's sarcoma accounts for roughly 6% of all malignant bone tumors. Approximately 4% of Ewing's sarcomas have arisen in the bones of the head and neck, with 1% occurring in the jaws. Most involve the bones of the lower extremity or pelvis. When the jaws are involved, there is a predilection for the ramus of the mandible, with few cases reported in the maxilla. Because Ewing's sarcoma has a propensity to metastasize to other bones, the possibility that jawbone involvement represents metastatic disease from another skeletal site should always be considered.

Clinical Features. Ninety percent of Ewing's sarcomas occur between the ages of 5 and 30 years, and over 60% affect males. The mean age of occurrence for primary tumors involving the bones of the head and neck is 10.9 years. Pain and swelling are the most common presenting symptoms. Involvement of the mandible or maxilla may result in facial deformity, destruction of alveolar bone with loosening of teeth, and mucosal ulcers (Fig. 14–16). Radiographic findings in the jaws are non-specific and may simulate an infectious process as well as a malignant process. The most characteristic appearance is that of a moth-eaten destructive radiolucency of medulla and erosion of cortex with expansion (Fig. 14–17). A variable periosteal "onion-skin" reaction may also be seen. A significant number of patients additionally have a soft tissue mass.

Histopathology. With an adequate tissue biopsy, Ewing's sarcoma is recognized microscopically as a proliferation of uniform, closely

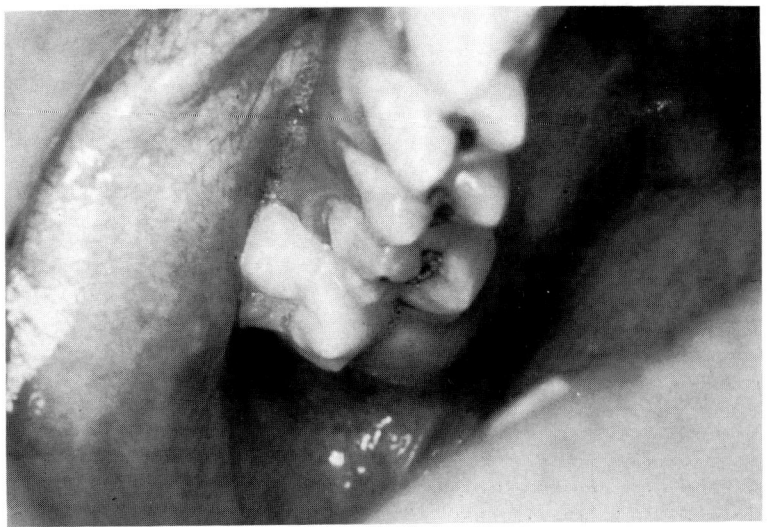

Figure 14–16. Ewing's sarcoma of the maxilla causing displacement of second molar.

418 MALIGNANT NON-ODONTOGENIC NEOPLASMS OF THE JAWS

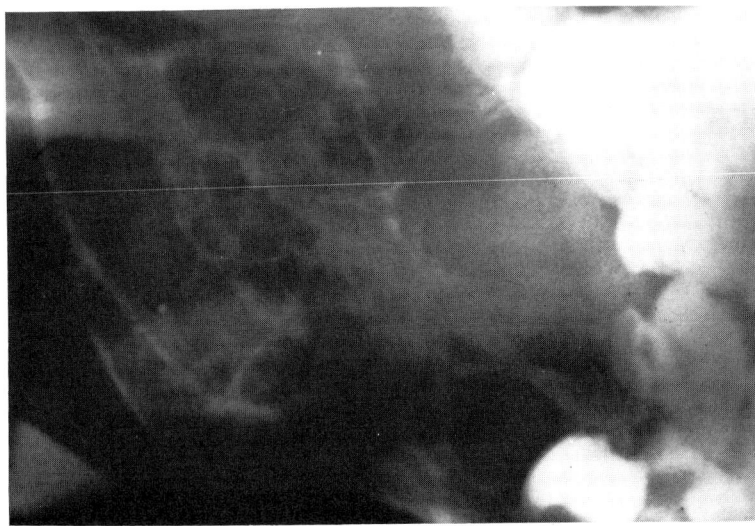

Figure 14–17. Lateral jaw radiogram of Ewing's sarcoma of the ramus of the mandible in a 4-year-old male. Condyle in upper left and posterior teeth in lower right.

packed cells that may be compartmentalized by fibrous bands (Fig. 14–18). The round to oval nuclei have finely dispersed chromatin and inconspicuous nucleoli. The cytoplasm characteristically stains with the periodic acid–Schiff stain, indicating the presence of glycogen. Although glycogen staining by this technique is helpful in diagnosis, some otherwise histologically acceptable cases of Ewing's sarcoma have yielded negative results. In addi-

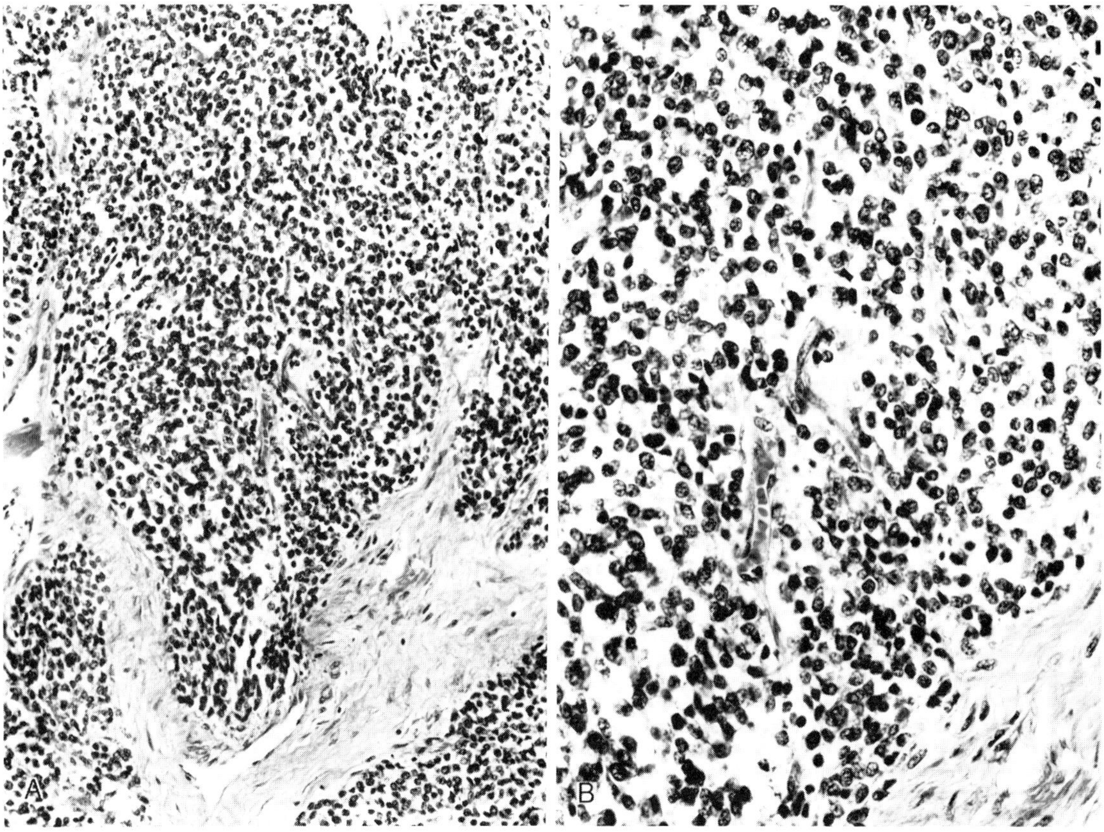

Figure 14–18. *A*, Low-power micrograph of Ewing's sarcoma with compartmentalizing fibrous bands. *B*, High-power micrograph of undifferentiated small cell proliferation in Ewing's sarcoma.

tion, other tumors that mimic Ewing's sarcoma may contain glycogen.

Differential Diagnosis. Microscopically, Ewing's sarcoma is sufficiently undifferentiated or anaplastic that its appearance is readily simulated by other so-called small round cell tumors common to childhood and adolescence. This differential diagnosis includes lymphoma/leukemia, metastatic neuroblastoma, mesenchymal chondrosarcoma, small cell osteosarcoma, and although rare for this age group, metastatic carcinoma. Routine light microscopy can often be used to discriminate between these similar-appearing neoplasms, but frequently electron microscopy or immunohistochemistry must be employed to reach a conclusive diagnosis. By electron microscopy, the cells of Ewing's sarcoma are characterized by pools of cytoplasmic glycogen, sparse organelles, and rare primitive intercellular junctions. By immunohistochemistry, all Ewing's sarcomas contain abundant vimentin intermediate filaments. The presence of other classes of intermediate filaments has been recently demonstrated in frozen tissue specimens. The heterogeneity of antigenic expression in these primitive neoplasms suggests that Ewing's sarcoma is a true blastoma, derived from primitive totipotential cells that may differentiate along numerous lines.

Treatment and Prognosis. The highly malignant nature of this sarcoma is reflected in its propensity for metastasis, especially to lungs, other bones, and lymph nodes. Multiple-method treatment protocols, involving surgery or radiation for local control and chemotherapy for systemic micrometastases, have dramatically improved the formerly dismal 10% five-year survival. With these newer intensive therapies, 79% two-year disease-free survival and 60% five-year actuarial survival rates have been reported. Clinical features associated with poor prognosis include presentation below age 10, the presence of metastatic disease, systemic symptoms, a high erythrocyte sedimentation rate, elevated serum lactate dehydrogenase value, and thrombocytosis. In addition, the site of involvement appears to be of prognostic significance in Ewing's sarcomas—patients with mandibular tumors are noted to have a more favorable overall survival than those with any other bone site of origin.

BURKITT'S LYMPHOMA

Burkitt's lymphoma is a high-grade non-Hodgkin's lymphoma that is endemic in Africa and occurs only sporadically in North America. It was first recognized by Dennis Burkitt in Uganda in 1958 as a jaw sarcoma occurring with high frequency in African children. By 1961, further reports demonstrated the distinctive clinical and pathologic features of this tumor, by then confirmed to be a malignant lymphoma. Subsequently, non-endemic forms of Burkitt's lymphoma were recognized in the United States. The African and American forms of Burkitt's lymphoma are histologically and immunophenotypically identical. Clinical differences, however, between the African and American forms exist.

Both American and African forms of Burkitt's lymphoma are characterized by a translocation of the distal part of chromosome 8 to chromosome 14. The former is the site of the c-myc oncogene and the latter, the immunoglobulin heavy chain locus. This translocation may be directly involved in the enhanced tumor cell proliferation of Burkitt's lymphoma, which has been shown to have the highest proliferation rate of any neoplasm in humans, with a potential doubling time of 24 hours and a growth fraction of nearly 100%.

Clinical Features. In Africa, malignant lymphoma accounts for 50% for all childhood malignancies, but it composes only 6 to 10% of childhood malignancies in the United States and Europe. Whereas the African form of Burkitt's lymphoma has a peak incidence between 3 and 8 years of age and a 2 to 1 male predominance, the American form affects a slightly older age group, with a mean age of 11 years, and has no gender predilection. The overwhelming majority (77%) of American Burkitt's lymphoma occurs in whites.

African Burkitt's lymphoma typically involves the mandible, maxilla, and abdomen, with extranodal involvement of retroperitoneum, kidneys, liver, ovaries, and endocrine glands. The incidence of jaw tumors in African Burkitt's lymphoma is related to the age of the patient, with 88% of those under 3 years of age and only 25% of those older than 15 years showing jaw involvement. Involvement of the jaws is relatively uncommon in the American form of this disease, with a 16% incidence at presentation. The American Burkitt's lymphoma presents most often as an abdominal mass involving the mesenteric lymph nodes or ileocecal region, often with an intestinal obstruction. Involvement of the retroperitoneum, gonads, and other viscera occurs less frequently. Although predominantly an extranodal disease, involvement of cervical lymph nodes or bone marrow has also been noted. A

420 MALIGNANT NON-ODONTOGENIC NEOPLASMS OF THE JAWS

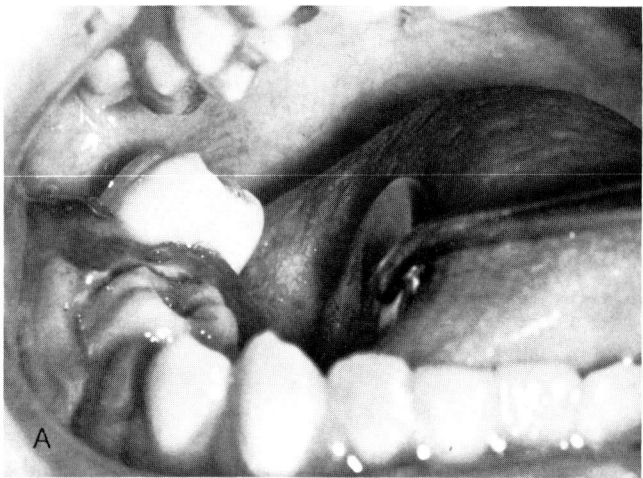
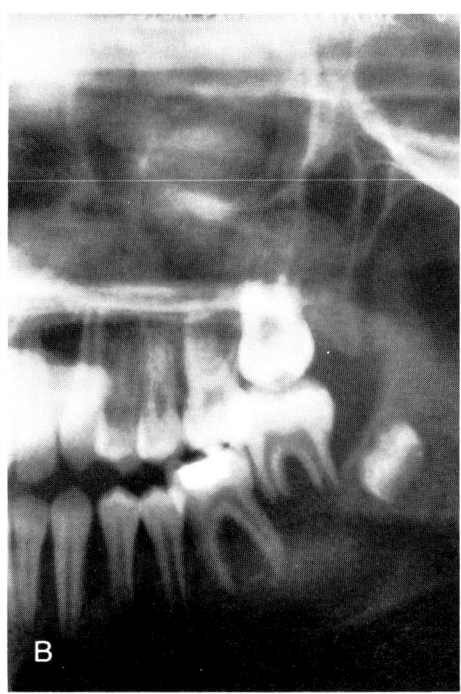

Figure 14–19. *A*, Burkitt's lymphoma of the mandible resulting in extrusion of second molar. *B*, Radiograph showing ill-defined diffuse lucency in the molar area. (Courtesy of Dr. R. Robert.)

notable difference between the endemic (African) and non-endemic (American) forms of Burkitt's lymphoma is that the Epstein-Barr virus genome can be detected in 90% of the African cases but in only 10% of the American cases.

When the mandible and maxilla are involved, the initial focus is usually in the posterior region, more commonly in the maxilla than the mandible (Fig. 14–19). The tumors in the American population appear more localized, whereas, in the African form, they more commonly involve all four quadrants. The usual signs associated with jaw lesions are an expanding intraoral mass and mobility of teeth. Pain and paresthesia are occasionally present. In addition to a facial mass, in the American population, toothache is a common complaint as well as paresthesia of the lip. Burkitt's lymphoma has also been noted to invade the dental pulp, especially in developing teeth. Radiographically, there is a moth-eaten, poorly margined destruction of bone. The cortex may be expanded, eroded, or perforated, with soft tissue involvement.

Histopathology. Burkitt's lymphoma is a neoplastic B cell proliferation that contains cell-surface B-lineage differentiation antigens and monoclonal surface immunoglobulin. Although the lymphoma may be nodular, most often it is a diffuse proliferation of small transformed or non-cleaved follicular center cell lymphocytes that are considered undifferentiated in the Rappaport classification. The proliferation is extremely monomorphic, composed of intermediate-sized lymphocytes with round nuclei and three to five small basophilic nuclei. Throughout the lymphoid proliferation are numerous scattered macrophages containing pyknotic debris, contributing the so-called starry-sky appearance (Fig. 14–20). The narrow rim of cytoplasm is pyroninophilic with the methyl green-pyronine stain. In touch imprints, cytoplasmic vacuoles containing lipid can be demonstrated.

The histologic differential diagnosis includes other subtypes of non-Hodgkin's lymphoma, undifferentiated carcinoma and sarcoma, metastatic neuroblastoma, and acute leukemia.

Treatment and Prognosis. Burkitt's lymphoma was at one time invariably fatal within 4 to 6 months of diagnosis. However, because of its high proliferation rate, Burkitt's lymphoma has proved to be extremely sensitive to combination chemotherapy and, therefore, potentially curable. The African and American forms of Burkitt's lymphoma show similar complete response rates to chemotherapy, with similar rates of relapse and survival. With combination chemotherapy, the overall 2-year

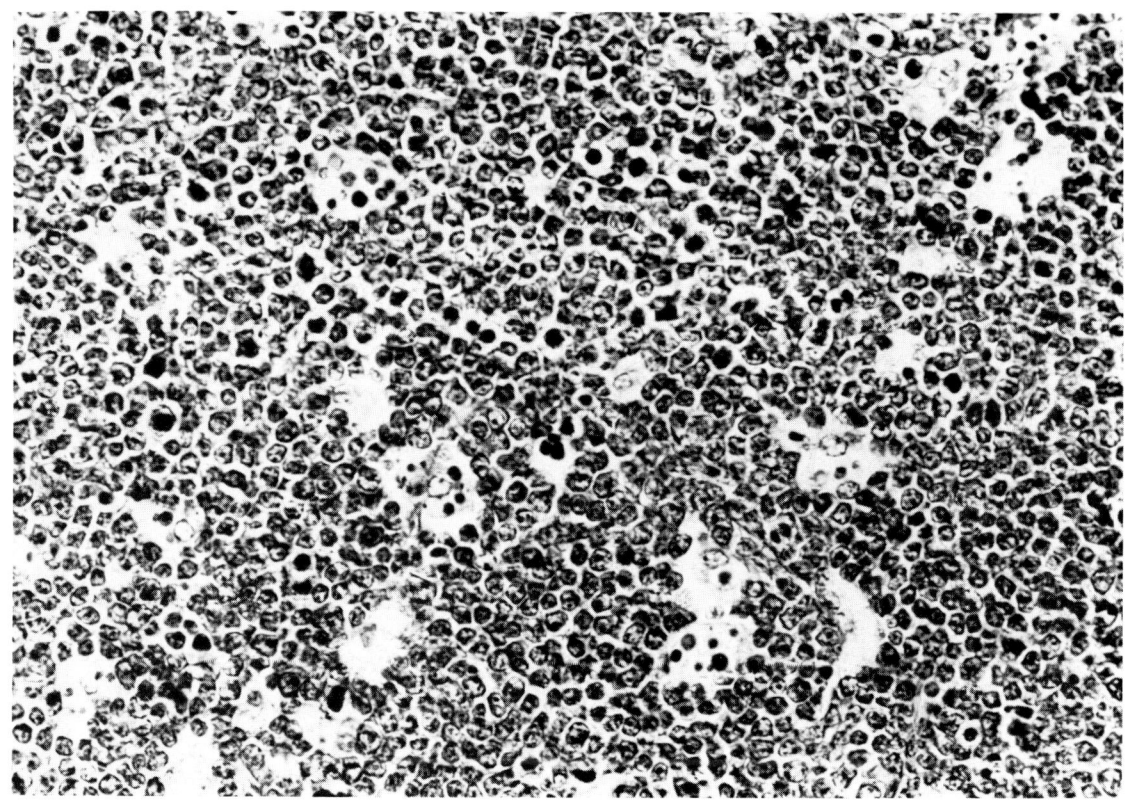

Figure 14–20. Burkitt's lymphoma showing a monotonous proliferation of small non-cleaved lymphocytes with interspersed macrophages containing engulfed pyknotic debris lending a "starry-sky" appearance.

survival is 54%, with a range of 80% for low-stage disease and 41% for advanced-stage disease.

PLASMA CELL NEOPLASMS

Multiple Myeloma

Plasma cell neoplasms are derived from bone marrow stem cells of B lymphocyte lineage, and they are functionally differentiated in their ability to produce and secrete immunoglobulin. Because these tumors are derived from a single neoplastic clone, they are associated with the production of monoclonal immunoglobulin components, with the immunoglobulin light chain restricted to either the kappa or the lambda type. These tumors may present in soft tissue as extramedullary plasmacytoma, in bone as a solitary lytic lesion known as a plasmacytoma of bone, or most commonly, as part of the multifocal disseminated disease multiple myeloma. Eighty percent of the extramedullary plasmacytomas involve the head and neck region, with a predilection for the nasopharynx, nasal cavity, paranasal sinuses, and tonsils. The tumors have also been reported in gingiva, palate, floor of the mouth, and tongue. Solitary plasmacytoma of bone is rare in the jaws; it more commonly appears in the ileum, femur, humerus, thoracic vertebrae, and skull. Multiple myeloma is a disease of the hematopoietic marrow–bearing bone of the skeleton, but 70 to 95% of these patients have also had radiographic involvement of the bones of the maxilla or mandible.

Clinical Features. Rarely seen before the fifth decade, multiple myeloma appears at a mean age of 63 years. There is a slight male predominance. Involvement of the jaws may be asymptomatic or may produce pain, swelling, expansion, numbness, mobility of teeth, or pathologic fracture. Rarely is there an associated soft tissue mass. Some patients may exhibit weakness, weight loss, anemia, and hyperviscosity syndromes. Roughly 10% of patients with multiple myeloma develop systemic amyloidosis. Eighty-five percent of patients with multiple myeloma have an abnormal skeletal radiographic survey. Although the remaining patients have an apparently normal radiographic series, they demonstrate plasmacytosis on marrow aspirate or biopsy.

The most common peripheral blood abnormality is anemia, with rouleau formation and, rarely, circulating plasma cells. The production of monoclonal immunoglobulin components by the neoplastic plasma cells results in an excess of abnormal protein that circulates in serum and can often be detected in urine. By serum protein electrophoresis, most patients with myeloma have a decreased quantity of normal immunoglobulin and an abnormal monoclonal immunoglobulin protein peak known as an M spike. The immunoglobulin is usually of the IgG or IgA class, with a monoclonal light chain component. Some plasma cell neoplasms may secrete only a monoclonal light chain. These monoclonal immunoglobulin components can be demonstrated by immunoelectrophoresis of both serum and urine in 91 to 97% of patients with myeloma. Urinary monoclonal light chains, so-called Bence Jones proteinuria, may be detected by a less sensitive heat test in roughly half of myeloma patients. Two percent of myeloma cases are non-secretory, although monoclonal immunoglobulin may be demonstrated within plasma cell cytoplasm by the immunoperoxidase method.

The radiographic appearance of myeloma can vary. Typically, there are multiple sharply "punched-out" but non-corticated radiolucent areas of bone destruction in the jaws and in many of the hematopoietic marrow–containing bones of the skeleton (Fig. 14–21). Plasma cell tumors in the jaws may be expansile and on rare occasions may be osteosclerotic. The finding of a solitary plasma cell tumor in the jaws is more often a manifestation of systemic disease than is a solitary plasmacytoma of bone.

Histopathology. Histologically, all clinical manifestations of plasma cell tumors are similar. Tumors are composed of a monotonous proliferation of pure plasma cells. The neoplastic plasma cells may display a wide range of differentiation, from mature-appearing plasma cells (Fig. 14–22) to less differentiated forms resembling immunoblastic large cell lymphomas. The abundant plasma cells within bone marrow can be distinguished from plasma cells of a chronic osteomyelitis or periapical granuloma by the associated proliferation of small vessels and fibroblasts with admixed neutrophils and macrophages in the reactive lesions. In addition, with the immunoperoxidase technique, a monoclonal intracytoplasmic immunoglobulin light chain can be demonstrated in nearly all plasma cell neoplasms, whereas reactive plasma cell infiltrates are uniformly polyclonal.

Differential Diagnosis. Although the "punched-out" lytic appearance is characteristic, the radiographic differential diagnosis of these jaw lesions includes other malignant neoplasms of the jaws, such as metastatic carcinoma, lymphoma, and idiopathic histiocytosis. Therefore diagnosis must be confirmed by tissue biopsy or aspirate. Histologically, very poorly differentiated plasma cell neoplasms may simulate other relatively undifferentiated malignant neoplasms, such as lymphoma, leukemia, undifferentiated carcinoma, metastatic malignant melanoma, and neuroblastoma. These entities can be distinguished by immunoperoxidase detection of the leukocyte common antigen in lymphoma/leukemia, cytokeratin in carcinomas, S-100 protein and melanoma-associated antigens in melanoma, and neuron-specific enolase in neuroblastoma.

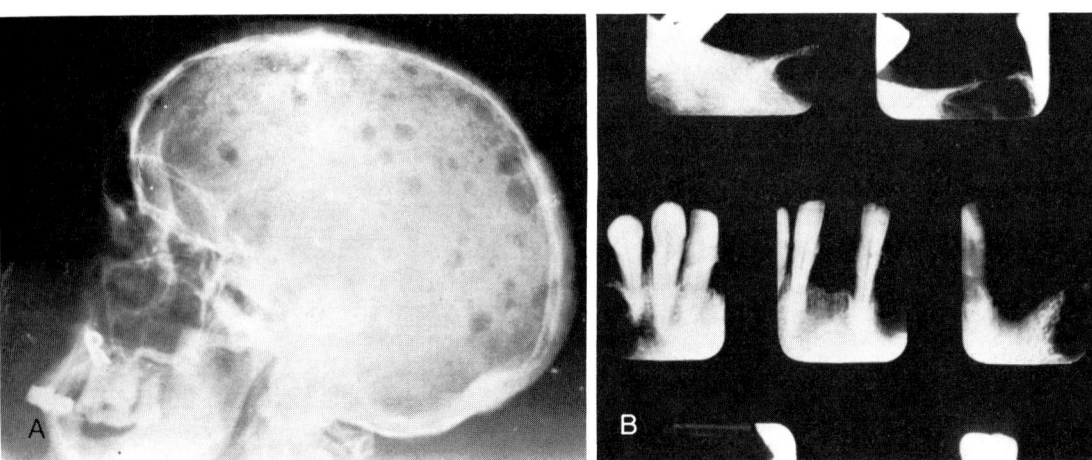

Figure 14–21. *A* and *B*, Multiple myeloma of the skull and mandible consisting of multiple "punched-out" radiolucencies.

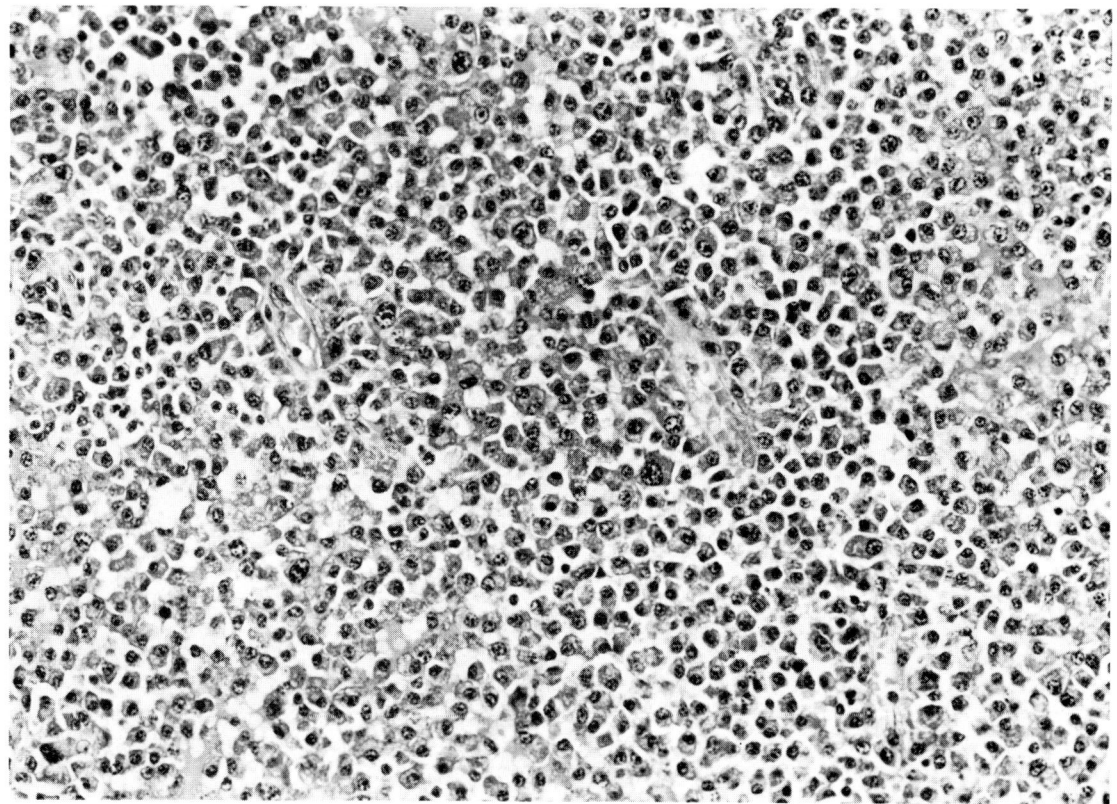

Figure 14–22. This well-differentiated plasma cell myeloma in jaws is a monotonous proliferation of readily recognizable neoplastic plasma cells.

Plasma cell tumors do not express these antigens.

Treatment and Prognosis. Most patients with myeloma die of infection and, less commonly, of renal failure, disseminated myeloma, cardiac complications, and hematologic complications of hemorrhage or thrombosis. Multiple myeloma is treated with chemotherapeutic alkylating agents and steroids, with local radiation directed to painful bone lesions. The overall mean survival is 20 months, with only 18% of patients surviving 5 years. Indicators of poor prognosis are severe azotemia, hypercalcemia, and anemia.

Solitary Plasmacytoma of Bone

Like multiple myeloma, solitary plasmacytoma of bone is a disease of adulthood, with a mean age of 50 years at presentation and a predominance in males. Solitary plasmacytomas rarely occur in the jaws, but, when they do, they are often located in the angle of the mandible. For a diagnosis of solitary plasmacytoma to be obtained, a radiologic bone survey and random bone marrow aspirate and biopsy should reveal no evidence of plasmacytosis in other areas of the body. However, 32 to 75% of patients diagnosed with solitary plasmacytoma of bone eventually progress to multiple myeloma. It is not possible to predict which patients will develop disseminated disease and which will not. As with multiple myeloma, the clinical symptoms include pain, swelling, and pathologic fracture.

Radiographically, solitary plasmacytoma is a well-defined lytic lesion that may be multilocular, resembling the appearance of central giant cell granuloma. Solitary plasmacytomas may destroy the cortical bone and spread into adjacent soft tissue. Unlike those with multiple myeloma, patients with solitary plasmacytoma of bone have a normal peripheral blood picture and a normal differential and clinical chemistry profile. In 17 to 25% of cases of solitary plasmacytoma of bone, a monoclonal immunoglobulin can be demonstrated in serum or urine. Biopsy of solitary plasmacytoma of bone reveals an identical histologic appearance to that of multiple myeloma, with a monotonous proliferation of neoplastic plasma cells producing monoclonal immunoglobulin components.

Solitary plasmacytoma of bone is treated primarily by local radiotherapy. Accessible lesions may be surgically excised, followed by radiation therapy. In 10 to 15% of patients, there is local recurrence of the solitary plasmacytoma, and small numbers of patients may develop an additional solitary plasmacytoma of bone. Despite the fact that a significant proportion progress to multiple myeloma, the overall survival of patients with solitary plasmacytoma is 10 years, in contrast to the 20-month mean survival of patients initially diagnosed with multiple myeloma. This appears to indicate that many solitary plasmacytomas are biologically low-grade but slowly progressive forms of multiple myeloma.

METASTATIC CARCINOMA

The most common malignancy affecting skeletal bones is metastatic carcinoma. However, metastatic disease to the mandible and maxilla is unusual; it is estimated that 1% of malignant neoplasms metastasize to these sites. Metastases to the jaws most commonly originate from primary carcinomas of the breast, kidney, lung, colon, prostate, and thyroid gland, in decreasing order of frequency.

Clinical Features. Individuals most likely to be affected by metastatic carcinoma of the jaws are in the older age groups, with an average age of 56 years reflecting the greater prevalence of malignancy in this population. The mechanism of spread to the jaws is usually hematogenous from the primary visceral neoplasm or from lung metastases. Within the jaw, the angle and body of the mandible are more commonly involved by metastatic disease. Bone pain, loosening of teeth, lip paresthesia, bone swelling, gingival mass (Fig. 14–23), and pathologic fracture may be clinically evident.

The radiographic appearance of most jaw metastases are poorly marginated, radiolucent, irregular, moth-eaten, expansile defects (Fig. 14–24). Some metastatic carcinomas, notably prostate and thyroid, are often characterized by an osteoblastic process. Although the appearance of osteomyelitis is also a moth-eaten radiolucency, it rarely expands the cortical bone.

Histopathology. The histologic appearance of metastatic carcinoma can be extremely variable, reflecting tumor type and grade of tumor differentiation. A prominent desmoplastic stromal response is often present. The diagnosis of metastatic carcinoma in difficult cases can be verified with an immunoperoxidase stain for cytokeratin, which is present in all carcinoma cells. In addition, immunoperoxidase staining to identify tissue-specific markers such as prostate-specific antigen, prostatic alkaline phosphatase, thyroglobulin, and calcitonin can indicate a primary origin in the prostate or thyroid gland. Antibodies to tumor type–specific antigens that are reactive in formalin-fixed paraffin-embedded material and capable of pointing to primary sites in lung, breast, colon, or kidney are not as yet available. It is anticipated that, with advances in monoclonal antibody development, this technique will be very useful in identifying carcinomas of unknown metastatic origin.

Differential Diagnosis. The differential diagnosis of poorly differentiated carcinoma in-

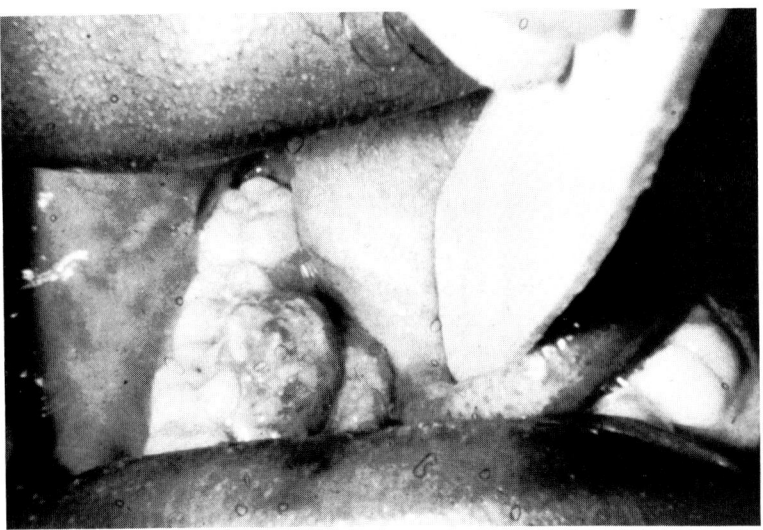

Figure 14–23. Undifferentiated carcinoma metastatic to the mandible and presenting as a gingival mass.

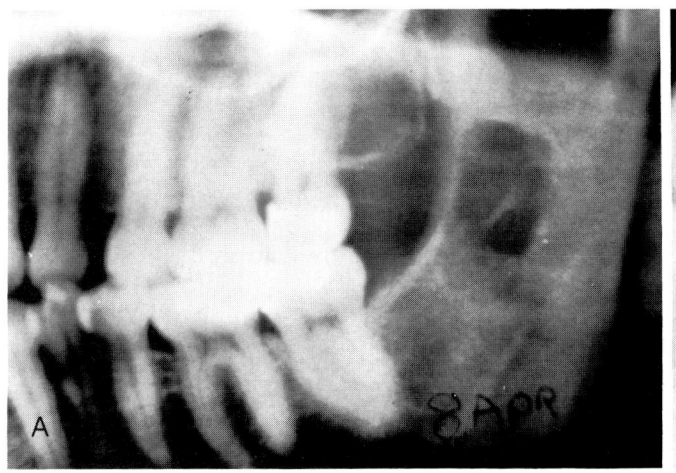 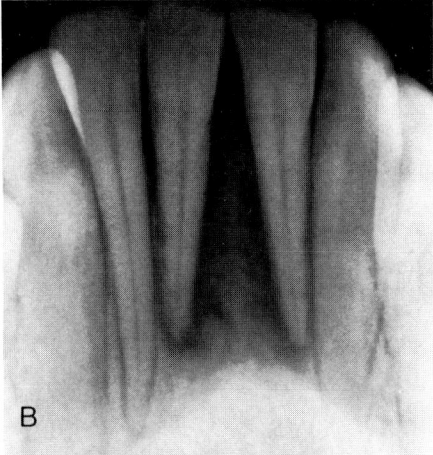

Figure 14–24. *A*, Carcinoma of the breast metastatic to the mandible. *B*, Metastatic disease of the mandibular anterior alveolar process. (Courtesy of Dr. R. Courtney.)

cludes anaplastic sarcoma, lymphoma, and amelanotic melanoma. The very rare primary intraosseous carcinoma of probable odontogenic origin was considered in Chapter 11. The presence of cytokeratin within the tumor cells is diagnostic of carcinoma. Immunoperoxidase stains for the leukocyte common antigen verify a diagnosis of lymphoma/leukemia, whereas immunoreactivity with melanoma-associated antigens and S-100 protein indicate a diagnosis of melanoma. Although many of these sophisticated diagnostic techniques can be used to indicate the nature of an anaplastic neoplasm, there is no substitute for an accurate medical history and physical examination, especially in the diagnosis of metastatic carcinoma.

Treatment and Prognosis. Metastatic carcinoma to the jaws requires further work-up to identify the primary site and to stage the degree of metastatic involvement. This is useful in identifying whether the jaw metastasis represents a solitary focus or, as is often the case, is merely the clinical sign of disseminated skeletal disease. A single focus may be treated by surgical excision or chemoradiotherapy. Generalized skeletal metastases are usually an ominous event and treated palliatively. The prognosis for patients with metastatic carcinoma to the jaws is grave, with a dismal 10% four-year survival and over two thirds dead within a year.

Bibliography

Osteosarcoma

Ahuja S, Villacin A, Smith J, et al. Juxtacortical (parosteal) osteogenic sarcoma. Histologic grading and prognosis. J Bone Joint Surg 59A:632–647, 1977.

Banerjee S. Juxtacortical osteosarcoma of mandible: review of literature and report of case. J Oral Surg 39:535–538, 1981.

Bras J, Donner R, van der Kwast W, et al. Juxtacortical osteogenic sarcoma of the jaws. Review of the literature and report of a case. Oral Surg 50:535–544, 1980.

Caron A, Hajdu S, Strong E. Osteogenic sarcoma of the facial and cranial bones. A review of 43 cases. Am J Surg 122:719–725, 1971.

Chambers R, Mahoney W. Osteogenic sarcoma of the mandible. Current management. Am Surg 36:463–471, 1970.

Clark J, Krishnan K, Unni M, et al. Osteosarcoma of the jaw. Cancer 51:2311–2316, 1983.

Dahlin D. Bone Tumors. General Aspects and Data on 6,221 Cases. 3rd ed. Charles C Thomas, Springfield, Ill, 1978, pp 226–273.

DeSantos L, Murray J, Finklestein J, et al. The radiographic spectrum of periosteal osteosarcoma. Radiology 127:123–129, 1978.

Gardner D, Mills D. The widened periodontal ligament of osteosarcoma of the jaws. Oral Surg 41:652–656, 1976.

Garrington G, Scofield H, Cornyn J, et al. Osteosarcoma of the jaws. Analysis of 56 cases. Cancer 20:377–391, 1967.

Schajowicz F. Juxtacortical chondrosarcoma. J Bone Joint Surg 59B:473–480, 1977.

Scranton P, DeCicco F, Totten R, et al. Prognostic factors in osteosarcoma. A review of 20 years' experience at the University of Pittsburgh Health Center Hospitals. Cancer 36:2179–2191, 1975.

Unni K, Dahlin D, Beabout J, et al. Periosteal osteogenic sarcoma. Cancer 37:2476–2485, 1976.

Unni K, Dahlin D, Beabout J, eta l. Parosteal osteogenic sarcoma. Cancer 37:2466–2475, 1976.

Zarbo R, Regezi J, Baker S. Periosteal osteogenic sarcoma of the mandible. Oral Surg 57:643–647, 1984.

Chondrosarcoma

Arlen M, Tollefsen H, Huvos A, et al. Chondrosarcoma of the head and neck. Am J Surg 120:456–460, 1970.

Evans H, Ayala A, Romsdahl M. Prognostic factors in chondrosarcoma of bone: a clinicopathologic analysis with emphasis on histologic grading. Cancer 40:818–831, 1977.

Fu Y, Perzin K. Non-epithelial tumors of the nasal cavity, paranasal sinuses, and nasopharynx: a clinicopathologic study. 3. Cartilaginous tumors (chondroma, chondrosarcoma). Cancer 34:453–463, 1974.

Salvador A, Beabout J, Dahlin D. Mesenchymal chondrosarcoma: observations on 30 new cases. Cancer 28:605–615, 1971.

Sato K, Nukaga H, Horikoshi T. Chondrosarcoma of the jaws and facial skeleton: a review of the Japanese literature. J Oral Surg 35:892–897, 1977.

Ewing's Sarcoma

Graham-Poole J. Ewing's sarcoma: treatment with high dose radiation and adjuvant chemotherapy. Med Pediatr Oncol 7:1–8, 1979.

Moll R, Inchul L, Gould V, et al. Immunocytochemical analysis of Ewing's tumors. Patterns of expression of intermediate filaments and desmosomal proteins indicate cell type heterogeneity and pluripotential differentiation. Am J Pathol 127:288–304, 1987.

Pomeroy T, Johnson R. Prognostic factors for survival in Ewing's sarcoma. Am J Roentgenol Radium Ther Nucl Med 123:598–606, 1975.

Pritchard D, Dahlin D, Dauphine R, et al. Ewing's sarcoma. A clinicopathological and statistical analysis of patients surviving five years or longer. J Bone Joint Surg 57A:10–16, 1975.

Rosen G, Caparros B, Nirenberg A, et al. Ewing's sarcoma: ten-year experience with adjuvant chemotherapy. Cancer 47:2204–2213, 1981.

Siegal G, Oliver W, Reinus W, et al. Primary Ewing's sarcoma involving the bones of the head and neck. Cancer 60:2829–2840, 1987.

Som P, Krespi Y, Hermann G, et al. Ewing's sarcoma of the mandible. Ann Otol Rhinol Laryngol 89:20–23, 1981.

Telles N, Rabson A, Pomeroy T. Ewing's sarcoma: an autopsy study. Cancer 41:2321–2329, 1978.

Burkitt's Lymphoma

Adatia A. Radiology of dental changes in Burkitt's lymphoma. In Proceedings of the Third International Congress of Maxillofacial Radiologists, Tokyo. Japan Science Press, Tokyo, 1974, pp 405–414.

Berard C, Greene M, Jaffe E, et al. A multidisciplinary approach to non-Hodgkin's lymphomas. Ann Intern Med 94:218–235, 1981.

Grogan T, Warnke R, Kaplan H. A comparative study of Burkitt's and non-Burkitt's "undifferentiated" malignant lymphoma: immunologic, cytochemical, ultrastructural, cytologic, histopathologic, clinical, and cell culture features. Cancer 49:1817–1828, 1982.

Levine P, Kamaraju L, Connelly R, et al. The American Burkitt's lymphoma registry. Eight years' experience. Cancer 49:1016–1022, 1982.

Sariban E, Donahue A, MaGrath I. Jaw involvement in American Burkitt's lymphoma. Cancer 53:1777–1782, 1984.

Ziegler J. Burkitt's lymphoma. N Engl J Med 305:735–745, 1981.

Ziegler J. Treatment results of 54 American patients with Burkitt's lymphoma are similar to the African experience. N Engl J Med 297:75–80, 1977.

Plasma Cell Neoplasms

Alexanian R, Balcerzak S, Bonnet J, et al. Prognostic factors in multiple myeloma. Cancer 36:1192–1201, 1975.

Bataille R, Sany J. Solitary myeloma: clinical and prognostic features of a review of 114 cases. Cancer 48:845–851, 1981.

Corwin J, Lindberg R. Solitary plasmacytoma of bone vs extramedullary plasmacytoma and their relationship to multiple myeloma. Cancer 43:1007–1013, 1979.

Kapadia S. Multiple myeloma. A clinicopathologic study of 62 consecutively autopsied cases. Medicine (Baltimore) 59:380–392, 1980.

Kyle R. Multiple myeloma. Review of 869 cases. Mayo Clin Proc 50:29–40, 1975.

Meyer J, Schulz M. "Solitary" myeloma of bone. A review of 12 cases. Cancer 34:438–440, 1974.

Regezi J, Zarbo R, Keren D. Plasma cell lesions of the head and neck: immunofluorescent determination of clonality from formalin-fixed paraffin-embedded tissue. Oral Surg 56:616–621, 1983.

Woodruff R, Malpas J, White F. Solitary plasmacytoma. 2. Solitary plasmacytoma of bone. Cancer 43:2344–2347, 1979.

Metastatic Carcinoma

Batsakis J. Tumors of the Head and Neck. Clinical and Pathological Considerations. 2nd ed. Williams & Wilkins, Baltimore, 1979, p. 241.

Chapter 15

Metabolic and Genetic Jaw Diseases

Paul Crespi

METABOLIC CONDITIONS
Paget's Disease
Hyperparathyroidism
Hyperthyroidism
Hypophosphatasia
Infantile Cortical Hyperostosis
Phantom Bone Disease
Acromegaly
GENETIC ABNORMALITIES
Cherubism
Osteopetrosis
Osteogenesis Imperfecta
Cleidocranial Dysplasia
Crouzon's Syndrome (Craniofacial Dysostosis)
Treacher Collins Syndrome (Mandibulofacial Dysostosis)
Pierre Robin Syndrome
Marfan's Syndrome
Ehlers-Danlos Syndrome
Down Syndrome (Trisomy 21)
Hemifacial Atrophy
Hemifacial Hypertrophy
Clefts of the Lip and Palate
Fragile X Syndrome

METABOLIC CONDITIONS

Paget's Disease

Etiology and Pathogenesis. Paget's disease, or osteitis deformans, is a chronic, slowly progressive condition of unknown etiology. Numerous theories of origin have been postulated since the early concept of a chronic inflammatory process. These included autoimmunity, an endocrine abnormality related to hyperthyroid disease, an inborn error of connective tissue metabolism, an autonomic nervous system–mediated vascular disorder, a paramyxovirus infection, and more recently a slow virus–type infection.

The disease may be broken down into three stages. The initial phase is the bone resorptive phase. The second or vascular phase appears with concomitant haphazard osteoblastic repair. In this phase symptoms become evident and often cause the patient to seek treatment. The final phase is an appositional or sclerosing phase in which mineralization of previously deposited bony matrix occurs, with a diminution of the overall cellularity and vascularity of the lesions.

Clinical Features. The maxilla and mandible are involved in approximately 17% of cases, with involvement usually being bilateral and symmetric. The maxilla is affected approximately twice as often as the mandible. Enlargement of the maxilla or mandible as well as the skull is common. At initial presentation, symptoms often relate to deformity or pain in the affected bones. Neurologic complaints—including headache, auditory or visual disturbances, facial paralysis, vertigo, and weakness—may be related, in large part, to narrowing of skull foramina, resulting in compression of vascular and neural elements.

Classically, the dental patient who wears complete dentures may complain of newly acquired poor prosthetic adaptation and function as the maxilla progressively enlarges. Ultimately, the alveolar ridge widens, with a rel-

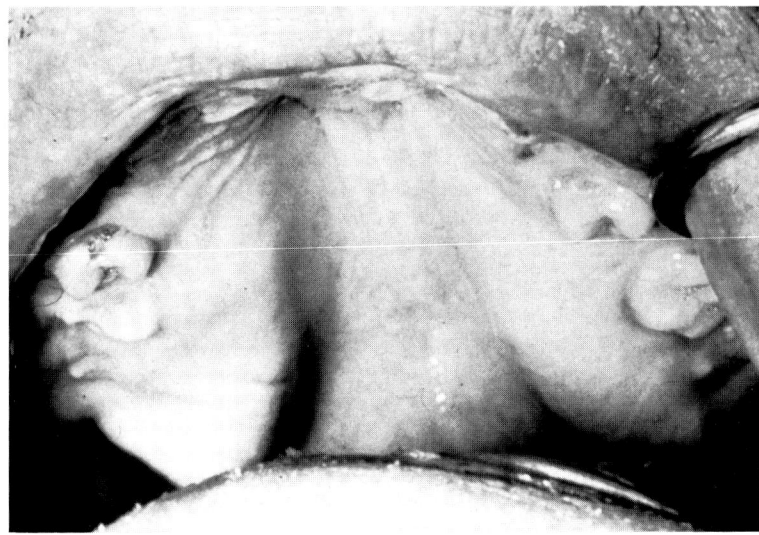

Figure 15–1. Paget's disease of the maxilla. Note bilateral enlargement of ridges.

ative flattening of the palatal vault (Fig. 15–1). When teeth are present, increased spacing as well as loosening is noted (Fig. 15–2). In severe cases, continued enlargement of the maxilla or mandible can make closure of the lips difficult or impossible.

The classic radiographic findings in later stages of Paget's disease relate to a haphazard arrangement of newly formed bone providing a patchy radiopaque pattern termed "cotton wool" by many (Fig. 15–3). In the jaws, this pattern of bone change may be associated with hypercementosis of tooth roots, loss of lamina dura, obliteration of the periodontal ligament space, and resorption of roots (Fig. 15–4).

Histopathology. Histologically, in the initial, resorptive phase, random osteoclastic bone resorption is evident. The osteoclasts contain large numbers of nuclei. Resorbed bone is replaced by dense, vascularized connective tissue, which is often seen in direct apposition to eroded bony spicules. The second phase represents a dynamic composite of osteolysis and osteogenesis (Fig. 15–5). Broad osteoid bands or seams that are in the process of mineralization are evident. A classic histologic pattern develops; it is known as a mosaic because of irregular bone formation with numerous cemental or reversal lines. In the final, sclerotic phase, a decrease in osteoclastic activity and an increase in osteoblastic function are seen (Fig. 15–6).

The laboratory can provide important information regarding the diagnosis of Paget's disease. Normal serum calcium and serum phosphate levels are present in the face of

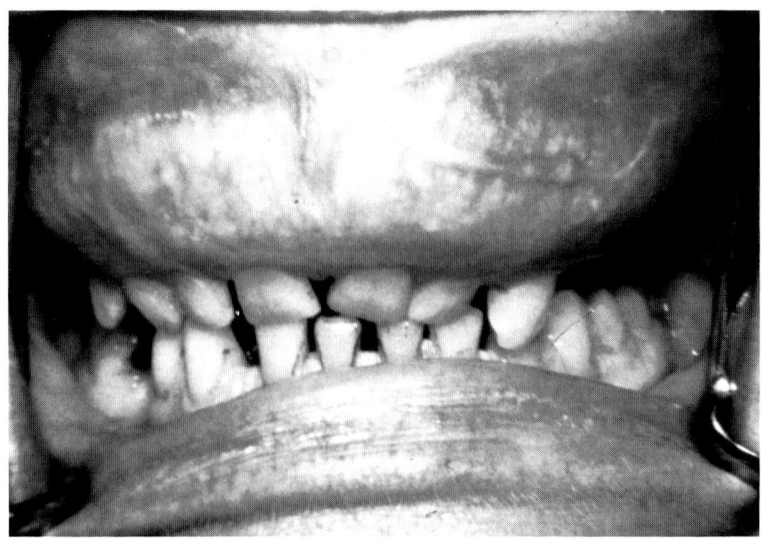

Figure 15–2. Paget's disease causing increased spacing of teeth.

METABOLIC AND GENETIC JAW DISEASES 429

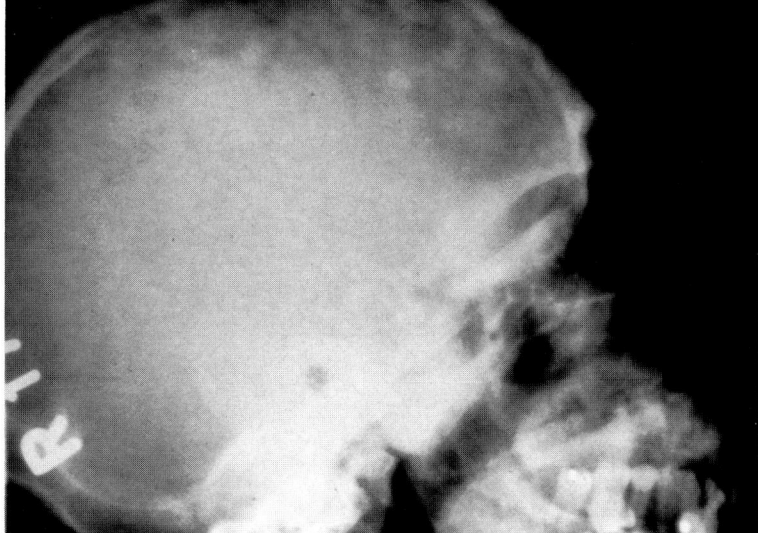

Figure 15–3. Paget's disease of the skull showing patchy opaque pattern ("cotton wool").

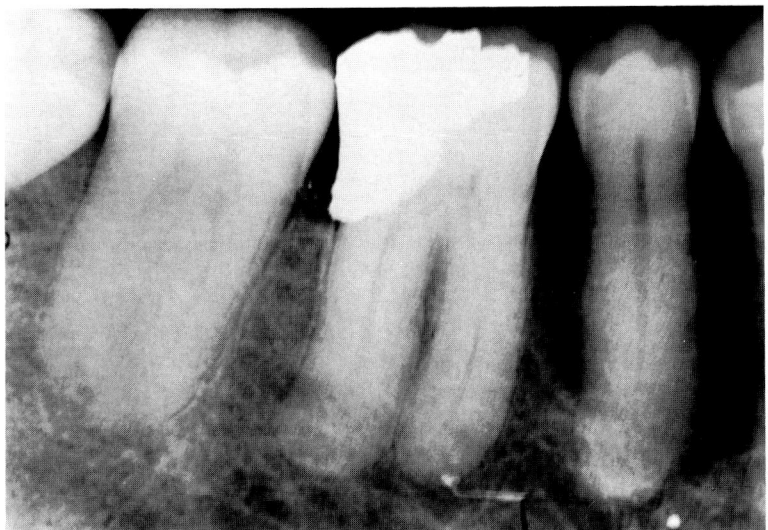

Figure 15–4. Hypercementosis of Paget's disease.

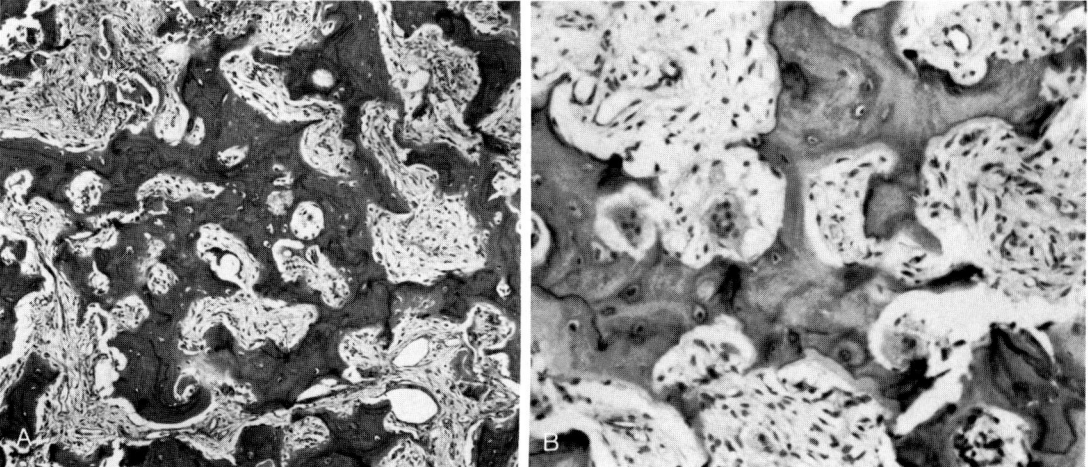

Figure 15–5. *A* and *B*, Paget's disease exhibiting intense osteoblastic and osteoclastic activity. Note reversal lines.

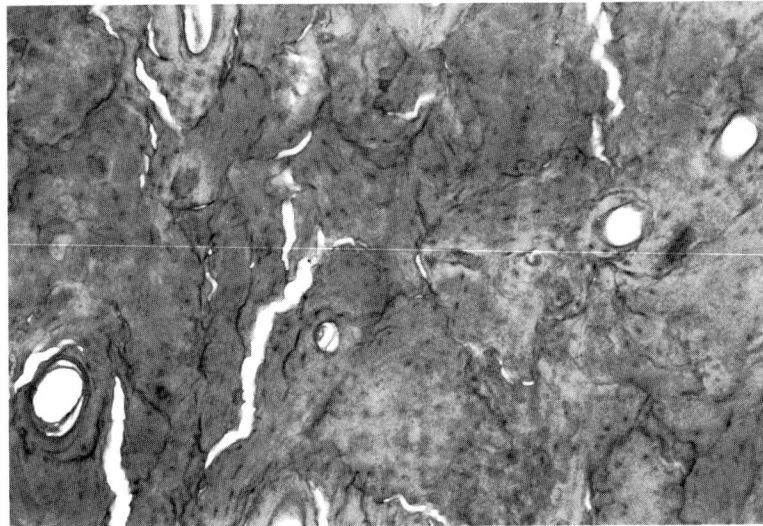

Figure 15–6. Late stage of Paget's disease showing dense sclerotic bone.

sometimes markedly elevated alkaline phosphatase. The intense osteoblastic activity in this metabolically active bone is believed to be responsible for the elevated alkaline phosphatase. The amount of bone resorption may be correlated to increases in urinary calcium and hydroxyproline levels. The differential diagnosis in Paget's disease may include acromegaly, florid osseous dysplasia, sclerosing osteomyelitis, osteosarcoma, and possibly the adult or acquired form of osteopetrosis.

Treatment. Therapy is essentially symptomatic, with analgesics utilized for pain control. Recently, use of calcitonin or bisphosphonate as parathormone antagonists has been effective. Both suppress bone resorption and deposition as reflected in reduction in the biochemical indexes, including alkaline phosphatase and urinary hydroxyproline levels.

Unfortunately, Paget's disease is a slowly progressive disorder. It is seldom fatal. Complications relate to deformity, weakened bones, neurologic damage, and pathologic fracture. In a small percentage of cases, malignant transformation into osteosarcoma is well documented. Depending upon the series reported, this has ranged from 1 to 15%.

Hyperparathyroidism

Primary hyperparathyroidism is characterized by hypersecretion of parathyroid hormone from hyperplastic parathyroid glands, a parathyroid adenoma, or less commonly, an adenocarcinoma. In the hyperplastic state, there is usually an increase in the total amount of parathyroid tissue represented by an increase in both size and number of cells. The most consistent abnormal findings are elevated parathormone levels and hypercalcemia, with the hypersecreting parathyroid glands being less sensitive to the suppressive or negative feedback effects of increased extracellular or serum calcium levels.

The finding of elevated or normal serum parathyroid hormone levels in the presence of elevated serum calcium confirms the diagnosis of hyperparathyroidism. The primary form is defined as occurring from intrinsic disease within the gland, and the secondary form is defined as a compensatory response to hypocalcemia, as may be seen in renal failure.

Etiology. In most instances, the etiology of primary hyperparathyroidism is unknown. It has been suggested that prior irradiation may be a possible cause. Because the disease is more common in postmenopausal women, the possibility that diminished levels of estrogen may be partially responsible for this disease has also been suggested. In a small percentage of cases, the disease may be hereditary, occurring in patients with one of the multiple endocrine neoplasia syndromes.

Clinical Features. The disease spectrum of primary hyperparathyroidism ranges from asymptomatic cases, which are diagnosed by routine serum calcium determinations, to severe cases manifesting as lethargy and occasionally coma. Early symptoms include fatigue, weakness, nausea, anorexia, polyuria, thirst, depression, and constipation. Frequently, bone pain and headaches are present.

There are several clinical features associated with the primary form of this disease, classically described as "stones, bones, groans, and moans." Lesions of the kidneys, skeletal system, gastrointestinal tract, and nervous system are responsible for this syndrome complex. The renal component includes the presence of renal calculi or, more rarely, nephrocalcinosis.

Severe osseous changes (called, in the past, osteitis fibrosa cystica) result from significant bone demineralization, with fibrous replacement producing radiographic changes that appear cyst-like. The latter are of chief importance as far as the maxilla and especially the mandible are concerned. In long bones, fractures may occur, and in the vertebrae, collapse may be seen (Fig. 15–7).

Gastrointestinal manifestations include peptic ulcer, secondary to the increase in gastric acid, pepsin, and serum gastrin levels. Rarely, pancreatitis may develop, secondary to obstruction of the smaller pancreatic ducts by calcium deposits.

Finally, the neurologic manifestations may become evident when serum calcium levels are very high, exceeding 16 to 17 mg per dl. In such instances, coma or parathyroid crisis may supervene. Loss of memory and depression are common, and rarely, true psychosis may occur. Some of the neurologic findings may be attributed to ectopic calcium deposits in the brain. Metastatic calcifications of the oral mucosa may rarely be seen in hyperparathyroidism. This is to be distinguished from dystrophic calcification, which occurs at sites of previous tissue injury in the presence of normal levels of serum calcium and phosphorus.

The chief oral finding is the appearance of well-defined cystic radiolucencies of the jaw, which may be monolocular or multilocular (Fig. 15–8). Less obvious radiographic pathology may include an osteoporotic appearance of the mandible and maxilla, reflecting a more generalized condition. Loosening of the teeth may also occur as well as corresponding obfuscation of trabecular detail and overall cortical thinning. Partial loss of lamina dura is seen in a minority of patients with hyperparathyroidism (Fig. 15–9).

Histopathology. The bone lesions of hyperparathyroidism, although not specific, are important in establishing the diagnosis. The bony trabeculae exhibit osteoclastic resorption as well as formation of osteoid trabeculae by large numbers of osteoblasts (Fig. 15–10). In these areas, large numbers of capillaries and endothelium-lined spaces are seen, with multinucleated giant cells scattered within a delicate fibrocellular stroma. Accumulations of hemosiderin and extravasated red blood cells also are present. The lesions are microscopically identical to central giant cell granulomas.

Treatment. Management of primary hyperparathyroidism is aimed at eliminating the parathyroid pathology. Surgery is the treatment of choice in most instances, since it offers the best opportunity for long-term cure. Individuals with hypercalcemia greater than 11 mg per dl or those with signs or symptoms are candidates for surgery. It has been observed that long-term hypercalcemia can be associated with increased morbidity, usually as a result of worsening renal function.

Treatment of secondary hyperparathyroidism due to increased parathyroid function as a result of chronic renal failure is aimed at management of kidney disease. The dental and

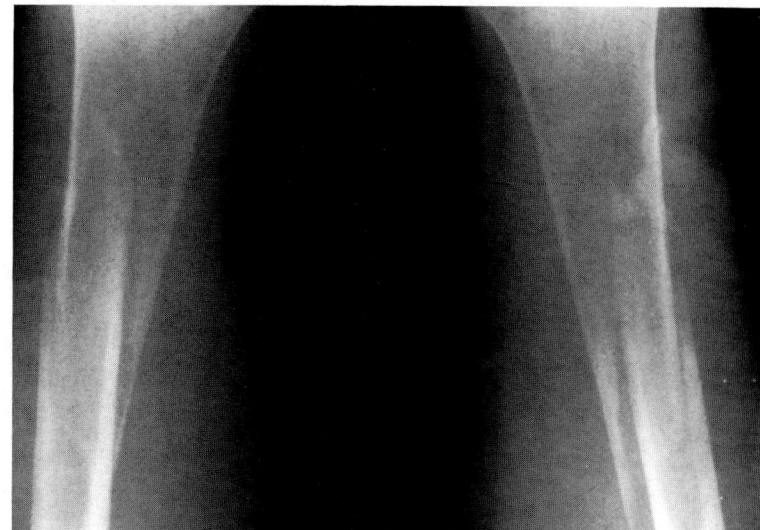

Figure 15–7. Bilateral fractures in primary hyperparathyroidism.

432   METABOLIC AND GENETIC JAW DISEASES

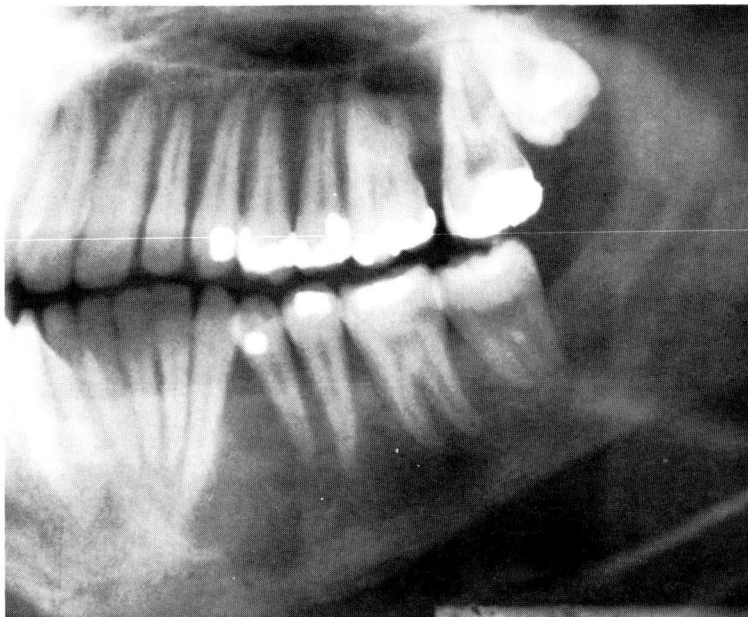

Figure 15–8. Radiolucencies of hyperparathyroidism.

oral considerations in this form of hyperparathyroidism may be identical to those in the primary form of the disease.

Hyperthyroidism

Hyperfunction of the thyroid gland, or hyperthyroidism, is characterized by excessive amounts of thyroid hormones T_3 (triiodothyronine) and T_4 (thyroxine) or by increased levels of thyroid-stimulating hormones (TSH). In adults, hyperthyroidism occurs with an incidence of 3 cases per 10,000 per year, with a distinct female preponderance of approximately 5 to 1. This disease is rare in children, with most cases in the pediatric age group occurring between 10 and 14 years.

The most common disorder leading to clinical hyperthyroidism is Graves' disease. The exact etiology of this particular process is obscure but appears to be related to production of abnormal thyroid stimulator (long-acting thyroid stimulator, LATS), which differs chemically and functionally from TSH. LATS acts similar to TSH but over a longer period

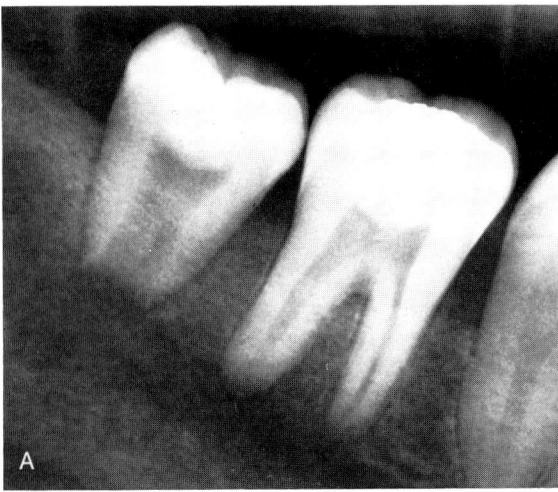
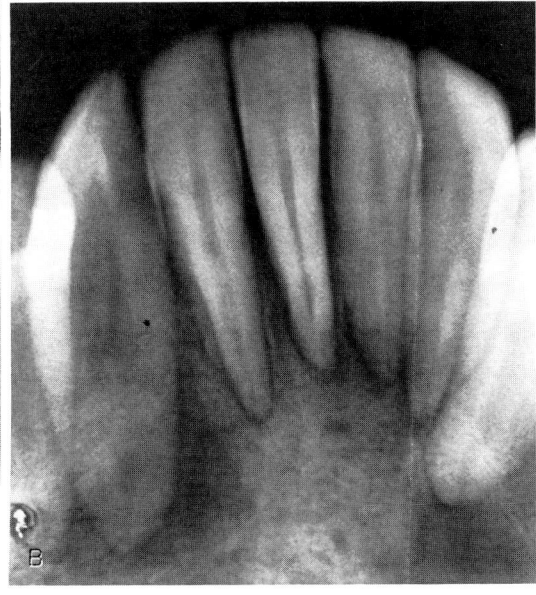

Figure 15–9. *A* and *B*, Hyperparathyroidism showing radiolucencies and loss of lamina dura.

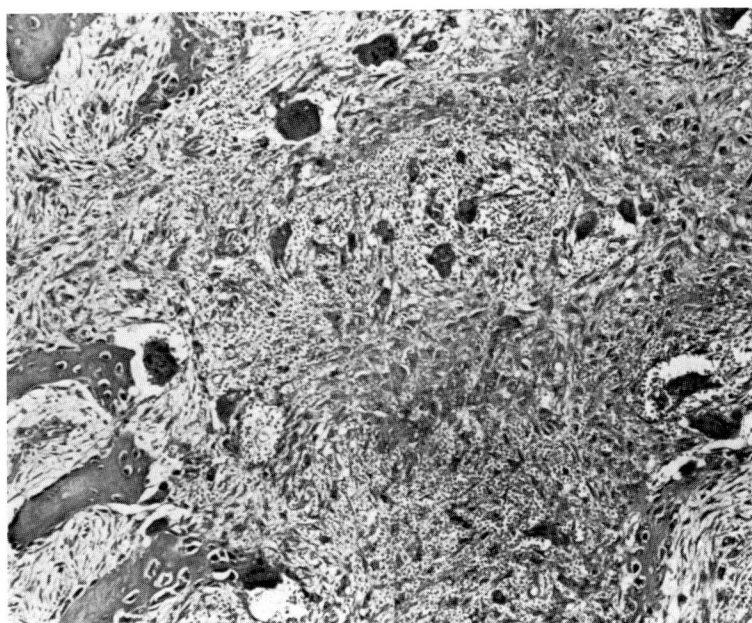

Figure 15-10. Hyperparathyroidism showing bone replacement by fibrous tissue and giant cells.

of time. The LATS substance is an IgG produced by B lymphocytes, which is capable of inducing thyroid hyperplasia and increasing iodine uptake by the thyroid, free of any pituitary gland influence.

Hyperhidrosis is a common finding. Patients complain of altered complexion, which is often ruddy. Thinning and brittle hair is a frequent finding. Palmar erythema is also common. Ocular changes include upper lid retraction and so-called lid lag on normal blinking. The bright-eyed stare that often results from upper lid retraction may be further accentuated by exophthalmos.

Cardiac manifestations are among the earliest and most consistent features of this disease. The increased metabolic activity places greater demand on the cardiovascular system; accordingly, increases in stroke volume, pulse rate, and cardiac output are usually observed.

Although the oral manifestations of this condition are not characteristic, they are consistent. In children, premature or accelerated exfoliation of deciduous teeth and concomitant rapid eruption of permanent teeth are often noted. In adults osteoporosis of the mandible and maxilla may be found. On occasion, patients may complain of burning of the tongue as well as other non-specific symptoms. Of interest is a reported threefold increase in the incidence of dental erosion in comparison with euthyroid control subjects.

Treatment consists of thyroid-suppressive drug therapy or radioactive iodine administration, which essentially inactivates the hyperfunctional thyroid tissue. Thyroid-suppressive drugs include thiocarbamides such as propylthiouracil and methimazole. These drugs inhibit iodine oxidation and iodination of tyrosyl residues, two steps in the synthesis of thyroid hormones. Surgical therapy remains an option, although the potential for parathyroid gland removal and subsequent hypoparathyroidism is a risk.

Of clinical importance is the need to reduce stress to minimize the risk of precipitating a thyroid crisis in patients with this disease. Use of certain drugs such as epinephrine and atropine is contraindicated because they may precipitate a thyroid storm.

Hypophosphatasia

Hypophosphatasia indicates a deficiency of alkaline phosphatase. This hereditary disorder is transmitted in an autosomal recessive manner. Of chief importance is that this unusual genetic metabolic disease is one of the main causes of premature loss of the primary dentition. (Other conditions in which premature tooth exfoliation may be seen include cyclic neutropenia, idiopathic histiocytosis, juvenile periodontitis, acrodynia, rickets, and Papillon-Lefèvre syndrome.)

The chief clinical features and characteristics of hypophosphatasia include enlarged pulp chambers of the primary teeth, alveolar bone loss with a predisposition for the anterior portion of the mandible and maxilla, and hypoplasia or true aplasia of cementum over the root surface. Root formation may be deficient, especially toward the apex. The crowns of the involved teeth demonstrate rickets-like changes, chiefly characterized by hypoplastic enamel defects.

In addition to the oral manifestations, long bones show inadequate levels of mineralization. Serum chemistry studies indicate a reduction in alkaline phosphatase levels, with concomitant urinary findings of detectable phosphoethanolamine. Tissue levels of alkaline phosphatase are likewise decreased in this disorder.

Four clinical types of hypophosphatasia have been recognized. The congenital type demonstrates at least a 75% rate of neonatal mortality. The early infantile type appears within the first 6 months of life, with an associated mortality rate of 50%. Renal calcinosis may be seen with this disease as well as significant risk of cranial synostosis, delayed motor development, and premature loss of teeth. The late infantile or childhood type begins between 6 and 24 months of age. Skeletal findings tend to be less pronounced, but abnormalities of long bone structures, in particular at the metaphysis, may be seen along with rickets-type changes at the costochondral junctions. Of importance in this form of the disease is premature loss of the anterior primary teeth, often the first sign of the illness. Finally, the adult type, although distinctly uncommon, is characterized by bone pain, pathologic fractures, and a childhood history of rickets.

No successful treatment is known, apart from controlling the hypercalcemia resulting from the hypophosphatasia. Large doses of vitamin D have occasionally produced partial improvement, although hypercalcemia and soft tissue calcinosis may result from such an approach. Genetic counseling of the family as well as early diagnosis is of great value.

Infantile Cortical Hyperostosis

Infantile cortical hyperostosis, or Caffey's disease, is a self-limited, short-lived process characterized by cortical thickening of various bones. In addition to the osseous changes, there is usually swelling of the overlying soft tissues.

There are no gender, racial, or geographic predilections. The characteristic age of onset is usually by the seventh month of life, with the average age of onset being 9 weeks.

Many feel that genetic factors are involved in the origin of this disease process. An autosomal dominant mode of inheritance with incomplete penetrance and variable expressivity has been cited. Sporadic cases also occur, suggesting possibilities that include an infectious agent, immunologic disorder, nutritional aberrations, allergy, trauma, hormonal disturbances, and disorders of collagen metabolism.

Clinically, the involvement of the mandible, maxilla, or other bones is characterized by firm, tender swelling with rather deep-seated edema. Pain, fever, and hyperirritability may precede or develop concurrently with the swelling. From 75 to 90% of cases demonstrate mandibular involvement, typically over the angle and ascending ramus. Sporadic cases of infantile cortical hyperostosis almost always show mandibular involvement, with familial cases demonstrating such involvement approximately 60% of the time.

Radiographically, an expansile hyperostotic process is visible over the cortical surface, with rounding or blunting of the mandibular coronoid process. Initially, the hyperostotic element is separated from the underlying bone by a thin radiolucent line.

Diagnosis may be facilitated by the use of technetium (^{99m}Tc) scans, which are often positive before routine radiographic detection is made. Laboratory findings that are also helpful in establishing the diagnosis include an elevated erythrocyte sedimentation rate, increased phosphatase levels, anemia, leukocytosis, and occasionally, thrombocytopenia or thrombocytosis.

Infantile cortical hyperostosis is usually a self-limiting process, with treatment generally directed at supportive care. Systemic corticosteroids and, more recently, non-steroidal anti-inflammatory drugs have been utilized with some success. There is a tendency for this disease to follow an uneven though predictable course, with relapses and remissions possible. The resolution phase ranges from 6 weeks to 23 months, with the average time being 9 months. Radiographic and histologic resolution may take up to several years, with a generally excellent prognosis in spite of the possibility of recurrences and occasional residual effects, such as severe malocclusion and mandibular asymmetry.

Phantom Bone Disease

Phantom bone disease, also known as massive osteolysis, is an unusual process characterized by slow, progressive, localized destruction of bone. It is a non-neoplastic condition characterized by a proliferative vascular and connective tissue response. This is a rare entity, with approximately 60 cases reported since its initial description in 1838. The process has been described in virtually every bone in the body, with 15 cases reported in the maxillofacial region.

No ethnic or gender predilection has been noted. There appears to be no genetic basis for transmission. Various studies, including metabolic, endocrine, and neurologic tests, have proved not to be helpful in determining the etiology of phantom bone disease.

In most patients, the disease develops prior to the fourth decade of life, although it has been described in patients ranging from 18 months to 72 years of age. The onset of the disease is insidious, with pain usually not a feature unless there is concomitant pathologic fracture of the involved bone. Although most cases involve a single bone, the disease may also be polyostotic, affecting usually contiguous bones. This disease is progressive but variable—over time the bone may completely disappear, or it may spontaneously stabilize. Significant regeneration has not been reported.

The earliest radiographic evidence of the disease has been reported as one or more intermedullary subcortical radiolucencies of variable size, usually with indistinct margins and thin radiopaque borders. In time, these foci enlarge and coalesce and eventually involve the cortex (Fig. 15–11). A characteristic tapering ultimately occurs when long bones are affected.

Laboratory studies fail to detect biochemical abnormalities. Microscopically, replacement of bone by connective tissue with many dilated capillaries and anastomosing vascular channels is noted (Fig. 15–12). As the disease progresses, dissolution of both medullary and cortical bony elements is seen, with a fibrotic band remaining—thought to represent residual periosteum.

There is no effective treatment for phantom bone disease. Limited success has been seen with bone grafts and implants.

Acromegaly

Acromegaly is an uncommon condition with a prevalence of approximately 40 cases per million population and an incidence of 3 cases per million per year. This disease is characterized by bony and soft tissue overgrowth and metabolic disturbances secondary to chronic hypersecretion of growth hormone subsequent to the closure of the epiphyseal plates.

Etiology. The etiology in over 90% of cases is hypersecretion of growth hormone from a benign pituitary adenoma or so-called somatotropinoma. Occasionally, the pituitary tumor may produce prolactin along with growth hormone or other hormones, including TSH or adrenal corticotropic hormone (ACTH). Such adenomas, although most common in the pituitary gland itself, may also arise in ectopic

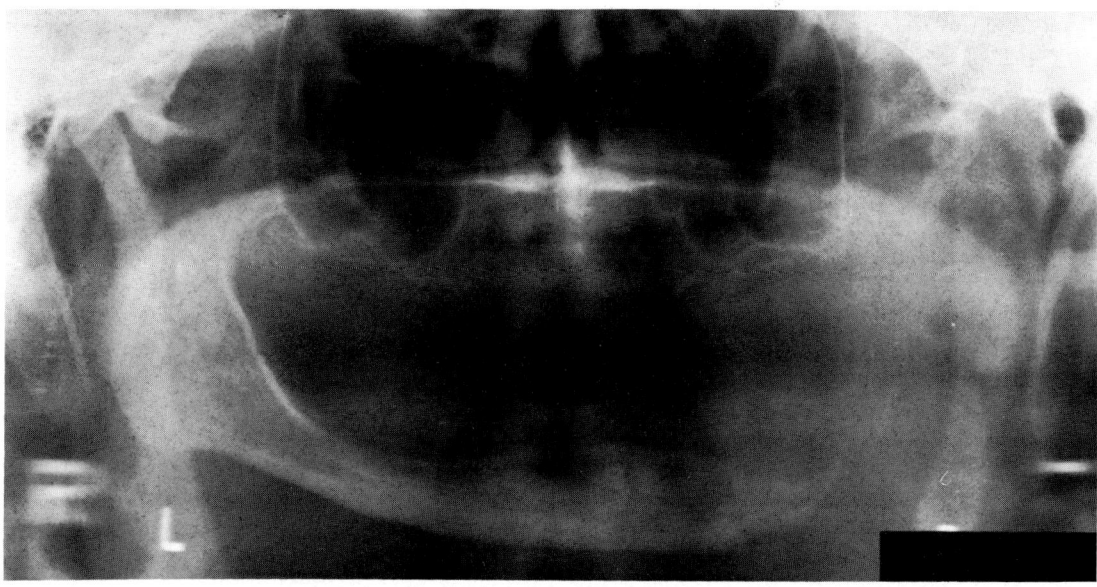

Figure 15–11. Phantom bone disease, right mandible. (Courtesy of Dr. D. Frederickson.)

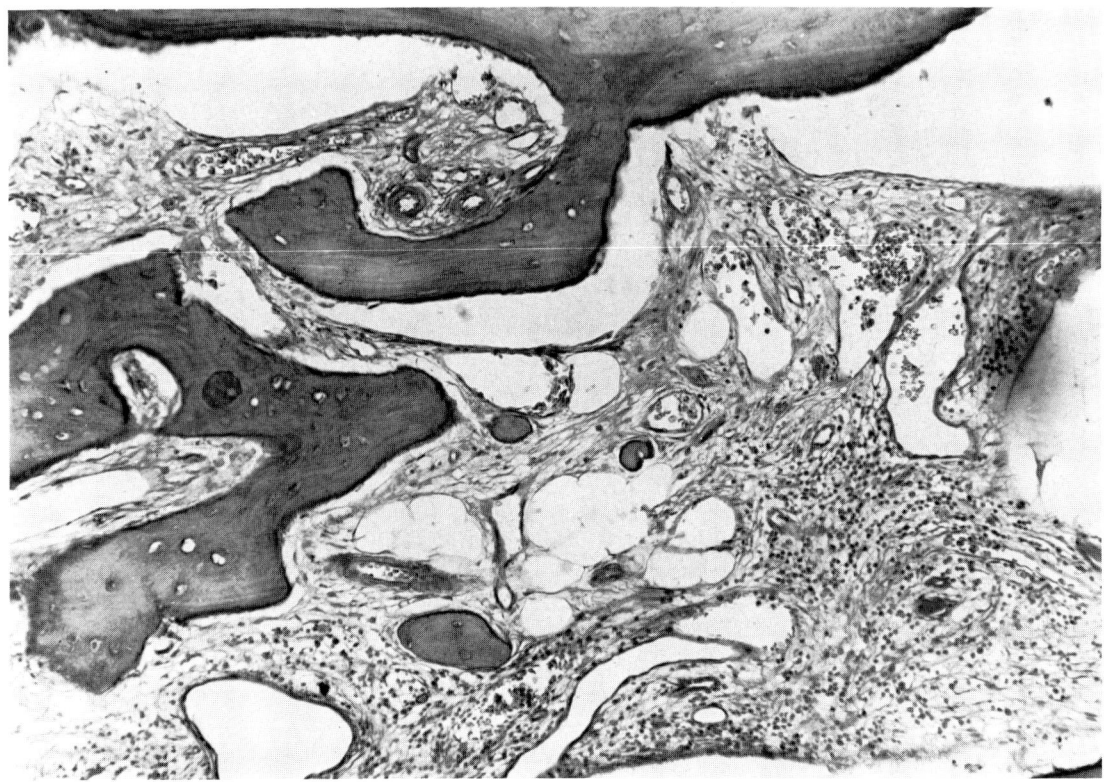

Figure 15–12. Phantom bone disease showing fibrous replacement of bone.

locations along the migration path of Rathke's pouch. Rarely, a condition that is indistinguishable clinically from acromegaly may be found in individuals with normal basal and dynamic growth hormone levels with no detectable pituitary or other secreting type of lesion. Such patients possess a unique growth-promoting factor, with the diagnosis classified as acromegaloidism. In general, growth hormone levels correlate proportionally to the size of the adenoma as well as the overall severity of the disease.

Clinical Features. Acromegaly presents most frequently in the fourth decade, with an even gender distribution and no racial or geographic predominance. This disorder is of insidious onset, with diagnosis often delayed for many years.

Individuals present with hyperhidrosis; muscle weakness; paresthesia, especially carpal tunnel syndrome; dysmenorrhea; and decreased libido. In the facial bones and the jawbones, new periosteal bone formation may be seen as well as cartilaginous hyperplasia and ossification. The resultant orofacial changes include frontal bossing, nasal bone hypertrophy, and relative mandibular prognathism or prominence. Enlargement of the paranasal sinuses as well as secondary laryngeal hypertrophy produces a rather deep, resonant voice, which is typical of acromegaly. Overall coarsening of facial features is noted, secondary to connective tissue hyperplasia (Fig. 15–13). Microadenomas of the pituitary may also produce secondary hypothyroidism, hypogonadism, and adrenal insufficiency as well as headache, visual disturbances, and cranial neuropathies.

Oral manifestations include enlargement of the mandible and maxilla, with secondary separation of teeth due to alveolar overgrowth. Condylar hyperplasia with concomitant bone formation at the anterior portion of the mandible and a distinct increase in the bony angle produces a rather typical dental malocclusion and prognathism. Complete posterior crossbite is a common finding in such a circumstance. Thickened oral mucosa, increased salivary gland tissue, and macroglossia as well as prominent lips will also be noted in most instances. It has been reported that, with the concomitant changes in mandibular structure, myofascial pain dysfunction syndrome and speech abnormalities may result. The specific diagnostic tests include demonstration of growth hormone levels that are non-suppressible by glu-

METABOLIC AND GENETIC JAW DISEASES 437

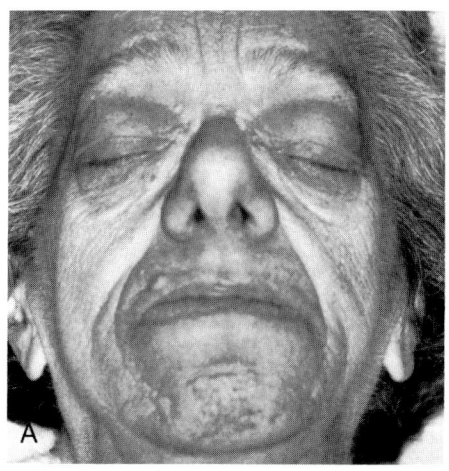 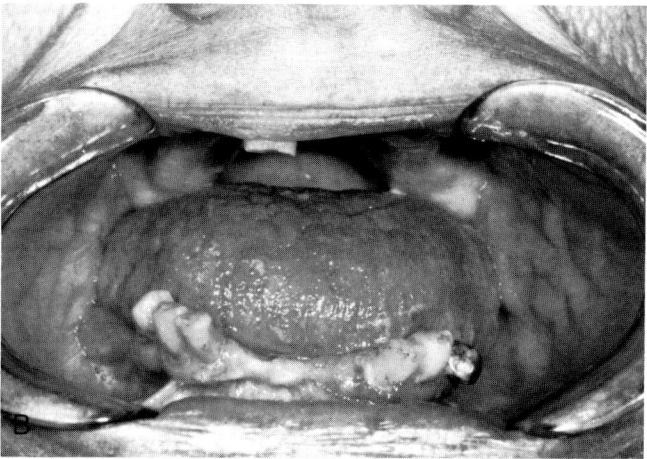

Figure 15–13. *A* and *B*, Acromegaly. Note tipping of teeth due to macroglossia *(B)*.

cose loading. Computed tomography of the sella turcica should be performed to supplement the biochemical criteria. Radioimmunoassay studies of somatomedin C may also be used as a routine screening test as well as for establishing correlation between disease activity and other tests.

Treatment. Treatment relates to a normalization of growth hormone levels, with concomitant preservation of normal pituitary function. The most frequently employed treatment is transsphenoidal surgery; a rapid therapeutic response is usually noted. Conventional radiotherapy to this area over a 4- to 6-week period carries a 70% rate of normalization of pituitary function, although hypopituitarism may be an unfavorable sequela. Current medical therapy utilizes bromocriptine, a dopamine agonist, as an adjunctive agent but not as a primary modality.

Successful management may be reflected in reversal of soft tissue abnormalities, although many of the facial deformities may persist. In such instances, corrective oral and maxillofacial surgery may be indicated, including mandibular osteotomy and partial glossectomy.

GENETIC ABNORMALITIES

Cherubism

Cherubism is a benign hereditary condition of the maxilla and mandible, usually found in children by 5 years of age. The term "cherubism" was chosen to describe three siblings presenting with marked fullness of the jaws and cheeks and upwardly gazing eyes. A characteristically round and symmetrically full face was suggestive of a cherub (Fig. 15–14).

Etiology and Pathogenesis. Cherubism usually occurs as an autosomal dominant disorder, with 100% penetrance in males and 50 to 75% penetrance in females, with a 2 to 1 male predominance. Sporadic cases have also been reported.

Mesenchymal alteration during the development of the jaw bones as a result of reduced

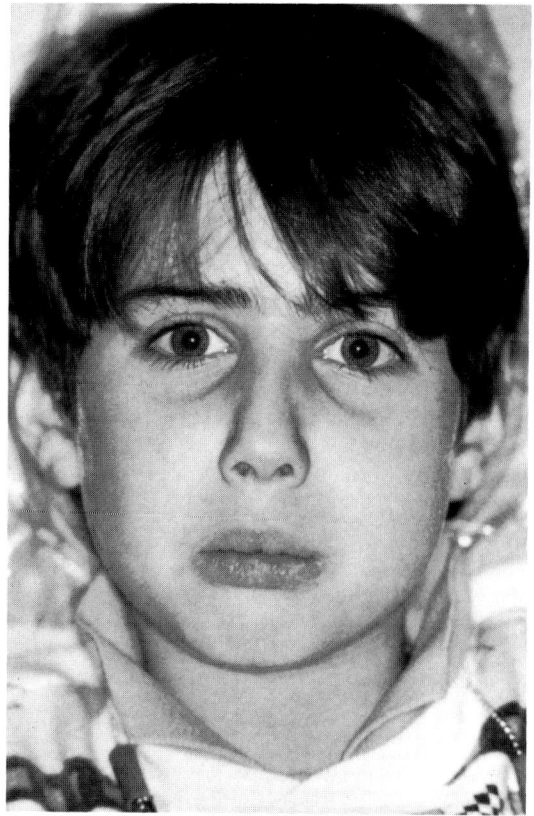

Figure 15–14. This patient exhibits the bilateral symmetric facial expansion often seen in cherubism.

oxygenation secondary to perivascular fibrosis has been suggested as a possible cause. It is usually a self-limiting disease, with rapid progression during childhood, often beginning by 2 years of age, through puberty. At this time, the bony lesions begin to regress, often to the degree that only a minor residual deformity may be present by age 30.

Clinical Features. The mandibular angle, ascending ramus, retromolar region, and posterior maxilla are most often affected. The coronoid process can also be involved, but the condyles are always spared. The vast majority of cases occur only in the mandible. The bony expansion is most frequently bilateral, although unilateral involvement has been reported.

Typically, patients present with a painless symmetric enlargement of the posterior region of the mandible, with expansion of the alveolar process and ascending ramus. The clinical appearance may vary from a barely discernible posterior swelling of a single jaw to marked anterior and posterior expansion of both jaws, resulting in masticatory, speech, and swallowing difficulties. Intraorally, a hard, non-tender swelling can be palpated in the affected area.

With maxillary disease, involvement of the orbital floor and anterior wall of the antrum occurs. Superior pressure on the orbit results in an increasing prominence of sclera and the appearance of upturned eyes. The palatal vault may be reduced or obliterated. Maxillary involvement usually results in the greatest deformity. All four quadrants of the jaws may be simultaneously involved. Premature exfoliation of the primary dentition may occur as early as 3 years of age. Displacement of developing tooth follicles results in poor development of selective permanent teeth and ectopic eruption. Permanent teeth may be missing or malformed, with the mandibular second and third molars most often affected. Significant malocclusions can be anticipated even with unifocal involvement.

Reactive regional lymphadenopathy, particularly of submandibular lymph nodes, usually subsides after 5 years of age. Intelligence is unaffected. Serum calcium and phosphorus levels are within normal limits, but alkaline phosphatase levels may be elevated.

Radiographic surveys may provide the only signs of disease. The radiographic lesions characteristically appear as multiple, well-defined, multilocular radiolucencies of the jaws (Fig. 15–15). The borders are distinct and divided by bony trabeculae. In the mandible, there is expansion and thinning of the cortical plate,

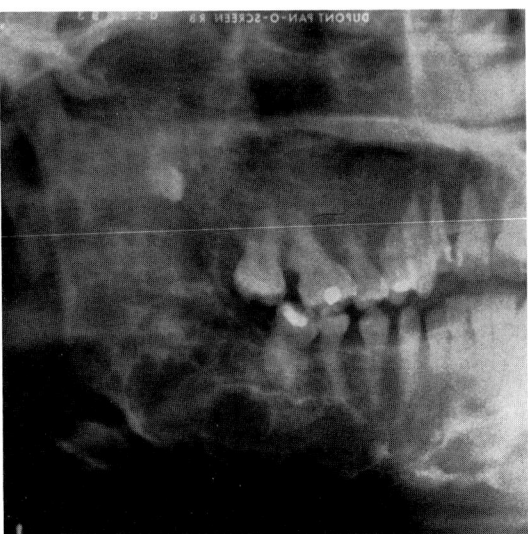

Figure 15–15. Well-defined multilocular radiolucencies of the mandible and maxilla characteristic of cherubism.

with occasional perforation; there may be displacement of the inferior alveolar canal. An occlusal radiograph of the maxilla may give a soap bubble–like picture with maxillary antrum obliteration. Unerupted teeth are often displaced and appear to be floating in the cyst-like spaces.

Histopathology. Histologically, the lesions bear a close resemblance to those seen in central giant cell granulomas (Fig. 15–16). There is a highly vascularized fibrous stroma, often arranged in a whorled pattern. Numerous fibroblasts and multinucleated giant cells with prominent nuclei and nucleoli are noted. In mature lesions, there are a large amount of fibrous tissue and fewer giant cells. A distinctive feature is eosinophilic perivascular cuffing of collagen surrounding small capillaries throughout the lesion. Although this is not always present, perivascular collagen cuffing is regarded as pathognomonic for cherubism.

Differential Diagnosis. Clinical differential diagnosis of bilateral jaw swelling should include hyperparathyroidism, infantile cortical hyperostosis, and multiple odontogenic keratocysts. Unilateral swelling in children requires inclusion of fibrous dysplasia, central giant cell granuloma, histiocytosis, and odontogenic tumors.

Treatment and Prognosis. The prognosis is relatively good, particularly if the disease is limited to only one jaw—especially the mandible. The disease is usually self-limiting and regressive. Lesions of the maxilla act in a more aggressive manner and occasionally pose serious anatomic considerations. Although it is

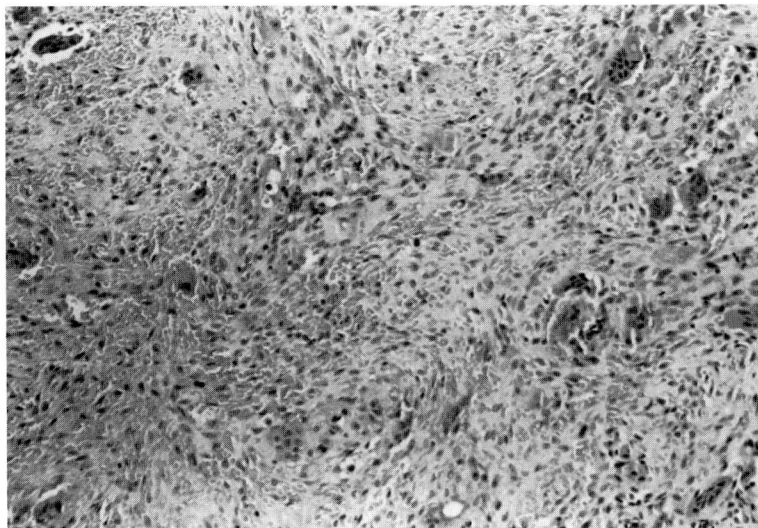

Figure 15–16. Cherubism. Note giant cells in a fibrous stroma.

generally accepted that spontaneous regression begins at puberty, with relatively good resolution by age 30, no long-term follow-up of spontaneous resolution has been documented. Surgical intervention must be based on the need to improve function, prevent debilitation, and satisfy aesthetic considerations. If necessary, conservative curettage of the lesion with bone recontouring may be done.

Osteopetrosis

Osteopetrosis is an uncommon hereditary bone condition characterized by a generalized symmetric increase in skeletal density and abnormalities of bone resorption remodeling. In 1904, the first case of generalized sclerosis of the skeleton was reported by Albers-Schönberg.

Osteopetrosis is generally divided into two main types. The infantile (malignant, congenital) type is the most severe form of the disease; it is characterized by skeletal, hematologic, and neurologic abnormalities. The adult (benign, tarda) form, which is usually diagnosed in the third or fourth decade of life, is limited predominantly to skeletal anomalies; it carries a more favorable prognosis. A mild intermediate form also exists and appears to be more common than previously recognized.

Etiology and Pathogenesis. The adult form is inherited as an autosomal dominant trait; the infantile variety, with its fulminating course, is inherited as an autosomal recessive trait. The recently recognized intermediate form, with its mild and variable clinical presentation, is also inherited as an autosomal recessive trait. There is no reported gender or racial predilection.

The characteristic feature of osteopetrosis is an absence of physiologic bone resorption owing to reduced osteoclastic activity. Animal studies have shown that osteoclasts do not respond appropriately to the presence of parathyroid hormone or to physiologic stimuli that normally promote bone resorption. The osteoclasts fail to undergo membrane elaboration to form the so-called ruffled border and allow release of lysosomal enzymes at the bone cell interface. The lack of bone resorption manifests itself in skeletal disturbances, including bone cavity occlusion, decreased hematopoietic activity, and growth retardation. Cranial nerve compression may result in blindness, deafness, anosmia, ageusia, and sometimes facial paralysis. Normal cortical and cancellous bone is replaced by a dense, poorly structured bone that is fragile and has a propensity for pathologic fracture.

Delayed dental eruption is due to bony ankylosis, absence of alveolar bone resorption, and formation of pseudo-odontomas during apicogenesis. Premature exfoliation may be due to a defect in the periodontal ligament.

Clinical Features. Infantile osteopetrosis is the most severe form of the disease. It is usually present at birth and is diagnosed within the first few months of life (Fig. 15–17). Patients with this condition rarely survive adolescence, and death is usually the result of infection or anemia. Hematologic manifestations result from a decrease in the marrow compartment causing anemia, thrombocytopenia, and pancytopenia. Hepatosplenomegaly, secon-

440 METABOLIC AND GENETIC JAW DISEASES

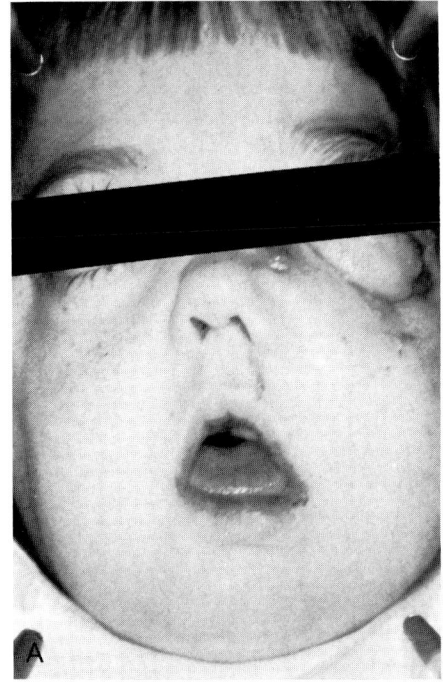
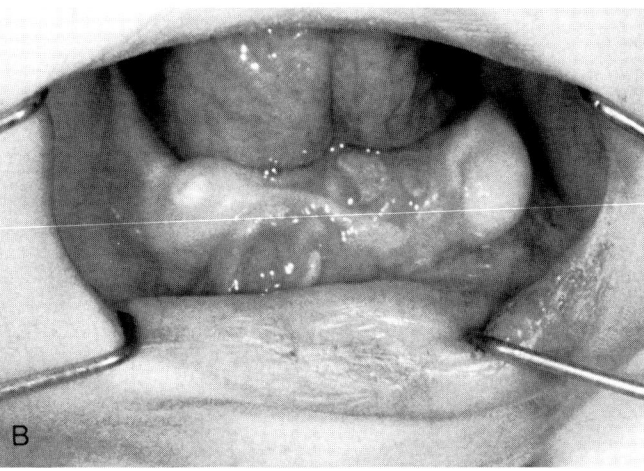

Figure 15–17. *A,* A child with osteopetrosis exhibiting multiple draining sinuses in the left infraorbital region. *B,* Osteopetrosis showing malformed teeth with enamel hypoplasia and dental caries.

dary to compensatory extramedullary hematopoiesis, is often present.

The clinically benign adult form develops later in life and may not be diagnosed until the third or fourth decade. Bone involvement is similar to that seen in the malignant recessive type. Optic and facial nerve impairment is frequently present owing to narrowing of cranial foramina and resultant pressure on the nerves. Often the first sign of the disease is pathologic fracture.

Dental findings include delayed eruption, congenitally absent teeth, unerupted and malformed teeth, and enamel hypoplasia. Decreased alveolar bone production, defective and abnormally thickened periodontal ligament, and marked mandibular prognathism have been reported. An elevated caries index may be secondary to enamel hypoplasia. This has serious implications owing to the propensity for development of osteomyelitis resulting from inadequate host response because of the diminished vascular component of osteopetrotic bone. Osteomyelitis is a serious complication of the disease; it occurs most frequently in the mandible and occasionally in the maxilla, scapula, and extremities.

Radiographic findings are characteristic of this disease. The classic "bone within bone" radiographic presentation is due to a defect in metaphyseal bone remodeling resulting in greatly thickened cortices and medullary space obliteration. Generally the skeletal density is greatly increased owing to a uniform diffuse sclerosing of all bones (Fig. 15–18). The mandible is less frequently involved than are other bones. Loss of the distinct interface between the cortex and medulla appears along with clubbing of the long bones with transverse peripheral banding.

Histopathology. Osteopetrosis is histologically characterized by normal production of bone with absence of physiologic bone resorption (Fig. 15–19). There is disruption in the pattern of endochondral bone formation with a decrease in osteoclastic function and a compensatory increase in numbers of osteoclasts. This results in failure to develop normal lamellar structure in the bone and an absence of definable marrow cavities. Biopsies of endochondral bone exhibit a core of calcified cartilage surrounded by bone matrix.

Endosteal bone has been described as exhibiting three distinct patterns: a pattern with a tortuous arrangement of lamellar trabeculae, an amorphous pattern, and an osteophilic pattern. An abundance of multinucleated osteoclasts and aggregated bony lacunae void of cellular components is often noted.

Unerupted teeth demonstrate areas of ankylosis at the cementum-bone interface in a jigsaw-puzzle pattern. There is disruption in the continuity of the periodontal membrane in ankylosed teeth. The periodontal ligament is often composed of fibrous connective tissue, running parallel to the two surfaces, and an

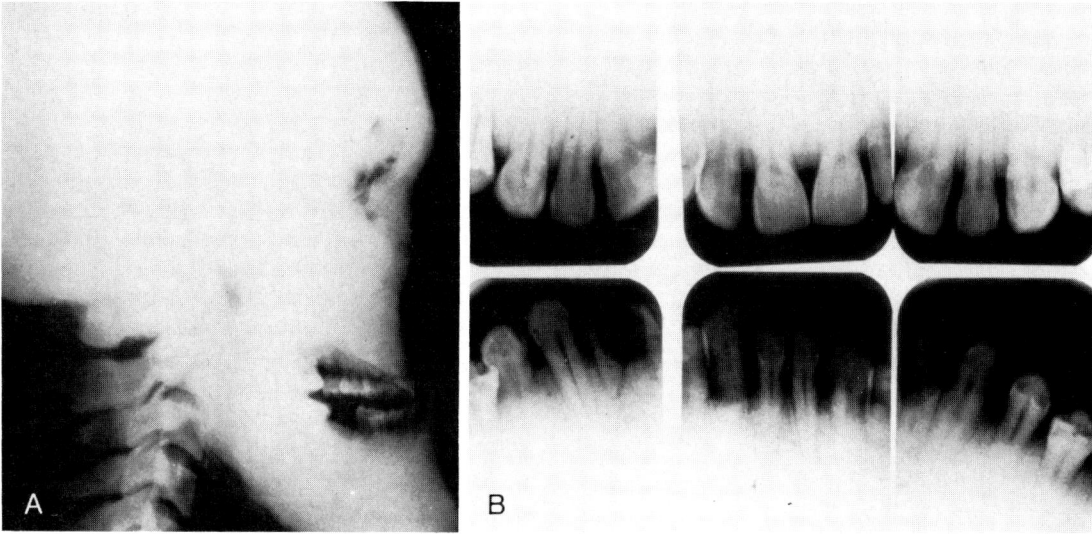

Figure 15–18. *A* and *B*, Radiographs of late stage of osteopetrosis.

associated inflammatory infiltrate. In regions where osteomyelitis develops, marrow spaces appear fibrotic and contain chronic inflammatory cells.

Treatment and Prognosis. The prognosis for infantile osteopetrosis is poor, with patients rarely surviving adolescence. Death results from secondary infection or anemia. The adult variety is more variable and insidious. Bone involvement is similar to the infantile recessive type but is usually less severe. Often, the diagnosis is not made until a pathologic fracture occurs.

Management should be directed at recognition and treatment of complications, with frequent testing of visual fields and sight acuity and periodic radiographic examination of the optic foramina. Transfusion may be required for anemia, and splenectomy may be useful in some patients. Therapy is often directed at controlling the hematologic component of the disorder with systemic steroids.

Owing to the high risk of developing osteomyelitis, initiation of dental preventive regimens, similar to those for patients at risk for osteoradionecrosis, should be considered. This includes the implementation of frequent dental evaluations, topical and systemic fluorides, and fastidious home care programs.

Osteogenesis Imperfecta

Osteogenesis imperfecta represents a genetically heterogeneous group of heritable defects of connective tissue. Classically, the syndrome

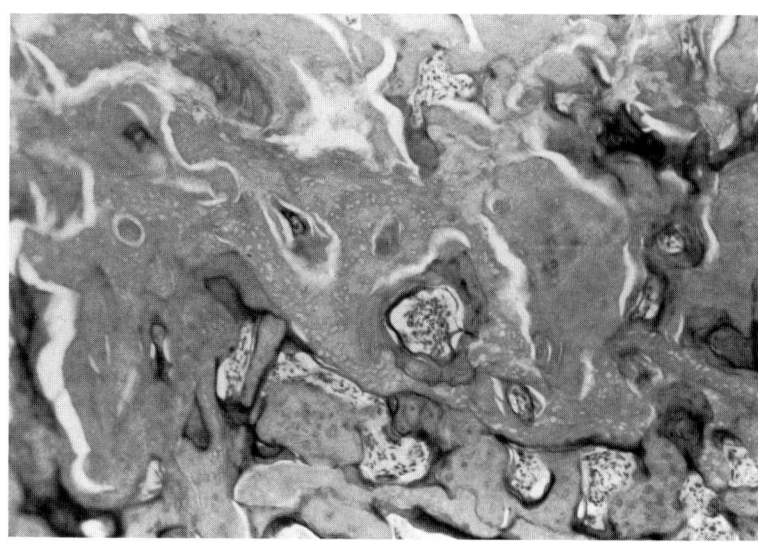

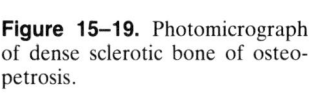

Figure 15–19. Photomicrograph of dense sclerotic bone of osteopetrosis.

is characterized by fragile bones, blue sclera, ligamentous laxity, hearing loss, or dentinogenesis imperfecta, or a combination of these features. Some affected patients exhibit extreme bone fragility with numerous fractures and die during the perinatal period; others manifest mild bone fragility and live a normal life span. Four distinct types have been identified: two inherited as autosomal dominant traits, one inherited as autosomal recessive traits and one inherited as both autosomal dominant and autosomal recessive traits. The presence of numerous fractures early in life with dentinogenesis imperfecta or blue sclera, or both, is sufficient to establish the diagnosis. Early hearing loss in a patient or a member of a family with a history of fragile bones is highly suggestive of the disorder.

Etiology and Pathogenesis. Osteogenesis imperfecta is probably the most common inherited bone disease. It is estimated that approximately 30,000 individuals in the United States have osteogenesis imperfecta, and owing to its variable clinical expression, many mildly affected patients remain undiagnosed. Osteogenesis imperfecta type I is the most common variety; it has an incidence of about 1 in 30,000 live births. It is a mild to moderately severe disorder with an autosomal dominant mode of inheritance. There is considerable variability in the inheritance. Type II is the most severe form; it has a reported incidence of 1 in 100,000 deliveries. It has an autosomal recessive transmission, although spontaneous cases are reported. Type III, which has both an autosomal dominant and an autosomal recessive mode of inheritance, and type IV, which is transmitted autosomal dominantly, are intermediate in severity.

Biochemical findings suggest that osteogenesis imperfecta syndromes are a result of inborn errors of collagen metabolism. Most forms of the disease are believed to be caused by mutations in the structural genes for the collagen protein. The specific molecular defect in most patients with osteogenesis imperfecta has not been identified, and the phenotypic heterogeneity may be due to mutations in genes required for the assembly and maintenance of bone and connective tissues.

Clinical Features. Osteogenesis imperfecta type I is characterized by osteoporosis, bone fragility, blue sclera, and conductive hearing loss in adolescents and adults. The sclera is distinctive, and it is described as having a deep blue-black hue. Fractures may be present at birth in 10% of patients or commence during infancy or childhood. There is considerable variability in the age of onset, frequency of fractures, and degree of skeletal deformity. Generally, birth weight and height are normal. Mild short stature is postnatal in onset and relates to the degree of involvement of the limbs and spine. Long bone deformities tend to be mild, with bowing of the limbs and angulation deformities occurring at previous fracture sites. Progressive kyphoscoliosis is seen in 20% of adults and may be severe. Hyperlaxity of ligaments of the hands, feet, and knees is common in children. Hearing impairment, which usually begins in the second decade of life, is present in 35% of adults. Dentinogenesis imperfecta is present in some type I patients.

Type II osteogenesis imperfecta is a lethal syndrome, with half of all patients stillborn. It has a reported incidence of 1 in 100,000 deliveries. It has an autosomal recessive mode of transmission, although spontaneous cases are reported. It is characterized in infancy by low birth weight, short stature, and broad thighs extending at right angles to the trunk. The limbs are short, curved, and grossly deformed. The skin is thin and frail and may be torn during delivery. Cranial vault ossification is lacking, and the facies is notable for hypotelorism, small beaked nose, and a triangular shape. Defects in skeletal ossification lead to extreme bone fragility and frequent fractures, even during delivery. Dental abnormalities have been found, including atubular dentin with a lace-work of argyrophilic fiber structures, an absence of predentin, and an abundance of argyrophilic fibers in the coronal pulp.

Type III osteogenesis imperfecta has both an autosomal dominant and an autosomal recessive mode of inheritance. It is a rare disorder, characterized in the newborn by severe bone fragility, multiple fractures, and progressive skeletal deformity. The sclera is blue at birth, but the color diminishes with age; adolescents and adults exhibit normal sclera coloration. Childhood mortality is high owing to cardiopulmonary complications, and prognosis is poor because of severe kyphoscoliosis. Individuals with type III exhibit the shortest stature of all patients with osteogenesis imperfecta. Dentinogenesis imperfecta is found in some patients with type III osteogenesis imperfecta. Hearing impairment has not been reported in these children.

Osteogenesis imperfecta type IV is a dominantly inherited osteopenia leading to bone fragility, without the other classic features associated with the osteogenesis imperfecta syndromes. The sclera is bluish at birth only.

Onset of fractures ranges from birth to adulthood, and the skeletal deformities are extremely variable. Bowing of the lower limbs at birth may be the only feature of this syndrome, and progressive deformities of the long bones and vertebral column may occur without fractures. Spontaneous improvement often occurs with puberty. Dentinogenesis imperfecta is seen in some type IV patients. The frequency of hearing impairment in adults is low.

Dentinogenesis imperfecta associated with osteogenesis imperfecta is described as a blue, brown, or amber opalescent discoloration of teeth. The primary teeth are more severely affected than is the permanent dentition (Fig. 15–20). There is considerable variation in expression of the discoloration, ranging from all teeth being affected to only a few. Teeth that are discolored are more prone to enamel wear and fracture. The crowns are described as shortened and bell-shaped, with a cervical constriction. The roots are narrow and short, and partial or complete pulpal obliteration occurs. A high frequency of class II malocclusions and a high incidence of impacted first and second molars have been reported.

Treatment and Prognosis. There is no specific treatment for this condition. Management of fractures may be a significant orthopedic challenge. With the onset of puberty, the severity of this problem frequently lessens. When dentinogenesis imperfecta is present, management is focused around the preservation of the teeth. To prevent wear and improve aesthetic appearance, full crown coverage may be necessary.

Because of the wide variation in clinical expression, prognosis ranges from very good (dominant form) to very poor (recessive form).

Cleidocranial Dysplasia

This syndrome is notable for aplasia or hypoplasia of the clavicles, characteristic craniofacial malformations, and the presence of multiple supernumerary and unerupted teeth.

Etiology and Pathogenesis. The etiology and pathogenesis are not well understood, although the disease has been described as a manifestation of both dominant and recessive inherited traits. Cases of sporadic occurrences have also been reported. It occurs with equal frequency among males and females; there is no racial predilection. Most patients with the disease exhibit normal intelligence.

Intramembranous and endochondral bones in the skull are affected, resulting in a sagittally diminished cranial base, transverse enlargement of the calvarium, and delayed closure of the fontanelles. Hydrocephalic pressure on unossified regions of the skull, especially the fontanelles, causes biparietal and frontal bossing and extension of the cranial vault. The deficiency of the clavicles is responsible for the long appearance of the neck and the narrow shoulders. The combined abnormalities of the middle third of the face and the dental alveolar complex result in the characteristic facial appearance.

The cause of delayed or failed eruption of the teeth has been associated with lack of cellular cementum. It is postulated that failure of cementum formation may be due to me-

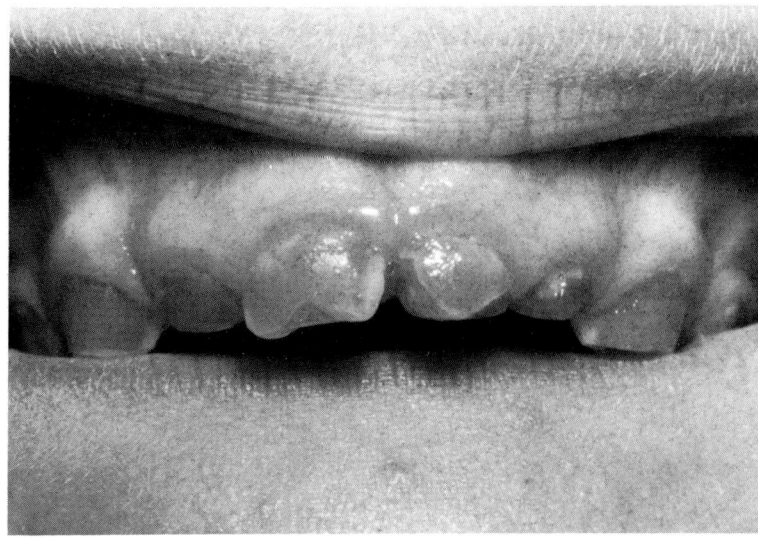

Figure 15–20. Primary teeth of a child with osteogenesis imperfecta exhibiting the classic opalescent discoloration.

chanical resistance to eruption by the dense alveolar bone overlying the unerupted teeth.

Clinical Features. The clinical appearance of cleidocranial dysplasia is so distinct as to be pathognomonic. The stature is unusually short, with the neck appearing long and narrow and the shoulders markedly drooped. Complete or partial absence of clavicular calcification results in hypermobility of the shoulders, allowing for variable levels of approximation in an anterior plane (Fig. 15–21A).

The head is large and brachycephalic. There is pronounced frontal, parietal, and occipital bossing. The facial bones and paranasal sinuses are hypoplastic, giving the face a small and short appearance. The nose is broad based, with a depressed nasal bridge. Ocular hypertelorism is frequently present. The entire skeleton may be affected, with defects of the pelvis, long bones, and fingers.

Maxillary hypoplasia gives the mandible a relatively prognathic appearance. The palate is narrow and highly arched, and there is an increased incidence of submucosal clefts and complete or partial clefts of the palate involving the hard and soft tissues.

The deciduous dentition is usually normal, although occasionally it may be delayed in eruption and exfoliation. The permanent dentition is severely delayed, and many teeth fail to erupt. Unerupted supernumerary teeth are frequently present in the premolar region (Fig. 15–21B). The over-retention of deciduous teeth, failure of eruption of permanent teeth, multiple supernumerary teeth, and maxillary hypoplasia result in severe malocclusion.

Radiographic findings of clinical significance pertain to the abnormalities of the craniofacial region, dentition, clavicles, and pelvis. Radiographs of the skull classically exhibit patent fontanelles and wormian bones, broad and anomalous cranial sutures, and underdeveloped paranasal sinuses. The clavicles may be aplastic unilaterally or bilaterally, or hypoplastic, appearing as small fragments attached to the sternum or acromial process. The mandible and maxilla contain many unerupted teeth, which are often malpositioned. Supernumerary teeth are most remarkable, occurring usually in the premolar region.

Treatment. There is no specific treatment for the patient with cleidocranial dysplasia. Genetic counseling is most important. The current mode of therapy for the dental anomalies combines early surgical intervention with orthodontic therapy. Extraction of supernumerary teeth and over-retained primary teeth, when the root formation of succedaneous teeth is greater than 50%, is followed by surgical exposure of unerupted teeth and orthodontic treatment. Early surgical exposure of unerupted teeth has resulted in stimulation of cementum formation and eruption of the dentition with normal root formation. Orthog-

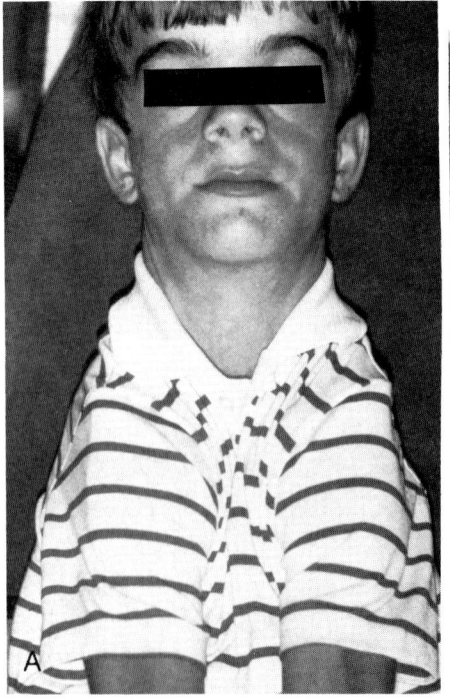
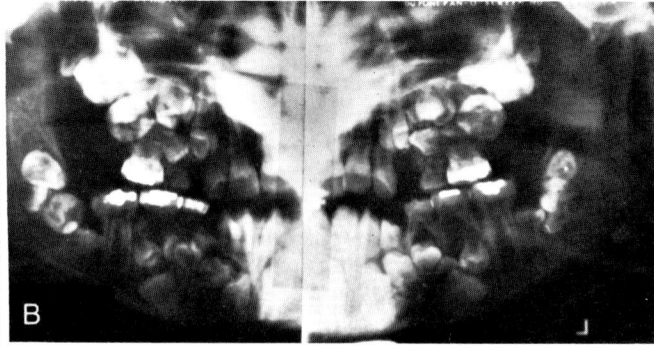

Figure 15–21. *A,* This patient with cleidocranial dysplasia is able to approximate his shoulders in this classical pose owing to hypoplasia of the clavicles. *B,* Multiple unerupted and malpositioned teeth are evident. The premolar regions are remarkable for numerous supernumerary teeth.

nathic surgery for correction of the dental-facial deformity, post-surgical orthodontics, and prosthetics can be anticipated.

Crouzon's Syndrome (Craniofacial Dysostosis)

Crouzon's syndrome is characterized by variable cranial deformity, maxillary hypoplasia, and shallow orbits with exophthalmos and divergent strabismus. The character of the cranial deformity depends upon the sutures affected, the degree of involvement, and the sequence of sutural fusion. Systemic complications include mental retardation, hearing loss, speech and visual impairment, and convulsions.

Etiology and Pathogenesis. Craniofacial dysostosis is inherited in an autosomal dominant mode, with complete penetrance. About one third of the cases reported arise spontaneously. There is increasing severity of expression of the disease in successive siblings, with the youngest child most severely affected.

Craniosynostosis results when premature fusion of the cranial sutures occurs. The etiology is not known, but premature closure of these sutures can initiate changes in the brain, secondary to increased intracranial pressure.

The deformities of the cranial bones and orbital cavities are the result of the fusion of sutures and increased intracranial pressure. Exophthalmos and reduced orbital volume are noted. Hypertelorism is accentuated by a downward and forward displacement of the ethmoid plate. Abnormalities of the bony orbit account for several functional ocular abnormalities. Severe distortion of the cranial base leads to reduced maxillary growth and nasopharyngeal hypoplasia with potential upper airway restriction.

Clinical Features. Patients with Crouzon's syndrome have a characteristic facies often described as "frog-like." Mid-face hypoplasia and exophthalmos are striking (Fig. 15–22). There is relative mandibular prognathism, with the nose resembling a parrot's beak. The upper lip and philtrum are usually short, and the lower lip often droops. The cranial deformity is dependent upon which sutures are involved. Proptosis with strabismus and orbital hypertelorism is common. Optic nerve damage is seen in 80% of cases.

Oral findings include severe maxillary hypoplasia, resulting in a narrowing of the maxillary arch and a compressed, high-arched palate. Bilateral posterior lingual crossbites are common. Premature posterior occlusion as a result of the inferiorly positioned maxilla results in an anterior open bite.

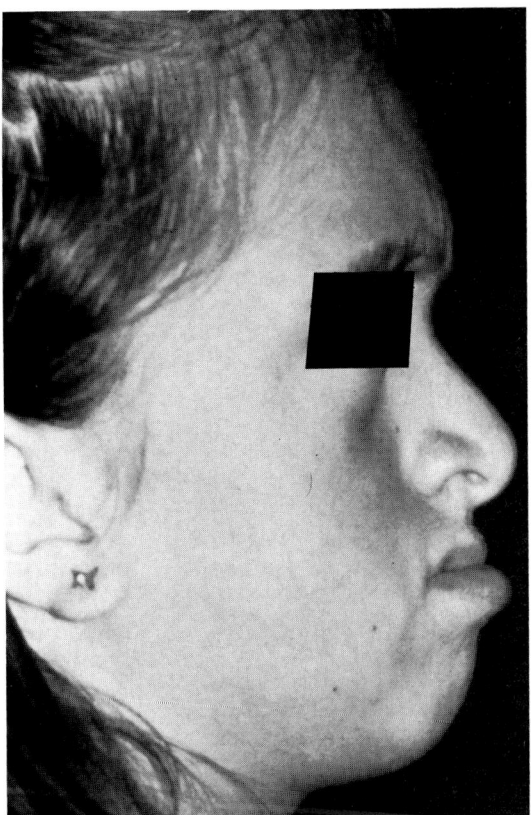

Figure 15–22. Severe maxillary hypoplasia, proptosis, and a short philtrum are noted in this patient with Crouzon's syndrome. (Courtesy of Dr. A. Shanske.)

Radiographs of the skull reveal obliterated suture lines with obvious bony continuity. A "hammered-silver" appearance is often seen in regions of the skull where compensatory deformity cannot occur. Lordosis of the cranial base is apparent on lateral skull projections, and angular deformities with vertical sloping of the anterior cranial fossa can be visualized. A large calvarium with hypoplasia of the maxilla, shallow orbits, and a relatively large mandible is common.

Treatment and Prognosis. The age of onset and the degree of craniosynostosis influence the severity of the complications, which range from craniofacial dystrophy to hearing loss, speech and visual impairment, and mental retardation. With a high degree of suspicion, the condition is often identifiable at birth. Early recognition is essential to guide growth and development of the face and cranium. Surgical intervention may be necessary if progressive exophthalmos exists, optic nerve damage or visual acuity is impaired, evidence of developing mental deficiency is noted, or intracranial pressure continues to rise. Treatment includes the surgical placement of artificial sutures to allow growth of the brain while minimizing intracranial pressure and secondary calvarial deformities.

Treacher Collins Syndrome (Mandibulofacial Dysostosis)

Treacher Collins syndrome primarily affects structures developing from the first branchial arch, but it also involves the second branchial arch, to a minor degree. It is generally a bilateral anomaly with a characteristic facies including downward sloping of the palpebral fissures, colobomas of the lower eyelid, mandibular and midface hypoplasia, and deformed pinnas.

Etiology and Pathogenesis. Treacher Collins syndrome is transmitted by an autosomal dominant mode of inheritance, although about half the cases are due to spontaneous mutation. The gene has a high degree of penetrance, with little intersibling variability. This disorder is relatively rare, with an incidence between 0.5 and 10.6 cases per 10,000 births.

It is believed that the embryologic and morphologic defects that result in the phenotypic expression of this syndrome begin as early as the sixth to seventh embryonic week. Evidence of a defect in the stapedial artery during embryogenesis may be responsible for the anatomic deficits seen. Stapedial artery dysfunction will give rise to defects of the stapes and incus and the first arch vessels supplying the maxilla. Failure of the inferior alveolar artery to develop an ancillary vascular supply will give rise to mandibular abnormalities. Improper orientation and hypoplasia of the mandibular elevator muscles, resulting from an aplastic or hypoplastic zygomatic arch, may also be contributory.

Mandibular retrognathia and midface vertical excess may be accentuated by the pull of abnormally oriented mandibular elevator muscles causing a backward rotation in mandibular growth pattern. The syndrome seems to be limited to defects of the bones and soft tissue of the face. Vascularization of the posterior portion of the second visceral arch by the stapedial artery seems unimpaired.

Clinical Findings. Treacher Collins syndrome is a manifestation of combined developmental anomalies of the second and, mainly, first branchial arch. It includes varying degrees of hypoplasia of the mandible, maxilla, zygoma, and external and middle ear (Fig. 15–23). In the fully expressed syndrome, the facial appearance is characteristic and is often described as "bird-like" or "fish-like."

Notched or linear colobomas of the outer third of the lower eyelids are found in 75% of patients. The lower eyelashes are absent medial to the colobomas in about 50% of patients. Antimongoloid obliquity or downward slanting of the palpebral fissures is striking.

Congenital atresia of the external auditory canal and microtia are often present. The ears are low set, with deformed, crumpled, or absent pinnae. Middle ear defects include fibrous bands of the long process of the incus, mal-

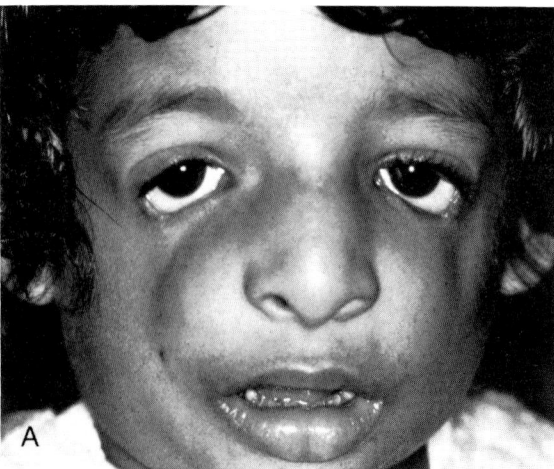
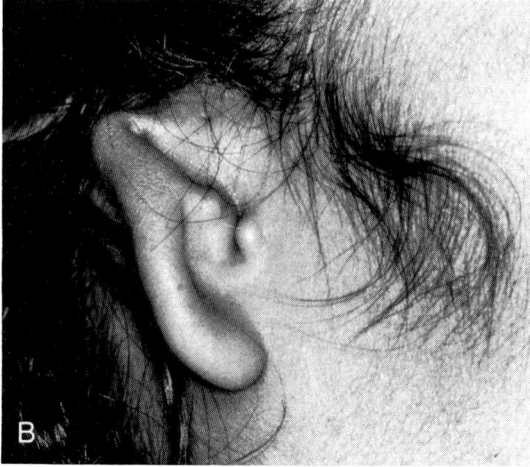

Figure 15–23. *A,* Treacher Collins syndrome. Note characteristic facial appearance, including downward sloping of the palpebral fissures and colobomas of the lower eyelids. *B,* Microtia, or underdeveloped ear, and a narrow extension of hair over the preauricular region, known as a "hair lick," are common in patients with Treacher Collins syndrome.

formed and fixed stapes and malleus, and accompanying conductive hearing loss. Ear tags and blind fistulas are often located between the pinna and the commissures of the mouth.

Atypical hair growth in the shape of a tongue-like process extends from the hairline toward the cheeks. Other associated anomalies such as skeletal deformities and facial clefts may be concomitant.

Oral findings include cleft palate in about 30% of patients and macrostomia in 15% of patients. High-arched palate and dental malocclusion consisting of apertognathia and widely separated and displaced teeth are common. Severe mandibular hypoplasia is most characteristic. The underdeveloped zygomaticomaxillary complex leads to a clinically severe midface deficiency.

Treacher Collins syndrome is notable for characteristic radiographic findings including downward sloping floors of the orbits, peaked bony nasal contour, aplastic or hypoplastic zygomatic process of the temporal bone, and obtuse mandibular angle. Lateral cephalograms demonstrate antigonial notching and broad curvature of the mandible. The condyle and coronoid processes are frequently flattened or aplastic.

Treatment and Prognosis. Treatment is directed at correction or reconstruction of the existing deformities. Neutralization of conductive hearing loss through surgery and hearing aids is helpful. Ophthalmologic surgery to correct eye deformities by orbital reconstruction is often performed. Extensive orthodontic treatment prior to orthognathic surgical reconstruction of the mandible and maxilla can be anticipated.

Pierre Robin Syndrome

The clinical presentation of micrognathia, glossoptosis, and high-arched or cleft palate in the neonate has been termed the Pierre Robin syndrome. This malformation complex can occur as an isolated finding or as a component of various syndromes or developmental anomalies. The mandibular retrognathia and hypoplasia is considered the primary malformation. Respiratory and feeding problems are prevalent and may result in episodic airway obstruction, with infant hypoxia and malnutrition.

Etiology and Pathogenesis. The incidence of Pierre Robin syndrome is 5.3 to 22.7 per 100,000 births, with 39% of the infants exhibiting no additional abnormalities. Of the remaining infants, 25% have known syndromes, and 36% have one or more anomalies that are not part of a known syndrome.

Fetal malposition and interposition of the tongue between the palatal shelves have long been considered the etiologic catalysts for palatal deformity and micrognathia. Arrest of mandibular development may prevent descent of the tongue and failure of palatal shelf elevation and fusion. Recent evidence suggests that the primary defect may be due to genetically influenced metabolic growth disturbances of the maxilla and mandible rather than to mechanical obstruction by the tongue during embryogenesis. Organogenetic differences lead to the variable presentation of micrognathia and cleft palate.

Clinical Features. Infants present with severe micrognathia and mandibular hypoplasia (Fig. 15–24). A U-shaped cleft palate is a common but not constant feature, and in some instances, the palate is highly arched. Glossoptosis is the result of the retropositional attachment of the genioglossus muscle because of the retrognathic mandible. The geniohyoid muscle is foreshortened, so that support to the hyoid bone and strap muscles of the larynx is also compromised.

Treatment and Prognosis. Respiratory and feeding problems are frequent in the immediate postnatal and neonatal periods. Constant medical supervision may be necessary to prevent airway obstruction and hypoxia, malnutrition, aspiration, bronchopneumonia, and exhaustion. In most cases, conservative repositioning of the infant and frequent prone posture are sufficient to prevent upper airway

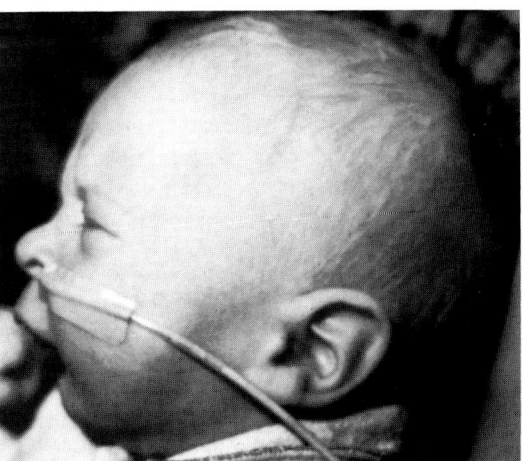

Figure 15–24. Infant with Pierre Robin syndrome exhibiting severe micrognathia of the mandible. (Courtesy of Dr. A. Shanske.)

obstruction, by making optimal use of the effects of gravity during resting and feeding. In severe cases with frequent cyanotic episodes, intraoral or nasal pharyngeal airway placement, some form of tongue and lip adhesion, and even tracheostomy may be considered. The feeding of infants with mandibular hypoplasia requires expertise and patience.

The growth of the mandible is remarkable during the first 4 years of life, and often a normal profile is achieved between 4 to 6 years of age. Some patients have a residual mild mandibular retrognathia requiring treatment later in life.

Marfan's Syndrome

Marfan's syndrome is a heritable disorder of connective tissue, characterized by abnormalities of the skeletal, cardiovascular, and ocular systems. It is currently estimated that 23,000 Americans have Marfan's syndrome. The disorder is notable for a number of sudden catastrophic deaths that have occurred in affected (undiagnosed) athletes.

Etiology and Pathogenesis. Marfan's syndrome is an autosomal dominant–inherited disorder that affects 1 in 10,000 individuals. There are no ethnic, racial, or gender predilections. The condition exhibits complete but extremely variable penetrance, with the offspring of an affected individual having a 50% chance of acquiring the disorder. Approximately 15 to 35% of cases arise spontaneously, as a result of gamete gene mutation in the ovum or sperm; a greater number occur with increasing paternal age. The Marfan gene is believed to produce a change in one of the proteins that provides strength to a component of connective tissue, probably collagen. Early diagnosis is difficult, with no specific laboratory tests available. Diagnosis is based on characteristic abnormalities of the musculoskeletal, ocular, and cardiovascular systems and a positive family history. Because most features progress with age, the diagnosis is often more obvious in older persons.

Clinical Features. Patients characteristically possess a tall, slender stature with relatively long legs and arms, large hands with long fingers, and loose joints. The arms, legs, and digits are disproportionately long compared with the patient's trunk. Chest deformities include a protrusion or indentation of the breast bone (pectus carinatum, pectus excavatum). Often the normal thoracic kyphosis is absent, leading to a straight back. Varying degrees of scoliosis are present. Oral findings include a narrow, high-arched palate and dental crowding. The face appears long and narrow.

The cardiovascular system is affected in nearly all persons. Mitral valve prolapse occurs in 75 to 85% of affected patients, and a small percentage develop mitral regurgitation. Ascending aortic dilatation may result in aortic regurgitation and heart failure. Progressive dissection of the aorta may lead to aneurysms, placing the patient at great risk for a catastrophic episode.

Ocular findings include dislocation of the lens (ectopia lentis), which occurs in half these patients. The most common eye anomaly, however, is myopia (nearsightedness). Retinal detachment occurs infrequently, but it is more prevalent following lens removal.

Treatment and Prognosis. Morbidity and mortality are directly related to the degree of connective tissue abnormality in the involved organ systems. The cardiovascular abnormalities of ascending aorta dilatation and mitral valve prolapse, subluxation of the lens of the eye, chest cavity deformities and scoliosis, and potential for pneumothorax are serious prognostic indicators.

Treatment of the Marfan syndrome patient consists of annual medical examinations with a cardiovascular emphasis, frequent ophthalmologic examination, scoliosis screening, and echocardiography. Often, physical activity is restricted and redirected in an attempt to protect the aorta.

Antibiotic prophylaxis has been recommended for infective endocarditis, regardless of the clinical evidence of valvular disease. Beta blockers such as propranolol are often used to reduce aortic stress and have been shown to significantly reduce both the rate of aortic dilatation and the risk of serious complications. The prognosis for untreated ascending aorta aneurysm is extremely poor.

Ehlers-Danlos Syndrome

The Ehlers-Danlos syndrome is an uncommon inherited disorder of connective tissue, clinically characterized by joint hypermobility and skin hyperextensibility. The clinical manifestations of the disease are due to inherited defects in collagen metabolism. In addition to the skin and joint anomalies, severe cardiovascular and gastrointestinal complications may occur and coexist.

Etiology and Pathogenesis. Various subtypes of Ehlers-Danlos syndrome are inherited as autosomal dominant, autosomal recessive, and X-linked traits. The disease is relatively uncommon.

A defect in the synthesis or structure of type III collagen has been suggested in some cases. This theory is supported by the occurrence of spontaneous rupture of the aorta or intestines, tissues rich in type III collagen.

A deficiency of the enzyme lysyl hydroxylase, resulting in decreased amounts of collagen hydroxylysine, has also been reported in some patients with Ehlers-Danlos syndrome. Others may have a defect in collagen metabolism, preventing the conversion of procollagen to collagen. Also, a disorder of copper metabolism has been noted in some patients.

Clinical Features. Classic clinical features include marked hyperelasticity of the skin and extreme laxity of the joints (Fig. 15–25). The skin may be stretched for several centimeters, but when released, it resumes its former contours. Skin manifestations include a velvety appearance with a high degree of fragility and bruisability. Minor trauma may produce ecchymoses, bleeding, and large gaping wounds with poor healing tendencies and "cigarette paper" scar formation, especially evident on the forehead and lower legs and over pressure points. Other cutaneous findings include molluscoid pseudotumors, redundant skin on the palms and soles, and subcutaneous lipid-containing cysts, which may calcify.

Articular hypermobility is variable. It may be of sufficient severity to cause spontaneous dislocation of the joints. Extreme joint laxity leads to genu recurvatum (back knee), flat feet, habitual joint dislocation, kyphoscoliosis, and other skeletal deformities.

Severe cardiovascular, gastrointestinal, and pulmonary manifestations may be present. Cardiovascular anomalies include dissecting aortic aneurysm, mitral valve prolapse, and rupture of major blood vessels. The majority of patients have a bleeding diathesis that may consist of a tendency to bruise, or may be severe, with hematoma formation and bleeding from the nose, gut, lungs, and urogenital tract.

Rupture of the bowel and bladder may occur. Pulmonary problems include spontaneous pneumothorax and respiratory impairment, secondary to chest wall deformities. Hernias, gastrointestinal diverticula, and ocular defects may exist.

Orofacial features include a narrow maxilla and wide nasal bridge. Marked extensibility of the tongue, enabling contact with the tip of the nose, has been described.

Treatment and Prognosis. Prognosis is dependent on the severity of the systemic manifestations. The cardiovascular status of all patients should be evaluated and closely monitored. Sudden death in youth or early adult life may occur owing to dissecting aneurysms and ruptured arteries.

Surgical intervention must be tempered in light of connective tissue fragility. Joint ligament repair is often unsuccessful owing to suture failure. Wound healing is usually de-

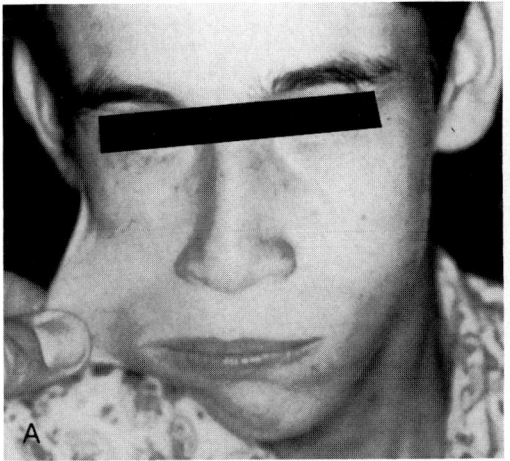 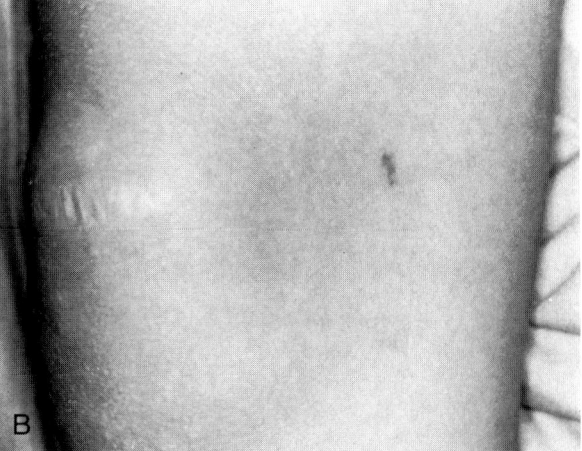

Figure 15–25. *A*, Patient with Ehlers-Danlos syndrome exhibiting marked extensibility of the facial skin. (Courtesy of Dr. H. Diner.) *B*, Minor trauma may produce cigarette-paper scar formation as seen on the knee of this patient with Ehlers-Danlos syndrome.

layed, and prolonged bleeding may occur following injury. Osteoarthritis is a common complication in patients with repeated dislocations.

Down Syndrome (Trisomy 21)

Down syndrome is a common and easily recognizable chromosomal aberration. The incidence is reported to be 1 in 600 to 1 in 700 live births; however, more than half of the affected fetuses spontaneously abort during early pregnancy. Approximately 10 to 15% of all institutionalized patients have Down syndrome.

Most cases of trisomy 21 (94%) are caused by nondisjunction, resulting in an extra chromosome. The remaining patients with Down syndrome have various chromosomal abnormalities. The translocation type occurs in 3%, mosaicism occurs in 2%, and rare chromosomal aberrations make up the remaining 1% of cases. This condition is also associated with increasing maternal age.

Etiology and Pathogenesis. Possible etiologies for Down syndrome include undetected mosaicism in a parent, repeated exposure to the same environmental insult, genetic predisposition to nondisjunction, an ovum with an extra 21 chromosome, or a preferential survival *in utero* of trisomy 21 embryos and fetuses with increasing maternal age. Parents of any age who have had one child with trisomy 21 have a significant risk (about 1%) of having a similarly affected child, a risk of recurrence equivalent to that affecting births to a mother over 45 years of age. There appear to be no racial, social, economic, or gender predilections.

Clinical Features. Patients with Down syndrome present with numerous characteristic clinical findings and a variety of common systemic manifestations. A number of common phenotypic findings in children with Down syndrome have been identified; these can assist in establishing a diagnosis.

Variable degrees of mental retardation exist in all patients with Down syndrome. Most mildly affected individuals are highly functioning and are able to perform well in a workshop environment. Dementia affects about 30% of patients with Down syndrome, and early aging is common. After age 35, nearly all individuals develop the neuropathologic changes analogous to those found in Alzheimer disease, although 70% exhibit no clinically detectable behavioral changes. These two disorders have many neuropathologic and neurochemical similarities, and an increased risk for Down syndrome has been found in families with a predilection for Alzheimer disease.

In Down syndrome, the skull is brachycephalic, with a flat occiput and prominent forehead (Fig. 15–26). A third or fourth fontanelle is present, and all the fontanelles are large and have extended patency. Sagittal suture sepa-

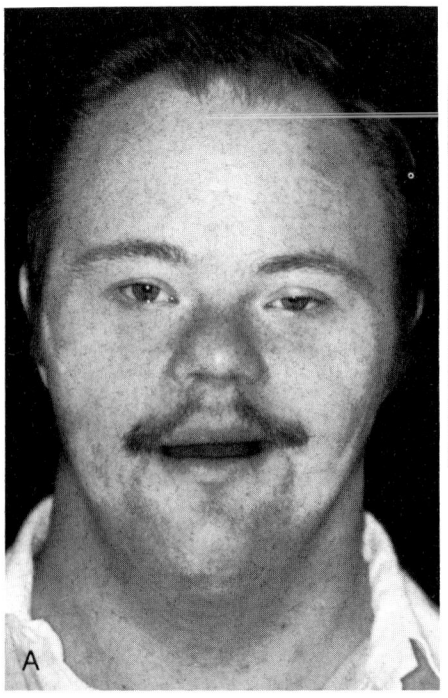
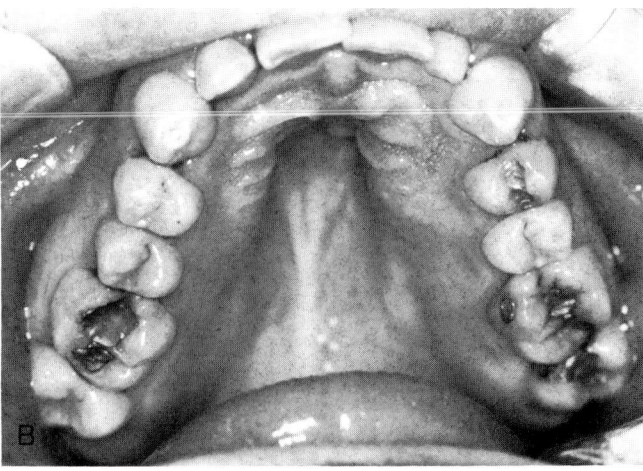

Figure 15–26. *A*, Typical facies of patient with Down syndrome. Note oblique palpebral fissures, prominent forehead, flat nasal bridge, and open mouth posture. *B*, The palate is highly vaulted, with decreased width and length.

ration greater than 5 mm is present in 98% of affected individuals. Frontal and sphenoid sinuses are absent, and the maxillary sinus is hypoplastic in over 90% of patients. Midface skeletal deficiency is quite marked, with ocular hypotelorism, flattened nasal bridge, and relative mandibular prognathism.

The eyes are almond-shaped, with upward-slanting palpebral fissures, epicanthic folds, and Brushfield spots of the iris frequently noted. Other ocular anomalies include convergent strabismus, nystagmus, refractive errors, keratoconus, and congenital cataracts.

Congenital heart disease is present in 30 to 45% of all patients with Down syndrome. Anomalies include complete atrioventricular canal, partial endocardial cushion abnormalities, and ventricular septal defects. Tetralogy of Fallot, patent ductus arteriosus, and secundum atrial septal defects are seen less frequently.

It appears that T cell and probably B cell function is aberrant, with some affected children being more susceptible to infectious diseases. Thyroid dysfunction occurs in upward of 50% of all patients. There is also an increased incidence of acute lymphocytic leukemia.

Skeletal problems include hypoplasia of the maxilla and sphenoid bones, rib and pelvic abnormalities, hip dislocation, and patella subluxation. Of particular concern is the presence of atlantoaxial instability in 12 to 20% of persons with Down syndrome, owing to the increased laxity of the transverse ligaments between the atlas and the odontoid process. Delay in recognizing this condition may result in irreversible spinal cord damage, which might occur during manipulation of the neck in patients undergoing dental therapy or general anesthesia.

Oral manifestations of Down syndrome are common. The tongue is often fissured, and macroglossia is usually relative to the small oral cavity, although true macroglossia may exist. Open mouth posture is common, owing to a narrow nasopharynx and hypertrophied tonsils and adenoids causing upper airway compromise. A protruding tongue and frequent mouth breathing result in drying and cracking of the lips. Palatal width and length are significantly decreased, and bifid uvula and cleft lip and palate are occasionally observed. Elevated concentrations of sodium, calcium, and bicarbonate ion have been demonstrated in parotid saliva.

The dentition exhibits a number of characteristic anomalies, and periodontal disease is prevalent. The incidence of dental caries, however, appears to be no greater than in normal individuals. Considering the existence of poor oral hygiene, this may reflect the greater buffering capacity of the saliva or the ability to control dietary intake in institutional and home settings.

Eruption of both the primary and the permanent dentitions is delayed in 75% of cases. Abnormalities in eruption sequence occur frequently. Hypodontia occurs in both dentitions, and microdontia is often seen. Developmental tooth anomalies, including crown and root malformations, are often present. Almost 50% of Down syndrome patients exhibit three or more dental anomalies. Enamel hypocalcification occurs in about 20% of patients.

Occlusal disharmonies consisting of mesioclusion owing to a relative prognathism, posterior crossbites, apertognathia, and severe crowding of the anterior teeth are common. Posterior crossbites are of maxillary basal bone origin, whereas anterior open bites are due to dental-alveolar discrepancies.

Treatment and Prognosis. Infants with Down syndrome that includes significant congenital heart disease have a poor prognosis. Causes of death frequently include cardiopulmonary complications, gastrointestinal malformations, and acute lymphoblastic leukemia.

Recent technologic advances in cardiovascular diagnosis have brought about a marked improvement in prognosis. Newborns require chest x-rays, electrocardiograms, echocardiograms, and subsequent pediatric cardiac consultation if cardiovascular anomalies are detected.

Regular ophthalmologic and audiologic follow-ups are extremely important. They can intercept early visual and hearing problems that may affect learning and development. Detection of atlantoaxial instability may prevent a catastrophic spinal injury.

Dental therapy is directed at prevention of dental caries and periodontal disease. Frequent follow-up and institution of stringent home care regimens are critical. Highly functioning children may be candidates for orthodontic intervention and subsequent maxillofacial surgery, if required. Guidelines established by the American Heart Association for antibiotic prophylaxis should be followed for those patients with congenital heart disease.

Hemifacial Atrophy

This is a rare disorder that represents a progressive unilateral atrophy of the face. It may occasionally affect other regions on the same side of the body. The cause of this condition is totally unknown, although trauma, dysfunction of the peripheral nervous system, infection, and genetic abnormalities have been suggested.

Hemifacial atrophy typically appears during young adulthood. The condition affects both soft tissue and bone of the affected side. Orally, the tongue and lips may show hemiatrophy. Developing teeth may show incomplete root development and delayed eruption on the affected side.

The course of this disease is of several years' duration, but eventual stabilization is seen without medical or surgical intervention. Contralateral jacksonian epilepsy, trigeminal neuralgia, and eye and hair changes may also occur with this condition. There is no known treatment for this disfiguring problem.

Hemifacial Hypertrophy

Congenital hemihypertrophy is a rare disorder, characterized by gross body asymmetry. It may be simple, limited to a single digit; segmental, involving a specific region of the body; or complex, encompassing half the body. The enlargement is usually unilateral, although limited bilateral crossover does occur. All tissues in the region of abnormal growth may be involved, but occasionally, a selective number of tissues are affected. It classically presents as a unilateral, localized overgrowth of the facial soft tissues, bones, and teeth.

Etiology and Pathogenesis. Gross asymmetry has been found in 1 in 86,000 patients, with a 3 to 2 female preponderance. Almost all cases appear to be sporadic. There are equal numbers of segmental and complex forms, with neither side of the body exhibiting a greater incidence of involvement. Wilms' tumor is the most common neoplasm reported in association with hemihypertrophy.

Multiple etiologic factors have been implicated in the development of hemihypertrophy including anatomic and functional vascular or lymphatic abnormalities, endocrine dysfunction, altered intrauterine environment, central nervous system disturbances, chromosomal abnormalities, and asymmetric cell division. Etiologic heterogeneity may be responsible for the varied clinical presentation, affecting single or multiple systems, and the degree of tissue involvement.

Clinical Features. The varieties and complexities of hemihypertrophy have resulted in a wide range of reported dental-facial findings. In some patients, the face is involved solely, but often unilateral facial enlargement is associated with hypertrophy of a portion of the body. Frequently, the tissues involved are not affected uniformly, accentuating the variable clinical presentation.

Craniofacial findings include asymmetry of the frontal bone, maxilla, palate, mandible, alveolar process, condyles, and associated overlying soft tissue (Fig. 15–27). The skin may be thickened, with excessive secretions by sebaceous and sweat glands and hypertrichosis. The pinna is often remarkably enlarged. Unilateral enlargement of one of the cerebral hemispheres may be responsible for mental retardation in 15 to 20% of patients and for the occurrence of seizure disorders.

The oral findings are quite striking, affecting the dentition and tongue to a significant degree. The tongue is unilaterally hyperplastic and often distorted in appearance, with a distinct midline demarcation. The fungiform papillae are usually enlarged and resemble soft polypoid excrescences. Dysgeusia has been reported. Intraoral soft tissues are thickened and anatomically enlarged, often being described as overabundant and lying in soft velvety folds.

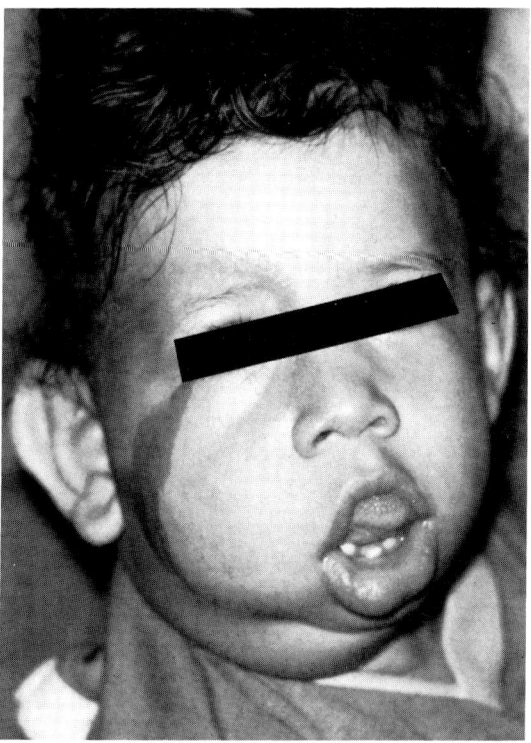

Figure 15–27. Child with hemifacial hypertrophy (as part of epidermal nevus syndrome).

Dental findings include abnormalities in crown size and root size and shape as well as precocious development and eruption. The permanent canines, premolars, and first molars are most frequently enlarged. When the primary dentition is affected, abnormalities are limited to the second molars and, less frequently, the canines. Unilateral macrodontia approaches but does not exceed a 50% increase in crown dimension in mesiodistal and buccolingual diameters. Root size and shape are proportionately enlarged or uncommonly shortened, and there is usually premature apical development. Early eruption of the affected permanent teeth by age 4 or 5 years has been reported.

Dental malocclusions are common owing to asymmetric growth of the maxilla, mandible, and alveolar process and abnormalities of tooth morphology and eruption patterns. Midline deviations, severely canted occlusal planes, and open bites are common.

Lateral and posterior anterior cephalograms demonstrate pronounced bony asymmetry and facial bone hypertrophy as well as evidence of hypertrophied soft tissues, such as tonsillar enlargement. Root anomalies, crown enlargement, and evidence of premature eruption are easily identifiable by panoramic or periapical radiography.

Differential Diagnosis. The diagnosis of true congenital hemifacial hypertrophy rests on the presence of unilateral hypertrophy of the craniofacial structures and associated soft tissue, including the dentition. Angio-osteohypertrophy (Klippel-Trenaunay-Weber syndrome) can be ruled out by the absence of an overlying cutaneous nevus flammeus. Neurofibromatosis may cause gross enlargement of the soft tissue and skeleton of half the face, but it does not affect tooth size and eruption sequence. Lymphangioma and hemangioma are characterized by soft tissue enlargement; they do not affect tooth morphology. Acromegaly produces symmetric bilateral jaw enlargement.

Other syndromes and conditions that produce soft and hard tissue hypertrophy and asymmetry include Russell's, or Silver's, syndrome, Beckwith-Wiedemann syndrome, congenital lymphedema, arteriovenous aneurysms, multiple exostoses, and facial tumors of childhood.

Treatment and Prognosis. During infancy and childhood, the patient should be examined frequently to facilitate early identification of potential neoplasms involving the liver, adrenal glands, and kidneys. Growth and development should be observed closely for evidence of mental impairment or abnormalities of sexual development.

Abnormalities during the mixed dentition phase relate to tooth size–arch size discrepancies and abnormalities in eruption sequence. Asymmetric growth of the craniofacial complex and dental alveolus will require early orthodontic intervention, including space maintenance, minor tooth movement, and functional appliances. Surgical reconstruction of hard and soft tissue anomalies to improve function and aesthetics must be anticipated.

The frequent association of congenital hemihypertrophy with vascular anomalies, embryonal neoplasms, and mental retardation requires a multidisciplinary team of dental and medical specialists.

Clefts of the Lip and Palate

Clefts of the lip and palate are frequently encountered congenital anomalies that often result in severe functional deficits of speech, mastication, and deglutition. Frequently, there is an increased prevalence of associated congenital malformations as well as learning disabilities secondary to hearing deficits.

Generally, clefts of the lip and palate are classified into four major types: (1) cleft lip, (2) cleft palate, (3) unilateral cleft lip and palate, and (4) bilateral cleft lip and palate. Other clefts of the lip and mouth include lip pits, linear lip indentations, submucosal clefts of the palate, bifid uvula and tongue, and numerous facial clefts extending through the nose, lips, and oral cavity. Clefting deformities are extremely variable in nature; they may range from furrows in the skin and mucosa to extensive cleavages involving muscle and bone. A combination of cleft lip and palate is the most common clefting deformity seen.

Etiology and Pathogenesis. Cleft lip and palate account for approximately 50% of all cases, whereas isolated cleft lip and isolated cleft palate each occur in about 25% of cases. The incidence of cleft lip and cleft palate has been reported to be between 1 in 700 and 1 in 1000 births, with variable racial predilection. Isolated cleft palate is less common, with an incidence between 1 in 1500 and 1 in 3000 births. Cleft lip with or without cleft palate is more frequent in males, and cleft palate alone is more common in females.

The majority of cases of cleft lip or cleft palate, or both, can be explained by the multifactorial threshold hypothesis. The multifactorial inheritance theory implies that many contributory risk genes interact with one another and the environment and collectively determine whether a threshold of abnormality is breached, resulting in a defect in the developing fetus. Multifactorial or polygenic inheritance explains the transmission of isolated cleft lip or palate, and it is extremely useful in predicting occurrence risks of this anomaly among family members of an affected individual.

Disruption of normal patterns of facial growth, including deficiencies of any of the facial processes, may lead to maldevelopment of the lips and palate. Cleft lip generally occurs at about the sixth to seventh week *in utero*; it is a result of failure of the epithelial groove between the medial and the lateral nasal processes to be penetrated by mesodermal cells.

Cleft palate is a result of epithelial breakdown at about the eighth week of embryonic development, with ingrowth failure of mesodermal tissue and lack of lateral palatal segment fusion. Most embryologists believe that true tissue deficiencies exist in all clefting deformities, and that actual anatomic structures are absent. Varying degrees of cleft lip and palate may occur, ranging from mild notching of the vermilion border or bifid uvula to severe bilateral complete clefts of the lip, alveolus, and entire palate.

Clinical Features. The Veau system of classification for cleft lip and palate is widely used by clinicians; it helps to describe the variety of lip and palatal clefts seen. The system classifies cleft lip and cleft palate separately into four major categories, with emphasis on the degree of clefting present.

Cleft lip may vary from a pit or small notch in the vermilion border to a complete cleft extending into the floor of the nose (Fig. 15–28). Using the Veau classification, a class I cleft of the lip is a unilateral notching of the vermilion border that does not extend into the lip. If the unilateral notching of the vermilion extends into the lip but does not involve the floor of the nose, it is designated as a class II cleft. Class III lip clefts are unilateral clefts of the vermilion border extending through the lip into the floor of the nose. Any bilateral cleft of the lip, exhibiting incomplete notching or a complete cleft, is classified as a class IV cleft.

Clefting deformities of the palate can also be divided into four clinical types using the Veau system (Fig. 15–29). A cleft limited to the soft palate is a class I palatal cleft. Class II clefts are defects of the hard and soft palate; they extend no further than the incisive foramen and, therefore, are limited to the secondary palate only. Clefts of the secondary palate may be complete or incomplete. A complete cleft includes the soft and hard palate to the incisive foramen. An incomplete cleft involves the velum and a portion of the hard palate, not extending to the incisive foramen. Complete unilateral clefts extending from the uvula to the incisive foramen in the midline and the alveolar process unilaterally are designated as class III palatal clefts. Class IV clefts are complete bilateral clefts involving the soft and hard palate and the alveolar process on both sides of the premaxilla, leaving it free and often mobile.

Submucosal clefts are not included in this system of classification, but they can be identified clinically by the presence of a bifid uvula, palpable notching of the posterior portion of the hard and soft palate, and the presence of a zona pellucida or a thin translucent membrane covering the defect.

Clefts of the soft palate, including submu-

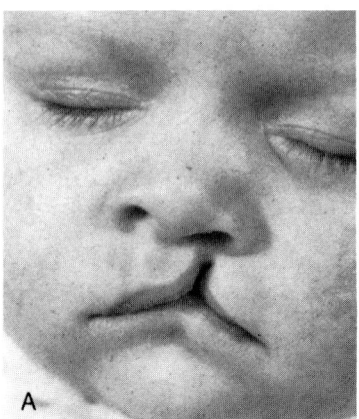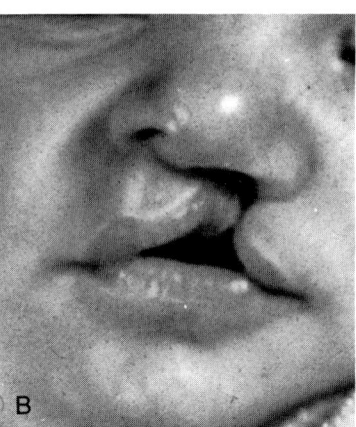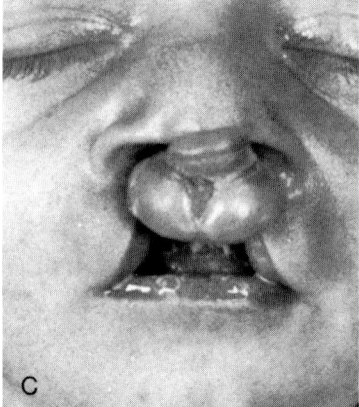

Figure 15–28. Cleft lip. *A*, Unilateral soft tissue cleft. *B*, Complete unilateral cleft extending through alveolus into floor of nose. *C*, Complete bilateral cleft lip.

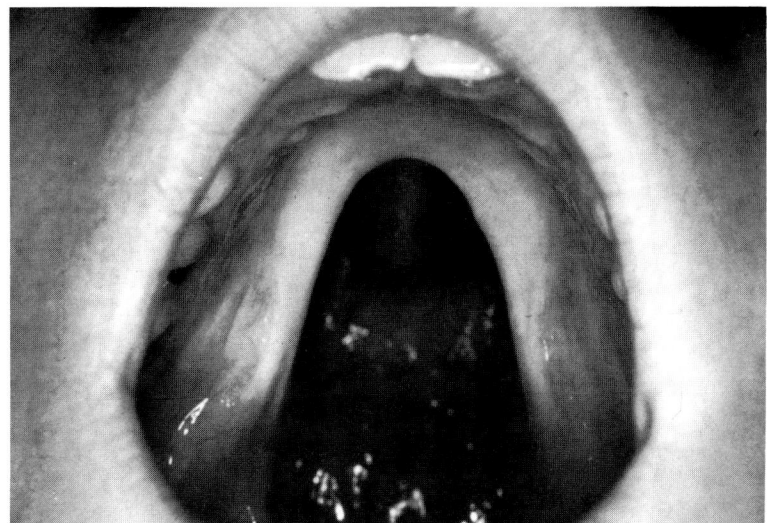

Figure 15–29. Complete cleft of the palate.

cosal clefts, are often associated with velopharyngeal incompetence or eustachian tube dysfunction. Recurrent otitis media and hearing deficits are common complications. Palatal pharyngeal incompetence results from failure of the soft palate and pharyngeal wall to make contact during swallowing and speech, thus preventing the necessary muscular seal between the nasal and the oral pharynx. Speech is often characterized by air emission from the nose and has a hypernasal quality.

The prevalence of dental anomalies associated with cleft lip and palate is remarkable (Fig. 15–30). Abnormalities of tooth number, size, morphology, calcification, and eruption have been well described. Both deciduous and permanent dentitions may be affected. The lateral incisor in the vicinity of the cleft is often involved, but teeth outside the cleft area exhibit developmental defects to a greater degree than is seen in unaffected patients.

There is a high incidence of congenitally missing teeth, especially deciduous and permanent maxillary lateral incisors adjacent to the alveolar cleft. The prevalence of hypodontia increases directly with the severity of the cleft. Complete unilateral and bilateral alveolar clefts are often associated with supernumerary teeth as well, usually the maxillary lateral incisors. Tooth formation is often delayed, and enamel hypoplasia, microdontia or macrodontia, and fused teeth are seen frequently.

Treatment and Prognosis. Prognosis is dependent on the severity of the clefting disorder. Aesthetic considerations and hearing and speech deficits often result in significant developmental problems.

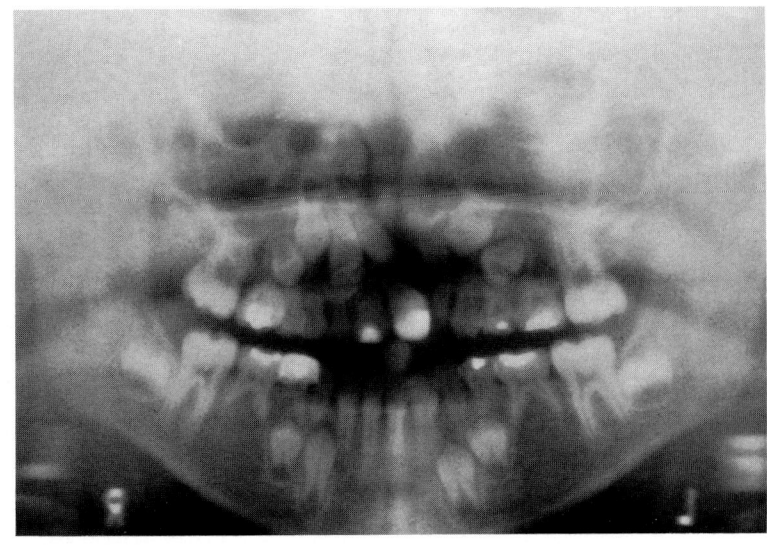

Figure 15–30. Panographic radiograph (Panorex) of a patient with a unilateral maxillary dental alveolar cleft. Note the alveolar bone defect and malpositioned teeth.

Treatment is chronologically sequenced and often requires a multidisciplinary team concept, owing to the extensive nature of the problem and its impact on the child and the immediate family. Craniofacial or cleft palate teams are made up of dental, medical, and surgical specialists, with the assistance of allied health professionals in social services, child development, and hearing and speech therapy.

Generally, cleft lip repair is accomplished during early infancy when the child is stable, weighs at least 10 pounds, and has hemoglobin levels of 10 mg per dl. Cheiloplasty is often required later in life. Closure of soft palate defects with sliding or pharyngeal flaps is often recommended at approximately 1 year of age to promote normal speech development. Palatal obturators are often fabricated for infants with cleft palate disorders who are having difficulty feeding or are regurgitating food or liquids through the nasal cavity. Early audiologic and speech evaluation is highly recommended, and hearing aids are often indicated to prevent associated learning problems seen in children with cleft palate who have frequent episodes of otitis media.

Preventive dental services are extremely important, since an intact dentition is the foundation for future orthodontic therapy. Treatment is often required to correct developmental dental defects. Orthodontic treatment is sometimes initiated during the primary dentition to correct unilateral and bilateral posterior maxillary crossbites and to retract an anterior displaced premaxillary segment.

Once into the mixed dentition phase of development, conventional orthodontic therapy is initiated to establish a normal maxillary arch form (Fig. 15–31). Often this is done in preparation for an autogenous bone graft to the alveolar cleft to re-establish maxillary arch continuity. It is recommended that the grafting procedure be performed when root formation of the unerupted permanent tooth associated with the alveolar defect (usually the maxillary canine) has reached one-quarter to one-half completion. These teeth have been shown to successfully erupt passively or mechanically through the graft site, consolidating the arch and re-establishing alveolar competency.

Further orthodontic treatment, followed by orthognathic surgery, is often required for those patients with significant dental-facial deformities. Frequent plastic surgical procedures to correct the aesthetics and function of the vermilion border, lip, philtrum, and nose can be anticipated.

Fragile X Syndrome

It has long been recognized in the general population that more males than females are mentally deficient. The large percentage of mentally disabled males and historical documentation of families with affected male and unaffected female children is highly suggestive of an X-linked inheritance pattern. Since the report in 1943 of a family with 11 severely retarded males delivered to an apparently unaffected mother, multiple case reports have been presented that have identified a syndrome (fragile X syndrome) characterized by X-linked mental retardation, macro-orchidism, and a characteristic phenotypic presentation.

Etiology and Pathogenesis. The fragile X

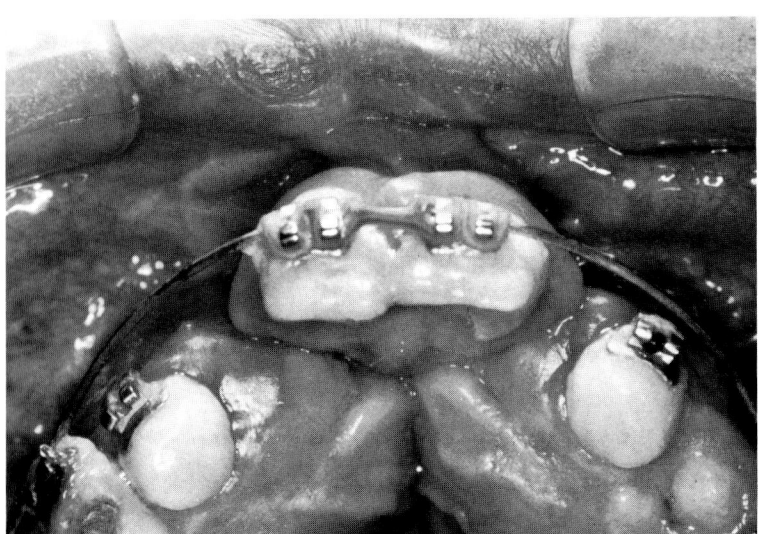

Figure 15–31. Patient with bilateral dental alveolar cleft and cleft of the palate undergoing early orthodontic treatment.

syndrome, believed to account for 30 to 50% of all families with X-linked mental retardation, takes its name from an identifiable fragile site on the X chromosome that is a reliable diagnostic marker. It is now recognized that X-linked mental retardation may be as common as Down syndrome in males; it accounts for approximately 25% of all mentally disabled males, with an incidence of 1 affected child per 500 male births. The finding of 20 to 30% of female carriers with varying degrees of mental retardation may be explained by lyonization or random inactivation of one of the X chromosomes.

The family history remains the primary tool for recognition of patients with X-linked mental retardation. In the fragile X syndrome, specific cytogenetic studies can aid in the diagnosis. In 30 to 50% of patients tested for chromosomal changes, an abnormal secondary constriction near the terminal end of the long arm (q) of the X chromosome is identifiable. Often this segment is broken, and it has been termed the fragile site. Abnormalities of speech have also been noted in the fragile X syndrome, and it has been theorized that major genes related to verbal function are located on the X chromosome and are disrupted at the fragile site.

Clinical Features. The classic clinical presentation is that of a mentally retarded male with postpubescent macro-orchidism, large ears, prognathism, and a long narrow face with a high forehead and prominent supraorbital ridges (Fig. 15-32). The patients have a characteristic repetitive jocular speech and may exhibit hyperactive behavior or autism. Often the hands are large and fleshy, and the iris may be pale. Oral findings include a high-arched palate, prominent lateral palatine ridges, anterior and posterior dental crossbites, and increased occlusal attrition. A high-normal birth weight is common, and increased head circumference during infancy and childhood is noted.

The degree of mental retardation is variable, even among affected siblings. Testicular biopsies and endocrine function tests are found to be within normal limits.

Treatment and Prognosis. The significance of identification of X-linked retardation in families cannot be overemphasized. Since the syndrome is inherited as an X-linked trait and the fragile X site can be identified in 30 to 50% of families with X-linked mental retardation, early diagnosis and genetic counseling are imperative.

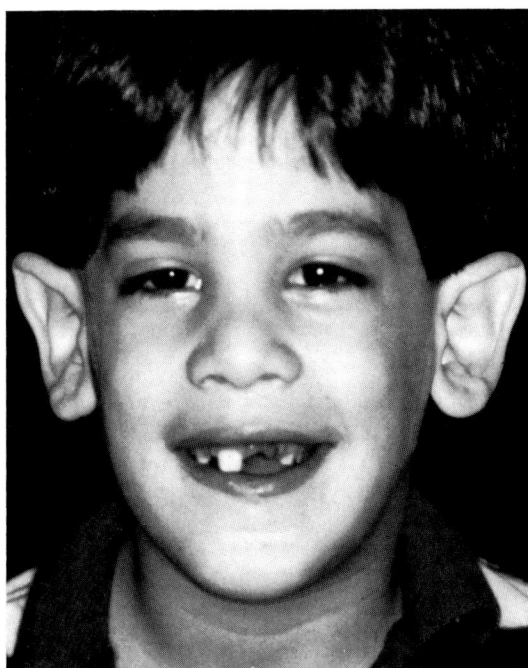

Figure 15-32. This mentally retarded male child with fragile X syndrome demonstrates the typical clinical features, including a long narrow face and large ears.

Fragile X syndrome screening of the mentally retarded population has proved to be cost-effective. Genetic counseling of families with positive histories may help to advise potential or proven carriers of the risks of bearing an affected child. The fragile X chromosome has been identified in amniotic fluid cells, which may provide for eventual prenatal screening.

Bibliography

Metabolic Conditions

Basle MF, Rebel A, Fournier JG, et al. On the trail of paramyxoviruses in Paget's disease of bone. Clin Orthop 217:9-14, 1987.

Broadus AE, Rasmussen H. Clinical evaluation of parathyroid function. Am J Med 70:475-478, 1981.

Ellis G, Connole P. Diffuse mandibular enlargement caused by osteitis deformans. Ear Nose Throat J 64:466-477, 1985.

Frederiksen NL, Wesley RK, Sciubba JJ, et al. Massive osteolysis of the maxillofacial skeleton. A clinical, radiographic, histologic, and ultrastructural study. Oral Surg 55:470-480, 1983.

Goepferd SJ. Advanced alveolar bone loss in the primary dentition. J Periodontol 52:753-757, 1981.

Hampton RE. Acromegaly and resulting myofascial pain and temporomandibular joint dysfunction. J Am Dent Assoc 114:625-631, 1987.

Heyman E, Laver J, Beer S. Prostaglandin synthetase inhibitor in Caffey's disease. J Pediatr 101:314, 1982.

Jadresic A, Banks LM, Child DF, et al. The acromegaly syndrome: relation between clinical features, growth hormone values, and radiological characteristics of the pituitary tumors. Q J Med 51:189–204, 1982.

Kjellman M, Oldfelt V, Nordenram A, et al. Five cases of hypophosphatasia with dental findings. Int J Oral Surg 2:152–158, 1973.

Lederman DA. Oral radiographic manifestations of systemic disease: bone disorders. Clin Prev Dent 5:22–26, 1983.

Melmed S, Fagin JA. Acromegaly update—etiology, diagnosis, and management. West J Med 146:328–333, 1987.

Murphy JB, Doker HC, Carter BC. Massive osteolysis: phantom bone disease. J Oral Surg 36:318–322, 1978.

Preston CJ, Yates AJP, Beneton MNC, et al. Effective short-term treatment of Paget's disease with oral etidronate. Br Med J 292:79–80, 1986.

Saul RA, Lee WH, Stevenson RE, et al. Caffey's disease revisited: further evidence of autosomal dominant inheritance with incomplete penetrance. Am J Dis Child 136:56–60, 1982.

Shear M, Copelyn M. Metastatic calcification of the oral mucosa in renal hyperparathyroidism. Br J Oral Surg 42:81–87, 1966.

Stafne EC, Austin LT. A study of dental roentgenograms in cases of Paget's disease (osteitis deformans), osteitis fibrosa cystica, and osteoma. J Am Dent Assoc 25:1202–1214, 1938.

Xhonga FA, Herle AV. The influence of hyperthyroidism on dental erosion. Oral Surg 36:349–357, 1973.

Zachariades N, Skordalaki A, Papanicolaou S, et al. Infantile cortical hyperostosis: report of two cases. J Oral Maxillofac Surg 44:644–648, 1986.

Genetic Abnormalities

Abbas KA, Majid W. Ehlers-Danlos syndrome: a case report. J Pakistan Med Assoc 31:130–132, 1981.

Beighton AP, Lord J, Dickson E. Variants of the Ehlers-Danlos syndrome: clinical, biochemical, hematological, and chromosomal features of 100 patients. Ann Rheum Dis 28:228–244, 1969.

Bell RA, McTigue DJ. Complex congenital hemihypertrophy: a case report and literature review. J Pedodontics 8:300–313, 1984.

Bhatia R, Deka RC. Treacher-Collins syndrome with deviated nasal septum. Indian J Pediatr 51:739–741, 1984.

Bjorvtan K, Gilhuus-Moe O. Oral aspects of osteopetrosis. Scand J Dent Res 87:245–252, 1979.

Braun TW, Sotereanos GC. Alveolar reconstruction in adolescent patients with cleft palates. J Oral Surg 39:510–517, 1981.

Braun TW, Sotereanos GC. Orthognathic surgical reconstruction of cleft palate deformities in adolescents. J Oral Surg 39:255–263, 1981.

Byers PH, Bonadio JF, Steinmann B. Invited editorial comment: osteogenesis imperfecta: update and perspective. Genetics 17:429–435, 1984.

Caputo PJ, Walter JH Jr. Osteogenesis imperfecta. J Am Podiatr Med Assoc 73:456–460, 1983.

Carpenter NJ, Leichtman LG, Say B. Fragile X-linked mental retardation. Am J Dis Child 136:392–398, 1982.

Christian J, Gorlin RJ, Anderson VE. The syndrome of pits of the lower lip and cleft lip and/or palate, genetic considerations. Clin Genet 2:95–103, 1971.

Chu N. Marfan syndrome and epilepsy: report of two cases and review of the literature. Epilepsia 24:49–55, 1983.

Cohen MM Sr, Cohen M Jr. The oral manifestations of trisomy 21 (Down's syndrome). Birth Defects 7:241–251, 1971.

Cutter NR, Heston LL, Davies P, et al. Alzheimer's disease and Down's syndrome: new insights. Ann Intern Med 103:566–578, 1985.

Dean DH, Hiramoto RN. Osteogenesis imperfecta congenita: dental features of a rare disease. J Oral Med 39:119–121, 1984.

El Deeb M, Messer LB, Lehnert MW, et al. Canine eruption into grafted bone in maxillary alveolar cleft defects. Cleft Palate J 19:9–16, 1982.

Dicks JL, Dennis ES. Down's syndrome and hepatitis: an evaluation of carrier status. J Am Dent Assoc 114:637–639, 1987.

Edwards JRG, Newall DR. The Pierre Robin syndrome reassessed in the light of recent research. Br J Plast Surg 38:339–342, 1985.

Fraser FC. The genetics of cleft lip and cleft palate. Am J Hum Genet 22:336–352, 1970.

Friedman E, Eisenbud L. Surgical and pathological considerations in cherubism. Int J Oral Surg 10 (Suppl 1):52–57, 1981.

Gahlo SR, Jethra SS, Goyal RK, et al. Ehlers-Danlos syndrome. J Assoc Physicians India 30:855–856, 1982.

Geormaneanu M, Iagaru N, Popescu-Miclosanu SP, et al. Congenital hemihypertrophy. Tendency to association with other abnormalities and/or tumors. Morphol Embryol (Bucur) 29:39–45, 1983.

Gott VL, Pyeritz RE, Macgovern GJ Jr, et al. Surgical treatment of aneurysms of the ascending aorta in the Marfan syndrome. N Engl J Med 314:1070–1074, 1986.

Henessy WT, Cromie WJ, Duckett JW. Congenital hemihypertrophy and associated abdominal lesions. Urology 18:576–579, 1981.

Horton WA, Schimke RN, Iyama T. Osteopetrosis: further heterogeneity. J Pediatr 97:580–585, 1980.

Hume WJ. Hemifacial hypertrophy associated with endocrine disharmony. Br Dent J 139:16–20, 1975.

Kahler SG, Burns JA, Aylsworth AS. A mild autosomal recessive form of osteopetrosis. Am J Med Genet 17:451–464, 1984.

Koch PE, Hammer WB. Case reports: cleidocranial dysostosis: review of literature and report of case. J Oral Surg 36:39–42, 1978.

Kwon HJ, Waite DE, Stickel FR, et al. The management of alveolar cleft defects. J Am Dent Assoc 102:848–853, 1981.

Levin LS, Salinas CF, Jorgenson RJ. Classification of osteogenesis imperfecta by dental characteristics. Lancet 1(8059):332–333, 1978.

Loh HS. Congenital hemifacial hypertrophy. Br Dent J 153:111–112, 1982.

McIntee RA, Moore IJ, Yonkers AJ. A general review of maxillofacial cleft deformities with emphasis on dental anomalies. Ear Nose Throat J 65:286–290, 1986.

Miekicki CM. Marfan's syndrome. AANA J 51:142–145, 1983.

Mixon JC, Dev VG. Understanding the fragile X syndrome. Ala J Med Sci 21:284–286, 1984.

Miyamato RT, House WF. Neurologic manifestations of the osteopetroses. Arch Otolaryngol 106:210–214, 1980.

Monasky GE, Winkler S, Icenhower JB, et al. Cleidocranial dysostosis—two case reports. NY State Dent J 49:236–238, 1983.

Pasyayan HM, Lewis M. Clinical experience with the Robin sequence. Cleft Palate J 21:270–276, 1984.

Pyeritz RE, McKusick V. Basic defects in the Marfan syndrome. N Engl J Med 305:1011–1012, 1981.

Ranta R. Incomplete median cleft of the lower lip associated with cleft palate, the Pierre Robin anomaly or hypodontia. Int J Oral Surg 13:555–558, 1984.

Reade P, McKellar G, Radden B. Unilateral mandibular cherubism: brief review and case report. J Maxillofac Surg 22:189–194, 1984.

Rintala A, Ranta R, Stegars T. On the pathogenesis of cleft palate in the Pierre Robin syndrome. Scand J Plast Reconstr Surg 18:237–240, 1984.

Rosen HM, Witaker LA. Cranial base dynamics in craniofacial dysostosis. J Maxillofac Surg 12:56–61, 1984.

Sandham A. Classification of clefting deformity. Early Hum Dev 12:81–85, 1985.

Scarbrough PR, Cosper P, Finley SC, et al. Fragile X syndrome—an overview. Ala J Med Sci 21:68–72, 1984.

Sculerati N, Jacobs JB. Congenital facial hemihypertrophy: report of a case with airway compromise. Head Neck Surg 8:124–128, 1985.

Shellhart WC, Casamassimo PS, Hagerman RJ, et al. Oral findings in fragile X syndrome. Am J Med Genet 23:179–187, 1986.

Shprintzen RJ, Siegel-Sadewitz VL, Amato J, et al. Anomalies associated with cleft lip, cleft palate, or both. Am J Med Genet 20:585–595, 1985.

Steiner M, Gould AR, Means WR. Osteomyelitis of the mandible associated with osteopetrosis. J Oral Maxillofac Surg 41:395–405, 1983.

Stewart RE, Barber TK, Troutman KC, et al. (eds). Pediatric Dentistry: Scientific Foundations and Clinical Practice. CV Mosby Co, St Louis, 1982.

Sunderland EP, Smith CJ. The teeth in osteogenesis and dentinogenesis imperfecta. Br Dent J 149:287–289, 1980.

Svoboda PJ, Mendieta C, Reeve CM. Albers-Schönberg disease complicated with periodontal disease. J Periodontol 54:10:592–597, 1983.

Trimble LD, West RA, McNeil RW. Cleidocranial dysplasia: comprehensive treatment of the dentofacial abnormalities. J Am Dent Assoc 105:661–666, 1982.

Trusler S, Beatty-DeSana J. Fragile X syndrome: a public health concern. Am J Public Health 75:771–772, 1985.

Turvey TA, Vig K, Moriarty J, et al. Delayed bone grafting in the cleft maxilla and palate: a retrospective multidisciplinary analysis. Am J Orthod 86:244–256, 1984.

Whyte M, Murphy W, Fallon M, et al. Osteopetrosis, renal tubular acidosis and basal ganglia calcification in three sisters. Am J Med 69:64–74, 1980.

Winship IM. Ehlers-Danlos syndrome in the Western Cape. S Afr Med J 67:509–511, 1985.

Younai F, Eisenbud L, Sciubba JJ. Osteopetrosis: a case report including gross and microscopic findings in the mandible at autopsy. Oral Surg Oral Med Oral Pathol 65:214–221, 1988.

Zachariades N, Papanicolaou S, Xypolyta A, et al. Cherubism. Int J Oral Surg 14:138–145, 1985.

Chapter 16

Abnormalities of Teeth

ALTERATIONS IN SIZE
Microdontia
Macrodontia
ALTERATIONS IN SHAPE
Gemination
Fusion
Concrescence
Dilaceration
Dens Invaginatus
Dens Evaginatus
Taurodontism
Supernumerary Roots
Enamel Pearls
Attrition, Abrasion, Erosion
ALTERATIONS IN NUMBER
Anodontia
   Impaction
Supernumerary Teeth
DEFECTS OF ENAMEL
Environmental Defects of Enamel
Amelogenesis Imperfecta
DEFECTS OF DENTIN
Dentinogenesis Imperfecta
Dentin Dysplasia
DEFECTS OF ENAMEL AND DENTIN
Regional Odontodysplasia
ABNORMALITIES OF DENTAL PULP
Pulp Calcification
Internal Resorption
External Resorption
ALTERATIONS IN COLOR
Exogenous Stains
Endogenous Stains

ALTERATIONS IN SIZE

Microdontia

Generalized microdontia is a term used to indicate that all teeth in the dentition appear smaller than normal. Teeth may actually be measurably smaller than normal, as in pituitary dwarfism, or they may be relatively small in comparison with a large mandible and maxilla.

Focal or localized microdontia refers to a single tooth that is smaller than normal (Fig. 16–1). The shape of these microdonts is also often altered with the reduced size. This phenomenon is most commonly seen with maxillary lateral incisors in which the tooth crown appears cone- or peg-shaped prompting the designation *peg lateral* (Fig. 16–2). An autosomal dominant inheritance pattern has been associated with this condition. Peg laterals are of no significance, other than cosmetic appearance. The second most commonly seen microdont is the maxillary third molar, followed by supernumerary teeth.

Macrodontia

Generalized macrodontia is a term used to indicate the appearance of enlarged teeth throughout the dentition. This may be absolute, as seen in pituitary gigantism, or it may

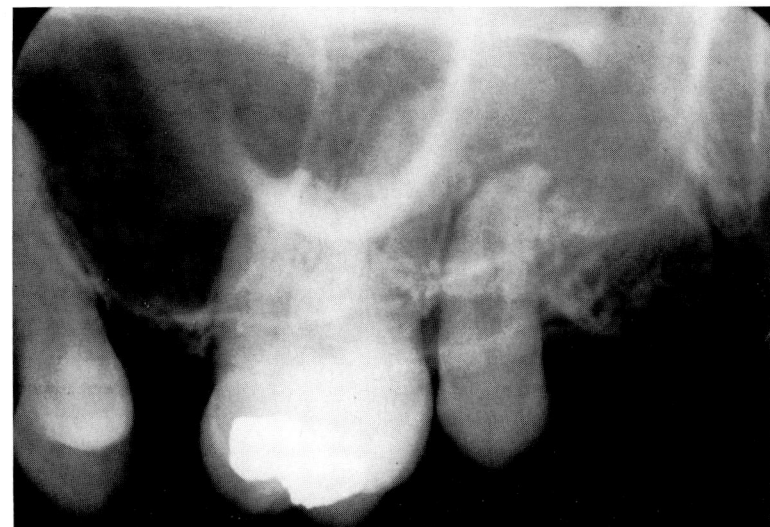

Figure 16–1. Microdont in third molar position.

be relative owing to a disproportionately small maxilla and mandible. The latter results in crowding of teeth and possibly an abnormal eruption pattern because of insufficient arch space.

Focal or localized macrodontia refers to an abnormally large tooth or group of teeth (Fig. 16–3). This relatively uncommon condition is usually seen with mandibular third molars. In the rare condition known as hemifacial hypertrophy, teeth on the affected side are abnormally large compared with the unaffected side.

ALTERATIONS IN SHAPE

Gemination

Gemination is defined as the attempt to make two teeth from a single enamel organ (Fig. 16–4). The typical result is partial cleavage, with the appearance of two crowns that share the same root canal. Occasionally, complete cleavage or twinning occurs, resulting in two teeth from one tooth germ. Although trauma has been suggested as a possible cause,

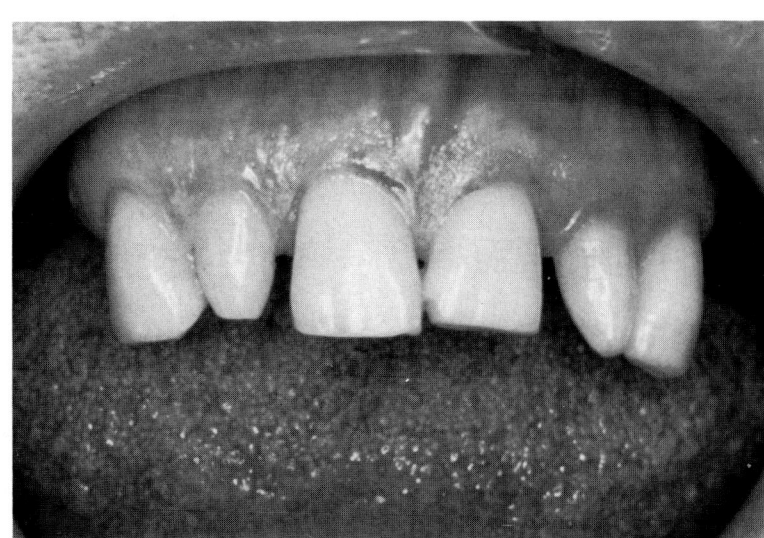

Figure 16–2. Peg laterals.

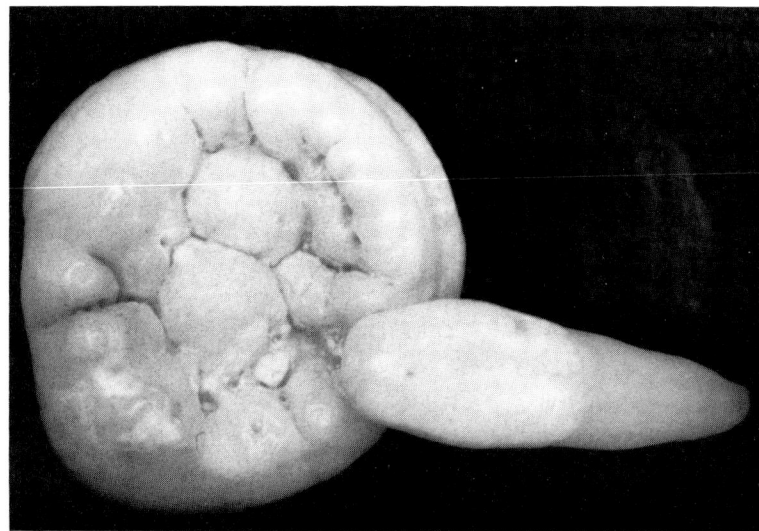

Figure 16–3. Occlusal view of a macrodont (molar) and a peg lateral.

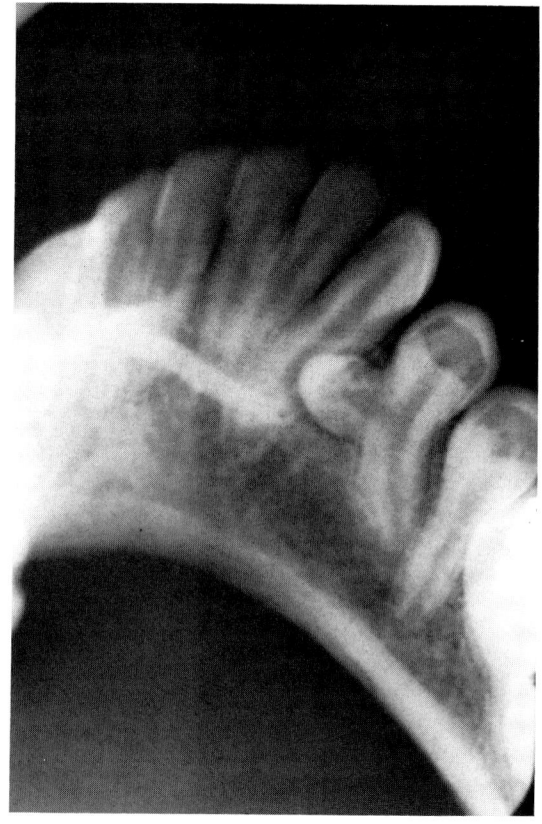

Figure 16–4. Gemination of mandibular first premolar. (Courtesy of Dr. R. Courtney.)

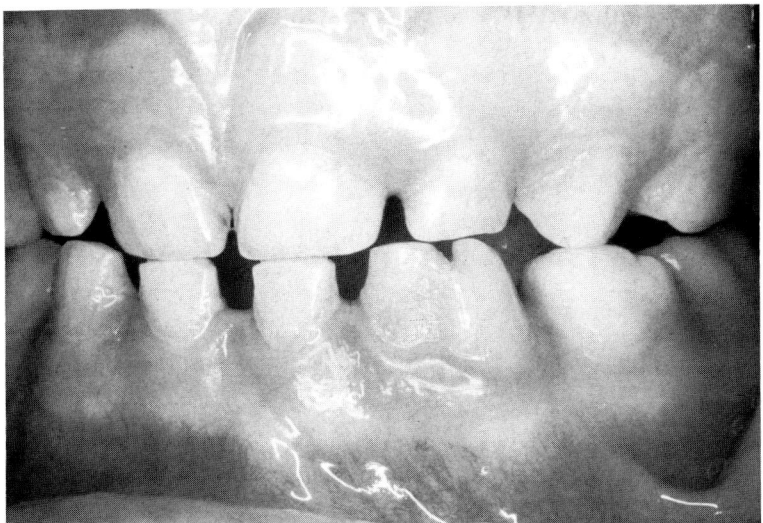

Figure 16–5. Fusion of primary incisor and cuspid.

the etiology of gemination is unknown. These teeth may be cosmetically unacceptable and may cause crowding.

Fusion

Fusion is defined as the joining of two developing tooth germs, resulting in a single large tooth structure (Fig. 16–5). The fusion process may involve the entire length of the teeth, or it may involve the roots only, in which case cementum and dentin are shared. Root canals may also be separate or shared. It may be impossible to differentiate fusion of normal and supernumerary teeth from gemination.

The cause of this condition is unknown, although trauma has been suggested.

Concrescence

Concrescence is a form of fusion in which the adjacent already-formed teeth are joined by cementum (Fig. 16–6). This may take place before or after eruption of teeth and is believed to be related to trauma or overcrowding. Concrescence is most commonly seen in association with the maxillary second and third molars. This condition is of no significance, unless one of the teeth involved requires extraction. Surgical sectioning may be required to save the other tooth.

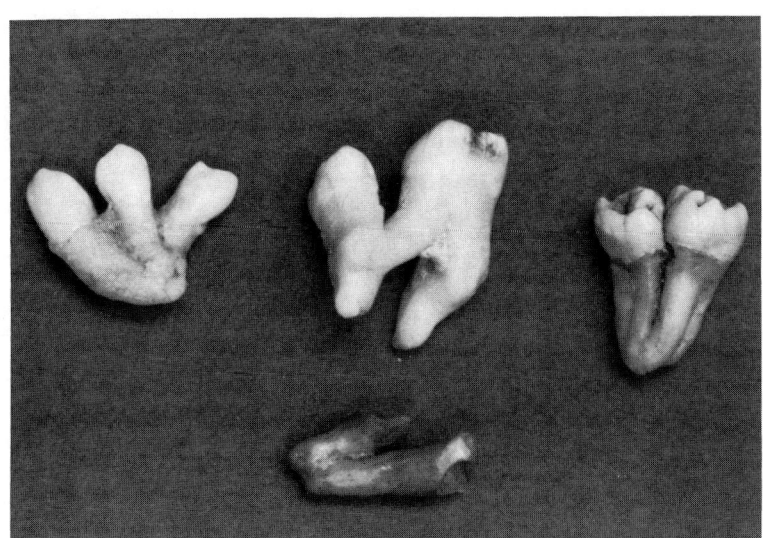

Figure 16–6. Concrescence.

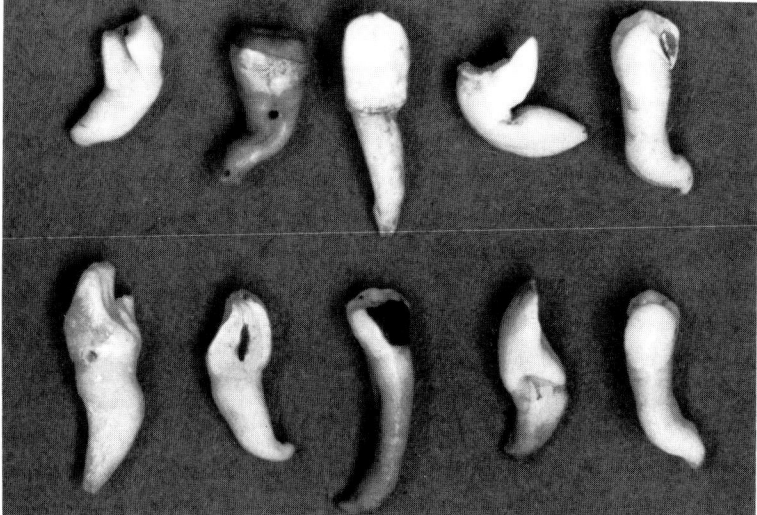

Figure 16–7. Dilaceration.

Dilaceration

Dilaceration refers to the extraordinary curving or angulation of tooth roots (Fig. 16–7). The cause of this condition has been related to trauma during root development. Movement of the crown, or of the crown and part of the root from the remaining developing root, may result in sharp angulation after the tooth completes development. Hereditary factors are believed to be involved in a small number of cases. Eruption generally continues without problems. However, extraction may be difficult. Obviously, if root canal fillings are required in these teeth, the procedure is challenging.

Dens Invaginatus

Also known as dens in dente or tooth within a tooth, dens invaginatus is an uncommon tooth anomaly that represents an exaggeration or accentuation of the lingual pit (Fig. 16–8). This defect ranges in severity from superficial, in which only the crown is affected, to deep,

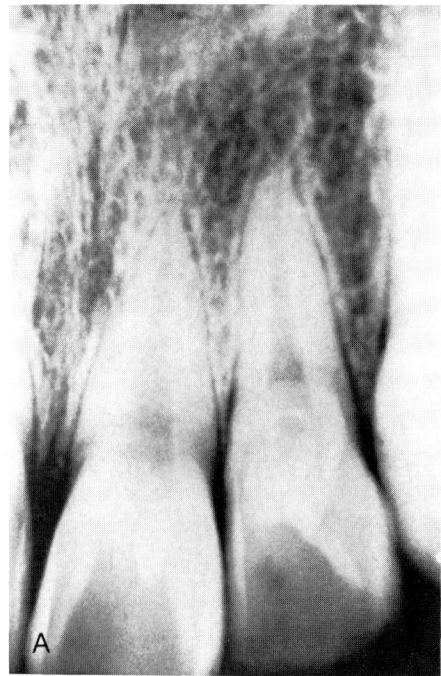
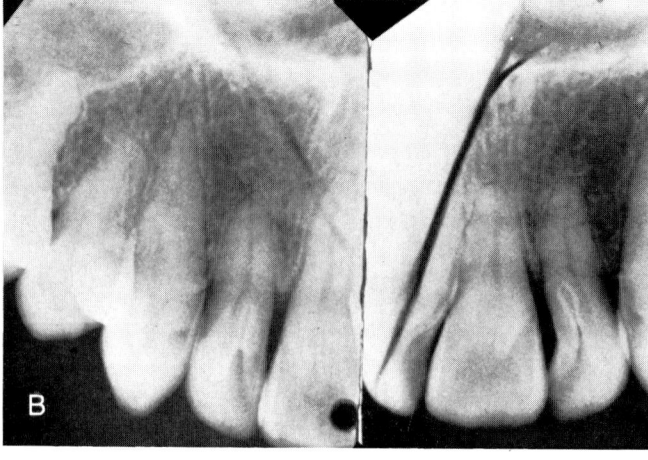

Figure 16–8. *A* and *B*, Dens invaginatus of maxillary lateral incisors.

ABNORMALITIES OF TEETH 465

in which both the crown and the root are involved. The permanent maxillary lateral incisors are most commonly involved, although any anterior tooth may be affected. Bilateral involvement is frequently seen. The etiology of this developmental condition is unknown. Genetic factors are believed to be involved in only a small percentage of cases.

Because the defect cannot be kept free of plaque and bacteria, dens invaginatus predisposes the tooth to early decay and subsequent pulpitis. Prophylactic filling of the pit is recommended to avoid this complication. Because the defect may often be identified on radiographic examination before tooth eruption, the patient can be prepared in advance of the procedure. In cases in which pulpitis has led to non-vitality, endodontic procedures may salvage the affected tooth.

Dens Evaginatus

This is a relatively common developmental condition affecting predominantly premolar teeth. It has been reported almost exclusively in individuals of the Mongoloid race (Asians, Eskimos, Native Americans) (Fig. 16–9). The defect, frequently bilateral, is an anomalous tubercle or cusp located in the center of the occlusal surface. Because of occlusal abrasion, the tubercle wears relatively quickly, causing early exposure of an accessory pulp horn that extends into the tubercle. This may result in periapical pathology in young caries-free teeth, often before completion of root development and apical closure, making root canal fillings more difficult. Judicious grinding of the opposing tooth or the accessory tubercle to stimulate secondary dentin formation may prevent

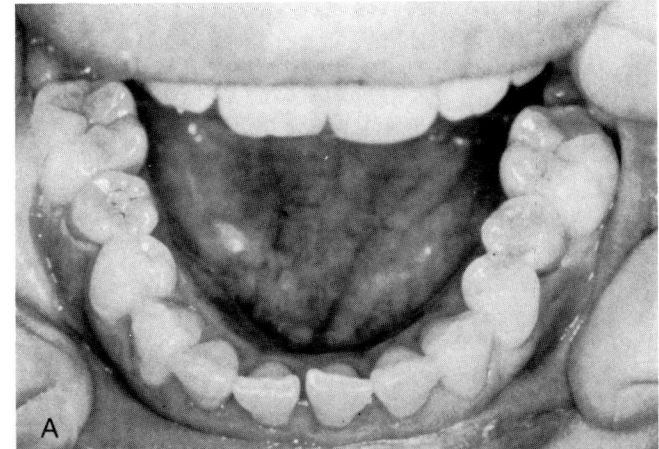

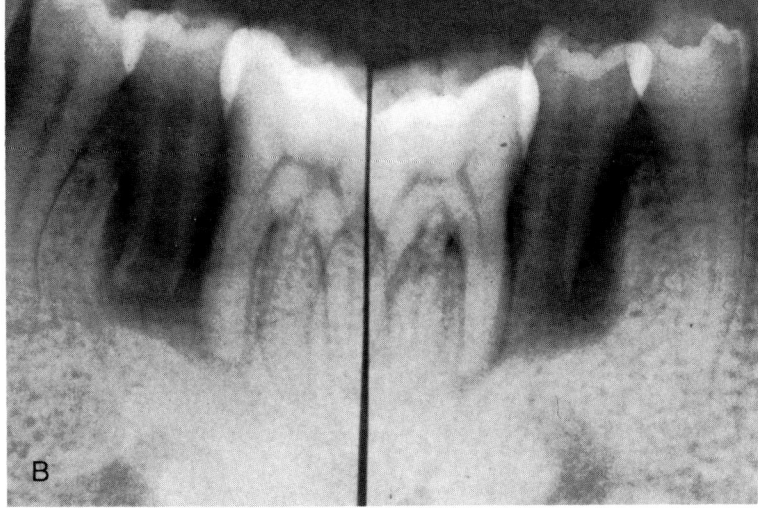

Figure 16–9. *A* and *B*, Dens evaginatus of second premolars. Note apical lucencies resulting from pulp exposures. (Courtesy of E. S. Senia.)

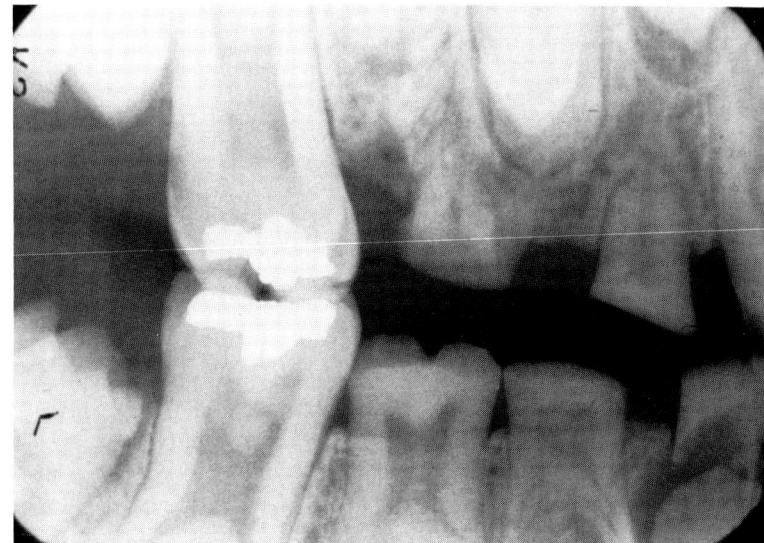

Figure 16–10. Taurodontism.

Taurodontism

This term refers to teeth that have elongated crowns or apically displaced furcations, resulting in pulp chambers that have increased apical-occlusal height (Fig. 16–10). Because this abnormality resembles teeth in bulls and other ungulates, the term "taurodontism" was coined. Varying degrees of severity may be seen, but subclassifications that have been developed to describe them appear to be of academic interest only. Taurodontism may be seen as an isolated incident, in families, in association with syndromes such as Down's and Klinefelter's, and in past primitive populations such as Neanderthals. Although taurodontism is generally an uncommon finding, it has been reported to have a relatively high prevalence in Eskimos, and it has been reported to be as high as 11% in a Middle Eastern population. Other than a possible relationship to other genetically determined abnormalities, taurodontism is of little clinical significance. No treatment is required.

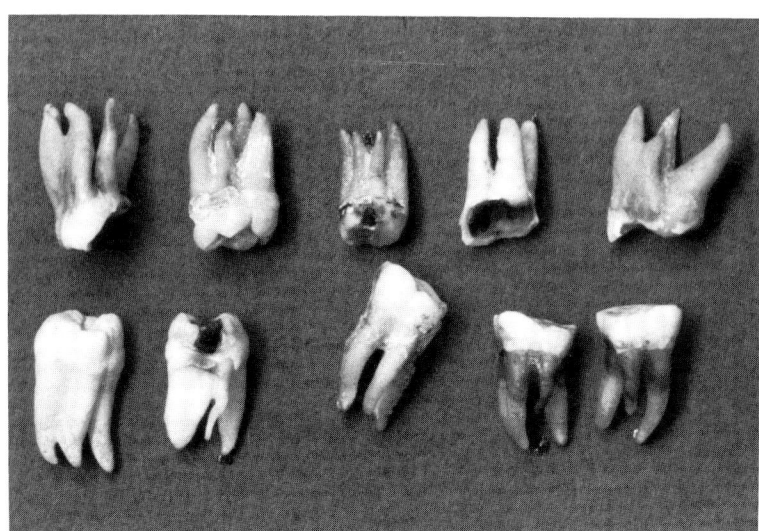

Figure 16–11. Supernumerary roots.

Supernumerary Roots

Accessory roots are most commonly seen in mandibular canines, premolars, and molars (especially third molars). They are rarely found in upper anterior teeth and mandibular incisors (Fig. 16–11). Radiographic recognition of an extraordinary number of roots becomes important when extractions or root canal fillings are necessary.

Enamel Pearls

Droplets of ectopic enamel or so-called enamel pearls may occasionally be found on the roots of teeth (Fig. 16–12). They occur most commonly in the bifurcation or trifurcation of teeth but may appear on single-rooted premolar teeth as well. Maxillary molars are more frequently affected than are mandibular molars. These deposits are occasionally supported by dentin and rarely have a pulp horn extending into them. This developmental disturbance of enamel formation may be detected on radiographic examination. It is generally of little significance, except when located in an area of periodontal disease. In such cases, it may contribute to the extension of a periodontal pocket, since periodontal ligament attachment would not be expected, and hygiene would be more difficult.

Attrition, Abrasion, Erosion

Attrition is the physiologic wearing of teeth resulting from mastication. It is an age-related process and varies from one individual to another. Factors such as diet quality, dentition, jaw musculature, and chewing habits can significantly influence the pattern and extent of attrition.

Abrasion is the pathologic wearing of teeth as a result of an abnormal habit or abnormal use of abrasive substances orally. Pipe smoking, tobacco chewing, aggressive tooth brushing, and use of abrasive dentifrices are among the more common causes (Figs. 16–13 and 16–14). The location and pattern of abrasion is directly dependent upon the cause, with so-called toothbrush abrasion along the cementoenamel junction an easily recognized pattern.

Erosion is the loss of tooth structure from a non-bacterial chemical process (Fig. 16–15). Most commonly, acids are involved in the dissolution process from either an external or an internal source. Externally, the acid may be found in the work environment (e.g., battery manufacturing) or in the diet (e.g., excessive use of citrus fruits). The internal source of acid is most probably from gastric contents following regurgitation. This may be seen in any disorder in which chronic vomiting is a part. Self-induced vomiting as a component of anorexia nervosa or bulimia syndrome has become an increasingly important cause of dental erosion and other oral abnormalities. The pattern of erosion associated with vomiting is usually generalized tooth loss on lingual surfaces. However, all surfaces may be affected, especially in individuals who compensate for fluid loss by excessive intake of fruit juices. In many cases of tooth erosion, no cause is found.

ALTERATIONS IN NUMBER

Anodontia

Absence of teeth is known as anodontia. It is further qualified as complete anodontia,

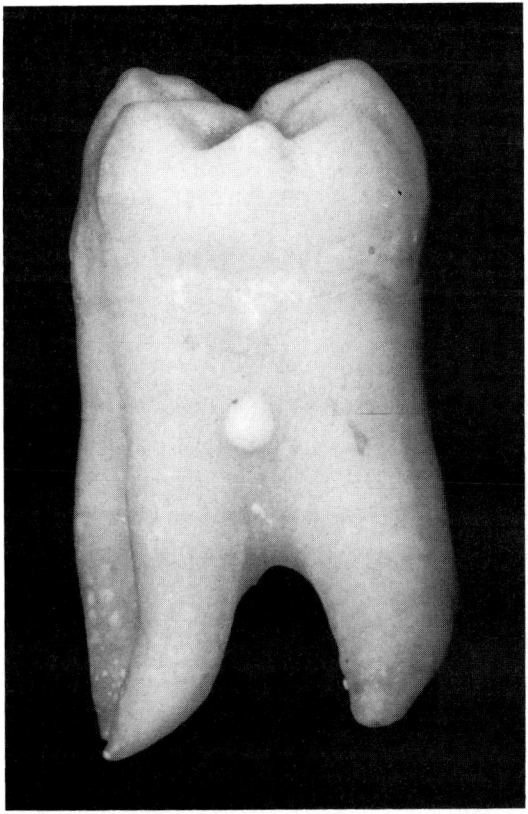

Figure 16–12. Enamel pearl.

468 ABNORMALITIES OF TEETH

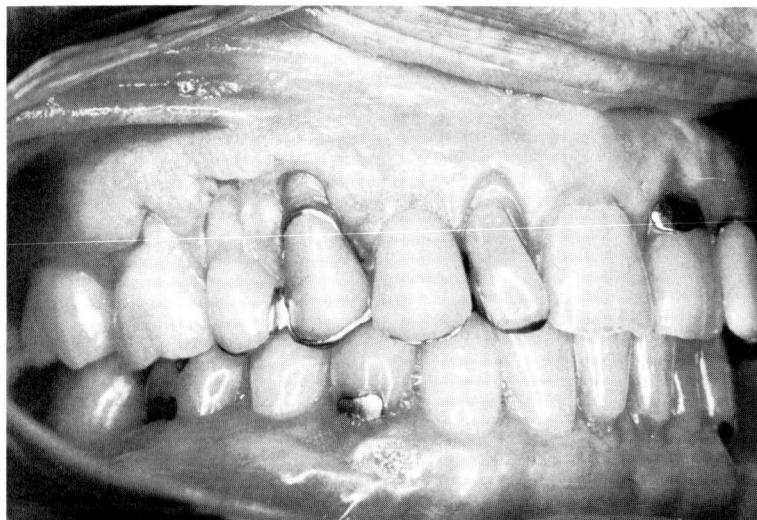

Figure 16–13. Toothbrush abrasion of cervical zone of maxillary teeth.

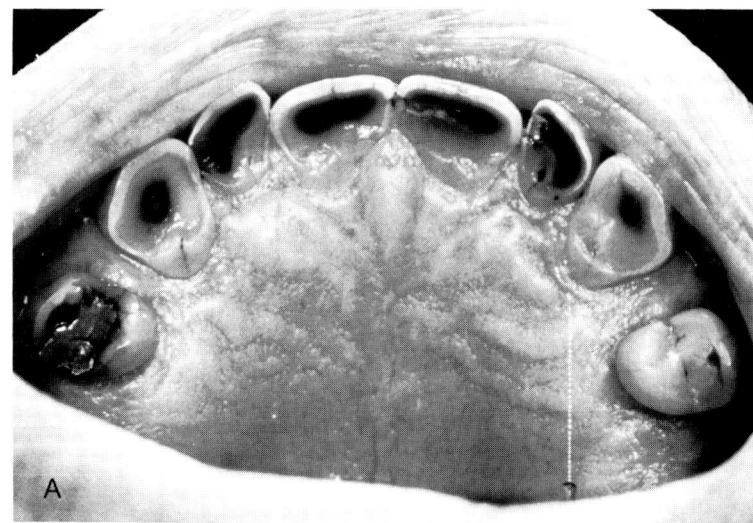

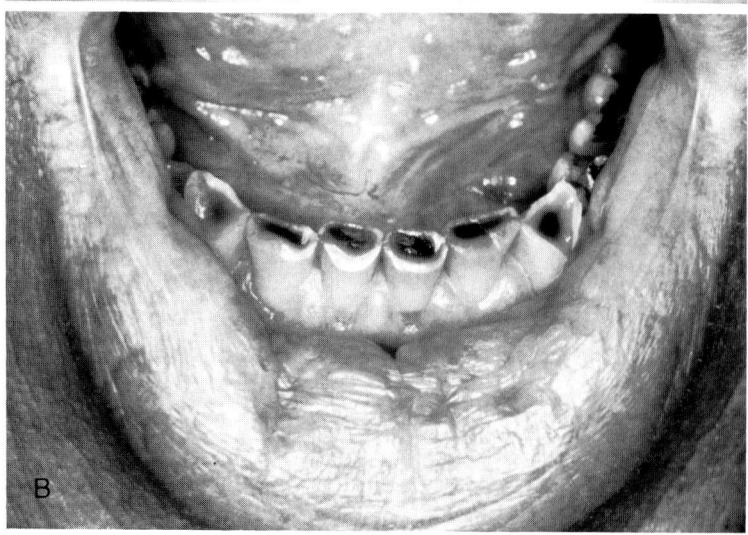

Figure 16–14. *A* and *B*, Tooth abrasion from cigar chewing.

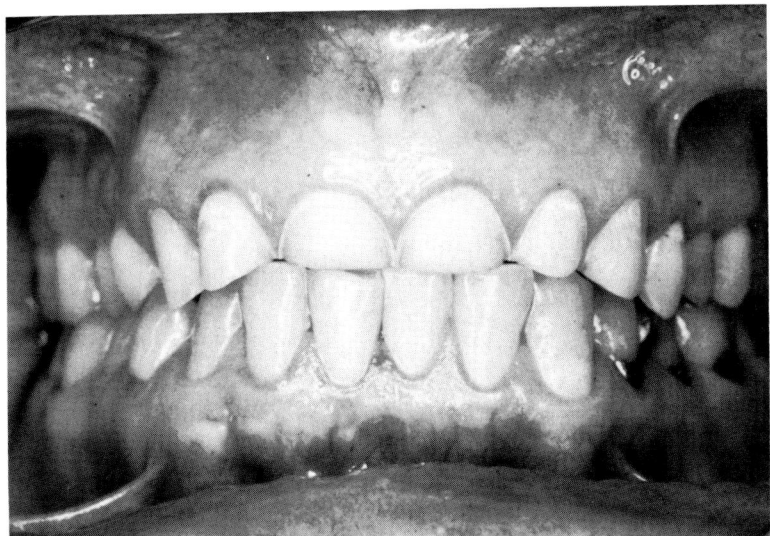

Figure 16-15. Erosion of maxillary anterior teeth.

when all teeth are missing; as partial anodontia, when one or several teeth are missing; as pseudoanodontia, when teeth are absent clinically because of impaction or delayed eruption; and as false anodontia, when teeth have been exfoliated or extracted. Partial anodontia is relatively common. Congenitally missing teeth are usually third molars, followed by maxillary lateral incisors and second premolars (Fig. 16-16). The cause of partial anodontia is unknown, although hereditary factors are frequently involved. Complete anodontia is rare but is often associated with a syndrome known as hereditary ectodermal dysplasia, which is usually transmitted as an X-linked recessive disorder. Partial anodontia is more typical of this syndrome, however (Fig. 16-17). The few teeth that are present are usually conical.

Impaction

Impaction of teeth (pseudoanodontia) is a common event that most frequently affects the mandibular third molars and maxillary cuspids (Fig. 16-18). Less commonly, premolars, mandibular cuspids, and second molars are involved. It is very rare to see impactions of incisors and first molars. Impaction occurs because of obstruction from crowding or from some other physical barrier. Occasionally, it may be due to an abnormal eruption path, presumably because of unusual orientation of

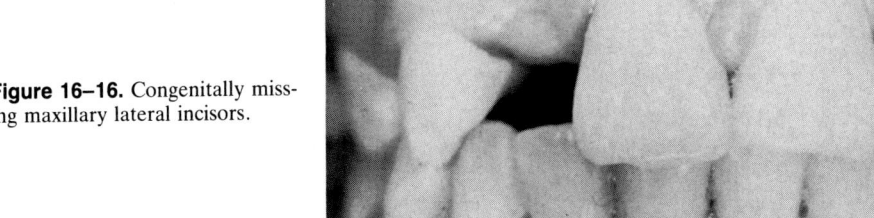

Figure 16-16. Congenitally missing maxillary lateral incisors.

470 ABNORMALITIES OF TEETH

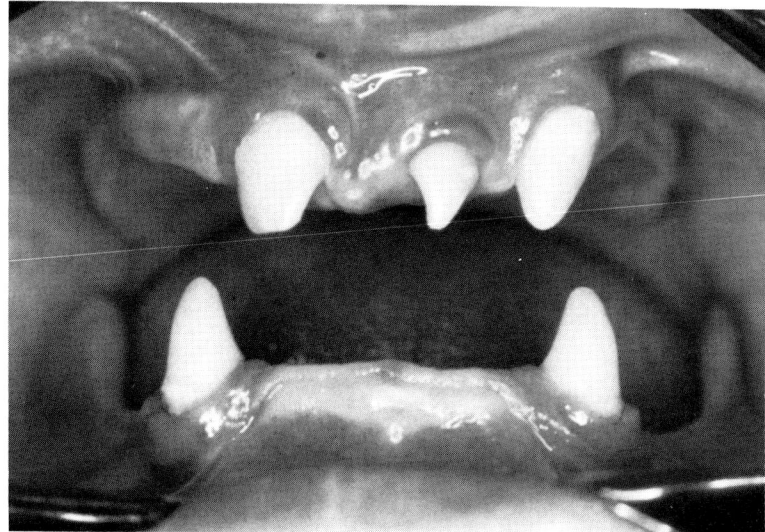

Figure 16–17. Partial anodontia in a patient with hereditary ectodermal dysplasia.

Figure 16–18. Impaction of maxillary third molar. Note supernumerary microdont and pulp stones.

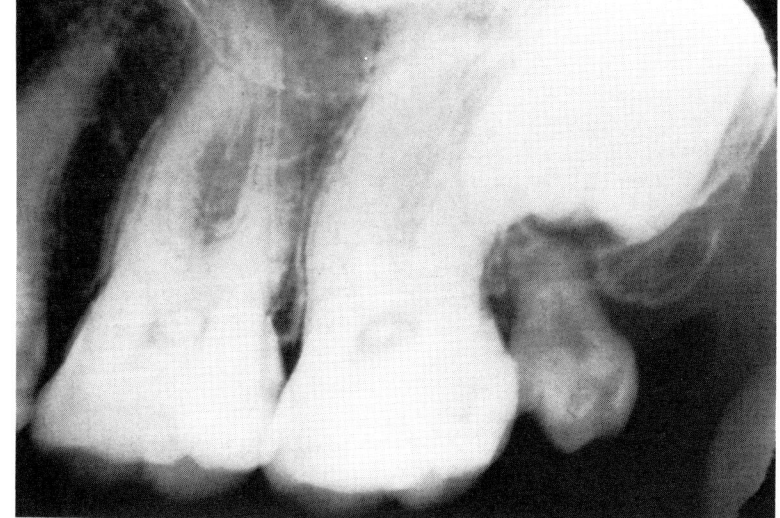

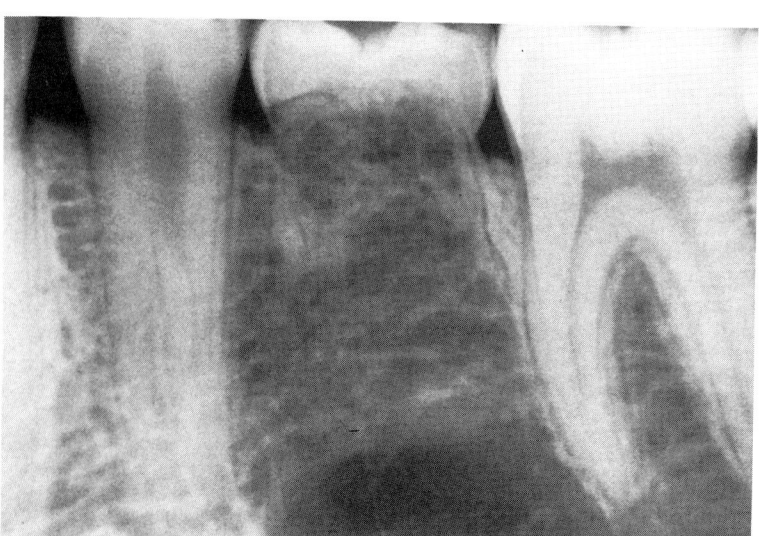

Figure 16–19. Ankylosis of primary molar tooth. Note congenitally missing subjacent permanent tooth.

ABNORMALITIES OF TEETH 471

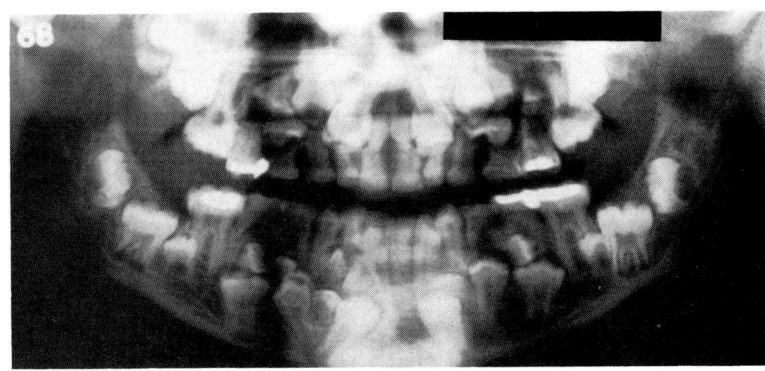

Figure 16–20. Supernumerary and impacted teeth in a patient with cleidocranial dysplasia.

the tooth germ. *Ankylosis*, the fusion of a tooth to surrounding bone, is another cause of impaction. This usually occurs in association with erupted primary molars (Fig. 16–19). This may result in impaction of a subjacent permanent tooth. The reason for ankylosis is unknown, but it is believed to be related to periapical inflammation and subsequent bone repair. With the focal loss of the periodontal ligament, bone and cementum become inextricably mixed, causing "fusion" of tooth to alveolar bone.

Supernumerary Teeth

Extra or supernumerary teeth in the dentition most probably result from continued proliferation of the permanent or primary dental lamina to form a third tooth germ. The resulting teeth may have a normal morphology or may be rudimentary and miniature. Most are isolated events, although some may be familial, and others may be syndrome associated (Gardner's syndrome and cleidocranial dysplasia [Fig. 16–20]). Supernumerary teeth are found more often in the permanent than in the primary dentition and are much more frequently seen in the maxilla than in the mandible (10:1) (Fig. 16–21). The anterior midline of the maxilla is the most common site, in which case the supernumerary tooth is known as a mesiodens (Fig. 16–22). The maxillary molar area (fourth molar or paramolar) is the second most common site. The significance of supernumerary teeth is that they occupy space. When they are impacted, they may block the eruption of other teeth, or they may cause delayed eruption or maleruption of adjacent teeth. If supernumerary teeth erupt, they may may cause malalignment of the dentition, and they may be cosmetically objectionable.

Supernumerary teeth appearing at the time of birth, known as *natal teeth*, are believed to

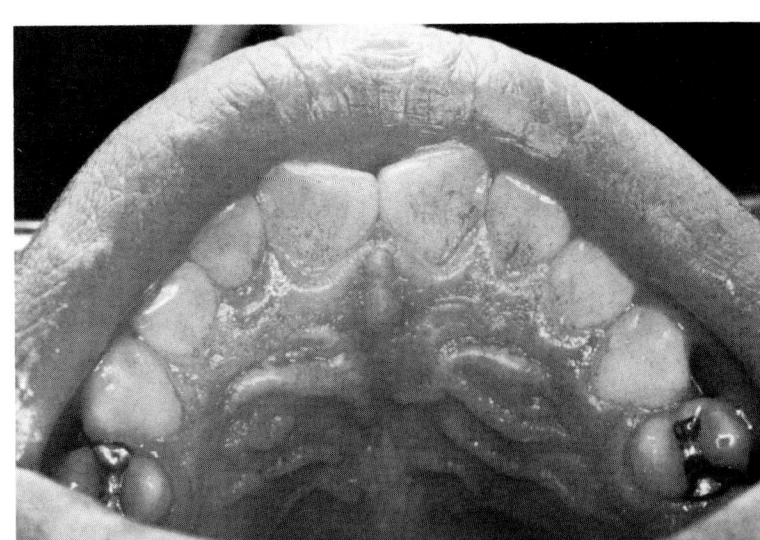

Figure 16–21. Supernumerary incisor teeth.

ABNORMALITIES OF TEETH

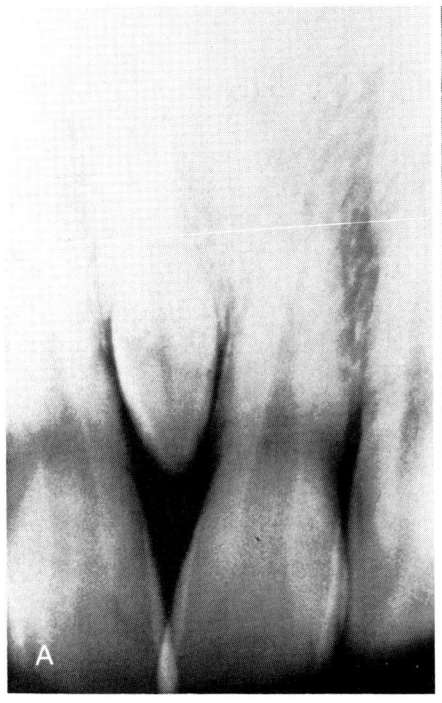

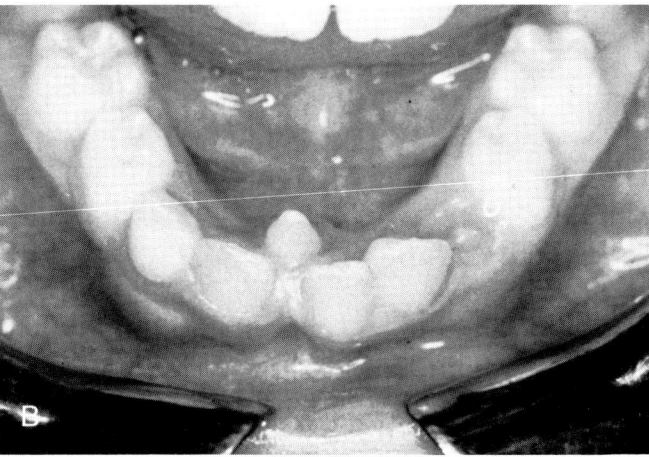

Figure 16–22. *A* and *B*, Mesiodens.

be a rare event (Fig. 16–23). More commonly seen are prematurely erupted deciduous teeth. Not to be confused with both these phenomena is the appearance of the common gingival or dental lamina cysts of the newborn.

Supernumerary teeth appearing after the loss of the permanent teeth are known as *postpermanent dentition*. This is generally regarded as a rare event. Most cases of teeth appearing after extraction of the permanent teeth are believed to be due to the eventual eruption of previously impacted teeth.

DEFECTS OF ENAMEL

Environmental Defects of Enamel

During enamel formation, ameloblasts are susceptible to various external factors that may be reflected in erupted teeth. Metabolic injury, if severe enough and long enough, can cause defects in quantity and shape of enamel or in the quality and color of enamel. Quantitatively defective enamel, when of normal hardness, is known as enamel hypoplasia. Qualitatively de-

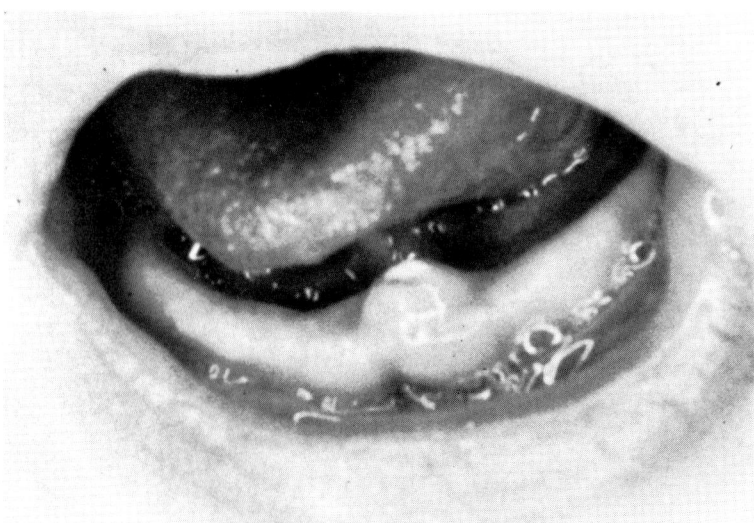

Figure 16–23. Natal tooth.

fective enamel, in which normal amounts of enamel are produced but are hypomineralized, is known as enamel hypocalcification. In this defect, the enamel is softer than normal. The extent of the enamel defect is dependent upon three conditions: (1) the intensity of the etiologic factor, (2) the duration of the factor's presence, and (3) the time at which the factor occurs during crown development. The factors that lead to ameloblast damage are highly varied, although the clinical signs of defective enamel are the same.

Etiologic factors may occur locally, affecting only a single tooth, or they may act systemically, affecting all teeth in which enamel is being formed. Local trauma or abscess formation can adversely affect the ameloblasts overlying a developing crown, resulting in enamel hypocalcification or hypoplasia. Affected teeth may have areas of coronal discoloration, or they may have actual pits and irregularities. This is most commonly seen in permanent teeth in which the overlying deciduous tooth becomes abscessed or is physically forced into the enamel organ of the permanent tooth. The resulting hypoplastic or hypocalcified permanent tooth is sometimes known as Turner's tooth (Fig. 16–24).

For systemic factors to have an effect on developing permanent teeth, they must generally occur after birth and before the age of 6 years. During this time the crowns of all permanent teeth (with the exception of the third molars) develop. Because most enamel defects affect anterior teeth and first molars, systemic factors will have occurred predominantly during the first year and a half of life (Fig. 16–25). Primary teeth and possibly the

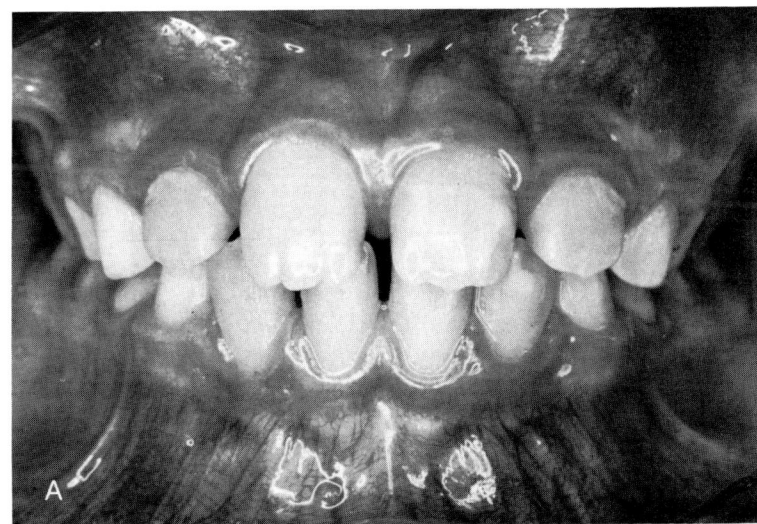
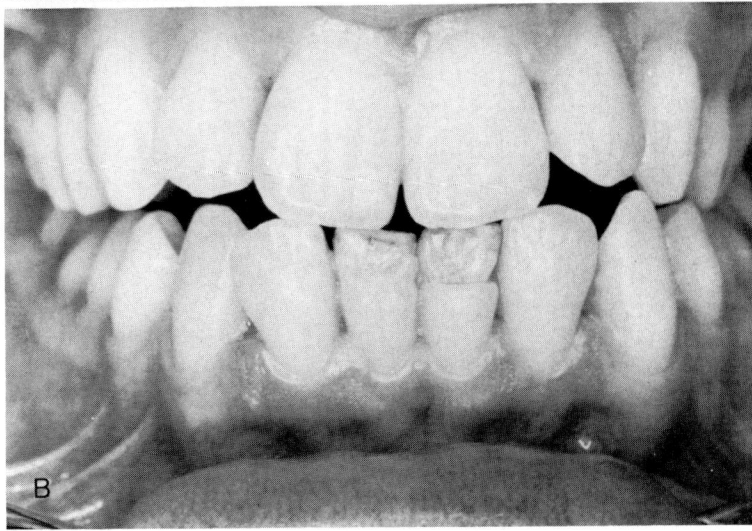

Figure 16–24. *A,* Hypocalcified maxillary left-central incisor (Turner's tooth). *B,* Hypoplastic mandibular central incisors.

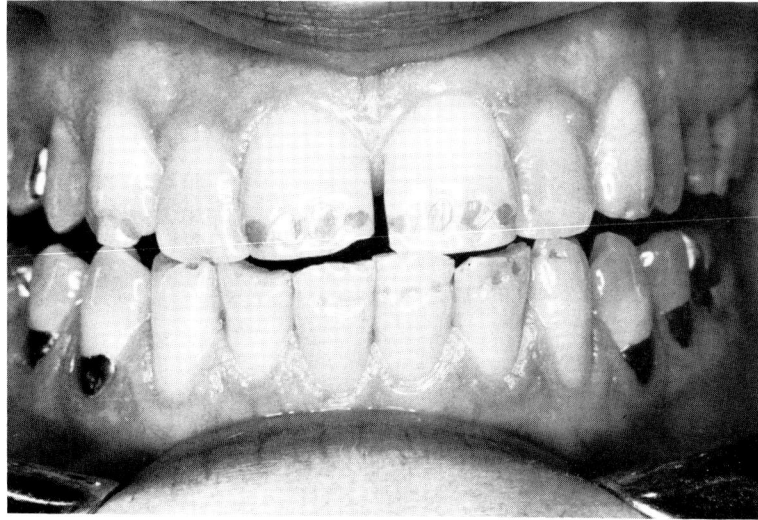

Figure 16–25. Environmental hypoplasia of anterior teeth.

tips of first permanent molars and permanent central incisors may reflect ameloblast dysfunction occurring *in utero,* as these are the teeth undergoing enamel calcification during this period. The specific causes of systemically induced enamel defects are often obscure but are usually attributed to childhood infectious diseases. This, however, has not been well substantiated with research data. Other cited causes of enamel hypoplasia or hypocalcification include nutritional defects such as rickets (Fig. 16–26), congenital syphilis, birth trauma (neonatal line in primary teeth), fluoride, and idiopathic factors. The enamel hypoplasia that may be seen with congenital syphilis is rather characteristic. The *in utero* infection by *Treponema pallidum* affects the developing permanent incisors and first molars (Fig. 16–27). The incisors, also known as Hutchinson's incisors, are tapered incisally and are notched centrally on the incisal edge. The molars, also known as mulberry molars, show a lobulated or crenated occlusal surface.

Ingestion of drinking water containing fluoride at levels greater than 1 part per million during the time crowns are being formed may result in enamel hypoplasia or hypocalcification, also known as fluorosis (Fig. 16–28). Endemic fluorosis is known to occur in areas where the drinking water contains excessive naturally occurring fluoride. As with other causative agents, the extent of damage is dependent upon duration, timing, and intensity or concentration. Mild to moderate fluorosis

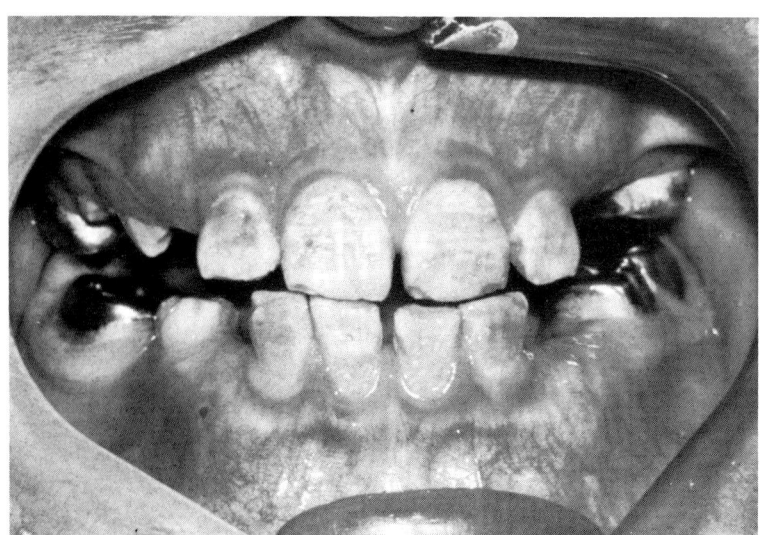

Figure 16–26. Enamel hypoplasia due to rickets.

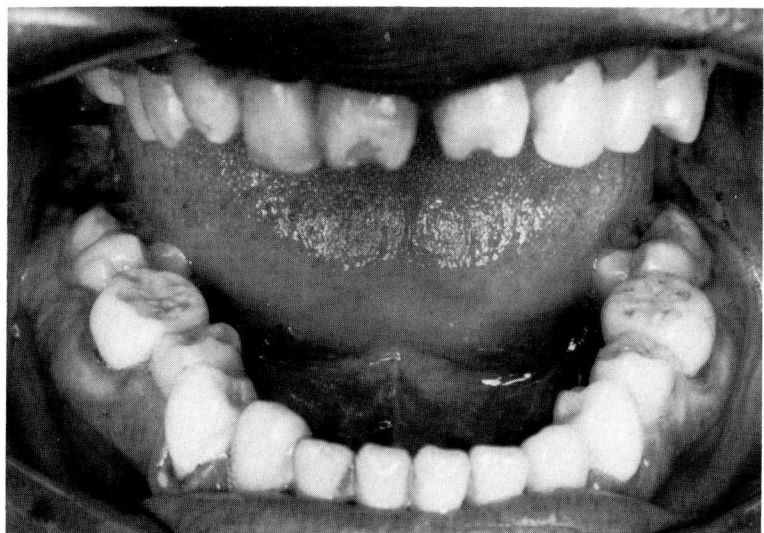

Figure 16–27. Notched incisors and mulberry molars resulting from congenital syphilis.

ranges clinically from white enamel spots to "mottled" brown and white discolorations. Severe fluorosis appears as pitted, irregular, and discolored enamel. Although fluoride-induced enamel hypoplasia or hypocalcification is caries resistant, it may be cosmetically objectionable, making aesthetic dental restorations desirable.

Amelogenesis Imperfecta

Amelogenesis imperfecta refers to a group of similar-appearing hereditary disorders of enamel formation in both dentitions. Most cases fall into one of two major types, hypoplastic or hypocalcified. Recently, a third type known as hypomaturation has been added to the list. Numerous subtypes of the three major groups are also recognized; these are based on different inheritance patterns and clinical appearances. The hereditary patterns range from autosomal dominant or recessive to X-linked dominant or recessive.

In the hypoplastic type, teeth erupt with insufficient amounts of enamel (Fig. 16–29), ranging from pits and grooves in one patient to complete absence (aplasia) in another. Because of reduced enamel thickness in some cases, abnormal contour and absent interproximal contact points may be evident. In the hypocalcified type, the quantity of enamel is normal, but it is soft and friable, so that it fractures and wears readily (Fig. 16–30). The color of the teeth varies from tooth to tooth

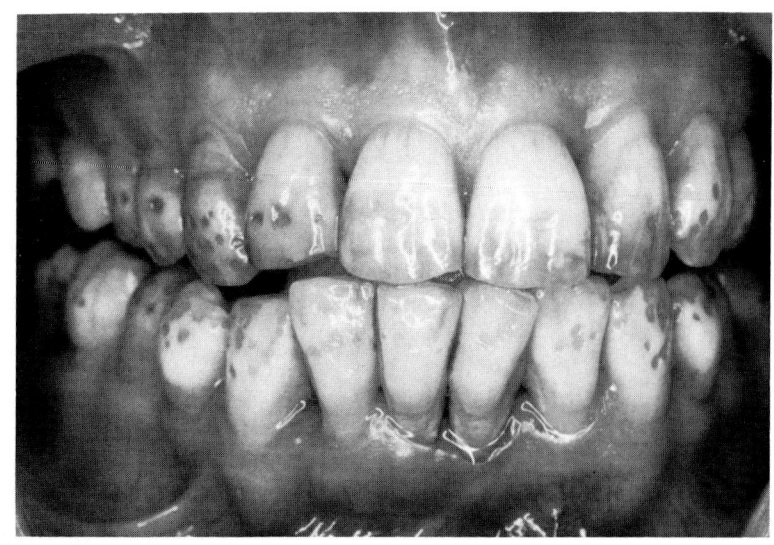

Figure 16–28. Enamel hypoplasia (fluorosis) resulting from excessive levels of fluoride in drinking water.

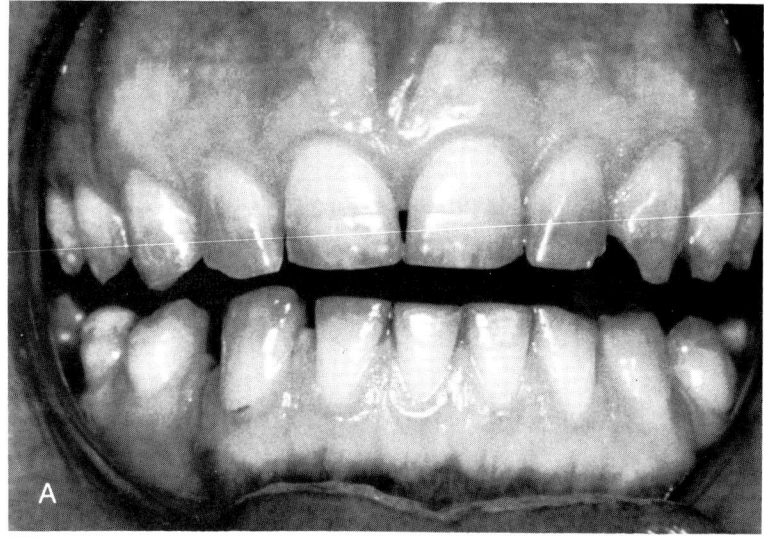
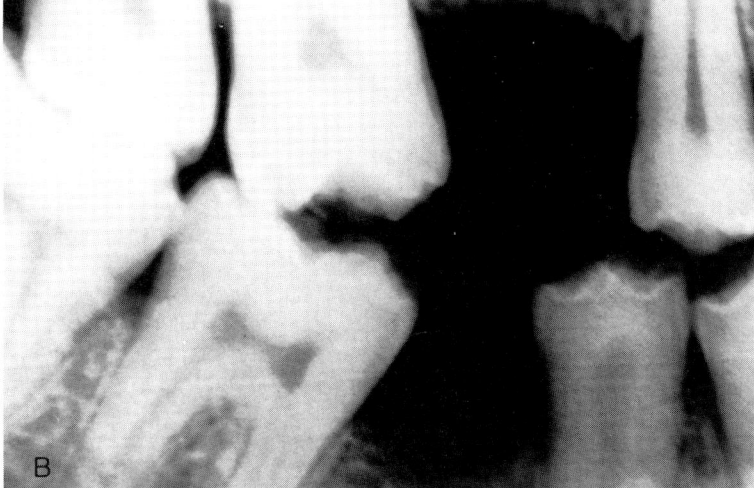

Figure 16–29. *A* and *B*, Amelogenesis imperfecta, hypoplastic type.

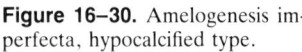

Figure 16–30. Amelogenesis imperfecta, hypocalcified type.

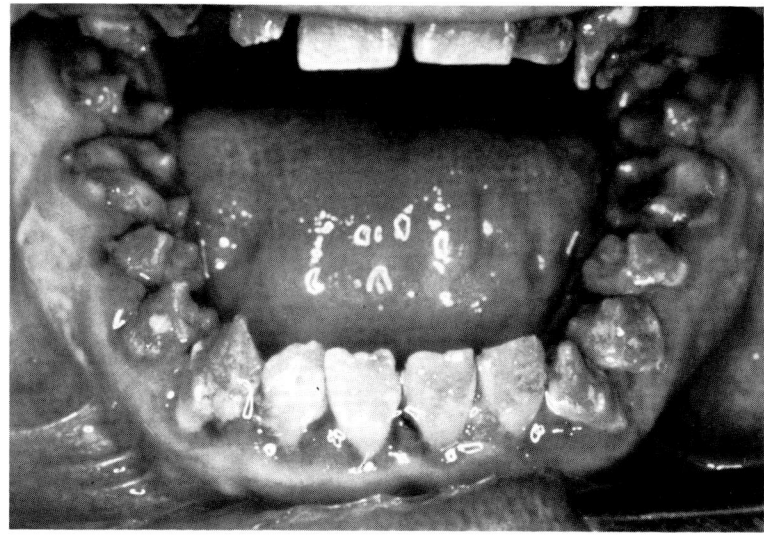

and patient to patient. Color ranges from white opaque to yellow to brown. Teeth also tend to darken with age, owing to exogenous staining. Radiographically, enamel appears reduced in bulk, often showing a thin layer over occlusal and interproximal surfaces. Dentin and pulp chambers appear normal. Other than cosmetic restoration, no treatment is necessary. Although the enamel is soft and irregular, teeth are not caries prone.

DEFECTS OF DENTIN

Dentinogenesis Imperfecta

Dentinogenesis imperfecta is an autosomal dominant trait with variable expressivity. It affects dentin of both the primary and the permanent dentition. Because of the clinical discoloration of teeth, this condition has also been known as (hereditary) opalescent dentin.

Dentinogenesis imperfecta has been divided into three types: type I, in which the dentin abnormality occurs in patients with concurrent osteogenesis imperfecta. In this form, primary teeth are more severely affected than permanent teeth. In type II, patients have only dentin abnormalities and no bone disease (Figs. 16–31 and 16–32). In type III or Brandywine type (discovered in the triracial Brandywine isolate in Maryland), only dental defects occur, similar to type II but with some clinical and radiographic variations (Fig. 16–33). Features of type III that are not seen in types I and II include multiple pulp exposures, periapical radiolucencies, and a variable radiographic appearance.

Clinically, all three types share numerous features. In both dentitions, teeth exhibit an

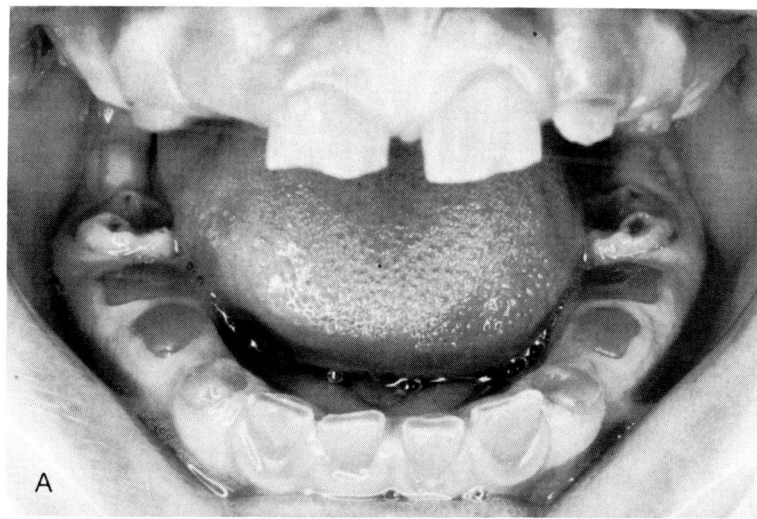
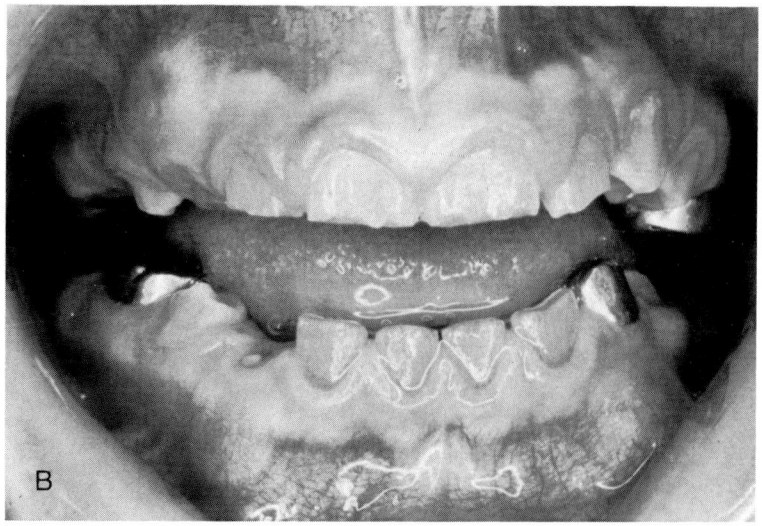

Figure 16–31. *A* and *B,* Dentinogenesis imperfecta in two brothers. Note severe wear and abnormal color.

478 ABNORMALITIES OF TEETH

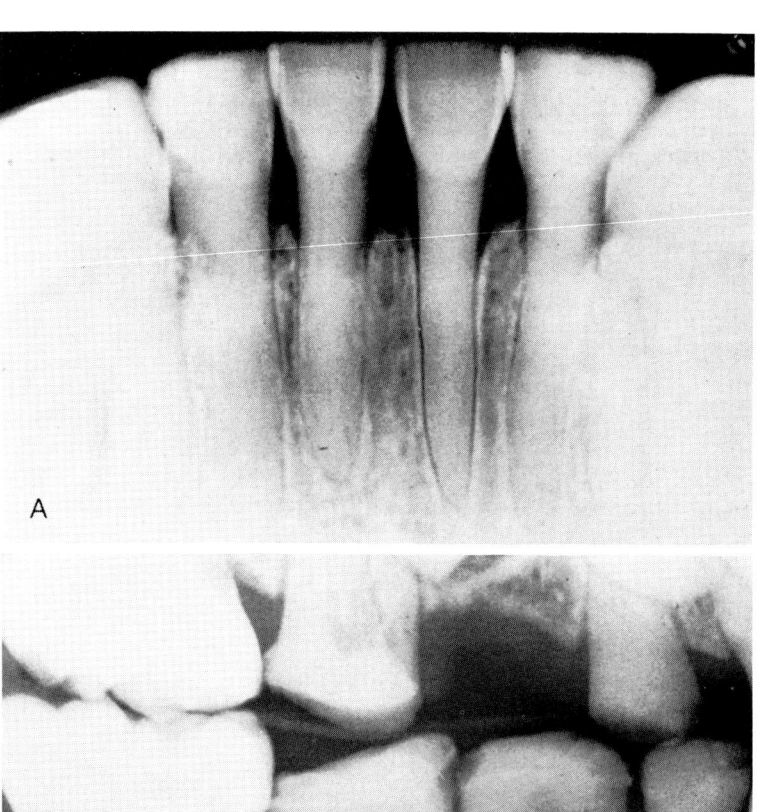

"Tulip Teeth"

Figure 16-32. *A* and *B*, Dentinogenesis imperfecta. Note obliterated pulps, bell-shaped crowns, and short roots.

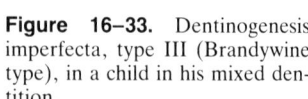
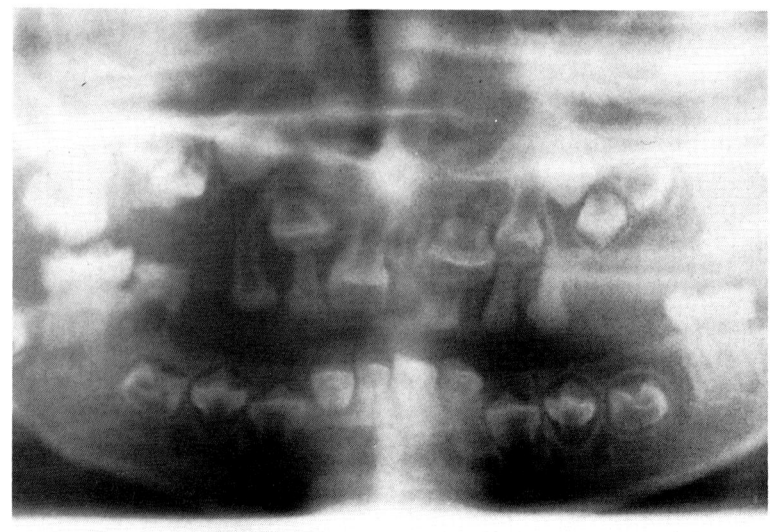

Figure 16-33. Dentinogenesis imperfecta, type III (Brandywine type), in a child in his mixed dentition.

unusual translucent, opalescent appearance with color variation from yellow-brown to gray. The entire crown appears discolored owing to the abnormal underlying dentin. Although the enamel is structurally and chemically normal, it fractures easily, resulting in rapid wear. The enamel fracturing is believed to be due to the poor support provided by the abnormal dentin and possibly to the absence of the microscopic scalloping normally seen between dentin and enamel that is felt to help mechanically lock the two hard tissues together. Overall tooth morphology is unusual in that there is excessive constriction at the cementoenamel junction, giving the crowns a tulip or bell shape. Roots are shortened and blunted. The teeth do not exhibit any greater susceptibility to caries, and they may in fact show some resistance because of the rapid wear and absence of dentinal tubules.

Radiographically, types I and II exhibit identical changes. Opacification of dental pulps occurs owing to continued deposition of abnormal dentin. The short roots and the bell-shaped crowns are also obvious on radiographic examination. In type III, the dentin appears thin, and the pulp chambers and root canals are extremely large, giving the appearance of thin dentin shells, hence the previous designation of shell teeth.

Microscopically, the dentin of teeth in dentinogenesis imperfecta contains fewer but larger and irregular dentinal tubules. The pulpal space is nearly completely replaced over time by the irregular dentin. Enamel appears normal, but the dentinoenamel junction is smooth instead of scalloped.

Treatment is directed toward protecting tooth tissue from wear and toward improving the aesthetic appearance of the teeth. Generally, fitting with full crowns at an early age is the treatment of choice. In spite of the qualitatively poor dentin, support for the crowns is adequate. These teeth should not be used as abutments, because the roots are prone to fracture under stress.

Dentin Dysplasia "Rootless Teeth"

Dentin dysplasia is another autosomal dominant trait that affects dentin. This is a rare condition that has been subdivided into type I or radicular type (Figs. 16-34 and 16-35) and a more rare type II or coronal type that varies slightly in its clinical presentation. In type II dentin dysplasia, the color of the primary dentition is opalescent, and the permanent dentition is normal; in type I, both dentitions are of normal color. The coronal pulps in type II are usually large ("thistle tube") and are filled with globules of abnormal dentin. Also, periapical lesions are not a regular feature of type II as they are in type I.

Clinically, the crowns in dentin dysplasia type I appear to be normal in color and shape. Premature tooth loss may occur because of short roots or periapical inflammatory lesions. Teeth show greater resistance to caries than do normal teeth.

Radiographically, in type I dentin dysplasia, roots appear extremely short, and pulps are almost completely obliterated. Residual fragments of pulp tissue appear typically as horizontal lucencies (chevrons). Periapical lucencies are typically seen; they represent chronic abscesses, granulomas, or cysts. In type II dentin dysplasia, deciduous teeth are similar in radiographic appearance to type I, but permanent teeth exhibit enlarged pulp chambers

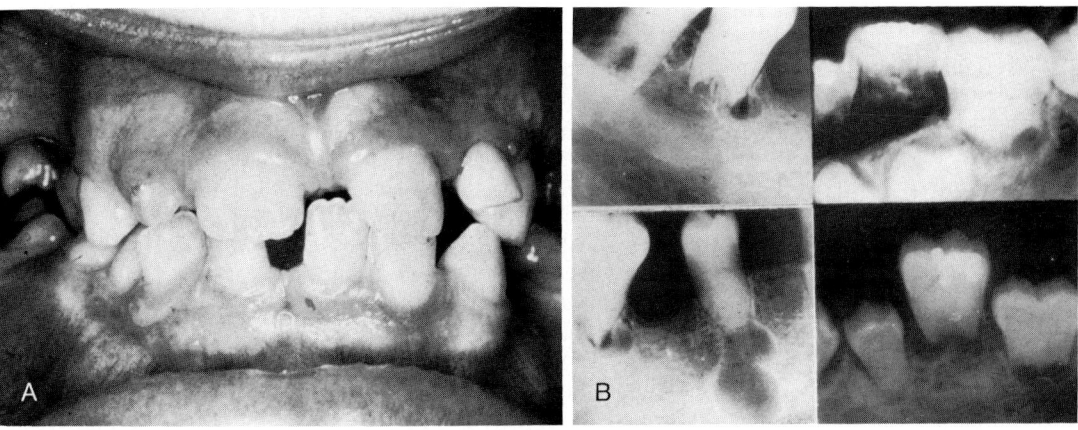

Figure 16-34. *A* and *B*, Dentin dysplasia, type I (radicular type). Note normal color of teeth.

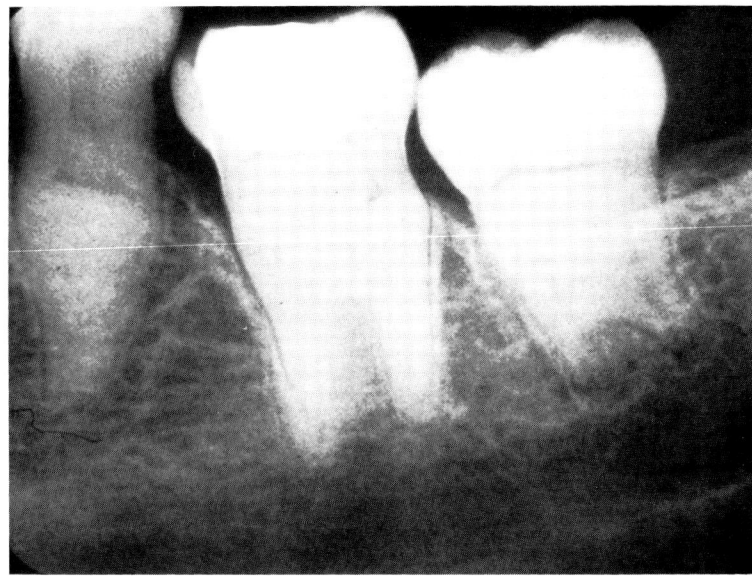

Figure 16–35. Dentin dysplasia, type I, with intrapulpal calcification and short roots. Note thin zone of pulp tissue in the coronal area of the molars.

that have been described as "thistle tube" in appearance.

Microscopically, the enamel and the immediately subjacent dentin appear normal. Deeper layers of dentin show atypical tubular patterns, with amorphous, atubular areas and irregular organization. On the pulpal side of the normal-appearing mantle of dentin, globular or nodular masses of abnormal dentin are seen.

Treatment is directed toward retention of teeth for as long as possible. However, because of the short roots and periapical lesions, the prognosis for prolonged retention is poor. This dental condition has not been associated with any systemic connective tissue problems.

DEFECTS OF ENAMEL AND DENTIN

Regional Odontodysplasia

This dental abnormality involves the hard tissues that are derived from both epithelial (enamel) and mesenchymal (dentin and cementum) components of the tooth-forming apparatus. The teeth in a region or quadrant of the maxilla or mandible are affected to the extent that they exhibit short roots, open apical foramina, and enlarged pulp chambers (Fig. 16–36). The thinness and poor mineralization quality of the enamel and dentin layers have given rise to the term "ghost teeth." The permanent teeth are affected more than the primary teeth, and the maxillary anterior teeth are affected more than other teeth. Eruption of the affected teeth is delayed or does not occur.

The cause of this rare dental abnormality is unknown, although numerous etiologic factors have been suggested, including trauma, nutritional deficiencies, infections, metabolic abnormalities, systemic diseases, and genetic influences.

Because of the poor quality of the affected teeth, their removal is usually indicated. The resulting edentulous zone can then be restored with a prosthesis.

ABNORMALITIES OF DENTAL PULP

Pulp Calcification

This is a rather common phenomenon that occurs with increasing age for no apparent reason. There appears to be no relation to inflammation, trauma, or systemic disease. Pulp calcification may be microscopic in size, or it may be large enough to be detected radiographically (Fig. 16–37). Calcifications may be either diffuse (linear) or nodular (pulp stones). The diffuse or linear deposits are typically found in the root canals and generally are parallel to the blood vessels. Pulp stones are usually found in the pulp chamber. When they are composed predominantly of dentin, they are referred to as true denticles; when they represent foci of dystrophic calcification, they are referred to as false denticles. Pulp stones are occasionally subdivided into attached and free types, depending on whether

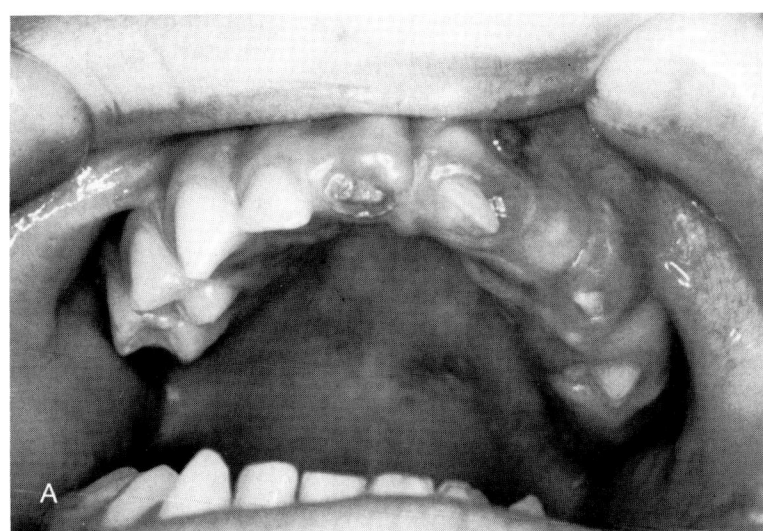
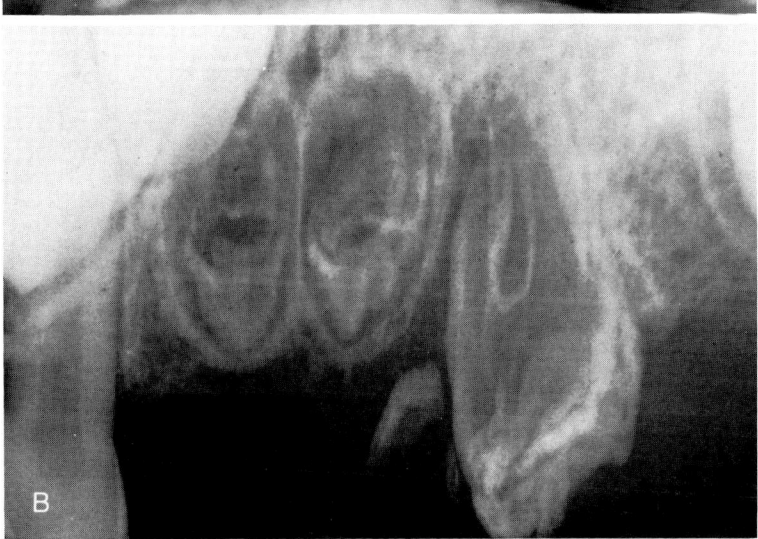

Figure 16–36. *A* and *B*, Regional odontodysplasia of maxilla.

they are incorporated into the dentin wall or are surrounded by pulpal tissue.

Pulp stones appear to have no clinical significance. They are not believed to be a source of pain and are not associated with any forms of pulpitis. They may, however, be problematic during endodontic therapy of non-vital teeth.

Internal Resorption

Resorption of the dentin of the pulpal walls may be seen as part of an inflammatory response to pulpal injury, or it may be seen in cases in which no apparent trigger can be identified (Fig. 16–38). The resorption occurs as a result of the activation of osteoclasts or dentinoclasts on internal surfaces of the root or crown. Resorption lacunae are seen, containing these cells and chronic inflammatory cells. Reversal lines may also be found in the adjacent hard tissue indicating attempts at repair. In time, the root or crown will be perforated by the process, making the tooth useless.

Any tooth may be involved, and usually only a single tooth is affected, although cases in which more than one tooth is involved have been described. In advanced cases, teeth may appear pink owing to the proximity of pulp tissue to the tooth surface. Until root fracture or communication with a periodontal pocket occurs, patients generally have no symptoms.

The treatment of choice is root canal therapy before perforation. Once there is communication between pulp and periodontal ligament,

482 ABNORMALITIES OF TEETH

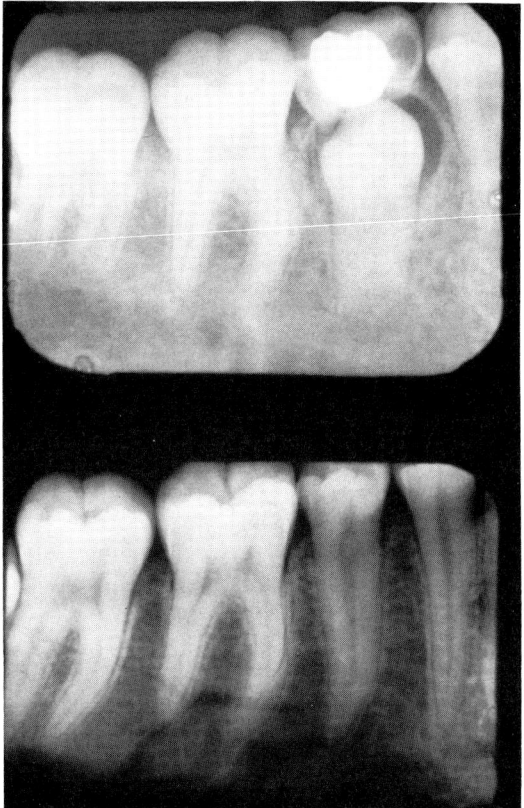

Figure 16–37. Pulp stone in erupting second premolar (top) and erupted tooth in the same patient.

the prognosis of saving the tooth is very poor. Occasionally, the process may spontaneously arrest for no apparent reason.

External Resorption

Resorption of teeth from external surfaces may have one of several causes. This change may be the result of an adjacent pathologic process, such as (1) chronic inflammatory lesions, (2) cysts, (3) benign tumors, and (4) malignant neoplasms. The pathogenesis of external resorption from these causes has been related to release of chemical mediators, increased vascularity, and pressure. External resorption of teeth may also be seen in association with (1) trauma, (2) reimplantation or transplantation of teeth, and (3) impactions (Fig. 16–39). Trauma that causes injury to or necrosis of the periodontal ligament may initiate resorption of tooth roots. This trauma may be from a single event, from malocclusion, or from excessive orthodontic forces. Because reimplanted and transplanted teeth are nonvital and have no surrounding viable periodontal ligament, they are eventually resorbed and replaced by bone. This is basically a natural physiologic process in which the calcified collagen matrix of the tooth serves as a frame-

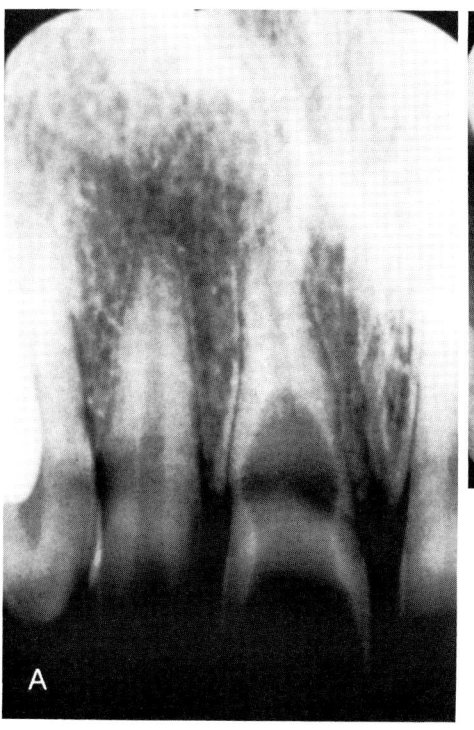
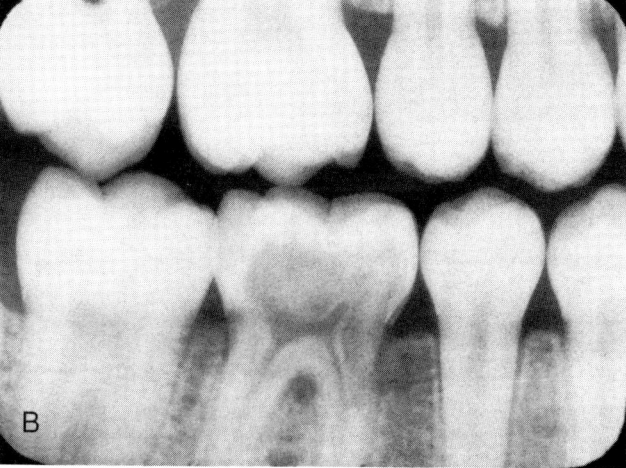

Figure 16–38. Internal resorption in a maxillary incisor *(A)* and a mandibular molar *(B)*.

ABNORMALITIES OF TEETH 483

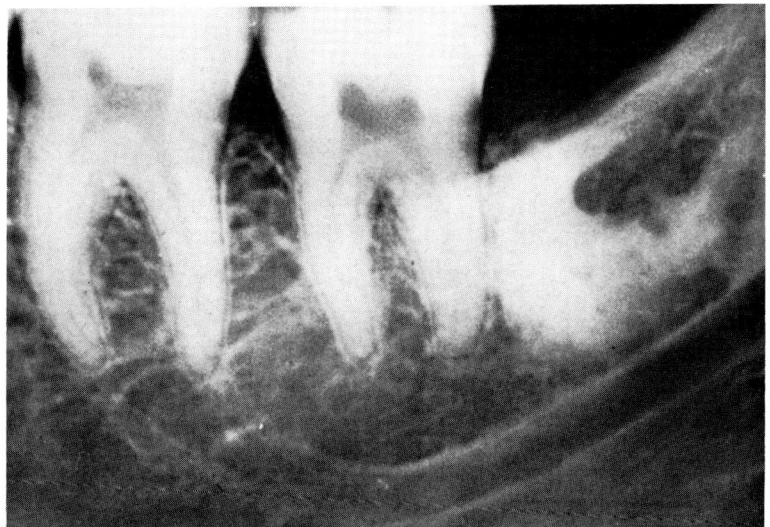

Figure 16–39. Resorption of an impacted third molar.

work for the deposition of new viable bone. Impacted teeth, when they impinge or exert pressure on adjacent teeth, may cause root resorption of the otherwise normally erupted tooth. Occasionally, impacted teeth themselves may undergo resorption. The cause of this phenomenon is unknown, although it is believed to be related to a partial loss of the protective effect of the periodontal ligament or reduced enamel epithelium.

Finally, external resorption of erupted teeth may be idiopathic. This may occur in one or more teeth. Any tooth may be involved, although molars are least likely to be affected. One of two patterns may be seen. In one, resorption occurs immediately apical to the cementoenamel junction, mimicking a pattern of caries associated with xerostomia (Fig. 16–40). In external resorption, however, the lesions occur on root surfaces below the gingival epithelial attachment. In the other pattern of external resorption, the process starts at the

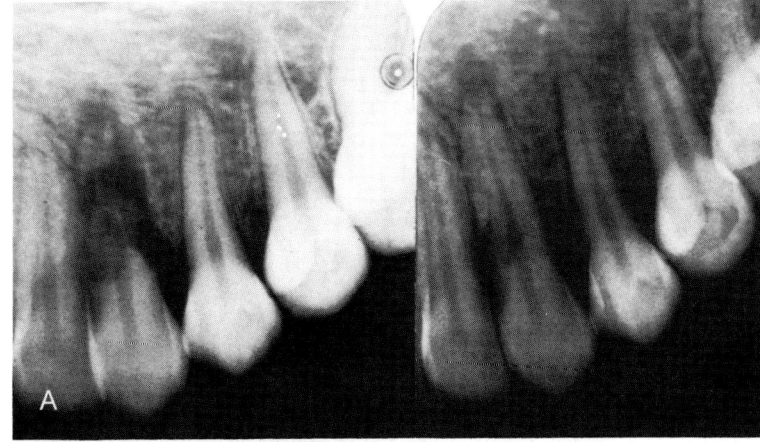

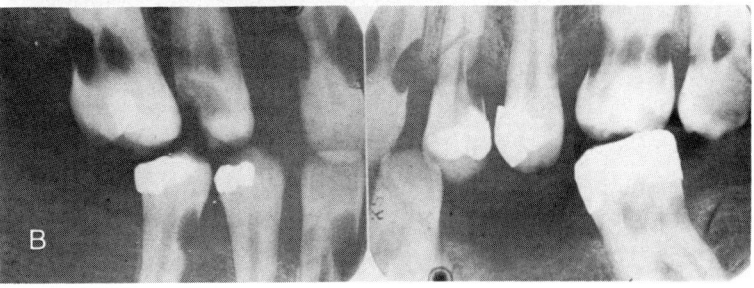

Figure 16–40. *A* and *B*, External resorption in the cervical areas of permanent teeth.

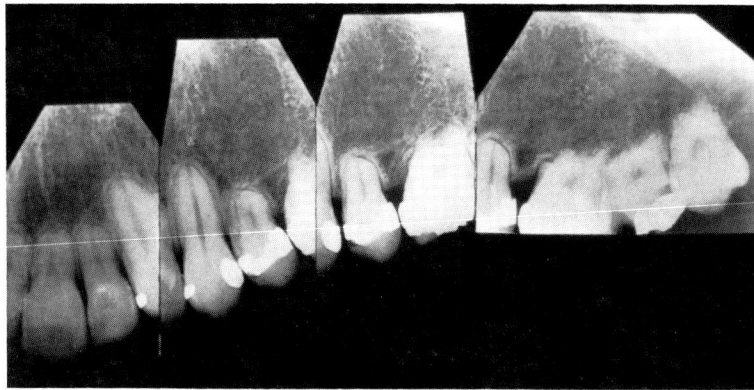

Figure 16–41. External resorption beginning at the apices of permanent teeth.

tooth apex and progresses occlusally (Fig. 16–41).

External resorption is a particularly frustrating type of dental abnormality for both patient and practitioner, because there is no plausible or evident explanation for the condition and no effective treatment. Over an extended clinical course, resorption eventually causes loss of the affected tooth.

ALTERATIONS IN COLOR

Exogenous Stains

Stains on the surface of teeth that can be removed with abrasives are known as exogenous or extrinsic stains. The color change may be caused by pigments in dietary substances (e.g., coffee, tobacco) or by the colored byproducts of chromogenic bacteria in dental plaque. Chromogenic bacteria are believed to be responsible for brown, black, green, and orange stains seen predominantly in children. Brown and black stains are typically seen in the cervical zone of teeth, either as a thin line along the gingival margin or as a wide band (Fig. 16–42). This type of stain is also often found on teeth adjacent to salivary duct orifices. Green stain is tenacious and is usually found as a band on the labial surfaces of the maxillary anterior teeth (Fig. 16–43). Blood pigments are thought to contribute to the green color. Orange or yellow-orange stains appear on the gingival third of teeth in a small percentage of children. These are generally easily removed.

Endogenous Stains

Discoloration of teeth resulting from deposits of systemically circulating substances during tooth development is defined as endogenous or intrinsic staining.

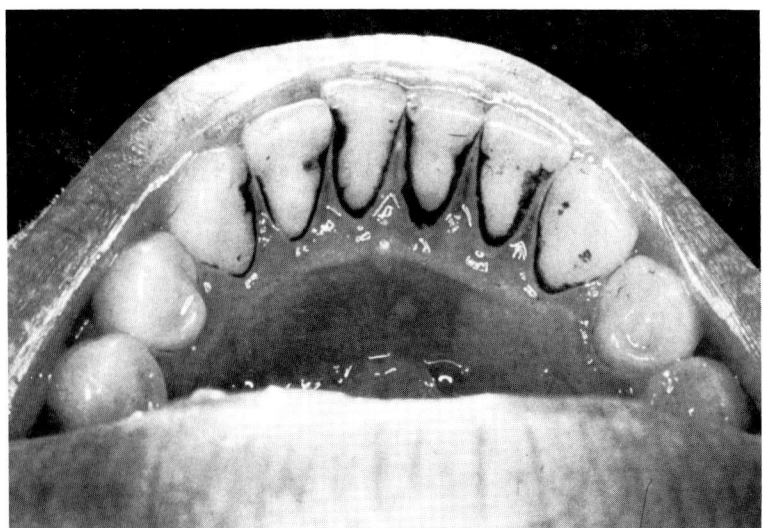

Figure 16–42. Black stain.

ABNORMALITIES OF TEETH 485

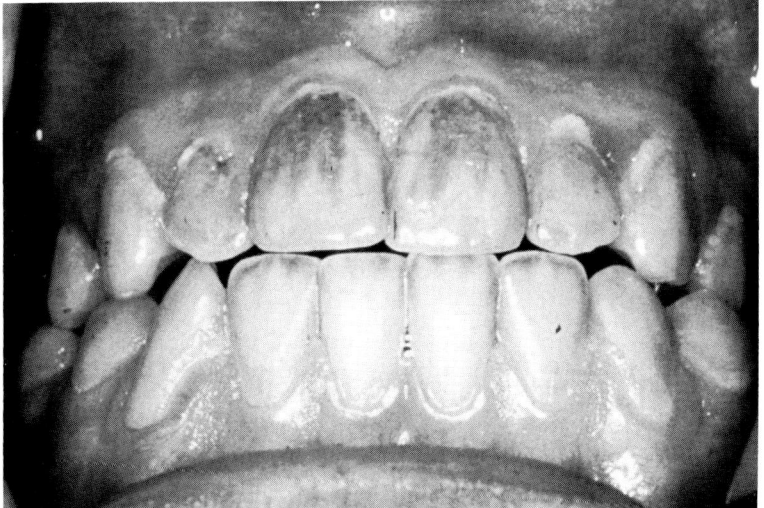

Figure 16–43. Green stain.

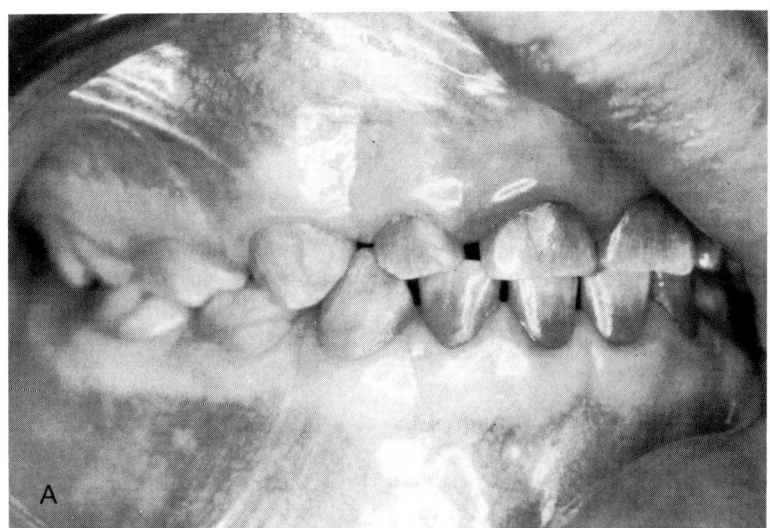

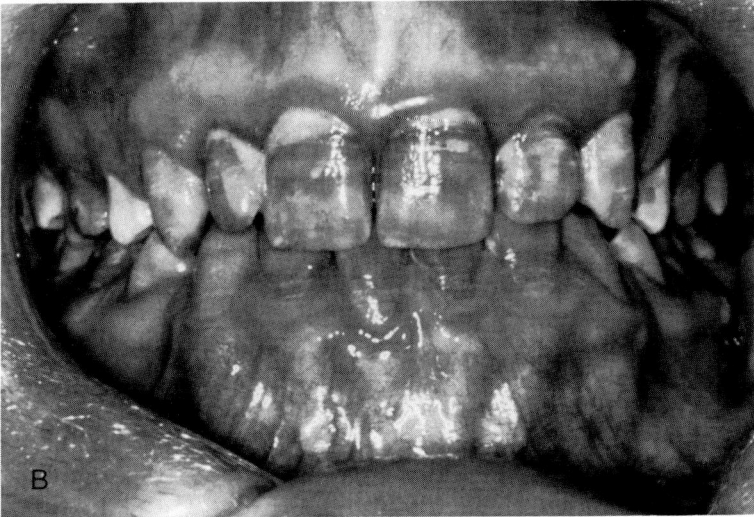

Figure 16–44. *A* and *B*, Tetracycline stain. Note dark (gray) staining of anterior teeth due to oxidization of tetracycline.

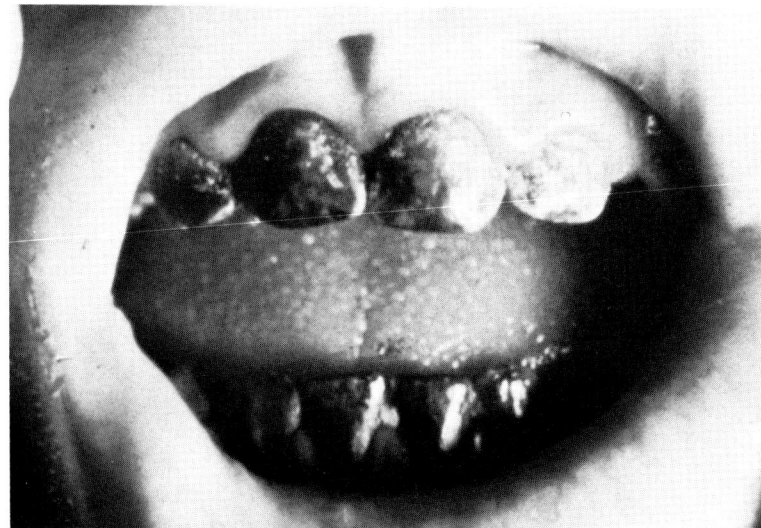

Figure 16–45. Porphyrin stain.

Systemic ingestion of *tetracycline* during tooth development is a well-known cause of endogenous staining of teeth. Tetracycline has an affinity for teeth and bones and will be deposited in these sites during metabolic activity. The drug's bright yellow color is reflected in the subsequently erupted teeth (Fig. 16–44). The fluorescent property of tetracycline can be demonstrated with an ultraviolet light in clinically erupted teeth. With time, the tetracycline oxidizes, resulting in a color change from yellow to gray or brown with the loss of its fluorescent quality. Because tetracycline can cross the placenta, it may stain primary teeth if taken during pregnancy. If administered between birth and age 6 or 7 years, permanent teeth may be affected. Only a small minority of children given tetracycline for various bacterial diseases, however, will exhibit clinical evidence of discoloration. Staining is directly proportional to the age at which the drug is administered and the dose and duration of drug usage.

The significance of tetracycline staining lies in its cosmetically objectionable appearance. Because other equally effective antibiotics are available, tetracycline should not be prescribed for children under 7 years of age, except in unusual circumstances.

It should be noted that minocycline, a semisynthetic derivative of tetracycline, can stain the roots of adult teeth. It also may stain skin and mucosa in a diffuse or patchy pattern (see Chapter 5).

Rh incompatibility (erythroblastosis fetalis) has been cited as a cause of endogenous staining in primary teeth. Because of red blood cell hemolysis resulting from maternal antibody destruction of fetal red blood cells, blood breakdown products (bilirubin) are deposited in developing primary teeth. The teeth appear green to brown. Treatment is not required, because only primary teeth are affected.

Congenital porphyria, one of several inborn errors of porphyrin metabolism, is also a potential cause of endogenous pigmentation (Fig. 16–45). This autosomal recessive trait is also associated with photosensitivity, vesiculo-bullous skin eruptions, red urine, and splenomegaly. Teeth may appear red to brown, because of deposition of porphyrin in the developing teeth. Affected teeth will fluoresce red with ultraviolet light.

Liver disease, *biliary atresia* and *neonatal hepatitis,* may produce discoloration of the primary dentition. In biliary atresia, the teeth may assume a green discoloration; a yellowish-brown color will be noted in cases of neonatal hepatitis. This is secondary to the deposition or incorporation of bilirubin in developing enamel and dentin.

Bibliography

Brady W. The anorexia nervosa syndrome. Oral Surg Oral Med Oral Pathol 50:509–516, 1980.

Congleton J, Burkes E. Amelogenesis imperfecta with taurodontism. Oral Surg Oral Med Oral Pathol 48:540–544, 1979.

Escobar V, Goldblatt L, Bixler D. A clinical, genetic, and ultrastructural study of snowcapped teeth: amelogenesis imperfecta, hypomaturation type. Oral Surg Oral Med Oral Pathol 52:607–614, 1981.

Ferguson F, Friedman S, Frazzetto V. Successful apexification technique in an immature tooth with dens in dente. Oral Surg Oral Med Oral Pathol 49:356–359, 1980.

Gorlin R, Goldman H. Toma's Oral Pathology. 6th ed. CV Mosby Co, St Louis, 1970, Chaps 3 and 4.

Grover P, Carpenter W, Allen G. Panographic survey of United States' Army recruits: analysis of dental health status. Milit Med 147:1059–1061, 1982.

Grover P, Lorton L. Gemination and twinning in the permanent dentition. Oral Surg Oral Med Oral Pathol 59:313–318, 1985.

Grover P, Lorton L. The incidence of unerupted permanent teeth and related clinical cases. Oral Surg Oral Med Oral Pathol 59:420–425, 1985.

Heimler A, Sciubba J, Lieber E, et al. An unusual presentation of opalescent dentin and Brandywine isolate hereditary opalescent dentin in an Ashkenazic Jewish family. Oral Surg Oral Med Oral Pathol 59:608–615, 1985.

Jaspers M. Taurodontism in the Down syndrome. Oral Surg Oral Med Oral Pathol 51:632–636, 1981.

Jaspers M, Witkop C. Taurodontism, an isolated trait associated with syndromes and x-chromosomal aneuploidy. Am J Hum Genet 32:396–413, 1980.

Levin L, Leaf S, Jelmini R, et al. Dentinogenesis imperfecta in the Brandywine isolate (DI type III): clinical, radiologic, and scanning electron microscopic studies of the dentition. Oral Surg Oral Med Oral Pathol 56:267–274, 1983.

Lin L, Chance K, Skribner J, et al. Dens evaginatus: a case report. Oral Surg Oral Med Oral Pathol 63:86–89, 1987.

Rotstein I, Stabholz A, Friedman S. Endodontic therapy for dens invaginatus in a maxillary second premolar. Oral Surg Oral Med Oral Pathol 63:237–240, 1987.

Rubin M, Nevins A, Berg M, et al. A comparison of identical twins in relation to three dental anomalies: multiple supernumerary teeth, juvenile periodontosis, and zero caries incidence. Oral Surg Oral Med Oral Pathol 52:391–394, 1981.

Ruprecht A, Batniji S, El-Neweihi E. The incidence of taurodontism in dental patients. Oral Surg Oral Med Oral Pathol 63:743–747, 1987.

Sclare R. Hereditary opalescent dentin (dentinogenesis imperfecta). Br Dent J 84:164–166, 1984.

Spyropoulos N, Patsakas A, Angelopoulos A. Simultaneous presence of partial anodontia and supernumerary teeth. Oral Surg Oral Med Oral Pathol 48:53–56, 1979.

Witkop C. Hereditary defects of dentin. Dent Clin North Am 19:25–45, 1975.

Witkop C, Jaspers M. Teeth with short, thin, dilacerated roots in patients with short stature: a dominantly inherited trait. Oral Surg Oral Med Oral Pathol 54:553–559, 1982.

Chapter 17
Dental Caries*

Nathaniel Rowe

CLINICAL FEATURES
Age and Sex
Race and Economic Status
Location of Dental Caries Lesions
Classification
MICROSCOPIC FEATURES
Relationships between Lesion Location on the Tooth and Anatomic Shape and Size
Pathophysiologic Dynamics of the Caries Process
  Demineralization
  Remineralization
CAUSATION
Essential Factors
  Natural Teeth
  Dental Plaque
  Diet
Modifying Factors

Dental caries is one of the most common diseases of humans. This disease is expressed as focal degradation of dental hard tissues. Cavitation of the clinical crown of the tooth is the *sine qua non* of the process. Carious lesions are the result of mineral dissolution from the dental hard tissues by the acid metabolic end products of those bacteria capable of fermenting carbohydrates, primarily sugars.

Until recently, both prevalence and incidence of dental caries have steadily increased. In general, the increase correlated well with the advance of civilization. The steady increase in dental caries experience up until about 1970 is exemplified by a study from the University of Minnesota; this indicated that over a 20-year period (1929–1949) entering college freshmen exhibited a 14% increase in the number of teeth that had experienced dental caries. By 1970, it was reported by the National Institutes of Health that the average child in the United States had three decayed teeth upon entering school at age 5. Eleven teeth had evidence of dental caries by age 15. Preschool children had a lesser dental caries incidence, but even so, 10% of children aged 1½ to 2 years and 60% of children aged 3 to 3½ years had experienced dental caries. By the early 1980s, it was recognized that in the industrialized nations, a change was taking place—dental caries was no longer increasing in prevalence but, in fact, was decreasing. Today, approximately one third of United States school children are completely free of experience with dental caries. The numbers of both missing teeth and fillings in the remainder of these children have diminished as well.

With the exception of the past decade, there has been a steady and dramatic increase in dental caries over the last 400 years. Although epidemiologic studies of human diseases are usually limited to contemporary populations, preservation of mineralized tissues, especially the dentition, permits examination of the prevalence of this disease over an extended period of time. Studies of human remains from burial sites in Warwickshire, England, revealed that the dental caries rate of 8% in the Iron Age had increased to 48% in the modern population living in the same area. Distribution of carious lesions within the dentition had also changed. Early skeletal remains as well as non-human primates studied in the field display lesions located primarily at the cervical junc-

---

*Text taken in modified form from G T Charbeneau, et al. Principles and Practice of Operative Dentistry. 2nd ed. Lea & Febiger, Philadelphia, 1981. Reprinted by permission of Lea & Febiger.

tion of enamel and cementum. In contrast, occlusal and interproximal lesions predominate in modern human populations.

The dental caries rate at the present time is recognized to be higher in people living in industrialized countries than in people living in underdeveloped countries. Dental caries activity in various groups of people living in underdeveloped countries drastically increased when the foods and cultural influence of people from industrialized societies were substituted for their previous diet and patterns of life. Dental caries experience clearly is best attributed to factors related to "civilization," not evolution. The most conspicuous factor distinguishing the low–dental caries groups (both ancient "primitive" and modern "primitive" people) from the high–dental caries group (modern, "industrialized" people) is conversion of the diet from "primitive" to "civilized." Dental caries experience in a population appears to be a function of the degree of dietary conversion from raw and unrefined foods to highly processed, sugar-sweetened, soft, retentive foodstuffs.

CLINICAL FEATURES

Age and Sex

When ages are equal, young girls have a slightly higher dental caries rate than boys. The difference is attributed to the earlier eruption of teeth in girls (i.e., longer exposure to the cariogenic oral environment). By the middle of the second decade of life, the small, gender-dependent dental caries difference disappears. In the United States, cumulative experience with the disease increases with age until the third decade of life, when most teeth at risk have already been afflicted, if such is to be their fate. Dental caries is the greatest cause of tooth loss before age 35 years.

Race and Economic Status

Different races exhibit wide variations in dental caries experience. Cultural and dietary influences play such an overwhelming role in determining dental caries incidence that it has been difficult to quantify the genetic impact. Data on dental caries derived from the Ten-State Nutrition Survey of 1968 to 1970 are of particular relevance. These data are especially useful because they are unique with regard to (1) sample size, including more than 10,000 individuals between the ages of 5 and 20 years; (2) income range considered (primarily individuals with lower income, who, as a socioeconomic group, in many instances are encumbered with a greater load of health-related problems); and (3) the wealth of data on the two largest racial groupings, whites and blacks, who differ in many important health-related respects.

The data show a consistent, dramatic, and meaningful difference in dental caries experience between black and white children at all ages. This difference transcends socioeconomic grouping, nutritional level, and developmental status. This study also has shown an apparently protective effect of poverty insofar as dental caries is concerned. Children from lower income families had experienced less dental caries activity than had children from higher income families.

Location of Dental Caries Lesions

Not all dentitions, nor all teeth in any one dentition, nor even all surfaces on individual teeth within one dentition are equally prone to develop dental caries. Some individuals have little or no dental caries during their lifetime. On the other hand, some individuals experience rapid, severe carious destruction of virtually the entire dentition at an early age (Fig. 17–1). The former persons have been described as caries "immune," whereas the latter are described as having "rampant" dental caries. The time-honored custom of using the term "caries immune" is unfortunate. This term increasingly is being recognized as nonapplicable as a consequence of the advance of our understanding of immunity and the immune system over the past 2 decades. For example, those unfortunate individuals who have experienced a severe disintegration of their immune systems in midlife after being infected with the human immunodeficiency virus (acquired immunodeficiency syndrome, AIDS) are not more susceptible to dental caries. Variability of individual experience with dental caries appears to be the rule. The basis for this variation among individuals will be discussed later, when we examine the multiple factors related to the causation of the disease.

In general, the maxillary arch experiences more dental caries than does the mandibular arch. The maxillary and mandibular first permanent molars are the most susceptible individual teeth. The mandibular incisors are the

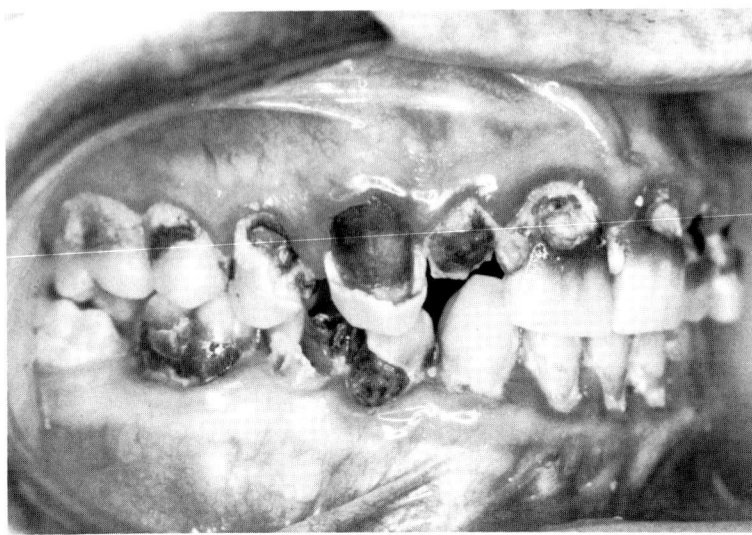

Figure 17-1. Rampant caries.

most resistant. Lesion distribution within the dentition is highly symmetric.

The occlusal surface of teeth is by far the most susceptible. Dental caries involvement of the occlusal surfaces is approximately equal to the caries experience of all the other surfaces combined.

Classification

Dental caries is classified in several ways, the most common one being according to the location of the lesion on the tooth. The process occurs in two principal locations: the occlusal *pits and fissures*, and the *smooth surfaces* of the facial, lingual, and interproximal areas immediately apical to the contact area.

Some investigators believe that the facial and lingual smooth-surface carious lesions should be further subdivided, according to their location relative to the cervical line, into *enamel* caries and *cemental* caries. They believe that, because the age group and the physical features of cervical cemental caries differ sufficiently from those of cervical enamel caries, the process should be considered distinctly different from the same disease process in the other location.

On an environmental level, dental caries of different areas of a tooth represents the similar macroscopic end result of somewhat different microscopic and chemical interactions. Dental caries of smooth surfaces and dental caries of fissures are caused by quite different conditions. In the former, synthesis of a proteinaceous matrix adherent to the tooth surface appears essential. In the latter, physical impaction of food particles into occlusal fissures and pits causes retention without an adherent matrix. Similarly, the chemical requirements differ. Smooth-surface plaque requires relatively small, diffusible, fermentable molecules to initiate caries activity. The retentiveness of pits and fissures provides the time necessary for conversion of large polysaccharide molecules of starch into acid. So although the end result, clinical lesions of dental caries, is the same for both smooth surfaces and pits and fissures, the biologic requirements and interactions are quite different. Because each type of tooth location presents special microbial, chemical, and physical conditions, any one type of anticaries activity (e.g., toothbrushing) may have its principal, if not exclusive, effect upon only one type of caries.

Although dental caries is most often classified according to location, occasionally it is classified according to the rate of lesion progression into *acute, chronic,* or *arrested* caries. The progression rate is a function of several variables. In addition to less important intrinsic (tooth-related) variables, such as degree of tissue mineralization and amount of matrix protein, rate of lesion development and progression depends primarily upon variables external to the tooth. These include the cariogenicity of the plaque microbiota, the availability (quality and frequency of ingestion) of acidogenic substrate, and the remineralizing capability of the oral fluids. Frequent snacks, especially sweets, coupled with newly erupted, immature enamel and poor oral hygiene provide optimal conditions for carious destruction of dental hard tissues. These conditions are more likely to be present in young persons. The result is rapid progression of caries ("acute"), affecting many teeth within the dentition simultaneously. Such widespread dental caries attack within the dentition may be termed "rampant" dental caries to signify distribution. In adults, whose hygiene is usually better or whose diet is directed away from sweets and snacks, dental caries activity in existing lesions will by comparison be slower ("chronic" caries) and may even eventually cease to progress. When this occurs, the lesions are termed "arrested" dental caries. Arrested carious lesions are found most often in the premolar region of mandibular teeth in the cervical areas, usually in cementum.

MICROSCOPIC FEATURES

Relationships between Lesion Location on the Tooth, and Anatomic Shape and Size

A new or inexperienced, dental practitioner may be surprised, upon probing a deep, dark occlusal fissure in a young patient, to have the explorer sink nearly out of sight. An extremely large carious lesion is thereby revealed, despite the fact that, outwardly, only slight deviation from the normal occlusal surface appearance was noted. An understanding of the direction and speed of lesion progression is predicated upon knowledge of the microscopic and chemical events that produce the carious lesion. This is most easily examined first at the macroscopic or clinical level.

Dental caries always begins at the tooth surface. The lesion progresses from the surface into the deeper tooth tissues. The speed of penetration is determined by a combination of external and intrinsic factors. The intrinsic factors include the spatial relationship and proximity of the crystallites to one another as well as the relative proportions of inorganic to organic phases. Within each of the dental hard tissues, the degree of mineralization is relatively homogeneous; *between* them, for example, enamel compared with dentin, differences are noteworthy. Enamel is more mineralized (96%) than is dentin (70%), and it is destroyed more slowly by the carious process. It would be an erroneous oversimplification to assume that dental caries is simply acid dissolution of the mineral crystallites in teeth, however, since when a tooth is dropped *in vitro* into acid, the enamel experiences more rapid destruction than does the dentin. The proteinaceous components of dentin add another dimension to the caries process. They serve as a source of nutriment for certain bacterial species and correspondingly favor their selection and growth. Structurally, the arrangement of protein within the dentinal tubules provides, upon lysis, pathways for more rapid bacterial invasion. Greater access to the more widely spaced mineral crystallites is also afforded the by-products of the acidogenic bacteria that invade dentin.

The direction of lesion progression is determined not only by the point source of the acid formed by food fermentation but also by the microscopic structure of the dental hard tissues involved. Carious penetration into enamel smooth surfaces tends to be cone-shaped, with the point or apex toward the deep (pulpal) aspect (Fig. 17–2). In enamel pit or fissure caries, a marked difference in the penetration pattern compared with the smooth-surface lesion occurs because of the different orientation

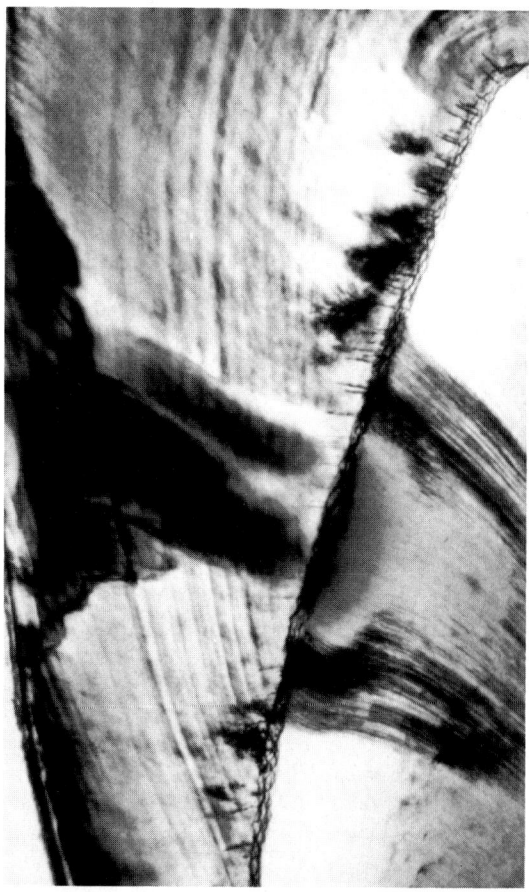

Figure 17–2. This early carious lesion of the interproximal smooth surface exhibits the typical fan-shaped penetration pattern. The base is at the enamel surface, and the apex or point is at the dentinoenamel junction. Spread into the dentin and along the dentinoenamel junction has begun.

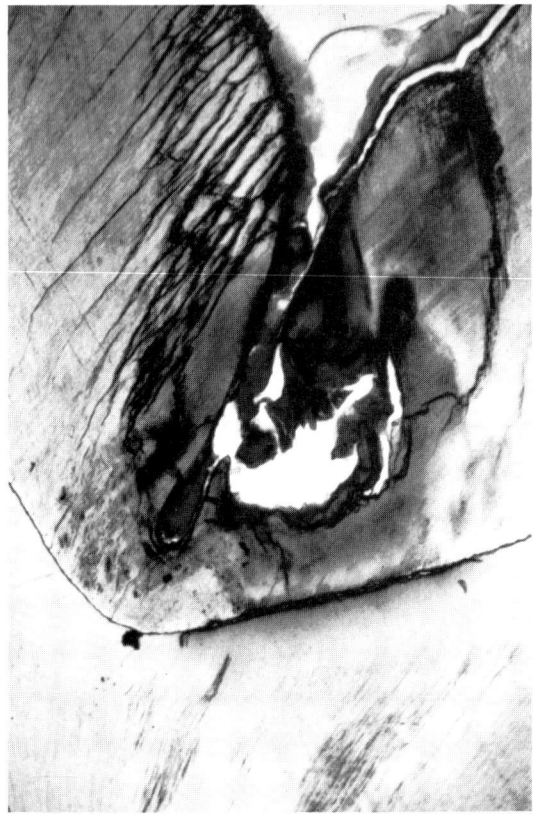

Figure 17–3. This early carious lesion of an occlusal fissure in a molar exhibits the typical inverted fan-shaped penetration pattern. The apex or point is at the enamel surface, and the base is at the dentinoenamel junction. Dental caries and its spread along the dentinoenamel junction have begun.

Once dentin is reached, however, the dentinoenamel junction and the tubular microstructure coupled with decreased levels of mineralization enhance carious degradation and lesion extension. The pattern characteristic of caries in dentin is cone-shaped, with the base at the dentinoenamel junction and the blunt point toward the pulp chamber. This shape is the result of the dentinal tubules that originate at the dentinoenamel junction and course in a gentle sigmoid curve basically parallel to one another as they progress toward the pulp. Lateral spread along the dentinoenamel junction occurs at a rate faster than lateral spread within the enamel; therefore, once dental caries reaches the dentinoenamel junction, it quickly undermines sound enamel. Retrograde enamel destruction results from extension along the dentinoenamel junction beneath otherwise sound enamel. Both dentin and enamel become carious, extending laterally along the dentinoenamel junction well beyond the borders of the visible surface-enamel lesion. This is why, once the enamel has been completely penetrated and dentinal caries has been initi-

of the enamel rods at this location (Fig. 17–3). Compared with those of the smooth surface, the rods in the areas of a pit or fissure diverge as they radiate inward from the tooth surface toward the dentinoenamel junction. In enamel in other than pit and fissure areas, the rods either are parallel or converge slightly as they move from the tooth surface inward to the dentinoenamel junction. This markedly different enamel microanatomy in the pit and fissure area gives rise to the peculiarly shaped, cross-sectional destruction pattern, which diverges or becomes larger as it penetrates deeper into the enamel—just the opposite of the lesional shape that results when smooth surfaces are attacked. For this reason, a relatively small external opening of a carious pit or fissure on an occlusal surface may be the only clinical evidence of a much larger subsurface lesion (Fig. 17–4). Conversely, smooth-surface lesions in enamel are largest at the surface and become progressively smaller as they penetrate into the enamel.

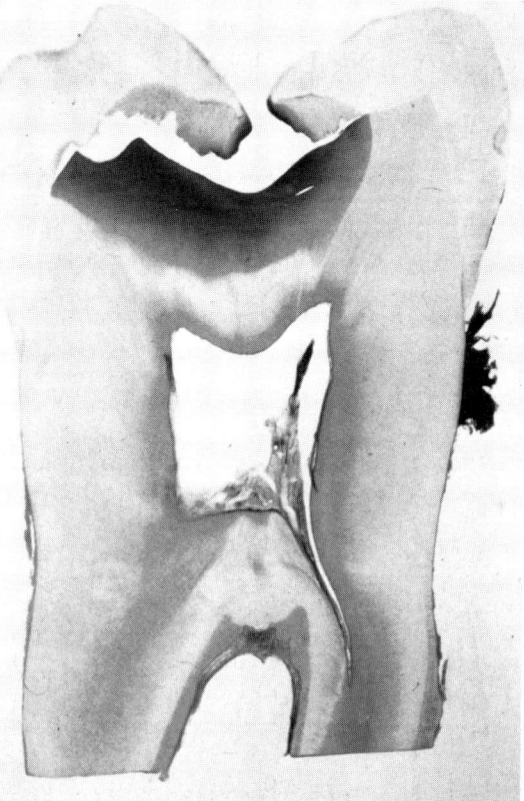

Figure 17–4. This advanced carious lesion shows a small external opening but extensive enamel undermining and dentin destruction.

ated, the dentinal lesion rapidly becomes larger laterally than is evidenced at the deep aspect of the enamel lesion. This, coupled with the special invasion pattern in enamel below pits and fissures, explains why dentinal involvement is often so much more extensive below pits and fissures than one might suspect.

The time required for development of a clinically evident carious lesion is, as might be expected, somewhat variable. Lesions resembling incipient caries have been produced experimentally in less than 1 month when oral hygiene procedures were discontinued and high-sucrose solution rinses were instituted several times per day. The average speed of carious penetration of interproximal enamel has been determined by serial radiographs in adolescent children. Penetration of the outer half of enamel on the mesial surface of the first permanent molars required approximately 1.5 years in the absence of special dietary or hygiene manipulation.

Clinically, the earliest evidence of disease is a chalky-white etch on an otherwise translucent tooth enamel surface. Measured by microhardness testing, this altered enamel is softer than sound enamel. Microscopic tissue alterations combine to produce the clinically observable lesion. When the incipient lesion is examined in greater detail by scanning electron microscopy, the tooth surface appears covered with a multitude of tiny pits, resembling a honeycomb. Transmission electron microscopy at right angles to the surface reveals that the mineral crystallite density is reduced not only at the surface but also to an even greater extent immediately beneath the surface.

Knowledge of the microstructure of enamel is essential to an understanding of the natural history of dental caries. Enamel, viewed at right angles by light microscopy, is composed of multitudes of somewhat parallel, segmented, rod-like structures that follow a gentle spiral course from the dentinal junction outward to the tooth surface. Each enamel rod is composed of myriads of tightly packed hydroxyapatite crystallites whose long axes are, in general, oriented parallel to the direction of the rod. The boundaries between adjacent rods (interstices) exhibit considerable variation in crystallite orientation. Crystallites are packed tightly against one another within a sparse matrix of structural protein, *enamelin*. Enamelin composes only a minute portion of mature enamel (less than 1%). The matrix serves initially to orient crystallite deposition during enamel formation. Following eruption of the fully formed tooth, the enamelin continues to serve as a matrix for reception, orientation, and retention of additional crystallites deposited from the oral fluid that bathes the tooth surface.

Initial decalcification, which occurs beneath the dental plaque at the plaque-enamel interface, assaults the enamel along its surface, dissolving individual hydroxyapatite crystallites. Thinning and shortening of individual crystallites is the initial evidence of decalcification. Decalcification in time penetrates into the enamel. The mineral loss is particularly apparent within the striae of Retzius, better termed planes of Retzius. Acids dissolve crystallites to create microcavities. If the process continues, the micro-cavities enlarge and coalesce laterally across adjacent rods to form tunnels or interconnecting channels. The surface layer of enamel (50–100 μm thick) remains relatively intact until it is almost completely undermined by the coalescence of the multiple interconnecting channels and microcavities within the subsurface enamel. Loss of the intact surface layer is, therefore, a late event in the induction of the incipient carious lesion.

Pathophysiologic Dynamics of the Caries Process

Minerals are continually exchanged between the enamel surface and its adjacent oral environment. The direction of mineral movement in general depends upon the relative mineral concentrations and the pH at the interface.

Demineralization

Excess movement of minerals from the enamel into the adjacent environment for prolonged periods of time produces the incipient lesion described earlier. Both *in vivo* and *in vitro*, the lesion at this stage may be reversed under appropriate conditions. The critical stage at which reversal is no longer possible is believed to be the point at which the amount of crystallites removed compromises the integrity of the structural protein matrix. Collapse of the matrix initiates the irreversible lesion, cavitation, which requires dental restorative procedures. Until such a time, minerals are able to ebb and flow both from the enamel surface into the oral fluids and from the oral fluids into the enamel without cavity production and subsequent need for dental restoration.

Remineralization

During the remineralization phase, crystallites are re-formed within the microcavities that were created during demineralization. Complete remineralization of the surface and near-to-the-surface microcavities prematurely chokes off crystallite formation in the deeper microcavities. This results in a hypermineralized enamel surface "skin" a few microns deep. The hypermineralized surface layer retards somewhat the effect of transient cariogenic influences. It also maintains the remineralization potential of the structural unit even while crystallites some distance from the surface are being degraded. Saliva is the source of minerals for the remineralization process. The critical role of intact, functional salivary glands cannot be overemphasized. When the salivary glands are compromised, resulting in xerostomia, rapid and widespread dental caries follows unless special therapy is instituted to prevent carious destruction of the dentition.

CAUSATION

Causative factors responsible for the development of dental caries are multiple and can be divided into two main groups. *Essential factors*, three in number, must all be present at the same time for dental caries to occur: (1) natural teeth with susceptible surfaces exposed to the oral environment; (2) the complex indigenous oral bacterial flora adherent to the tooth surface (dental plaque); and (3) diet—food ingested by mouth. *Modifying factors*, although more numerous, exert their effects in more subtle ways, primarily affecting location of dental caries within the dentition. Dental caries lesion initiation, progression, or reversal is the clinically evident result of the interactions of obvious as well as obscure multiple causative factors.

Essential Factors

Natural Teeth

The requirement of natural teeth with susceptible surfaces exposed to the oral environment seems so obvious that it hardly needs mentioning as a prerequisite. Yet it should be remembered that sometimes teeth are formed that do not erupt into the oral cavity—for example, impacted third molars or unerupted teeth formed within ovarian dermoid cysts. These unerupted teeth do not develop dental caries. Complete coverage of the crown of a tooth by dental restorative material also isolates the susceptible tooth tissue from what might otherwise be a highly cariogenic environment and thereby prevents carious attack. Isolation of susceptible sites from the oral cavity is the principle upon which the practice of "prophylactic odontotomy" (conservative occlusal restorations of deep pits and fissures prior to caries development) and the use of "sealants" (adherent materials placed upon the occlusal surfaces of teeth) to prevent dental caries are based.

Dental Plaque

Dental plaque is the term applied to the aggregate of bacteria, salivary glycoproteins, and inorganic salts that accumulates on the tooth surface. The presence of microorganisms in contact with susceptible tooth surfaces has been proved essential for the production of dental caries in laboratory animals. Rodents with cariogenic oral bacteria fed a cariogenic diet develop dental caries, whereas gnotobiotic (virtually germ-free) rodents identical in every other way and fed the same diet do not. Many types of plaque bacteria, including several strains of streptococci, lactobacilli, and actinomyces, have been demonstrated to be able to cause dental caries in rats. It is logical to assume, although conclusive evidence is lacking, that dental caries in humans is also a consequence of cariogenic microorganism activity. It is expected that, as in laboratory animals, several different organisms may, under different environmental conditions, be etiologically related to dental caries (Table 17-1).

The usual clinical appearance of dental plaque is white, soft, adherent to tooth surface, and film-like. Although inspection with the unaided eye might suggest that all dental plaques are identical, microscopic, biochemical, and pathologic examinations readily dispel this misconception. Although the specific details of the indigenous oral microbiota related to cariogenicity lie beyond the scope of this chapter, it is sufficient to say that selection factors are constantly at work in the oral cavity to determine the pathogenicity (or lack of it) of dental plaque for the patient's teeth. Some of the conspicuous factors that determine the *qualitative* character of the plaque are the type and frequency of substrate introduction (dietary composition and intake frequency). Among those that determine the *quantitative* character are the efficiency and frequency of various oral hygiene procedures.

Table 17-1. SOME HUMAN ISOLATES THAT CAUSE DENTAL CARIES WHEN INTRODUCED AS MONOCONTAMINANTS IN GNOTOBIOTIC RATS

Isolate		Affected Tooth Surface		
Bacterium	*Strain*	Fissures	Smooth	Root
Streptococcus mutans	GS5, LM7, AHT	+	+	
	6715	+	+	+
	NCTC 10449		+	
S. salivarius	1A	+	+	+
	SS2	+		+
	H-1	+		
S. sanguis	OMZ9	+	+	
S. fecalis	ND547	+		
Lactobacillus casei	ATCC 4646	+		
Actinomyces viscosus	M100			+
	X_1	+		
A. naeslundii	I			+
	X_1, X_3	+		
A. israelii	X_4	+		

Modified from Shaw J. Causes and control of dental caries. Reprinted, by permission of The New England Journal of Medicine 317:996–1004, 1987.

The relationship between dental plaque and dental caries was postulated long ago. Simply stated, in those locations where plaque accumulates, carious lesions are likely to develop. Conversely, in those locations where plaque does not aggregate, carious lesions are unlikely to occur. The mere presence of dental plaque does not necessarily spell doom for the continued integrity of the tooth surface. For example, "primitive" Eskimos examined by early dental investigators were found to be virtually caries free, and yet the crowns of their entire dentitions were encased within a lifetime accumulation of plaque and calculus, since oral hygiene procedures were unknown to them. Great variation in plaque pathogenicity for dental hard tissues is thus evident.

The ability of oral microorganisms to initiate dental caries depends upon several bacterial characteristics, including the ability to adhere to tooth surfaces, acidogenicity (the ability to rapidly form lactic, formic, and other acids rapidly from C_{12} and C_6 sugars), and aciduricity (the ability to survive in a low-pH environment). Bacterial adhesion characteristics determine the nature of the initial dental plaque. Later, adhesive interactions between bacterial strains and differences in growth rates revise the bacterial species composition. Dental plaque varies in composition from site to site within the dentition and even upon a single tooth. Cariogenic risk similarly varies from site to site, depending upon the character of the plaque indigenous to the specific site. The constant microbial adaptations within the plaque select for strain differences that express themselves as differences in pathogenicity for dental hard tissues, ranging from harmless to highly destructive.

Dental plaque speciation and, consequently, pathogenicity are greatly influenced by plaque and diet relationships. In general, dental plaque pathogenicity, with respect to dental caries, is largely a function of bacterial selection mediated by dietary manipulation. A high-protein and low-sucrose diet selectively discriminates against growth of the odontolytic organisms within the plaque, whereas a low-protein and high-sucrose diet predisposes to growth of odontolytic organisms, particularly when food intake is frequent. The dental hard tissue organic and inorganic phases are less transitory than the other intraoral selection pressures and, therefore, exert a stabilizing influence that favors those organisms that can utilize the minerals and proteins provided by odontolysis. Those organisms capable of destroying the teeth as a means of deriving their own nutrient supply would seem best able to survive and adapt to environmental variations.

A systematic search for a single causative organism of dental caries by the application of scientific bacteriologic principles and Koch's postulates began with W. D. Miller shortly before the turn of the twentieth century. Investigators since that time have shared Miller's frustration and disappointment at being unable to identify any single organism as the one specific etiologic agent. In the 1920s and especially during the following 3 decades, *Lac-*

tobacillus acidophilus appeared to be the prime candidate. Large numbers of this organism were consistently found in the mouths of patients who exhibited rampant dental caries. The presence of these bacteria preceded the appearance of dental carious lesions with impressive regularity, and their capacity to survive and produce acid even in a low-pH environment was amply demonstrated. As time passed, data were acquired that blunted the thrust of the earlier reports. Isolation of *L. acidophilus* in mouths of caries-free individuals was perhaps the strongest argument against the hypothesis that dental caries resulted specifically from infection by this organism.

Streptococcus mutans, an organism capable of utilizing sucrose to synthesize a sticky insoluble polysaccharide (polyglucans) that serves as a structural matrix for attachment of plaque organisms to tooth surfaces, received renewed attention in the 1960s. *S. mutans* is an acidogenic and aciduric organism that has been epidemiologically associated with human dental caries experience in several areas of the world. Laboratory rodents whose oral flora was suppressed by antibiotics developed rapid carious destruction of their dentition when they were infected with certain streptococci and then fed diets high in sugar. As a consequence of the habit of coprophagy (feces eating), cariogenic streptococci were able to be transmitted from infected mothers to their progeny and also by caries-active infected rodents to their originally uninfected cage mates. Dental caries followed infection when high-sugar diets were fed. This demonstrated the transmissibility of the disease process in rodents. It should be noted, however, that the transmissibility occurred only under highly manipulated conditions in coprophagic rodents, conditions not at all analogous to the human situation. When the glucans (polymers of glucose) produced by *S. mutans* were digested by the enzyme dextranase, caries activity in the rodents ceased. Attempts to duplicate this feat in humans have failed consistently. It has been found that at least three different polyglycans are synthesized in human plaque. Consequently, a single specific polyglucanolytic enzyme would not bring about the same result as in rodents.

Increasingly, the importance of *S. mutans* in the etiology of human dental caries has become uncertain. Although it is the most common oral microorganism that produces polyglucans, the evidence purporting to show that colonization by *S. mutans* precedes caries development in a specific site is inconsistent. Although many studies provide evidence of a positive association, other studies have demonstrated a lack of correlation. Although the prevalence of both lactobacilli and *S. mutans* at sites of incipient dental caries is increased, careful inspection suggests that the caries process might have already been under way. Because it is difficult to decide at which point dental caries actually begins, a cause-and-effect association between *S. mutans* and dental caries may in reality be artifactual. It might be that this organism is neither responsible for initiating carious lesions nor essential to the caries process.

Dental caries is regarded by some as the consequence of a specific infection. Whether the disease can be considered "specific" when several different types of organisms, such as *S. mutans*, and certain species of *Lactobacillus* and *Actinomyces*, all have a demonstrated association with it remains an open question. Additionally, since all three microorganisms are indigenous to the oral cavity irrespective of whether dental caries is present, attention is focused on the fact that although all persons may be infected, not all are diseased. *It is especially important to distinguish between "infection" and "disease" and to recognize that they are not synonymous.* The disease dental caries does not result from infection by a specific organism in the same way that other infectious diseases, such as measles or tuberculosis, do. Thus, the etiologic complexity of the disease dental caries is underscored, and the importance of bacteria-substrate relationships in the multifactorial causation is emphasized.

Diet

Ingestion of food by mouth is essential for development of dental caries. It has been demonstrated that a highly cariogenic diet tube-fed to susceptible animals does not produce dental caries.

The term "diet" is more applicable than "nutrition" because a relationship between nutritional status and caries, although aggressively sought, has not been substantiated. On the other hand, certain dietary constituents, primarily sugars, have consistently been correlated with dental caries activity. The introduction of honey and figs into the human diet ushered the disease dental caries into common experience. Since early times, attention has focused upon the relationship between diet and dental caries.

In England during the 2000 years from the

Iron Age to the medieval era, coarse black bread, made from rye or barley, was the principal item in the diet. It was not until the twelfth century AD that sucrose became obtainable, and small amounts were imported. Evidence suggests that when the more "civilized" conditions of the Roman period were substituted, including eating bread made from finely ground wheat, an increase in the caries rate occurred.

The reverse situation was observed in the late 1800s following the isolation of a small number of British subjects on a little-known island in the Atlantic Ocean, Tristan da Cunha. Living away from the usual shipping routes, the inhabitants were forced to become independent of external commerce and live off the land. The dental caries rate in these people and their descendants dropped correspondingly. However, when the island residents were finally relocated in their original homeland, dental caries returned to a high level, similar to that of the indigenous British population.

At least three major changes have been identified that can be attributed to the transformation from low to high dental caries activity as diet is changed. (Less dramatic influences have also been recognized.) The three principal changes are

1. Deletion of *protective factors* from food during harvesting, processing, storage, or preparation.
2. Addition of *cariogenic factors* to food.
3. *Changes in dietary habits*. There has been a shift away from protein and toward carbohydrate as well as an increase in frequency of ingestion, typified by snacking.

That protective factors were deleted by the refinement of food was suspected as early as 1931, when it was reported that rats whose diets were rich in phosphorus developed fewer dental caries than did rats whose diet contained less phosphorus. A human counterpart was observed when a modern-day "primitive" people adopted European ways of living. In the South African Bantu, it was doubted that cereal and sugar per se could be responsible for the observed increase in dental caries activity. The volume intake of cereal did not increase when they became Europeanized; nor was sugar newly introduced, since they had chewed sugar cane regularly prior to Europeanization. Refinement of these two foods was the only difference that could be identified. It was postulated, and supported by careful but unsophisticated *in vitro* experiments, that in the natural or crude state, these carbohydrates were accompanied by a protective agent that had been removed by the refining process. Later, it was recognized that the "active principle" could be extracted in aqueous solution; it subsequently was identified as *phytate*, an organic soluble phosphate. Experiments with rats confirmed the significant anticaries, or protective, effect of phytate. Investigations conducted on Alaskan Eskimos revealed higher salivary phosphorus in those immune to caries than in those susceptible to the disease. Unfortunately, these findings have not been adequately confirmed. An extensive literature now exists that demonstrates the inverse relationship between level of dietary phosphate and dental caries activity in animal experiments. In humans, the protective action of dietary phosphate remains to be adequately demonstrated.

Sugar clearly heads the list of cariogenic foods. Data to support this contention are plentiful. Sucrose is the most cariogenic sugar. By virtue of its common use and the destruction of the dentition that attends its use, sucrose has been called the "arch criminal" of dental caries. Carefully conducted British studies of human skeletal remains demonstrated the connection between the commercial importance of sugar and the dental caries experience during various time periods.

The seventeenth century was a time of major change. Cane sugar began to be imported into England from the New World, where sugar industries were being established. Sugar became cheaper and more available. (In addition, improved methods of milling led to bread being made from increasingly refined flour.) Location of the lesions had also shifted from the cervical area, characteristic of ancient populations, to the occlusal surfaces and buccal fissures. The most common lesion site became the interproximal surface rather than the cementoenamel junction typical of earlier periods.

Two additional major changes took place in the mid-nineteenth century: the repeal of the Corn Laws in 1846; and reduced duties on sugar until their final removal in 1875. The former led to a rapid increase in wheat importation from North America, and the latter resulted in an increase in annual per capita sugar consumption from 10 or 20 pounds to 90 pounds by the end of the century. Dental caries increased greatly during that time, and by the end of the nineteenth century, the prevalence and distribution of caries was virtually the same as that found in the present-day British population. Introduction of refined sugar into the diet has been universally accompanied by the onset and acceleration of dental caries activity. When a caries-active population experienced a scarcity of sucrose (Norwegian and Channel Island children during World War II), dental caries activity decreased. After the war, when sucrose was reintroduced, dental caries activity increased in these populations—up to and beyond the levels experienced before the war.

One of the most informative studies of the influence of sucrose on dental caries was an experiment conducted over a 5-year period with patients in a mental institution in southern Sweden. This post–World War II study was designed to determine the influence of the quantity of ingested sugar versus the frequency of its ingestion upon dental caries activity. It was found that sucrose in liquid form consumed with meals caused virtually no increase in dental caries, even though approximately 10 times as much sugar was consumed. On the other hand, when sugar was ingested either between meals (frequent intake) or in a form that persisted in the oral cavity (sticky, retentive candies), dental caries activity increased dramatically. From this and other studies, it can be stated that instead of *quantity* of sucrose ingested, it is the *frequency* with which it is eaten that is important. In general, it can be said that the earlier in life sucrose ingestion is begun and the more frequent its intake, the more likely and the more devastating will be the disease dental caries.

It has been demonstrated experimentally in animals that sucrose, fructose, lactose, and glucose, in order of decreasing activity, predispose to dental caries. In humans, from both the theoretical point of view (as a glycosyl donor utilized by certain indigenous oral bacteria to produce an adhesive matrix for dental plaque and acid upon degradation) and the clinical point of view (associated with the introduction and acceleration of caries), sucrose remains the single most important dietary constituent.

Modifying Factors

In addition to food by mouth, dental plaque, and susceptible tooth surface, certain other factors act to enhance or diminish the probability of dental caries development. Some of these probably have an indirect effect by virtue of influencing one or more of the three essential factors. Certain systemic diseases have been reported to alter dental caries experience. The etiologic factors in each instance are not altogether clear. In patients institutionalized with neurologic diseases, the high level of dental caries might be attributed to an inability of the patient to carry out or secure adequate oral hygiene procedures. In patients with uncontrolled diabetes mellitus, increased levels of salivary sugars have been reported. Delayed tooth eruption is an important clinical feature of hypothyroidism. When children with this condition are compared with unaffected children of the same age, a difference in the length of time that the teeth have been exposed to intraoral cariogenic influences must be recognized.

A number of studies have been conducted to show what relationship, if any, exists between dental caries experience and heredity. Dental caries activity exhibits a narrower range of disease expression in monozygotic and dizygotic twins than in unrelated, comparably aged children. Children with Down's syndrome, whether institutionalized or living at home, are believed to have a lower-than-normal dental caries rate. A major problem in studying the relationship between heredity and dental caries is the difficulty of separating genetic from environmental influences. For example, very few studies have attempted to delineate inherited family patterns of caries susceptibility. It can be argued that environmental conditions in a household, rather than heredity, are of major importance. Husbands and wives, for example, constitute genetically unrelated individuals who live together and share a common diet. Data from the Ten-State Nutrition Survey of 1968 to 1970 were examined to find race-specific, spouse-pair DMFT (decayed, missing, or filled teeth) similarities. The husband-wife correlations became even stronger with advancing age. Parent-child correlations for DMFT in the same data base were also positive and statistically significant. Correlations were systematically higher for mother-child than for father-child pairs. The parent-child similarities were higher in blacks than they were in whites. Sibling similarities (brother-brother, sister-sister, and brother-sister) were also positive. These findings suggest that only part of the familial DMFT resemblances have a genetic basis. Twin studies have also demonstrated that environmental differences are capable of overriding hereditary similarities.

The role of saliva in determining susceptibility or resistance to caries is a very important one. Physical suspension and flushing of food particles (bacterial substrate) from the tooth surface, as well as flushing away of bacteria and their metabolites, constitute an important function. The buffering capacity and antibacterial substances within the saliva, such as IgA, are also important determinants of dental plaque cariogenicity. Additionally, saliva is a major source of mineral salts for the oral fluids that bathe the tooth surface. Soluble minerals, particularly phosphates, reduce enamel solubility by the common ion effect (when the concentration of the phosphate ions in oral fluid is higher than the solubility product of the phosphates in the mineral phase of the enamel, enamel dissolution is prevented). When salivary flow is reduced or eliminated, as in xerostomia, a marked increase in dental caries is commonly experienced.

The biochemical character of tooth substance itself is a modifying factor. In addition to anatomic tissue characteristics that distinguish the various dental hard tissues from one another, compositional differences within the mineral phase play a significant role. Nutritional deficiencies during tooth formation have been carefully explored to determine impact upon the final tissue's susceptibility. Foremost among those nutrients believed to play a role are the vitamins A and D and the minerals calcium, phosphate, and fluoride. Clinical confirmation of a major role for all but fluoride is either weak or non-existent. Fluoride, on the other hand, is an essential ion for formation of caries-resistant dental hard tissue.

The presence of fluoride in drinking water during the years of tooth mineralization results in formation of fluorapatite crystallites, which are less soluble and more caries resistant than the usual hard tissue mineral species, hydroxyapatite. This exerts a powerful anticaries influence upon the final mineralized hard tissue product. The systemic effect of fluoride in the drinking water in minute amounts (1 part per million) during primary mineralization of the dental hard tissues is associated with a dental caries reduction of approximately 60% in children. After primary mineralization is complete and the tooth has erupted into the oral cavity, continued fluoride uptake by the enamel, although slight, occurs by topical or surface interaction with fluoride-containing substances (fluoridated water, dentifrice, or prophylaxis paste). Incorporation of fluoride into the mineral phase is believed to occur in three stages: (1) uptake of fluoride into the hydration shell of the hydroxyapatite; (2) fixation of the fluoride on the surface of the crystallites; and eventually, (3) exchange of fluoride ions for hydroxyls in the crystal lattice. The magnitude of effect of the topical application of fluoride depends upon whether fluoride was present during tooth formation (an additive effect) or not (a substitutive effect). The former situation results in a greater increment of protection than does the latter.

Bibliography

Arends J, Christoffersen J. The nature of early caries lesions in enamel. J Dent Res 65:2–11, 1986.

Arnett R III, McKusick D, Sonnefeld S, Cowell C. Projections of health care spending to 1990. Health Care Finance Rev 7:1–36, 1986.

Arnold F Jr, Likins R, Russell A, Scott D. Fifteenth year of the Grand Rapids fluoridation study. J Am Dent Assoc 65:780–785, 1962.

Ast D, Bushel A, Wachs B, Chase H. Newburgh-Kingston caries-fluorine study. VIII. Combined clinical and roentgenographic dental findings after eight years of fluoride experience. J Am Dent Assoc 50:680, 1955.

Ast D, Fitzgerald B. Effectiveness of water fluoridation. J Am Dent Assoc 65:581–587, 1962.

Backer-Dirks O. The relation between the fluoridation of water and dental caries experience. Int Dent J 17:582–605, 1967.

Becks H, Jensen A, Millarr C. Rampant dental caries: prevention and prognosis; a five-year clinical survey. J Am Dent Assoc 31:1189, 1944.

Berkowitz R, Jordan H, White G. The early establishment of *Streptococcus mutans* in the mouths of infants. Arch Oral Biol 20:171–174, 1975.

Bibby B, Mundorff S, Zero D, Almekinder K. Oral food clearance and the pH of plaque and saliva. J Am Dent Assoc 112:333–337, 1986.

Birch R. The role of dietary supplements of fluoride in dental health programs for fluoride deficient areas. J Public Health Dent 29:170, 1969.

Black G. Susceptibility and immunity to dental caries. Dent Cosmos 41:826, 1899.

Blayney J. A report on 13 years of water fluoridation in Evanston, Illinois. J Am Dent Assoc 61:76–79, 1960.

Blayney J, Bradel S, Harrison R, Hemmens E. Continuous clinical and bacteriologic study of proximal surfaces of premolar teeth before and after the onset of caries. J Am Dent Assoc 29:1645, 1942.

Bohannan H. Caries distribution and the case for sealants. J Public Health Dent 43:200–204, 1983.

Bowen W, Genco R, O'Brien T (eds). Immunologic Aspects of Dental Caries. Information Retrieval, Arlington, Va, 1976.

Bransby E, Knowles E. A comparison of the effect of enemy occupation and postwar conditions on the incidence of dental caries in children in the Channel Islands in relation to diet and food supplies. Br Dent J 87:236, 1949.

Brewer H, Stookey G, Muhler J. A clinical study concerning the anticariogenic effects of NaH_2PO_4-enriched breakfast cereals in institutionalized subjects: results after two years. J Am Dent Assoc 80:121–124, 1970.

Brown W, McLaren H, Poplove M. The Brantford-Sarnia-Stratford fluoridation caries study—1959 report. Can Dent Assoc J 26:131–142, 1960.

Brown W, Konig K (eds). Cariostatic mechanisms of fluorides. Caries Res 11 (Suppl 1), 1977.

Brudevold F, Hein J, Bonner J, Nevin R, Bibby B, Hodge H. Reaction of tooth surfaces with one ppm of fluoride as sodium fluoride. J Dent Res 36:771–779, 1957.

Bunting R, Palmerlee F. The role of *Bacillus acidophilus* in dental caries. J Am Dent Assoc 12:381–413, 1925.

Burt B, Ismail A, Eklund S. Root caries in an optimally fluoridated and a high fluoride community. J Dent Res 65:1154–1158, 1986.

Carlos J. Epidemiologic trends in caries: impact on adults and the aged. *In* Guggenheim B (ed). Cariology Today. S Karger, Basel, 1984, pp 131–148.

Carlsson J, Egelberg J. Effect of diet on early plaque formation in man. Odont Rev 16:112, 1965.

Carlsson J, Sunderstrom B. Variations in composition of early dental plaque following ingestion of sucrose and glucose. Odont Rev 19:161, 1968.

Challacombe S, Russell M, Hawkes J. Passage of intact IgG from plasma to the oral cavity via crevicular fluid. Clin Exp Immunol 34:417–422, 1978.

Corbett M, Moore W. The distribution of dental caries in ancient British populations. IV. The 19th century. Caries Res 10:401–414, 1976.

Critchley P, Wood J, Saxton C, Leach S. The polymerisation of dietary sugars by dental plaque. Caries Res 1:112, 1967.

Czerkinsky C, Prince S, Michalek S, et al. IgA antibody producing cells in peripheral blood after antigen ingestion: evidence for a common mucosal immune system in humans. Proc Natl Acad Sci USA 84:2449–2453, 1987.

Dean H, McKay F, Elvove E. Mottled enamel survey of Bauxite, Arkansas, ten years after a change in the common water supply. Public Health Rep 53:1736, 1938.

Dean HT, Jay P, Arnold F Jr, Elvove E. Domestic water and dental caries. II. A study of 2,832 white children, aged 12 to 14 years, of eight suburban Chicago communities, including *Lactobacillus acidophilus* studies of 1,761 children. Public Health Rep 56:761–792, 1941.

Downer M. Changing patterns of disease in the western world. *In* Guggenheim B (ed). Cariology Today. S Karger, Basel, 1984, pp 1–12.

Doyle R, Ciardi J (eds). Glucosyltransferases, Glucans, Sucrose, and Dental Caries. National Institute for Dental Research Proceedings. Information Retrieval, Arlington, Va, 1983.

Edwardsson S. Bacteriological studies on deep areas of carious dentine. Odont Rev 25 (Suppl 32):1–143, 1974.

Englander H. Dental caries experience of teen-aged children who consumed fluoridated or fluoride deficient water continuously from birth. Int Dent J 14:497–504, 1964.

Englander H, Reuss R, Kesel R. Roentgenographic and clinical evaluation of dental caries in adults who consume fluoridated versus fluoride deficient water. J Am Dent Assoc 68:14–19, 1964.

Feagin F, Koulourides T, Pigman W. The characterization of enamel surface demineralization, remineralization, and associated hardness changes in human and bovine material. Arch Oral Biol 14:1407, 1969.

Finn S, Jamison H. The effect of a dicalcium phosphate chewing gum on caries incidence in children: 30-month results. J Am Dent Assoc 74:987–995, 1967.

Fitzgerald R, Jordan H, Stanley H. Experimental caries and gingival pathologic changes in the gnotobiotic rat. J Dent Res 39:923, 1960.

Fitzgerald R, Keyes P. Demonstration of the etiologic role of streptococci in experimental caries in the hamster. J Am Dent Assoc 61:9–19, 1960.

Fosdick L, Englander H, Hoerman K, Kesel R. A comparison of pH values of *in vivo* dental plaque after sucrose and sorbitol mouth rinses. J Am Dent Assoc 55:191–195, 1957.

Garn S, Cole P, Solomon M, Schaefer A. Relationships between sugar foods and the DMFT in 1968 to 1970. Ecology Food Nutr 9:135–138, 1980.

Garn S, Rowe N, Clark D. Parent-child similarities in dental caries rates. J Dent Res 55:1129, 1976.

Garn S, Rowe N, Cole P. Husband-wife similarities in dental caries experience. J Dent Res 56:186, 1977.

Garn S, Rowe N, Cole P. Sibling similarities in dental caries. J Dent Res 55:914, 1976.

Gibbons R, Banghart S. Synthesis of extracellular dextran by cariogenic bacteria and its presence in human dental plaque. Arch Oral Biol 12:11, 1967.

Gibbons R, Socransky S. Intracellular polysaccharide storage by organisms in dental plaques. Its relation to dental caries and microbial ecology of the oral cavity. Arch Oral Biol 7:73, 1962.

Gibbons R, van Houte J. On the formation of dental plaques. J Periodontol 44:347, 1973.

Gilmore N. The effect on dental caries activity of supplementing diets with phosphates; a review. J Public Health Dent 29:188, 1969.

Glass R. A two-year clinical trial of sorbitol chewing gum. Caries Res 17:365–368, 1983.

Glass R (ed). The first international conference on the declining prevalence of dental caries. J Dent Res 61:1304–1383, 1982.

Gray J, Francis M. Physical chemistry of enamel dissolution. *In* Sognnaes R (ed). Mechanisms of Hard Tissue Destruction. Washington, DC, American Association for the Advancement of Science, 1963, pp 213–260.

Gustafsson B, Quensel C, Lanke L, Lundqvist C, Grahnen H, Bonow B, Krasse B. The Vipeholm dental caries study. The effect of different levels of carbohydrate intake on caries activity in 436 individuals observed for five years. Acta Odontol Scand 11:232, 1954.

Harris R. Biology of the children of Hopewood House, Bowral, Australia. IV. Observations of dental caries experience extending over five years (1957 to 1961). J Dent Res 42:1387–1398, 1963.

Hefferren J (ed). Scientific consensus conference on methods for assessment of the cariogenic potential of foods. J Dent Res 65:1473–1543, 1986.

Hill T. Fluoride dentifrices. J Am Dent Assoc 59:1121–1127, 1959.

Holloway P, James P, Slack G. Dental disease in Tristan da Cunha. Br Dent J 115:19–25, 1963.

Horowitz A, Bawden J. Proceedings of National Institutes of Health Consensus Development Conference: Dental sealants in the prevention of tooth decay. J Dent Educ 48 (Suppl):1–34, 1984.

Isaac S, Brudevold F, Smith F, Gardner D. The relation of fluoride in the drinking water to the distribution of fluoride in enamel. J Dent Res 37:318–325, 1958.

Isaac S, Brudevold F, Smith F, Gardner D. Solubility rate and natural fluoride content of surface and subsurface enamel. J Dent Res 37:254–262, 1958.

Jay P. The reduction of oral *Lactobacillus acidophilus* counts by the periodic restriction of carbohydrate. Am J Orthodontics 33:162–184, 1947.

Jenkins G, Forster M, Speirs R, Kleinberg I. The influence of the refinement of carbohydrates on their cariogenicity. *In vitro* experiments on white and brown flour. Br Dent J 106:195–208, 1959.

Jensen M. Responses of interproximal plaque pH to snack foods and effect of chewing sorbitol containing gum. J Am Dent Assoc 113:262–266, 1986.

Johansson B. Remineralization of slightly etched enamel. J Dent Res 44:64–70, 1965.

Johnson C, Gross S, Hillman J. Cariogenic potential in

vitro in man and in vivo in the rat of lactate dehydrogenase mutants of *Streptococcus mutans*. Arch Oral Biol 25:707–713, 1980.

Katz R, Hazen S, Chilton N, Mumma R Jr. Prevalence and intraoral distribution of root caries in an adult population. Caries Res 16:265–271, 1982.

Keene H. History of dental caries in human populations: the first million years. *In* Tanzer J (ed). Animal Models in Cariology: Symposium Proceedings. Information Retrieval, Arlington, Va, 1981, pp 23–40.

Keyes P. The infectious and transmissible nature of experiemental dental caries. Arch Oral Biol 1:304, 1960.

Keyes P. Recent advances in dental caries research. Bacteriology. Int Dent J 12:443–464, 1962.

Keyes P, Fitzgerald R, Jordan H, White C. The effect of various drugs on caries and periodontal disease in albino hamsters. Arch Oral Biol 7 (Suppl):159–177, 1962.

Klein H. Dental effects of community water accidentally fluoridated for 19 years. II. Differences in the extent of caries reduction among different types of permanent teeth. Public Health Rep 63:563–573, 1948.

Kohler B, Andreen I, Jonsson B. The effect of caries preventive measures in mothers on dental caries and the oral presence of the bacteria *Streptococcus mutans* and lactobacilli in their children. Arch Oral Biol 29:879–883, 1984.

Kohler B, Bratthal D, Krasse B. Preventive measures in mothers influence the establishment of the bacterium *Streptococcus mutans* in their infants. Arch Oral Biol 28:225–231, 1983.

Konig K. Feeding regimens and caries. J Dent Res 49:1327–1332, 1970.

Koulourides T. Remineralization methods. Ann NY Acad Sci 153:84, 1968.

Krasse B. The effect of caries including streptococci in hamsters fed diets with sucrose or glucose. Arch Oral Biol 10:223–226, 1965.

Kristofferson K, Birkhed D. Effects of partial sugar restriction for six weeks on numbers of *Streptococcus mutans* in saliva and interdental plaque in man. Caries Res 21:79–86, 1987.

Littleton N. Dental caries and periodontal diseases among Ethiopian civilians. Public Health Rep 78:631–640, 1963.

Littleton N, White C. Dental findings from a preliminary study of children receiving extended antibiotic therapy. J Am Dent Assoc 68:520–526, 1964.

Loe H, Kleinman D (eds). Dental plaque control measures and oral hygiene practices. Information Retrieval, Alexandria, Va, 1986.

Mandel I. Effects of dietary modifications on caries in humans. J Dent Res 49:1201–1211, 1970.

Mandel I. Relation of saliva and plaque to caries. J Dent Res 53:246–266, 1974.

Marthaler T. Explanations for changing patterns of disease in the western world. *In* Guggenheim B (ed). Cariology Today. S Karger, Basel, 1984, pp 13–23.

McClure F, Likins R. Fluorine in human teeth studied in relation to fluorine in the drinking water. J Dent Res 30:172–176, 1951.

McKay F. The establishment of a definite relation between enamel that is defective in its structure, as mottled enamel, and the liability to decay. Dent Cosmos 71:747–755, 1929.

Mellanby H, Mellanby M. Dental structure and caries in five-year-old children attending London County Council schools. Result of five surveys (1929 to 1949). Br Med J 1:1341, 1950.

Michalek S, McGhee J, Shiota T, Devenyns D. Low sucrose levels promote *Streptococcus mutans* induced dental caries. Infect Immun 16:712–716, 1977.

Mitchell D, Holmes L. Topical antibiotic control of dentogingival plaque. J Periodontol 36:202–208, 1965.

Moore W, Corbett M. The distribution of dental caries in ancient British populations. III. The 17th century. Caries Res 9:163–175, 1975.

Muhlemann H, Meyer R, Konig K, Marthaler T. The cariostatic effects of some antibacterial inhibitors. J Dent Res 40:697, 1961.

Muhler J. Effect of a stannous fluoride dentifrice on caries reduction in children during a three-year study period. J Am Dent Assoc 64:216, 1962.

Navia J, Lopez H, Harris R. Cariostatic effects of sodium trimetaphosphate when fed to rats during different stages of tooth development. Arch Oral Biol 13:779, 1968.

Newbrun E. Sucrose, the arch criminal of dental caries. Odont Rev 18:373–386, 1967.

Nizel A, Harris R. The effects of phosphates on experimental dental caries: a literature review. J Dent Res 43:1123, 1964.

Osborn T, Noriskin J. The relation between diet and caries in the South African Bantu. J Dent Res 16:431–441, 1937.

Peterson J. North Dakota field test of cariostatic effect of 1% sodium dihydrogen phosphate and disodium hydrogen phosphate added to presweetened breakfast cereals. J Dent Res 49:1308, 1969.

Pigman W, Koulourides T, Cueto H. Rehardening of softened tooth enamel. Arch Oral Biol (Suppl):133–134, 1963.

Price W. Eskimo and Indian field studies in Alaska and Canada. J Am Dent Assoc 23:417, 1936.

Rogers A. The source of infection in the intrafamilial transfer of *Streptococcus mutans*. Caries Res 15:26–31, 1981.

Rosebury T, Waugh L. Dental caries among Eskimos of the Kuskokwim area of Alaska. Am J Dis Child 57:871, 1939.

Rowe N. Is dietary phosphate fortification of value as an anticaries agent? Ecology Food Nutr 1:173–177, 1972.

Rowe N (ed). Diet, Nutrition, and Dental Caries: Proceedings of Symposium. University of Michigan Press, Ann Arbor, 1979.

Rowe N, Garn S, Clark D, Guire K. The effect of age, sex, race, and economic status on dental caries experience of the permanent dentition. Pediatrics 57:457–461, 1976.

Rugg-Gunn A, Edgar W, Geddes D, Jenkins G. The effect of different meal patterns upon plaque pH in human subjects. Br Dent J 139:351–356, 1975.

Russell A, Leatherwood E, Le Van Hien, Van Reen R. Dental caries and nutrition in South Vietnam. J Dent Res 44:102–111, 1965.

Scheinin A, Makinen K, Ylitalo K. Turku sugar studies. V. Final report on the effect of sucrose, fructose, and xylitol diets on the caries incidence in man. Acta Odontol Scand 34:179–216, 1976.

Schlesinger E, Overton D, Chase H, Cantrell K. Newburgh-Kingston caries-fluorine study. XIII. Pediatric findings after ten years. J Am Dent Assoc 152:296–306, 1956.

Shaw J. Causes and control of dental caries. N Engl J Med 317:996–1004, 1987.

Shaw J. An evaluation in rats of the relationship between the frequency of providing food and the caries producing ability of diets. Arch Oral Biol 13:1003–1013, 1968.

Shaw J, Krumins I, Gibbons R. Comparison of sucrose, lactose, maltose, and glucose in the causation of experimental oral diseases. Arch Oral Biol 12:755–768, 1967.

Silverstone L. The significance of remineralization in caries prevention. Can Dent Assoc J 50:157–167, 1984.

Sognnaes R. An analysis of a wartime reduction of dental caries in European children, with special regard to observations from Norway. Am J Dis Child 75:792, 1948.

Sognnaes R. Histologic evidence of developmental lesions in teeth originating from Paleolithic, prehistoric, and ancient man. Am J Pathol 32:547–577, 1956.

Sreebny L. Sugar availability, sugar consumption, and dental caries. Community Dent Oral Epidemiol 10:1–7, 1982.

Stamm J, Banting D. Comparison of root caries prevalence in adults with lifelong residence in fluoridated and non-fluoridated communities (Abstract). J Dent Res 59:406, 1980.

Stiles H, Loesche W, O'Brien T (eds). Microbial Aspects of Dental Caries, Vols 1 and 2. Information Retrieval, Alexandria, Va, 1976.

Stookey G, Carroll R, Muhler J. The clinical effectiveness of phosphate enriched breakfast cereals on the incidence of dental caries in children: results after two years. J Am Dent Assoc 74:752–758, 1967.

Stralfors A. Disinfection of dental plaques in man. Odont Tidskr 70:183–203, 1962.

Swango P. The current status of research with xylitol: a review of dental caries in animals and human subjects. *In* Shaw J, Roussos G (eds). Sweeteners and Dental Caries. Information Retrieval, Alexandria, VA, 1978, pp 225–237.

Taubman M, Smith D, Ebersol J, Stack W, Tsukuda T, Trocme M. Caries immunity and immune responses to *Streptococcus mutans* glucosyltransferase. *In* Hamada S, Michalek S, Kiyono H, Menaker L, McGhee J (eds). Molecular Microbiology and Immunobiology of *Streptococcus mutans*. Elsevier Press, Amsterdam, 1986, pp 279–286.

Toverud G. Dental caries in Norwegian children during and after the Second World War. J Am Diet Assoc 26:673, 1950.

Van Houte J, Gibbons R, Banghart S. Adherence as a determinant of the presence of *Streptococcus salivarius* and *Streptococcus sanguis* on the human tooth surface. Arch Oral Biol 15:1025–1034, 1970.

Von der Fehr F, Loe H, Theilade E. Experimental caries in man. Caries Res 4:131–148, 1970.

Winter G. Sucrose and cariogenesis. A review. Br Dent J 124:407, 1968.

Zinner D, Aran A, Jablon J, Brust B, Saslaw M. Experimental caries induced in animals by streptococci of human origin. Proc Soc Exp Biol Med 118:766–770, 1965.

Chapter 18

Periodontal Disease

Frederick Burgett

ETIOLOGY AND PATHOGENESIS
PERIODONTAL EXAMINATION
GINGIVITIS
Simple Gingivitis
Hyperplastic Gingivitis
Acute Necrotizing Ulcerative Gingivitis
PERIODONTITIS
Acute Periodontitis
Chronic Periodontitis
Juvenile Periodontitis
Papillon-Lefèvre Syndrome

Inflammatory periodontal disease is the other major oral disease that, along with dental caries, represents the chief oral health threat to Americans. Dental caries damages the tooth itself; the supporting structures for the tooth—gingiva, cementum, alveolar bone, and periodontal membrane—are affected by periodontal disease.

Periodontal disease refers to the full spectrum of inflammatory diseases of the periodontium. Classically, the natural history of periodontal disease is described as a continuum:

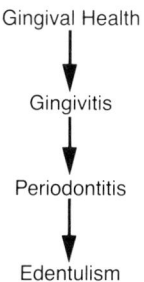

Periodontal disease strongly relates to age. Many children are free from gingivitis despite the presence of dental plaque. During puberty, general susceptibility to gingivitis occurs. Over 65% of American teenagers have significant gingivitis. Periodontal pockets and the loss of periodontal attachment commence in the 20s and 30s. Over 65% of American adults have periodontal pockets. About one half of those over the age of 70 are edentulous. Dental caries and periodontal disease are the major causes of edentulism. These prevalence figures come from cross-sectional epidemiologic data (National Center for Health Statistics, 1973).

The detrimental result of periodontal disease activity can be determined directly through measurement of attachment levels—the distance between the probing depth of the periodontal pocket and the cementoenamel junction (Fig. 18–1). Tooth extraction, regardless of cause, also results in the loss of periodontal support. Recent national epidemiologic studies utilizing attachment level measurements and tooth loss estimate an average loss of 1.9 mm of periodontal support for the mean of 24 teeth of employed American adults (National Center for Health Statistics, 1973). These averages represent a loss of more than 25% of the total periodontal support of the complete dentition of 28 teeth with no periodontal attachment loss. For Americans over age 65, estimated mean attachment loss exceeds 3 mm, with a mean of 10 teeth remaining, a loss of about 75% of the periodontal support. Even so, compared with previous surveys of Americans, these findings show an improvement in oral health status.

Longitudinal epidemiologic studies provide strong support for the chronic disease model

Pocket Depth Attachment Loss

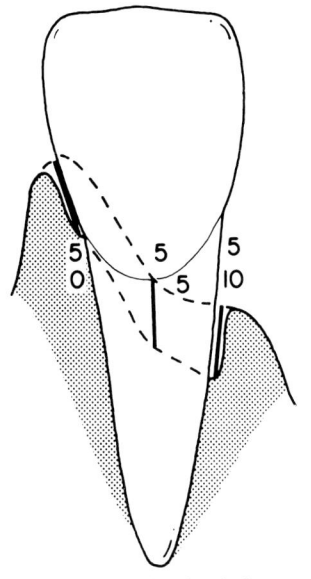

Figure 18–1. Attachment levels. A 5-mm pocket depth with no attachment loss (left); 5 mm of attachment loss (middle); and 10 mm of attachment loss (right).

of periodontal disease. In longitudinal epidemiologic studies, periodontal scoring is done repeatedly on the same individuals over time. Major differences in the rate of attachment loss occur between people of different cultures. Despite these differences, there is a trend toward gradual destruction of the periodontium starting prior to the age of 20. For each individual, there may be periods of slow progress and periods that show acceleration. By age 40, on average, people lose from about 1.5 mm of periodontal support to about 4.5 mm. Mean rate of loss of attachment is between 0.1 mm and 0.3 mm per year; it increases somewhat with increasing age.

In considering these figures, it is important to remember that the rate of attachment loss varies appreciably among individuals. Some people are significantly more susceptible and suffer greater periodontal destruction; others exhibit slight, if any, loss. One population has shown rapid loss of periodontal attachment in about 10% of the individuals followed longitudinally, no loss in about 10%, and a moderate rate of loss in the remaining 80%. The degree of progression also varies between different sites within an individual's dentition, although there is a tendency for bilateral symmetry in the distribution of attachment loss, bone loss, and tooth loss from periodontitis.

ETIOLOGY AND PATHOGENESIS

Inflammatory periodontal disease represents an equilibrium between the primary etiologic factor, dental plaque, and the host at the dentogingival junction. In this host-parasite balance, supragingival plaque and its constituents are responsible for gingivitis, and subgingival plaque and its constituents are responsible for the development of periodontitis. Although gingivitis is a precursor of periodontitis, it does not always progress to periodontitis. An individual with gingivitis remains at greater risk for the development of periodontitis. When the host is in balance, periodontal stability or homeostasis exists; when out of balance, tissue destruction occurs.

Periodontal status is very strongly related to the extent of dental plaque and to age. However, given a low plaque score, there is also a low periodontal score regardless of age. With increasing age, there is a greater periodontal reaction to the presence of plaque. The greater length of time of exposure to the irritant in older individuals is probably the reason for the difference in the response rather than a reduced periodontal resistance concomitant with aging.

Individuals respond differently to plaque accumulation. These changes can be followed in experimental gingivitis studies wherein subjects discontinue home care procedures. When oral hygiene procedures are discontinued, plaque-induced gingival bleeding inevitably occurs, but the time of development varies. It may take only 10 to 12 days to develop in more susceptible individuals, or it may take as long as 3 weeks in more resistant individuals. With reinstitution of oral hygiene, gingivitis resolves sooner in those individuals in whom it took longer to develop.

Changes in the microbiologic make-up of dental plaque occur as it accumulates over time and coincide with the inflammatory changes seen clinically. Young plaque, 1 to 3 days old, consists of gram-positive, facultative cocci and small rods, considered health-related plaque. Filamentous organisms such as *Actinomyces israelii* and *A. viscosus* dominate the plaque flora after 2 or 3 days without oral hygiene. At about 7 days and preceding the development of gingivitis, the proportion of vibrios and spirochetes increases. Gingivitis develops following a shift in the plaque flora from primarily gram-positive streptococci to primarily gram-negative forms and a marked increase in the proportion of motile microorganisms. A correlation exists between the proportion of motile forms in the plaque and the degree of inflammation. Plaque flora associated with health, with gingivitis, and with periodontitis have distinct and different compositions.

Local etiologic factors in addition to dental plaque are dental calculus, subgingival margins of restorations, overhanging restorations, food impaction, trauma from occlusion, faulty dental prostheses, malocclusion, and mouth breathing. Systemic factors that can influence or impair host response are malnutrition, immune system defects, certain drug therapies, endocrine dysfunctions, some hereditary diseases, and stress.

A patient with untreated periodontal disease usually demonstrates sites with varying levels of disease activity, distributed somewhat symmetrically within the mouth. Although there is a continuum of changes from health to disease, stages are described by the occurrence of major events in the disease's progression. In the development of gingivitis, microscopic changes precede clinically apparent inflammation.

In health, the lining of the gingiva within the dentogingival junction consists of a long junctional epithelium, which provides a seal against the tooth and a line of defense against plaque organisms (Fig. 18–2). The connective tissue is made up almost entirely of collagen fiber bundles and endothelium-lined blood vessels. The few inflammatory cells consist of lymphocytes, neutrophils, and macrophages.

Accumulation of dental plaque at the free gingival margin leads to the development of the initial lesion of periodontal disease. It is characterized by acute inflammatory changes within the gingiva—increased migration of inflammatory exudates, gingival crevicular fluid and leukocytes, into the gingival crevice. Some of the collagen fibers within the gingiva near the free gingival margin are destroyed and replaced by the inflammatory infiltrate and enlarged blood vessels. Chemotactic substances from the maturing dental plaque initiate the host response.

The early lesion of gingivitis evolves from the initial lesion after about 4 days; with the early lesion, some clinical signs such as redness and swelling may develop (Fig. 18–3). As plaque invades the crevice, the gingival sulcus deepens through reduction in length of the junctional epithelium, and an inflammatory reaction against the plaque is triggered near the free gingival margin. Predominant cell types are neutrophils in the junctional epithelium and T lymphocytes in the connective tissue. The junctional epithelial zone persists between the irritant and the principal fibers of the periodontal membrane. No loss of periodontal membrane attachment occurs in either the initial or the early lesion. Characteristics of the early lesion may persist for a few weeks of plaque development. During this time, the inflammatory changes become more pronounced, with increased flow of crevicular fluid and leukocytic migration into the sulcus, a further reduction in collagen fibers, and an increase in numbers of lymphocytes in the infiltrated connective tissue. The immune system response of delayed hypersensitivity can trigger changes similar to these found in the early lesion.

A significant part of the defense mechanism of the gingiva occurs within the sulcus. Gingival fluid acts as a flushing mechanism to lubricate and cleanse the sulcus; it contains enzymes and antibodies directed against bacteria. It also contains neutrophils and monocytes that phagocytose bacteria. A smooth tooth surface can facilitate the functioning of the host response at the dentogingival junction. The volume of

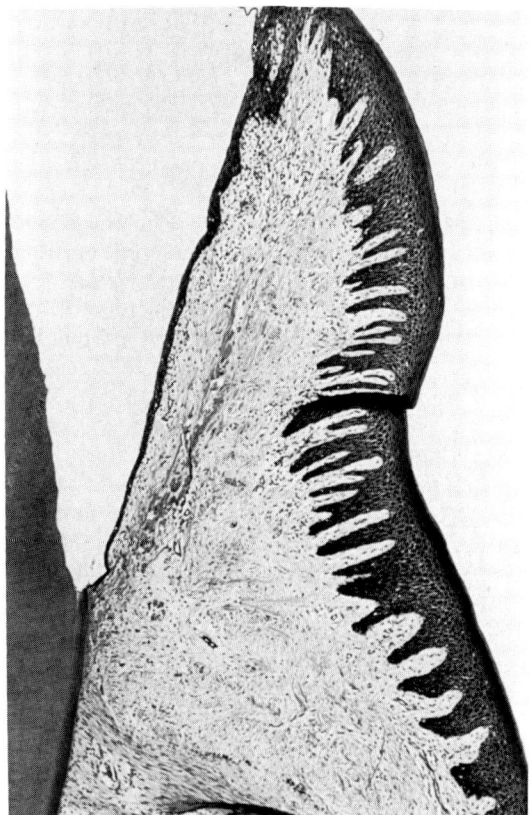

Figure 18–2. Decalcified histologic section of healthy gingiva. Enamel space to left and top.

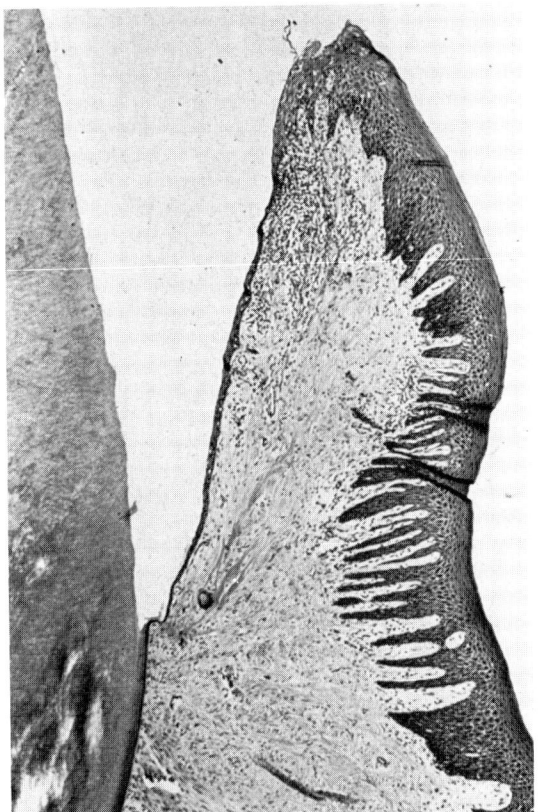

Figure 18-3. Decalcified histologic section of an early gingival lesion. Note inflammatory cells on crevicular side of the gingiva.

content of the gingiva by inflamed connective tissue, ulceration of the pocket epithelium, increased crevicular fluid production and purulence, a general destruction of the normal anatomy of the gingiva, and its replacement by elements of the inflammatory response. Plasma cells and T lymphocytes increase and B lymphocytes decrease, proportionally. The root surface is altered by the process; plaque and calculus adhere to the tooth surface and attach to irregularities in the cementum; the cementum is altered and absorbs endotoxins. A random mixture of clumps of different types of bacteria are scattered within the tissue. The junctional epithelium is short and extends apically as the principal fibers of the periodontal membrane are destroyed. Osteoclastic activity is induced by factors from the dental plaque or by the inflammatory response itself. Supporting bone for the teeth is lost. Episodes of acute inflammation within the advanced lesion may be necessary for periodontal destruction to occur.

At an individual site, pathogenesis proceeds as follows:

gingival fluid flow correlates directly with the extent of inflammation.

After several weeks, the established lesion of gingivitis develops from the early lesion, and with it, more obvious clinical signs develop—increase in swelling, crevicular bleeding, and exudates; and further color change (Fig. 18-4). In the established lesion, the predominating cell types in the infiltrate are plasma cells along with T and B lymphocytes. Junctional epithelium is changed to pocket epithelium characterized by cell proliferation, an increase in cell size, rete peg formation, and ulceration. There is an organization to the lesion: large numbers of neutrophils in the epithelium and sulcus, plasma cells located at the edge of the infiltrate, and macrophages just subjacent to the pocket epithelium. Mast cells are also present. The established lesion may exist for long periods of time, months or perhaps years, without progressing to the advanced lesion.

The advanced lesion involves an infection of plaque deep within the dentogingival junction, replacement of much of the collagen fiber

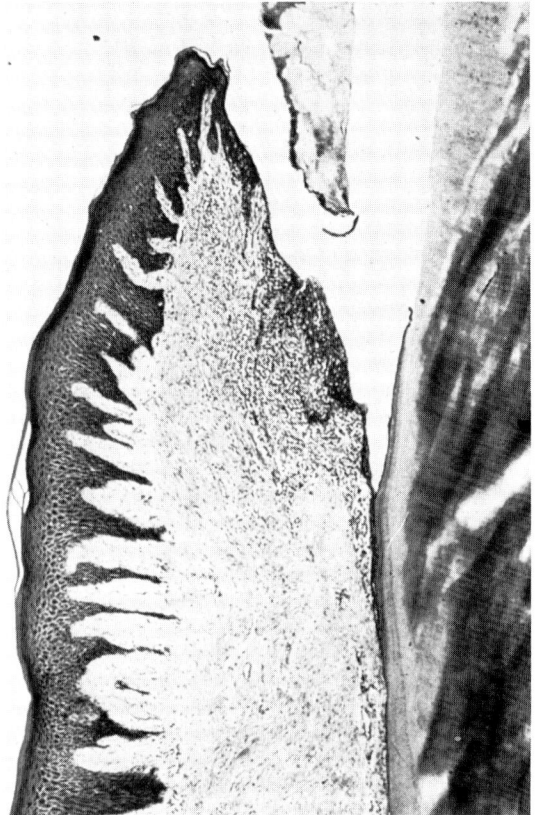

Figure 18-4. Decalcified histologic section of an established gingival lesion. Note plaque adjacent to enamel space and inflammatory cells on crevicular side of the gingiva.

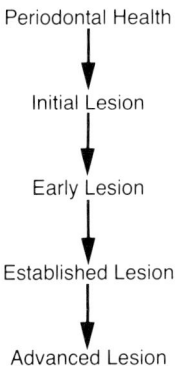

With treatment, the lesion resolves in the reverse order to that in which it develops.

Why the established lesion without attachment and bone loss progresses to the destructive advanced lesion is not known. It is not merely a matter of pocket depth, as depths greater than 3 mm can remain stable over time, with no progressive periodontal disease activity. From autopsy material, it is apparent that if plaque within the periodontal pocket is within 0.5 mm of the base of the junctional epithelium, bone loss will occur. If subgingival plaque is greater than 3 mm from the base of the junctional epithelium, no osteoclastic activity will occur within the alveolar crest. Between these two extremes, increasing bone loss occurs. The degree of destruction is determined by the depth of the infection, or rather the length of junctional epithelium apical to the infection, instead of by the depth of the periodontal pocket. Subgingival plaque produces a zone of inflammatory reaction in a radius of about 2 mm. If the periodontal membrane and alveolar bone lie within this zone, destruction occurs.

In addition to differences in microbiologic make-up, supragingival and subgingival plaque differ in their rates of colonization onto a tooth. Supragingival plaque builds up on the tooth surface within a few hours after removal. Plaque must overcome the host defense system to populate the gingival crevice. The rate of plaque growth along the tooth surface into the crevice may be as slow as 1 mm per year.

According to the chronic disease model, periodontitis develops as a sequel to chronic gingivitis, possibly secondary to the presence of opportunistic, non-specific bacteria or their products causing an injury sufficient to overpower the defense mechanisms of the periodontium.

Another theory of disease is that periodontitis develops in response to infection by specific bacteria. The specific plaque theory is based on the observation that plaque changes character as gingival disease develops. The specific plaque hypothesis suggests that adult periodontitis involves a specific infection. In addition to treatment directed at the elimination of local factors, the infection must be treated by antiseptics or antibiotics. The flora of dental plaque associated with periodontal disease is complex in adults, involving over 300 different microbial species, many of which are yet to be completely characterized. Microbiologically, the flora varies among patients, among teeth within a patient, and even among different sites on the same tooth. Putative periodontopathic organisms for adult periodontitis are *Actinobacillus actinomycetemcomitans* and two black-pigmented *Bacteroides* species, *intermedius* and *gingivalis*. Many other organisms have been implicated, as might be predicted if an opportunistic infection is involved.

Through experimental manipulation of the subgingival environment by alternating gold restorations without and with overhangs, the flora can be changed from health-related flora to a flora dominated by the putative pathogens. In other words, a pathogenic infection can develop following the placement of an overhanging restoration and be cured by removing the defective restoration. Local treatment can affect the infective component of periodontitis.

Since there is a change in plaque as disease develops, it has been suggested that quantification of the flora of the plaque might be used to diagnose periodontal disease. One approach recommends the use of phase-contrast microscopy to determine the presence of motile organisms in plaque to diagnose periodontitis. The proportion of motile organisms correlates to pocket depths but not to periodontal disease activity, as stable pockets can harbor plaque with high numbers of motile forms. Too many false positive tests result from the use of plaque motility criteria as determined by phase-contrast microscopy.

In summary, periodontitis is a chronic disease that progresses at an average rate of 0.2 mm per year. A host-parasite balance is involved, with components of subgingival plaque acting as the parasite. The cause is multifactorial, with both local etiologic factors and host defense factors playing significant roles. Disease activity represents episodes of imbalance between the host and the parasite—these may involve simultaneous breakdown occurring at several different sites within an individual's dentition or at a single site. It is the sequel to gingivitis. Given the present level of understanding of the disease, its activity can be determined only by evidence of increasing periodontal attachment loss, increasing pocket depth, bone loss, and tooth loss.

PERIODONTAL EXAMINATION

Since there are no objective tests that have adequate predictive value to be of use in the diagnosis of periodontal disease activity, a subjective evaluation of periodontal status is necessary. Periodontal examination involves visual assessment of the gingiva, probing assessment of the dentogingival junction, and radiographic assessment of bone support. The examination must be systematic. Each individual site, i.e., each tooth surface, needs to be assessed as to its status—healthy or diseased. Repeated examinations are needed to determine changes in pocket depth and attachment level. Attributes of the gingiva and the relationship between the gingiva and the tooth to be evaluated are (1) gingival color, form, and density; (2) ease of probing of dentogingival junction; (3) crevicular bleeding tendency; (4) crevicular exudates; (5) subgingival plaque; (6) subgingival calculus; (7) pocket depth; and (8) periodontal attachment level.

Healthy gingival and dentogingival junction characteristics are (1) coral-pink color, firm resilient density, knife-edged free gingival margins, papilla filling interproximal spaces; (2) significant resistance to probing; (3) no bleeding tendency; (4) no exudates; (5) no subgingival plaque; (6) no subgingival calculus; (7) no change in pocket depth over time; and (8) no change in attachment level over time.

Diseased gingival and dentogingival junction relationships are reflected by (1) reddening or bluish-red coloration, swollen edematous character, and spongy gingival density; (2) absence of resistance to probing; (3) crevicular bleeding tendency; (4) presence of exudates, especially purulence; (5) presence of subgingival plaque; (6) presence of subgingival calculus; (7) deepening of pocket depths; and (8) loss of periodontal attachment. Characteristics of established and advanced periodontal lesions are reflected clinically by gingival color change, no resistance to probing, crevicular bleeding tendency, intracrevicular exudates and plaque, and subgingival calculus. Only by repeated measurement over time can disease progression be monitored. Deepening pockets and loss of attachment differentiate the advanced lesion from the established lesion. Conversely, if these factors remain stable with repeated measurements, some positive findings for the other disease criteria may be tolerated. Treatment can return both the established lesion and the advanced lesion to health or periodontal stability.

Certain clinical relationships determined by the periodontal examination—pocket depths, periodontal attachment levels, plaque level, and bleeding tendency—should be recorded on the periodontal chart for comparing responses to treatment and to maintenance care.

A complete series of periapical radiographs and bite-wing radiographs complete the periodontal examination. They are used to evaluate alveolar bone (particularly at the alveolar crest and inter-radicular area), the lamina dura, periodontal membrane space, root form and length, presence of calculus, and fit of restorations.

Clinical and radiographic findings of the periodontal examination are considered in arriving at the appropriate diagnosis.

GINGIVITIS

Simple Gingivitis

Etiology and Pathogenesis. Simple gingivitis is the initial event in periodontal disease; unless treated, it can progress to periodontitis. With the maturation of dental plaque to include filamentous and motile microorganisms, gingivitis develops as the host response to the irritant. It is simple only in the sense that it is a reaction to local etiologic factors on the teeth and is uncomplicated by unusual local etiologic factors, such as mouth breathing, or host response features, such as diabetes mellitus.

Clinical Features. Inflammation causes changes in gingival color, form, and tone. Inflamed gingiva has a reddened or bluish-red appearance and a swollen, rolled character to the free gingival margins and to the gingival papilla, which may overfill the interproximal spaces. It also has a boggy or spongy density (Fig. 18–5). In addition to changes in appearance and resiliency of the gingiva, changes in the dentogingival junction occur that can best be determined by periodontal probing. There may be subgingival plaque and calculus, but crevicular bleeding is particularly significant. Bleeding tendency can be graded by how soon it occurs following probing and by its extent. Immediate, substantial bleeding on probing signifies a serious established gingival lesion. In simple gingivitis, the periodontal attachment level is on the enamel, although gingival

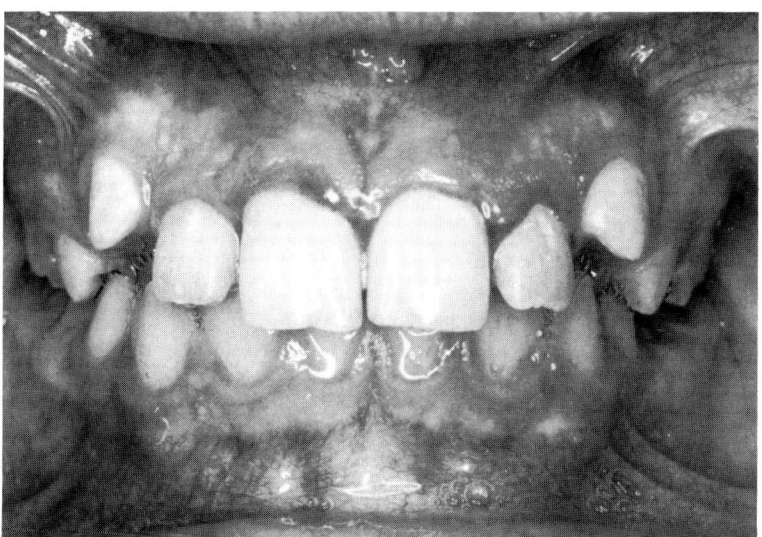

Figure 18–5. Simple gingivitis.

pockets may be present. Gingival bleeding on brushing is the symptom most often reported by the patient. Radiographic changes are absent in simple gingivitis.

Treatment and Prognosis. Treatment directed at elimination of local etiologic factors (including plaque, calculus, and overhangs from restorations) results in healing of the gingival lesions. A series of two to four visits for treatment and patient education should result in the restoration of gingival health. Prevention of recurrence can be accomplished through the patient's adoption of effective methods of daily personal oral hygiene. Participation in a dental care program involving periodic oral health examinations and tailored recall intervals for dental prophylaxis provides the best chance for oral health maintenance.

Hyperplastic Gingivitis

Etiology and Pathogenesis. Local factors (dental plaque and plaque retentive factors) must be present for gingivitis to develop. In hyperplastic gingivitis, the host response is dominated by tissue hyperplasia, perhaps because of an unusual local factor or because of the presence of a systemic modifying factor. Hyperplastic tissue can consist primarily of edema and inflammatory components, or it can consist of dense, fibrous tissue. Untreated hyperplastic gingivitis can develop into periodontitis.

Clinical Features. Findings in the periodontal examination are similar to those found in simple gingivitis, except for the striking feature of a marked increase in gingival bulk. Hyperplastic tissues dominated by inflammatory components are soft and edematous and bright red or cyanotic. They have a pronounced bleeding tendency (Fig. 18–6). When the tissue bulk is made up mostly of collagen fibers, the tissue is dense and fibrous (color change may be slight), and the crevicular bleeding tendency, though present, is less pronounced (Fig. 18–7). The gingival hyperplasia may be generalized or localized to an area or to a single papilla. With limited involvement, there may be etiologic agents that are unique to that particular area of the mouth, such as mouth breathing, gross calculus deposits, or overhanging restorations. Radiographic changes are absent in hyperplastic gingivitis.

Differential Diagnosis. Although no complicating factor may be established to explain hyperplastic gingivitis, suspicions should be aroused. Edematous hyperplastic gingivitis caused by mouth breathing ("mouth-breathing" gingivitis) can be diagnosed by the presence of a sharp demarcation or slight ridge between the gingiva irritated by drying and that portion protected by the lip (Fig. 18–8). The anterior palatal gingiva may be involved. Also helpful in arriving at the diagnosis is a report by the patient of a dry mouth on awakening.

Hormonal changes involved in puberty and pregnancy may contribute to the development of edematous hyperplastic gingivitis.

Leukemia, particularly acute monocytic and myelogenous types, superimposed on pre-existing gingival inflammation can cause gingival hyperplasia. The concomitant marked increase

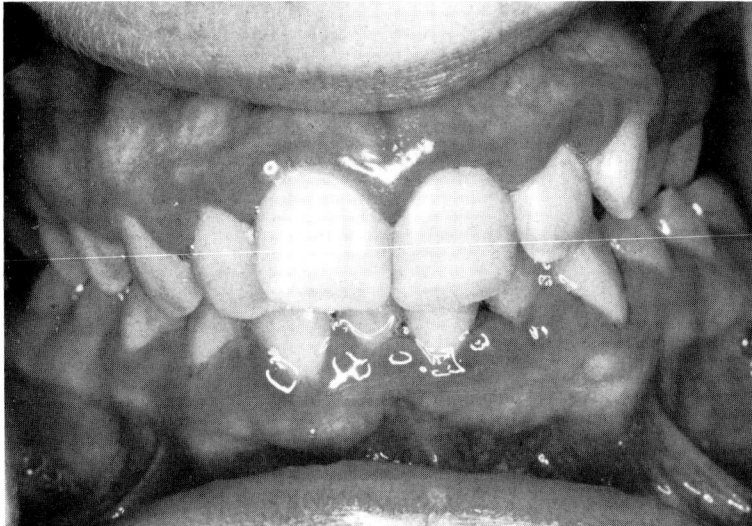

Figure 18–6. Hyperplastic gingivitis.

in gingival bleeding tendency may be the patient's first sign of the presence of a blood dyscrasia. Medical referral is indicated when systemic disease is suspected.

Generalized fibrous hyperplastic gingival lesions may result from drug therapy involving phenytoin (Dilantin), cyclosporine, or nifedipine. Phenytoin is used to control seizures, but it causes gingival hyperplasia in about 60% of patients using it. The gingival enlargement is composed primarily of dense connective tissue elements. Similar enlargements can be caused by cyclosporine, a powerful immunosuppressant drug used in organ transplant patients, and nifedipine, a drug used in patients with coronary insufficiency.

Massive fibrous gingival enlargements develop in idiopathic or hereditary gingival fibromatosis. Several forms of such conditions exist, each associated with different extraoral components.

Treatment and Prognosis. Uncomplicated hyperplastic gingivitis responds to treatment directed at elimination of local factors. Surgical reduction of extremely fibrous gingival enlargement may be necessary. Effective oral hygiene practices and regular dental visits, including prophylaxis, can prevent recurrence.

Patients with phenytoin-induced gingival hyperplasia usually require periodontal surgery; they should also have a 3-month recall interval for dental prophylaxis to minimize the potential for recurrence.

Mouth breathing–associated gingivitis often

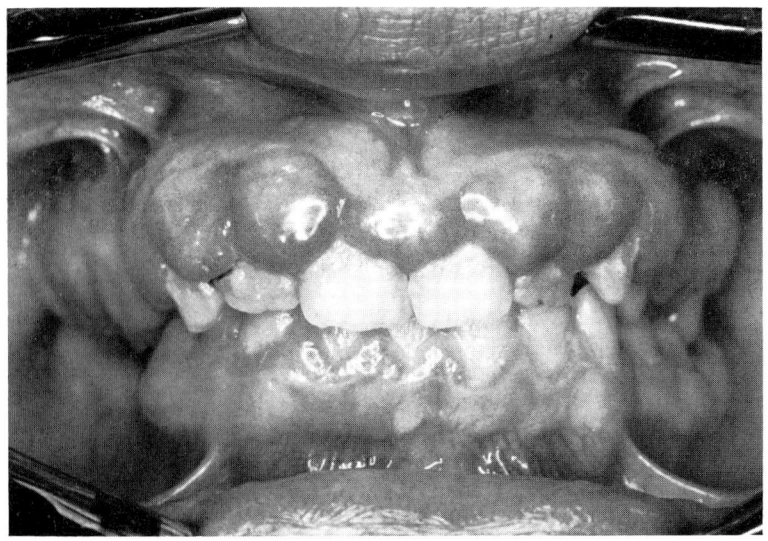

Figure 18–7. Fibrous hyperplastic gingivitis.

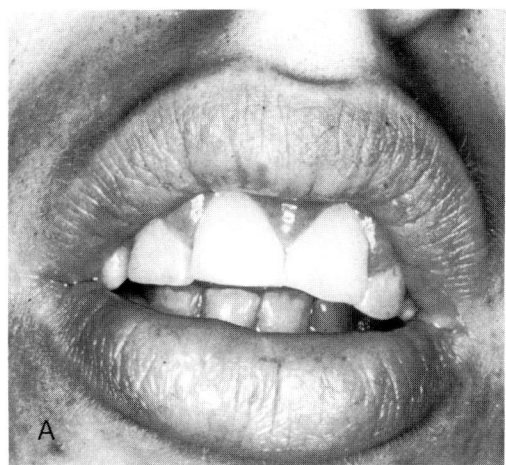 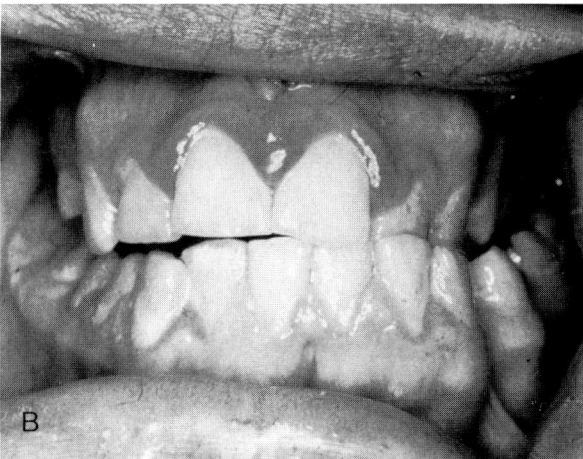

Figure 18-8. *A* and *B,* Mouth-breathing gingivitis.

cannot be resolved completely since drying of the tissue cannot be eliminated. It is important for the therapist and the patient to realize that plaque control alone will not eliminate the mild refractory gingivitis in the affected area. With good plaque control, however, the areas can remain stable and need not progress to a more destructive lesion.

Acute Necrotizing Ulcerative Gingivitis

Etiology and Pathogenesis. Acute necrotizing ulcerative gingivitis (ANUG) is a relatively rare condition clinically characterized by necrosis of the gingival tissue, starting interproximally at the tip of the papilla and proceeding circumferentially around the free gingival margin. The lower anterior region is usually affected first, but all gingiva may become involved. Progression is rapid, but periods of remission are possible. Development of the gingival lesions is accompanied by a marked increase in the proportion of fusiform bacilli and medium-sized spirochetes in the oral flora. An invasion of spirochetes in practically pure culture can be identified in the epithelium and connective tissue. Bone loss can result from long-standing necrotizing ulcerative gingivitis.

Attempts to transfer the disease through inoculation of infective material into healthy individuals have been unsuccessful, supporting the concept that the disease is not contagious.

Emotional stress and smoking have been implicated as predisposing factors in the initiation of the disease. Both can affect host defense mechanisms at local and systemic levels. Smoking can depress the chemotactic and phagocytic functions of lymphocytes. Individuals afflicted by Down's syndrome are more susceptible to ANUG-like infections and have reduced resistance to infections characterized by polymorphonuclear leukocytic chemotactic defects.

Clinical Features. ANUG presents a characteristic clinical picture of pain, necrosis of the gingival margins, cratering of the interdental papilla, and a marked bleeding tendency from the ulcerated tissue subjacent to the necrosis (Fig. 18-9). The lesions are covered by a "pseudomembrane" made up of necrotic material, inflammatory cells, and microorganisms. Calculus deposits often are present on the teeth in areas of the cratered papilla. Afflicted individuals have fetid breath. Involvement can be generalized and severe (Fig. 18-10). Those most commonly affected range in age from 15 to 30 years. Fever, lymphadenopathy, and malaise may accompany the lesions. The infection can involve the mucosa of the soft palate or the tonsils.

Differential Diagnosis. Primary herpetic gingivostomatitis can be differentiated from ANUG by the presence of ulcers in the mucosa away from the gingiva. Fever is prodromal in primary herpetic gingivostomatitis rather than concurrent as with ANUG. ANUG very rarely occurs prior to the onset of puberty; primary herpetic gingivostomatitis usually precedes puberty.

Erosive gingival lichen planus differs from ANUG in that it occurs away from the gingival margin and is associated with white striae. Lichen planus usually occurs in individuals over the age of 30.

Treatment and Prognosis. Reduction of acute symptoms of ANUG can be accom-

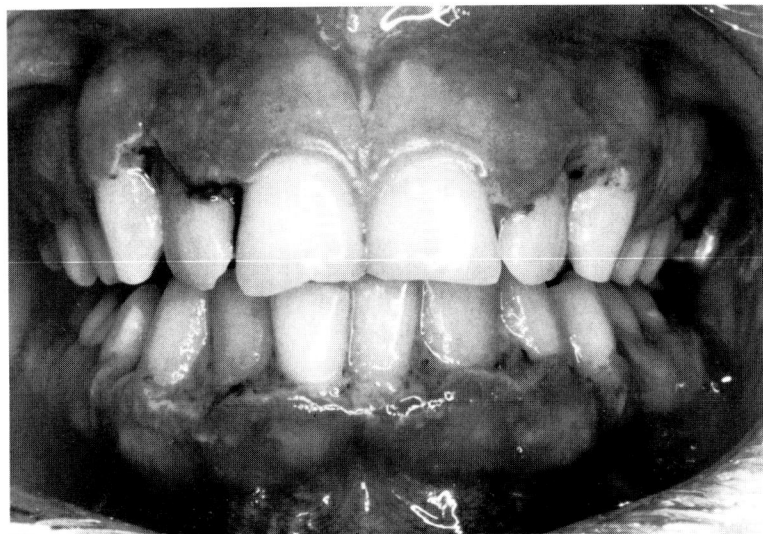

Figure 18–9. ANUG showing necrosis of interdental papillae and gingival margins.

plished by local débridement. Relief is often immediate and dramatic. With active lesions, the home care prescribed should involve use of a soft toothbrush and basswood toothpicks for interproximal cleansing, as the affected tissue can be very tender. As healing occurs, a multitufted toothbrush and dental floss may be substituted. Some patients find diluted hydrogen peroxide rinses helpful initially. Local retreatment of the patient on a weekly or bimonthly basis can allow complete restoration of the cratered papilla. Restoration of the papilla takes about 2 or 3 months. Surgery is rarely needed, if enough time is allowed for gingival healing to occur.

Recurrence commonly occurs following antibiotic therapy without local treatment—such management is inappropriate. In acutely ill patients, a course of antibiotics should be prescribed to supplement local therapy. For some patients, an episode of ANUG provides the impetus to develop effective personal oral health habits.

PERIODONTITIS

Acute Periodontitis

Etiology and Pathogenesis. Acute periodontitis or lateral periodontal abscess develops as a complication of gingival or periodontal pockets. Abscesses are caused by invasion of pyogenic bacteria through the pocket epithelium secondary to microtrauma or blockage of flow of inflammatory exudates from within the peri-

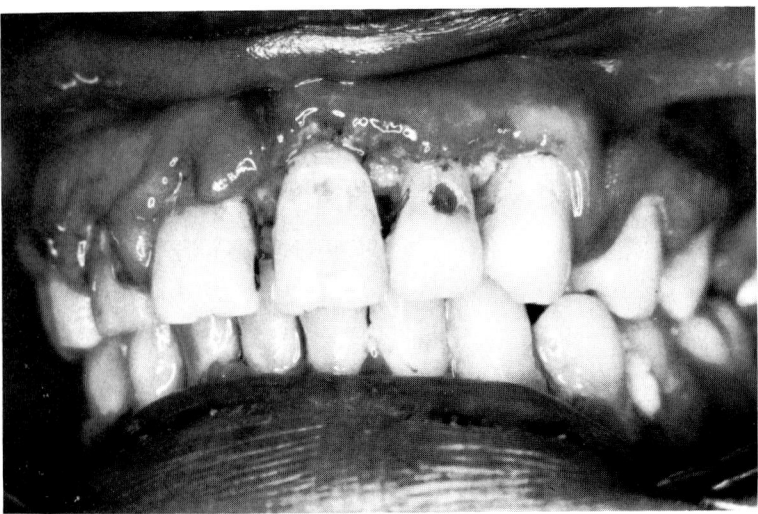

Figure 18–10. Severe ANUG with extensive necrosis.

odontal pocket. Entrapment of foreign bodies, such as seeds, popcorn husks, or toothbrush bristles, can initiate the problem. Inadvertent trauma associated with subgingival scaling may also initiate the problem. The onset is sudden. An acute inflammatory response (purulence) develops in which central tissue necrosis occurs. Several millimeters of periodontal attachment and alveolar bone can be lost within a few days. Drainage of pus may occur spontaneously, through the crevice or through the development of a sinus tract in the alveolar process.

Clinical Features. The periodontal abscess, "gum boil," or parulis is a painful gingival swelling with a red or yellowish-red color. It occurs anywhere around affected teeth (Fig. 18–11). Swelling can involve the vestibule or the cheek, since pus follows the path of least resistance. Depending on the severity of the infection, the patient may experience regional lymphadenitis, malaise, or fever. Such circumstances can represent a true emergency situation demanding immediate attention.

Differential Diagnosis. Proper management of a periodontal abscess requires identification of its cause. Periapical abscesses often drain along the root surface to mimic lateral periodontal abscesses. Lateral periodontal abscesses involving the palatal aspect of maxillary anterior teeth frequently drain through the labial gingiva or vestibule to mimic periapical abscesses. Periapical radiographs and vitality testing of the affected teeth are standard practice in the diagnosis of patients with abscesses. Complicating the clinical diagnosis are combined periodontal-pulpal lesions and partially necrotic pulps that may respond as vital to pulp testing. Other conditions to be considered are root perforations from restorative procedures or endodontic therapy and root fractures. In a patient with severe pain, fever, and malaise, who has several adjacent teeth sensitive to percussion, osteomyelitis may have developed as a complication of the acute infection.

Treatment and Prognosis. Drainage of a periodontal abscess should be attempted through the gingival crevice by introducing a flat instrument. Often a considerable amount of pus can be released and some immediate relief of symptoms obtained. This procedure should be done very gingerly, because of the painful nature of the abscess and on the chance that drainage may not be possible. Anesthesia should not be attempted by injection of anesthetic solution into the affected area, because of the hazard of spreading the infection. The pocket can be explored and débrided with a scaler. Occasionally, a foreign body or a plug of debris may be found. The pocket can be irrigated using a syringe with saline or antiseptic solution. Depending on the condition of the patient, i.e., the presence of fever, malaise, or pain, systemic antibiotics and pain medication can be prescribed. Most periodontal abscesses will resolve with local treatment only.

Patients with abscesses should be re-evaluated after 3 to 7 days to see that resolution of the acute problem has occurred. This is also the time for possible initiation of definitive treatment for patients with generalized periodontal problems. If the abscess does not resolve or recurs following its resolution, the diagnosis should be reconsidered; the possibility of the presence of a systemic condition such

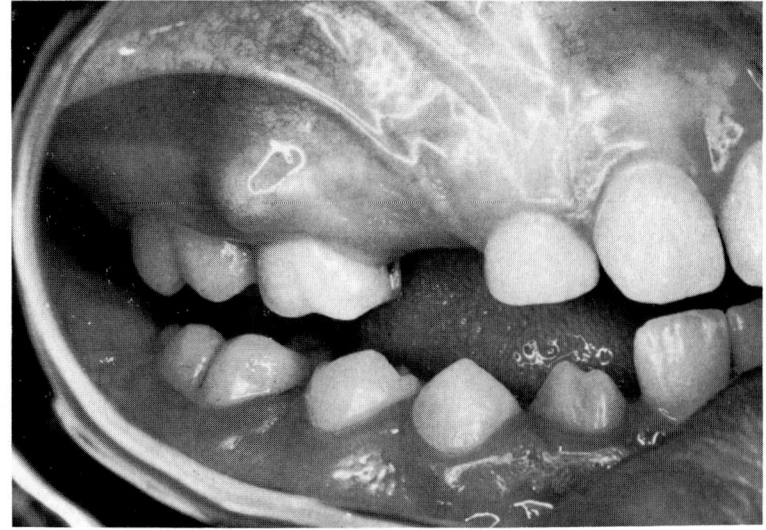

Figure 18–11. Acute periodontitis; an abscess involving the furcation area of the maxillary first molar.

as diabetes mellitus should be weighed. Periodontal pockets caused by the drainage of periapical abscesses through the periodontal membrane space and gingival crevice can heal completely following endodontic therapy. The decision to extract a tooth should be delayed until after resolution of the abscess, as remarkable healing of abscess-associated periodontal attachment loss and bone loss can occur. This type of healing may take 2 or 3 months. Acutely ill patients, including those in whom osteomyelitis is suspected, should be re-evaluated on a daily basis to ensure satisfactory response to treatment.

Chronic Periodontitis

Etiology and Pathogenesis. Chronic periodontitis is a slowly progressive disease of adults that destroys the supporting structures of the teeth. It involves a host-parasite balance of dental plaque and the body's reaction to it. When the equilibrium is disturbed, the disease progresses. When episodes of disease activity recur within an established periodontal lesion, it is termed an advanced lesion. No clear cause for the shift between these two lesion types is known. Although there may be periods of exacerbation and remission, the net effect of periodontitis without treatment is gradual destruction of the periodontium over a period of years or decades.

Clinical Features. With periodontitis, the gingiva may exhibit varying degrees of inflammation (Fig. 18–12). With deeper periodontal pockets, the gingiva often has a superficially relatively healthy appearance. Changes within the gingival tissue and the dentogingival junction can best be detected by periodontal probing. Characteristics of the established or advanced periodontal lesion are scant resistance to probing, pronounced bleeding tendency, intracrevicular exudates and plaque, and subgingival calculus. Crevicular bleeding tendency is always present, although it may at times be difficult to provoke because of extensive debris within the pocket. Purulent exudates represent a particularly serious finding. Only by repeated measurement over time can disease progression (deepening pockets and loss of periodontal attachment) be shown clinically and the advanced lesion be differentiated from the established lesion.

The number of missing teeth, tooth mobility, and the presence of occlusal trauma represent some other clinical findings that are part of periodontal evaluation and can influence the diagnosis.

The extent of alveolar bone loss can best be determined by radiographs. Bone loss should be judged in proportion to the length and shape of the roots. Absence of lamina dura over the alveolar crest suggests inflammation involving the bone in that area. The pattern of bone loss and loss involving the furcations

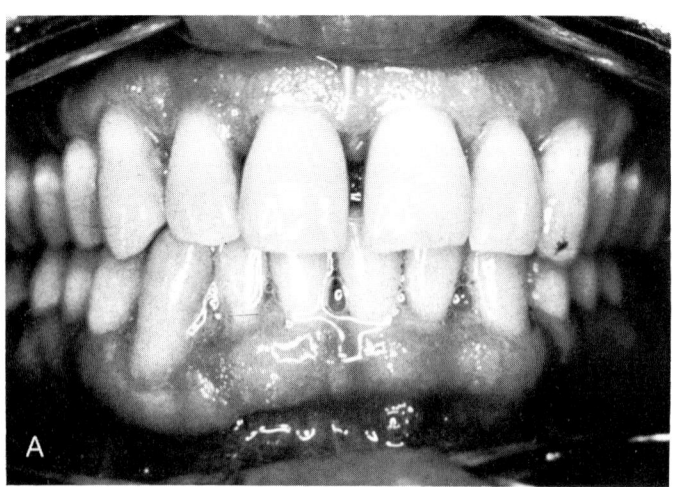
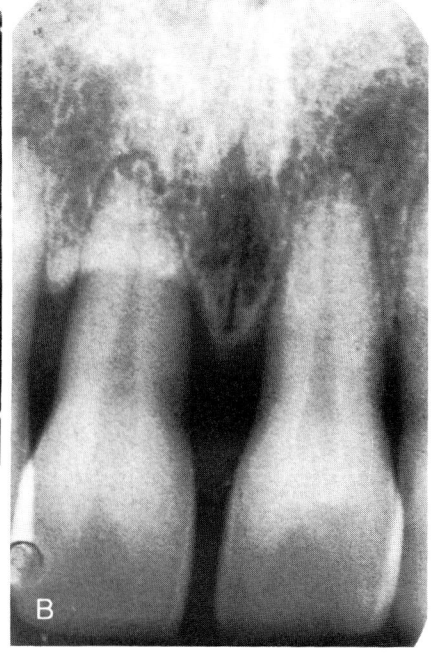

Figure 18–12. *A* and *B*, Chronic periodontitis with minimally apparent soft tissue inflammation.

of roots can be evaluated. Occlusal trauma can alter the appearance of the lamina dura and widen the periodontal membrane space. Calculus and overhanging restorations are other etiologic factors that can be assessed radiographically.

The findings from the various aspects of the periodontal examination are considered in arriving at the appropriate diagnosis. According to the degree of involvement, periodontitis is classified into stages: early or incipient, moderate, and advanced. Early periodontitis has moderate pocket depth, minor to moderate bone loss, and no tooth mobility (Fig. 18–13). Moderate periodontitis has moderate to deep pockets, moderate to severe bone loss, and slight tooth mobility (Fig. 18–14). Advanced periodontitis has deep pockets, severe bone loss, advanced tooth mobility patterns, and usually is complicated by missing or hopelessly involved teeth (Fig. 18–15).

Differential Diagnosis. Chronic periodontitis is usually found in individuals over the age of 35 years. It has been further divided into

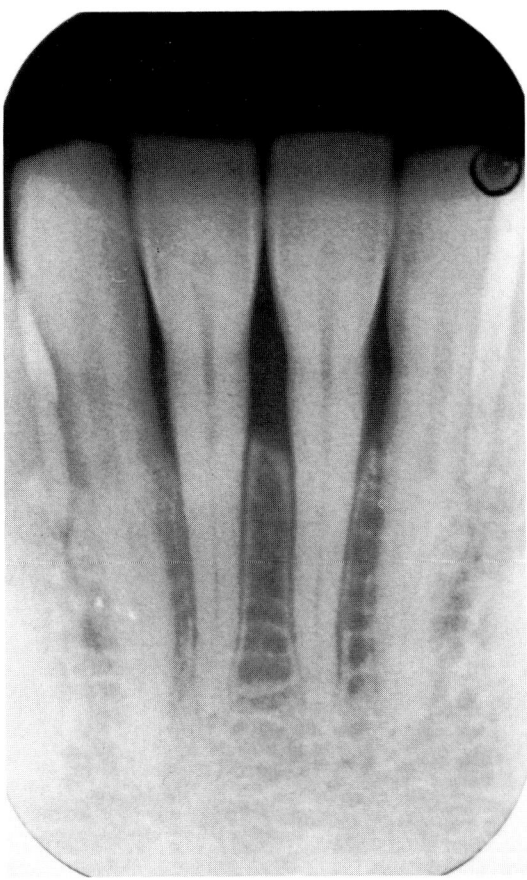

Figure 18–14. Radiograph showing moderate bone loss of moderately advanced periodontitis.

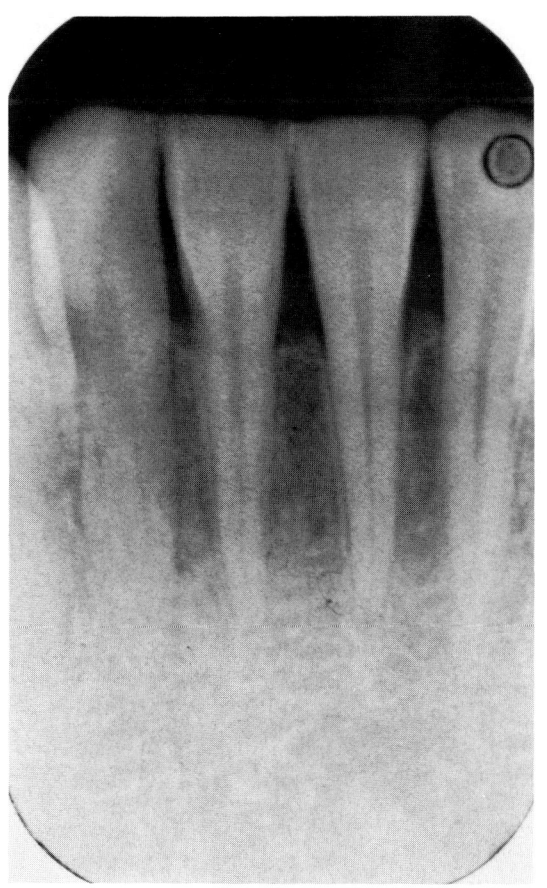

Figure 18–13. Radiograph showing incipient bone loss of early periodontitis.

simple and complex periodontitis. Simple periodontitis is caused by plaque and calculus, and it involves horizontal bone loss. Complex periodontitis refers to those situations in which the host response has been altered or those in which unusual local factors are involved. Periodontitis with vertical or angular bone loss and a marked difference in attachment loss between adjacent teeth or on different surfaces of the same tooth is termed complex periodontitis. Occlusal trauma is the complication that, along with local irritation, is considered to be involved in this form of periodontitis.

Treatment and Prognosis. Treatment of periodontitis follows four phases: systemic, initial or hygienic, corrective, and maintenance phases. In the systemic phase, attention is given to systemic factors, such as the control of diabetes mellitus, or the need for premedication, such as for patients with rheumatic heart disease. Steps in the hygienic phase are patient education, scaling and root planing, oral hygiene instruction, smoothing and polishing of the teeth, and restorations. These steps

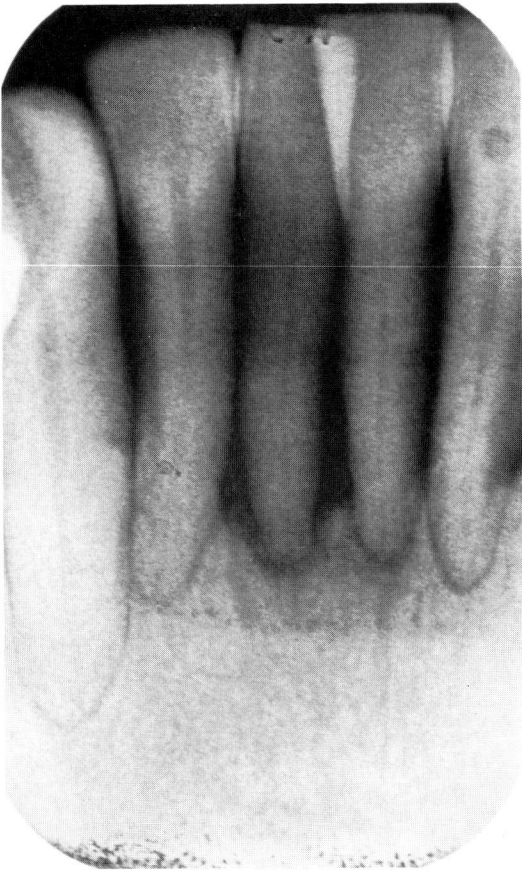

Figure 18–15. Radiograph showing severe bone loss of advanced periodontitis.

month recall intervals for periodontal prophylaxis to remain stable.

Juvenile Periodontitis

Etiology and Pathogenesis. Juvenile periodontitis (JP) is a rare condition typically affecting permanent first molars and possibly incisors in otherwise healthy adolescents. It is hypothesized that the disease is caused by an infection of specific microorganisms, such as *A. actinomycetemcomitans,* and that a host neutrophil dysfunction is involved. The periodontal breakdown progresses rapidly but often appears to become arrested. The typical pattern of JP involvement may be seen in older individuals—individuals in their 20s, 30s, or even 40s—with minimal periodontal breakdown elsewhere. Cessation of disease activity may occur because of replacement of the pathogens by other microorganisms in the oral flora.

are directed toward eliminating the local initiating factors (plaque, calculus, overhangs from restorations). Several visits are usually necessary to gain a good response. Healing from the initial treatment for periodontitis may continue for as long as 12 months. Occlusal therapy and periodontal surgery are done in the corrective phase. Sites that do not respond well initially require surgical access to help establish biologically acceptable tooth surfaces that are essential to healthy dentogingival junctions. Conservative surgical procedures designed to gain access for more complete root instrumentation are indicated rather than those directed at eliminating pockets or recontouring alveolar bone. The maintenance phase completes the periodontal treatment plan. With a favorable response to treatment, prevention of recurrence can be accomplished through the patient's adoption of effective methods of daily personal oral hygiene and participation in a maintenance program. No periodontal treatment has been shown to be effective without maintenance care. Many patients require 3-

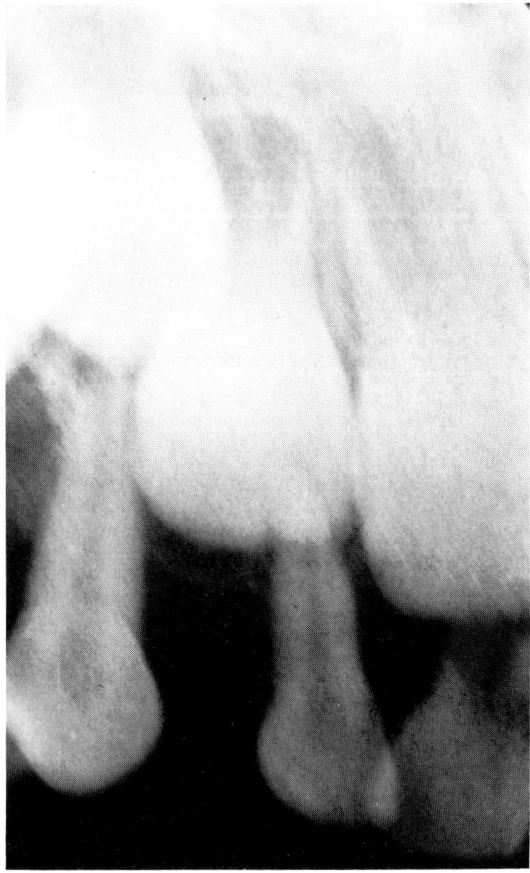

Figure 18–16. Radiograph showing bone loss from periodontitis involving primary teeth (prepubertal periodontitis).

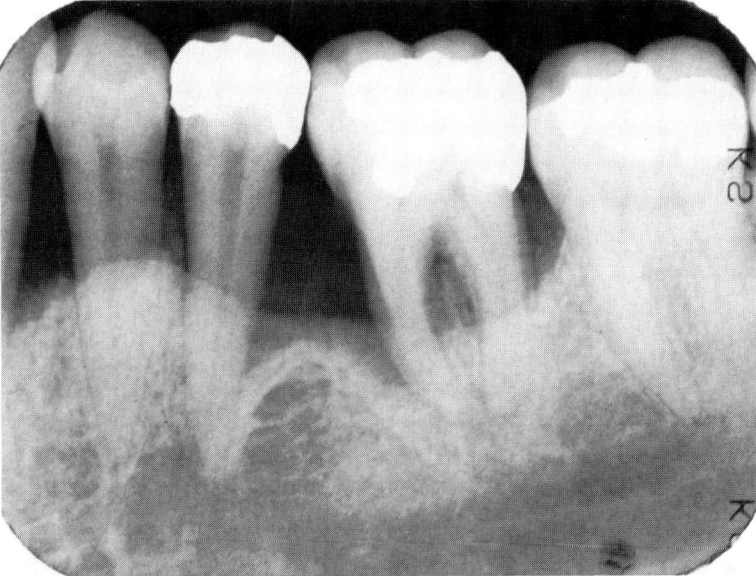

Figure 18–17. Radiograph showing severe horizontal bone loss in a 28-year-old patient (rapidly progressing periodontitis).

Severe periodontal involvement found in patients under the age of 35 years has been termed early onset periodontitis. In addition to JP, prepubertal periodontitis involves pockets and bone loss on primary teeth (Fig. 18–16); rapidly progressing periodontitis describes a condition of severe generalized periodontitis in adults under age 35 (Fig. 18–17). Signs of impaired host defense such as defects in leukocyte function have been reported in all three of these conditions. It has been postulated that the immune defect may be specific for putative periodontopathic organisms or that the organisms involved cause an immune defect. A familial tendency for early development of periodontitis has been found.

Clinical Features. The presence of deep periodontal pockets and angular bone loss on molars and incisors in adolescents is diagnostic for JP (Fig. 18–18). Periodontal pockets in this disease harbor minimal amounts of plaque and calculus. The disease is often not found until

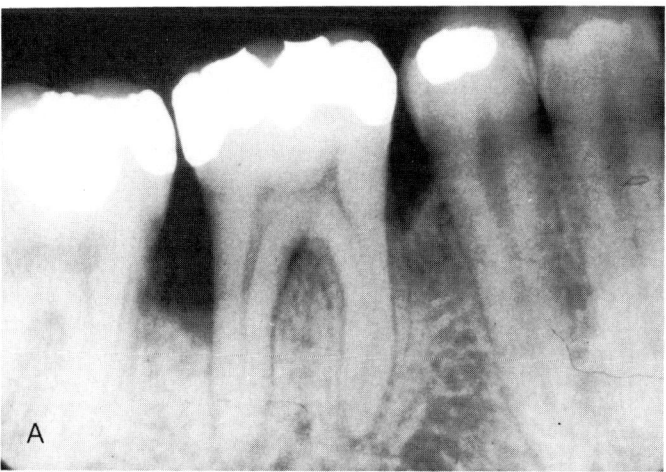
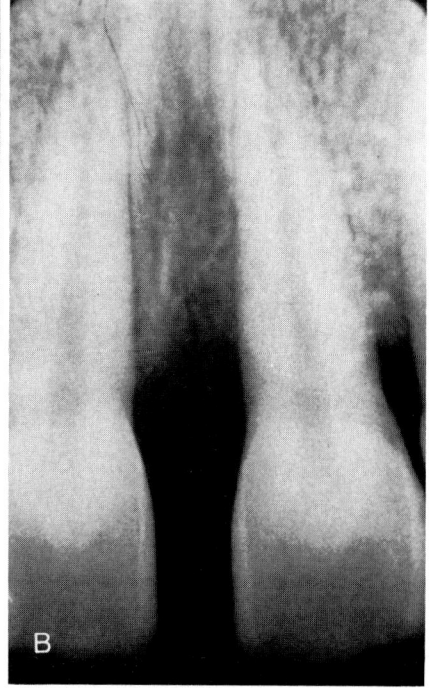

Figure 18–18. *A* and *B*, Radiograph of mandibular first molar and maxillary centrals of a patient with juvenile periodontitis.

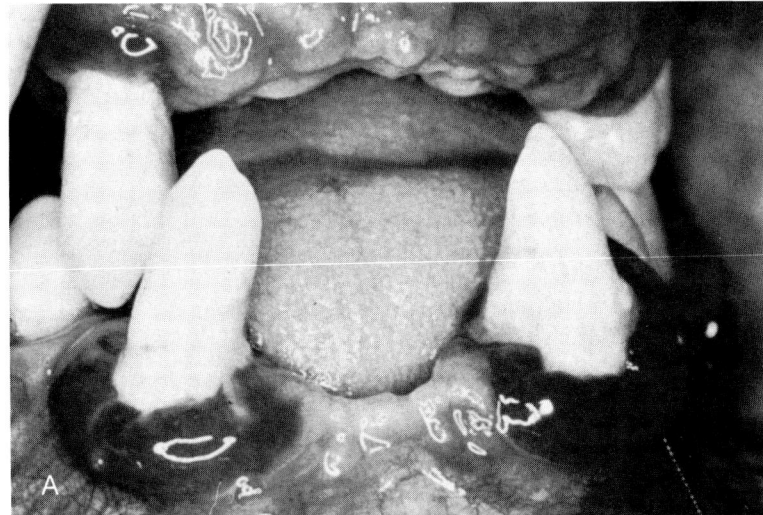
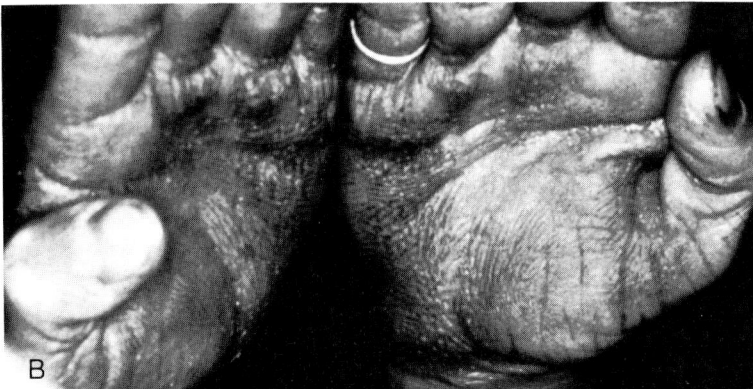

Figure 18–19. *A* and *B*, Patient with Papillon-Lefèvre syndrome showing gingival inflammation, tooth loss, and hyperkeratotic palms.

patients are beyond adolescence. There can be more general involvement of the dentition beyond the incisor and first molar teeth.

Treatment and Prognosis. Treatment should involve débridement of the diseased sites and institution of careful home care procedures. Periodontal surgery of the modified Widman flap type, to eliminate the soft tissue lining the pockets and instrumentation of the exposed root surfaces, is indicated. Antibiotic coverage with tetracycline hydrochloride, 250 mm, four times per day, for 2 or 3 weeks following the surgery, can assist during the restoration of some of the lost alveolar bone. With adequate maintenance care, prognosis is good in general for patients with local JP, although severely affected teeth may be lost over time.

Papillon-Lefèvre Syndrome

Etiology and Pathogenesis. Over 100 cases of Papillon-Lefèvre syndrome (hyperkeratosis palmoplantaris) have been reported. These patients lack resistance to periodontal disease. Hyperkeratotic lesions occur on the hands and feet of individuals with this autosomal recessive genetic disease. Immunologic abnormalities postulated to be involved are defective neutrophil chemotaxis and possibly an induced immunologic defect caused by an interaction between periodontal pathogens and pocket epithelium.

Severe periodontal attachment loss and bone loss around primary and permanent teeth in patients with hyperkeratotic lesions of the hands and feet characterize Papillon-Lefèvre syndrome (Fig. 18–19). Teeth may be lost within 2 to 3 years after their eruption.

No treatment has been shown to be effective for this syndrome. Prognosis for the teeth is hopeless. Vital submersion of the roots (vital root banking) of the teeth may stabilize alveolar bone height and contour and improve the prognosis for a lifetime of complete denture use.

Bibliography

Axelsson P, Lindhe J. Effect of controlled oral hygiene procedures on caries and periodontal disease in adults. J Clin Periodontol 5:133–151, 1978.

Axelsson P, Lindhe J. The significance of maintenance care in the treatment of periodontal disease. J Clin Periodontol 8:133–151, 1981.

Badersten A, Nilveus R, Egelberg J. Effect of non-surgical periodontal therapy. II. Severely advanced periodontitis. J Clin Periodontol 11:63–76, 1984.

Barak S, Engelberg I, Hiss J. Gingival hyperplasia caused by nifedipine-histopathologic findings. J Periodontol 58:639–642, 1987.

Bragd L, Dahlen G, Wikstrom M, et al. The capability of *Actinobacillus actinomycetemcomitans, Bacteroides gingivalis,* and *Bacteroides intermedius* to indicate progressive periodontitis; a retrospective study. J Clin Periodontol 14:95–99, 1987.

Genco R, Slots J. Host responses in periodontal diseases. J Dent Res 63:441–451, 1984.

Grant D, Stern I, Listgarten M. Periodontics. CV Mosby Co, St Louis, 1988, Chaps 8, 11, 17.

Hirschfeld L, Wasserman B. A long-term survey of tooth loss in 600 treated periodontal patients. J Periodontol 49:225–237, 1978.

Knowles J, Burgett F, Nissle R, et al. Results of periodontal treatment related to pocket depth and attachment level. Eight years. J Periodontol 50:225–233, 1979.

Lang N, Kiel R, Anderhalden K. Clinical and microbiological effects of subgingival restorations with overhangs or clinically perfect margins. J Clin Periodontol 10:563–578, 1983.

Lareau D, Baehni P, McArthur W. Human neutrophil migration under agarose to bacteria associated with the development of gingivitis. J Periodontol 55:540–549, 1984.

Lindhe J. Clinical Periodontology. Munksgaard, Copenhagen, 1985, Chaps 5, 6, 7.

Lindhe J, Westfelt E, Nyman S, et al. Healing following surgical/non-surgical treatment of periodontal disease, a clinical study. J Clin Periodontol 9:115–128, 1982.

Listgarten M. Pathogenesis of periodontitis. J Clin Periodontol 13:418–425, 1986.

Listgarten M. A reevaluation of selected diagnostic techniques: potential influence on the clinical practice of periodontics. Can Dent Assoc J 50:549–554, 1984.

Listgarten M, Lindhe J, Hellden L. Effect of tetracycline and/or scaling on human periodontal disease. J Clin Periodontol 5:246–271, 1978.

Löe H, Anerud A, Boysen H, et al. Natural history of periodontal disease in man. Rapid, moderate, and no loss of attachment in Sri Lankan laborers 14 to 46 years of age. J Clin Periodontol 13:431–440, 1986.

Löe H, Anerud A, Boysen H, et al. The natural history of periodontal disease in man. The rate of periodontal destruction before 40 years of age. J Periodontol 49:607–620, 1978.

Löe H, Theilade E, Jensen S. Experimental gingivitis in man. J Periodontol 36:177–187, 1965.

Miller A, Brunelle J, Carols J, et al. Oral health of United States' adults. The national survey of oral health in US employed adults and seniors: 1985–86. NIH Publication no 87-2868, 1987.

Moore L, Moore W, Cato E, et al. Bacteriology of human gingivitis. J Dent Res 66:989–995, 1987.

Morrison E, Ramfjord S, Hill R. Short-term effect of initial non-surgical periodontal treatment (hygienic phase). J Clin Periodontol 7:199–211, 1980.

National Center for Health Statistics. Related Dental Findings in Adults by Age, Race, and Sex: United States, 1960–1962, Vital and Health Statistics. Series 11, No. 7. DHEW Pub. No. (HRA) 74–1274. Health Resources Administration. US Government Printing Office, August 1973.

Page R. Gingivitis. J Clin Periodontol 13:345–355, 1986.

Page R, Schroeder H. Pathogenesis of inflammatory periodontal disease, a summary of current work. Lab Invest 33:235–249, 1976.

Page R, Schroeder H. Periodontitis in man and other animals. A comparative review. S Karger, New York, 1982.

Pihlstrom B, McHugh R, Oliphant T, et al. Comparison of surgical and non-surgical treatment of periodontal disease. A review of current studies and additional results after six and one half years. J Clin Periodontol 10:524–541, 1984.

Ramfjord S, Ash M. Periodontology and Periodontics. WB Saunders Co, Philadelphia, 1979, Chaps 7, 10, 17, 23.

Ramfjord S, Caffesse R, Morrison E, et al. Four modalities of periodontal treatment compared over five years. J Clin Periodontol 14:445–452, 1987.

Rosling B, Nyman S, Lindhe J. The effect of systemic plaque control on bone regeneration in infrabony pockets. J Clin Periodontol 3:38–53, 1976.

Schei O, Waerhaug J, Lovdal A, et al. Alveolar bone loss as related to oral hygiene and age. J Periodontol 30:7–16, 1959.

Seymour G, Powell R, Davies W. Conversion of a stable T-cell lesion to a progressive B-cell lesion in the pathogenesis of chronic inflammatory periodontal disease: an hypothesis. J Clin Periodontol 6:266–277, 1979.

Soderholm G. Effect of a dental care program on dental health conditions. A study of employees of Swedish shipyards. Thesis, University of Lund, Malmo, Sweden, 1979.

Waerhaug J. The infrabony pocket and its relationship to trauma from occlusion and subgingival plaque. J Periodontol 50:355–365, 1979.

Bibliography

Axelsson P, Lindhe J. Effect of controlled oral hygiene procedures on caries and periodontal disease in adults. J Clin Periodontol 5:133–151, 1978.

Axelsson P, Lindhe J. The significance of maintenance care in the treatment of periodontal disease. J Clin Periodontol 8:133–151, 1981.

Badersten A, Nilveus R, Egelberg J. Effect of non-surgical periodontal therapy. II. Severely advanced periodontitis. J Clin Periodontol 11:63–76, 1984.

Barak S, Engelberg I, Hiss J. Gingival hyperplasia caused by nifedipine-histopathologic findings. J Periodontol 58:639–642, 1987.

Bragd L, Dahlen G, Wikstrom M, et al. The capability of *Actinobacillus actinomycetemcomitans, Bacteroides gingivalis,* and *Bacteroides intermedius* to indicate progressive periodontitis; a retrospective study. J Clin Periodontol 14:95–99, 1987.

Genco R, Slots J. Host responses in periodontal diseases. J Dent Res 63:441–451, 1984.

Grant D, Stern I, Listgarten M. Periodontics. CV Mosby Co, St Louis, 1988, Chaps 8, 11, 17.

Hirschfeld L, Wasserman B. A long-term survey of tooth loss in 600 treated periodontal patients. J Periodontol 49:225–237, 1978.

Knowles J, Burgett F, Nissle R, et al. Results of periodontal treatment related to pocket depth and attachment level. Eight years. J Periodontol 50:225–233, 1979.

Lang N, Kiel R, Anderhalden K. Clinical and microbiological effects of subgingival restorations with overhangs or clinically perfect margins. J Clin Periodontol 10:563–578, 1983.

Lareau D, Baehni P, McArthur W. Human neutrophil migration under agarose to bacteria associated with the development of gingivitis. J Periodontol 55:540–549, 1984.

Lindhe J. Clinical Periodontology. Munksgaard, Copenhagen, 1985, Chaps 5, 6, 7.

Lindhe J, Westfelt E, Nyman S, et al. Healing following surgical/non-surgical treatment of periodontal disease, a clinical study. J Clin Periodontol 9:115–128, 1982.

Listgarten M. Pathogenesis of periodontitis. J Clin Periodontol 13:418–425, 1986.

Listgarten M. A reevaluation of selected diagnostic techniques: potential influence on the clinical practice of periodontics. Can Dent Assoc J 50:549–554, 1984.

Listgarten M, Lindhe J, Hellden L. Effect of tetracycline and/or scaling on human periodontal disease. J Clin Periodontol 5:246–271, 1978.

Löe H, Anerud A, Boysen H, et al. Natural history of periodontal disease in man. Rapid, moderate, and no loss of attachment in Sri Lankan laborers 14 to 46 years of age. J Clin Periodontol 13:431–440, 1986.

Löe H, Anerud A, Boysen H, et al. The natural history of periodontal disease in man. The rate of periodontal destruction before 40 years of age. J Periodontol 49:607–620, 1978.

Löe H, Theilade E, Jensen S. Experimental gingivitis in man. J Periodontol 36:177–187, 1965.

Miller A, Brunelle J, Carols J, et al. Oral health of United States' adults. The national survey of oral health in US employed adults and seniors: 1985–86. NIH Publication no 87–2868, 1987.

Moore L, Moore W, Cato E, et al. Bacteriology of human gingivitis. J Dent Res 66:989–995, 1987.

Morrison E, Ramfjord S, Hill R. Short-term effect of initial non-surgical periodontal treatment (hygienic phase). J Clin Periodontol 7:199–211, 1980.

National Center for Health Statistics. Related Dental Findings in Adults by Age, Race, and Sex: United States, 1960–1962, Vital and Health Statistics. Series 11, No. 7. DHEW Pub. No. (HRA) 74–1274. Health Resources Administration. US Government Printing Office, August 1973.

Page R. Gingivitis. J Clin Periodontol 13:345–355, 1986.

Page R, Schroeder H. Pathogenesis of inflammatory periodontal disease, a summary of current work. Lab Invest 33:235–249, 1976.

Page R, Schroeder H. Periodontitis in man and other animals. A comparative review. S Karger, New York, 1982.

Pihlstrom B, McHugh R, Oliphant T, et al. Comparison of surgical and non-surgical treatment of periodontal disease. A review of current studies and additional results after six and one half years. J Clin Periodontol 10:524–541, 1984.

Ramfjord S, Ash M. Periodontology and Periodontics. WB Saunders Co, Philadelphia, 1979, Chaps 7, 10, 17, 23.

Ramfjord S, Caffesse R, Morrison E, et al. Four modalities of periodontal treatment compared over five years. J Clin Periodontol 14:445–452, 1987.

Rosling B, Nyman S, Lindhe J. The effect of systemic plaque control on bone regeneration in infrabony pockets. J Clin Periodontol 3:38–53, 1976.

Schei O, Waerhaug J, Lovdal A, et al. Alveolar bone loss as related to oral hygiene and age. J Periodontol 30:7–16, 1959.

Seymour G, Powell R, Davies W. Conversion of a stable T-cell lesion to a progressive B-cell lesion in the pathogenesis of chronic inflammatory periodontal disease: an hypothesis. J Clin Periodontol 6:266–277, 1979.

Soderholm G. Effect of a dental care program on dental health conditions. A study of employees of Swedish shipyards. Thesis, University of Lund, Malmo, Sweden, 1979.

Waerhaug J. The infrabony pocket and its relationship to trauma from occlusion and subgingival plaque. J Periodontol 50:355–365, 1979.

Index

Note that page numbers in *italic* designate figures and those followed by t designate tables; page references to the Overview section are preceded by the letter "O-."

Abdominal mass, in Burkitt's lymphoma, 419
Abrasion, of teeth, 467, *468*
Abscess(es), actinomycotic, 40, *41*
　gingival, O-27, 122, *122*
　in pyostomatitis vegetans, 180
　in sporotrichosis, 45
　Munro, 140, *141*
　of palate, O-61, 394, *395*
　of periodontal pocket, 512–514, *513*
　of skin, odontogenic, 394, *395*
　periapical. See *Periapical abscess.*
　periodontal, 512–514, *513*
　pharyngeal, in scarlet fever, 145
　pulp, 391, *392*
Acantholysis, in follicular keratosis, 88, *89*
　in pemphigus vulgaris, 14, 16, *16*, 18
Acanthomatous ameloblastoma, 341
Acanthosis, O-18
　in condyloma latum, 169
　in focal epithelial hyperplasia, 174, *175*
　in hereditary benign intraepithelial dyskeratosis, 87, *87*
　in leukoedema, 85
　in pyostomatitis vegetans, 180
　in white sponge nevus, 85
Accessory roots, *466*, 467
Accessory teeth, 471, *471*, *472*
Acetylsalicylic acid, and oral ulcers, 31
Acids, and dental erosion, 467
Acinic cell(s), of salivary gland, 248, *249*
Acinic cell carcinoma, 263t, 272, *272*, *273*
Acne therapy, and mucosal pigmentation, 166
Acoustic neuromas, 215
Acquired immunodeficiency syndrome, candidiasis in, 111, 115
　caries in, 489
　condyloma acuminatum in, 172
　hairy leukoplakia in, 99, *100*, 102
　Kaposi's sarcoma in, 137–139, *137*, 137t, *138*
　oral manifestations of, 99t
Acral-lentiginous melanoma, 161, *162*
Acromegaloidism, 436
Acromegaly, *O-102*, O-103, 435–437, *437*
　salivary gland enlargement in, 243
Actinic cheilitis, *O-22*, O-23, 93, *94*
Actinomyces species, and caries, 496
　in periodontal disease, 504, 507, 516

Actinomycosis, O-11, 40, *41*
Acyclovir, for herpes infection, 8
　for varicella-zoster infections, 11
Adamantinoma, of tibia, 348
Addison's disease, 153t, 154, *155*
Adenoameloblastoma, 352
Adenocarcinoma(s), of maxillary sinus, 81
　of palate, 74, 76
　of salivary gland, 263t, 279
　terminal duct, 276, *277*, 277t, *279*
Adenocystic carcinoma, 263t, 268–272, *269–271*
Adenoid basal cell carcinoma, 69
Adenoma(s), membranous, of parotid gland, 253, 254, *255*, 256
　of salivary glands, basal cell, 253–256, 253t, *254–256*
　　monomorphic, 249t, 253–258, 253t
　　pleomorphic, 249–253, 249t, *250–252*
　oxyphilic, 256, *257*
　pituitary, 435
Adenomatoid odontogenic tumor, *O-80*, O-81, 338t, 351–353, *353–355*
Adolescents, periodontitis in, 516–518, *516*
Adrenal cortical insufficiency, and freckles, 153t, 154, *155*
Adrenal tumor, 215, 217
Adrenocorticotropic suppression, with steroid therapy, 50, *51*
Age, and caries, 489
　and periodontal disease, 503, 504
Age spots, 155, *155*
AIDS. See *Acquired immunodeficiency syndrome.*
Airway obstruction, in Pierre Robin syndrome, 447, 448
Albers-Schonberg syndrome, *O-104*, O-105, 439–441, *440*, *441*
Albright's syndrome, 153t, 156
　fibrous dysplasia in, O-87, 372
Alcohol consumption, and oral cancer, 72
Alcoholism, and salivary gland enlargement, 243
Alkaline phosphatase deficiency, 433
Allergic gingivostomatitis, 145, *146*, 147
Allergy(ies), contact, *O-14*, O-15, 64–66, *65*, *66*
　and red-blue lesions, 146
　intravascular oral lesions in, *O-34*, O-35
　to drugs, O-15, 62–64, 62t, *63–65*

521

Alopecia, cyclosporine for, 189
  in discoid lupus, 58, *58*
  radiation-induced, 78
Alveolar bone loss, in chronic periodontitis, 514–516, *515*, *516*
  in sarcoidosis, 241
Alveolar cleft, 455, *455*, *456*, *457*
Alveolar cyst, median, 321
Alveolar process, tumor invasion of, 81
Alveolar ridge, cysts of, *O-26*, 120, *121*, 122
Alzheimer disease, 450
Amalgam fillings, and white lesions, 98
Amalgam tattoo, *O-40*, O-41, 157t, 163, *164*, *165*
Ameloblast(s), damage to, 472, *473*
  dysfunction of, *in utero*, 474
Ameloblastic carcinoma, 346, *347*
Ameloblastic fibroma, *O-82*, O-83, 338t, 364–368, *366*
Ameloblastic fibro-odontoma, *O-82*, O-83, 338t, 364–368, *365*, *367*
Ameloblastic fibrosarcoma, 367, *367*
Ameloblastic odontoma, 363
Ameloblastoma, *O-80*, O-81, 337–348, 338t
  acanthomatous, 341
  basal cell, 341
  clinical features of, 338, *338–341*
  cystic, 341, *343*
  differential diagnosis of, 345, *346*
  extraosseous peripheral, 340
  follicular, 341, *342*
  ghost cell keratinization in, 344, *344*
  granular cell, 341, *343*
  histological types of, 340–345, *342–345*
  malignant, 346
  mandibular, *338–341*
  metastases from, 346–348, *347*, *348*
  of maxilla, 345, *346*
  peripheral (gingival), *342*
  plexiform, 341
  regional distribution of, 338, *340*
  related lesions, 346, 348, *348*
  spindle, 341
  treatment of, 345–348
  unicystic vs. multicystic, 344, *345*, 346
  vs. dentigerous cyst, 308, 309, 345
  with calcifying odontogenic cyst, 317, 318
  with dentigerous cyst, *341*
Amelogenesis imperfecta, 475–477, *476*
Ampicillin allergy, 64
Amyloid, in calcifying epithelial odontogenic tumor, 350, *351*, *352*
Amyloidosis, in multiple myeloma, 421
ANA test, in lupus erythematosus, 57, 60, 60t, 61t
Analgesics, in mucosal burns, 117
Anemia, in multiple myeloma, 422
  in osteopetrosis, 439–441
  iron deficiency, O-33, 143
  pernicious, O-33, 142, *142*
Anergy, in sarcoidosis, 241
Anesthetic(s), in mucosal burns, 117
Aneurysm, aortic, 448, *449*
Aneurysmal bone cyst, *O-76*, O-77, 323–325, *324*, *326*
Angina. See also *Pain*.
  Ludwig's, 394
Angioedema, 63, *63*
Angiofibroma, juvenile nasopharyngeal, 195, *195*

Angiolymphoid hyperplasia with eosinophilia, 286
Angiomatosis, encephalotrigeminal, 126, *128*
Angio-osteohypertrophy syndrome, 126, 129, 453
Angiosarcoma, 205, *206*
Angiotensin-I converting enzyme, in sarcoidosis, 242, 243
Angular cheilitis, 112, *113*
Ankylosed teeth, in osteopetrosis, 439, 440
Ankylosis, *470*, 471
Ann Arbor staging, of Hodgkin's disease, 287, 288t
  of non-Hodgkin's lymphoma, 293
Anodontia, 467, *469*, *470*
Anorexia nervosa, and parotid gland enlargement, 243
  dental erosion in, 467
Antholetrithione, 238
Antibiotic glossitis, 111
Antibiotic prophylaxis, in Marfan's syndrome, 448
Antibiotic stomatitis, 111
Antibiotic therapy, and candidal superinfection, 111
  and hairy tongue, 102
  for aphthous ulcers, 51
  for osteomyelitis, 395, 398
  for periapical abscess, 394
  in acute necrotizing ulcerative gingivitis, 512
Antibody(ies). See also *Autoantibody(ies)*.
  anti–*Candida albicans*, 286
  monoclonal, in lymphoma, 297
    in metastatic bone carcinoma, 424
  pemphigus, 14, 17, *17*, 18
  Sjögren's syndrome, 58, 60
  in burning mouth syndrome, 144
Antibody testing, in lupus erythematosus, 57, 58, 60, 60t, 61t
Anticonvulsive agents. See *Phenytoin*.
Antifungal therapy, in papillary hyperplasia, 168
Antigen(s), bullous pemphigoid, 22
  drugs as, 62
  histocompatibility, in dermatitis herpetiformis, 24
    in geographic tongue, 103
    in sarcoidosis, 241
    in Sjögren's syndrome, 246
  human leukocyte, in aphthous ulcers, 46
  in keratoacanthoma, 177
  in metastatic bone carcinoma, 424
Antigen challenge test, in tuberculosis, 38
Antigenic markers, in idiopathic histiocytosis, 384, 385
Antinuclear antibody test, in lupus erythematosus, 57, 60, 60t, 61t
Antoni tissue, 211, *213*, 214
Antral carcinoma, 81, 82
Antral cyst(s), 234, *234*
Antral mucocele, 230, 233
Antral polyps, 235
Antrectomy, for maxillary sinus mucocele, 234
Antrum, maxillary. See *Maxillary sinus*.
Aortic aneurysm, in Ehlers-Danlos syndrome, 449
  in Marfan's syndrome, 448
Aphthous stomatitis, 7, 8t, 18, 47, *49*
  treatment of, 50
  vs. pemphigus, 18

Aphthous ulcer(s), *O-12*, O-13, 46–53
  clinical forms of, *O-12*, O-13, 47, *48–50*, 48t
  herpetiform, 48, 48t, *50*
  treatment of, 50–53, 51t, 52t
  vs. herpes simplex virus infection, 7, 8t, 47, 48, 50
  vs. pemphigoid, 18
Apical periodontal cyst. See *Periapical cyst(s)*.
Apicoectomy, for periapical cyst, 306
Appliances, prosthetic. See *Denture(s)*; *Prosthetic devices*.
Argyrosis, focal, *O-40*, O-41, 157t, 163, *164*, *165*
Arsenic deposits, mucosal, 165
Arteriole embolization, for hemangiomas, 130
Arteriovenous malformation, and aneurysmal bone cyst, 324
Arthritis, of temporomandibular joint, 139
  rheumatoid, with Sjögren's syndrome, 245, 246, 248
Articular hypermobility, 449
Artificial saliva. See *Saliva substitutes*.
Artificial tears, 248
Aspirin, and iron deficiency anemia, 143
  and mucosal sloughing, 117
  and oral ulcers, 31
Atlantoaxial instability, 451
Atopy, and geographic tongue, 103
Atrophic candidiasis, *O-34*, O-35, 145
Atrophic gastritis, in pernicious anemia, 143
Atrophic lichen planus, 105, *107*, 108, 110
Atrophic tongue, in vitamin B deficiency, 142, *142*, 143
Atrophy, epithelial, in submucous fibrosis, 118, *118*
  hemifacial, 451
Attrition, of teeth, 467
Atypia, cellular, definition of, 96
  in leukoplakia, 95, 97
Auspitz sign, 139, 140
Autoantibody(ies), in aphthous ulcers, 46
  in bullous pemphigoid, 22, 24
  in lupus erythematosus, 57, 58, 60
  in pemphigus vulgaris, 14, 17, *17*, 18
  in Sjögren's syndrome, 246
Autoimmune disorder(s). See also *Immunodeficiency states* and specific diseases.
  cicatricial pemphigoid, *O-6*, O-7, 19–22, 19t, *20–23*, 23t
  lichen planus. See *Lichen planus*.
  lupus. See *Lupus erythematosus*.
  pemphigus vulgaris in, 16
  Sjögren's syndrome. See *Sjögren's syndrome*.
Avian-associated infections, 42, 43t, *44*
Axillary freckles, 156, *156*
  in neurofibromatosis, 215

B lymphocyte(s). See also *Plasma cell(s)*.
  transformed, 294
B lymphocyte hyperactivity, in Sjögren's syndrome, 245
B_{12} deficiency, 141, 142, *142*
Bacteremia, and osteomyelitis, 394
Bacteria, chromogenic, and tooth stains, 484, *484*
  in cariogenesis, 494, 495t
  in plaque, 490, 494–496, 495t, 504, 505, 507
Bacterial conditions, actinomycosis, O-11, 40, *41*
  and geographic tongue, 103

Bacterial conditions *(Continued)*
  and oral cancer, 72
  gonorrhea, O-11, 37
  in periodontitis, 504–508, 512–518
  leprosy, O-11, 39
  noma, O-13, 41, *42*
  scarlet fever, 145
  syphilis, *O-10*, O-11, 34–37, *34–36*
  tuberculosis, *O-10*, O-11, 38, *38*, *39*
  ulcerative, 34–42
Bacterial overgrowth, and hairy tongue, 102
Bacterial sialadenitis, 240
Basal cell(s), destruction of, in lichen planus, 105, 108, *109*
Basal cell adenoma, of salivary gland, 253–256, 253t, *254–256*
Basal cell ameloblastoma, 341
Basal cell carcinoma, *O-16*, O-17, 68–70, *69*, *70*
  keratotic, 69
Basal cell nevus syndrome, 69, 314, 316
Behçet's syndrome, O-13, 48t, *53*, 53
Bence Jones proteinuria, 422
Beta blocker therapy, in Marfan's syndrome, 448
Betel nut chewing, and oral cancer, 72
  and submucous fibrosis, 117
Bifid uvula, 454
Biliary atresia, and tooth staining, 486
Bilirubin, and teeth staining, 486
Biopsy, labial salivary gland, 246–248
Birbeck granules, 385, *386*
Bismuth deposits, mucosal, 165
Bisphosphonate, 430
Biting, mucosal, *O-20*, O-21, 29, *30*, 85, 89, *90*
Black stain, of teeth, 484, *484*
Blastomycosis, 42, 43t, *44*
Bleeding, Auspitz sign, 139, 140
  gingival. See *Gingival bleeding*.
  in iron deficiency anemia, 143
  in Rendu-Osler-Weber syndrome, 129
  intranasal. See *Epistaxis*.
  prolonged, in blood dyscrasias, 148, 149
Bleeding tendency, in chronic periodontitis, 514
  in Ehlers-Danlos syndrome, 449
  in periodontal disease, 506, 508, 510
Blister(s), *O-2*, 29. See also *Bulla(e)*; *Vesiculobullous disease(s)*.
  fever, 3
  in cicatricial pemphigoid, 19
  in epidermolysis bullosa, 26, *26*
  intraepithelial, in pemphigus vulgaris, 14, 16, *16*, 18
Blood dyscrasia, and hyperplastic gingivitis, 509, 510
  extravascular lesions in, 148, *148*, 148t, 149, *149*
  oral, *O-34*, O-35
Blue lesions. See also *Red-blue lesions*.
  gingival cyst, 312
  in nasopharyngeal angiofibroma, 195
  mucocele, 226
  ranula, 231
Blue nevus, 158, *159*
Blue sclera, 442
Blunderbuss foramen, 215
Bohn's nodules, 120, 313
Boil, gingival, 122, *122*, 512–514, *513*
Bone(s), fragile, in osteogenesis imperfecta, 442
  hemangioma of, *O-88*, O-89, 382, *382*, *383*
  in angio-osteohypertrophy syndrome, 126, 129

Bone(s) *(Continued)*
  in myositis ossificans, 219
  progressive destruction of, 434, 435, *435, 436*
  solitary plasmacytoma of, 297, *300*, 421, 423
Bone cyst(s), aneurysmal, O-76, O-77, 323–325, *324, 326*
  static, *O-76, O-77*, 328, *329*
  traumatic (simple), *O-76, O-77*, 325, *327, 328*
Bone destruction, in verrucous carcinoma, 178, *179*
Bone disease, phantom, O-103, 434, *435, 436*
Bone lesions, in Paget's disease. See *Paget's disease.*
  in sarcoidosis, 241
  of jaws. See *Jaw(s); Mandible; Maxilla.*
Bone loss, in advanced gingivitis, 506, 507
  in chronic periodontitis, 514–516, *515, 516*
  in juvenile periodontitis, 517, *517*
  in Papillon-Lefèvre syndrome, 518, *518*
Bone marrow defect, focal osteoporotic, *O-76, O-77*, 329, *330*
Bone marrow hyperplasia, 329
Bone marrow inflammation, 390. See also *Osteomyelitis.*
Bone marrow neoplasms, 417–424
  Burkitt's lymphoma, *O-96, O-97*, 419–421, *420, 421*
  Ewing's sarcoma, O-97, 417–419, *417, 418*
  metastatic carcinoma, O-98, O-99, 424, *424, 425*
  myeloma, *O-98, O-99*, 297, *299*, 421–423, *422, 423*
  plasma cell tumors, *O-98, O-99*, 297, *299, 300*, 421–424, *422, 423*
  plasmacytomas, 297, *300*, 423
Bone necrosis. See *Osteonecrosis.*
Bone resorption, in Paget's disease, 428, *429*
  in peripheral giant cell granuloma, 132, 133, *134*
  physiologic, absence of, 439–441, *441*
Bone tumors, fibro-osseous. See *Jaw(s), benign non-odontogenic tumors of.*
  fibrosarcoma, 196, 197t, 199, *199*, 200
  fibrous histiocytoma, 196, 197t, 199, 200t, 201, *201–203*
  giant cell, 381
  myelomas, 297, *299*
  neurogenic sarcoma, 217
  of jaws. See *Jaw(s).*
  osteosarcoma. See *Osteosarcoma(s).*
  plasma cell, *O-98, O-99*, 297, *299, 300*, 421–424, *422, 423*
  solitary plasmacytoma, 297, *300*, 423
Bony nodules, O-89, 386, *387, 388*. See also *Exostoses; Torus(i).*
  in mucosa, *O-50*, O-51
Bony overgrowth, in acromegaly, 435
Bony scar, 402
Botryoid odontogenic cyst, 312
Bowel disease, inflammatory, and pyostomatitis vegetans, 180
Bowen's disease, 136, *136*
Branchial cleft cyst, *O-64*, O-65, 329, 330, *330–332*
Breast cancer, metastatic to jaws, O-99, 424, *425*
Breath, fetid, 511
Brown macules (café-au-lait), O-39, 153t, *156*, 156
Bruisability. See also *Ecchymosis.*
  in Ehlers-Danlos syndrome, 449

Bruit, 324, 325
  in hemangioma of bone, 382
  in vascular malformations, 126
Brushfield spots, 451
Buccal lesions, in cicatricial pemphigoid, 19, *20*
  in measles, 14
  in pemphigus vulgaris, 14, *15*
Buccal lymph node, hyperplastic, 285
Buccal mucosa, carcinoma of, 74, *75, 76*
  fibrosarcoma of, *199*
  Fordyce's granules of, 118, *119*
  hemangiomas of, *127*
  hemangiopericytoma of, *205*
  in hereditary benign intraepithelial dyskeratosis, O-21, 86
  in lichen planus, 105
  leukoedema of, O-21, 84, *85*
  leukoplakia of, 95
  lipoma of, *222*
  lymphangioma of, *204*
  swellings of, *O-56,* O-57
  ulcers of. See also *Ulcer(s); Ulcerative conditions.*
    in allergic reactions, *65*
  white sponge nevus of, 85, *86*
Bulimia, and parotid gland enlargement, 243
  dental erosion in, 467
Bulla(e), *O-2*
  in lichen planus, 107
Bullous disease(s). See also *Vesiculo-bullous disease(s).*
  epidermolysis bullosa, *O-6, O-7*, 26, *26*, 27
  pemphigoid, O-7, 19, 22–24, 23t, *24*
Burkitt's lymphoma, *O-96, O-97*, 2, 297, *297*, *298*, 419–421, *420, 421*
Burn(s), and oral ulcers, 31, *31*, 32, *32*
  electrical, 116, 117
  mucosal, *O-26, O-27*, 31, *31*, 32, *32*, 116, *117*
Burning, intraoral, in plasma cell gingivitis, 146
Burning mouth syndrome, O-35, 143–145
Butterfly rash, 58

Café-au-lait macules, O-39, 153t, 156, *156*
  in MEN III syndrome, 215
  in neurofibromatosis, 214
Caffey's disease, 434
Calcification(s), in sinus mucocele, 233
  mucosal, in hyperparathyroidism, 431
  of enamel, defective, 473–475, *473, 476*
  of fibroma, 185, *185*, 186, *186*, 369–371, *370, 371*
  of pulp, 480, *482*
Calcifying epithelial odontogenic tumor, O-81, 338t, 348–351, *350–352*
Calcifying epithelioma of Malherbe, 318
Calcinosis, renal, 431, 434
Calcitonin, 430
Calcium loss, in caries, 493
Calculus(i), renal, 431
  salivary. See *Sialoliths.*
Caldwell-Luc procedure, 234
Cancer. See also *Carcinoma(s); Neoplasm(s); Tumor(s).*
  of head and neck. See *Head and neck cancer* and specific types.
  of skin. See *Skin cancer.*
  oral, incidence and survival in, 70, *70, 71*
  oropharyngeal. See *Oropharyngeal cancer.*

Cancrum oris, 41, *42*
Candida albicans antibody, 286
Candidal leukoplakia, 113, 115
Candidal superinfection(s), in hairy leukoplakia, 100
　in lichen planus, 108
Candidiasis, *O-24*, O-25, 110–116, *112–114, 116*
　acute atrophic, 111, *112*
　and papillary hyperplasia, 167, 168
　atrophic, *O-34*, O-35, 145
　chronic, 113
　　and burning mouth syndrome, 143, 144
　circumoral, 113
　classification of, 110, 111t
　clinical features of, 111–115, *112–114*
　denture-related, 112, *113*, 114
　differential diagnosis in, 115
　endocrinopathy and, 114, 115
　etiology and pathogenesis of, 110, 111t
　familial, 114, 115
　histopathology of, 115, *116*
　hyperplastic/hypertrophic, 113, *114*, 115
　in AIDS, 111, 115
　in hairy leukoplakia, 100
　in lichen planus, 108
　iron deficiency in, 115
　laboratory findings in, 115
　median rhomboid glossitis in, 113, *114*
　mucocutaneous, 114, *114*, 115
　palatal papillary, 114, *114*
　predisposing factors in, 111t
　pseudomembranous (thrush), 111, *112*, 115
　secondary, in median rhomboid glossitis, 134, *134, 135*
　superinfection with, 111, 115
　treatment and prognosis of, 116
　ulcers in, 111, 115
　with myositis and thymoma, 115
Canker sore. See *Aphthous ulcer(s).*
Capillary hemangioma, 125, *130*, 139
Carcinogen(s), 71, 72
　tobacco. See *Tobacco.*
Carcinoma(s). See also *Cancer; Neoplasm(s); Tumor(s).*
　acinic cell, 263t, 272, *272, 273*
　adenocarcinomas. See *Adenocarcinoma(s).*
　adenocystic, 263t, 268–272, *269–271*
　ameloblastic, 346, *347*
　antral, 81, 82
　basal cell, *O-16*, O-17, 68–70, *69, 70*
　cervical, herpes infection and, 4
　epimyoepithelial, of intercalated ducts, 274–276, *276*
　leukoplakia and, 95–97, *97*
　lymph node metastasis in, *O-64*, O-65
　medullary, 215, 217
　metastatic. See also *Metastatic carcinoma(s).*
　　to jaws, *O-98*, O-99, 424, *424, 425*
　mucoepidermoid, 262t, 263–268, *264–267*
　nasopharyngeal. See *Nasopharyngeal carcinoma.*
　of breast, metastatic to jaws, O-99, 424, *425*
　of buccal mucosa, 74, *75, 76*
　of floor of mouth, 73, *75*
　of gingiva, 74, *75*
　of lips, 72, *73*
　of maxillary sinus, O-17, 81, 82
　of salivary gland duct, 279, *280, 281*
　of tongue, 72, *74*
　　in syphilis, 72
　primary intraosseous, 346

Carcinoma(s) *(Continued)*
　small cell, of salivary gland, 278
　spindle cell, 76
　squamous cell. See *Squamous cell carcinoma.*
　terminal duct, 276, *277*, 277t, *279*
　verrucous, *O-46*, O-47, 72, 74, *76*, 77, 98, *178, 178*, 178t, *179*, 180
Carcinoma ex-mixed tumor of salivary glands, 263t, 273, *274, 275*
Carcinoma *in situ*, in erythroplakia, 136, *136*
　in leukoplakia, 95–97, *97, 98*
Cardiac myxoma, 193
Cardiovascular disorders, in Ehlers-Danlos syndrome, 449
　in Marfan's syndrome, 448
Caries, 488–499
　age and gender factors in, 489
　and pulpitis, 390, 391, *392*
　arrested, 490, *491*
　causes of, 494–499
　　essential factors as, 494–498
　　modifying factors as, 494, 498
　changes in prevalence and incidence of, 488, 489
　classification of, 490
　clinical features of, 489–491, *490*
　decalcification in, 493
　demineralization in, 493, 499
　diet and, 496–498
　enamel and cemental, 490
　in Down syndrome, 451
　in natural teeth, 494
　in primitive man, 488, 489
　in Sjögren's syndrome, 246, *246*
　location of lesions, 489, 490, *490*
　　tooth anatomy and, 491–493, *491, 492*
　microscopic features of, 491–494, *491, 492*
　osteopetrosis and, 440, 441
　pathophysiologic dynamics in, 493, 494
　phytate and, 497
　plaque microbiota in, 490, 494–496, 495t
　prevention of, oral hygiene in, 490, 493, 494, 498
　　prophylactic odontotomy in, 494
　　sealants in, 494
　process of, 488, 490–494. See also *Cariogenesis.*
　race and economic factors in, 489
　radiation (cervical), 78, *79, 80*
　rampant, 489, *490*, 491
　rate of progression of, 490, 491
　remineralization in, 494
　resistance and susceptibility to, 489
　role of plaque in, 490, 494–496, 495t
　salivary gland irradiation and, 237, 238
　sugars and, 488, 495–498
　systemic diseases and, 498
　xerostomia and, 499
"Caries immunity," 489
Cariogenesis, 488, 490–494
　crystallites in, 491, 493, 494
　demographic factors in, 489
　infection vs. disease in, 496
　mineral exchange in, 488, 491, 493, 494
　rate of, 490, 491
　saliva in, 498
Cariogenic foods, 489–491, 496–498
Cariogenic risk, 495
Cariogenicity, 490
Carotid body tumor, O-65
Cartilage, tumors of, O-87, 377

Cataracts, 451
Catecholamine-producing tumor, 217
Cavernous hemangioma, 125, 130, *130*
Cavernous lymphangioma, 204
Cavernous sinus thrombosis, 394
Cavity medications, and oral ulcers, 31, *31*
Celiac disease, 24
Cell-mediated immunity. See *Immunity, cell-mediated.*
Cellulitis, 394, *395*
Cemental caries, 490
Cemental dysplasia, periapical, *O-82*, O-83, 338t, 361–363, *361, 362*
Cementifying fibroma, *O-80*, O-81, 338t, 359, *359, 360*, 369, 371
Cementoblastoma, *O-82*, O-83, 338t, 359–361
Cementoma, true, *O-82*, O-83, 359–361, *360*
Cementum, in advanced gingivitis, 506
Central giant cell granuloma, *O-88*, O-89, 379, *380, 381*
Central odontogenic fibroma, O-81, 356, *358*
Cervical caries, 78, *79, 80*
Cervical lymph nodes, non-Hodgkin's lymphoma of, *291*
Cervical lymphadenopathy, 289
Cervical lymphoepithelial cyst, 329, *330*
Cervicofacial actinomycosis, 40, *41*
Chancre (syphilitic), *O-10*, O-11, 34, *35*, 37
Cheek(s). See *Buccal mucosa.*
Cheek biting, *O-20*, O-21, 85, 89, *90*
  and hyperkeratosis, 85, 89, *90*
Cheilitis, angular, 112, *113*
  in plasma cell gingivitis, 146, *146*
  solar, *O-22*, O-23, 93, *94*
  vitamin B deficiency and, 142
Cheiloplasty, 456
Chemical burns, and mucosal necrosis, 116, *117*
Chemical erosion of teeth, 467
Chemical injury, and pulpitis, 391
Chemical irritants, and oral ulcers, 31, *31*, 32, *32*
Chemical mediators, in contact allergy, 64
  in drug reactions, 62, 63
Chemotherapy, antiviral, 2, 8, 11
  for non-Hodgkin's lymphoma, 295
  in Burkitt's lymphoma, 420
  in idiopathic histiocytosis, 385
Cherubism, *O-104*, O-105, 437–439, *437–439*
Chevrons, 479
Chewing, betel nut, 72, 117
  of oral mucosa, *O-20*, O-21, 29, *30*, 85, 89, *90*
Chewing gum, allergic reaction to, 65, *66*
  and allergic gingivostomatitis, 145, 146
Chewing tobacco. See *Tobacco.*
Chickenpox (varicella), 2, 9, *9, 10*
Chloroquine, for sarcoidosis, 243
Cholesterol clefts, in periapical cyst, 305, *305*
Chondroblastic osteosarcoma, 407, *408, 409*, 414
Chondroma, *O-87*, 377
Chondromatosis, synovial, 414
Chondrosarcoma, 378
  grading of, 414
  mesenchymal, 416
Chromogenic bacteria, and tooth staining, 484, *484*
Cicatricial pemphigoid, *O-6*, O-7, 19–22, 19t, *20–23*, 23t
  vs. lichen planus, 108
Cigar smoking. See also *Smoking.*
  and nicotine stomatitis, 92

Cigar smoking *(Continued)*
  and oral cancer, 71
  and tooth abrasion, *468*
"Cigarette paper" scar, 449, *449*
Cigarette smoking. See *Smoking.*
Cirrhosis, parotid gland enlargement in, 243
Citrus fruit, and dental erosion, 467
Civatte bodies, 108, 109
Clavicles, hypoplastic, 443, *444*
Clear cell tumors, 274, 275
  odontogenic, O-81, 351
Cleft(s), alveolar, 455, *455, 456, 457*
  submucosal, 454
Cleft lip, 453–456, *454*
Cleft palate, 453–456, *455, 456*
  in cleidocranial dysplasia, 443
  in Treacher Collins syndrome, 447
Cleidocranial dysplasia, 443–445, *444*
  accessory teeth in, 471, *471*
Clotrimazole, for candidiasis, 116
Clotting defects, and extravascular oral lesions, 148
C-myc oncogene, 419
Coagulative necrosis of mucosa, 116, 117
Coagulopathy(ies), and extravascular oral lesions, 148
Cobblestone palate, *O-44*, O-45, 167, *168*
Coccidioidomycosis, 42, 43t, *44*
Cold sores, 3
Colitis, and pyostomatitis vegetans, 180
Collagen cuffing, perivascular, 438
Collagen deficiency, in Ehlers-Danlos syndrome, 448–450
Collagen deposition, in fibroma, 185
  in gingival hyperplasia, 191
Collagen metabolism, inborn errors of, in Ehlers-Danlos syndrome, 448, 449
  in osteogenesis imperfecta, 442
Collagen overproduction, in traumatic fibroma, 191, *192*
Colobomas, 446
Complement component(s), in cicatricial pemphigoid, 19–21
  in lupus erythematosus, 61
  in pemphigus vulgaris, 14
Concrescence, of teeth, 463, *463*
Condensing osteitis, 402
Condyloma acuminatum, O-45, 172, *174*
Condyloma latum, *O-44*, O-45, 35, *36, 169*, 169
Congenital anodontia, 469, *469*
Congenital epulis, *O-52*, O-53
Congenital gingival granular cell tumor, 207–210, 209t, *210*
Congenital heart disease, in Down syndrome, 451
Congenital hemangiomas, 125, *126*, 126t, 130, *130*
  vs. lymphangioma, 204
Congenital hemihypertrophy, 452, *452*
Congenital hypophosphatasia, 434
Congenital porphyria, and teeth staining, 486, *486*
Congenital syphilis, 34, 35
  and enamel hypoplasia, 474, *475*
Congenital teeth, 471, *472*
Conjunctival adhesions, 22, *23*
Conjunctivitis, in Behçet's syndrome, 53
  in drug allergy, *64*
  in erythema multiforme, 55
  in hereditary benign intraepithelial dyskeratosis, O-21, 86, 87

Conjunctivitis *(Continued)*
  in herpes zoster, 10, *11*
  in Reiter's syndrome, 53
Connective tissue disorder*(s)*, Ehlers-Danlos syndrome as, 448–450, *449*
  Marfan's syndrome as, 448
  osteogenesis imperfecta as, 441–443, *443*
  with Sjögren's syndrome, 245, 246, 248
Connective tissue hyperplasia, in acromegaly, 436, *437*
Connective tissue lesions, 184–223. See also specific lesions.
  angiosarcoma, 205, *206*
  congenital hemangioma. See *Hemangioma(s)*.
  denture-induced fibrous hyperplasia, 193, *193*, *194*
  esthesioneuroblastoma, 218
  fibromatosis, 196t, 197t, 198, *198*
  fibrosarcoma, 196, 197t, 199, *199*, *200*
  fibrous, 184–201. See also *Fibrous proliferative disorders*.
  fibrous histiocytomas, 196, 197t, 199, 200t, 201, *201–203*
  gingival hyperplasia, *O-52*, O-53, 187–191, *188–191*. See also *Gingival hyperplasia*.
  granular cell tumors, *O-58*, O-59, 207–210, *209–213*, 209t
  granulomas, *O-50*, O-51, 185
  hemangiopericytoma, 205, *205*, *206*
  juvenile nasopharyngeal angiomatosis, 195, *195*
  leiomyoma and leimyosarcoma, 219, *220*
  lipoma and liposarcoma, *222*, 223
  lymphangioma, *O-66*, O-67, 204, *204*
  mucosal neuromas of MEN III syndrome, 212t, 215, *216*
  myositis ossificans, 219
  myxomas, 193, *194*, 195t
  neoplastic. See also *Neoplasm(s)* and specific lesions.
    fibrous, 193–201
    neural, 207–218, 212t
    of muscle and fat, 219–223, *220–222*
    vascular, 205–207, *205*, *206*
  neural, 207–218. See also *Neural lesions*.
  neurofibroma, *O-58*, O-59, 212t, 214, *214*, 215, *216*. See also *Neurofibromatosis*.
  neurogenic sarcoma, 217, *217*
  nodular fasciitis, 196, 196t, *197*, 197t
  of muscle and fat, 219–223, *220–222*
  peripheral fibromas, *O-58*, O-59, 185, *185*, *186*
  peripheral giant cell granuloma, 132–134, *133*, *134*
  pyogenic granuloma, 131, *131*, *132*
  reactive. See also *Reactive lesions*.
    hyperplastic, 184–193. See also *Reactive hyperplasia(s)*.
    neural, 207, *208*
    of muscle and fat, 219
    vascular, 201
  rhabdomyoma and rhabdomyosarcoma, 219, *220*, *221*
  schwannoma, 210–214, 212t, *213*
  traumatic fibroma, *O-56*, O-57, 191
  traumatic neuroma, 207, *208*
  vascular, 201, 204–207, *204–206*
  venous varix. See *Varix(ces)*.
Connective tissue–epithelial junction, in lichen planus, 108, *109*
  nevi of, 158, *159*, 160

Contact allergy, *O-14*, O-15, *O-34*, O-35, 64–66, *65*, *66*
  and red-blue lesions, 146
Convulsion therapy. See *Phenytoin*.
Copper metabolism, in Ehlers-Danlos syndrome, 449
Corneal inflammation, in syphilis, 35
Coronoid process, hyperplasia of, O-89, 387–389
Corps ronds/grains, 88
Cortical hyperostosis, infantile, O-103, 434
Corticosteroid(s), and hairy tongue, 102
  for aphthous ulcers, 50–53, 51t, 52t
  for cicatricial pemphigoid, 21
  for erythema multiforme, 57
  for lichen planus, 109
  for lupus erythematosus, 61
  for pemphigus vulgaris, 18
  for sarcoidosis, 243
  intraoral use of, 51, 52t
  systemic, 50, 51t
  topical, 51, 52t
"Cotton roll" ulcers, 31, *31*
Coxsackie virus infection(s), 11, *12*, 13, *13*
Cranial sutures, premature closure of, 445
Craniofacial deformities, in cleidocranial dysplasia, 443, 444
  in Crouzon's syndrome, 445, *445*
  in hemifacial hypertrophy, 452, *452*
  in osteogenesis imperfecta, 442
  in Paget's disease, 427
Craniofacial dysostosis, 445, *445*
Craniofacial fibrous dysplasia, 372
Craniopharyngioma, 346, 348, *348*
Craniosynostosis, in Crouzon's syndrome 445
CREST syndrome, 129
Crohn's disease, and pyostomatitis vegetans, 180
  vs. sarcoidosis, 241, 243
Crouzon's syndrome, 445, *445*
Crowe's sign, 156, *156*, 215
Cryptococcosis, 42, 43t
Crystallites, caries-resistant, 499
  in cariogenesis, 491, 493, 494
Cushing's syndrome, 50, 51
Cusp, anomalous, 465, *465*
Cutaneous abscess, odontogenic, 394, *395*
Cutaneous lesion(s). See also *Blister(s); Bulla(e); Plaque(s); Ulcer(s); Ulcerative conditions;* and *Vesiculo-bullous disease(s)*.
  in bullous pemphigoid, 23, *24*
  in cicatricial pemphigoid, 19
  in dermatitis herpetiformis, 24, *25*
  in discoid lupus, 58, *58*, 61
  in drug reactions, 63, *63*, 64
  in Ehlers-Danlos syndrome, 449
  in erythema multiforme, 54, *54*
  in follicular keratosis, 87, 88
  in hand, foot, and mouth disease, 11, *12*
  in herpes simplex infections, *O-4*, 4–6, *5–7*
  in Kaposi's sarcoma, 137
  in lichen planus, 98, 108, *108*
  in measles, 13
  in nevoid basal cell carcinoma syndrome, 316
  in pemphigus vegetans, 18, *18*
  in psoriasis, 139, 140, *140*
  in sarcoidosis, 241
  in varicella-zoster infection, 9, *10*, *11*
Cutaneous lichen planus, 108, *108*
Cutaneous lupus erythematosus, subacute, 57, 58, *59*
Cutaneous macular pigmentation. See *Pigmentation(s)*.

Cutaneous melanomas. See *Melanoma(s)*.
Cutaneous verruca vulgaris, 169
Cutaneous warts, 169
Cyclosporine, and gingival hyperplasia, 189, 510
Cyst(s), 301–335
    aneurysmal bone, *O-76*, O-77, 323–325, *324, 326*
    antral, 234, *234*
    botryoid odontogenic, 312
    branchial cleft, *O-64*, O-65, 329, 330, *330–332*
    calcifying, *O-75*, 317, 318, *318, 319*
    cervical lymphoepithelial, 329, *330*
    dental lamina, 310–313
    dentigerous (follicular), *O-72*, O-73, 306–309, *307–310*
    dermoid, 330, *332, 333*
    developmental, 330, 331
    epidermal, O-67
    eruption, *O-52*, O-53, 310, *311*
    focal osteoporotic bone marrow defect, *O-76, O-77*, 329, *330*
    gingival, *O-26*, O-27, *O-52*, O-53, 120–122, *121*
        of adulthood, 310–313, *312*
        of newborn, O-27, *O-72*, O-73, 313, *313*
    "globulomaxillary," *O-74*, O-75, 319
    incisive canal, *O-74*, O-75, 321–323, *322, 323*
    keratinizing, 120, 122, 305, 306, 313
    keratocyst, *O-74*, O-75, 313–317, *314–317*
    lateral periodontal, *O-72*, O-73, 310–313, *311, 312*
    lymphoepithelial, *O-54*, O-55, 119, 286, 329, *330, 331*
    median alveolar, 321, *321*
    median mandibular, *O-75*, 320
    mucus retention. See *Mucus retention cyst*.
    nasolabial, *O-75*, 320
    nasopalatine canal, *O-74*, O-75, 321–323, *322, 323*
    non-odontogenic, *O-74*, O-75, 319–323. See also *Non-odontogenic cysts*.
    odontogenic, 301–318, O-72–O-75, *O-72, O-74*. See also *Odontogenic cysts*.
        gingival, *O-26*, O-27, 120–122, *121*
    of alveolar ridge, *O-26*, 120, *121*, 122
    of neck, 329–335. See also *Soft tissue cysts*.
        developmental, 330, 331
    of palatine papilla, 321
    oral lymphoepithelial, 329, *331*
    palatal midline, 120
    periapical. See *Periapical cyst(s)*.
    primordial, 306, 313, 321, 323
    pseudocysts. See *Pseudocyst(s)*.
    radicular. See *Periapical cyst(s)*.
    residual periapical, 302, 306, *307*
    retention. See *Mucus retention cyst*.
    soft tissue. See *Soft tissue cysts*.
    static bone, *O-76*, O-77, 328, *329*
    thyroglossal tract, *O-66*, O-67, 331–335, *333, 334*
    tooth-containing, *O-72*, O-73, 306–309, *307–310*
    traumatic (simple) bone, *O-76*, O-77, 325, *327, 328*
Cystadenoma, papillary (Warthin's tumor), 249t, 257, *258, 259*
Cystic ameloblastoma, 341, *343*
Cystic fibrosis, and sinus mucocele, 233
Cystic hygroma, 204
Cytokeratin, 424, 425

Cytomegalic inclusion disease, 239
Cytomegalic sialadenitis, 239
Cytomegalovirus, 2
   and oral cancer, 72
Cytotoxicity, in lichen planus, 105

Dapsone, in lichen planus, 110
Darier's (Darier-White) disease, O-21, 87–89, *88, 89*
   vs. papillary hyperplasia, 168
   vs. squamous papilloma, 171
Deafness, in congenital syphilis, 35
Decalcification, in caries, 493
Dementia, 450
Demineralization, in caries, 488, 493
Demographic factors in cariogenesis, 489
Dens evaginatus, 465, *465*
Dens in dente, 464, *464*
Dens invaginatus, 464, *464*
Dental abnormalities. See also *Teeth, abnormalities of*.
   in congenital syphilis, 35, *36*
Dental caries. See *Caries*.
Dental erosion. See *Erosion(s), of teeth*.
Dental impression material,
   and oral ulcers, 32, *32*
Dental lamina cysts, 310–313
Dental personnel, mercury intoxication of, 165, 166
Dental plaque. See *Plaque (dental)*.
Dental pulp. See *Pulp*.
Dental roots. See *Root(s)*.
Denticles, true vs. false, 480
Dentifrice, abrasive, 467
Dentigerous cyst, *O-72*, O-73, 306–309, *307–310*
   ameloblastoma in, *341*
Dentin, defects of, 477–480, *477–481*
   in carious process, 491–493, *491, 492*
   in dentinogenesis imperfecta, 477–479, *477, 478*
   in regional odontoplasia, 480, *481*
   opalescent, 477
Dentin dysplasia, 479, *479, 480*
Dentin shells, 479
Dentinoenamel junction, in carious process, *491, 492, 492*
Dentinogenesis imperfecta, 442, 443, *443*, 477–479, *477, 478*
Dentition, post-permanent, 472
   premature loss of, 433
Dentogingival junction, examination of, 505, 508
Denture(s). See also *Prosthetic device(s)*.
   after radiation therapy, 80
   allergic reaction to, 65
   and burning mouth syndrome, 143, 144
   and fibrous hyperplasia, 193, *193, 194*
   and frictional hyperkeratosis, 89, *90*
   and palatal nodules, 114, *114*
   and papillary hyperplasia, 167
   and traumatic ulcers, 29, *30*
   in Paget's disease, 427
Denture sore mouth, 112
Depigmentation, in vitiligo, O-39, 156, *158*
Dermal analogue tumor, 253, 254, *255*, 256
Dermatitis, in niacin deficiency, 142
Dermatitis herpetiformis, O-7, 24–26, *25*
Dermoid cyst, of floor of mouth, O-55, *O-66*
   of neck, *O-66*, O-67, 330, *332, 333*

Desquamative gingivitis, 107, *107*
Developmental cysts, of neck, 330, 331
Developmental disorders, of teeth, 464–467, *464–467*. See also *Teeth, abnormalities of*.
Developmental lesions, lymphoid, 286
Diabetes insipidus, 383
Diabetes mellitus, caries in, 498
  parotid gland enlargement in, 243
  phycomycosis in, 45, *46*
Diet, and caries, 496–498
Dietary acids, and dental erosion, 467
Dietary deficiency(ies), and aphthous ulcers, 47
  and burning mouth syndrome, 143–145
  and caries, 499
  and iron deficiency anemia, 143
  and pernicious anemia, 142, *142*
  and salivary gland enlargement, 243
  of vitamin B, 141, 142, *142*
Dietary factor(s), in submucous fibrosis, 117
Diffuse sclerosing osteomyelitis, *O-92*, *O-93*, 399–402, *401*
Digital herpes, *O-4*, *O-5*, 5, *7*
Dilaceration, 464, *464*
Dilantin. See *Phenytoin*.
Discoid lupus erythematosus, 57, 58, *58*, *59*, 60, 60t, 61
  vs. white lesions, 97, 98
Discoloration of teeth, 472, 473, 475, 477, *477*, 479
  exogenous and endogenous stains, 484, *484–486*
DNA hybridization studies, in hairy leukoplakia, 99, *100*
DNA viruses, in papilloma, 169–171, *170*
Down syndrome, 450, *450*, 451
  caries in, 498
  gingivitis in, 511
Draining sinus tract, in periapical abscess, 394, *394*
Drug(s), and gingival hyperplasia, 188–190, *189*
  causing mucosal pigmentations, 166
  intraoral, and ulceration, 31, *31*
Drug reaction(s), and red-blue lesions, 146
  causing oral ulcers, O-15, 62–64, 62t, *63–65*
  intravascular oral lesions in, *O-34*, O-35
  lichen planus, 108
Drug-induced staining of teeth, 484, *485*, 486
Dry eyes, 245, 248
Dry mouth. See *Xerostomia*.
Duct(s), salivary. See *Salivary gland duct(s)*.
Dyscrasias, blood. See *Blood dyscrasia*.
Dysgeusia, 144
Dyskeratoma, warty, 88, 171. See also *Darier's disease*.
Dyskeratosis, hereditary benign intraepithelial, O-21, 86, *87*
Dysostosis, craniofacial, 445, *445*
  mandibulofacial, 446, *446*
Dysplasia, cleidocranial, 443–445, *444*
  dentin, 479, *479*, *480*
  epithelial. See *Epithelial dysplasia*.
  erythroplakia, 135–137, *136*
  fibrous, *O-86*, *O-87*, 371, 372–375, *373*, *374*, 375t
  florid osseous, O-83, 361, 401
  hereditary ectodermal, 469, *470*
  periapical cemental, *O-82*, *O-83*, 338t, 361–363, *361*, *362*

Ear, enlarged, in fragile X syndrome, 457, *457*
Ear defects, in Treacher Collins syndrome, 446, *446*
Ecchymosis(es), 146–148, *148*
  in blood dyscrasias, *O-34*, O-35, 148, *148*, 148t
  in Ehlers-Danlos syndrome, 449
  of palate, *148*
  traumatic, *O-34*, O-35, 148, *148*
  vs. hemangioma, 125
Ectodermal dysplasia, hereditary, 469, *470*
Ectopia lentis, 448
Ectopic enamel, 467, *467*
Ectopic eruption of dentition, 438
Ectopic lymphoid tissue, *O-26*, *O-27*, 119, *120*, 284, 285
Ectopic sebaceous glands, *O-26*, *O-27*, 118, *119*
  and keratoacanthoma, 175
Edema, buccal, in leukoedema, 84, *85*
Edentulism, prevalence of, 503
Ehlers-Danlos syndrome, 448–450, *449*
Electrical burns, 116, 117
Electrogalvanically induced keratosis, 98
Embolization, arteriole, for hemangiomas, 130
Embryonal rhabdomyosarcoma, 22, 219
Enamel, defects of, 472–477, *473–476*, 480, *481*
  ectopic, 467, *467*
  fracturing of, 479
  hypomaturation of, 475
  in amelogenesis imperfecta, 475–477, *476*
  in carious process, 491–493, *491*, *492*
  in regional odontoplasia, 480, *481*
Enamel caries, 490
Enamel hypocalcification, environmental factors in, 473–475, *473*
  hereditary, 475, *476*
Enamel hypoplasia, environmental, 472–475, *473–475*
  hereditary, 475, *476*
  in rickets, *474*
Enamel organ, cystic degeneration of, 306, 313
Enamel pearls, 467, *467*
Encephalotrigeminal angiomatosis, 126, *128*
Endocrine disorders. See *Endocrinopathy(ies)*.
Endocrine neoplasia syndrome, multiple, 212t, 215, *216*
Endocrine tumors, 215, 217
Endocrinopathy(ies), and candidiasis, 114, 115
  and diffuse intravascular lesions, 141–145
  salivary gland enlargement in, 243
Enteropathy, gluten-sensitive, 24, 26
Enterovirus, 11
Eosinophilia, with angiolymphoid hyperplasia, 286
Eosinophilic granuloma, O-89, 383
Ephelis(ides), *O-36*, *O-38*, *O-39*, 153–155, *154*, *155*
Epidermal cyst, O-67
Epidermal nevus syndrome, *452*
Epidermolysis acquisita, 26
Epidermolysis bullosa, *O-6*, *O-7*, 26, *26*, 27
Epilepsy, 452
Epimyoepithelial carcinoma of intercalated ducts, 274–276, *276*
Epimyoepithelial islands, 244, *245*, 247
Epistaxis, in Ehlers-Danlos syndrome, 449
  in esthesioneuroblastoma, 218
  in nasopharyngeal angiofibroma, 195
  in Rendu-Osler-Weber syndrome, 129

Epithelial atrophy, and red lesions, O-28, *O-28*
    in submucous fibrosis, 118, *118*
Epithelial basal cells. See *Basal cell(s)*.
Epithelial dysplasia, definition of, 96
    in leukoplakia, 95, 96, *97*
Epithelial hyperplasia, focal, *O-46*, O-47, 174, *175*
    in candidiasis, 113, 115
    in psoriasis, 139–141, *141*
Epithelial tumors, *O-80*, O-81, 337–353
    adenomatoid odontogenic, *O-80*, O-81, 338t, 351–353, *353–355*
    ameloblastoma. See *Ameloblastoma*.
    calcifying odontogenic (Pindborg), O-81, 338t, 348–351, *350–352*
    clear cell odontogenic, O-81, 351
    mixed with mesenchymal tumors, *O-82*, *O-83*, 363–368, *364–367*
    squamous odontogenic, O-81, 348, *349*
Epithelial–connective tissue interface, in lichen planus, 108, *109*
Epithelioma, calcifying, of Malherbe, 318
Epstein-Barr virus, 2, 2t
    and hairy leukoplakia, 99–102, *101*
    and oral cancer, 72
    in Burkitt's lymphoma, 420
Epstein's pearls, 120, 313
Epulis, congenital, *O-52*, O-53, 207–210, 209t, *210*
Epulis fissuratum, 193
Erosion(s), mucocutaneous, 29. See also *Ulcer(s)*.
    of teeth, 467, *469*
    in hyperthyroidism, 433
Erosive gingival lichen planus, 511
Erosive lichen planus, *O-24*, 107, 108, *110*
Eruption of dentition, delayed, in cleidocranial dysplasia, 443, 444, *444*
    in Down syndrome, 451
    in osteopetrosis, 439, 440
    ectopic, 438
Eruption cyst, *O-52*, O-53, 310, *311*
Eruption hematoma, 310
Eruptions. See *Vesiculo-bullous disease(s)*.
Erythema migrans. See *Geographic tongue*.
Erythema multiforme, *O-14*, O-15, 54–57, *54–56*, 57t
    vs. herpes infections, 55, 57, 57t
    vs. herpetic gingivostomatitis, 7
Erythematous drug reaction, 63, *64*
Erythroblastosis fetalis, and teeth staining, 486
Erythroplakia, *O-32*, O-33, 97, 135–137, *136*
    penile, 136
    smokeless tobacco and, 91
    speckled, *O-33*
    vs. lupus (speckled), 61
Erythroplasia of Queyrat, 136
Esthesioneuroblastoma, 218, *218*
Estrogen deficiency, in hyperparathyroidism, 430
Ewing's sarcoma, *O-97*, 417–419, *417*, *418*
Exocrinopathy, in Sjögren's syndrome, 245
Exophthalmos, in Crouzon's syndrome, 445
    in Hand-Schüller-Christian disease, 383
    in hyperthyroidism, 433
Exophytic growths, mucosal, 167. See also *Verrucal-papillary lesions*.
Exostoses, *O-50*, O-51, O-89, 386, 387, *388*
    vs. osteomas, 379
Extractions. See *Tooth extractions*.
Extramedullary plasmacytoma, 297, 421

Extravascular lesions, intraoral, 146–149, *148*, *149*
    vs. hemangiomas, 125
Eye(s). See also *Ocular* entries.
    dry, 245, 248
    herpes zoster infection of, 10, *11*
    herpetic infection of, 8
    protruding. See *Exophthalmos*.
    upturned, 438
Eyelid. See *Lid* entries.

Facial asymmetry, 451, 452, *452*
Facial atrophy, 451
Facial deformities, in acromegaly, 436
    in nevoid basal cell carcinoma syndrome, 316
Facial expansion, in cherubism, 437, *437*, 438
Facial hypertrophy, 452, *452*
Facial hypoplasia, in Crouzon's syndrome, 445
Facial lymph node, hyperplastic, 285
Facial necrosis, in noma, 41, *42*
Facial nerve, preservation of, in parotidectomy, 253, 271
Facial nerve damage, in mucoepidermoid carcinoma, 263
    in osteopetrosis, 440
Facial pain, in neurofibromatosis, 215
    in traumatic neuroma, 207
Facial paralysis, in Paget's disease, 427
Factitial injury(ies), mucosal chewing, *O-20*, O-21, *30*, 85, 89, *90*
    ulcers, 29, *30*, 31
Familial mucocutaneous candidiasis, 115
Fasciitis, nodular, 196, 196t, *197*, 197t
    pseudosarcomatous, 196
Fat, neoplasms of, 219–223, *220–222*. See also specific types.
    reactive lesions of, 219
Fat malabsorption, and dermatitis herpetiformis, 24
Fetal cytomegalovirus infection, 239
Fetid breath, 511
Fever, rheumatic, 145
    scarlet, O-35, 145
    uveoparotid, 241
Fever blisters, 3
Fibroblastic osteosarcoma, 407, 409, *409*
Fibroblasts, herringbone, 196, 197t, 199, *200*
Fibroma(s), ameloblastic, *O-82*, *O-83*, 338t, 364–368, *366*
    cementifying, *O-80*, O-81, 338t, 359, *359*, *360*, 369, 371
    central odontogenic, O-81, 356, *358*
    giant cell, 186, *187*, *188*
    irritation, 191, *192*, 193
    ossifying, *O-86*, *O-87*, 185, *185*, 186, *186*, 359, 369–372, *370*, *371*, 375t
        juvenile active, 372
        vs. fibrous dysplasia, 371, 373, 375t
    peripheral, *O-50*, O-51, 185, *185*, *186*
    peripheral odontogenic, 186, *187*
    traumatic, *O-56*, O-57, 191
Fibromatosis, 196t, 197t, 198, *198*
    hereditary gingival, 190, *191*, 510
Fibro-odontoma, ameloblastic, *O-82*, *O-83*, 338t, 364–368, *365*, *367*
Fibro-osseous lesions, of jaws. See *Jaw(s), benign nonodontogenic tumors of*.
    vs. chronic osteomyelitis, 396, *396*, *398*

Fibrosarcoma, 196, 197t, 199, *199, 200*
  ameloblastic, 367, *367*
Fibrosis, submucous, O-27, 117, *118*
Fibrous dysplasia, *O-86*, O-87, 372–375, *373, 374,* 375t
  vs. ossifying fibroma, 371, 373, 375t
Fibrous histiocytoma, benign, 196, 197t, 199, 200t, *201, 202*
  malignant, 199, 200t, 201, *203*
Fibrous hyperplasia, denture-induced, 193, *193, 194*
Fibrous hyperplastic gingivitis, 509, *510*
Fibrous proliferative disorders, 184–201
  clinical features of, 196, 197t
  denture-induced fibrous hyperplasia, 193, *193, 194*
  fibromatosis, 196t, 197t, 198, *198*
  fibrosarcoma, 196, 197t, 199, *199, 200*
  fibrous histiocytomas, 196, 197t, 199, 200t, 201, *201–203*
  gingival hyperplasia. See *Gingival hyperplasia.*
  granulomas, 185, *O-50,* O-51. See also *Giant cell granuloma; Pyogenic granuloma.*
  juvenile nasopharyngeal angiofibroma, 195, *195*
  myxomas, 193, *194,* 195t
  neoplastic, 193–201
  nodular fasciitis, 196, 196t, *197,* 197t
  peripheral fibroma, *O-50,* O-51, 185, *185, 186*
  reactive hyperplasias, 184–193. See also *Reactive hyperplasia(s).*
  traumatic fibroma, *O-56,* O-57, 191
Finger(s), herpetic infection of, *O-4,* O-5, 5, 7
  in hand, foot, and mouth disease, 12, *12*
Fingernails. See *Nail(s).*
Fissured tongue, 103
Fistula(s), oral-antral, 81
Fite stain, 40
Fixed drug reaction, 63, *64*
Floating teeth, 384, *384*
Floor of mouth, carcinoma of, 73, 75
  dermoid cyst of, *O-55, O-66,* 330, *332*
  erythroplakia of, 135, *136*
  leukoplakia of, *O-22,* 94, 95, *98,* 99
  lipoma of, *122*
  mucocele (ranula) of, 231–233, *232, 233*
  swellings of, *O-54,* O-55
Florid osseous dysplasia, O-83, 361
  vs. diffuse sclerosing osteomyelitis, 401
Fluorapatite crystallites, caries-resistant, 499
Fluoride, anticaries effect of, 499
Fluorosis, 474, *475*
Foam cells, 181, *181*
Focal periapical osteomyelitis, 402, *402*
Focal sclerosing osteomyelitis, *O-93, O-92,* 402–404, *402, 403*
Foliate papillae, 284
Folic acid deficiency, 142
Follicular ameloblastoma, 341, *342*
Follicular cyst, *O-72, O-73,* 306–309, *307–310*
Follicular keratosis, O-21, 87–89, *88, 89*
Follicular lymphoid hyperplasia, 285
Foods, cariogenic, 489–491, 496–498
Foot, hand, and mouth disease, O-5, 11–13, *12*
Fordyce's granules, *O-26,* O-27, 118, *119*
Foreign body, in acute periodontitis, 513
Fracture(s), in hyperparathyroidism, 431, *431*
  in osteogenesis imperfecta, 442, 443
  in osteopetrosis, 440
Fragile X syndrome, 456, *457*

Freckles, *O-36, O-38,* O-39, 153–155, *154, 155*
  axillary, 156, *156*
  in neurofibromatosis, 215
Frenum, lingual, squamous papilloma of, *172*
Frictional hyperkeratosis, *O-20,* O-21, 89, *90*
  vs. leukoplakia, 97
Fungal disease(s), O-13, 42–46
  and geographic tongue, 103
  candidiasis. See *Candidiasis.*
  deep, *O-12,* O-13, 42, 43t, *44*
  opportunistic, O-13, 45, *46*
  subcutaneous, O-13, 45
Fungal overgrowth, and hairy tongue, 102
Fusion, of teeth, 463, *463*

Galvanic keratosis, 98
Gangrenous stomatitis, 41, *42*
Gardner's syndrome, accessory teeth in, 471
  osteoma in, O-89, 378, *378, 379*
Garré's osteomyelitis, *O-92,* O-93, 399, *399, 400*
Gastritis, atrophic, in pernicious anemia, 143
Gemination, 461, *462*
Genetic counseling, in cleidocranial dysplasia, 444
  in fragile X syndrome, 457
Genetic disorders, *O-104,* O-105, 437–457
  cherubism, *O-104,* O-105, 437–439, *437–439*
  cleft deformities, 453–456, *453–456.* See also *Cleft palate.*
  cleidocranial dysplasia, 443–445, *444*
  Crouzon's syndrome (craniofacial dysostosis), 445, *445*
  Down syndrome, 450, *450,* 451
  Ehlers-Danlos syndrome, 448–450, *449*
  fragile X syndrome, 456, *457*
  hemifacial atrophy, 451
  hemifacial hypertrophy, 452, *452*
  Marfan's syndrome, 448
  osteogenesis imperfecta, 441–443, *443*
  osteoporosis, *O-104,* O-105, 439–441, *440, 441*
  Pierre Robin syndrome, 447, *447*
  Treacher Collins syndrome (mandibulofacial dysostosis), 446, *446*
Genital herpes, 2, 4, 8
Genital infection(s), gonorrhea, 37
  syphilis, 35
Genital lesion(s), condyloma acuminatum, 172
  in condyloma latum, 169
  white sponge nevus, 85
Genital ulcers, 34, *35,* 37
  in Behçet's syndrome, 53, *53*
Genokeratoses (genodermatoses), *O-20,* O-21, 84–89, *85–89*
Geographic tongue, *O-22, O-23, O-32, O-33,* 54, 103, *104,* 139, *139*
German measles, 13
Ghost cell keratinization, 317, 318, *319*
  in ameloblastoma, 344, *344*
  in craniopharyngioma, *348*
  in odontomas, 363
Ghost cell tumor, odontogenic, *O-75,* 317, 318, *318, 319*
Ghost teeth, 480
Giant cell(s), Langhans'. See *Langhans' giant cells.*
Giant cell fibroma, 186, *187, 188*
Giant cell granuloma(s), O-51
  central, *O-88,* O-89, 379, *380, 381*
  peripheral, *O-30,* O-31, 132–134, *133, 134*

Giant cell tumor, 381
  vs. central giant cell granuloma, 380, 381
Giant osteoid osteoma, 375
Gingiva, carcinoma of, 74, 75
  follicular keratosis of, 88, 88
  healthy, 505, 505, 508
  lichen planus of, 105, 107
  necrosis of, in noma, 41, 42
Gingival abscess(es), O-27, 122, 122
Gingival ameloblastoma, 342
Gingival bleeding, in gingivitis, 508, 509, 511
  in hemangioma of bone, 382
  spontaneous, 149
Gingival boil, 122, 122
Gingival cyst(s), O-26, O-27, O-52, O-53, 120–122, 121
  of adulthood, 310–313, 312
  of newborn, O-27, O-72, O-73, 120, 121, 122, 313, 313
Gingival enlargement. See also Gingival hyperplasia.
  generalized, 187
  in blood dyscrasias, 149, 149
Gingival fibromatosis, hereditary, 190, 191, 510
Gingival fluid, 505
Gingival granular cell tumor, congenital, 207–210, 209t, 210
Gingival hyperplasia, 509–511, 510, 511
  Dilantin (phenytoin) and, 126, 188, 189, 189
  drug-induced, 188–190, 189
  focal, O-48–O-53, O-50, O-52
  generalized, O-52, O-53, 187–191, 188–191
  idiopathic, 190, 191
  in peripheral giant cell granuloma, 132, 133, 134
  in pregnancy, 131, 132
  in pyogenic granuloma, 131, 131, 132
  leukemia and, 509
Gingival lichen planus, erosive, 511
Gingival mass, in metastases to jaw, 424, 424
Gingival stippling, 151, 152
Gingival swellings, O-48, O-49. See also Gingival hyperplasia.
Gingival ulcers, in cicatricial pemphigoid, 19, 20, 21
  in herpes simplex infection, O-4, O-5, 5, 6
  in histoplasmosis, 44
  in varicella, 9, 10
Gingivitis, 508–512. See also Periodontal disease.
  acute necrotizing ulcerative (Vincent's infection), 7
  advanced, 506
  and risk for periodontal disease, 504
  bleeding in, 508, 509, 511
  desquamative, 107, 107
  early lesion in, 505, 506
  established lesion of, 506, 506
  experimental, 504
  hyperplastic, 509–511, 510, 511
  inflammatory changes in, 505, 506, 506
  mouth breathing and, 509, 510, 511
  overhanging restorations and, 509
  plasma cell, O-35, 145, 146, 147
  refractory, in blood dyscrasia, 149
  simple, 508, 509
  susceptibility to, 503
Gingivosis, 19
Gingivostomatitis, allergic, 145, 146, 147
  herpetic, O-4, O-5, 2–4, 5, 6–9, 511

Gland(s), lacrimal, dysfunction of, 245
  parotid. See Parotid gland.
  salivary. See Salivary gland(s).
  sebaceous, ectopic, O-26, O-27, 118, 119, 175, 331, 333
  thyroid. See Thyroid gland entries.
"Globulomaxillary" cyst, O-74, O-75, 319
Glomerulitis, necrotizing, 66
Glomerulonephritis, scarlet fever and, 145
Glomerulopathy, in lupus erythematosus, 60
Glossitis, antibiotic therapy and, 111
  Hunter's (Moeller's), 143
  in plasma cell gingivitis, 145, 146
  in scarlet fever, 145
  median rhomboid, O-32, O-33, 113, 114, 134, 134, 135
  migratory. See Geographic tongue.
  syphilitic, 35
  vitamin B deficiency and, 142, 142, 143
Glucocorticoid(s). See also Corticosteroids.
  systemic effects of, 50, 51t
Gluten-sensitive enteropathy, 24, 26
Gold therapy, for pemphigus vulgaris, 19
Gonococcal infection, pharyngeal, 37
Gonorrhea, O-11, 37
Grading, in salivary gland biopsy, 248
  of chondrosarcomas, 414
  of squamous cell carcinoma, 80, 81t
Granular cell ameloblastoma, 341, 343
Granular cell tumors, O-58, O-59, 207–210, 209–213, 209t
Granulation tissue, exuberant, 184, 191. See also Granuloma(s); Reactive hyperplasia(s).
  tumors of. See Granuloma(s).
Granule(s), Birbeck, 385, 386
  Fordyce's, O-26, O-27, 118, 119
Granuloma(s), eosinophilic, O-89, 383
  giant cell central, O-88, O-89, 379, 380, 381
  peripheral, O-30, O-31, O-51, 132–134, 133, 134
  in sarcoidosis, 241, 242, 242
  in sporotrichosis, 45
  midline, O-16, O-17, 67, 67t, 68
  periapical, 301, 302, 302, 306, 393
  pyogenic. See Pyogenic granuloma.
  traumatic, 32
  tubercular, 39, 39
Granulomatosis, Wegener's, O-15, 66, 67t, 67
Granulomatous disease(s), chronic, O-17, 68
Granulomatous inflammation, fungal, 42, 43t, 44
Granulomatous vasculitis, Wegener's, 66
Graves' disease, 432
Green stain, of teeth, 484, 485
Growth hormone hypersecretion, 435
Gum, chewing. See Chewing gum.
Gum boil, 122, 122, 512–514, 513
Gumma, syphilitic, 34, 35, 36, 37
Gums. See Gingiva.
Gut-associated lymphoid tissue, 287, 290

Hair lick, 446, 447
Hair loss. See Alopecia.
Hairy leukoplakia, O-22, O-23, 99–102, 99t, 100, 101
Hairy tongue, O-23, 102, 102
Hamartoma syndrome, multiple, 168
Hand-Schüller-Christian syndrome, O-89, 383
Hansen's disease, 39

Hard palate. See *Palate.*
Head and neck, actinomycotic infections of, 40, *41*
　fibromatosis of, 198
　nodular fasciitis of, 196
　phycomycosis of, 45
Head and neck cancer, See also *Carcinoma(s); Neoplasm(s); Tumor(s)* and specific types.
　basal cell carcinoma in, 68–70, *69, 70*
　fibrosarcoma in, 196, 197t, 199, *199, 200*
　fibrous histiocytoma in, 199, 200t, 201, *203*
　leiomyoma and leiomyosarcoma in, 219, *220*
　lesions of muscle and fat in, 219–223, *220–222*
　lipoma and liposarcoma in, *222,* 223
　lymphomas in. See *Lymphoma(s).*
　melanomas in, 160–163. See also *Melanoma(s).*
　myelomas in, *O-98,* O-99, 297, *299, 300,* 421–423, *422, 423*
　of jaws. See *Jaw(s), non-odontogenic malignancies of.*
　of salivary glands. See *Salivary gland tumors.*
　plasma cell tumors in, *O-98,* O-99, 297, *299, 300,* 421–423, *422, 423*
　plasmacytomas in, 297, *300,* 423
　radiation therapy for. See also *Radiation therapy.*
　and oral ulcers, 32, *33*
　rhabdomyoma and rhabdomyosarcoma in, 219, *220, 221*
　verrucous carcinoma in, *O-46, O-47, 178,* 178, 178t, *179,* 180
Head and neck cysts. See *Cyst(s).*
Hearing loss, in cleft deformities, 455, 456
　in osteogenesis imperfecta, 442
Heart disease, congenital, in Down syndrome, 451
　rheumatic, periodontal therapy in, 515
Heart failure, in Marfan's syndrome, 448
Heat burns, 116, 117
　and oral ulcers, 31, 32, *32*
Heavy-metal pigmentations, O-41, 165, *165*
Heck's disease, *O-46, O-47,* 174, *175*
Heerfordt's syndrome, 241
Hemangioma(s), *O-30,* O-31, 125–130, 126t
　capillary, 130, *130*
　cavernous, 130, *130*
　congenital, 125, *126,* 126t, 130, *130*
　　vs. lymphangioma, 204
　histiocytic, 286
　in angio-osteohypertrophy syndrome, 126, 129
　in Rendu-Osler-Weber syndrome, 129, *129*
　in Sturge-Weber syndrome, 126, *128*
　of bone, *O-88,* O-89, 382, *382, 383*
　port-wine stain, 126, *128*
　telangiectasias, 129, *129*
　treatment of, 130
　vascular malformations, 125, 126, 126t, *127–129,* 129
　venous varices, 129, *129*
　vs. ecchymoses, 125
Hemangiopericytoma, 205, *205, 206*
Hematologic disorders, in osteopetrosis, 439–441
Hematoma, eruption, 310
Hematopoietic malignancy, and herpes zoster infection, 9
Hemifacial atrophy, 451
Hemifacial hypertrophy, 452, *452,* 461
Hemophilia, 148

Hemorrhage(s), in blood dyscrasias, 148, *148,* 148t, 149, *149*
　into soft tissue, 125, 146–149, *148*
　petechiae and ecchymoses, 125, 146–149, *148*
　spontaneous gingival, 149
Hemorrhagic spots, *O-34,* O-35, 146–149, *148*
Hemorrhagic telangiectasia, hereditary, *O-30,* O-31, 129, *129*
Hepatitis, neonatal, and teeth staining, 486
Hereditary angioedema, 63, *63*
Hereditary benign intraepithelial dyskeratosis, O-21, 86, *87*
Hereditary blood disorders, 148
Hereditary disease(s). See *Genetic disorders* and *Metabolic disorders.*
Hereditary ectodermal dysplasia, 469, *470*
Hereditary gingival fibromatosis, 190, *191,* 510
Hereditary granulomatous disease, 68
Hereditary hemorrhagic telangiectasia, *O-30,* O-31, 129, *129*
Hereditary keratotic disorders, *O-20,* O-21, 84–88, *85–89*
Hereditary opalescent dentin, 477
Herpangina, O-5, 13, *13*
Herpes keratitis, 8
Herpes simplex labialis, *O-4,* O-5, *5, 5,* 6, 8, *11*
Herpes simplex virus(es), 2, 2t
Herpes simplex virus infection(s), 2–9, *3–7*
　carcinogenic potential of, 4
　genital, 2, 4, 8
　histopathology of, 6, *7*
　of finger, *O-4,* O-5, *5, 7*
　pathogenesis of, 2–4, *4*
　primary gingivostomatitis, *O-4,* O-5, 4, *5*
　reactivation of virus in, 3, 4
　secondary infections, *O-4,* O-5, 3, 4, *5, 6*
　treatment of, 8
　ulcers in, *O-4,* O-5, 2–9, *5–7,* 8t
　vs. aphthous ulcers, 7, 8t, 47, 48, 50
　vs. erythema multiforme, 55, 57, 57t
　whitlow in, 5, *7*
Herpes simplex virus type II infection, 2, 4
Herpes zoster (shingles), O-5, 2, 9–11, *11*
Herpesvirus(es), cytomegalovirus, 2, 2t
　Epstein-Barr, 2, 2t
　herpes simplex. See *Herpes simplex virus infection(s).*
　types of, 1, 2, 2t
　varicella-zoster, O-5, 2, 9–11, *10, 11*
Herpetic gingivostomatitis, *O-4,* O-5, 2–4, 5, *6–9,* 511
Herpetic whitlow, *O-4,* O-5, *5, 7*
Herpetiform lesions, 24, *25*
　in aphthous ulceration, 48, 48t, *50*
Herringbone fibroblasts, 196, 197t, 199, *200*
Histiocyte(s), 294, 294t
Histiocytic hemangioma, 286
Histiocytoma, fibrous, 196, 197t, 199, 200t, 201, *201–203*
Histiocytosis, disseminated forms of, 383, 385
　idiopathic, *O-88,* O-89, 383–386, *384–386*
　sinus, 289
Histiocytosis X, 383
Histocompatibility antigens. See *Antigen(s), histocompatibility.*
Histoplasmosis, 42, 43t, *44*
HLA. See *Antigen(s), human leukocyte.*
Hodgkin's disease, 287, 288t
Hodgkin's lymphoma, 287–290, *288–290,* 288t, 289t

Homosexuals, hairly leukoplakia in, 99
Hormonal changes, and gingival hyperplasia, 187, 190, 509
Hormonal disorders, acromegaly, *O-102*, O-103, 435–437, *437*
  estrogen deficiency, 430
  hyperparathyroidism, *O-102*, O-103, 430–432, *431–433*
  hyperthyroidism, 432, 433
Hormonal imbalance, and burning mouth syndrome, 143
HPV. See *Papilloma virus.*
HSV. See *Herpes simplex virus.*
Human immunodeficiency virus infection, and AIDS. See *Acquired immunodeficiency syndrome.*
  and candidiasis, 111, 115
  caries in, 489
  salivary cytomegalovirus in, 240
Human leukocyte antigens. See *Antigen(s), human leukocyte.*
Human papilloma virus. See *Papilloma virus.*
Hunter's glossitis, 143
Hutchinson's incisors, 474, *475*
Hutchinson's triad, 35, *36*
Hyaline bodies, in periapical cyst, 305, *305*
Hybridization studies, DNA, in hairy leukoplakia, 99, 100
Hydrocolloid burn, and oral ulcers, 32, *32*
Hydrogen peroxide, and hairy tongue, 102
  and oral ulcers, 31
Hydroquinones, for vitiligo, 157
Hydroxyapatite crystallites, in caries, 491, 493, 494
Hygiene, oral, and caries, 490, 493, 494, 498
Hygroma colli, 204
Hyperbaric oxygen therapy, for diffuse sclerosing osteomyelitis, 402
  for osteoradionecrosis, 398
Hypercalcemia, 430, 431, 434
Hypercementosis, in Paget's disease, 428, *429*
Hyperelastic skin, 449
Hyperhidrosis, in acromegaly, 436
  in hyperthyroidism, 433
Hyperimmune response, in lichen planus, 105
  in midline granuloma, 67
  to drugs, 62–64
Hyperkeratosis(es). See also *Keratosis(es); White lesions.*
  and verrucous carcinoma, 178, 180
  frictional, *O-20*, O-21, 89, *90*
  hereditary, *O-20*, O-21, 84–89, *85–89*
  in pyostomatitis vegetans, 180
  in reactive ulcers, 32, *33*
  of palms and soles, 88, 518, *518*
  smokeless tobacco and, 90–92, *91, 92*
Hyperlipoproteinemia, and parotid gland enlargement, 243
Hyperostosis, cortical infantile, O-103, 434
Hyperparathyroidism, *O-102*, O-103, 380, 430–432, *431–433*
Hyperpigmentation, in dermatitis herpetiformis, 25
  in herpes zoster, 9
Hyperplasia(s), angiolymphoid with eosinophilia, 286
  connective tissue, in acromegaly, 436, *437*
  epithelial, in psoriasis, 140, *141*
  fibrous, denture-induced, 193, *193, 194*
  focal epithelial, *O-46*, O-47, 174, *175*

Hyperplasia(s) *(Continued)*
  gingival. See *Gingival hyperplasia.*
  lymphoid, reactive, 284, *285*, 293
  of coronoid processes, O-89, 387–389
  of parathyroid glands, 430
  papillary, *O-44*, O-45, 167, *168*
  pseudoepitheliomatous, 210, *211*
  reactive. See *Reactive hyperplasia(s).*
Hyperplastic chronic pulpitis, 392, *392*
Hyperplastic gingivitis, 509–511, *510, 511* See also *Gingival hyperplasia.*
Hyperplastic scar, 185, 191, 193. See also *Granuloma(s); Reactive hyperplasia(s).*
Hypersensitivity, of teeth, in pulpitis, 391
Hypersensitivity reaction(s), in allergic gingivostomatitis, 145
  in erythema multiforme, 54
  submucous fibrosis, O-27, 117, *118*
Hypertelorism, in Crouzon's syndrome, 445
Hyperthyroidism, 432, 433
Hypertrophic candidiasis, 113, *114*
Hypertrophy, hemifacial, 452, *452*, 461
  laryngeal, in acromegaly, 436
Hypocalcification, of enamel, 473–475, *473, 476*
Hypodontia, 451, 455
Hypoestrinism, and burning mouth syndrome, 143
Hypophosphatasia, 433
Hypoplasia, mid-face, 445
Hypoplastic clavicles, 443, *444*
Hypoplastic enamel, environmental factors in, 472–475, *473–475*
  hereditary, 475, *476*
Hypoplastic maxilla, in cleidocranial dysplasia, 443
  in Crouzon's syndrome, 445, *445*
Hypothyroidism, caries in, 498

Iatrogenic pigmentations, *O-40*, O-41, 157t, 163, *164, 165*
Idiopathic histiocytosis, *O-88*, O-89, 383–386, *384–386*
Idiopathic intravascular lesions, 139–141, *139–141*
Idiopathic leukoplakia. See *Leukoplakia, idiopathic.*
Idiopathic thrombocytopenic purpura, 148
Idiopathic verrucal-papillary lesions, O-47, 180–182, *181*
Idiopathic white lesions, 94–110. See also *White lesions.*
Idoxuridine, for herpes infection, 8
Immune complex vasculitis, in aphthous ulcers, 46, 50
  in erythema multiforme, 54, 55
Immune response, in drug reactions, 62, 63
Immune status, and caries, 489
Immunity, cell-mediated, in candidiasis, 115
  in follicular keratosis, 88
  in lichen planus, 105
Immunodeficiency states, acquired. See *Acquired immunodeficiency syndrome.*
  and aphthous ulcers. See *Aphthous ulcer(s).*
  and Behçet's syndrome, O-13, 48t, *53*, 53
  and bullous pemphigoid, O-7, 19, 22–24, 23t, *24*
  and candidiasis, 111, 115. See also *Candidiasis.*

Immunodeficiency states *(Continued)*
   and chronic granulomatous disease, O-17, 68
   and cicatricial pemphigoid, *O-6*, O-7, 19–22, 19t, *20–23*, 23t
   and contact allergy, *O-14*, O-15, 64–66, *65*, *66*
   and dermatitis herpetiformis, O-7, 24–26, *25*
   and diffuse intravascular lesions, 145, *146*, *147*
   and drug reactions. See *Drug reactions.*
   and erythema multiforme, *O-14*, O-15, 54–57, *54–56*, 57t
   and follicular keratosis, 88
   and Kaposi's sarcoma, 137–139, *137*, 137t, *138*
   and lupus erythematosus. See *Lupus erythematosus.*
   and midline granuloma, *O-16*, O-17, 67, 67t, 68
   and opportunistic fungal infections, 45
   and Papillon-Lefèvre syndrome, 518
   and pemphigus vulgaris, *O-6*, O-7, 14–19, *16–19*, 19t
   and plasma cell gingivitis, 145, *146*, *147*
   and Reiter's syndrome, O-13, 53
   and salivary gland disease, 243–247, *244–247*
   and ulcerative drug reactions, O-15, 62–64, 62t, *63–65*
   and Wegener's granulomatosis, O-15, 66, 67t, 67
   benign lymphoepithelial lesion, 243–245, *244*, *245*, 247
   caries in, 489
   Sjögren's syndrome. See *Sjögren's syndrome.*
   verruciform xanthoma in, 180–182
   viral infections in, 1, 2, 9
Immunofluorescence testing, in cicatricial pemphigoid, 19, 20, *22*
   in dermatitis herpetiformis, 26
   in lichen planus, 108, *109*
   in lupus erythematosus, 61
   in pemphigus vulgaris, 17, *17*, 18
Immunoglobulin(s), in cicatricial pemphigoid, 19–21
   in dermatitis herpetiformis, 24–26
   in lupus erythematosus, 61
   in pemphigus vulgaris, 14
   in Sjögren's syndrome, 246
Immunoglobulin component, monoclonal, in multiple myeloma, 421, 422
Immunohistochemical staining, in granular cell tumors, 207, 210
   in hairy leukoplakia, 100
   in lichen planus, 108, *109*
Immunologic defect. See *Immunodeficiency states.*
Immunomodulators, for sarcoidosis, 243
Immunosuppression, and herpes zoster, 9
Immunosuppressive therapy, and cytomegalovirus infection, 240
   and gingival hyperplasia, 189
   for cicatricial pemphigoid, 22
   for pemphigus vulgaris, 19
Impaction, mucus, 233
   of tooth. See *Teeth, abnormalities of, impaction.*
Impetigo, vs. oral herpes, 8
Inborn error of collagen metabolism, 442, 448, 449
Inborn error of porphyrin metabolism, 486
Incisive canal cyst, *O-74*, O-75, 321–323, *322*, *323*
Inclusion, of salivary gland, 328
Inclusion cyst of palate, 313

Infancy, neuroectodermal tumor of, *O-40*, O-41, 163, *163*, *164*
   gingival granular cell tumor of, 207–210, 209t, *210*
Infant(s). See *Neonate(s).*
Infantile cortical hyperostosis, O-103, 434
Infantile osteopetrosis, 439, *440*
Infection(s), actinomycosis, O-11, 40, *41*
   and diffuse intravascular lesions, 145
   and geographic tongue, 103
   and intravascular lesions, 145
   atrophic candidiasis. See *Candidiasis.*
   bacterial. See *Bacterial conditions.*
   blastomycosis, 42, 43t, *44*
   candidiasis. See *Candidiasis.*
   cellulitis, 394, *395*
   coccidioidomycosis, 42, 43t, *44*
   Coxsackie virus, 11, *12*, 13, *13*
   cryptococcosis, 42, 43t
   cytomegalovirus, fetal, 239
   fungal, *O-12*, O-13, 42–46, 43t, *44*, *46*
   genital, 35, 37
   gonococcal, 37
   herpes simplex virus. See *Herpes simplex virus infection(s).*
   histoplasmosis, 42, 43t, *44*
   in periodontitis, 505–507, 512–518. See also *Periodontal disease; Periodontitis.*
   intrauterine, 9, 14
   leprosy, O-11, 39
   mucocutaneous. See *Ulcerative conditions; Vesiculo-bullous disease(s).*
   neck swellings in, O-65
   noma, O-13, 41, *42*
   of mucocele, 233
   of salivary glands, 239–243
   opportunistic. See also *Opportunistic infections.*
      fungal, 45, *46*
   osteomyelitis. See *Osteomyelitis.*
   papilloma virus, *O-44*, O-45, 169–172, 169t, *170–172*
   periapical abscess, 393, *393–395*
   periodontal. See *Periodontal disease.*
   scarlet fever, 145
   spirochete, 34–37, *34–36*
   streptococcal, 145
   superinfections, candidal, 100, 108
      in hairy tongue, 102
   syphilis, condyloma latum in, 169
   tuberculosis, *O-10*, O-11, 38, *38*, *39*
   varicella-zoster, O-5, 9–11, *10*, *11*
   venereal, 34–37, *34–37*
   Vincent's. See *Gingivitis.*
   viral. See *Viral disease(s)* and specific infections.
   vs. disease, in cariogenesis, 496
Infectious mononucleosis, 2
Inflammatory bowel disease, pyostomatitis vegetans in, 180
Inflammatory lesions, of bone marrow. See *Osteomyelitis.*
   of bone. See *Osteomyelitis.*
   of jaws, O-91–O-93, 390–404
   of pulp, 390–393
   periapical, 393, *393–395*. See also *Periapical abscess.*
Influenza virus, 2t
Interferon, for condyloma acuminatum, 174
   for lymphoma, 297
   for varicella-zoster infections, 11

Interleukins, in lichen planus, 105
Intestinal malabsorption, and dermatitis herpetiformis, 24–26
Intestinal polyposis, 153t, 154, 378
Intestinal rupture, 449
Intracranial pressure, increased, in Crouzon's syndrome, 445
Intraosseous carcinoma, primary, 346
Intrauterine infection(s), 9, 14
Intravascular lesions. See also *Red-blue lesions*.
  diffuse, 141–146
  focal, 125–141
Inverted duct papilloma, 258, 259, *261*
Involucrin, in keratoacanthoma, 177
Iodine therapy, 433
Ionizing radiation, effect on salivary glands, 236–239
Iris, Brushfield spots of, 451
Iris freckling, 215
Iris lesion, 54, *54*
Iron deficiency, and leukoplakia, 95
  and oral cancer, 72
  in candidiasis, 115
Iron deficiency anemia, O-33, 143
Irritants, chemical, and oral ulcers, 31, *31*, 32, *32*
Irritation fibroma, 191, *192*, 193
Ischemic necrosis of salivary gland, 235, *235–237*

Jaffe-Lichtenstein syndrome, O-87, 372
Jaw(s). See also *Mandible; Maxilla*.
  actinomycotic infection of, 40, *41*
  benign non-odontogenic tumors of, O-85–O-89, 369–389
    central giant cell granuloma, O-88, O-89, 379, *380*, *381*
    chondroma, O-87, 377
    coronoid process hyperplasia, O-89, 387–389
    exostoses, O-89, 386, 387, *388*
    fibrous dysplasia, O-86, O-87, 372–375, *373*, *374*, 375t
    giant cell tumor, 381
    hemangioma, O-88, O-89, 382, *382*, *383*
    idiopathic histiocytosis (Langerhans' cell disease), O-88, O-89, 383–386, *384–386*
    ossifying fibroma, O-86, O-87, 369–372, *370*, *371*, 375t
    osteoblastoma, O-86, O-87, 375–377, *376*
    osteoid osteoma, 377
    osteoma, O-88, O-89, 378, *378*, *379*
    tori, O-89, 386, 387, *387*, *388*
  cysts of, 301–335. See also *Cyst(s)*.
  enlarged, in acromegaly, 436
    in Paget's disease, 427
  expansion of, in cherubism, 437, *437*, 438
  genetic disorders, 437–457. See also *Genetic disorders*.
  inflammatory lesions of, O-91–O-93, 390–404
    acute osteomyelitis, O-93, 394, 395
    chronic osteomyelitis, *O-92*, O-93, 395–404, *396–398*. See also *Osteomyelitis*.
    periapical abscess, 393, *393–395*
    pulpitis, 390–393
  metabolic disorders of, 427–437. See also *Metabolic disorders*.
  metastases to, *O-98*, O-99, 424, *424*, *425*

Jaw(s) *(Continued)*
  non-odontogenic malignancies of, O-95–O-99, 405–425
    Burkitt's lymphoma, *O-96*, O-97, 419–421, *420*, *421*
    chondrosarcoma, 413–417, *415*, *416*
    Ewing's sarcoma, O-97, 417–419, *417*, *418*
    mesenchymal chondrosarcoma, 416
    metastatic carcinoma, *O-98*, O-99, 424, *424*, *425*
    multiple myeloma, *O-98*, O-99, 297, *299*, *300*, 421–423, *422*, *423*
    of bone marrow, 417–424
    osteosarcoma, 405–413, *O-96*, O-97. See also *Osteosarcoma(s)*.
    plasma cell tumors, *O-98*, O-99, 297, *299*, *300*, 421–424, *422*, *423*
    plasmacytomas, 297, *300*, 423
  odontogenic, epithelial, 337–353, O-80, O-81. See also *Epithelial tumors*.
  odontogenic tumors of, O-80–O-83, 337–368, 338t. See also *Odontogenic tumors*.
    mesenchymal, 353–363, *O-80*, O-81. See also *Mesenchymal tumors*.
    mixed, *O-82*, O-83, 363–368, *364–367*
  protruding. See *Prognathism*.
  rhabdomyosarcoma of, 219
Joint laxity, 449
Junctional nevus, 158, *159*, 160
Juvenile active ossifying fibroma, 372
Juvenile nasopharyngeal angiofibroma, 195, *195*
Juvenile parotitis, 240
Juvenile periodontitis, 516–518, *516*
Juxtacortical osteosarcoma, 410, 411

Kaposi's sarcoma, O-33, 137–139, *137*, 137t, *138*, 205, 207
Keratin layer, altered, O-18, 84. See also *Hyperkeratosis; Keratosis(es); White lesions*.
Keratin loss, in candidiasis, 111, 112
  in geographic tongue, 103, *104*
Keratin pearls, in leukoplakia, 97
  in palatal carcinoma, 76
Keratin plug, 176, *177*
Keratinization. See also *Hyperkeratosis(es); White lesions*.
  ghost cell. See *Ghost cell keratinization*.
  in hairy tongue, 102
  in nicotine stomatitis, 91
  of cysts, 305, 306, 313
Keratinizing cyst(s), 120, 122
Keratinocyte(s), disorders of. See *Keratosis(es)*.
  hyperproliferation of, in psoriasis, 139
  in erythroplakia, 136
  in lichen planus, 105
Keratitis, herpes, 8
  in congenital syphilis, 35
Keratoacanthoma, *O-46*, O-47, 175–177, *176*, *177*
Keratoconjunctivitis sicca, 245, 248
Keratocyst(s), odontogenic, *O-74*, O-75, 69, 313–317, *314–317*
  dentigerous, 308, 309
  in nevoid basal cell carcinoma syndrome, 314, 316
  orthokeratotic, 314, *316*
Keratosis(es). See also *Hyperkeratosis; White lesions*.

Keratosis(es) *(Continued)*
  electrogalvanically induced, 98
  follicular, O-21, 87–89, *88, 89*
  frictional, vs. leukoplakia, 97
  hereditary, *O-20, O-21,* 84–89, *85–89*
  in lupus erythematosus, 58, *59, 60,* 61
  subungual, 88
  wart-like, 98
Keratotic basal cell carcinoma, 69
Keratotic striae, in lichen planus, 61, 105, *106,* 107, 109
Ketoacidotic diabetes. See *Diabetes* entries.
Kidney lesions, in hyperparathyroidism, 431
  in lupus erythematosus, 60
  in Wegener's granulomatosis, 66
Kimura's disease, 286
Klippel-Trenaunay-Weber syndrome, 453
Koebner's phenomenon, 139
Koilonychia, iron deficiency and, 143
Koplik's spots, 13, 14
Kveim test, 242
Kyphoscoliosis, 442

Labia. See *Lip(s)*.
Labial salivary gland biopsy, 246–248
Lacrimal gland dysfunction, 245
Lactobacilli, and caries, 495, 496
Langerhans' cell(s), in contact allergy, 64
  in lichen planus, 105, 108, *109*
  in plasma cell gingivitis, 146
  in verruciform xanthoma, 180, 182
Langerhans' cell disease, *O-88,* O-89, 383–386, *384–386*
Langhans' giant cells, 39, *39*
  in sarcoidosis, 242, *242*
Laryngeal hypertrophy, in acromegaly, 436
Lateral, peg, 460, *461, 462*
LE cell test, 57, 60, 60t, 61t
Lead intoxication, and pigmented mucosa, 165, *165*
Leiomyoma, 219, *220*
Leiomyosarcoma, 219
Lens dislocation, 448
Lentigo, *O-38, O-39,* 155, *155*
Lentigo maligna melanoma, 161
Leprosy, O-11, 39
Leptomeninges, venous malformations of, 126
Letterer-Siwe syndrome, O-89, 383
Leukemia(s), and extravascular oral lesions, 148, *149*
  and gingival hyperplasia, 190, *190,* 191
  and hyperplastic gingivitis, 509
  in Down syndrome, 451
Leukoedema, O-21, 84, *85*
  vs. leukoplakia, 85, 98
Leukoplakia, and verrucous carcinoma, 178, 180
  candidal, 113, 115
  definition of, 94, 95
  friction-induced, 85, 89
  hairy, *O-22, O-23,* 99–102, 99t, *100, 101*
  idiopathic, *O-22, O-23,* 94–99, *96–98*
    biopsy in, 95–97, *97, 98,* 99
    differential diagnosis of, 97–99
    etiologic associations in, 95
    histologic spectrum of, 94–97, *97*
    malignant transformation of, 95–97, *97, 98*
    premalignant, 95
    treatment and prognosis of, 99
    vs. leukoedema, 85, 98

Leukoplakia *(Continued)*
  of tongue, and cancer, 73
  proliferative verrucous, 96, 98
  simplex, 96
  speckled, 95
Lichen planus, *O-24, O-25,* 105–110, *106–110*
  atrophic, 105, *107,* 108, 110
  bullous, 107
  cutaneous, 108, *108*
  drug-induced, 108
  erosive, *O-24,* 107, 108, 110
  erosive gingival, 511
  etiology and pathogenesis of, 105
  malignant potential of, 110
  plaque form, 105, *106, 107*
  reticular, 105, *106*
  treatment of, 109, *110*
  vs. cicatricial pemphigoid, 108
  vs. keratoses, 86, 87
  vs. leukoplakia, 98
  vs. lupus erythematosus, 61, 61t, *62*
Lichenoid drug reaction, 63, *65*
Lid colobomas, 446
Lid lag, 433
Lingual carcinoma, 72, *74*
Lingual frenum, squamous papilloma of, *172*
Lingual lesions. See *Tongue*.
Lingual thyroid, O-59, 331, *334*
Lingual tonsil, 119, 284
Lingual ulcers. See *Tongue, ulcers of*.
Lip(s), angioedema of, 63, *63*
  carcinoma of, 72, *73*
  cleft, 453–456, *454*
  granular cell tumor of, *209*
  hemangiomas of, *128*
  herpetic lesions of, *O-4,* O-5, *5, 6, 8, 11*
  in cheilitis. See *Cheilitis*.
  in hereditary benign intraepithelial dyskeratosis, O-21, 86
  in solar cheilitis, *O-22, O-23,* 93, *94*
  leukoplakia of, 95
  lymphangioma of, 204
  pemphigus vegetans of, 18, *18*
  swellings of, O-56, O-57
  ulcers of, in dermatitis herpetiformis, 25
    in histoplasmosis, 44
    radiation-induced, *33*
  varices of, 129, *129*
Lip biting, and hyperkeratosis, 89
  and ulcers, 30, *30*
Lip licking, and candidiasis, 113
Lipoma(s), *222,* 223
  clinical features of, O-27, *122,* 123
  of floor of mouth, *122*
Liposarcoma, *222,* 223
Liquefaction necrosis, in pulpitis, 391, *392*
Lisch spots, 215
Liver disease, and tooth staining, 486
Liver spots, 155, *155*
Ludwig's angina, 394
Lukes-Butler classification, 288, 289t
Lung(s), fungal infections of, 42, 43t, *44*
Lung lesions, in Wegener's granulomatosis, 66
Lung metastases, in adenocystic carcinoma, 268, 272
Lupus erythematosus, *O-14,* O-15, 57–62
  antibody testing in, 57, 58, 60
  discoid, 57, 58, *58, 59,* 60, 60t, 61
    vs. leukoplakia, 97, 98
  subacute cutaneous, 57, 58, *59*
  systemic, 57, 60–62, *60,* 60t

Lupus erythematosus *(Continued)*
  treatment of, 61
  vs. erythroplakia, 61
  vs. lichen planus, 61, 61t, *62*
Lupus pernio, 241
Lymph node(s), cervical, non-Hodgkin's lymphoma of, *291*
  enlarged. See *Lymphadenopathy.*
  facial (buccal), hyperplastic, 285
Lymph node metastasis, O-64, O-65
Lymphadenitis, O-65
Lymphadenopathy, cervical, 289
  in Hodgkin's disease, 287
  in non-Hodgkin's lymphoma, 290, *291*
  in syphilis, 34, 35
  phenytoin and, 289
Lymphangioma, O-66, O-67, 204, *204*
Lymphocyte(s), cytotoxic, in lichen planus, 105, 108, *109*
  in aphthous ulcers, 46–48
  in follicular keratosis, 88
  in lupus erythematosus, 57
  in sarcoidosis, 241
Lymphocytic sialadenitis, 243, 244, *244*, 247
Lymphoepithelial cyst, O-54, O-55, 119, 286
  cervical, 329, *330*
  oral, 329, *331*
Lymphoepithelial lesion, benign, 243–245, *244, 245*, 247
Lymphoid cells, in non-Hodgkin's lymphoma, 294
Lymphoid hyperplasia, reactive, 284, *285*, 293
Lymphoid lesions, 284–300
  angiolymphoid hyperplasia with eosinophilia, 286
  Burkitt's lymphoma. See *Lymphoma(s), Burkitt's.*
  developmental, 286
  lymphoepithelial cyst, 286
  lymphoid hyperplasia, 284, *285*, 293
  lymphomas. See *Lymphoma(s).*
  myelomas, 297, *299, 300*, 421–424, *422, 423*
  neoplastic, 287–300
  plasmacytomas, 297, *300*, 423
  reactive, 284–286, *285*
Lymphoid malignancies, and herpes zoster infection, 9
Lymphoid tissue, ectopic, O-26, O-27, 119, *120*, 284, 285
  gut-associated, 287, 290
  normal sites of, 284
Lymphoid tumors. See *Lymphoma(s).*
Lymphokines, in candidiasis, 115
  in contact allergy, 64
  in lichen planus, 105
Lymphoma(s), 287–297
  Burkitt's, O-96, O-97, 297, *297, 298*, 419–421, *420, 421*
  Hodgkin's, 287–290, *288–290*, 288t, 289t
  non-Hodgkin's, 290–297, 290t, *291–298*, 294t. See also *Non-Hodgkin's lymphoma.*
  of neck, O-64, O-65
  of palate, O-60, O-61
Lymphoproliferative disease of hard palate, 285, *292, 293, 293*
Lymphoproliferative disorders. See *Lymphoid lesions.*

Macrocheilia, lymphangioma and, 204
Macrodontia, 460, *462*
  unilateral, 453
Macroglossia, in acromegaly, 436, *437*
  lymphangioma and, 204
Macro-orchidism, 457
Macular pigmentation. See *Pigmentation(s).*
Macule(s), café-au-lait, O-39, 153t, 156, *156*
  in neurofibromatosis, 214
  melanotic, oral, O-38, O-39, 155, 156, 157t, *157*
Maculopapular rash, in drug reactions, 63
  in hand, foot, and mouth disease, 12, *12*
  in herpes zoster, 10
  in measles, 13, 14
  in Reiter's syndrome, 53
  in syphilis, 34, *36*
Malabsorption, intestinal, and dermatitis herpetiformis, 24–26
Malassez, rests of, 301, 310, 311, 338, 348
Malherbe, calcifying epithelioma of, 318
Malignancy(ies). See also *Cancer; Carcinoma(s); Neoplasm(s); Tumor(s).*
  and herpes zoster infection, 9
  of paranasal sinuses, 81
Malnutrition, and noma, 41
Malocclusion, in acromegaly, 436
  in cherubism, 438
  in Down syndrome, 451
  in fibrous dysplasia, 372
  in hemifacial hypertrophy, 453
Mandible. See also *Jaw(s).*
  ameloblastoma of, 338–341
  central giant cell granuloma of, *380*
  coronoid hyperplasia of, O-89, 387–389
  hemangioma of, 382, *382*
  idiopathic histiocytosis of, 384, *384*
  in neurofibromatosis, 215
  Kaposi's sarcoma of, *137*
  metastatic carcinoma to, O-99, 424, *424, 425*
  mucoepidermoid carcinoma of, 264
  ossifying fibroma of, *370*
  osteosarcoma of, *406, 407*, 409
  torus of, O-61, 387, *388*
  traumatic cyst of, 325, *327*
Mandibular cyst, median, O-75, 320
Mandibular hypoplasia, in Pierre Robin syndrome, 447, *447*
  in Treacher Collins syndrome, 447
Mandibular movement, limited, 387
Mandibular mucosa, leukoplakia of, 95
Mandibulofacial dysostosis, 446, *446*
Mantoux test, 38
Marfan's syndrome, 448
Marrow. See *Bone marrow* entries.
Massive osteolysis, O-103, 434, *435, 436*
Mast cell activation, in drug reaction, 62, 63
Maxilla. See also *Jaw(s).*
  ameloblastoma of, 345, *346*
  central giant cell granuloma of, *381*
  neoplasms of, O-61
  neuroectodermal tumor of, 163, *163*
  osteosarcoma of, *406*
  rhabdomyosarcoma of, *221*
Maxillary hypoplasia, in cleidocranial dysplasia, 443
  in Crouzon's syndrome, 445, *445*

Maxillary sinus(es), angiosarcoma of, 205, 206
  carcinoma of, O-17, 81, 82
  mucocele of, 230, 233
  mucus retention cyst of, 234, *234*
  neoplasm of, O-61
  non-Hodgkin's lymphoma of, *292*
  pseudocyst of, 234
  pyocele of, 233
Maxillofacial deformity, in leprosy, 40
Measles, German (rubella), 13
  rubeola, O-5, 13
Median alveolar cyst, 321
Median mandibular cyst, O-75, 320
Median palatine cyst, 321
Median rhomboid glossitis, *0-32, 0-33*, 113, *114*, 134, *134, 135*
Mediators, chemical. See *Chemical mediators.*
Medullary carcinoma of thyroid, 215, 217
Melanocyte(s), O-36, *O-36*, 151, *152*
  loss of, in vitiligo, 156
Melanocyte-stimulating hormone, 154
Melanocytic nevus. See *Nevus(i).*
Melanocytogenic lesions. See also *Pigmentation(s).*
  benign, *O-38*, O-39, 151–157, *152–158*, 153t, 157t
  malignant, *O-40*, O-41, 157–163, *158, 159, 161–164*
Melanoma(s), *O-40*, O-41, 160–163, *161, 162*
  acral-lentiginous, 161, *162*
  lentigo maligna, 161
  nodular, 160, *161*
  superficial spreading, 160, *161*
  vs. benign pigmented lesions, 152, 153, 156, 157t, 160, 162, 164
Melanosis, oral focal, *O-38*, O-39, 156, *157*
  smoking and, *O-39*, 153, *154*
Melanosome(s), 151, *152*
  giant, 156
Melanotic macule, oral, *O-38*, O-39, 155, 156, 157t, *157*
MEN III syndrome, 212t, 215, *216*
Mental retardation, in Crouzon's syndrome, 445
  in Down syndrome, 450
  in fragile X syndrome, 456
  in hemifacial hypertrophy, 452
Mercury deposits, mucosal, 165
Mercury intoxication, chronic, 165, *166*
Mesenchymal chondrosarcoma, 416
Mesenchymal tumors, O-55, *O-80, O-81, O-82*, O-83, 353–363
  cementifying fibroma, *O-80, O-81*, 338t, 359, *359, 360*
  cementoblastoma, *O-82, O-83*, 338t, 359–361, *360*
  central odontogenic fibroma, O-81, 356, *358*
  mixed with epithelial tumors, *O-82, O-83*, 363–368, *364–367*
  odontogenic myxoma, *O-80, O-81*, 338t, 353, 356–358, *356*
  periapical cemental dysplasia, *O-82, O-83*, 338t, 361–363, *361, 362*
Mesiodens, 471, *472*
  degradation of, and primordial cysts, 321, 323
Metabolic disorders, *O-102*, O-103, 427–437
  acromegaly, *O-102*, O-103, 435–437, *437*
  and diffuse intravascular lesions, 141–145, *142*

Metabolic disorders *(Continued)*
  and enamel defects, 472
  and salivary gland enlargement, 243
  hyperparathyroidism, *O-102*, O-103, 430–432, *431–433*
  hyperthyroidism, 432, 433
  hypophosphatasia, 433
  infantile cortical hyperostosis, O-103, 434
  Paget's disease, *O-102*, O-103, 427–430, *428–430*. See also *Paget's disease.*
  phantom bone disease, O-103, 434, *435, 436*
Metal deposits, mucosal, O-41, 165, *165*
Metallic restorations, and white lesions, 98
Metastatic carcinoma(s), adenocystic, to lung, 268, 272
  mucoepidermoid, *265*
  to jaws, O-98, O-99, 424, *424, 425*
Microbial overgrowth, and hairy tongue, 102
Microdontia, 451, 460, *461, 462*
Micrognathia, mandibular, 447, *447*
Microtia, 446, *446*
Midline granuloma, *O-16*, O-17, 67, 67t, *68*
Mikulicz's disease, 243–245, *244, 245*, 247
Mineral(s), anticariogenic, 499
Mineral exchange, in cariogenesis, 488, 491, 493, 494
Mineralization, of teeth, fluoride and, 499
Minocycline pigmentation, O-41, 166, *166*, 486
Mitral valve prolapse, 448
Mixed tumors, ameloblastic fibroma and fibro-odontoma, *O-82, O-83*, 338t, 364–368, *365–367*
  epithelial and mesenchymal, *O-82, O-83*, 363–368, *364–367*
  odontoma, *O-82, O-83*, 338t, 363, *364, 365*
  of salivary gland, benign, 249–253, 249t, *250–252*
  malignant, 263t, 273, *274, 275*
Moeller's glossitis, 143
Molars, mulberry, 35, *36*, 474, *475*
Moles. See *Nevus(i).*
Monoclonal antibodies, for lymphoma, 297
  in metastatic bone carcinoma, 424
Monoclonal immunoglobulin component, in multiple myeloma, 421, 422
Monostotic fibrous dysplasia, 372, *373*
Mouth, denture sore in, 112
  dry. See *Xerostomia.*
  floor of. See *Floor of mouth.*
  open, in Down syndrome, 451
Mouth breathing, and gingivitis, 509, 510, *511*
  in Down syndrome, 451
Mouth, hand, and foot disease, O-5, 11–13, *12*
Mouth rinses, oxygenating, and hairy tongue, 102, 103
Mucin pooling, 226, *227*, 228, *228*
Mucinosis, focal, 195, 195t
Mucocele, O-57, 226–229, *227, 229*
  antral, 230, 233
  infected, 233
  of floor of mouth (ranula), 231–233, *232, 233*
  of maxillary sinus, 230, 233
  of paranasal sinuses, 233
  superficial, 226, *227*
Mucocutaneous candidiasis, 114, *114*, 115
Mucocutaneous infections. See *Ulcerative conditions; Vesiculo-bullous disease(s);* and individual types.

Mucocutaneous lesions, in lichen planus. See *Lichen planus.*
　in Reiter's syndrome, 53
　in Rendu-Osler-Weber syndrome, 129
　in scarlet fever, 145
　in syphilis, 34, 35
　pyostomatitis vegetans, 180
　white. See *White lesions.*
Mucoepidermoid carcinoma, 262t, 263–268, *264–267*
Mucormycosis, 45, *46*
Mucosa. See *Mucous membranes.*
Mucosal burns. See *Burn(s).*
Mucosal neuromas of MEN III syndrome, 212t, 215, *216*
Mucosal plaques. See *Plaque(s) (mucosal).*
Mucosal sloughing. See *Sloughing.*
Mucositis, radiation-induced, 78, *78*
Mucous membranes. See also *Soft tissue* entries.
　bony nodules in, O-50, O-51
　exophytic growths of, 167. See also *Verrucal-papillary lesions.*
　focal argyrosis of, O-40, O-41, 157t, 163, *164*, *165*
　lesions of. See also specific types.
　　pigmented, O-36–O-41, 151–166
　　red-blue, O-28–O-35, 125–149
　　ulcerative. See *Ulcer(s); Ulcerative conditions.*
　　verrucal-papillary, O-42–O-47, 167–182
　　vesiculo-bullous, O-3–O-7, O-2, O-8, 1–27
　　white, O-18–O-27, 84–123
　metal deposits in, O-41, 165, *165*
　oral, ulceration of. See *Ulcer(s); Ulcerative conditions; Vesiculo-bullous disease(s).*
Mucus extravasation phenomenon, O-56, O-57, 226–232, *226–229*
Mucus impaction tumor, 233
Mucus retention cyst, 0-57, 226, *226*, 229–232, *230, 231*
　of maxillary sinus, 234, *234*
Mucus retention phenomenon, O-54, O-55
Mulberry molars, 35, *36*, 474, *475*
Multiple endocrine neoplasia syndrome (type III), 212t, 215, *216*
Multiple myeloma, O-98, O-99, 297, *299*, 421–423, *422*, *423*
　vs. solitary plasmacytoma of bone, 423, *424*
Mumps, 239
Munro microabscesses, 140, *141*
Muscle(s), neoplasms of, 219–223, *220–222*. See also specific types.
　ossification of, 219
　proliferative myositis of, 196
　reactive lesions of, 219
　skeletal, reactive lesions of, 219
　smooth, tumors of, 219, *220*
Mycosis(es). See *Fungal disease(s).*
Myeloma, multiple, O-98, O-99, 297, *299*, 421–423, *422*, *423*
Myoblastoma, granular cell. See *Granular cell tumor.*
Myoepithelial cells, of salivary gland, 248, 249
Myoepithelioma, 249, 261, *261*, *262*
Myofascial pain dysfunction syndrome, 436
Myopia, 448
Myositis, proliferative, 196
　with candidiasis, 115
Myositis ossificans, 219
Myxofibroma, 353

Myxoma(s), 193, *194*, 195t
　cardiac, 193
　nerve sheath, 195
　odontogenic, *O-80*, O-81, 338t, 353, *356–358*, 356
　soft tissue, 193, *194*

Nail(s), in follicular keratosis, 88
　in mucocutaneous candidiasis, 114
　melanomas of, 161
　thickening of, 86, 87
Nasal deformity, in congenital syphilis, 35
Nasal obstruction, nasolabial cyst and, 320
Nasal polyp(s), in esthesioneuroblastoma, 218
Nasal septum, perforation of, in midline granuloma, 67
Nasal sinus(es), fungal infection of, 45
　necrosis of, in Wegener's granulomatosis, 66
Nasolabial cyst, O-75, 320
Nasopalatine canal cyst, O-74, O-75, 321–323, *322, 323*
Nasopharyngeal angiofibroma, juvenile, 195, *195*
Nasopharyngeal carcinoma, Epstein-Barr virus and, 2
Natal teeth, 471, *472*
Neck, actinomycotic infections of, 40, *41*
　branchial cleft cyst of, 329, 330, *330–332*
　cancer of. See also *Head and neck cancer; Tumor(s);* and specific types.
　　radiotherapy for, and oral ulcers, 32, *33*
　dermoid cyst of, *O-66*, O-67, 330, *332, 333*
　developmental cysts of, 330, 331
　lymphangioma of, 204
　lymphoma of, *O-64*, O-65
　phycomycosis of, 45
　soft tissue cysts of, 329–335
　swellings of, O-63—O-67, *O-64, O-66*
　thyroglossal tract cyst of, 331–335, *333, 334*
Neck dissection, radical. See *Radical neck dissection.*
Necrosis, coagulative, in mucosal burns, 116, 117
　in phycomycosis, 45, *46*
　liquefaction, in pulpitis, 391, *392*, 393
　of bone. See *Osteonecrosis.*
　orofacial (noma), 41, *42*
Necrotizing sialometaplasia, 32, 235, *235–237*
Necrotizing ulcerative gingivitis, 41
　acute, 511, 512, *512*
Necrotizing vasculitis, in Wegener's granulomatosis, 66
Neonatal gingival cyst(s), O-27, 120, *121*, 122
Neonatal hepatitis, and teeth staining, 486
Neonate(s), cytomegalic inclusion disease of, 239
　epulis of, *O-52*, O-53, 207–210, 209t, *210*
　gingival cyst of, *O-72*, O-73, 312, 313, *313*
　neuroectodermal tumor of, *O-40*, O-41, 163, *163, 164*
　palatine cyst of, 313
Neoplasia syndrome, multiple endocrine, 212t, 215, *216*
Neoplasm(s). See also *Cancer; Carcinoma(s); Tumor(s).*
　angiosarcoma, 205, *206*
　basal cell carcinoma, *O-16*, O-17, 68–70, *69, 70*
　erythroplakia, 135–137, *136*

Neoplasms(s) *(Continued)*
　esthesioneuroblastoma, 218
　fibromatosis, 196t, 197t, 198, *198*
　fibrosarcoma, 196, 197t, 199, *199, 200*
　fibrous, 193–201
　fibrous histiocytomas, 196, 197t, 199, 200t, 201, *201–203*
　granular cell tumors, *O-58*, O-59, 207–210, *209–213*, 209t
　hemangiopericytoma, 205, *205, 206*
　juvenile nasopharyngeal angiofibroma, 195, *195*
　Kaposi's sarcoma, O-33, 137–139, *137*, 137t, *138*, 205, 207
　keratoacanthoma, *O-46*, O-47, 175–177, *176, 177*
　leiomyoma, 219, *220*
　leiomyosarcoma, 219
　lipomas, *222*, 223
　liposarcoma, *222*, 223
　lymphoid, 287–300. See also *Lymphoma(s); Myeloma(s).*
　maxillary sinus carcinoma, O-17, 81, 82
　melanocytogenic, *O-40*, O-41, 157–163, *158, 159, 161–164*
　melanomas. See *Melanoma(s).*
　mesenchymal, O-55
　mucosal neuromas of MEN III syndrome, 212t, 215, *216*
　multiple endocrine neoplasia syndrome type III, 212t, 215, *216*
　myelomas. See *Myeloma(s).*
　myxomas, 193, *194*, 195t
　neural, 207–218, 212t
　neuroectodermal tumor of infancy, *O-40*, O-41, 163, *163, 164*
　neurofibroma, *O-58*, O-59, 212t, 214, *214*, 215, *216*. See also *Neurofibromatosis.*
　neurogenic sarcoma, 217, *217*
　nevi. See *Nevus(i).*
　nodular fasciitis, 196, 196t, *197*, 197t
　of bone marrow, 417–424. See also *Bone marrow neoplasms.*
　of bone. See *Bone tumors.*
　of maxillary sinus, O-61
　of salivary glands. See *Salivary gland tumors.*
　of smooth muscle, 219, *220*
　of soft tissue. See *Soft tissue tumors* and specific types.
　plasmacytomas. See *Plasmacytomas.*
　rhabdomyoma, 219, *220*
　rhabdomyosarcoma, 219, *221*
　schwannoma, 210–214, 212t, *213*
　squamous cell carcinoma. See *Squamous cell carcinoma.*
　ulcerative, 68–82
　vascular, 125–130, 205–207, *205, 206*. See also *Hemangioma(s).*
　verrucal-papillary, *O-46*, O-47, 175–180, *176–179*
　verrucous carcinoma, *O-46*, O-47, *178*, 178, 178t, *179*, 180
Neoplastic transformation, in viral infection, 1
Nephrocalcinosis, 431, 434
Nephrolithiasis, 431
Nerve(s). See also *Neural* entries and individual nerves.
　trigeminal, in latent herpes, 3, 4
Nerve damage, in leprosy, 40

Nerve sheath myxoma, 195, 195t
Neural involvement, in viral infections, 3, 4, 9, 10
Neural lesions, esthesioneuroblastoma, 218
　granular cell tumors, *O-58*, O-59, 207–210, *209–213*, 209t
　mucosal neuromas in MEN III syndrome, 212t, 215, *216*
　neoplasms, 207–218, 212t
　neurofibroma, *O-58*, O-59, 212t, 214, *214*, 215, *216*. See also *Neurofibromatosis.*
　neurogenic sarcoma, 217, *217*
　of connective tissue, 207–218
　reactive, 207, *208*
　schwannoma, 210–214, 212t, *213*
　traumatic neuroma, 207, *208*
Neural syphilis, 34, 35
Neuralgia, post-herpetic, 9–11
　trigeminal, 452
Neurilemmoma, 210–214, 212t, *213*
Neuroblastoma, olfactory, 218, *218*
Neuroectodermal defect, and mucosal neuroma, 215
Neuroectodermal tumor of infancy, *O-40*, O-41, 163, *163, 164*
Neurofibroma, *O-58*, O-59, 212t, 214, *214*, 215, *216*
　plexiform, 215, *216*
Neurofibromatosis, 153t, 156, *156*, 214, *214*, 215, *216*
　schwannomas in, 211
Neurogenic sarcoma, 217, *217*
Neurologic disorders, in hyperparathyroidism, 431
　in nevoid basal cell carcinoma syndrome, 317
　in Paget's disease, 427
Neuroma(s), acoustic, 215
　mucosal, in MEN III syndrome, 212t, 215, *216*
　traumatic, 207, *208*
Nevoid basal cell carcinoma syndrome, 314, 316
Nevus(i), *O-40*, O-41, 157–160, *158, 159*
　blue, 158, *159*
　flammeus (port-wine), 126, *128*
　junctional, 158, *159*, 160
　strawberry, 125, *125*, 130, *130*
　types of, 158, *159*
　white sponge, 85, *86*, 98
Nevus cell(s), *O-36*, 151, 157, *159*
Nevus syndrome, epidermal, *452*
Niacin deficiency, 142
Nicotine stomatitis, *O-20*, O-21, 92, *93*
　vs. papillary hyperplasia, 168
Nifedipine, and gingival hyperplasia, 510
Nikolsky sign, 14, 19, *21*
Nocardia asteroides infection, 40
Nodular fasciitis, 196, 196t, *197*, 197t
Nodule(s), Bohn's, 120, 313
　bony, O-89, 386, 387, *387, 388*
　in mucosa, *O-50*, O-51
Noma, O-13, 41, *42*
Non-Hodgkin's lymphoma, 290–297, 290t, *291–298*, 294t
　Burkitt's, *O-96*, O-97, 297, *297, 298*, 419–421, *420, 421*
　classification of, 293, 294t
　diffuse, 293, 294, 294t, *295*
　histiocytic, 294t, 295, *296*
　lymphocytic, 294t, 295, *296*

Non-Hodgkin's lymphoma *(Continued)*
  lymphoproliferative disease of hard palate, 285, 292, 293, *293*
  nodular, 293, 294, *294*, 294t
  sites of, 290t
  staging of, 293
  treatment and prognosis in, 295
Non-odontogenic cysts, "globulomaxillary," *O-74*, *O-75*, 319
  median mandibular, O-75, 320
  nasolabial, O-75, 320
  nasopalatine canal, *O-74*, *O-75*, 321–323, *322*, *323*
Non-odontogenic tumors, benign, *O-85–O-89*, 369–389. See also *Jaw(s), benign non-odontogenic tumors of.*
  malignant, *O-95–O-99*, 405–425. See also *Jaw(s), non-odontogenic malignancies of.*
Nose. See also *Nasal* entries.
  saddle, in syphilis, 35
Nutritional deficiency. See *Dietary deficiency(ies).*
Nystatin, for candidiasis, 116

Occlusal defects, restoration for, 494
Occlusal stress, and exostoses, 387
Occlusal trauma, and chronic periodontitis, 514, 515
Occupational exposure to heavy metals, and pigmentation, *O-41*, 165, *165*
Ocular changes, in hyperthyroidism, 433
Ocular herpes, 8
Ocular herpes zoster, 10, *11*
Ocular inflammation, in Behçet's syndrome, 53
  in erythema multiforme, 55
Odontogenic cyst(s), botryoid, 312
  calcifying, O-75, 317, 318, *318*, *319*
  dentigerous (follicular), *O-72*, *O-73*, 306–309, *307–310*
  eruption, 310, *311*
  ghost cell tumor, O-75, 317, 318, *318*, *319*
  gingival, *O-26*, *O-27*, 120–122, *121*
  of newborn, *O-72*, *O-73*, 313, *313*
  keratocyst, *O-74*, *O-75*, 69, 313–317, *314–317*
  lateral periodontal, *O-72*, *O-73*, 310–313, *311*, *312*
  radicular. See *Periapical cyst(s).*
Odontogenic fibroma(s), peripheral, 186, *187*
Odontogenic skin abscess, 394, *395*
Odontogenic tumors, O-80—O-83, 337–368, 338t
  adenomatoid, *O-80*, *O-81*, 338t, 351–353, *353–355*
  ameloblastic fibroma, *O-82*, *O-83*, 338t, 364–368, *366*
  ameloblastic fibro-odontoma, *O-82*, *O-83*, 338t, 364–368, *365*, *367*
  ameloblastoma. See *Ameloblastoma.*
  calcifying epithelial (Pindborg), O-81, 338t, 348–351, *350–352*
  cementifying fibroma, *O-80*, *O-81*, 338t, 359, *359*, *360*
  cementoblastoma, *O-82*, *O-83*, 338t, 359–361, *360*
  central fibroma, O-81, 356, *358*
  clear cell, O-81, 351
  epithelial, *O-80*, *O-81*, 337–353. See also *Epithelial tumors.*

Odontogenic tumors *(Continued)*
  mesenchymal, *O-80*, *O-81*, 353–363. See also *Mesenchymal tumors.*
  mixed epithelial and mesenchymal, *O-82*, *O-83*, 363–368, *364–367*
  myxoma, *O-80*, *O-81*, 338t, 353, *356–358*, 356
  odontoma, *O-82*, *O-83*, 338t, 363, *364*, *365*
  periapical cemental dysplasia, *O-82*, *O-83*, 338t, 361–363, *361*, *362*
  squamous, O-81, 348, *349*
  typical features of, 338t
Odontolytic organisms, in plaque, 490, 494–496, 495t
Odontoma(s), *O-82*, *O-83*, 338t, 363, *364*, *365*
  ameloblastic, 363
  with calcifying odontogenic cyst, 317, 318
Odontoplasia, regional, 480, *481*
Odontotomy, prophylactic, 494
Olfactory neuroblastoma, 218, *218*
Oncocytes, 256
Oncocytic tumors, of salivary gland, 249t, 256–258, *257–259*
Oncocytoma, 249t, 256, *257*
Oncogene, c-myc, 419
Opalescent dentin, 477
Opportunistic infection(s), condyloma acuminatum, O-45, 172, *174*
  fungal, 45, *46*
  candidal. See *Candidiasis.*
  in periodontitis, 507
  viral, hairy leukoplakia, 99
Optic nerve damage, in Crouzon's syndrome, 445
  in osteopetrosis, 440
Orabase, 51
Oral cancer. See also *Carcinoma(s); Neoplasm(s); Tumor(s).*
  carcinogens in, 71, 72
  incidence and survival in, 70, *70*, *71*
  metastatic to lymph nodes, *O-64*, *O-65*
Oral flora, effect of restorations on, 507
  in juvenile periodontitis, 516
Oral hygiene, and caries, 490, 493, 494, 498
Oral pigmented lesions. See *Pigmentation(s).*
Oral tonsil, 284, 285
Oral ulcer(s). See *Ulcer(s); Ulcerative conditions.*
Oral warts, 74, *76*
Oral-antral fistula, and maxillary sinus carcinoma, 81
Orange stain, of teeth, 484
Orbital deformities, in Crouzon's syndrome, 445
Orchitis, in mumps, 239
Orofacial necrosis (noma), 41, *42*
Oropharyngeal cancer, incidence and survival in, 70, *70*, *71*
Orthodontia, in cleft deformity, 456
Orthokeratotic odontogenic keratocyst, 314, *316*
Osseous dysplasia, florid, *O-83*, 361, 401
Ossification, of muscle, 219
Ossification defect, in osteogenesis imperfecta, 442
Ossifying fibroma, *O-86*, *O-87*, 185, *185*, 186, *186*, 359, 369–372, *370*, *371*, 375t
  juvenile active, 372
  vs. fibrous dysplasia, 373, 375t
Osteitis, condensing, 402
Osteitis deformans. See *Paget's disease.*
Osteitis fibrosa cystica, 431
Osteoblastic osteosarcoma, 407, *408*

Osteoblastoma, *O-86*, O-87, 375–377, *376*
  vs. osteoid osteoma, 375–377
  vs. osteosarcoma, 377
Osteoclastic activity, in periodontal disease, 506, 507
Osteogenesis imperfecta, 441–443, *443*, 477
Osteohypertrophy, with vascular malformation, 129
Osteoid osteoma, 377
  giant, 375
  vs. osteoblastoma, 375–377
Osteolysis, massive, O-103, 434, *435*, *436*
Osteoma, *O-88*, O-89, 378, *378*, *379*
  osteoid, giant, 375
  vs. osteoblastoma, 375–377
Osteomyelitis, actinomycosis and, 40, 41
  acute, O-93, 394, 395
  chronic, *O-92*, O-93, 395–404, *396–398*
    after tooth extraction, 396, 397
  diffuse sclerosing, *O-92*, O-93, 399–402, *401*
  focal periapical, 402, *402*
  focal sclerosing, *O-92*, O-93, 402–404, *402*, *403*
  Garré's, *O-92*, O-93, 399, *399*, *400*
  in acute periodontitis, 513, 514
  osteopetrosis and, 440, 441
  radiation therapy and, 396, *396*, 398
  sequestrum in, 395, 396, *398*
  treatment for, 395, 398
  vs. fibro-osseous lesions, 396, 397, 398
  vs. periapical cemental dysplasia, 361–363
Osteonecrosis, in osteomyelitis, 395, 396
  radiation-induced, 78, *80*
Osteopetrosis, infantile, 439, *440*
Osteoporosis, *O-104*, O-105, 439–441, *440*, *441*
  in hyperthyroidism, 433
Osteoporotic bone marrow defect, focal, *O-76*, O-77, 329, *330*
Osteoradionecrosis, 396, *396*, 398
Osteosarcoma(s), *O-96*, O-97, 405–412, *406–414*
  chondroblastic, 407, *408*, 409, 414
  clinical features of, 405–407, *406*, *407*
  differential diagnosis of, 409
  fibroblastic, 407, 409, *409*
  histopathology of, 407, *408*, 409
  juxtacortical, 410, 411
  osteoblastic, 407, *408*
  parosteal, 410, *410*, *411*
  periosteal, 410–413, *412–414*
  radiation therapy and, 405
  telangiectatic, 407, 409
  treatment and prognosis in, 409
  vs. osteoblastoma, 377
Otitis media, 455, 456
Oxygen therapy, for diffuse sclerosing osteomyelitis, 402
  for osteoradionecrosis, 398
Oxygenating mouth rinses, and hairy tongue, 102, 103
Oxyphilic adenoma, 256, 257

Pachyonychia congenita, vs. keratoses, 86, 87
Paget's disease, *O-102*, O-103, 427–430, *428–430*
  giant cell tumor in, 381
  vs. fibrous dysplasia, 374
  vs. periapical cemental dysplasia, 361
Pain, in acute necrotizing ulcerative gingivitis, 511

Pain *(Continued)*
  in acute periodontitis, 513
  in aneurysmal bone cyst, 324
  in burning mouth syndrome, 143
  in erythema multiforme, 54, 55
  in hand, foot, and mouth disease, 12
  in mumps, 239
  in neurofibromatosis, 215
  in osteoblastoma, 375
  in osteoid osteoma, 375, 377
  in Paget's disease, 427, 430
  in periapical abscess, 393
  in traumatic neuroma, 207
  nocturnal, 375, 377
  post-herpetic, 9–11
  referred, in maxillary sinus carcinoma, 81
  in pulpitis, 390
Pain dysfunction syndrome, myofascial, 436
Palatal obturators, 456
Palate, abscess of, O-61, 394, *395*
  adenocarcinoma of, 74, 76
  adenocystic carcinoma of, 268, *269*
  blue, in nasopharyngeal angiofibroma, 195
  burns of, 31, 116
  cleft, 443, 447, 453–456, *455*, *456*
  denture-related lesions of, 112, 114, *114*
  extravascular lesions of, *148*, 149
  follicular keratosis of, 88, *88*
  follicular lymphoid hyperplasia of, 285, *285*, 293
  inclusion cyst of, 313
  leukoplakia of, 95
  lymphoma of, *O-60*, O-61
  lymphoproliferative disease of, 285, *292*, 293, *293*
  midline cysts of, 120
  minocycline pigmentation of, 166, *166*
  mixed tumor of, 250, *250*
  mucoepidermoid carcinoma of, *264*
  myoepithelioma of, *261*
  necrotizing sialometaplasia of, 235, *235*
  non-Hodgkin's lymphoma of, 290t, *292*, *293*
  papillomatosis of, *O-44*, O-45, 167, *168*
  perforation of, in fungal infection, 45, *46*
    in midline granuloma, 67
    in Wegener's granulomatosis, 66
  squamous papilloma of, *171*
  swellings of, *O-60*, O-61
  torus of, O-61, 387, *387*
  ulcers of, chronic, 32
    herpetic, 4, 5, *6*, 7
    in cicatricial pemphigoid, 19, *20*
    in herpangina, 13, *13*
    in histoplasmosis, *44*
    in pemphigus vulgaris, 14, *15*
    in sinus tumor extension, 81
    tuberculous, 39, *39*
Palatine cyst, median, 321
  of newborn, 313
Palatine papilla cyst, 321
Palatopharyngeal incompetence, 455, 456
Palms, hyperkeratotic, 518, *518*
Palpebral fissures, oblique, *450*, 451
  sloping, 446, *446*
Pancreatitis, and salivary gland enlargement, 243
Papilla(e), filiform, in geographic tongue, 103, *104*
  in hairy tongue, 102, *102*
  foliate, 284
Papillary cystadenoma lymphomatosum, 249t, 257, *258*, *259*

Papillary hyperplasia, *O-44*, O-45, 167, *168*
  palatal, in candidiasis, 114, *114*
Papillary lesions. See *Verrucal-papillary lesions.*
Papilloma, inverted duct, 258, 259, *261*
  squamous, *O-44*, O-45, 169–172, 169t, *170–172*
Papilloma virus(es), 1, 2t
  carcinogenic, 72
  lesions associated with, 169t
Papilloma virus infection(s), and condyloma acuminatum, 172
  and hairy leukoplakia, 99, 100
  and oral verruca vulgaris, *O-44*, O-45, 169–172, 169t, *170*, *173*
  and squamous papilloma, *O-44*, O-45, 169–172, 169t, *170–172*
Papillomatosis, palatal, *O-44*, O-45, 167, *168*
Papillon-Lefèvre syndrome, 518, *518*
Papovavirus(es), 2t, 169
Papule(s), in focal epithelial hyperplasia, 174
  in follicular keratosis, 88, *88*
  in keratoacanthoma, 176
  in lichen planus, 108, *108*
Para-aminobenzoic acid, 94, 95t
Parakeratin, loss of, in geographic tongue, 103, *104*
Parakeratosis(es), in focal epithelial hyperplasia, 174, *175*
  in follicular keratosis, 88
  in leukoedema, 85
  in white sponge nevus, 85
  shaggy, in hairy leukoplakia, 100, *100*
  smokeless tobacco and, 91
Paralysis, facial, in Paget's disease, 427
Paramyxovirus, 2t, 13
  in mumps, 239
Paranasal sinus(es), fungal infection of, 45
  in acromegaly, 436
  malignancy of, 81
  maxillary. See *Maxillary sinus(es).*
  mucocele of, 233
Parathormone antagonists, 430
Parathyroid crisis, 431
Parathyroid glands, hyperplastic, 430
Parathyroid hormone hypersecretion, 430
Paresthesia(s), in herpes zoster, 9
  in maxillary sinus carcinoma, 81
  in osteosarcoma, 406
Parosteal osteosarcoma, 410, *410*, *411*
Parotid gland(s). See also *Salivary gland(s).*
  swelling of, in mumps, 239
    in sarcoidosis, 241
    metabolic disorders and, 243
Parotid lesion(s), *O-64*, O-65
Parotidectomy, facial nerve in, 253, 271
  for benign tumors, 253, 256, 257, 262
  for malignant tumors, 271, 275
Parotitis, juvenile variant of, 240
  suppurative, 239, 240
Parulis, O-27, *O-50*, O-51, 122, *122*, 512–514, *513*
  in periapical abscess, *394*
Paterson-Kelly syndrome, and leukoplakia, 95
Peg lateral, 460, *461*, *462*
Pellagra, 142
Pemphigoid, bullous, O-7, 19, 22–24, 23t, *24*
  cicatricial, *O-6*, O-7, 19–22, 19t, *20–23*, 23t
  vs. lichen planus, 108
Pemphigus vegetans, 18, *18*
Pemphigus vulgaris, *O-6*, O-7, 14–19, *16–18*, 19t

Penicillin, and hairy tongue, 102
  for bacterial sialadenitis, 240
  for gonorrhea, 37
  for scarlet fever, 145
  for syphilis, 34, 37
Penicillin allergy, *64*
Penile erythroplakia, 136
Penile ulcers, in Behçet's syndrome, *53*
Periadenitis mucosa necrotica, 47
Periapical abscess, 393, *393–395*
  extension of, O-61, 394, *394*, *395*
  vs. periodontal abscess, 513, 514
Periapical cemental dysplasia, *O-82*, O-83, 338t, 361–363, *361*, *362*
Periapical cyst(s), *O-72*, O-73, 301–306, *302–305*
  residual, 302, 306, *307*
Periapical granuloma, 393
  vs. cyst, 301, 302, *302*, 306
Periapical inflammation, sequelae of, 393, *393*
Periapical osteomyelitis, focal, 402, *402*
Peridex, for aphthous ucers, 52
Periodontal abscess, 512–514, *513*
Periodontal attachment, loss of, 503, 504, 508
Periodontal cyst(s), lateral, *O-72*, O-73, 310–313, *311*, *312*
Periodontal disease, 503–518
  age and, 503, 504
  and edentulism, 503
  and parulis, O-27, 122, 123
  and pulpitis, 391
  bleeding tendency in, 506, 508, 510
  chronic, and diffuse sclerosing osteomyelitis, 399
  disease models in, 507
  epidemiological data on, 503, 504
  etiology and pathogenesis of, 504–508
  examination for, 508
  gingivitis. See *Gingivitis.*
  in Down syndrome, 451
  initial lesion in, 505
  natural history of, 503
  osteoclastic activity in, 506, 507
  periodontal attachment loss in, 503, *504*, 508
  periodontitis. See *Periodontitis.*
  plaque in, 504–508
  plaque microbiota and, 504, 505, 507
  prevalence of, 503
  salivary gland irradiation and, 237, 238
  smokeless tobacco and, 71, 90–92, *91*, *92*
Periodontal examination, 508
Periodontal pocket(s), abscess of, 512–514, *513*
  and parulis, O-27, 122, 123
  examination of, 503, *504*, 508
  in adolescents, 517
  measurement of, 503, *504*
  prevalence of, 503
Periodontitis, 512–518. See also *Periodontal disease.*
  acute, 512–514, *513*
  bacterial conditions in, 504–508, 512–518
  chronic, 514–516, *514–516*
  in Papillon-Lefèvre syndrome, 518, *518*
  juvenile, 516–518, *516*
  local factors in, 505
  prepubertal, *516*, 517
  rapidly progressive, 517, *517*
  specific plaque theory in, 507
  systemic factors in, 505
Periodontium, age-related destruction of, 504
Perioral pigmentations. See *Pigmentation(s).*

Periosteal osteosarcoma, 410–413, *412–414*
Periosteum, invasion of, in verrucous carcinoma, 178, *179*
Periostitis, 399, *399, 400*
Peripheral giant cell granuloma, O-30, O-31, O-51, 132–134, *133, 134*
Perlèche, 112, *113*
Pernicious anemia, O-33, 142, *142*
Pernio, lupus, 241
Petechia(e), O-35, 146–148, *148*
Peutz-Jeghers syndrome, 153t, 154, *154*
Phantom bone disease, O-103, 434, *435, 436*
Pharyngeal abscess(es), in scarlet fever, 145
Pharyngeal incompetence, 455, 456
Pharyngitis, in herpangina, 13
 in scarlet fever, 145
 streptococcal. See *Streptococcal pharyngitis.*
Pharynx, gonococcal infection of, 37
 ulcers of, in tuberculosis, 39
Phenobarbital allergy, *64*
Phenol, and oral ulcers, 31, *31*
Phenytoin, and gingival hyperplasia, 126, 187, 189, *189*, 510
 and lymphadenopathy, 289
Pheochromocytoma, 215, 217
Phosphate, dietary, and caries, 497
Phosphoric acid, and oral ulcers, 31
Phycomycosis, 45, *46*
Phytate, anticaries effect of, 497
Picornavirus, 2t, 11
Pierre Robin syndrome, 447, *447*
Pigment(s), and tooth discoloration, 484, *484*
Pigmentation(s), amalgam tattoo/focal argyrosis, *O-40*, O-41, 157t, 163, *164, 165*
 benign melanocytic, *O-38*, O-39, 151–157, *152–158*, 153t, 157t
 vs. early melanoma, 156, 157t
 café-au-lait macules, *O-39*, 153t, 156, *156*
 cutaneous macular, 153–157, 153t
 drug-induced, 166
 ephelides (freckles), *O-36, O-38, O-39*, 153–155, *154, 155*
 exogenous deposits, *O-40*, O-41, 163–166, *164–166*
 gingival stippling, 151, *152*
 heavy-metal deposits, O-41, 165, *165*
 iatrogenic, 163, *164, 165*
 in neurofibromatosis, 156, *156*, 215
 lentigo, *O-38, O-39*, 155, *155*
 loss of, in vitiligo, 156
 malignant melanocytogenic, 157–163, *158, 159, 161–164*
 melanomas, *O-40*, O-41, 160–163, *161, 162.* See also *Melanoma(s).*
 melanotic macule, *O-38, O-39*, 155, 156, *157*, 157t
 minocycline therapy and, O-41, 166, *166*, 486
 neoplasms, *O-40*, O-41, 157–164, *158, 159, 161–163*
 neuroectodermal tumor of infancy, *O-40*, O-41, 163, *163, 164*
 nevi, *O-40*, O-41, 157–160, *158, 159.* See also *Nevus(i).*
 oral and perioral, *O-36--O-41*, 151–166
 physiologic, *O-38, O-39*, 151, *152, 153*, 157t
 post-inflammatory, 152, *153*
 process of, *O-36*, 151, *152*
 smoking-associated melanosis, *O-39*, 153, *154*
 syndromes associated with, 153t
 vitiligo, *O-39*, 156, *158*

Pigmentation(s) *(Continued)*
 with fibrous dysplasia, 372
 with myxoma, 193
Pigmented lesions. See *Pigmentation(s).*
Pilocarpine, 238, 248
Pilomatricoma, 318
Pindborg tumor, O-81, 338t, 348–351, *350–352*, 409
Pinpoint bleeding, in psoriasis, 139, 140
 petechiae, 146–148, *148*
Pipe smoking. See also *Smoking.*
 and nicotine stomatitis, 92
 and oral cancer, 71, 72
Pituitary adenoma, 435
Pituitary-adrenal axis suppression, with steroid therapy, 50, 51
Pizza burns, and oral ulcers, 31, 116
Plaque (dental), 490, 494–496, 495t
 in periodontal disease, 504–508
 specific plaque theory, 507
 maturation of, 504, 508
 polyglycans in, 496
 subgingival, 504, 507, 508
Plaque microbiota, 490, 494–496, 495t, 504, 505, 507
 shift in, 504, 505, 507
Plaque motility testing, 507
Plaque-enamel interface, in caries, 493
Plaque(s) (mucosal), candidal, 111, *112*, 115
 in lichen planus, 105, *106, 107*
 red, intraoral. See *Erythroplakia.*
 syphilitic, 35, *36*
 white. See *Leukoplakia; White lesions.*
Plasma cell(s), 297, 299
Plasma cell gingivitis, O-35, 145, *146, 147*
Plasma cell tumors, *O-98, O-99*, 297, *299, 300*, 421–424, *422, 423*
Plasmacytoma(s), 297, *300*
 extramedullary, 297, 421
 solitary, of bone, 297, *300*, 421, 423
Platelet defects, and extravascular oral lesions, 148
Pleomorphic adenoma of salivary gland, 249–253, 249t, *250–252*
Plexiform ameloblastoma, 341
 unicystic, 344, *345*
Plummer-Vinson syndrome, O-33
 and leukoplakia, 95
 and oral cancer, 72
 iron deficiency in, 143
Pocket. See *Periodontal pocket.*
Polyglycans, in plaque, 496
Polyostotic fibrous dysplasia, 372
Polyp(s), nasal, in esthesioneuroblastoma, 218
 sinus, 235
Polyposis, intestinal, 153t, 154, 378
Porphyrin stain of teeth, 486, *486*
Port-wine stain, 126, *128*
Prednisone. See also *Corticosteroid(s).*
 for aphthous stomatitis, 50
 for cicatricial pemphigoid, 21
 for pemphigus vulgaris, 18
Pregnancy, and congenital syphilis, 34, 35
 and tetracycline staining of teeth, 486
 gingival hyperplasia in, 131, *132*, 187, 509
 pyogenic granuloma in, 131
 viral infections during, 9, 14
Prepubertal periodontitis, *516*, 517
Prickle cells. See *Keratinocytes.*
Primordial cyst(s), 306, 313, 321, 323

Prognathism, in acromegaly, 436
  in Down syndrome, 451
Proliferative disorders, fibrous. See *Fibrous proliferative disorders.*
  lymphoid. See *Lymphoid lesions.*
Proliferative myositis, 196
Proptosis, in Crouzon's syndrome, *445*
Prosthetic device(s). See also *Denture(s).*
  after radiation therapy, 80
  and burning mouth syndrome, 143, 144
  and papillary hyperplasia, 167
Protein(s), S-100, 207, 210
Proteinuria, Bence Jones, 422
Pseudoanodontia, 469, *470*
Pseudocyst(s), *O-76, O-77,* 323–329
  aneurysmal bone cyst, *O-76, O-77,* 323–325, *324, 326*
  focal osteoporotic bone marrow defect, *O-76, O-77,* 329, *330*
  of maxillary sinus, 234, *234*
  traumatic (simple) bone cyst, *O-76, O-77,* 325, *327, 328*
Pseudoepitheliomatous hyperplasia, in granular cell tumor, 210, *211*
Pseudohyphae, in candidiasis, 111, 115
Pseudosarcomatous fasciitis, 196
Psoralens, for vitiligo, 157
Psoriasis, *O-33,* 103, 139–141, *140, 141*
Psychogenic burning mouth, 143, 144
Psychogenic ulcers, 29
Pulp, abnormalities of, 480–484, *481–484*
  exposure of, in dens evaginatus, 465, *465*
  in dentinogenesis imperfecta, 477
  in internal and external resorption, 481, 482, *482–484*
  opacification of, 479
  thistle tube, 479, *480*
Pulp abscess, 391, *392*
Pulp calcification, 480, *482*
Pulp necrosis, 391, *393*
Pulp stones, 480, 481, *482*
Pulpitis, 390–393
  acute, 391, *392*
  chronic, 391
  chronic hyperplastic, 392, *392*
  focal reversible, 391
  pathways of, 391, *391*
Purified protein derivative test, 38
Purpura, idiopathic thrombocytopenic, 148
Pustule(s), in pyostomatitis vegetans, 180
Pyocele, of maxillary sinus, 233
Pyogenic granuloma, *O-30,* O-31, *O-50,* O-51, 131, *131, 132*
  mature, 185
Pyostomatitis vegetans, O-47, 180

Queyrat, erythroplasia of, 136
Quid (pan), 72, 117

Race, and caries, 489
Radiation caries, 78, *79, 80*
Radiation therapy, and hairy tongue, 103
  and oral ulcers, 32, *33,* 78, *78*
  and osteosarcoma, 405
  and salivary gland disease, 236–239, 238t
  and xerostomia, 238

Radiation therapy *(Continued)*
  for ameloblastoma, 346
  for idiopathic histiocytosis, 385
  for midline granuloma, 68
  for mucositis, 78, *78*
  for non-Hodgkin's lymphoma, 295
  for squamous cell carcinoma, 77, *78–80,* 78t
  for verrucous carcinoma, 180
  side effects of, 78, 78t, *79,* 80, *80*
Radical neck dissection, for malignant mixed tumors, 274
  for mucoepidermoid carcinoma, 268
  for salivary duct carcinoma, 278
Radicular cyst. See *Periapical cyst(s).*
Radioactive iodine therapy, 433
Radium needle therapy, for mandibular osteosarcoma, 409
Ramsay Hunt syndrome, 10
Ranula, *O-54, O-55,* 231–233, *232, 233*
  plunging, 232, *233*
Rappaport classification, 293, 294t
Rash(es), in lupus erythematosus (butterfly), 58
  in measles, 13, 14
  in scarlet fever, 145
  in varicella, 9
  maculopapular. See *Maculopapular rash.*
Raspberry tongue, 145
Rathke's pouch, 348
Reactive hyperplasia(s), 131–134, *131–134,* 184–193
  denture-induced fibrous hyperplasia, 193, *193, 194*
  general features of, 184
  gingival. See *Gingival hyperplasia.*
  granulomas, 185, *O-50,* O-51. See also *Giant cell granuloma; Pyogenic granuloma.*
  of connective tissue, 131–134, *131–134*
  peripheral fibromas, *O-50,* O-51, 185, *185, 186*
  traumatic fibroma, *O-56,* O-57, 191
Reactive lesions, central giant cell granuloma, 379
  condyloma acuminatum, O-45, 172, *174*
  condyloma latum, *O-44,* O-45, 169, *169*
  focal epithelial hyperplasia, *O-46,* O-47, 174, *175*
  focal frictional hyperkeratosis, *O-20,* O-21, 89, *90*
  hyperplastic. See *Reactive hyperplasia(s).*
  intravascular, 131–135, *131–135*
  lymphoid, 284–286, *285*
  median rhomboid glossitis, 113, *114,* 134, *134, 135*
  myositis ossificans, 219
  neural, 207, *208*
  nicotine stomatitis, *O-20,* O-21, 92, *93*
  of muscle and fat, 219
  of salivary glands, maxillary sinus retention cyst and pseudocyst, 234, *234*
    mucocele of maxillary sinus, 230, 233
    mucus extravasation phenomenon, 226–232, *226–229*
    mucus retention cyst, 226, *226,* 229–232, *230, 231*
    necrotizing sialometaplasia, 235, *235–237*
    radiation-induced, 236–239, 238t
    ranula (mucocele), 231–233, *232, 233*
  papillary hyperplasia, *O-44,* O-45, 167, *168*
  peripheral giant cell granuloma, 132–134, *133, 134*

Reactive lesions *(Continued)*
  pyogenic granuloma, 131, *131*, *132*
  smokeless tobacco and, *O-20*, O-21, 90–92, *91*, *92*
  solar cheilitis, *O-22*, O-23, 93, *94*
  squamous papilloma, *O-44*, O-45, 169–172, 169t, *170–172*
  traumatic neuroma, 207, *208*
  ulcerative, *O-10*, O-11, 29–34, *30–33*
  vascular, 201
  venous varix, O-31, 129, *129*, 201
  verruca vulgaris, *O-44*, O-45, 169–172, 169t, *170*, *173*
  verrucal-papillary, *O-44*, O-45, *O-46*, O-47, 167–175
  white, *O-20*, O-21, *O-22*, O-23, 89–94, *90–94*, 95t
Red lesions, O-28. See also *Red-blue lesions.*
Red patch, intraoral. See *Erythroplakia.*
Red stain, of teeth, 486
Red tumescence, parulis. See *Parulis.*
  granuloma. See *Granuloma(s).*
Red-blue lesions, O-28–O-35, 125–149
  atrophic candidiasis, *O-34*, O-35, 145
  burning mouth syndrome, O-35, 143–145
  contact allergies, *O-34*, O-35, 146
  diffuse intravascular, *O-32*, O-33, *O-34*, O-35, 141–146
    immunologic abnormalities, 145, *146*, *147*
    infectious conditions, 145
    metabolic-endocrine conditions, 141–146, *142*
  drug reactions, *O-34*, O-35, 146
  erythroplakia, *O-32*, O-33, 61, 91, 135–137, *136*
  extravascular, *O-34*, O-35, 146–149
  focal intravascular, *O-30*, O-31, *O-32*, O-33, 125–141
    developmental, 125–130. See also *Hemangioma(s).*
    idiopathic, 139–141, *139–141*
    neoplasms, 135–139, *136–138*, 137t
    reactive, 131–135
  geographic tongue, *O-22*, O-23, *O-32*, O-33, 54, 103, *l04*, 139, *139*
  hemangiomas. See *Hemangioma(s).*
  in scarlet fever, 145
  iron deficiency anemia, O-33, 143
  Kaposi's sarcoma, O-33, 137–139, *137*, 137t, *138*, 205, 207
  median rhomboid glossitis, *O-32*, O-33, 113, *114*, 134, *134*, *135*
  peripheral giant cell granuloma, *O-30*, O-31, 132–134, *133*, *134*
  pernicious anemia, O-33, 142, *142*
  petechiae and ecchymoses, O-35, 146–149, *148*, *149*
  plasma cell gingivitis, O-35, 145, 146, *147*
  psoriasis, O-33, 139–141, *140*, *141*
  pyogenic granuloma, *O-30*, O-31, 131, *131*, *132*
  vitamin B deficiencies, *O-32*, O-33, 141, 142, *142*
Reed-Sternberg cells, 288, *288*
Regional odontoplasia, 480, *481*
Reimplanted teeth, 482
Reiter's syndrome, O-13, 53
Remineralization, in caries, 494
Renal calcinosis, 431, 434
Renal failure, in Wegener's granulomatosis, 66, 67
Renal stones, 431

Rendu-Osler-Weber syndrome, O-31, 129, *129*
Repair, exuberant. See *Granuloma(s); Reactive hyperplasia(s).*
Residual periapical cyst, 302, 306, *307*
Resorption, external, of teeth, 482, *483*, *484*
  of bone. See *Bone resorption.*
  of dentin, 481, *482*
Respiratory distress, in angioedema, 63
Restoration(s), and iatrogenic pigmentation, 163, *165*
  and pulpitis, 391
  for occlusal defects, 494
  overhanging, effect on oral flora, 507
    in gingivitis, 509
Rests of Malassez, 301, 310, 311, 338, 348
Rests of Serres, 120, 228
Retention cyst. See *Mucus retention cyst.*
Retinoids, for aphthous ulcers, 52
  for follicular keratosis, 89
  for leukoplakia, 99
  for lichen planus, 109, *110*
  systemic, 109, 110
Retrognathia, mandibular, 447
Retrovirus(es), 1
Retzius, planes of, 493
Rh incompatibility, and tooth staining, 486
Rhabdomyoma, 219, *220*
Rhabdomyosarcoma, 219, *220*
Rheumatic fever, 145
Rheumatic heart disease, periodontal therapy in, 515
Rheumatoid arthritis, in Sjögren's syndrome, 245, 246, 248
Rhinorrhea, in esthesioneuroblastoma, 218
Rhomboid glossitis, median, *O-32*, O-33, 113, *114*, 134, *134*, *135*
Riboflavin deficiency, 142
Rickets, enamel hypoplasia in, *474*
Rodent ulcer, 69
Root(s), abnormal angulation of, 464, *464*
  cysts of. See *Periapical cyst(s).*
  dilaceration of, 464, *464*
  shortened, *478*, *479*, *480*
  supernumerary, *466*, 467
Root banking, 518
Root resorption, of impacted teeth, 482, 483
Round cell sarcoma, O-97, 417–419, *417*, *418*
Rubella, 13
Rubeola (measles), O-5, 13
Rushton bodies, 305, *305*
Russell bodies, 305

S-100 protein, 207, 210
Saddle nose, 35
Saliva, accumulated, and angular cheilitis, 112, *113*
  artificial. See *Saliva substitutes.*
  herpesvirus in, 4, 5
  in cariogenesis, 498
  in herpangina, 13
  reduction of. See also *Xerostomia.*
    in bacterial sialadenitis, 240
    sialogogues for. See *Sialogogues.*
Saliva ejector, and oral ulcers, 31
Saliva substitutes, in burning mouth syndrome, 145
  in radiation-induced xerostomia, 239
  in Sjögren's syndrome, 248

Salivary gland(s). See also *Parotid gland(s)*.
  development of, 248
  effect of radiation on, 236–239, 238t
  infarction of, 235
  inflammation of, in nicotine stomatitis, 91
    with smokeless tobacco, 91, 92
  necrosis of, 32
  neoplasia of. See *Salivary gland tumors*.
Salivary gland biopsy, in Sjögren's syndrome, 248
Salivary gland diseases, 225–278
  associated with immune defects, 243–248, *244–247*
  bacterial sialadenitis, 240
  benign lymphoepithelial lesion, 243–245, *244, 245*, 247
  cytomegalic sialadenitis, 239
  infectious conditions, 239–243
  maxillary sinus retention cyst and pseudocyst, 234, *234*
  metabolic conditions, 243
  mucocele of maxillary sinus, 230, 233
  mucus extravasation phenomenon, 226–232, *226–229*
  mucus retention cyst, 226, *226*, 229–232, *230, 231*
  mumps, 239
  necrotizing sialometaplasia, 235, *235–237*
  neoplasms. See *Salivary gland tumors*.
  radiation-induced, 236–239, 238t
  ranula, 231–233, *232, 233*
  reactive lesions, 226–239. See also *Reactive lesions*.
  sarcoidosis, 240–243, *242*, 242t
  Sjögren's syndrome, 245–248, *246, 247*, 247t
  viral, 239, 240
Salivary gland duct(s), carcinoma of, 278, *280, 281*
  intercalated, carcinoma of, 274–276, *276*
  obstruction of, and mucus retention cyst, 229, 230, *230, 231*
    and ranula, 231, *232, 233*
  radiation-induced changes in, 236–239
  severance of, 226, *226*
  squamous metaplasia of, 235, 236, *236, 237*
Salivary gland enlargement, conditions associated with, 242t
  in bacterial sialadenitis, 240
  in benign lymphoepithelial lesion, 243
  in cytomegalovirus infection, 239
  in endocrinopathies, 243
  in mumps, 239
  in sarcoidosis, 241, *242*
  in Sjögren's syndrome, 246, *247*
  metabolic disorders and, 243, 243
  neoplastic. See *Salivary gland tumors*.
Salivary gland inclusion, 328
Salivary gland stones. See *Sialolith(s)*.
Salivary gland tumors, O-55, 248–278
  acinic cell carcinoma, 263t, 272, *272, 273*
  adenocarcinomas, 263t, 278
  adenocystic carcinoma, 263t, 268–272, *269–271*
  basal cell adenomas, 253–256, 253t, *254–256*
  benign, 248–262, 249t
  benign mixed tumor (pleomorphic adenoma), 249–253, 249t, *250–253*
  carcinoma ex-mixed tumor, 263t, 273, *274, 275*
  clear cell, 274, *275*

Salivary gland tumors *(Continued)*
  epimyoepithelial carcinoma of intercalated ducts, 274–276, *276*
  inverted duct papilloma, 258, 259, *261*
  malignant, 263–278, 263t
  monomorphic adenomas, 249t, 253–258, 253t
  mucoepidermoid carcinoma, 262t, 263–268, *264–267*
  myoepithelioma, 249, 261, *261, 262*
  oncocytic, 249t, 256–258, *257–259*
  papillary cystadenoma lymphomatosum (Warthin's tumor), 249t, 257, *258, 259*
  salivary duct carcinoma, 278, *280, 281*
  sebaceous tumors, 256
  sialadenoma papilliferum, 258, *260*
  small cell carcinoma, 278
  squamous cell carcinoma, 263t, 278. See also *Squamous cell carcinoma*.
  terminal duct carcinoma, 276, *277*, 277t, *279*
  vs. mucus retention cyst, 230
Salivary gland unit, 248, *248*
Salivary sugars, and caries, 498
Sarcoidosis, 240–243, *242*, 242t
  clinical features of, 241
Sarcoma(s), chondrosarcoma, 413–417, *415, 416*
  mesenchymal, 416
  Ewing's (round cell), O-97, 417–419, *417, 418*
  Kaposi's, O-33, 137–139, *137*, 137t, *138*, 205, 207
  neurogenic, 217, *217*
  osteosarcomas. See *Osteosaroma(s)*.
  spindle cell, 219
Scar, bony, 402
  "cigarette paper," 449, *449*
  hyperplastic, 185, 191, 193. See also *Granuloma(s); Reactive hyperplasia(s)*.
Scarlet fever, O-35, 145
Scarring, in cicatricial pemphigoid, 19
  in epidermolysis bullosa, 27
  in mucosal burns, 117
  vs. submucous fibrosis, 118
Schwann cell(s), in granular cell tumor, 207
Schwannoma, 210–214, 212t, *213*
  ancient, 214
Sclera, blue, 442
Sclerosant therapy, for hemangiomas, 130
Sclerosing osteomyelitis, diffuse, O-92, O-93, 399–402, *401*
  focal, O-92, O-93, 402–404, *402, 403*
Sclerosis, diffuse, in osteopetrosis, 440, *441*
  in Paget's disease, 427, 428, *430*
Scoliosis, 448
Sealants, to prevent caries, 494
Sebaceous gland(s), ectopic, O-26, O-27, 118, *119*
  and keratoacanthoma, 175
  in dermoid cyst, 331, *333*
Sebaceous tumors, of salivary gland, 256
Secretory cyst. See *Mucus retention cyst*.
Seizure disorders, 452
Seizure therapy. See *Phenytoin*.
Sensory nerves, accidental transection of, 207
  in herpes zoster, 9
Sequestrum, in osteomyelitis, 395, 396, *398*
Serres, rests of, 120, 338
Serum sickness, 63
Sexually transmitted disease(s), 34–37, *34–36*
Shell teeth, 479
Shingles (herpes zoster), O-5, 2, 9–11, *11*
Shoulders, drooping, 443, 444, *444*

Sialadenitis, bacterial, 240
  cytomegalic, 239
  lymphocytic, 243, 244, *244*, 247
  viral, 239
  with use of smokeless tobacco, 91, 92
Sialadenoma papilliferum, 258, *260*
Sialectasia, punctate, 246, *247*
Sialogogues, in radiation-induced xerostomia, 238
  in Sjögren's syndrome, 248
Sialography, in bacterial sialadenitis, 240
  in Sjögren's syndrome, 246, *247*
Sialolith(s), 231
  and mucus retention, O-55, O-57
  and mucus retention cyst, 230, *230*, *231*
  and ranula, 231, *232*
  removal of, 233
  vs. mumps, 239
Sialometaplasia, necrotizing, 32, 235, *235–237*
Sicca syndrome. See also *Xerostomia.*
  in Sjögren's syndrome, 245, 246, 248
  with salivary gland enlargement, 243
Sinus(es), mucocele of, 233
  nasal. See *Nasal sinus(es).*
  paranasal. See *Paranasal sinus(es).*
  tumors of, 81, 82
Sinus histiocytosis, 289
Sinus polyps, 235
Sinus thrombosis, cavernous, 394
Sinus tract, in actinomycosis, 40, *41*
Sinusitis, in maxillary sinus carcinoma, 81
  in Wegener's granulomatosis, 66
Sjögren's syndrome, 245–248, *246*, *247*, 247t
  benign lymphoepithelial lesion in, 243, 247
  neck swelling in, O-65
  systemic findings in, 247t
Sjögren's syndrome antibodies, 58, 60
  in burning mouth syndrome, 144
Skeletal anomalies, in osteogenesis imperfecta, 442
  in osteopetrosis, 439
Skeletal muscle, reactive lesions of, 219
Skin, hyperelastic, 449
  pigmentations of. See *Pigmentation(s).*
Skin cancer, melanomas, 160–163. See also *Melanoma(s).*
  nevi, 157–160. See also *Nevus(i).*
Skin lesions. See *Cutaneous lesion(s); Vesiculobullous disease(s).*
Skin testing, in contact allergy, 66
  in tuberculosis, 38, 39
SLE. See *Lupus erythematosus.*
Sloughing, mucosal, aspirin and, 117
  in burn injury, 116, 117
  vs. candidiasis, 115
Small cell carcinoma of salivary glands, 278
Smokeless tobacco. See *Tobacco, smokeless.*
Smoking. See also *Tobacco.*
  and gingivitis, 511
  and hairy tongue, 102
  and leukoplakia, 95
  and melanosis, O-39, 153, *154*
  and nicotine stomatitis, 92
  and squamous cell carcinoma, 71, 72
  reverse, 71, 93
Smooth muscle tumors, 219, *220*
Snuff, 90, 91. See also *Tobacco.*
  and squamous cell carcinoma, 71
Soft palate. See *Palate.*
Soft tissue. See also *Mucous membranes.*

Soft tissue cysts, eruption, 310, *311*
  nasolabial, 320
  of neck, 329–335
    branchial cleft, 329, 330, *330–332*
    dermoid, 330, *332*, *333*
    thyroglossal tract, 331–335, *333*, *334*
  palatine papilla, 321, 322
Soft tissue disease(s). See also under individual types.
  connective tissue lesions, 184–223
  lymphoid lesions, 284–300
  mucosal lesions. See *Mucous membranes, lesions of.*
  salivary gland diseases, 225–278
  submucosal swellings, 284–299
Soft tissue hemorrhage(s), 125, 146–149, *148*
Soft tissue injury, iatrogenic, and ulcers, 29, 31, *31*
Soft tissue myxoma, 193, *194*, 195t
Soft tissue pigmentations. See also *Pigmentation(s).*
  iatrogenic, 163, *164*, *165*
Soft tissue tumors, extramedullary plasmacytoma, 421
  fibrosarcoma, 196, 197t, 199, *199*, 200
  fibrous histiocytoma, 196, 197t, 199, 200t, 201, *201–203*
  leiomyoma and leiomyosarcoma, 219, *220*
  lipoma and liposarcoma, *222*, 223
  lymphomas. See *Lymphoma(s).*
  mesenchymal chondrosarcoma, 416
  neurogenic sarcoma, 217, *217*
  of muscle and fat, 219–223, *220–222*
  plasmacytomas, 297
  rhabdomyoma and rhabdomyosarcoma, 219, *220*, *221*
Solar cheilitis, O-22, O-23, 93, *94*
Solitary plasmacytoma of bone, 297, *300*, 421, 423
Somatomedin C assay, 437
Somatotropinoma, 435
Sore(s). See also *Ulcer(s).*
  canker. See *Aphthous ulcer(s).*
  cold, 3
Sore mouth, denture, 112
Southern blot hybridization studies, 99, 100
Specific plaque theory, 507
Speckled erythroplakia, O-33
Speckled leukoplakia, 95
Speech deficits, in cleft deformity, 455, 456
Spindle ameloblastoma, 341
Spindle cell carcinoma, 76
Spindle cell sarcoma(s), 219
Spirochete infection, 34–37, *34–36*
Sponge nevus, white, 85, *86*
  vs. leukoplakia, 98
Spore inhalation, and fungal infections, 42, 43t, *44*
Sporotrichosis, 45
Sprue (celiac), 24
Squamous cell carcinoma, O-16, O-17, 70–81
  clinical features of, 72–76, *73–77*
  differential diagnosis of, 77
  etiology of, 71
  in submucous fibrosis, 118
  incidence and survival in, 70, *70*, 71
  leukoplakia and, 95–97, *97*
  of maxillary sinus, 81
  of salivary glands, 263t, 279
  prognosis in, 80, 81t

Squamous cell carcinoma *(Continued)*
second primary lesion in, 81
treatment of, 77–80
and oral ulcers, 32
radiation regimens and complications in, 77, 78–80, 78t
tumor grading and staging in, 80, 81t
verrucous, 178
vs. granular cell tumor, 210
vs. keratoacanthoma, 176, 177, *177*
vs. necrotizing sialometaplasia, 235, 236
Squamous metaplasia, of salivary gland duct, 235, 236, *236, 237*
Squamous odontogenic tumor, O-81, 348, *349*
Squamous papilloma, *O-44*, O-45, 169–172, 169t, *170–172*
Staging, in Hodgkin's disease, 287, 288t
Staging system for tumors, 80, 81, 81t
Stains, of teeth, 484, *484–486*
Static bone cyst, *O-76*, O-77, 328, *329*
Stensen's duct, in mumps, 239
Steroid(s). See *Corticosteroid(s); Glucocorticoid(s).*
Stevens-Johnson syndrome, 55
Stippling, gingival, 151, *152*
Stomatitis, antibiotic therapy and, 111
aphthous. See *Aphthous stomatitis.*
gangrenous, 41, *42*
gingival, herpetic, *O-4*, O-5, 2–4, *5, 6–9*
nicotine, *O-20*, O-21, 92, *93*
vs. papillary hyperplasia, 168
Stone(s), in salivary duct. See *Sialolith(s).*
pulp, 480, 481, *482*
renal, 431
Strawberry nevus, 125, *125*, 130, *130*
Strawberry tongue, 145
Streptococcal infection, and scarlet fever, 145
Streptococcal pharyngitis, vs. herpangina, 13
vs. herpetic gingivostomatitis, 7
Streptococcus mutans, in cariogenesis, 495t, 496
Stress, and gingivitis, 511
Stria(e), Wickham's, 61, 105, *106*, 107, 109
Sturge-Weber syndrome, O-31, 126, *128*
Submucosal clefts, 454
Submucous fibrosis, O-27, 117, *118*
Sucrose, and caries, 488, 495–498
Sudden death, in Ehlers-Danlos syndrome, 449
in Marfan's syndrome, 448
Sugars, and caries, 488, 495–498
Sulfonamides, for aphthous ulcers, 52
Sulfur granules, in actinomycosis, 40
Sun exposure, and basal cell carcinoma, 68, 70
and cheilitis, 93, *94*
and freckles, 153
and keratoacanthoma, 175
and lentigo, 155
and lip varices, 129
and melanomas, 160, 161
protection against, 94, 95t
Sunscreens, 94, 95t
Supernumerary roots, *466*, 467
Supernumerary teeth, 471, *471, 472*
in cleidocranial dysplasia, 443, 444, *444*
Sutton's disease, 47
Sutures, artificial, 446
cranial, premature closure of, 445
Swelling(s), gingival, *O-48*, O-49. See also *Gingival hyperplasia.*
of floor of mouth, *O-54*, O-55
of lip and buccal mucosa, *O-56*, O-57

Swelling(s) *(Continued)*
of neck, O-63–O-67, *O-64, O-66*
of palate, *O-60*, O-61
of tongue, *O-58*, O-59
submucosal, in Hodgkin's disease, 287
Symblepharon, 22, *23*
Synovial chondromatosis, 414
Syphilis, *O-10*, O-11, 34–37, *34–36*
condyloma latum in, *O-44*, O-45, 169, *169*
congenital, 34, 35
and enamel hypoplasia, 474, *475*
neural, 34, 35
tongue carcinomas in, 72
Systemic lupus erythematosus. See *Lupus erythematosus.*

T lymphocytes. See also *Lymphocyte(s).*
in sarcoidosis, 241
Tabes dorsalis, 35
Taste, altered, 144
Tattoo, amalgam, *O-40*, O-41, 157t, 163, *164, 165*
Taurodontism, 466, *466*
Tear substitutes, in Sjögren's syndrome, 248
Teeth. See also *Dentition; Tooth.*
abnormalities of, 460–486
abrasion, 467, *468*
amelogenesis imperfecta, 475–477, *476*
anodontia, 467, *469, 470*
attrition, 467
color, 484–486, *484–486*
concrescence, 463, *463*
defects of dentin, 477–480, *477–481*
defects of enamel, 472–477, *473–476*, 480, 481. See also *Enamel.*
dens evaginatus, 465, *465*
dens invaginatus, 464, *464*
dentin dysplasia, 479, *479, 480*
dentinogenesis imperfecta, 477–479, *477, 478*
dilaceration, 464, *464*
enamel pearls, 467, *467*
environmental effects on enamel, 472–475, *473–475*
erosion, 467, *469*
exogenous stains, 484, *484, 485*
external resorption, 482, *483, 484*
fusion, 463, *463*
gemination, 461, *462*
impaction, 469, *470*
adenomatoid tumor and, 352, *353*
and resorption, 483
internal resorption, 481, *482*
macrodontia, 460, *462*
microdontia, 460, *461, 462*
number, 467–472, *469–472*
pulp, 480–484, *481–484*
pulp calcification, 480, *482*
regional odontoplasia, 480, *481*
shape, 461–467, *462–469*
size, 460, *461, 462*
supernumerary roots, *466*, 467
supernumerary teeth, 471, *471, 472*
taurodontism, 466, *466*
trauma and, 461, 463, 464
absence of, 467, *469, 470*
ankylosed, in osteopetrosis, 439, 440
caries of. See *Caries.*

Teeth *(Continued)*
  discolored, 472, 473, 475, 477, *477*, 479
    in osteogenesis imperfecta, 442, 443, *443*
  enlarged, 453, 460, *462*
    in hemifacial hypertrophy, 461
  erosion of, in hyperthyroidism, 433
  floating, 384, *384*
  ghost, 480
  hypersensitivity of, in pulpitis, 391
  natal, 471, *472*
  natural, caries in, 494
  overcrowded, 463
  post-permanent, 472
  premature loss of, 433
  primary, periodontitis of, *516*, 517
  shell, 479
  stained, 484, *484–486*
  supernumerary. See *Supernumerary teeth.*
  transplanted/reimplanted, 482
  unerupted, in cleidocranial dysplasia, 443, 444, *444*
    in dentigerous cyst, *O-72*, O-73, 306–309, *307–310*
Telangiectasia, hereditary hemorrhagic, *O-30*, O-31, 129, *129*
Telangiectatic osteosarcoma, 407, 409
Temporomandibular joint, arthritis of, 139
  chondromatosis of, 414
Terminal duct carcinoma, 276, *277*, 277t, *279*
Testicular enlargement, 457
Testicular inflammation, in mumps, 239
Tetracycline, allergic reaction to, 64
  and tooth staining, *485*, 486
  for aphthous ulcers, 51
Thermal injury, and oral ulcers, 31, 32, *32*
  and mucosal burns, 116, *117*
Thistle tube pulp, 479, *480*
Thrombocytopenic purpura, idiopathic, 148
Thrombosis, cavernous sinus, 394
Thrush, 111, *112, 115*. See also *Candidiasis.*
Thymoma, with candidiasis, 11
Thyroglossal tract cyst, *O-66*, O-67, 331–335, *333, 334*
Thyroid, lingual, O-59, 331, *334*
Thyroid carcinoma, 215, 217
Thyroid dysfunction, and candidiasis, 114, 115
Thyroid gland hyperfunction, 432, 433
Thyroid gland tumor, O-67
Thyroid hormone hypersecretion, 432
Thyroid stimulator, abnormal, 432
Thyroid storm, 433
Tibia, adamantinoma of, 348
  Garré's osteomyelitis of, 399
Tine test, 38
Tissue repair, exuberant. See *Granuloma(s); Reactive hyperplasia(s).*
TNM staging system, 80, 81, 81t
Tobacco. See also *Smoking.*
  and erythroplakia, 135
  and hairy tongue, 102
  and leukoplakia, 95
  and nicotine stomatitis, *O-20*, O-21, 92, *93*
  and squamous cell carcinoma, 71, 72
  and tooth discoloration, 484, *484*
  and verrucous carcinoma, 178
  smokeless, and oral cancer, 71, 72
    and submucous fibrosis, 117
    and white lesions, *O-20*, O-21, 90–92, *91, 92*
Toenails. See *Nail(s).*

Togavirus, 13
Tongue. See also *Lingual* entries.
  atrophic, in vitamin B deficiency, 142, *142*, 143
  benign fibrous histiocytoma of, *201*
  burning, 143–145
  carcinoma of, 72, *74*
  distorted, 452
  enlarged, in acromegaly, 436, *437*
  erythroplakia of, *136*
  fissured, 103
  geographic, *O-22*, O-23, *O-32*, O-33, 54, 103, *104*, 139, *139*
  granular cell tumor of, *209*
  hairy, O-23, 102, *102*
  hairy leukoplakia of, 100, *100*
  herpetic ulcers of, 5
  hyperextensible, 449
  in candidiasis, 111
  in median rhomboid glossitis, *O-32*, O-33, 113, *114*, 134, *134*, 135
  inflammation of. See *Glossitis.*
  leukoplakia of, 95, *97*
    and cancer, 73
  lichen planus of, *O-24*, 105, *106*
  lymphangioma of, 204
  mucoepidermoid carcinoma of, *264*
  neurofibroma of, *214*
  strawberry, 145
  swellings of, *O-58*, O-59
  ulcers of, chronic, 32, *33*
    in allergic reactions, 65
    in histoplasmosis, *44*
    in pemphigus vulgaris, 15, *16*
  varices of, 129, *129*
Tonsil(s), enlarged, in Hodgkin's disease, 287
  lingual, 119, 284
  non-Hodgkin's lymphoma of, 290t, *291*
  oral, 284, 285
Tooth, anatomy of, and location of caries, 491–493, *491, 492*
  Turner's, 473, *473*
Tooth anomalies. See *Teeth, abnormalities of.*
Tooth extraction(s), after radiation therapy, 78, 80, *80*
  and chronic osteomyelitis, 396, *397*
  and osteoporotic bone marrow defect, 329
  and traumatic neuroma, 207
  poor healing after, tumor and, 81
Toothache, referred, in maxillary sinus carcinoma, 81
Toothbrush abrasion, 467, *468*
Tooth-containing cyst, *O-72*, O-73, 306–309, *307–310*
Torus(i), O-61, O-89, 386
  mandibularis, 387, *388*
  palatinus, 387, *387*
Toxic metals, and mucosal pigmentations, 165, *165*
Toxins, erythrogenic, 145
Transplanted teeth, 482
Trauma, and dental abnormalities, 461, 463, 464
  and ecchymoses, *O-34*, O-35, 148, *148*
  and enamel defects, 473
  and hyperkeratosis, *O-20*, O-21, 89, *90*
  and necrotizing sialometaplasia, 235, *235*
  and pulpitis, 391
  and reactive hyperplasia, 184. See also *Reactive hyperplasia(s).*
  and tooth resorption, 482

Trauma *(Continued)*
  as co-carcinogen, 72
  in Ehlers-Danlos syndrome, 449, *449*
  occlusal, and periodontitis, 514, 515
  post-irradiation, and osteonecrosis, 78, *80*
  to salivary gland, and mucocele, 226–233, *226*
Traumatic fibroma, *O-56*, O-57, 191
Traumatic granuloma, 32
Traumatic keratosis, *O-20*, O-21, 89, *90*
  vs. leukoplakia, 97
Traumatic myositis ossificans, 219
Traumatic neuroma, 207, *208*
Traumatic (simple) bone cyst, *O-76*, O-77, 325, *327, 328*
Traumatic ulcers, 29, *30*
Treacher Collins syndrome, 446, *446*
Treponema pallidum infection, 34–37, *34–36*
  condyloma latum in, *O-44*, O-45, 169, *169*
Trigeminal ganglion, in herpes zoster, 9
  in latent herpes, 3, 4
Trigeminal nerve involvement, in neurofibromatosis, 215
Trigeminal neuralgia, 452
Trismus, in bacterial sialadenitis, 240
  in submucous fibrosis, 118
Trisomy 21 (Down syndrome), 450, *450, 451*
Tuberculoid leprosy, 40
Tuberculosis, *O-10*, O-11, 38, *38, 39*
  vs. sarcoidosis, 242
Tumor(s). See also *Cancer; Carcinoma(s); Neoplasm(s)*.
  carcinoma ex-mixed, 263t, 273, *274, 275*
  carotid body, O-65
  chondromas, 377
  chondrosarcoma, 378, 413–417, *415, 416*
    mesenchymal, 416
  clear cell, 274, *275*
  dermal analogue, 253, 254, *255,* 256
  endocrine, 215, 217
  ghost cell, O-75, 37, 318, *318, 319*
  granular cell, *O-58*, O-59, 207–210, *209–213*, 209t
  lymphoid. See *Lymphoma(s)*.
  mixed. See *Mixed tumors*.
  mucus impaction, 233
  neuroectodermal, of infancy, *O-40*, O-41, 163, *163, 164*
  of cartilage, 377, 378, 413–417, *415, 416*
  of jaws, benign non-odontogenic, O-85–O-89, 369–389. See also *Jaw(s), benign non-odontogenic tumors of*.
    non-odontogenic malignant, O-95–O-99, 405–425. See also *Jaw(s), non-odontogenic malignancies of*.
  of salivary glands. See *Salivary gland tumors*.
  of sinus(es), 81, 82
  of thyroid gland, O-67
  oncocytic, of salivary gland, 249t, 256–258, *257–259*
  Pindborg, O-81, 338t, 348–351, *350–352*, 409
  plasma cell, *O-98*, O-99, 297, *299, 300*, 421–424, *422, 423*
  sebaceous, of salivary gland, 256
  vascular, 205–207, *205, 206*. See also individual lesions.
  Warthin's, O-65, 249t, 257, *258, 259*
  Wilms', 452
Tumor grading and staging, in squamous cell carcinoma, 80, 81t
Tumor-associated viruses, 1

Turner's tooth, 473, *473*
Twins, caries in, 498
Tzanck cells, 16, *16*

Ulcer(s), *O-2, O-4*, O-5, *O-6*, O-7, *O-8*. See also *Ulcerative conditions; Vesiculo-bullous disease(s)*.
  aphthous. See *Aphthous ulcer(s)*.
  chemical irritants and, 31, *31*, 32, *32*
  chronic reactive, 32, *33*
  cotton roll–induced, 31, *31*
  crateriform, 32
  definition of, 29
  dental materials causing, 31, *31*, 32, *32*
  factitial, 29, *30*, 31
  fungal, *O-12*, O-13, 42–46, 43t, *44, 46*
  genital, 34, *35*, 37
  gonorrheal, 37
  iatrogenic, 29, 31, *31*
  in candidiasis, 111, 115
  in cicatricial pemphigus, 19, *20*
  in dermatitis herpetiformis, 25, *25*
  in hand, foot, and mouth disease, O-5, 11–13, *12*
  in herpes simplex infections, *O-4*, O-5, 2–9, *5–7*, 8t
  in pemphigus vulgaris, *O-6*, O-7, 14–19, *16–18*
  in varicella-zoster infections, O-5, 9–11, *10, 11*
  infectious, O-8, 2–6, 9, 11, 13
  necrotic, in midline granuloma, 67, *68*
    in Wegener's granulomatosis, 66, *67*
  penile, in Behçet's syndrome, *53*
  pharyngeal, in tuberculosis, 39
  psychogenic, 29
  radiation-induced, 32, *33*, 78, *78*
  reactive, *O-10*, O-11, 29–34, *30–33*
  rodent, 69
  self-induced, 29, *30*, 31
  syphilitic chancre, *O-10*, O-11, 34, *35*
  thermal burns and, 31, 32, *32*
  traumatic, 29, *30*
  tubercular, *O-10*, O-11, 39, *39*
Ulcerative colitis, and pyostomatitis vegetans, 180
Ulcerative conditions, 29–82. See also *Ulcer(s); Vesiculo-bullous disease(s)*.
  actinomycosis, O-11, 40, *41*
  aphthous ulcers. See *Aphthous ulcer(s)*.
  associated with immunologic defects, 46–68
  bacterial conditions, 34–42. See also *Bacterial conditions*.
  basal cell carcinoma, *O-16*, O-17, 68–70, *69, 70*
  Behçet's syndrome, O-13, 48t, *53*, 53
  chronic granulomatous disease, O-17, 68
  contact allergy, *O-14*, O-15, 64–66, *65, 66*
  drug reactions, O-15, 62–64, 62t, *63–65*
  erythema multiforme, *O-14*, O-15, 54–57, *54–56*, 57t
  fungal diseases, *O-12*, O-13, 42–46, 43t, *44, 46*
  gonorrhea, O-11, 37
  leprosy, O-11, 39
  lupus erythematosus. See *Lupus erythematosus*.
  maxillary sinus carcinoma, O-17, 81, *82*
  midline granuloma, *O-16*, O-17, 67, 67t, *68*

Ulcerative conditions *(Continued)*
  neoplasms, O-17, 68–82
  noma, O-13, 41, *42*
  peripheral giant cell granuloma, 133
  pyogenic granuloma, 131
  reactive lesions, *O-10*, O-11, 29–34, *30–33*
  Reiter's syndrome, O-13, 53
  squamous cell carcinoma. See *Squamous cell carcinoma.*
  syphilis, *O-10*, O-11, 34–37, *34–36*
  tuberculosis, *O-10*, O-11, 38, *38, 39*
  vesiculo-bullous. See *Vesiculo-bullous disease(s).*
  Wegener's granulomatosis, O-15, 66, *67*, 67t
Ulcerative gingivitis, acute necrotizing, 511, 512, *512*
Ultraviolet light exposure, and basal cell carcinoma, 69
  and cheilitis, 93
  and freckles, 153
  and lentigo, 155
  and melanomas, 160, 161
  and squamous cell carcinoma, 72
  blocking agents in, 94, 95t
Urethritis, in Reiter's syndrome, 53
Urticaria, in drug reactions, 63
Uveitis, in Behçet's syndrome, 53
  in erythema multiforme, 55
  in Reiter's syndrome, 53
Uveoparotid fever, 241
Uvula, bifid, 454

Vaccine, mumps, 239
Varicella (chickenpox), O-5, 2, 9–11, *9, 10*
Varicella-zoster infection(s), O-5, 9–11, *10, 11*
Varicella-zoster virus, 2, 9
Varicosity(ies), 129, *129*
Varix(ces), O-31, 129, *129*, 201
Vascular dilatation, abnormal, 129, *129*
Vascular leiomyoma, 219
Vascular lesion(s), angiolymphoid hyperplasia with eosinophilia, 286
  congenital, *O-66*, O-67, 204, *204*
  hemangiomas. See *Hemangioma(s).*
  lymphangiomas, *O-66*, O-67, 204, *204*
  of connective tissue, 201, 204–207, *204–206*
  reactive. See *Reactive lesion(s).*
  venous varices, O-31, 129, *129*, 201
Vascular malformation(s), 125, 126, 126t, *127–129*, 130
Vascular tumors, 125–130, 205–207, *205, 206*. See also *Hemangioma(s).*
Vasculitis, immune complex, in aphthous ulcers, 46, 50
  in erythema multiforme, 54, 55
  necrotizing, in Wegener's granulomatosis, 66
Veau classification of cleft deformities, 454
Velopharyngeal incompetence, 455, 456
Venereal infection(s), gonorrhea, 37
  syphilis, 34–37, *34–36*
Venous varices, O-31, 129, *129*, 201
Vermilion. See also *Lip(s).*
  epidermization of, 93
  Fordyce's granules of, 118
  melanotic macules of, 156, *157*
Vermilionectomy, in solar cheilitis, 94
Verocay body, 211

Verruca vulgaris, 98
  cutaneous, 169
  oral, *O-44*, O-45, 169–172, 169t, *170, 173*
Verrucal-papillary lesions, O-42–O-47, *O-42*, 167–182
  condyloma acuminatum, O-45, 172, *174*
  condyloma latum, *O-44*, O-45, 169, *169*
  focal epithelial hyperplasia, *O-46*, O-47, 174, *175*
  idiopathic, O-47, 180–182, *181*
  keratoacanthoma, *O-46*, O-47, 175–177, *176, 177*
  neoplasms, *O-46*, O-47, 175–180, *176–179*
  papillary hyperplasia, *O-44*, O-45, 167, *168*
  pyostomatitis vegetans, O-47, 180
  reactive, *O-44*, O-45, *O-46*, O-47, 167–175
  squamous papilloma, *O-44*, O-45, 169–172, 169t, *170–172*
  verruca vulgaris, *O-44*, O-45, 169–172, 169t, *170, 173*
  verruciform xanthoma, O-47, 180–182, *181*
  verrucous carcinoma, *O-46*, O-47, 178, *178*, 178t, *179*, 180
Verruciform xanthoma, O-47, 180–182, *181*
Verrucous carcinoma, *O-46*, O-47, 72, 74, 76, 77, 98, 178, *178*, 178t, *179*, 180
Verrucous lesions, in follicular keratosis, 88
Verrucous leukoplakia, proliferative, 96, 98
Vesicle(s), *O-2*. See also *Vesiculo-bullous disease(s).*
Vesiculo-bullous disease(s), O-3–O-7, *O-2, O-8*, 1–27. See also *Blister(s); Bulla(e); Ulcer(s); Ulcerative conditions.*
  associated with immunologic defects, *O-4*, O-7, 14–26
  bullous pemphigoid, O-7, 19, 22–24, 23t, *24*
  cicatricial pemphigoid, *O-6*, O-7, 19–22, 19t, *20–23*, 23t
  dermatitis herpetiformis, O-7, 24–26, *25*
  pemphigus vulgaris, *O-6*, O-7, 14–19, *16–19*, 19t
  epidermolysis bullosa, *O-6*, O-7, 26, *26, 27*
  hereditary, 26, *26, 27*
  viral, *O-4*, O-5, 1–14, 2t
    hand, foot, and mouth disease, O-5, 11–13, *12*
    herpangina, O-5, 13, *13*
    herpes simplex infections, 2–9, *3–7*. See also *Herpes simplex virus infections.*
    measles (rubeola), O-5, 13
    varicella-zoster infections, O-5, 9–11, *10, 11*
Vidarabine, for herpes infections, 8
  for varicella-zoster infections, 11
Vincent's infection. See *Gingivitis.*
Viral disease(s), *O-4*, O-5, 1–14, 2t
  and oral cancer, 72
  during pregnancy, 9, 14
  hairy leukoplakia, *O-22*, O-23, 99–102, 99t, *100, 101*
  hand, foot, and mouth disease, O-5, 11–13, *12*
  herpangina, O-5, 13, *13*
  herpes simplex infections, 2–9, *3–7*
  measles (rubeola), O-5, 13
  of salivary glands, cytomegalovirus infection, 239
  mumps, 239
  varicella-zoster infections, O-5, 9–11, *10, 11*
  verruca vulgaris, 98
Viral sialadenitis, 239

Virus(s), 1, 2t
  Coxsackie, 2t, 11
  DNA, in papilloma, 169–171, *170*
  enterovirus, 11
  Epstein-Barr, 2, 2t, 420
    and oral cancer, 72
    in hairy leukoplakia, 99–102, *101*
  genital infections with, 2, 4, 8
  herpesviruses, 2–11, 2t. See also *Herpes simplex virus infection(s)*; *Varicella-zoster infection(s)*.
  infections due to. See *Viral disease(s)*.
  influenza, 2t
  latency of, 1–4
  papilloma, 1, 2t, 169–171, 169t, *170*
  papovavirus, 2t, 169
  paramyxovirus, 2t, 13, 239
  picornaviruses, 2t, 11
  replication of, 1, 2, 8
  retroviruses, 1
  togavirus, 13
  tumor-associated, 1
  varicella-zoster, 2, 9
Virus particle, 1, 3
Virus-host cell interaction, 1, *3*
Virus-like particles, in focal epithelial hyperplasia, 174
  in keratoacanthoma, 175
Vital root banking, 518
Vitamin A derivatives, for aphthous ulcers, 52
  for follicular keratosis, 89
  for leukoplakia, 99
  for lichen planus, 109, *110*
  systemic retinoids, 109, 110
Vitamin B deficiencies, O-32, O-33, 141, 142, *142*
Vitamin deficiency(ies), and aphthous ulcers, 47
  and caries, 499
Vitiligo, O-39, 156, *158*
Vomiting, and erosion of teeth, 467
von Recklinghausen's disease. See *Neurofibromatosis*.

Waldeyer's ring, 287, 290
Wart(s). See also *Verrucous* entries.
  cutaneous, 169
Warthin-Finkeldey giant cells, 14
Warthin's tumor, O-65, 249t, 257, 258, 259
Wart-like keratoses, 98
Wart-like lesions, intraoral, 74, *76*
Warty dyskeratoma, 88, 171. See also *Darier's disease*.
Wegener's granulomatosis, O-15, 66, 67t, *67*
White hairy tongue, O-23, 102, *102*
White lesions, O-18–O-27, 84–123
  diagnostic approach to, O-18, 84. See also *Keratosis(es)* and specific lesions.
  focal frictional hyperkeratosis, O-20, O-21, 89, *90*
  follicular keratosis, O-21, 87–89, *88, 89*
  general features of, O-18, 84

White lesions *(Continued)*
  hereditary benign intraepithelial dyskeratosis, O-21, 86, *87*
  hereditary keratotic disorders, O-20, O-21, 84–89, *85–89*
  idiopathic, 94–110. See also *Leukoplakia*; *Lichen planus*.
    geographic tongue, O-22, O-23, *O-32, O-33*, 54, 103, *104*, 139, *139*
    hairy tongue, O-23, 102, *102*
  leukoedema, O-21, 84, *85*, 98
  metallic restorations and, 98
  nicotine stomatitis, O-20, O-21, 92, *93*
  non-epithelial white-yellow. See *White-yellow lesions, nonepithelial*.
  reactive, O-20, O-21, *O-22, O-23*, 89–94, *90–94*, 95t. See also *Reactive lesions*.
  smokeless tobacco and, O-21, *O-20*, 71, 72, 90–92, *91, 92*
  solar cheilitis, *O-22, O-23*, 93, *94*
  sponge nevus, 85, *86*
  tobacco and, *O-20, O-21*, 90–93, *91–93*
White plaques. See *Leukoplakia*; *White lesions*.
White sponge nevus, 85, *86*
  vs. leukoplakia, 98
White-yellow lesions, non-epithelial, O-24, O-25, O-26, O-27, 110–123
  candidiasis. See *Candidiasis*.
  ectopic lymphoid tissue, O-26, O-27, 119, *120*
  Fordyce's granules (ectopic sebaceous glands), O-26, O-27, 118, *119*
  gingival cysts. See *Gingival cyst(s)*.
  lipoma. See *Lipoma(s)*.
  mucosal burns, O-26, O-27, 31, *31*, 32, *32*, 116, *117*
  parulis (gingival boil), O-27, 122, *122*
  submucous fibrosis, O-27, 117, *118*
Whitlow, herpetic, O-4, O-5, 5, *7*
Wickham's striae, 61, 105, *106*, 107, 109
Wilms' tumor, 452
Wound healing, in Ehlers-Danlos syndrome, 449

Xanthomas, verruciform, O-47, 180–182, *181*
Xerophthalmia, in Sjögren's syndrome, 245, 248
Xerostomia, and caries, 499
  differential diagnosis of, 238t
  in burning mouth syndrome, 143, 144
  in Sjögren's syndrome, 245, 246, *246*, 248
  radiation-induced, 78, *79*, 238
X-linked mental retardation, 456

Yeast infection(s), candidal. See *Candidiasis*.
Yellow-orange stain, of teeth, 484
Yellow-white non-epithelial lesions. See *White-yellow lesions, nonepithelial*.

Ziehl-Neelsen stain, 38, 39
Zoster, herpes, O-5, 2, 9–11, *11*